Grieve's Modern Manual Therapy

In memory of Gregory Peter Grieve, 11 December 1918 – 24 April 2001

For Churchill Livingstone:

Editorial Director, Health Professions: Mary Law
Project Development Manager: Claire Wilson
Project Manager: Ailsa Laing
Illustrations: PCA Creative
Design: Judith Wright

Grieve's Modern Manual Therapy

The Vertebral Column

THIRD EDITION

Edited by

Jeffrey D. Boyling MSc (Lond) BPhty (Hons) (Qld) GradDipAdvManipTher (SAIT) MAPA MCSP MErgS MMPA

Chartered Physiotherapist and Ergonomist, Hammersmith, London, UK

Gwendolen A. Jull MPhty GradDipManipTher PhD FACP

Professor and Head, Division of Physiotherapy, The University of Queensland, Australia

Foreword by

Professor Lance T. Twomey BAppSc BSc PhD TTC MAPA

Vice-Chancellor, Curtin University of Technology, Perth, Australia

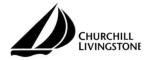

CHURCHILL
LIVINGSTONE

EDINBURGH   LONDON   NEW YORK   OXFORD   PHILADELPHIA   ST LOUIS   SYDNEY   TORONTO   2004

CHURCHILL LIVINGSTONE
An imprint of Elsevier Limited

First edition 1986
Second edition 1994
Third edition 2004

ISBN 0443 071551

British Library Cataloguing in Publication Data
A catalogue record for this book is available from the British Library

Library of Congress Cataloging in Publication Data
A catalog record for this book is available from the Library of Congress

Note
Every effort has been made by the Editors and the Publishers to ensure that the descriptions of the
techniques included in this book are accurate and in conformity with the descriptions published by
their developers. The Publishers and the Editors do not assume any responsibility for any injury
and/or damage to persons or property arising out of or related to any use of the material contained
in this book. It is the responsibility of the treating practitioner, relying on independent experience
and knowledge of the patient, to determine the best treatment and method of application for the
patient, to make their own evaluation of their effectiveness and to check with the developers or
teachers of the techniques they wish to use that they have understood them correctly.

The Publisher

The
Publisher's
policy is to use
**paper manufactured
from sustainable forests**

ELSEVIER your source for books,
journals and multimedia
in the health sciences
www.elsevierhealth.com

Contents

Contributors

Priscilla J. Barker BAppSc(Physio)
Department of Anatomy and Cell Biology, University of Melbourne, Victoria, Australia

Kim Bennell BAppSc(Physio) PhD
Associate Professor, Centre for Health, Exercise and Sports Medicine, School of Physiotherapy, University of Melbourne, Victoria, Australia

Jill Binkley MCISc(PT) FAAOMPT FCAMT
Assistant Professor (PT), McMaster University, Hamilton, Ontario, Canada; Director, Sentinel Associates, Alpharetta, Georgia, USA

Jeffrey J. W. Boyle BSc(Phty) GradDipManipTher
Lecturer, Centre for Musculoskeletal Studies, School of Surgery and Pathology, University of Western Australia, Australia

Jeffrey D. Boyling MSc(Lond) BPhty(Hons)(Qld) GradDipAdvManip Ther (SAIT) MAPA MCSP MergS MMPA
Chartered Physiotherapist and Ergonomist, Hammersmith, London, UK

Christopher A. Briggs DipEd BSc MS PhD
Department of Anatomy and Cell Biology, University of Melbourne, Victoria, Australia

Lucie Brosseau PhD
Associate Professor, School of Rehabilitation Sciences, University of Ottawa, Ontario, Canada

Bert M. Chesworth PhD FCAMT
Research Director, Ontario Joint Replacement Registry, London Health Sciences Centre, London, Ontario, Canada

Jacek Cholewicki PhD
Associate Professor, Biomechanics Research Laboratory, Department of Orthopaedics and Rehabilitation, Yale University School of Medicine, Connecticut, USA

Nicole Christensen MAppSc PT OCS FAAOMPT
Assistant Professor, Orthopaedic Curriculum Coordinator, Department of Physical Therapy, Mount St Mary's College, and Clinical Faculty, Kaiser Permanente Los Angeles Manual Therapy Fellowship, Los Angeles, USA

Angela M. Downing MSc MCSP DipTP CertEd
Senior Lecturer, School of Allied Health Professions, Faculty of Health and Social Care, University of the West of England, Bristol, UK

Stephen J. Edmondston DipPT AdvDipPT(ManTher) PhD
Associate Professor of Musculoskeletal Physiotherapy, School of Physiotherapy, Curtin University of Technology, Perth, Australia

Ian Edwards PhD GradDipPhysio(Ortho) MAPA
Physiotherapist, The Brian Burdekin Clinic, and Lecturer, School of Health Sciences, University of South Australia, Adelaide, Australia

Mark Elkins BPhty
Centre for Evidence-Based Physiotherapy, The University of Sydney, and Royal Prince Alfred Hospital, Sydney, Australia

Robert L. Elvey BAppSc(Physio) GradDipManipTher
Manipulative Physiotherapist, Senior Lecturer in Manipulative Physiotherapy, Curtin University of Technology, Perth, Western Australia

Deborah Falla BPhty(Hons) PhD
Research Officer, Department of Physiotherapy, University of Queensland, Brisbane, Australia

Peter Fazey BAppSc(Physio) GradDipManipTher
Lecturer, Centre for Musculoskeletal Studies, School of Surgery and Pathology, University of Western Australia; Private Practitioner, Perth, Australia

Mary Galea BAppSc(Physio) BA GradDipPhysio(Neuro) GradDipNeurosciences PhD
Professor of Clinical Physiotherapy, School of Physiotherapy, The University of Melbourne, Victoria, Australia

Ian D. Graham PhD MA BA
Associate Professor, School of Nursing, University of Ottawa; Senior Social Scientist, Associate Director, Clinical Epidemiology Program, Ottawa Health Research Institute; Associate Professor, Medicine and Epidemiology and

Community Medicine, University of Ottawa, Canada; CIHR
New Investigator

Jane Greening PhD MSc MCSP MMACP
Consultant Physiotherapist, Dartford, Gravesend and Swanley
Primary Care Trust, NHS Kent; Senior Honorary Research
Fellow, Physiology Department, University College London;
Research Fellow, London South Bank University, UK

Anita Gross MSc BHScPT GradDipManipTher FCAMT
Associate Clinical Professor, School of Rehabilitation Sciences,
McMaster University, Hamilton, Ontario, Canada

Toby M. Hall MSc GradDipManipTher
Manipulative Physiotherapist, Adjunct Senior Teaching Fellow,
School of Physiotherapy, Curtin University of Technology;
Director, Manual Concepts, Perth, Australia

Hannu Heikkilä MD PhD
Specialist in Family Medicine and Physical Medicine &
Rehabilitation, Department of Otorhinolaryngology, Northern
Sweden University Hospital, Umea, Sweden

Robert D. Herbert PhD BAppSc MAppSc(ExSpSc)
School of Physiotherapy, Faculty of Health Sciences, University
of Sydney, Sydney, Australia

Julie A. Hides, BPhty MPhtySt PhD
Senior Lecturer, Department of Physiotherapy, The University of
Queensland, Brisbane, Australia

Paul W. Hodges PhD MedDr BPhty(Hons)
Professor and NHMRC Senior Research Fellow, Department of
Physiotherapy, The University of Queensland, Brisbane, Australia

Jan Lucas Hoving PhD MSc PT MT
Senior Research Fellow, Department of Epidemiology and
Preventive Medicine, Monash University, Melbourne, Australia

D. Glenn Hunter MSc MCSP SRP CertEd
Principal Lecturer, School of Allied Health Professionals,
Faculty of Health and Social Care, University of the West of
England, Bristol, UK

Laurie Hurley BSc PT MSc
Lecturer, Department of Physical Therapy, University of
Toronto, Ontario, Canada

Mark Jones BSc(Psych) PT GradDipAdvanManipTher MAppSc
Senior Lecturer, Director, Master of Musculoskeletal and Sports
Physiotherapy, School of Health Sciences, Physiotherapy
Discipline, University of South Australia, Adelaide, Australia

Gwendolen A. Jull MPhty GradDipManipTher PhD FACP
Professor and Head, Division of Physiotherapy, The University
of Queensland, Brisbane, Australia

Susannah Kelley BPhty MPhtySt
Musculoskeletal Physiotherapist, Performance Rehab, Brisbane,
Australia

Roger Kerry MSc MCSP MMACP
Lecturer, Division of Physiotherapy Education, University of
Nottingham, Nottingham, UK

Emily A. Keshner PT EdD
Senior Clinical Research Scientist, Sensory Motor Performance
Program, Rehabilitation Institute of Chicago; Research Professor,
Department of Physical Medicine and Rehabilitation, Feinberg
School of Medicine, Northwestern University, Chicago, USA

Bart Koes PhD
Professor of General Practice, ErasmusMC, University Medical
Center, Rotterdam, The Netherlands

Eythor Kristjansson PT PhD ManipTher BSc MNFF
Private Practitioner, Reykjavik, Iceland

Judy Larsen BPhty
Physiotherapist and private practitioner, Wesley Hydrotherapy
Centre and St Andrew's Hydrotherapy Centre, Brisbane,
Queensland, Australia

Diane Lee BSR(Hons) FCAMT
Education and Clinical Consultant, Ocean Pointe
Physiotherapy Consultants, White Rock, British Columbia,
Canada

Jenny McConnell BAppSci(Phty) GradDipManipTher MBiomedE
Director, McConnell and Clements Physiotherapy, Mosman,
Australia

Christopher G. Maher PhD GradDipAppSc BAppSc
Associate Professor, School of Physiotherapy, Faculty of Health
Sciences, The University of Sydney, Australia

Susan Mercer BPhty(Hons) MSc PhD FNZCP
Senior Lecturer, Department of Anatomy and Structural
Biology, University of Otago, Dunedin, New Zealand

Steve Milanese BAppScGrad Cert(Sports Physiotherapy) MAppSc GradDip
(Ergonomics)
Ergonomist, Rankin Occupational Safety and Health, Mile End,
South Australia; Senior Research Officer, Centre for Allied
Health Research, University of South Australia, Adelaide,
Australia; Clinical Specialist – Musculoskeletal, St Mary's
Hospital, London, UK

Anne M. Moseley PhD GradDipAppSc
Rehabilitation Studies Unit, The University of Sydney,
Australia

G. Lorimer Moseley PhD BAppSc(Phty)(Hons)
NHMRC Clinical Research Fellow, Senior Lecturer, School of
Physiotherapy, The University of Sydney, Australia

Kenneth R. Niere BAppSc(Physio) GradDipManipTher MManipPhysio
Lecturer, School of Physiotherapy, La Trobe University, Victoria,
Australia

Shaun O'Leary BPhty(Hons) MPhtySt
Department of Physiotherapy, University of Queensland,
Brisbane, Australia

Peter B. O'Sullivan DipPhysio GradDipManipTher PhD
Senior Lecturer, Manipulative Physiotherapist, School of
Physiotherapy, Curtin University of Technology, Perth, Australia

Rob A. B. Oostendorp PhD MScPT MT
Professor in Allied Health Care, Centre for Quality of Care Research, University Medical Centre, Catholic University of Nijmegen, Nijmegen; Research Director, Dutch Institute of Allied Health Care, Amersfoort, Netherlands

Carolyn A. Richardson BPhty(Hons) PhD
Associate Professor and Reader, Department of Physiotherapy, University of Queensland, Brisbane, Australia

Darren A. Rivett BAppSc(Phty) GradDipManipTher MAppSc (ManipPhty) PhD
Associate Professor, Discipline of Physiotherapy, Faculty of Health, University of Newcastle, Australia

Sally Roberts PhD BSc FIMLS
Director of Spinal Research, Centre for Spinal Studies, Robert Jones and Agnes Hunt Orthopaedic Hospital NHS Trust, Oswestry, and Reader, Institute of Science and Technology in Medicine, Faculty of Health, Keele University, UK

Ruth Sapsford AUA DipPhty
Pelvic Floor Physiotherapist, Mater Misericordiae Hospital, Brisbane, Australia

Catherine Sherrington BAppSc(Physio) MPH PhD
Research Fellow, Prince of Wales Medical Research Institute, University of New South Wales, Sydney, Australia

Debra Shirley BSc(UNSW) GradDipPhty(Cumb) GradDipManipTher (Cumb) PhD(USYD)
Lecturer, School of Physiotherapy, Faculty of Health Sciences, The University of Sydney, Australia

Sheri P. Silfies PhD PT OCS
Assistant Professor, Department of Rehabilitation Sciences, Drexel University, Philadelphia, USA

Kevin P. Singer PhD MSc PT
Associate Professor and Head, Centre for Musculoskeletal Studies, School of Surgery and Pathology, The University of Western Australia, Perth, Australia

Tina Souvlis BPhty(Hons) PhD
Lecturer, Division of Physiotherapy, The University of Queensland, Brisbane, Australia

Valerie Sparkes PhD MPhty BA MCSP SRP MMACP
Lecturer, Department of Physiotherapy Education, University of Wales College of Medicine, Cardiff, Wales, UK

Michele Sterling BPhty GradDipManipTher MPhty PhD
Lecturer, Division of Physiotherapy, The University of Queensland, Brisbane, Australia

Raymond A. H. M Swinkels MSc PT MT
Medical Centre Coevering, Geldrop; Manual Therapy, Faculty of Medicine and Pharmacology, Free University, Brussels, Belgium; Lecturer, University of Genoa, Italy; Lecturer, MSc Physical Therapy, Breda, The Netherlands

Alan J. Taylor MSc MCSP SRP
Physiotherapy Manager, Nottingham Nuffield Hospital, Nottingham, UK

Julia Treleaven BPhty
Division of Physiotherapy, The University of Queensland, Brisbane, Australia

Jocelyn P. Urban PhD DIC
Physiology Laboratory, Oxford University, Oxford, UK

Bill Vicenzino PhD MSc BPhty GradDipSportsPhty
Senior Lecturer and Director, Musculoskeletal Pain and Injury Research Unit, Department of Physiotherapy, The University of Queensland, Brisbane, Australia

Andry Vleeming PhD
Chairman of the Advisory Board for the Spine and Joint Centre, Rotterdam, Netherlands

Paul J. Watson PhD MSc BSc(Hons) DipPT MCSPg
Senior Lecturer, Department of Health Sciences, University of Leicester, UK

Anthony Wright BSc(Hons) GradCertEduc MPhtySt PhD MMPA
Professor and Head of School, School of Physiotherapy, Curtin University of Technology, Perth, Australia

Max Zusman DipPhysio GradDipHlthSc MAppSc
Lecturer, School of Physiotherapy, Curtin University of Technology, Perth, Australia

Foreword

Modern Manual Therapy of the Vertebral Column had a major impact when it was first published in 1986. It was a huge book, almost 900 pages long, containing scholarly and clinical information from important international practitioners within or associated with the rapidly evolving discipline of manual therapy. The second edition (1994) was similarly large with two-thirds of the chapters containing new material, while the remainder was substantially revised and updated. The third edition is entirely new and truly demonstrates not only the evolution in the thinking and practice within this discipline, but also highlights a 'changing of the guard' as the early eminent authorities properly give way to younger scholars and clinicians. Along the way, this ensures that manual therapy continues to forge ahead into the 21st century with the vigour and vitality which were a hallmark of its beginnings.

Only 11 of the 52 authors involved in the second edition have contributed to the third, and *all* of these have presented different topics to before. It is particularly sad to note that three major authors and world figures that presented their seminal work in the first two editions are now deceased. They were Greg Grieve from the United Kingdom, David Lamb from Canada and Brian Edwards from Australia. All three were charismatic leaders and educators, pre-eminent in their field, enthusiastic in their promotion of the discipline and truly wonderful men. As an international community, we are much the poorer for their loss. Nevertheless, their legacy is demonstrated in the continued growth of and regard for manual therapy worldwide, which is well demonstrated by this third volume. Many of the new wave of authors have studied and worked with Greg, David and Brian, each of whom would have been delighted to see their life's work so well amplified and extended.

Manual therapists are problem solvers. Each patient presents a unique occasion for therapists to use their understanding of science and behaviour to work toward the satisfactory resolution of spinal problems. While this volume provides an up-to-date account of the clinical skills and practices available to therapists, it does so in the context of science and evidence-based practice. It is in these latter areas that knowledge has expanded so dramatically in recent years. Science now provides a much more complete knowledge of the structure, function, movement behaviour and pathology of the vertebral column than it ever did in the past. At the same time, there is a greater understanding of the physiology and manifestation of pain from vertebral structures and the behaviour of people affected by spinal pain and movement disorders. It is this reliance on science and evidence-based practice that so distinguishes the manual therapy of today from that of the mid-20th century.

In developing this third edition, the editors have not made the mistake of staying with the tried and trusted format of the past. This is a bold book. It moves the discipline forward and, although it pays due respect to the past, it proudly strides into the future with new authors, good science, great ideas and soundly based practice. I suspect that Gregory Grieve would have loved the ways in which his passion for the discipline and practice of manual therapy have been made manifest in this third edition.

Perth, 2005   L.T.T.

Preface to the third edition

Since the second edition of this book was published the world has changed. Only future generations will be able to judge whether it was in general for the better or for the worse. However, in the world of manual therapy the changes that have taken place have been for the better.

This third edition comes some 9 years after the second and 17 years after the first. Some readers may consider the gaps between the three editions to be long but in reality change does not take place overnight. The pauses reflect the time taken for further maturity to occur within the field of manual therapy. Research that was being considered at the time of the second edition has now been undertaken and the results considered. Readers of this new edition will be able to benefit from that research. At the same time, however, previous editions are not obsolete but remain a valuable reference tool and, with the passage of time, will provide a useful barometer of how the focus of the profession has changed and matured.

Churchill Livingstone were the publishers of the first and second editions of *Modern Manual Therapy*. In the intervening period the Churchill Livingstone imprint first became part of Harcourt Health Sciences and then, more recently, part of Elsevier Limited. Fortunately, the same team has been able to assist the editors to compile this edition. All the chapters are new and the line-up of authors has been changed to reflect retirements as well as new aspiring manual therapists at the forefront of research and practice.

Sadly, Greg Grieve is no longer with us to share in the publication of this edition. However, his quest for knowledge and for answers to questions lives on. On reflection it is clear to see that his thirst for knowledge was the forerunner of evidence-based practice. His publications in the field of manual therapy are proof of this. However, his attention to clinical detail should not be overlooked since it reinforced the reality of practice-based evidence. It is to be hoped that the reader will find a balance between evidence-based practice and practice-based evidence as they appear in this edition of *Grieve's Modern Manual Therapy: The Vertebral Column*.

London and Brisbane, 2005

J. D. B.
G. A. J.

Preface to the second edition

The retirement of Gregory Grieve left Churchill Livingstone with a superb text to be continued as well as with the task of finding a replacement editor. The fact that the second edition has been a joint effort is a reflection on the immense contribution to physiotherapy, and manual therapy in particular, that Gregory Grieve has made.

The first edition reflected the leading edge of practice in the early 1980s, and it is to be hoped that this edition reflects the views of manual therapists in the early 1990s. This text is by no means meant to be exhaustive or representative of the full spectrum of work being undertaken. That task represents a dream of past and present editors.

The challenge to validate work has been taken up and it is reflected in the research work included in this text, as well as in the change of emphasis on examination as shown by the appropriate chapters. It is also pleasing to see new material developed by physiotherapists being added to the knowledge base.

It is fitting that this new edition of *Modern Manual Therapy* is being published in the centenary year of the oldest physiotherapy association, the Chartered Society of Physiotherapy. The very roots of the profession are steeped in manual therapy, and it is pleasing that one of the core skills is still at the heart of physiotherapy practice.

It is almost 10 years since the first edition, which is still regarded as the standard text in the subject area, was published. Consequently, the second edition is completely new, with the inclusion of representatives of a new generation of manual therapists keen to display their philosophies and techniques. In addition, long-standing and established practitioners have been able to completely review their contributions as the result of continuing practice and research. The practical application and scientific basis of manual therapy marches on.

Clinical problem-solving has become part of every therapist's repertoire and this, linked to the need for rigorous quality assurance measures, has increased the need for research to support the use of manual therapy in a cost conscious world.

The authors of the chapters have all produced outstanding work, which allows this book to remain at the forefront of physiotherapy practice. No doubt, by the time the next edition is produced yet another group of aspiring manual therapists will be ready to share their professional expertise. The progress of manual therapy moves ever onward.

In conclusion, it is to be hoped that this text will be useful to undergraduates, to practising manual therapists and to the ever-increasing number of therapists completing higher degrees.

J. D. B.
London and Cardiff, 1994
N. P.

Preface to the first edition

Churchill Livingstone's invitation to compile and edit a text on *Modern Manual Therapy* prompted my first concept of a rich and comprehensive totality. Constraints of the possible soon whittled down that version, yet the chapters are, I hope, a fair representation of what physiotherapists were thinking and doing in the mid-1980s, together with authoritative accounts of some contexts of that work.

I have enjoyed the privilege of being associated with the sixty authors, whose views I may not necessarily share of course.

Together with excellent contributions from British colleagues, the manifest overseas presence reflects my abiding links with those energetic and restless countries whose citizens have contributed much sound, realistic advancement.

This is not an exhaustive text on technique, nor even a representative vocabulary. Technique is not of prime importance, since technique springs most naturally from the fullest grasp of the nature of the musculo-skeletal problem. More arduous than learning the various ways to push this or tweak and pull that is the task of educating oneself in understanding the problem. This is infinitely worthwhile and rewarding, because this also teaches when not to handle the patient.

Improvement of clinical competence is a demanding business. Ultimately, clinical effectiveness is directly related to the strength of the individual's desire to *be* clinically effective, and it is pointless beseeching deaf heaven, 'Will somebody please tell me what to think', since always there are those only too happy to do this. Workers who seek to improve their clinical efficacy need discrimination and lively ability to distinguish fact from fancy.

We derive from each other, as the painter Sickert (1860–1942) has expressed it: '. . . the language of paint, like any other language, is kneaded and shaped by all the competent workmen labouring at any given moment; it is, with all its individual variations, a common language and not one of us would have been exactly what he is but for the influence and experience of all the other competent workmen of the period.' Many recent advances in basic knowledge, and alternative ways of thinking about old problems, have already made our yesterdays seem centuries ago, yet we need to recognize sterile propaganda and plain advertisement. Novelty is not progress.

By its nature, manipulative medicine does not enjoy the same scientific basis as anatomy, physiology, molecular biology, pathology or pharmacology, for example. We cannot take the bits apart to see what we are doing, or why we need to do it. Much of what we do is simply what has *been proven on the clinical shop floor* to be effective in getting our patients better – we do not always know precisely why.

We continue to sound as though we know so much, when we know comparatively little. It might be a good thing to admit to this. We make much of clinical science, enthusiastically referring to this or that part of the massive mountain of literature which best serves our particular interest, yet Oliver Sacks (1982), who researched the effects of L-dopa on Parkinson's disease, puts the matter clearly: 'We rationalise, we dissimilate, we pretend; we pretend that modern medicine is a rational science, all facts, no nonsense and just what it seems. But we have only to rap its glossy veneer for it to split wide open and reveal to us its roots and foundations, the old dark heart of metaphysics, mysticism, magic and myth.'

As astrology is to the science of astronomy, pure science tends to fall by the wayside as wishful thinking, therapeutic likes, dislikes and old loyalties push to the fore. While it is ordinary common sense to work in the way in which one feels most comfortable, and most effective, we cannot thereby make a scientific virtue out of expediency.

Professor Lewis Thomas, of the State University of New York at Stony Brook, recently mentions (in *Late Night Thoughts* 1984 OUP): 'Medicine, the newest and youngest of all the sciences, bobs along in the wake of biology, indeed not yet sure that it *is* all that much of science, but certain that if there is to be a scientific future for medicine it can come only from basic biomedical research.'

Manual therapists may have a long road to travel before we talk an agreed common language, founded on scientific fact, but we can enjoy some solid progress towards that end and are now travelling with confidence.

Halesworth, Suffolk, 1986   G. P. G.

Acknowledgements

Publications of the size and quality of the third edition of *Grieve's Modern Manual Therapy: The Vertebral Column* cannot come to fruition without the work of many individuals.

As Editors, we would like to thank most particularly the contributors to this text. They not only gave of their time to write the chapters, but the written material presented in this text reflects the contributors' lifelong work and dedication to enhancing the sciences and clinical practices of today's modern manual therapies. The contributors are to be congratulated on their outstanding work, their impressive research and cutting edge applications to clinical practices. The text represents literally hundreds of years of experience and reveals the leadership of physiotherapists in the musculoskeletal field.

Thanks are also given to the publishers, Elsevier, and in particular to Mary Law, Barbara Muir, Dinah Thom, Claire Wilson and Ailsa Laing whose untiring work and, at many times, patience has brought this third edition to print. Stephanie Pickering is also to be thanked for her attention to detail in copy-editing the manuscript. Any errors remaining are naturally those of the Editors.

Finally, we would like to acknowledge the tolerance of our respective families and friends. We thank them for their patience and support during the preparation of this publication.

J. D. B.
G. A. J

SECTION 1

Introduction to modern manual therapy

Chapter 1

The future scope of manual therapy

J. D. Boyling, G. A. Jull

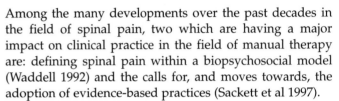

Among the many developments over the past decades in the field of spinal pain, two which are having a major impact on clinical practice in the field of manual therapy are: defining spinal pain within a biopsychosocial model (Waddell 1992) and the calls for, and moves towards, the adoption of evidence-based practices (Sackett et al 1997).

Placing spinal pain in the context of a biopsychosocial model has improved understanding of the multidimensional nature of pain and disability and has underpinned shifts and expansions in management approaches. Practising within this model has had undoubted benefits for back and neck pain patients. Nevertheless there are still challenges ahead. Even with the adoption of this model, there does not appear to have been any lessening in the lifetime incidence of neck and back pain, neither is there evidence that there has been any substantial success in preventing the transition from an initial acute episode of pain to a recurrent or chronic pain state.

One of the historic problems in this field has been the difficulty in obtaining a definitive patho-anatomical diagnosis for the vast majority of patients with an episode of neck or back pain. Working within a patho-anatomical model, researchers and clinicians still have to contend with such diagnoses as non-specific back pain, idiopathic neck pain, or neck pain following a whiplash injury. This in itself is unsatisfactory, but as is well appreciated clinically, possession of a definitive diagnostic label such as a 'discal injury' may not be much more helpful in directing treatment. Under such a diagnosis many different clinical presentations are possible, which often require different management approaches.

Given this situation, there are shifts in the paradigm of research in the medical literature. The shift is towards trying to better understand the processes in the pain, neuromuscular and psychological systems underlying patients' pain, disability and functional problems and their interaction. Health practitioners such as physiotherapists are well positioned to contribute to this research, as this is their model of practice. Historically, from the patient interview and physical examination, the manual therapy clinician has aimed to understand the patient as a person and how their spinal pain is affecting them personally and functionally, and to elucidate the nature of impairments in the articular, muscular and neural systems that are associated with the patient's problem. It is therefore pleasing to observe that the basic and applied clinical sciences of manual or musculo-skeletal therapy have undergone rapid development in the past decade in this mechanistic model of research. As is evident in the third edition of this text, researchers from the disciplines of manual therapy are involved in the basic and applied clinical sciences to better define the processes in spinal pain and disability. The outcomes of this research are indicating that quite specific problems occur in the various systems and the changes can be variable in nature and degree. Such changes in the pain and neuro-motor systems, with their attendant psychological responses, appear to occur simultaneously and interdependently. The outcomes of such mechanistic basic sciences research have the potential to indicate the type of treatment that is likely to be most suitable to reverse a certain problem. What has become evident from this research, and well known to clinicians, is that back and neck pain are not homogenous conditions. Researchers in the applied clinical sciences are testing the effectiveness and efficacy of these research directed interventions, but the current challenge is to better understand the precise nature of the changes and, most importantly, to be able to identify and classify the disorders and recognize patients who are more likely to be responsive to certain treatment approaches. The World Health Organization (WHO) has provided a starting point with two publications. The first is the International Statistical Classification of Diseases and Related Health Problems (ICD-10) (World Health Organization 2003a). Second, and of more interest, is the International Classification of Functioning, Disability and Health (ICF) (World Health Organization 2003b).

Manual therapy practices have changed over the past decade in response to new knowledge, and they will continue to undergo change and refinement. The continuing coalescence of the science and clinical practices of manual therapy will further strengthen the approach embraced in evidence-based practice. Not surprising, given the verification of multisystem involvement in neck and back pain, the evidence is pointing towards the greater efficacy of multi-modal therapies, particularly inclusive of exercise in the management of neck and back pain. However, the evidence of efficacy is not as yet unequivocal for any conservative management method and this is placing tensions on all in the healthcare sector internationally. Many reasons can be offered for this current state but perhaps the more important need is future directions which will assist the advancement of clinical evidence to assist the community to obtain optimal health care for neck and back pain. Clinicians need to play a major role and the nature of their participation is illustrated in Figure 1.1:

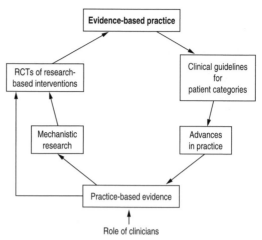

Figure 1.1 The clinician's contribution to evidence-based practices.

The evidence gained from clinicians treating patients is an important driver for research, and for the further development and implementation of evidence-based practices.

- further identification of physical and psychosocial processes in spinal pain patients
- recognition of recurring patterns of processes – diagnostic groups
- responses to interventions – evidence with patient-centred outcomes and outcomes of physical impairment and functioning, documentation of relationships
- responsiveness to treatment – identification of responders and non-responders
- data on patients' values, experiences and opinions of treatments.

This means that musculoskeletal physiotherapists, be they clinicians or researchers, need to look at outcomes. An outcome is that which comes out of something – a visible or practical result, effect or product. There are a number of fundamental questions. What should be measured? How do I measure the outcome? How do I use the measurement to analyse the efficacy or efficiency of the rehabilitation? The ICF provides a conceptual framework to understand the consequences of disease including spinal pain. The consequences act at the level of impairment, activity limitation and participation as well as at the level of quality of life. Haigh et al (2001) have reported that the majority of outcome measurement is at the impairment level, with some at the activity limitation level and very little at the quality of life level. It is worth remembering that musculoskeletal physiotherapy acts at more than the impairment level and therefore measures of outcome should reflect this. However, evidence-based practice is shaped by what forms of knowledge are counted as evidence. In view of this, Gibson & Martin (2003) have highlighted the role of qualitative research in evidence-based physiotherapy practice.

The destiny of manual therapy must be controlled by its clinicians, researchers and consumers. The third edition of *Modern Manual Therapy* has changed direction from previous editions, to highlight developments in the field. It embraces the biopsychosocial model of back pain and evidence-based practices and highlights the basic and applied clinical sciences underpinning current practices. Foremost, it should improve practice and open avenues for critical thought and appraisal to drive future research and clinical practice in manual therapy.

KEYWORDS	
biopsychosocial model	classification
evidence-based practices	outcome
practice-based evidence	

References

Gibson B E, Martin D K 2003 Qualitative research and evidence-based physiotherapy practice. Physiotherapy 89(6): 350–358

Haigh R, Tennant A, Biering-Sorensen F et al 2001 The use of outcome measures in physical medicine and rehabilitation in Europe. Journal of Rehabilitation Medicine 33: 273–278

Sackett D L, Richardson W S, Rosenberg W, Haynes R B 1997 Evidence-based medicine: how to practice and teach EBM, 1st edn. Churchill Livingston, New York

Waddell G 1992 Biopsychosocial analysis of low back pain. Baillière's Clinical Rheumatology 6: 523–557

World Health Organization 2003a International statistical classification of diseases and related health problems (ICD-10), 10th edn. World Health Organization, Geneva

World Health Organization 2003b International classification of functioning, disability and health (ICF). World Health Organization, Geneva

SECTION 2

Foundation sciences for manual therapy

Chapter **2**

Comparative anatomy of the spinal disc

S. Mercer

THE INTERVERTEBRAL DISC

The vertebral column acts as the central flexible rod of the trunk. Therefore each intervertebral disc, interposed between adjacent vertebrae, has several functions. Primarily it acts to separate the vertebral bodies allowing them to move relative to each other and thereby promoting motion at each interbody joint. Additionally, a disc must sustain the load of the body above it and the action of any surrounding muscles when they act. In order to carry out these functions an intervertebral disc must be pliable yet strong (Bogduk 1994).

Each section of the vertebral column must also meet specific regional demands. The cervical spine must ensure balance and free movement of the head. The thoracic spine provides for suspension of the ribs and therefore support of the thoracic cavity. The lumbar spine, opposite the abdominal cavity, ensures mobility between the thoracic portion of the trunk and the pelvis while withstanding the higher loads of the trunk above.

The morphology of the vertebrae of each section of the spine reflects these regional differences in function. In the lumbar spine the superior and inferior surfaces of the vertebral bodies are comparatively large and flat reflecting their load transfer function (Bogduk 1997). On the other hand, the superior surfaces of cervical vertebrae 2–7 have uncinate processes reflecting the need for multidirectional mobility of the neck and also the need for stability (Penning 1988). The vertebral bodies of thoracic vertebrae 2–10 increase in size and change shape down the vertebral column and, importantly, each has two demi-facets for the attachment of ribs (Breathnach 1965). This association of the thoracic vertebrae with the ribcage results in a more rigid region of the spine (Takeuchi et al 1999).

The notion of form and function when considering the bony morphology of regional or individual vertebrae is not unusual as musculoskeletal physiotherapists are familiar with these changing shapes and sizes of vertebrae reflecting the regional changes in function within the vertebral column. Yet, when the morphology of the intervertebral disc is considered, a fairly uniform structure is typically portrayed. The archetypal intervertebral disc is depicted as a nucleus pulposus encircled by an annulus fibrosus, interposed between a superior and an inferior end-plate (Williams et al 1995). However, this description is based on the anatomy of a lumbar disc, the region where most research concerned with the spine has occurred and from which many authors have extrapolated the anatomy to all intervertebral discs. More recently, studies of the cervical intervertebral discs have demonstrated that these discs are distinctly different to lumbar discs and that these differences are evident from birth (Mercer & Bogduk 1999, Oda et al 1988, Pooni et al 1986, Scott et al 1994, Taylor 1974, Tondury 1972). Little is currently available in the literature regarding thoracic disc morphology

LUMBAR INTERVERTEBRAL DISC

In the lumbar region the nucleus pulposus consists of a central core of proteoglycan matrix surrounded by fibrocartilage. In infancy the nucleus pulposus is a soft gel and occupies three-quarters of the anterior–posterior dimension of the disc (Taylor et al 2000). Although dehydrating with age, the healthy adult nucleus pulposus is still a semi-fluid mass of mucoid material. Taylor et al (2000) found that even in cadaveric material of older adults the nucleus still demonstrates the ability to imbibe water (Fig. 2.1).

The lumbar annulus fibrosus consists of approximately 10–20 concentric lamellae of collagen fibres which surround the nucleus pulposus. Collagen fibres within each lamella run in parallel at an angle of approximately 65 degrees to the vertical but for each pair of lamellae the direction of the fibres alternates. Such an arrangement enhances the capacity of the lumbar annulus to restrain different movements in diverse directions (Bogduk 1997). Alternating the direction of fibres in each lamella is vital in the disc resisting twisting (Hickey & Hukins 1980).

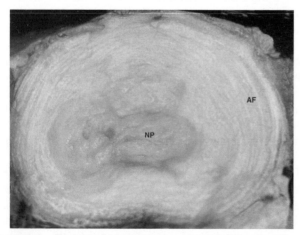

Figure 2.1 Photograph showing a top view of a 39-year-old lumbar intervertebral disc. The annulus fibrosus (AF) is thick and surrounds the nucleus pulposus (NP).

Typically the lamellae are depicted in diagrammatic form with each one completely encircling the nucleus pulposus and being of fairly uniform thickness. However, the thickness of each lamella varies with location and each one does not necessarily form a complete ring around the disc (Marchand & Ahmed 1990). The lamellae closer to the nucleus pulposus are thicker. Furthermore the anterior and lateral lamellae are thick while the posterior lamellae are thinner and more closely packed (Marchand & Ahmed 1990). When viewed from above the posterior portion of the lumbar annulus fibrosus is therefore narrower than the anterolateral aspects (see Fig. 2.1). Incomplete lamellae, that is lamellae that fail to pass around the circumference of the disc, are normal anatomy. They have been noted to be more common in the mid-portion of the disc (Tsuji et al 1993). Marchand & Ahmed (1990) report that within any quadrant of the disc about 40% of the lamellae are incomplete while in the posterolateral corners some 50% are incomplete. When incomplete, the lamella will fuse or approximate with the lamellae superficial or deep to it.

On the basis of attachment sites two portions of the annulus fibrosus may be identified. The outermost lamellae insert into the ring apophysis of the upper and lower vertebrae. These fibres, attaching bone to bone, may be considered as ligaments and as such are designed primarily to limit motion between adjacent vertebrae. The inner lamellae do not attach to bone, rather they attach to the superior and inferior cartilaginous end-plates. These more cartilaginous, proteoglycan-rich lamellae form an envelope around the nucleus pulposus (Taylor et al 2000) and so resist any radial expansion of it (Bogduk 1997).

The cartilaginous end-plates bind the disc to the vertebral bodies and act in the transmission of load. They cover the central area of the vertebral body encircled by the ring apophysis. Closer to its vertebral surface the end-plate is composed of hyaline cartilage while its discal surface is fibrocartilage (Peacock 1951). The inner fibres of the annulus fibrosus are strongly attached to the vertebral end-plates while the end-plates are only weakly attached to the vertebral body. Consequently the end-plates are considered part of the intervertebral disc rather than as part of the lumbar vertebral body (Coventry 1969, Taylor 1975). Such morphology renders the disc susceptible to avulsion from the vertebral body in some forms of trauma.

CERVICAL INTERVERTEBRAL DISC

Detailed study of the normal cervical intervertebral disc has only recently been undertaken and the results indicate that the anatomy of the cervical disc is distinctly different to that of the lumbar intervertebral disc (Mercer & Jull 1996).

From birth the nucleus pulposus of the cervical disc comprises a much smaller portion of the disc, some 25% rather than the 50% seen for the lumbar nucleus (Taylor 1974). In addition the nucleus, even in infancy and childhood, has a higher collagen content than the thoracic or lumbar nucleus

(Scott et al 1994, Taylor et al 1992). Furthermore, by adolescence or adulthood the nucleus is no longer mucoid in nature but is characterized by fibrocartilage (Oda et al 1988, Tondury 1959, 1972). Bland & Boushey (1990) state that, by 40 years of age, there is no gelatinous nucleus pulposus; rather this central region of the cervical disc is composed of fibrocartilage, islands of hyaline cartilage and tendon-like material. Anatomical studies to date indicate that a gelatinous nucleus pulposus is only to be expected in children and young adults. The adult cervical nucleus pulposus is characterized by fibrocartilage (Fig. 2.2).

Examination of the three-dimensional anatomy of the cervical intervertebral disc reveals that it does not mirror the morphology of the lumbar disc (Mercer & Bogduk 1999). The annulus fibrosus is not a ring-like structure of lamellae. Rather it is a discontinuous structure which comprises two distinct portions. The anterior annulus, found running anteriorly between the uncinate processes, is crescentic in shape. It is well developed and thick at the midline, tapering laterally and posteriorly as it approaches the anterior margin of the uncinate processes (Fig. 2.2). The orientation of the collagen fibres within the anterior annulus is also dissimilar to the lumbar annulus fibrosus. In the cervical disc the fibres of the anterior annulus converge superiorly towards the lower anterior edge of the vertebral body above. The anterior annulus may therefore be considered as an interosseous ligament, arranged like an inverted 'V' whose apex is located at the axis of axial rotation (Bogduk & Mercer 2000, Mercer & Bogduk 2001). What we may consider the posterior annulus is a small structure represented by a few vertically oriented fibres located close to the median plane at the posterior aspect of the disc. It is a thin lamina, being no more than 1 mm in depth (see Fig. 2.2). The posterolateral aspects of the cervical disc therefore lack

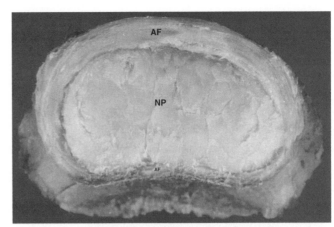

Figure 2.2 Photograph showing the top view of a 39-year-old cervical intervertebral disc. The anterior annulus fibrosus (AF) is thick and fibrous, tapering posteriorly towards the uncinate region. Posteriorly the thin annulus fibrosus (AF) is found only towards the midline. Centrally the nucleus pulposus (NP) appears as a fibrocartilaginous core.

the support of an annulus fibrosus. Only the posterior longitudinal ligament covers the majority of the posterior disc. Posterolaterally the uncovertebral clefts are overlaid by periosteofascial tissue (Fig. 2.3). This unorganized fibrous connective tissue embedded with fat and a large number of blood vessels is continuous with the periosteum of the vertebral body and pedicles (Mercer & Bogduk 1999).

Centrally, the nucleus pulposus of the adult cervical disc is fibrocartilaginous in nature (Bland & Boushey 1990, Oda et al 1988, Tondury 1972). The clefts, which extend into this fibrocartilaginous core, open under the periosteofascial tissue (Mercer & Bogduk 1999). These clefts begin developing

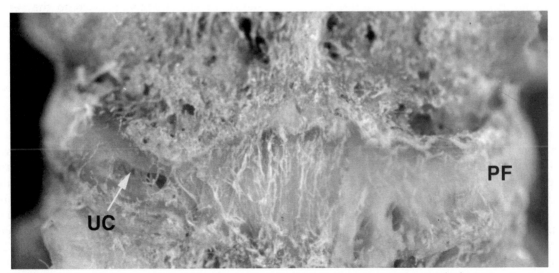

Figure 2.3 Photograph of cervical intervertebral disc from behind. On the left the uncovertebral cleft (UC) which extends into the fibrocartilaginous core. On the right the periosteofascial tissue (PF) which covers the uncovertebral cleft.

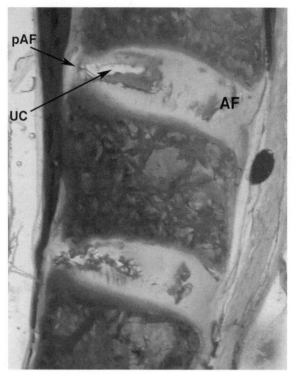

Figure 2.4 Photograph of a sagittal section through cervical intervertebral discs C2/C3 and C3/C4. Note the anterior annulus fibrosus (AF) and narrower posterior annulus fibrosus (pAF). The uncovertebral clefts (UC) have transected the posterior two-thirds of the intervertebral discs.

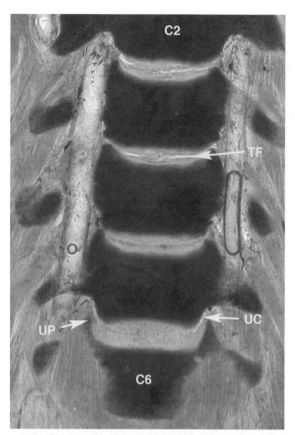

Figure 2.5 Photograph of a coronal section through cervical intervertebral discs. The section through the C5/C6 intervertebral disc reveals the uncinate processes (UP) and uncovertebral cleft (UC). The coronal sections through the higher discs are further posterior and reveal the penetration of the clefts towards the midline to transect the posterior disc.

between 9 and 14 years of age when the uncinate processes reach their maximum height (Ecklin 1960, Tondury 1959). With increasing age the clefts penetrate more medially into the core until they completely transect the posterior two-thirds of the disc, occasionally leaving a small isolated bar of fibrocartilage just deep to the posterior annulus (Ecklin 1960, Mercer & Bogduk 1999, Tondury 1972) (Figs 2.4, 2.5). These clefts are normal anatomy of a cervical disc which, together with the absence of a substantial posterior annulus, facilitate axial rotation (Bogduk & Mercer 2000, Mercer & Bogduk 2001).

THORACIC INTERVERTEBRAL DISC

Very little is known of the detailed morphology of the thoracic intervertebral disc. Pooni et al (1986) reported that in cross-section thoracic discs were more circular than either cervical or lumbar discs, which were more elliptical in shape. In addition thoracic discs were less wedge-shaped.

Although depicted in a variety of texts as similar in gross structure to lumbar discs (Kapandji 1974, Woodburne & Burkel 1988), Zaki (1973) described the annulus fibrosus of the thoracic disc to be a discontinuous two-part structure, with the fibres of the posterior annulus being of vertical orientation. He gave no indications regarding the transition of morphology from cervical to thoracic disc or thoracic to

lumbar disc, or of transitions within the thoracic spine. In addition Lee (1994) postulated the presence of transverse fissures in the thoracic disc.

Recent preliminary work regarding the three-dimensional anatomy of the thoracic intervertebral disc has indicated that the thoracic discs through to the T9/T10 level exhibit a morphology similar to the cervical disc (Mercer 2001). The anterior annulus fibrosus is crescentic, thicker anteriorly towards the midline, and tapering laterally and posteriorly to the costal region (Fig. 2.6). The central fibres of the radiate ligament pass horizontally anterior to the annulus fibrosus, to be covered by the fibres of the anterior longitudinal ligament. Posteriorly the fibres of the thin, centrally placed posterior annulus fibrosus are vertical, being covered by the central longitudinal fibres and lateral extensions of the posterior longitudinal ligament. Posterolaterally, from T1/T2 to T9/T10 the head of the rib articulates with the upper and lower demi-facets and with the intervertebral disc via the intra-articular ligament (Fig. 2.7). At these levels the anterior annulus has tapered prior to the costovertebral joints. Within the fibrocartilaginous core, fissures and clefts are ubiquitous and normal (Figs 2.8, 2.9).

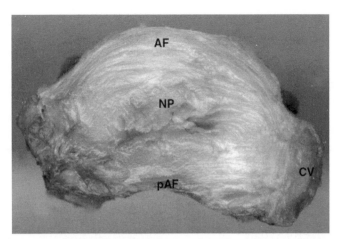

Figure 2.6 Photograph of a top view through a transverse section of a T2/T3 intervertebral disc. The anterior annulus fibrosus (AF) is much thicker than the posterior annulus fibrosus (pAF) tapering laterally towards the costovertebral joint (CV). The nucleus pulposus (NP) is located centrally.

At lower levels, where the head of the rib is articulating with only one vertebral body and not with the disc, the thoracic intervertebral disc adopts a lumbar-type three-dimensional morphology (Mercer 2001). Beginning at the T10/T11 level, the annulus fibrosus is free to pass around the circumference of the disc as seen in the lumbar spine (Fig. 2.10). Here the nucleus pulposus, upon sectioning, would show signs of swelling or weeping as has been reported for lumbar discs.

The typical thoracic disc appears to have been adapted from a cervical design rather than from a lumbar design. The annulus fibrosus of the cervical intervertebral disc morphology has a posterolateral deficiency where the rib can gain access to the fibrocartilaginous core without having to negotiate a posterolateral annulus fibrosus. The transition occurs from this morphology to a lumbar disc morphology at the

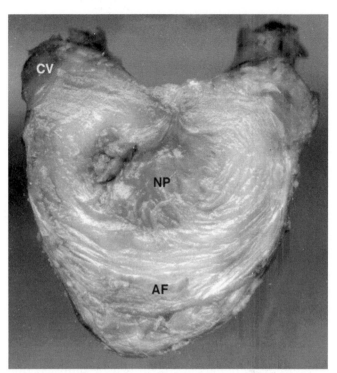

Figure 2.7 Photograph of a top view through a transverse section of a T5/T6 intervertebral disc. The anterior annulus fibrosus (AF) tapers as it approaches the costovertebral joint (CV) to surround the nucleus pulposus (NP) anteriorly and laterally.

level where the rib is no longer associated with the intervertebral disc and articulates solely with the vertebral body.

BLOOD SUPPLY

As there are no major arterial branches directly supplying each intervertebral disc, a disc may be considered as an

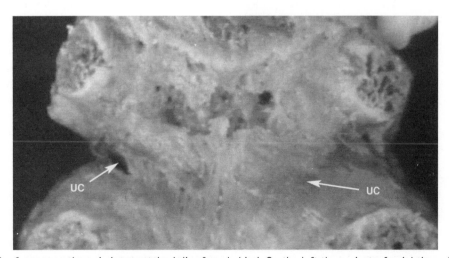

Figure 2.8 Photograph of an upper thoracic intervertebral disc from behind. On the left the periosteofascial tissue has been resected to reveal the uncovertebral cleft (UC). On the right the periosteofascial tissue has been left in situ to demonstrate the uncovertebral cleft (UC) opening beneath it.

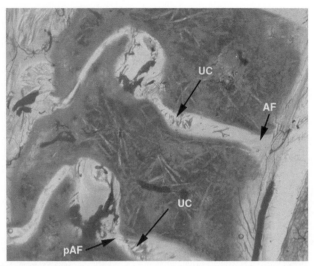

Figure 2.9 Photograph of a sagittal section through the upper thoracic spine. Uncovertebral clefts (UC) are present posteriorly. The posterior (pAF) is very thin while the anterior annulus fibrosus (AF) is relatively thick.

avascular mass of cartilage nourished by diffusion from blood vessels around its perimeter (Taylor et al 2000). Nutrients must therefore diffuse through the annulus fibrosus or through the vertebral end-plate to reach the nucleus pulposus.

As demonstrated in the lumbar spine, the outermost fibres of the annulus fibrosus receive small branches from the metaphyseal arteries, which are anastomosing over its surface (Maroudas et al 1975). In the subchondral bone

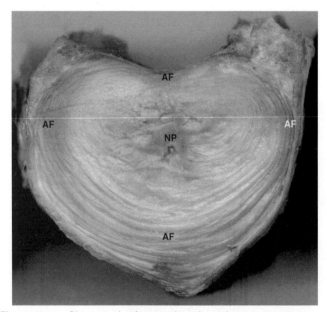

Figure 2.10 Photograph of a top view through a transverse section of a T11/T12 intervertebral disc. The annulus fibrosus (AF) is now surrounding the nucleus pulposus (NP). Note that the anterior section of the annulus fibrosus is thicker than the posterior section of the annulus fibrosus.

underlying the end-plates and in the base of the vertebral end-plate, the terminal branches of the metaphyseal arteries and the nutrient arteries of the vertebra form a dense capillary network. Nutrients are then able to diffuse through the permeable central portions of the vertebral end-plates (Urban et al 1978).

In the cervical spine Oda et al (1988) observed calcification within the cartilaginous end-plate to begin in early adulthood. These authors postulated that such a process leads to a reduction of the nutritional route through the vertebral end-plates leading to the early fibrotic changes observed in the nucleus pulposus.

INNERVATION

Extensive plexuses cover the anterior, lateral and posterior aspects of all intervertebral discs. These plexuses arise from the sympathetic trunks, gray rami communicantes, vertebral nerve and ventral rami and send nerve fibres which penetrate the outer annulus fibrosus at all levels of the spine (Bogduk et al 1981, 1988, Groen et al 1990).

Nerve fibres and nerve endings have been identified in the outer third to half of the lumbar annulus fibrosus (Ashton et al 1994, Bogduk et al 1981, Hirsch & Schajowicz 1952, Malinsky 1959, Palmgren et al 1999, Rabischong et al 1978, Roofe 1940, Taylor & Twomey 1979, Yoshizawa et al 1980). Much less work has been carried out elsewhere in the spine. In the cervical region, nerve fibres have been demonstrated in the outer third of the annulus fibrosus (Bogduk et al 1988) or less specifically in the outer layers (Ferlic 1963). A more extensive pattern of innervation was described by Mendel et al (1992) who reported the presence of nerve fibres throughout the annulus, particularly in the middle third of the disc. These three studies indicate that the cervical intervertebral disc, like the lumbar disc, is innervated. However, precise anatomy of this innervation is lacking.

Based on these findings for the cervical and lumbar intervertebral discs and the presence of extensive plexuses covering all intervertebral discs (Bogduk et al 1981, 1988, Groen et al 1990), it is reasonable to assume that the thoracic intervertebral disc has a similar pattern of innervation. However, the precise anatomy of this innervation awaits further study. Current evidence for innervation of the thoracic discs lies in clinical studies where pain is evoked with provocation discography (Wood et al 1999).

CLINICAL IMPLICATIONS

An appreciation of the differing anatomy of the intervertebral discs throughout the spine is important when developing clinical models. The models developed for the lumbar intervertebral disc, such as internal disc disruption, radial and circumferential annular tears and disc herniation (Bogduk 1991, Moneta et al 1994, Vanharanta et al 1987), are based on the structure of the lumbar intervertebral disc. As the structure and function of the cervical and thoracic intervertebral discs are different to the lumbar disc the models developed for injury or the mechanism by which pain is produced in the lumbar disc are therefore not necessarily applicable to models developed for the cervical and thoracic discs.

KEYWORDS

lumbar intervertebral disc	annulus fibrosus
cervical intervertebral disc	nucleus pulposus
thoracic intervertebral disc	

References

Ashton I K, Roberts S, Jaffray D C, Polak S M, Eisenstein S M 1994 Neuropeptides in the human intervertebral disc. Journal of Orthopaedic Research 12: 186–192

Bland J, Boushey D R 1990 Anatomy and physiology of the cervical spine. Seminars in Arthritis and Rheumatism 20: 1–20

Bogduk N 1991 The lumbar disc and low back pain. Neurosurgery Clinics of North America 2: 791–806

Bogduk N 1994 Anatomy of the spine. In: Klippel J H, Dieppe P A (eds) Rheumatology. Mosby, Sydney

Bogduk N 1997 Clinical anatomy of the lumbar spine and sacrum, 3rd edn. Churchill Livingstone, Edinburgh

Bogduk N, Mercer S R 2000 Biomechanics of the cervical spine. I: Normal kinematics. Clinical Biomechanics 15: 633–648

Bogduk N, Tynan W, Wilson A S 1981 The nerve supply to the human lumbar intervertebral discs. Journal of Anatomy 132: 39–56

Bogduk N, Windsor M, Inglis A 1988 The innervation of the cervical intervertebral discs. Spine 13: 2–8

Breathnach A S 1965 Frazer's Anatomy of the human skeleton. J&A Churchill Ltd, London

Coventry M B 1969 Anatomy of the intervertebral disk. Clinical Orthopaedics and Related Research 67: 9–15

Ecklin U 1960 Die altersveranderungen der halswirbelsaule. Springer Verlag, Berlin

Ferlic D C 1963 The nerve supply of the cervical intervertebral disc in man. Bulletin of the Johns Hopkins Hospital 113: 347–351

Groen G J, Baljet B, Drukker J 1990 Nerves and nerve plexuses of the human vertebral column. American Journal of Anatomy 188: 282–296

Hickey D S, Hukins D W L 1980 Relation between the structure of the anulus fibrosus and the function and failure of the intervertebral disc. Spine 5: 100–116

Hirsch C, Schajowicz F 1952 Studies on structural changes in the lumbar annulus fibrosus. Acta Orthopaedica Scandinavica 22: 184–189

Hirsch C, Ingelmark B E, Miller M 1963 The anatomical basis for low back pain. Acta Orthopaedica Scandinavica 33: 1–17

Kapandji I A 1974 The physiology of the joints. Vol 3: The trunk and the vertebral column. Churchill Livingstone, Edinburgh

Lee D 1994 Manual therapy for the thorax: a biomechanical approach. DOPC, Vancouver

Malinsky J 1959 The ontogenetic development of nerve terminations in the intervertebral discs of man. Acta Anatomica 38: 96–113

Marchand F, Ahmed A M 1990 Investigation of the laminate structure of lumbar disc anulus fibrosus. Spine 15: 402–410

Maroudas A, Nachemson A, Stockwell R, Urban J 1975 Some factors involved in the nutrition of the intervertebral disc. Journal of Anatomy 120: 113–130

Mendel T, Wink C S, Zimny M L 1992 Neural elements in human cervical intervertebral discs. Spine 17: 132–135

Mercer S R 2001 Transitions between cervical and lumbar intervertebral disc morphology. In: Proceedings of the 12th Biennial Conference, Musculoskeletal Physiotherapy Australia 31, Adelaide

Mercer S R, Bogduk N 1999 The ligaments and anulus fibrosus of human adult cervical intervertebral discs. Spine 24: 619–628

Mercer S R, Bogduk N 2001 The joints of the cervical vertebral column. Journal of Orthopaedic and Sports Physical Therapy 31: 174–182

Mercer S R, Jull G A 1996 Morphology of the cervical intervertebral disc: implications for manual therapy. Manual Therapy 1(2): 76–81

Moneta G B, Videman T, Kaivanto K et al 1994 Reported pain during lumbar discography as a function of annular ruptures and disc degeneration: a re-analysis of 833 discograms. Spine 19: 1968–1974

Oda J, Tanaka H, Tsuzuki N 1988 Intervertebral disc changes with aging of human cervical vertebra: from neonate to the eighties. Spine 13: 1205–1211

Palmgren T, Gronblad M, Virri J, Kaapa E, Karaharju E 1999 An immunohistochemical study of nerve structures in the anulus fibrosus of human normal lumbar intervertebral discs. Spine 24: 2075–2079

Peacock A 1951 Observations on the pre-natal development of the intervertebral disc in man. Journal of Anatomy 85: 260–274

Penning L 1988 Differences in anatomy, motion, development and aging of the upper and lower cervical disk segments. Clinical Biomechanics 3: 37–47

Pooni J S, Hukins D W L, Harris P F, Hilton R C, Davis K E 1986 Comparison of the structure of human intervertebral discs in the cervical, thoracic, and lumbar regions of the spine. Surgical Radiological Anatomy 8: 175–182

Rabischong P, Louis R, Vignaud J, Massare C 1978 The intervertebral disc. Anatomica Clinica 1: 55–64

Roofe P G 1940 Innervation of anulus fibrosus and posterior longitudinal ligament. Archives Neurology and Psychiatry 44: 100–103

Scott J, Bosworth T, Cribb A, Taylor J 1994 The chemical morphology of age related changes in human intervertebral disc glycosaminoglycans from cervical, thoracic and lumbar nucleus pulposus and anulus fibrosus. Journal of Anatomy 180: 137–141

Takeuchi T, Abumi K, Shono Y, Oda I, Kaneda K 1999 Biomechanical role of the intervertebral disc and costovertebral joint in stability of the thoracic spine: a canine model study. Spine 21: 1423–1429

Taylor J R 1974 Growth and development of the human intervertebral disc. PhD Thesis, University of Edinburgh

Taylor J R 1975 Growth of the human intervertebral discs and vertebral bodies. Journal of Anatomy 120: 49–68

Taylor J R, Twomey L T 1979 Innervation of lumbar intervertebral discs. Medical Journal of Australia 2: 701–702

Taylor J R, Scott J E, Cribb A M, Bosworth T R 1992 Human intervertebral disc acid glycosaminoglycans. Journal of Anatomy 180: 137–141

Taylor J, Twomey L, Levander B 2000 Contrasts between cervical and lumbar motion segments. Critical Reviews in Physical and Rehabilitation Medicine. 12: 345–371

Tondury G 1959 La colonne cervicale, son développement et ses modifications durant la vie. Acta Orthopaedica Belgica 25: 602–625

Tondury G 1972 The behaviour of the cervical discs during life. In: Hirsch C, Zotterman Y (eds) Cervical pain. Pergamon Press, Oxford

Tsuji H, Hirano N, Ohshima H, Ishihara H, Terahata N, Motoe T 1993 Structural variation of the anterior and posterior anulus fibrosus in the development of human lumbar intervertebral disc: a risk factor for intervertebral disc rupture. Spine 18: 204–210

Urban J P G, Holm S, Maroudas A 1978 Diffusion of small solutes into the intervertebral disc. Biorheology 15: 203–223

Vanharanta H, Sachs B L, Spivey M A et al 1987 The relationship of pain provocation to lumbar disc degeneration as seen by CT/discography. Spine 12: 295–298

Williams P L, Bannister L H, Berry M M et al 1995 Gray's Anatomy: the anatomical basis of medicine and surgery, 38th edn. Churchill Livingstone, Edinburgh

Wood K B, Schellhas K P, Garvey T A, Aeppli D 1999 Thoracic discography in healthy individuals: a controlled prospective study of magnetic resonance imaging and discography in asymptomatic and symptomatic individuals. Spine 24: 1548–1555

Woodburne R T, Burkel W E 1988 Essentials of human anatomy. Oxford University Press, Oxford

Yoshizawa H, O'Brien J P, Thomas-Smith W, Trumper M 1980 The neuropathy of intervertebral discs removed for low-back pain. Journal of Pathology 132: 95–104

Zaki W 1973 Aspect morphologique et fonctionnel de l'anulus fibrosus du disque intervertebrale de la colonne dorsale. Archives Anatomie Pathologie 21: 401–403

Chapter **3**

Comparative anatomy of the zygapophysial joints

K. P. Singer, J. J. W. Boyle, P. Fazey

INTRODUCTION

The design specification for the human vertebral column is the provision of structural stability, affording full mobility, as well as protection of the spinal cord and axial neural tissues. While achieving these seemingly disparate objectives for the axial skeleton, the spine also contributes to the functional requirements of gait and to the maintenance of static weight-bearing postures.

At a component level, the paired zygapophyses of the human vertebral column are synovial joints within the 'functional mobile segment'. This term was coined by the German radiologist Herbert Junghanns (Schmorl & Junghanns 1971) to represent the union of two adjacent vertebrae, their intervening intervertebral disc (IVD) and articulations formed between the posterior elements. The regulation of compressive, shear and tensile forces applied to this 'triad' of disc and paired zygapophysial joints defines its functional role within the skeletal system, both at the segmental level and within the spine overall.

Understanding the variable structure and function of the human zygapophysial joints is an important requirement in manual therapy during the assessment and management of individuals with mechanical spinal pain disorders. Although in life, function of the mobile segment cannot separate out consideration of the intervertebral disc, this chapter will focus primarily on the development, form, function and variations in zygapophysial joints throughout the vertebral column. In some literature, the zygapophysial joints are referred to as facets, interlaminar joints, or the grouped term, posterior elements, is used. The most cranial zygapophysial joints are located between the second and third cervical levels, and the most caudal at the level of the lumbosacral junction. For reference to the specialized anatomy of the suboccipital region as well as the atlanto-occipital and atlanto-axial joints, the comprehensive review by Prescher is recommended (Prescher 1997).

DEVELOPMENT OF THE ZYGAPOPHYSIAL JOINTS

The ossification of the posterior arches occurs separately from the vertebral body centrum and disc (O'Rahilly et al 1980). The paired neural arches unite to enclose the spinal canal and cord, from which stem the respective superior articular processes (SAP) and inferior articular processes (IAP), plus mammillary processes (MP), transverse, and spinous processes (Reichmann 1971, Rickenbacher et al 1985). There is an organized appearance of primary ossification centres for each vertebral element (Bagnall et al 1977), which proceeds in a caudal direction and is generally complete by the fourth month in utero (Christ & Wilting 1992). According to Med (1977), during gestation the articular surfaces of the thoracic zygapophysial joints are relatively flat, with the cervical and lumbar joints showing greater rates of remodelling. Impairment in normal development, often in the first 4 weeks of gestation, has been speculated to contribute to joint configuration anomalies (Med 1980), in addition to segmentation anomalies, which can result in hemivertebra and block vertebra (Christ & Wilting 1992, Saada et al 2000).

The rudimentary zygapophysial joint cavity and capsule is complete in embryos of 70 mm crown–rump length, and by birth the IAP and SAP of the zygapophyes are incompletely ossified (O'Rahilly et al 1980). During development the IAPs, projecting inferiorly from the inferolateral aspect of the neural arch, engage with their respective SAPs to provide a congruent, symmetrical coupling. In the lumbar spine, the SAP is typically J-shaped, producing a coronally orientated medial component which acts to resist anterior shear strain, and a longer, more sagittal posterior part which acts to constrain rotation or torsion applied to the segment (Adams & Dolan 1995).

The posteromedial margin of the SAP is given by Reichmann to show the most marked change, in particular the formation of the sagittal joint expansion (Reichmann 1971). The ossification of the lateral margin of the SAP is protracted during the first year of life with the expanding lateral cartilaginous cap lost to ossification until the definitive form of the SAP is achieved by 7–9 years of age. This lateral element comprises the MP and projects posteriorly from the SAP to offer attachment to the multifidus muscle, which then ascends obliquely and medially, via tendinous slips, towards the superior two vertebral spinous processes (Macintosh et al 1986).

The secondary ossification centres, at the tips of each of the articular, spinous, transverse, mammillary and accessory processes, variously fuse during the first two decades of life (Singer & Breidahl 1990), taking their direction and shape according to the tensile forces applied to them from the attaching musculature and ligaments (Lutz 1967). Indeed, anomalous development of the multifidus muscle, originating from the MP of the SAP, is given by Odgers (1933) to account for asymmetric configuration of lumbar zygapophyses – termed 'articular tropism' by some authors.

The early prenatal configuration of the spinal zygapophyses is essentially similar throughout the spine in that they are aligned predominantly on the frontal plane (Lewin et al 1962), although the precursors for their eventual adult form are already evident in some individuals (Reichmann 1971). During the first postnatal year, the shape of the paired zygapophysial joints changes as functional and regional demands are imposed. The specifications for the cervical and lumbar regions, through the relatively greater vertical dimension of the IVD, confer greater mobility on these segments. In contrast the thoracic discs, which account for only a fifth of the vertical dimension of this region, predispose less segmental sagittal plane motion (Gregersen & Lucas 1967). The regional variations in morphology of the cervical, thoracic and lumbar vertebrae and their respective zygapophysial joints are depicted in Figure 3.1.

There is considerable variation in the alignment and shape of the zygapophyses throughout the spine, despite the tendency in modern anatomy textbooks to depict symmetry (Grieve 1981). At the transitional junctions, where developmental and pathological anomalies predominate (Schmorl & Junghanns 1971), there may be marked morphological differences between right and left zygapophysial joints (Singer et al 1989a) (Fig. 3.2). Even in areas remote from the transitional junctions there may also be marked joint asymmetry (Burkus 1988), providing an important caution against always inferring abnormal mechanical behaviour from passive motion assessment of spinal segments.

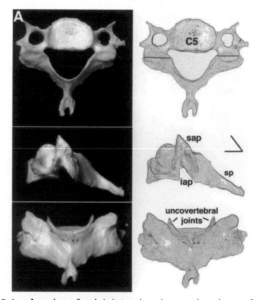

Figure 3.1   A series of axial, lateral and posterior views of mid-cervical (A), thoracic (B) and lumbar (C) vertebrae to depict the primary configuration of their respective zygapophysial joints. In the cervical region, these joints lie lateral to the neural axis compared with the thoracic and lumbar joints. The typical thoracic segment (B) shows the more vertical and coronal alignment whereas the lumbar vertebrae (C) show the 'J'-shaped zygapophyses with their coronal and sagittal elements.

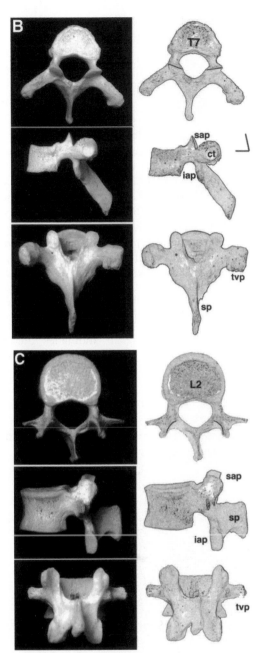

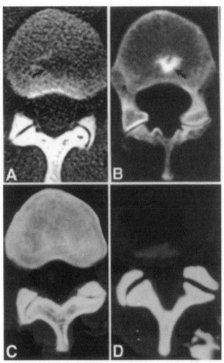

Figure 3.2 Four transverse CT images depicting articular asymmetry, or tropism, of the paired zygapophysial joints. Where tropism occurs at one transitional junction, this and other anomalies may be found at adjacent transitions. The lower images are of a 35-year-old male, with a similar asymmetry pattern of T11–12 (C) and also at L4–5 (D).

Figure 3.1 *Contd*

The eventual adult configuration and shape of the zygapophyses is influenced by the exertional forces applied during early gestation and immediate postnatal motor development. Using in utero ultrasound, Boszczyk et al (2002) have speculated that prenatal morphological changes in zygapophysial joint shape occur in response to spinal torsion putatively induced from muscle actions. During early postnatal development, as the child adopts weight-bearing postures and commences crawling then walking, there is an intensified loading on the lateral margins of the joint which contributes to the sagittalization of the lumbar zygapophysial joints, as seen in the adult form (Lutz 1967). In the apex and lateral region of the lumbar

SAP, there is typically a thicker cartilage in response to these lateral forces (Putz 1985) (Fig. 3.3).

ZYGAPOPHYSIAL JOINT MORPHOLOGY

The articular surfaces are covered in hyaline cartilage and, like most synovial joints, have small fatty or fibrous synovial meniscoid-like fringes (Fig. 3.3) which project between the joint surfaces from the margins (Singer et al 1990). These intra-articular synovial folds (IASF) are found at all levels of the spine (Tondury 1972, Singer et al 1990, Mercer & Bogduk 1993) and are most developed within the polar regions, acting as space fillers during joint displacements and actively assisting dispersal of synovial fluid within the joint cavity.

Occasionally, the cartilage forms a non-articulating 'bumper' wrapping around the posteromedial aspect of the IAP of the joint, typically with a well-developed posterior expansion of the capsular ligament (Fig. 3.4). Often, these bumper cartilage formations are associated with evidence of articular cartilage degeneration and fissuring, ossification of the ligamentum flavum and reactive hyperplasia at the posterior joint margins (refer to Fig. 3.5). The joint cavity is closed anteromedially and reinforced by the ligamentum flavum, which assists in approximation of the articular surfaces and, through its elastic properties, maintains the lumen

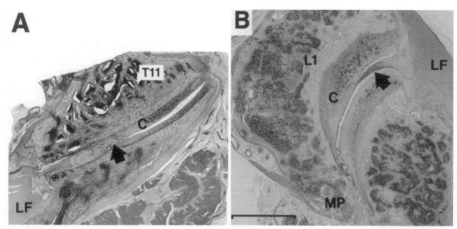

Figure 3.3 Photomicrograph of 100 µm thick transverse sections cut in the plane of the superior vertebral end plate at T11–12 showing a long, finger-like intra-articular synovial protrusion formed within the medial joint cavity, filling this void (A). In the T12–L1 joint (B), a fibro-fatty fold arising from the ligamentum flavum is depicted in the medial joint space projecting between the articular surfaces. In this instance, the SAP forms into an extended mammillary process, which wraps around the IAP. Note the uniform appearance of articular cartilage on all facets, with normal chondrocyte density evenly distributed, particularly with the apex of the lumbar joint (B). Adapted from Singer et al 1990. (C – articular cartilage; MP – mammillary processes; SAP – superior articular process; IAP – inferior articular process; LF – ligamentum flavum.)

of the vertebral canal (Ponseti 1995). Considerable ossification within the ligamentum flavum may be associated with degeneration of the articular triad, although this tends to predominate in the region of the lower thoracic and upper lumbar segments (Malmivaara et al 1987, Maigne et al 1992).

The articular processes of all zygapophysial joints comprise a cortical exterior containing trabecular bone with a thick subchondral region immediately adjacent to the articular cartilage. In regions of highest loading, for example the apex of the concavity of the biplanar lumbar SAP of the zygapophysial joints (see Fig. 3.3), the subchondral bone is most dense, in response to shear and torsional loading. In contrast, the more planar joints of the cervical and thoracic regions tend to show a uniform distribution of cartilage across the face of the facet (Fig. 3.4). The articular cartilage is approximately 1 mm thick with a smooth surface in a normal articular facet. There may be regions of chondrocyte aggregation with thickening at zones of highest joint stress (see Fig. 3.3B). Reactive changes may be identified within the cartilage as a result of minor injury or degenerative changes. Complete enurbation of the cartilage is relatively rare given the tendency for repair via hyperplastic changes within the joint and its constituents which delay direct joint debridement (Fig. 3.5).

In the cervical spine, the zygapophysial joints are relatively flat while progressively increasing their surface area, and tend towards 45 degrees to the horizontal (see Fig. 3.1A), which reflects an increased axial loading of the head through the lower part of the cervical lordosis (Pal & Routal 1986). In the thoracic region, the joints adopt an almost vertical direction while remaining essentially in a coronal orientation (see Fig. 3.1B), which facilitates axial rotation and resists anterior displacement (Gregersen & Lucas 1967). The zygapophysial joints in the lumbar spine are vertical, with

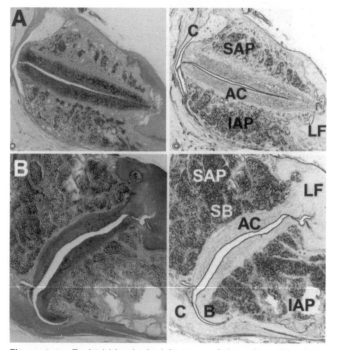

Figure 3.4 Typical histological features of thoracic and lumbar zygapophysial joints where the ligamentum flavum encloses the joint space medially and the lateral joint margin is closed by the capsular ligaments. The relative differences in capsular ligament thickness is noted with the thoracic joint (A) depicting a slight, loose arrangement, which accommodates the excursion of the SAP on the IAP during rotation displacements (A). Both sections illustrate healthy articular surfaces despite slight incongruity of the lumbar joint, which also demonstrates a bumper extension of the articular cartilage wraps around the lateral margin of the IAP (B). The respective elements labelled on the right. (AC – articular cartilage; MP – mammillary processes; SAP – superior articular process; IAP – inferior articular process; LF – ligamentum flavum; SB – subchondral bone; B – bumper cartilage; C – capsule.)

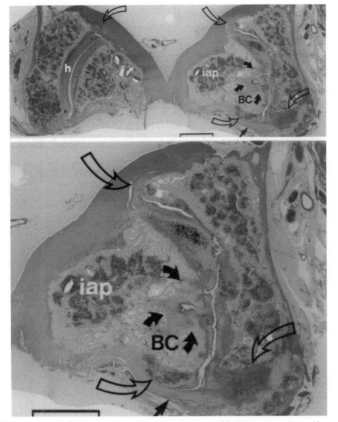

Figure 3.5 Photomicrograph of a 100 μm-thick transverse section cut in the plane of the superior vertebral end plate at L1-2 to highlight unilateral zygapophysial joint degeneration. A normal intact joint is shown in the upper inset figure (A) and, in contrast, the higher magnification of the right joint (B) shows histological evidence of focal degeneration adjacent to a subchondral bone cyst and remodelling of the coronal region of the joint. Hyperplastic reactive bumper cartilage on the posterior margin of the IAP with thickening of the capsular ligament is also evident. (H – articular cartilage; IAP – inferior articular process; LF – ligamentum flavum; BC – bone cyst.)

a curved, J-shaped surface predominantly in the sagittal plane (see Fig. 3.1C), which restricts rotation and also resists anterior shear. The change in shape of these joints between segments is generally progressive, although in some individuals there may be a more abrupt transition at the junctions between regions (Cihak 1981, Singer et al 1989a, Boyle et al 1996).

ZYGAPOPHYSIAL JOINT CAPSULE

The morphology of the synovial joint capsule varies across the spinal regions. In the lumbar joints the capsule is thick and strong posteriorly to moderate sagittal plane movements and resist torsion and extreme lateral flexion. This is in contrast to thoracic and cervical joints where it has a less robust composition (see Fig. 3.4) to permit the greater joint translations which occur in these regions, particularly rota-

tion in the thoracic region and composite motions in the cervical spine. In a fresh, unpreserved lumbar spine, with the zygapophysial joints sectioned horizontally at the level of the superior vertebral end-plate, the ligamentum flavum and posterior joint capsular ligaments hold the articular surfaces firmly apposed. Where disc or zygapophysial joint injury or degeneration is apparent there is often greater joint play, unless the degenerative change is advanced. The ligamentum flavum is a substantial structure which envelops the anterior aspect of both the IAP and SAP (see Fig. 3.4), and maintains their approximation. The ligamentum flavum has two primary fibre orientations. Fibres are principally orientated vertically between adjoining laminae, although some pass medially and obliquely onto the anterior aspect of the SAP, helping to form the posterior margin to the intervertebral foramen. Given the high proportion of elastin in this ligament (Tan et al 2003), its function is to maintain the lumen of the posterior wall of the vertebral canal and aid in elastic recoil of the spine back to its resting position, particularly after flexion motion (Ponseti 1995).

The posterior joint capsule may merge its attachment into the peripheral articular boundary of the SAP, and in turn is reinforced by the tendinous slips of multifidus, which can tension the posterior joint. Occasionally, small sections of the posterior articular cartilage appear to become displaced from the subchondral bone (Taylor & Twomey 1986), possibly arising from sudden shearing of the IAP across the SAP under compressive or torsional load. Such examples of minor internal derangement of the zygapophysial joints respond well to manual therapy.

NORMAL ZYGAPOPHYSIAL JOINT FUNCTION AND RESPONSE TO INJURY

Early descriptions of the role of the zygapophysial joints have defined their function as guides to direct and constrain segmental motion (Humphry 1858), a view endorsed by contemporary reviews of spinal biomechanics (Stokes 1988, Adams et al 2002). One of the more interesting perspectives on the functional role of the zygapophysial joints comes from the Canadian orthopaedist Harry Farfan, who conceptualized the 'spinal engine' (Farfan 1973). This mechanistic model employs the zygapophysial joints as cogs in a transmission to reciprocally transmit axial torque, generated by swinging the arms and shoulders, through the spinal segments to power the lower limbs for ambulation (Farfan 1995).

The cardinal role of the zygapophysial joints is to moderate the direction and extent of segmental motion which may be safely sustained. As regional spinal motion capacity is regulated also by the shape and height of the intervertebral disc, an intrinsic role of the zygapophysial joints is protection, especially against excessive torsion and shear (Pearcy 1997). Shear strain is a major force vector in the lower lumbar segments given the lumbosacral angle, hence the potential for the initiation of spondylolysis, which can develop through high compressive loading or repetitive dynamic loading (Swärd et al 1991). Thus the zygapophysial joints can act both to facilitate and to limit physiological motion.

Segmental axes of rotation vary correspondingly throughout the vertebral column moderated by the lordotic or kyphotic alignment and the physical shape and height of the intervertebral discs. At the thoracolumbar junction (TLJ) the interlocking morphology of the zygapophysial joints (Singer 1989), coined a 'mortice joint' by Davis (1955) (Fig. 3.6), limits motion mainly to sagittal plane movements and small gliding displacements. Caution is required by manual therapists when mobilizing TLJ and upper lumbar segments where rotation mobilization and manipulation may be strongly countered by the 'mortice-type' configuration of the zygapophysial joints (Singer 1989, Singer & Giles 1990).

ARTICULAR ASYMMETRY

Articular asymmetry, or 'tropism', of spinal joint facets has been attributed in earlier reports to left or right hand dominance (Whitney 1926), which may bias the movement preferences and body directions in which an individual habitually moves. Others have suggested this may be caused through imbalance in muscle actions exerted against the joint (Odgers 1933, Lutz 1967). The incidence of tropism of spinal joints is highest at the TLJ (see Fig. 3.2), typically the T11–12 level, where 41% show >10 degrees of difference and 19% show >20 degrees of horizontal plane variation (Singer et al 1988) (Fig. 3.7). Similarly, at the cervicothoracic junction (CTJ) almost a quarter of C6–7 joint pairs showed differences >10 degrees, while for C7–T1 and T1–2 the differences were 18 and 16% respectively (Boyle et al 1996). In contrast, asymmetry is less common in the lumbar zygapophysial joints; however, at the lumbosacral junction articular tropism may be demonstrated. Cihak has reported up to 10 degrees of asymmetry in 16% of cases (Cihak 1970), and several other reports have confirmed this tendency (Putti 1927, Cihak 1981, Kenesi & Lesur 1985). Farfan has proposed that there was a higher incidence of unilateral lumbosacral IVD prolapse on the side of the more coronal facing facet, which is disposed to torsion, compared to the side protected by a sagittal facing joint (Farfan et al 1972, Farfan 1983).

In some individuals, tropism may have a developmental origin, whereas in others an acquired facet tropism may occur following injury to the zygapophysial joint resulting in remodelling. However, considerable variation in the orientation and symmetry of the lumbar zygapophysial joints has been described in asymptomatic individuals, with much conjecture as to whether this contributes to late problems. As the lower lumbar motion segments are more fre-

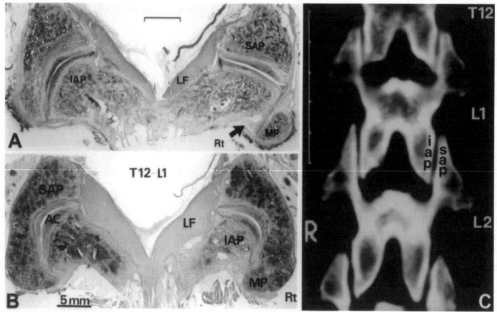

Figure 3.6 Photomicrograph of a 100 μm thick transverse section cut in the plane of the superior vertebral end plate at T11–12 illustrating a type I bilateral mortice joint (A) formed by the embracing mammillary processes which normally fuse with the lateral expansion of the superior articular process. Despite the articular asymmetry, the hyaline cartilage appears normal. A bilateral mortice type joint configuration at T12–L1 is depicted with both mammillary processes forming an enclosure to the respective IAPs (B). Note the uniform appearance of articular cartilage on all facets. A frontal plane CT image (C) demonstrates the medial taper effect of the IAPs, which would achieve a complete 'close-packed' position in axial weight-bearing postures and extension of these upper lumbar zygapophysial joints. Adapted from Singer 1989. (AC – articular cartilage; MP – mammillary processes; SAP – superior articular process; IAP – inferior articular process; LF – ligamentum flavum.)

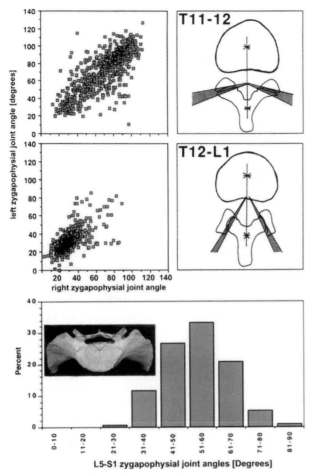

Figure 3.7 The great variability of thoracolumbar transitional zygapophysial joint configurations is clearly evident in plots of the right vs left joint angles at T11–12 and to lesser extent at T12–L1. The range of lumbosacral joint angles recorded by Cihak (1970) is depicted in the lower graph with the largest range of joint angles approximating the coronal compared to the sagittal plane. Adapted from Singer et al 1989a and Cihak 1970.

quently affected by injury and degeneration, joint tropism has been implicated as a possible aetiological feature. Cyron & Hutton (1980) observed that, when subjected to posteroanterior shear, motion segments with asymmetrical zygapophysial joints tend to rotate towards the more coronally aligned joint. Manual therapy passive motion segment testing requires a preparedness to accept that not all aberrant motion reflects underlying pathology (Grieve 1981). This reinforces the inadequacy of isolated testing and the necessity to consider all assessment findings, including imaging where available.

ZYGAPOPHYSIAL JOINT MECHANICS

In the middle to lower cervical regions, the dual requirements of stability and mobility are provisioned through zygapophysial joints, which permit a composite of sagittal and lateral plane motions (Milne 1993b), with C5–6 con-

tributing the greatest segmental mobility (Fig. 3.8). The middle segments have a zygapophysial joint angle of approximately 45 degrees to the long axis of the spine, which reduces more abruptly at the CTJ (Boyle et al 1996). The more caudal segments approaching the CTJ show a tendency for a smaller range of motion as the zygapophyses adopt a form more characteristic of the upper thoracic segments. It is here that axial loading is higher and the segmental mobility becomes markedly diminished as the thoracic cage commences (Bullough & Boachie-Adjei 1988, Boyle et al 1998). It is not unexpected that, with such an abrupt functional change at this transitional junction, severe fracture–dislocation injury can occur at this site, particularly in response to excessive applied forces as occur in motor vehicle roll-over accidents (Boyle et al 2004).

The uncinate processes, a unique feature of the cervical spine, whose form continues in the thoracic region as the paired costovertebral joints (Milne 1993a), strongly influences composite segmental motion, helping to prevent translation and, to some extent, lateral flexion (Bland & Boushey 1990, Milne 1991). The axes of rotation are commonly reported to be in the anterior region of the subjacent vertebra, with axial displacements progressively reducing towards the CTJ, corresponding with the change in inclination of the zygapophysial joints (Boyle et al 1996, 1998). In flexion, the upper cervical vertebra tilts and glides over the subjacent vertebra like an egg rolling in an egg cup. The composite cervical spine motion is represented in Figure 3.8 both schematically, from multiple CT slice superimpositions, and graphically from ex vivo cadaver studies (Milne 1993a). The consequence of increased segmental mobility is the tendency for higher levels of disc degeneration (Singer 2000).

Due to the oblique orientation of the cervical articular facets, the movements of rotation and lateral flexion are coupled within the cervical spine so that rotation is accompanied by ipsilateral lateral flexion. This motion can be considered to occur about a single axis, which is perpendicular to the plane of the zygapophysial joints as seen in the lateral projection (Penning & Wilmink 1987, Milne 1993b). As the lower cervical and thoracic articular facets become more vertical, the axis of coupled motion could be expected to become more horizontal, involving more lateral flexion. However, the interfacet angles have been shown to have a bearing on the axis of coupled motion (Milne 1993b). At C3 and C4 the interfacet angles are less than 180 degrees and the orientation of the axis of coupled motion is constrained to a narrow band perpendicular to the facets (see Fig. 3.8); while in the lower cervical and thoracic regions, where the interfacet angles are greater than 180 degrees, the orientation of the axis of coupled motion can vary greatly depending on whether the applied force was axial rotation or lateral flexion.

The articular surfaces of the cervical vertebrae not only regulate the direction and type of movement but, because of their oblique inclination, in a posteroanterior direction they also transmit the weight of the head (Med 1973). With

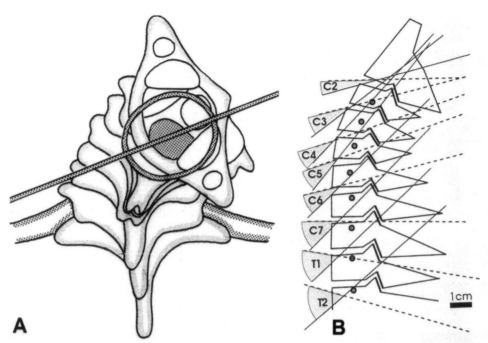

Figure 3.8   A reconstruction based on functional CT studies, to show the nature of composite rotation and side flexion occurring between the first cervical and the first thoracic segments (A). The axes of coupled lateral flexion and axial rotation in the cervicothoracic spine (C2–T2) are depicted schematically. Solid lines indicate the axes of coupled motion when the applied force was rotary, and the interrupted lines indicate the axes when the applied force was lateral bending. The lower three segment axes shown can take on a wide range of orientation, but the range of motion here is quite limited in contrast to the middle three segments which have the widest potential excursion. Adapted from Penning & Wilmink 1987 and Milne 1993b.

age-related changes in adult cervical spine posture, the load transfer role of the zygapophysial joints becomes increasingly important in resisting anterior shear (Boyle et al 2002).

The zygapophyses of the upper thoracic spine show some morphological features of the cervical region (Med 1972, 1973), and similarly the joints of the lower thoracic spine progressively approximate those of the upper lumbar region (Singer et al 1989a). The middle segments of the thoracic spine appear designed for less mobility as the thoracic cage articulations limit sagittal plane motion while accommodating axial displacements (Gregersen & Lucas 1967). The orientation of the articular facets in the thoracic spine changes only slightly throughout the middle region, approximating the coronal plane and thereby permitting some sagittal motion and axial rotation while, in concert with the thoracic cage, limiting lateral bending. The middle thoracic segments, according to measurements involving pin insertion into the spinous processes, showed the largest axial displacements compared with the upper and lower segments (Gregersen & Lucas 1967). There is an abrupt decrease in the range of axial rotation at the level of the TLJ, as the zygapophysial joints conform to the typically sagittal configuration of the upper lumbar region (Malmivaara et al 1987, Singer et al 1989c).

The axis of rotation for the thoracic spine has been described by Davis (1959) to lie in the region of the upper subjacent vertebral body, given the slight vertical inclina-

tion of the articular facets. In extension, the inferior pole of the articular facets can contact the laminae of the vertebra below which is believed to denote an important axial load transmission mechanism (Pal & Routal 1987). At the TLJ, there is a specialized mortice-like arrangement, which appears in weight-bearing positions, designed to embrace the IAPs into the recess formed by the paired SAPs (Singer 1989) (see Fig. 3.6). This anatomical lock is accentuated by the medial taper of the SAPs into which the tenon-like IAPs fit (Fig. 3.6C).

The zygapophyses of the lumbar spine are morphologically designed to prevent forward translation while allowing considerable sagittal plane and lateral bending motions. The characteristic function of the lumbar spine is to transmit axial load while providing stability and mobility of the trunk in relation to the lower limbs. A principal role of the upper lumbar zygapophysial joints is limitation of axial displacements (Fig. 3.9), in part to protect the disc from torsion (Farfan 1969), and to prevent anterior shear strain (Adams et al 2002). This requirement is well achieved in the upper lumbar spine, witnessed by the low rates of disc degeneration, prolapse or listhesis, in contrast to the lower segments where disc injury is one consequence of the increased capacity for torsional displacements or increased shear in response to listhesis.

Relative to disc height, there is a progressive increase in lumbar segmental mobility with the L4–5 and L5–S1 seg-

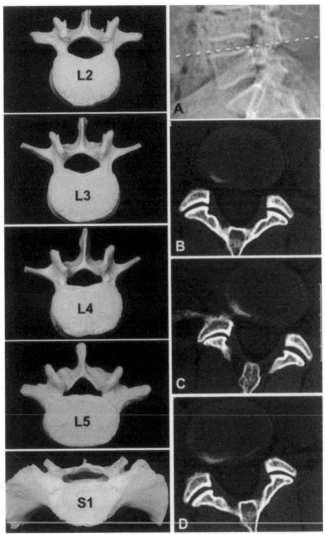

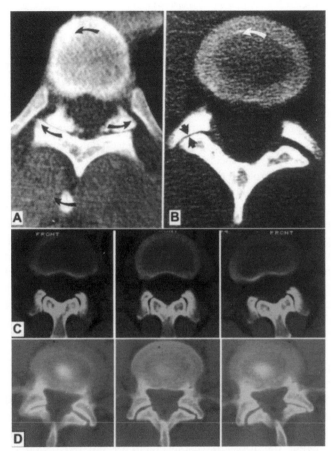

Figure 3.9   A series of functional CT images at L4–5 to compare the neutral and subsequent side posture rotation images of the same segment which highlights the ipsilateral compression of the tension joint with separation of the opposite side. The scan plane was referenced to the superior vertebral end plate at L4 (A–D). The typical change in configuration of the lumbar zygapophysial joints describes the more sagittal orientation in the upper region, especially L1–2, to a progressively more coronal configuration at L5–S1.

Figure 3.10   From in vivo functional CT of the thoracic and lumbar spine in normal subjects; there were distinct differences evident according to different zygapophysial joint morphologies, with evident axial displacement of the T10–11 thoracic segment (A) compared with the L4–5 lumbar segment (B). In contrast the upper lumbar segments with sagittal zygapophyses show little differences from right or left rotation postures (C), whereas at L4–5 there is a greater tendency for ipsilateral compression and separation during side posture rotation scans (D). Adapted from Singer et al 1989 and Singer et al 2001.

ments contributing the most to sagittal plane motion. Through the tendency in the caudal segments towards more coronally angled lumbar facets, slightly more axial plane motion may be achieved (Singer et al 2001) (Fig. 3.10). The anterior longitudinal ligament, which acts to passively constrain the lordotic postures, is a particularly well-developed structure in lumbar and cervical regions, more so than its posterior counterpart. The classic work of Rolander (1966) demonstrated that the axes of rotation in the sagittal plane are principally located in the anterior region of the disc. For axial displacements, the axis of rotation tends to be located within the posterior annulus. The morphological adaptation of the last lumbar vertebra acts to allow torsion, by the more coronal orientation of the zygapophyses, as a requirement for locomotion (Boszczyk et al 2001). One consequence of segments disposed to excess torsion is the tendency for higher rates of disc degeneration (Farfan & Sullivan 1967, Farfan 1969, Singer 2000).

In extension, the zygapophysial joints tend towards a close-packed position due to the apposition of the articular surfaces and the approximation of the inferior articular facet into the lamina below (Adams et al 1994). No difference was found in the range of lumbar rotation when subjects were tested in full flexion, compared to upright standing, although the range of rotation increased when tested in a mid-position (Pearcy & Hindle 1991). The rotational stiffness of an isolated motion segment is decreased by 40–60% following removal of the posterior elements (Markolf 1972). This emphasizes a key role of the lumbar zygapophysial joints in resisting rotation.

ZYGAPOPHYSIAL JOINT LOADING AND INJURY

The physiological 'S'-shaped curve of the human spine contributes to stability and to shock absorption, particularly during locomotion, in a manner analogous to a spring. However, the capacity for loading of these small joints varies depending upon their location. The cervical and lumbar zygapophyses are close to the line of gravity and consequently they contribute more to axial load transfer than the thoracic facets, which lie posterior to this line. This mechanical role of the zygapophyses and laminae as load-bearing constructs has been examined as a function of sagittal curve. Where the curvature is concave posteriorly, as in the cervical and lumbar regions, greater load was found to pass posteriorly (Pal & Routal 1986, 1987). Ex vivo mechanical studies of lumbar segments have confirmed that between 25 and 70% of the vertebral compressive load could be transmitted across the zygapophysial joints between adjacent vertebrae (Adams & Hutton 1980, Yang & King 1984). Sustained or dynamic compressive loading through the zygapophysial joints can increase significantly in loaded lordotic postures (Adams et al 2002), particularly those adopted in sports such as gymnastics and cricket bowling actions. In contrast, flexion loads are passed more anteriorly through the IVD, leaving the zygapophysial joints relatively unloaded. In this situation, anterior shear is resisted by the coronal portion of the SAP, which acts to prevent the forward displacement of the IAP. Such an anatomical restraint to flexion is important, as in full flexion there is quiescence of the extensor musculature (Kippers & Parker 1985).

There are typical sites where function is disturbed when excess force is applied, as in the case of spinal injury resulting in fracture dislocation. Often, such injury is focused at locations of greatest morphological change between regions (Singer et al 1989a, Boyle et al 2004), where the anatomy is least capable of dissipating the stress loading. The greater joint play associated with zygapophysial or disc injury has important implications for the concept of clinical instability. In the absence of reduced passive movement and symptoms consistent with instability, treatment decisions must be made with regard to the appropriate use of passive versus active stabilizing interventions.

INNERVATION PATTERN

The typical innervation pattern of the zygapophysial joints, lying so close to the spinal nerves, is via medial branches arising from the dorsal ramus, one of which descends around the SAP beneath the mammillo-accessory ligament to the inferior aspect of the same joint, with a descending branch to the superior aspect of the zygapophysis below (Groen & Stolker 2000) (Fig. 3.11). Thus each joint has a dual innervation, which is discretely unilateral in contrast to ventral structures, which possess a complex overlapping and bilateral innervation system (Groen & Stolker 2000). The zygapophysial joint capsule and IASFs (Giles & Harvey 1987) share this innervation, which may explain some types of segmental localized back pain syndromes which may be ameliorated by manipulation (Tondury 1971). Spasm of the multifidus muscle can be invoked with articular injury or entrapment of IASFs, given their shared innervation by branches of the dorsal ramus (Bogduk 1983, Bogduk & Marsland 1988, Groen et al 1990, Bogduk & Valencia 1994). The zygapophysial joints are therefore determinants of both quality and quantity of lumbar spine move-

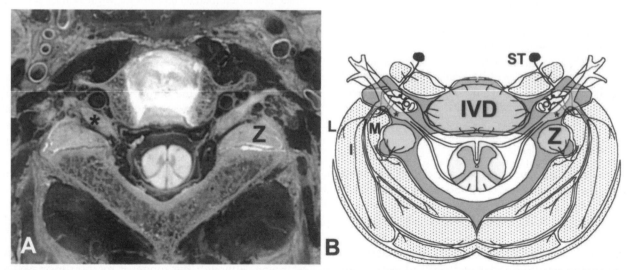

Figure 3.11 Horizontal plane section of the mid-cervical spine to illustrate the topographic anatomy of the paired zygapophysial joints (Z) situated in the plane of the vertebral canal. The spinal cord, dorsal root ganglia (*) and the emerging spinal nerves are clearly depicted (A). A schematic illustration to depict the innervation of the paired zygapophysial joints from the medial (M) branches of the dorsal ramus. The intermediate (I) branch supplying primarily muscle and the lateral (L) branch becoming cutaneous. Sympathetic trunk (ST). Permission to use these images was kindly provided by Professor Gerbrand Groen, MD, PhD, Universität Utrecht, and represent work in progress on the Human Spine CD project.

ments and are an important source of local and referred low back pain (Mooney & Robertson 1976, McCall et al 1979).

MANUAL THERAPY CONSIDERATIONS

The manual therapist commonly encounters zygapophysial joint related disorders in routine practice. As such, a clear understanding of their anatomy as it relates to clinical presentation is necessary as an aid to forming a diagnosis and classification before evaluating the most appropriate course of action. For example, zygapophysial joint orientation may contribute information relevant to clinical presentation. The sagittal orientation of the posterior part of lumbar zygapophysial joints, along with the posterior capsule, restrains rotation to afford protection to the disc. Forceful rotation may therefore dispose the articular cartilage and subchondral bone to compression injury, particularly in the lordosed or extended position when the articular processes are more fully engaged. As well, the posterior capsule may be injured. Clinically, symptoms may then be reproduced by applied forces and combinations of movements that either compress the injured joint surfaces, for example extension and/or ipsilateral lateral flexion, or stretch the capsule via flexion and/or contralateral lateral flexion. Compressive patterns of pain reproduction may therefore

be suggestive of zygapophysial joint articular cartilage involvement while stretch patterns may be more suggestive of capsular strain. This identification of the source of symptoms has implications for management with regard to encouragement of movement either towards or away from the pain-provoking direction. The same principles can be applied to cervical and thoracic regions with consideration of the movements constrained by either capsular tightness or articular process apposition.

Effective manual therapy utilizes clinical application of knowledge of zygapophysial joint form and function. Formulation of a diagnosis based upon the clinical reasoning process must also consider the neurology and biomechanics of these joints, and their relationships with IVDs, muscle and other extra-articular structures.

KEYWORDS	
zygapophysial joints	ligaments
spine	injury
vertebral column	trauma
development	biomechanics
morphology	innervation
joint capsule	manual therapy

References

Adams M A, Dolan P 1995 Recent advances in lumbar spinal mechanics and their clinical significance. Clinical Biomechanics 10: 3–19

Adams M A, Hutton W C 1980 The effects of posture on the role of the apophyseal joints in resisting intervertebral compressive forces. Journal of Bone and Joint Surgery 62-B: 358–362

Adams M A, McNally D S, Chinn H, Dolan P 1994 Posture and the compressive strength of the lumbar spine. Clinical Biomechanics 9: 5–14

Adams M, Bogduk N, Burton A K, Dolan P 2002 Biomechanics of back pain. Churchill Livingstone, Edinburgh

Bagnall K M, Harris P F, Jones P R M 1977 A radiographic study of the human fetal spine. 2. The sequence of development of ossification centres in the vertebral column. Journal of Anatomy 124: 791–798

Bland J H, Boushey D R 1990 Anatomy and physiology of the cervical spine. Seminars in Arthritis and Rheumatism 20: 1–20

Bogduk N 1983 The innervation of the lumbar spine. Spine 8: 286–293

Bogduk N, Marsland A 1988 The cervical zygapophysial joints as a source of neck pain. Spine 13: 610–617

Bogduk N, Valencia F 1994 Innervation and pain patterns of the thoracic spine. In: Grant R (ed) Physical therapy of the cervical and thoracic spine, 2nd edn. Churchill Livingstone, Edinburgh, pp 77–88

Boszczyk B M, Boszczyk A A, Putz R V 2001 Comparative and functional anatomy of the mammalian lumbar spine. Anatomical Record 264: 157–168

Boszczyk A A, Boszczyk B M, Putz R V 2002 Prenatal rotation of the lumbar spine and its relevance for the development of the zygapophyseal joints. Spine 27: 1094–1101

Boyle J J W, Singer K P, Milne N 1996 Morphological survey of the cervicothoracic junctional region. Spine 21: 544–548

Boyle J W W, Milne N, Singer K P 1998 Clinical anatomy of the cervicothoracic junction. In: Giles L, Singer K (eds) Clinical anatomy and management of cervical spine pain. Butterworth Heinemann, Oxford, pp 40–52

Boyle J W W, Milne N, Singer K P 2002 Influence of age on cervicothoracic spinal curvature: postural implications. Clinical Biomechanics 17: 361–367

Boyle J J W, Woodland P, Singer K P 2004 Patterns of fracture /dislocation at the cervicothoracic junctional region: an Australian perspective. Spine (forthcoming)

Bullough P G, Boachie-Adjei O 1988 Atlas of spinal disorders. Lippincott, Philadelphia

Burkus J 1988 Cervical facet asymmetry simulating facet dislocation. Spine 13: 118–120

Christ B, Wilting J 1992 From somites to vertebral column. Annals of Anatomy 174: 23–32

Cihak R 1970 Variations of lumbosacral joints and their morphogenesis. Acta Universitatis Carolinae Medica 16: 145–165

Cihak R 1981 Die Morphologie und Entwicklung der Wirbelbogengelenke. Die Wirbelsäule in Forschung und Praxis 87: 13–28

Cyron B, Hutton W 1980 Articular tropism and stability of the lumbar spine. Spine 5: 168–172

Davis P 1955 The thoraco-lumbar mortice joint. Journal of Anatomy 89: 370–377

Davis P R 1959 The medial inclination of the human thoracic intervertebral articular facets. Journal of Anatomy 93: 68–74

Farfan H 1969 The effects of torsion on the intervertebral joints. Canadian Journal of Surgery 12: 336–341

Farfan H 1973 Mechanical disorders of the low back. Lea and Febiger, Philadelphia

Farfan H 1983 The torsional injury of the lumbar spine. Spine 8: 53

Farfan H F 1995 Form and function of the musculoskeletal system as revealed by mathematical analysis of the lumbar spine. Spine 20: 1462–1474

Farfan H F, Sullivan J D 1967 The relation of facet orientation to intervertebral disc failure. Canadian Journal of Surgery 10: 179–185

Farfan H, Huberdeau R, Dubow H 1972 Lumbar intervertebral disc degeneration. The influence of geometrical features on the pattern of disc degeneration: a post mortem study. Journal of Bone and Joint Surgery 54-B: 492–510

Giles L, Harvey A 1987 Immunohistochemical demonstration of nociceptors in the capsule and synovial folds of human zygapophyseal joints. British Journal of Rheumatology 26: 362–364

Gregersen G, Lucas D 1967 An in vivo study of the axial rotation of the human thoracolumbar spine. Journal of Bone and Joint Surgery 49-A: 247–262

Grieve G 1981 Common vertebral joint problems. Churchill Livingstone, Edinburgh

Groen G J, Stolker R J 2000 Thoracic neural anatomy. In: Giles L, Singer K P (eds) Clinical anatomy and management of thoracic spine pain. Butterworth Heinemann, Oxford, pp 114–142

Groen G J, Baljet B, Drukker J 1990 Nerves and nerve plexuses of the human vertebral column. American Journal of Anatomy 188: 282–296

Humphry G M 1858 A treatise on the human skeleton. Macmillan, London

Kenesi C, Lesur E 1985 Orientation of the articular processes at L4, L5 and S1: possible role in pathology of the intervertebral disc. Anatomica Clinica 7: 43–47

Kippers V, Parker A W 1985 Electromyographic studies of erectores spinae: symmetrical postures and sagittal trunk motion. Australian Journal of Physiotherapy 31: 95–105

Lewin T, Moffett B, Viidik A 1962 The morphology of the lumbar synovial intervertebral joints. Acta Morphologica Neerlando Scandinavica 4: 299–319

Lutz G 1967 Die Entwicklung der kleinen Wirbelgelenke. Zeitschrift für Orthopädie und ihre Grenzgebiete 104: 19–28

McCall I W, Park W M, O'Brien J P 1979 Induced pain referral from posterior lumbar elements in normal subjects. Spine 4: 441–446

Macintosh J, Valencia F, Bogduk N, Munro R 1986 The morphology of the human lumbar multifidus. Clinical Biomechanics 1: 196–204

Maigne J Y, Ayral X, Guèrin-Surville H 1992 Frequency and size of ossifications in the caudal attachments of the ligamentum flavum of the thoracic spine: role of rotatory strains in their development. Surgical and Radiologic Anatomy 14: 119–124

Malmivaara A, Videman T, Kuosma E, Troup J D G 1987 Facet joint orientation, facet and costovertebral joint osteoarthrosis, disc degeneration, vertebral body osteophytosis and Schmorl's nodes in the thoracolumbar junctional region of cadaveric spines. Spine 12: 458–463

Markolf K L 1972 Deformation of the thoracolumbar intervertebral joints in response to external loads. Journal of Bone and Joint Surgery 54A: 511–533

Med M 1972 Articulations of the thoracic vertebrae and their variability. Folia Morphologica 20: 212–215

Med M 1973 Articulations of the cervical spine and their variability. Folia Morphologica 21: 324–327

Med M 1977 Prenatal development of thoracic intervertebral articulations. Folia Morphologica 25: 175–177

Med M 1980 Prenatal development of intervertebral articulation in man and its association with ventrodorsal curvature of the spine. Folia Morphologica 28: 264–267

Mercer S, Bogduk N 1993 Intra-articular inclusions of the cervical synovial joints. British Journal of Rheumatology 32: 705–710

Milne N 1991 The role of zygapophysial joint orientation and uncinate processes in controlling motion in the cervical spine. Journal of Anatomy 178: 189–201

Milne N 1993a Comparative anatomy and function of the uncinate processes of cervical vertebrae in humans and other mammals. PhD thesis, University of Western Australia, Perth

Milne N 1993b Composite motion in cervical disc segments. Clinical Biomechanics 8: 193–202

Mooney V, Robertson J 1976 The facet syndrome. Clinical Orthopaedics 115: 149–156

Odgers P 1933 The lumbar and lumbo-sacral diarthrodial joints. Journal of Anatomy 67: 301–317

O'Rahilly R, Muller F, Meyer D B 1980 The human vertebral column at the end of the embryonic period proper. 1. The column as a whole. Journal of Anatomy 131: 565–575

Pal G, Routal R 1986 A study of weight transmission through the cervical and upper thoracic regions of the vertebral column in man. Journal of Anatomy 148: 245–261

Pal G, Routal R 1987 Transmission of weight through the lower thoracic and lumbar regions of the vertebral column in man. Journal of Anatomy 152: 93–105

Pearcy M J 1997 Biomechanics of the lumbosacral spine. In: Giles L, Singer K P (eds) Clinical anatomy and management of low back pain. Butterworth Heinemann, Oxford, pp 165–172

Pearcy M J, Hindle R J 1991 Axial rotation of lumbar intervertebral joints in forward flexion. Proceedings of the Institute of Mechanical Engineers 205: 205–209

Penning L, Wilmink J T 1987 Rotation of the cervical spine. Spine 12: 732–738

Ponseti I V 1995 Differences in ligamenta flava among some mammals. Iowa Orthopaedic Journal 15: 141–146

Prescher A 1997 The craniovertebral junction in man, the osseous variations, their significance and differential diagnosis. Annals of Anatomy 179: 1–19

Putti V 1927 New conceptions on the pathogenesis of sciatic pain. Lancet 2: 53–60

Putz R 1985 The functional morphology of the superior articular processes of the lumbar vertebrae. Journal of Anatomy 143: 181–187

Reichmann S 1971 The postnatal development of form and orientation of the lumbar intervertebral joint surfaces. Zeitschrift für Anatomie Entwicklungsgeschichte 133: 102–123

Rickenbacher J, Landolt A M, Theiler K 1985 Applied anatomy of the back. Springer-Verlag, Berlin pp 30, 31

Rolander S D 1966 Motion of the lumbar spine with special reference to the stabilizing effect of posterior fusion. Acta Orthopedica Scandinavia 90 (Suppl.): 1–144

Saada J, Song S, Breidahl W H 2000 Developmental anomalies of the thoracic region. In: Giles L, Singer K P (eds) Clinical anatomy and management of thoracic spine pain. Butterworth Heinemann, Oxford, pp 83–99

Schmorl G, Junghanns H 1971 The human spine in health and disease. Grune and Stratton, New York

Singer K P 1989 The thoracolumbar mortice joint: radiological and histological observations. Clinical Biomechanics 4: 137–143

Singer K P 2000 Pathology of the thoracic spine. In: Giles L, Singer K P (eds) Clinical anatomy and management of thoracic spine pain. Butterworth Heinemann, Oxford, pp 63–82

Singer K P, Breidahl P D 1990 Accessory ossification centres at the thoracolumbar junction. Surgical and Radiologic Anatomy 12: 53–58

Singer K P, Giles L G F 1990 Manual therapy considerations at the thoracolumbar junction: an anatomical and functional perspective. Journal of Manipulative and Physiological Therapeutics 13: 83–88

Singer K P, Breidahl P D, Day R E 1988 Variations in zygapophyseal orientation and level of transition at the thoracolumbar junction: a preliminary CT survey. Surgical and Radiologic Anatomy 10: 291–295

Singer K P, Breidahl P D, Day R E 1989a Posterior element variation at the thoracolumbar transition: a morphometric study using computed tomography. Clinical Biomechanics 4: 80–86

Singer K P, Day R E, Breidahl P D 1989b In vivo axial rotation at the thoracolumbar junction: an investigation using low dose CT in healthy male volunteers. Clinical Biomechanics 4: 145–150

Singer K P, Willén J, Breidahl P D, Day R E 1989. The influence of zygapophyseal joint orientation on spinal injuries at the thoracolumbar junction. Surgical and Radiologic Anatomy 11: 233–239

Singer K P, Giles L G F, Day R E 1990 Intra-articular synovial folds of the thoracolumbar junction zygapophyseal joints. Anatomical Record 226: 147–152

Singer K P, Svansson G, Day R E, Breidahl W H, Horrex A 2001 The utility of diagnosing lumbar rotational instability from twist CT scans. Journal of Musculoskeletal Research 5: 45–51

Stokes I A F 1988 Mechanical function of facet joints in the lumbar spine. Clinical Biomechanics 3: 101–105

Swärd L, Hellström M, Jacobsson B, Nyman R, Peterson L 1991 Disc degeneration and associated abnormalities of the spine in elite gymnasts: MRI study. Spine 16: 437–443

Tan C I, Kent G N, Randall A G, Edmondston J, Singer K P 2003 Age-related changes in collagen, pyridinoline and deoxypyridinoline in normal human thoracic intervertebral discs. Journal of Gerontology: Biological Sciences 58(5B): 387–393

Taylor J R, Twomey L T 1986 Age changes in lumbar zygapophyseal joints: observations on structure and function. Spine 11: 739–745

Tondury G 1971 Functional anatomy of the small joints of the spine. Annales de Medecine Physique 15: 173–191

Tondury G 1972 Anatomie fonctionelle des petites articulations de rachis. Annales de Medecine Physique 15: 173–191

Whitney C 1926 Asymmetry of vertebral articular processes and facets. American Journal of Physical Anthropology 9: 451–455

Yang K, King A 1984 Mechanism of facet load transmission as a hypothesis for low back pain. Spine 9: 559–565

Chapter 4

Kinematics of the spine

S. Mercer

INTRODUCTION

An understanding of movement of the spine is essential to comprehension of its normal function. One of the most fundamental parameters of spinal motion is spinal range of motion, which is often used as an index of spinal function. The normative data against which impairment ratings are made have been collected from cadavers and from living individuals using a variety of techniques including external devices or radiography. Shortcomings of this normative data lie in the lack of generalizability of subjects, lack of reliability of the measuring instruments and lack of validity between external instruments and radiological techniques. In addition cadaver studies cannot be generalized to living individuals as the motion and resistance provided by muscles have been removed. But most importantly, measures of global range of motion do not reveal what is happening inside the neck or trunk.

Recognition of the shortcomings of these global range of motion studies led to studies examining segmental motion. These technically more difficult investigations have also examined cadavers and living individuals with external devices, radiographs and computed tomography (CT). They have provided data regarding segmental motion including patterns of coupled motion. The purpose of this chapter is to describe spinal kinematics in terms of segmental motion, highlighting the clinically relevant gaps in our knowledge.

ATLANTO-OCCIPITAL JOINT

The deep atlantal sockets of the atlas are designed to cradle the occiput and transmit forces from the head to the cervical spine. This design facilitates flexion and extension but impedes other movements (Mercer & Bogduk 2001). In living individuals the average mean motion is about 14–15 degrees (Table 4.1), although Fielding (1957) reported a much higher value of 35 degrees. However, the variability in range of motion in normal subjects is large, being 0–22 degrees (Kottke & Mundale 1959) or 0–25 degrees (Brocher 1955). Furthermore, Lind et al (1989) reported a mean of 14 degrees with a standard deviation of 15 degrees in normal subjects. Such wide variations in reported normal flexion and extension range of motion must be taken into account when making decisions about what constitutes normal or abnormal movement at the atlanto-occipital joint. These variations could be due to differences in the way in which the occipital flexion and extension movements were performed or to the paradoxical motion of the atlas that different postural strategies may induce (Bogduk & Mercer 2000).

Other more detailed information regarding the kinematics of the atlanto-occipital joints comes from studies on cadaveric material (Werne 1958, Worth 1985, Worth & Selvik 1986). Werne (1958) measured 13 degrees of flexion–extension and 0 degrees of axial rotation, although he was able to measure 8 degrees of axial rotation when the movement was forced. A more precise radiographic study described the mean range (SD) of flexion–extension at 18.6 degrees (0.6), axial rotation 3.4 degrees (0.4) and lateral flexion 3.9 degrees (0.6) (Worth 1985, Worth & Selvik 1986).

During flexion–extension negligible motion was observed in the other planes; however, during axial rotation 1.5 degrees of extension and 2.7 degrees of lateral flexion were recorded (Worth 1985, Worth & Selvik 1986). Therefore in cadavers axial rotation was artificially created through a combination of extension and lateral flexion. This pattern of coupling should not necessarily be accepted as the normal pattern of coupling as it could be the result of how and when the axial torque was applied to the cadavers (Bogduk & Mercer 2000). We do not know whether this is the pattern of coupling that occurs in vivo when muscles are active or whether posture would affect such patterns of coupled motion. When inducing lateral flexion, Worth & Selvik (1986) noted that this movement could be coupled with flexion, extension or axial rotation, with the pattern of coupling being dependent on the shape of the atlantal sockets. As individual anatomical variation may therefore influence the pattern of coupling and as there is a dearth of studies examining atlanto-occipital joint motion, particular rules for patterns of defined coupled motion are not supported by the current literature.

Table 4.1 Normal ranges of motion of in vivo flexion-extension at the atlanto-occipital joint

| Study | Mean | Range of motion (degrees) | |
		Range	SD
Brocher 1955	14.3	0–25	
Lewit & Krausova 1963	15.0		
Markuske 1971	14.5		
Fielding 1957	35.0		
Kottke & Mundale 1959		0–22	
Lind et al 1981	14.0		15

ATLANTO-AXIAL JOINT

Studies examining range of motion at the atlanto-axial joints in cadavers report 10 degrees of flexion–extension and 47 degrees of axial rotation (Werne 1958), and about 5 degrees of lateral flexion (Dankmeijer & Rethmeier 1943). A more recent study using CT scanning observed 32 degrees (SD, 10) of axial rotation to either side (Dvorak et al 1987a).

In living individuals the reported range of flexion–extension motion is highly variable, varying between 2 and 18 degrees (Table 4.2). Due to the difficulties in accurately determining from plain X-rays the range of axial rotation, most studies have only examined flexion–extension at the atlanto-axial joints.

Mimura et al (1989) used biplanar radiography to more accurately examine atlanto-axial joint motion. The total range of axial rotation (left to right) of the occiput relative to C2 was 75.2 degrees (SD, 11.8). This axial rotation was accompanied by 14 degrees (SD, 6) of extension and 24 degrees (SD, 6) of contralateral lateral flexion, although the authors reported that in some cases flexion would accompany the axial rotation rather than extension. This variability in coupling occurs because of the passive nature of the kinematics of the atlas (Mercer & Bogduk 2001). Whether the atlas flexes or extends during axial rotation depends on the geometry of the atlanto-axial joints and the precise direction of any forces acting through the atlas from the head (Bogduk & Mercer 2000).

Table 4.2 Normal ranges of motion at the atlanto-axial joint in living individuals

| Study | Ranges of motion (degrees) | | |
| | Flexion–extension | Axial rotation | |
		One side	Total
Brocher 1955	18 (2–16)		
Kottke & Mundale 1959	11		
Lewit & Krausova 1983	16		
Markuske 1971	21		
Lind et al 1989	13 (+/–5)		
Fielding 1957	15		90
Hohl & Baker 1964	(10–15)	30	

In normal living subjects imaged via CT scanning a mean of 43 degrees (SD, 5.5) of axial rotation was measured to each side at C1–2 with a left–right asymmetry of 2.8 (SD, 2) (Dvorak et al 1987b). This finding led these authors to suggest that 56 degrees is an upper limit of normal axial rotation.

LOWER CERVICAL SPINE

The general pattern of segmental motion during flexion and extension of the cervical spine has been described by van Mameren (1988). Flexion may be divided into three sequential phases. The initial phase begins in the lower cervical spine (C4–7) where C6–7 makes its maximum contribution followed by the C5–6 segment and then by C4–5. Motion in the second phase occurs initially at C0–2 followed by C2–3 and C3–4, the order of contribution of C2–3 and C3–4 being variable. During this phase slight extension occurs at C6–7 and in some individuals at C5–6. The third phase of motion occurs again at the lower cervical spine (C4–7) initially, with the C4–5 segment followed by C5–6 then C6–7 segment. Flexion in normal subjects is therefore initiated and terminated by C6–7, never by the mid-cervical segments. The C0–2 and C2–3, C3–4 segments contribute maximally during the middle phase of motion, but in a variable sequence (Bogduk & Mercer 2000).

Extension may also be divided into three phases (van Mameren 1988). The first phase is initiated in the lower cervical spine (C4–7) with no regular pattern to the sequence of segmental motion. In the middle phase, motion occurs at C0–2 and at C2–4 with the order of contribution being quite variable between C2 and C4. The third phase is characterized by a second contribution from the lower segments (C4–7) in which the individual segments move in a regular order C4–5, C5–6, then C6–7. Meanwhile motion of C0–2 attains its maximum range. This pattern of motion during flexion and extension was shown to be reproducible (van Mameren 1988).

Although many studies have been undertaken to determine normal ranges of segmental motion during flexion and extension of the cervical spine, few have included mean range and standard deviation of this motion. Two early studies (Aho et al 1955, Bhalla & Simmons 1969) provided raw data so that means and standard deviations can be calculated (Bogduk & Mercer 2000), while two more recent studies (Dvorak et al 1988, Lind et al 1989) also afford more meaningful normative data for clinicians (Table 4.3). However, only Lind et al (1989) and Dvorak et al (1988) also report the inter-observer error of their measurement technique, therefore providing the most reliable normative data. Examination of Table 4.3 reveals the largest range of flexion–extension motion at the C4–5 and C5–6 segments.

The work of van Mameren (van Mameren et al 1990) has highlighted the difficulties of using normative segmental motion data for clinical purposes. This study demonstrated that in normal subjects the total range of motion of the neck is not the arithmetical sum of its intersegmental ranges of motion. Further, segmental range of motion differs according to whether the motion is performed from flexion to extension or from extension to flexion resulting in differences of 10–30 degrees in total range of cervical motion. Finally, the ranges of motion are not stable over time (Bogduk & Mercer 2000). The clinical implication of this study is that normal motion must be considered as a fluctuating range of values and not as a single value.

At the segmental level, flexion is a movement composed of anterior sagittal rotation and anterior translation. The extent of coupling between the rotation and translation is determined by the height of the superior articular process (Nowitzke et al 1994). As the superior articular processes are shorter at higher cervical levels these segments exhibit relatively greater amplitude of translation, while at lower levels the taller superior articular processes impede translation resulting in a greater ratio of rotation to translation.

Using CT scanning in the conventional horizontal plane Penning & Wilmink (1987) determined the mean and ranges of axial rotation at each level within the cervical spine (Table 4.4). Due to the structure of the cervical spine, axial rotation in the horizontal plane is, however, inescapably coupled with ipsilateral lateral flexion. Consequently when axial rotation has been examined by CT scanning in the horizontal plane the ranges of axial rotation computed have been confounded by movement of the plane of view. Therefore the normal values provided in Table 4.6 are only an imprecise estimate of the range of segmental axial rotation within the cervical spine.

Table 4.3 Mean and standard deviation in degrees for segmental motion during cervical flexion and extension

Study	Mean values and (SD) of flexion and extension motion				
	C2–3	C3–4	C4–5	C5–6	C6–7
Aho et al 1955	12 (5)	15 (7)	22 (4)	28 (4)	15 (4)
Bhalla & Simmons 1969	9 (1)	15 (2)	23 (1)	19 (1)	18 (3)
Lind et al 1981	10 (4)	14 (6)	16 (6)	15 (8)	11 (7)
Dvorak et al 1988	10 (3)	15 (3)	19 (4)	20 (4)	19 (4)

Table 4.4   Mean and range of axial rotation of cervical motion segments (based on Penning & Wilmink 1987)

Level	Range of motion (degrees)	
	Mean	Range
Occ–C1	1.0	−2–5
C1–2	40.5	29–46
C2–3	3.0	0–10
C3–4	6.5	3–10
C4–5	6.8	1–12
C5–6	6.9	2–12
C6–7	2.1	2–10
C7–T1	2.1	−2–7

Mimura et al (1989) subsequently used trigonometric reconstruction of motion recorded via biplanar radiography to provide a more valid measurement of axial rotation and coupled motion within the cervical spine. The normal ranges of motion are provided in Table 4.5. Coupling of flexion with axial rotation was observed at C5–6 and C6–7 while extension was seen above C4–5. Ipsilateral lateral flexion coupled with axial rotation caudal from C3 to C4. However, what must be kept in mind are the large variations in normal motion as expressed in the standard deviations being much larger than the mean values of motion (Table 4.7).

If motion in the cervical spine is considered in terms of form and function rather than following the traditional convention of planes the pure movements available are flexion–extension around the coronal axis and axial rotation around an axis perpendicular to the facets of the zygapophysial joints (Bogduk & Mercer 2000). Axial rotation in the plane of the facet rather than in the horizontal plane results in the inferior articular processes gliding freely across the superior articular facets of the vertebra below while the superior vertebral body rotates within the concavity formed by the uncinate processes below (Bogduk & Mercer 2000, Mercer & Bogduk 2001). Bogduk & Mercer

(2000) calculated the range of axial rotation in the plane of the zygapophysial joints to be about 8 degrees for a range of 6 degrees of horizontal rotation.

THORACIC SPINE

The few studies describing motion in the thoracic spine have been undertaken on cadaveric material or on living individuals using external devices that have not been validated with regard to segmental motion. Consequently the research literature at present provides limited clinically useful data.

White (1969) measured range of motion in three planes on cadaveric thoracic spines (Table 4.6). Examination of Table 4.8 reveals the pattern of cephalocaudal variation in range of motion. There is a tendency for greater flexion–extension at lower levels of the thoracic spine, no particular pattern is evident for lateral flexion, while less axial rotation is found at lower vertebral levels.

Studies which have examined coupling in the thoracic spine have reported that lateral flexion may be coupled with ipsilateral (Gregersen & Lucas 1967, White 1969) or equally ipsilateral or contralateral axial rotation in the upper region (Willems et al 1996), while in the middle or lower regions of the thoracic spine lateral flexion may be coupled ipsilaterally or contralaterally with axial rotation (White 1969) or predominantly ipsilaterally (Gregerson & Lucas 1967, Willems et al 1996). The differences in methods and subjects in each of these few studies influence the variability in reported data. At present there exist insufficient data to support models of specific patterns of coupling within the thoracic spine.

LUMBAR SPINE

Flexion of the lumbar spine from erect standing involves an unfolding or straightening of the lumbar lordosis followed

Table 4.5   Normal ranges of axial rotation and coupled flexion (+) and extension (−), ipsilateral (+) and contralateral (−) lateral flexion associated with right or left axial rotation, mean degrees and (SD) (based on Mimura et al 1989)

Level	Coupled movement		
	Axial rotation	Flexion/extension	Lateral flexion
Occ–C2	75 (12)	−14 (6)	−2 (6)
C2–3	7 (6)	0 (3)	−2 (8)
C3–4	6 (5)	−3 (5)	6 (7)
C4–5	4 (6)	−2 (4)	6 (7)
C5–6	5 (4)	2 (3)	4 (8)
C6–7	6 (3)	3 (3)	3 (7)

Table 4.6   Means (SD) of segmental motion in degrees during total flexion–extension, lateral flexion and axial rotation (based on White 1969)

Vertebral level	Flexion–extension	Lateral flexion	Axial rotation
T1–2	2.8 (0.8)	6.0 (3.8)	
T2–3	2.6 (0.8)	4.8 (3.4)	4.0 (1.9)
T3–4	2.3 (1.7)	3.7 (2.1)	5.1 (3.4)
T4–5	1.8 (0.9)	5.0 (5.1)	3.9 (1.4)
T5–6	2.6 (1.0)	5.3 (2.9)	5.0 (2.1)
T6–7	2.3 (1.3)	4.2 (5.5)	4.1 (1.3)
T7–8	3.3 (1.7)	4.1 (3.0)	4.3 (1.7)
T8–9	3.2 (1.8)	3.7 (1.8)	5.5 (2.1)
T9–10	3.1 (1.4)	4.4 (1.8)	3.2 (1.7)
T10–11	3.9 (2.7)	4.4 (2.3)	3.4 (1.8)
T11–12	6.5 (4.7)	3.7 (3.6)	2.6 (0.3)

by at most a small reversal of the lordotic curve. Kanayama et al (1996) reported that motion usually begins in the upper lumbar region followed by the rest of the lumbar spine or else all segments move at the same time. Extension is essentially the reverse of flexion. However, Gatton & Pearcy (1999) observed no consistency in sequencing of segmental motion during flexion. Further, they found that normal subjects may use any of a variety of movement strategies to achieve flexion of the lumbar spine. When performing lumbar flexion twice some subjects used different movement sequences each time. While examining trunk extension from flexion Okawa et al (1998) also found no particular pattern of regional motion to occur.

The ranges for segmental motion during flexion and extension are shown in Table 4.7. These data come from the studies of Pearcy et al (1984) and Pearcy & Tibrewal (1984) who examined males 25–36 years of age. When considering motion in the sagittal plane all lumbar joints have a similar total range of motion; however, the highest and lowest joints have relatively greater range of extension while the middle joints exhibit a relatively greater range of flexion. However, what must be remembered is that these results may not necessarily be generalized to males of other ages or to females.

At the segmental level lumbar flexion occurs through anterior sagittal rotation and simultaneous anterior sagittal translation of each vertebra (Okawa et al 1998) while during extension posterior sagittal rotation and posterior translation occur. During flexion each vertebra rotates and translates from the backward tilted position adopted with the assumption of the lordosis to a neutral position where the superior and inferior surfaces of adjacent vertebrae become parallel. Additional movement in the upper lumbar region allows a reversal of the lordotic curve to occur with the upper vertebrae rotating further forwards

through anterior compression of the intervertebral discs (Bogduk 1997).

The ranges of motion for rotation and translation in each plane during flexion and extension are depicted in Table 4.8. For each level the ranges of the sagittal plane motion during flexion lie between 8 and 13 degrees of rotation and 1–3 mm of translation. In addition these movements are regularly associated with 1 degree of coronal and axial rotation and very small and variable amounts of lateral and vertical translation. During extension 1–5 degrees of sagittal plane rotation is coupled with 1 degree of translation while very small amounts of coronal and axial rotation in association with negligible amounts of vertical and lateral translation occur (Table 4.8). These very small ranges available in conjunction with the large amount of variation do not confirm specific patterns of coupled motion which have been postulated in the clinical literature.

During axial rotation the superior vertebrae will initially rotate about an axis located in the posterior annulus fibrosus (Cossette et al 1971). After about 3 degrees of axial rotation the zygapophysial joint contralateral to the direction of rotation impacts. Any further axial rotation occurs around

Table 4.7 Ranges of segmental motion during flexion, extension and flexion and extension

Segment	Mean range of motion in degrees (SD)		
	Flexion	Extension	Flexion and extension
L1–2	8 (5)	5 (2)	13 (5)
L2–3	10 (2)	3 (2)	13 (2)
L3–4	12 (1)	1 (1)	13 (2)
L4–5	13 (4)	2 (1)	16 (4)
L5–S1	9 (6)	5 (4)	14 (5)

Table 4.8 Motion coupled with flexion and extension (based on Pearcy et al. 1984)

Level	Coupled motion					
	Mean (SD) rotations (degrees)			Mean (SD) translations (mm)		
	Sagittal	Coronal	Axial	Sagittal	Coronal	Axial
Flexion						
L1	8 (5)	1 (1)	1 (1)	3 (1)	0 (1)	1 (1)
L2	10 (2)	1 (1)	1 (1)	2 (1)	1 (1)	1 (1)
L3	12 (1)	1 (1)	1 (1)	2 (1)	1 (1)	0 (1)
L4	13 (4)	2 (1)	1 (1)	2 (1)	0 (1)	0 (1)
L5	9 (6)	1 (1)	1 (1)	1 (1)	0 (1)	1 (1)
Extension						
L1	5 (1)	0 (1)	1 (1)	1 (1)	1 (1)	0 (1)
L2	3 (1)	0 (1)	1 (1)	1 (1)	0 (1)	0 (1)
L3	1 (1)	1 (1)	0 (1)	1 (1)	1 (1)	0 (1)
L4	2 (1)	1 (1)	1 (1)	1 (1)	0 (1)	1 (1)
L5	5 (1)	1 (1)	1 (1)	1 (1)	1 (1)	0 (1)

an axis that has now migrated to the impacted zygapophysial joint and so further rotation is at the expense of the intervertebral disc.

Ranges of axial rotation studied via biplanar radiography in 24–36-year-old males are depicted in Table 4.9 (Pearcy & Tribrewal 1984, Pearcy et al 1984). The small ranges of axial rotation available would appear to be similar at all levels and all fall within the 3 degree safe limit described in the biomechanical literature.

Axial rotation tends to couple with contralateral lateral flexion at upper lumbar levels but with ipsilateral lateral flexion at L5/S1. However, examination of Table 4.10 highlights the very small amounts of mean motion being discussed while the variation in size and direction of motion is large. Flexion or extension may couple with axial rotation resulting in the mean magnitude of coupled motion in the sagittal plane being zero.

Lateral flexion is a complex and highly variable movement. It involves lateral bending and rotatory movements of the interbody joints and a variety of movements at the zygapophysial joints (Bogduk 1997). Biplanar radiography in young male adults reveals the smaller range of lateral flexion at lower levels of the lumbar spine when compared with upper segments (Table 4.11) reflecting the bony and ligamentous anatomy of the L5 and to a lesser extent the L4 vertebrae (Pearcy & Tribrewal 1984, Pearcy et al 1984).

Table 4.9 Ranges of segmental motion in degrees during axial rotation (based on Pearcy et al 1984, Pearcy & Tribrewal 1984)

Segment	Mean range of motion in degrees	
	Left	Right
L1–2	1	1
L2–3	1	1
L3–4	1	2
L4–5	1	2
L5–S1	1	0

Table 4.11 Ranges of segmental motion in degrees during lateral flexion (based on Pearcy et al 1984, Pearcy & Tribrewal 1984)

Segment	Mean range of motion	
	Left	Right
L1–2	5	6
L2–3	5	6
L3–4	5	6
L4–5	3	5
L5–S1	0	2

The general pattern of coupled motion is for lateral flexion to be associated with contralateral axial rotation at upper lumbar levels but ipsilateral axial rotation at L5/S1 (Table 4.12). Lateral flexion may be accompanied by either flexion or extension but as extension occurs more frequently and at a larger magnitude, the results of this study suggest that lateral flexion is usually accompanied by extension (Pearcy & Tribrewal 1984).

The work by Pearcy and colleagues highlights the fact that the patterns of coupled motion in the lumbar spine are only general patterns that are subject to a high degree of variability both between subjects and between segments within the one individual. A normal subject may exhibit the general pattern of coupling at one level but may exhibit reverse coupling at other levels (Pearcy 1985). Consequently there is at present little evidence for strict rules of coupled motion that determine whether an individual has abnormal ranges or directions of coupling in the lumbar spine.

KEYWORDS	
kinematics	atlanto-occipital joint
spinal range of motion	atlanto-axial joint

Table 4.10 Coupled movements of lumbar spine rotation (based on Pearcy & Tribrewal 1984)

Level	Axial rotation (degrees)		Lateral flexion (degrees)		Flexion/extension (degrees)	
	Mean	Range	Mean	Range	Mean	Range
R L1	−1	(−2–1)	3	(−1–5)	0	(−3–3)
L L1	1	(−1–1)	−3	(−7 to −1)	0	(−4–4)
R L2	−1	(−2–1)	4	(1–9)	0	(−2–2)
L L2	1	(−1–1)	−3	(−5–0)	0	(−4–4)
R L3	−1	(−3–1)	3	(1–6)	0	(−2–2)
L L3	2	(0–1)	−3	(−6–0)	0	(−3–2)
R L4	−1	(−2–1)	1	(−7–0)	0	(−9–5)
L L4	2	(0–1)	−2	(−5–1)	0	(−7–2)
R L5	−1	(−2–1)	−2	(−7–0)	0	(−5–3)
L L5	0	(−2–1)	1	(0–2)	0	(−5–3)

Table 4.12 Coupled movements of the lumbar spine during lateral flexion (based on Pearcy & Tibrewal 1984)

Level	Lateral flexion (degrees)		Axial rotation (degrees)		Flexion/extension (degrees)	
	Mean	Range	Mean	Range	Mean	Range
R L1	−5	(−8 to −2)	0	(−3–1)	−2	(−5–1)
L L1	6	(4–10)	0	(−2–1)	−2	(−9–0)
R L2	−5	(−8 to −4)	1	(−1–1)	−1	(−3–1)
L L2	6	(2–10)	−1	(−3–1)	−3	(−4 to −1)
R L3	−5	(−11–2)	1	(−1–1)	−1	(−3–1)
L L3	5	(−3–8)	−1	(−4–1)	−2	(−4–3)
R L4	−3	(−5–1)	1	(0–1)	0	(−1–4)
L L4	3	(−3–6)	−1	(−4–1)	−1	(−4–2)
R L5	0	(−2–3)	0	(−1–1)	2	(−3–8)
L L5	−3	(−6–1)	−2	(−3–1)	0	(−5–5)

References

Aho A, Vartianen O, Salo O 1955 Segmentary antero-posterio mobility of the cervical spine. Annales Medicinae Internae Fenniae 44: 287–299

Bhalla S K, Simmons E H 1969 Normal ranges of intervertebral joint motion of the cervical spine. Canadian Journal of Surgery 12: 181–187

Bogduk N 1997 Clinical anatomy of the lumbar spine and sacrum, 3rd edn. Churchill Livingstone, Edinburgh

Bogduk N, Mercer S R 2000 Biomechanics of the cervical spine. I: Normal kinematics. Clinical Biomechanics 15: 633–648

Brocher J E W 1955 Die occipito-cervical-gegend: eine diagnostiche pathogenetische studie. Georg Thieme Verlag, Stuttgart

Cossette J W, Farfan H F, Robertson G H, Wells R V 1971 The instantaneous center of rotation of the third lumbar intervertebral joint. Journal of Biomechanics 4: 149–153

Dankmeijer J, Rethmeier B J 1943 The lateral movement in the atlanto-axial joints and its clinical significance. Acta Radiologica 24: 55–66

Dvorak J, Panjabi M, Gerber M, Wichmann W 1987a CT-functional diagnostics of the rotatory instability of upper cervical spine. 1: An experimental study on cadavers. Spine 12: 197–205

Dvorak J, Hayek J, Zehnder R 1987b CT-functional diagnostics of the rotatory instability of the upper cervical spine. 2: An evaluation on healthy adults and patients with suspected instability. Spine 12: 725–731

Dvorak J, Froehlich D, Penning L, Baumgartner H, Panjabi M M 1988 Functional radiographic diagnosis of the cervical spine: flexion/extension. Spine 13: 748–755

Fielding J W 1957 Cineradiography of the normal cervical spine. Journal of Bone and Joint Surgery 39: 1280–1288

Gatton M L, Pearcy M J 1999 Kinematics and movement sequencing during flexion of the lumbar spine. Clinical Biomechanics 14: 376–383

Gregersen G, Lucas D 1967 An in vivo study of the axial rotation of the human thoracolumbar spine. Journal of Bone and Joint Surgery 49A: 247–262

Hohl M, Baker H R 1964 The atlanto-axial joint. Journal of Bone and Joint Surgery 46A: 1739–1752

Kanayama M, Abumi K, Kaneda K, Tadano S, Ukai T 1996 Phase lag of the intersegmental motion in flexion-extension of the lumbar and lumbosacral spine: an in vivo study. Spine 21: 1416–1422

Kottke F J, Mundale M O 1959 Range of mobility of the cervical spine. Archives of Physical Medicine and Rehabilitation 40: 379–382

Lewit K, Krausova L 1963 Messungen von vor-und ruckbeuge in den kopfgelenken. Fortschrift Rontgenst 99: 538–549

Lind B, Sihlbom H, Nordwall A, Malchau H 1989 Normal range of motion of the cervical spine. Archives Physical Medicine and Rehabilitation 70: 692–695

Markuske H 1971 Untersuchungen zur statik und dynamik der kindlichen halswirbelsaule: der aussagewert seitlicher rontgenaufnahmen: die wirbelsaule in forschung und praxis. Hippokrates, Stuttgart

Mercer S R, Bogduk N 2001 The joints of the cervical vertebral column. Journal of Orthopaedic and Sports Physical Therapy 31: 174–182

Mimura M, Moriya H, Watanabe T, Takahashi K, Yamagata M, Tamaki T 1989 Three-dimensional motion analysis of the cervical spine with special reference to the axial rotation. Spine 14: 1135–1139

Nowitzke A, Westaway M, Bogduk N 1994 Cervical zygapophyseal joints: geometrical parameters and relationship to cervical kinematics. Clinical Biomechanics 9: 342–348

Okawa A, Shinomiyaw K, Komori H, Muneta T, Arai Y, Nakai O 1998 Dynamic motion study of the whole lumbar spine by videofluoroscopy. Spine 23: 1743–1749

Pearcy M J 1985 Stereo-radiography of lumbar spine motion. Acta Orthopaedica Scandinavica 212 (Suppl.): 1–41

Pearcy M J, Tibrewal S B 1984 Axial rotation and lateral bending in the normal lumbar spine measured by three-dimensional radiography. Spine 9: 582–587

Pearcy M, Portek I, Shepherd J 1984 Three-dimensional X-ray analysis of normal movement in the lumbar spine. Spine 9: 294–297

Penning L, Wilmink J T 1987 Rotation of the cervical spine: a CT study in normal subjects. Spine 12: 732–738

van Mameren H 1988 Motion patterns in the cervical spine. Thesis, University of Limberg, Maastricht

van Mameren H, Drukker J, Sanches H, Beursgens J 1990 Cervical spine motion in the sagittal plane. I: Range of motion of actually performed movements, an X-ray cinematographic study. European Journal of Morphology 28: 47–68

Werne S 1958 The possibilities of movement in the craniovertebral joints. Acta Orthopaedica Scandinavica 28: 165–173

White A A 1969 Analysis of the mechanics of the thoracic spine in man. Acta Orthopaedica Scandinavica 127 (Suppl.): 1–105

Willems J M, Jull G A, Ng J K-F 1996 An in vivo study of the primary and coupled rotations of the thoracic spine. Clinical Biomechanics 11: 311–316

Worth D 1985 Cervical spine kinematics. PhD Thesis, Flinders University of South Australia

Worth D, Selvik G 1986 Movements of the craniovertebral joints. In: Grieve G (ed) Modern manual therapy of the vertebral column. Churchill Livingstone, Edinburgh

Chapter 5

Chemistry of the intervertebral disc in relation to functional requirements

J. P. Urban, S. Roberts

INTRODUCTION

The intervertebral disc has a prominent role in the structure and function of the spine. It is able to transmit load and act as a joint. Although its mechanical behaviour in compression, extension, torsion and bending has been extensively investigated, little is yet known of how the composition and structure of the disc influence its mechanical behaviour. In this chapter, current ideas on the relationship between disc mechanical function and its chemical composition will be reviewed.

GROSS STRUCTURE OF THE DISC

The intervertebral disc is generally considered to consist of two distinct regions: the outer, firm, banded annulus fibrosus and the inner, soft, gelatinous nucleus pulposus. The cartilaginous end-plates are interposed between the bony vertebral bodies and the disc itself. Figure 5.1 illustrates the regions of the disc. Some useful reviews of disc structure and the changes found with age and with degeneration have been published (Coventry et al 1945, Peacock 1951, Buckwalter 1995, Urban & Roberts 1995).

The nucleus pulposus

The nucleus occupies the central region of the disc. Its composition and appearance change markedly throughout life. In children it is highly hydrated, being 85–90% water, and is white and translucent. There is a clear demarcation

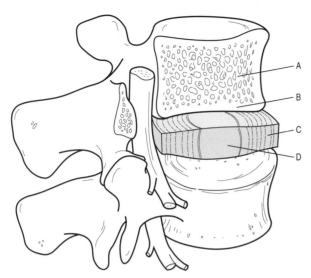

Figure 5.1   Schematic view of the disc and vertebral body showing (a) vertebral body, (b) cartilaginous end-plate, (c) nucleus pulposus, (d) annulus fibrosus.

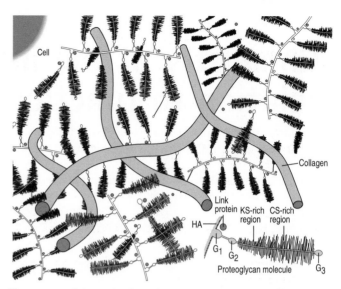

Figure 5.2   Schematic view of the disc extracellular matrix showing details of the aggrecan molecule.

between it and the surrounding annulus fibrosus. In adults the hydration drops markedly and, as the tissue becomes firmer and loses its translucency and becomes increasing yellow-brown, the boundary between nucleus and annulus becomes more difficult to distinguish. In old age the hydration of the nucleus approaches that of the annulus.

The annulus fibrosus

To the naked eye, the annulus fibrosus appears to consist of a series of concentric layers surrounding the nucleus pulposus (see Fig. 5.1). This banded appearance results from the intricate arrangement of fibrous lamellae, which will be discussed in more detail later. The annulus is less hydrated than the nucleus, and changes with age in this structure are not so apparent.

The cartilage end-plate

In children this region acts as a growth plate until skeletal maturity is reached, when the outer ring of 2–3 mm calcifies and fuses with the rim of the vertebral body. A plate of hyaline cartilage, approximately 1–2 mm in thickness, remains abutting the central region of the disc throughout adult life. Fibres from the disc continue into the end-plate where they align horizontally. At the bony interface there is a region of calcified cartilage. The composition of the end-plate resembles that of the disc, but with less water and a greater fibrous component (Roberts et al 1989).

THE CONSTITUENTS OF THE DISC

The matrix of the intervertebral disc is very similar in composition to that of articular cartilage. It consists of collagen fibres embedded in a proteoglycan–water gel (Fig. 5.2). Contained within this matrix are cells, the chondrocytes, which are actively maintaining and repairing it. The mean cell density in the disc is very low so that cells occupy only about 1–5% of the tissue volume. Because of the low cellularity, the mechanical properties of the disc depend chiefly on the constituents of the matrix. However, activity of the cells is vital for maintaining the integrity of the tissue.

Proteoglycans

Proteoglycans (PGs) are some of the largest and most complex molecular structures in mammalian tissue and consist of polysaccharide chains covalently bound to a central protein core. The number and type of polysaccharide chains and the organization, composition and size of the core protein are very variable. At present 30 different proteoglycans are known although not all occur in the disc. They fulfil a variety of different functions such as binding growth factors, regulating collagen fibril size and other properties, for example influencing transparency in the cornea (Iozzo & Murdoch 1996, Woods & Couchman 2001). However, in this chapter only the biophysical functions of the proteoglycans will be discussed. These relate principally to the response of the disc to mechanical load. As in all load-bearing cartilages, proteoglycans endow the matrix with a high osmotic pressure and a low hydraulic permeability and hence constitute the compression-resisting component of the disc.

Disc proteoglycans

Aggrecan. The main proteoglycan found in the disc is the large aggregating proteoglycan, aggrecan (Johnstone & Bayliss 1995). The protein core of aggrecan is able to attach at one end to hyaluronan (HA), a long unbranched polysaccharide. Aggrecan, when undegraded, thus exists in the tissue as very large aggregates consisting of a long chain of HA with many aggrecan molecules attached (see Fig. 5.2). The protein core of aggrecan has a second globular domain adjacent to the HA binding region followed by a long straight central domain. The glycosaminoglycan (GAG) chains of the polysaccharides chondroitin sulphate (CS) and keratan sulphate (KS) are covalently attached to the central domain of the protein core. Each intact aggrecan molecule has around 100 GAG chains attached to it (Iozzo & Murdoch 1996).

In situ in the disc, aggrecan molecules tend to be smaller than those from hyaline cartilages. Only about 30% of monomers found in the disc nucleus can form aggregates compared with about 80% in hip cartilage. Moreover, the aggregates from the nucleus are smaller, having a molecular weight of about 7 million compared to 100 million for aggregates found in bovine nasal septum. There are indications that the disc PGs are able to form aggregates when newly synthesized, but that they are degraded in the tissue and that their HA-binding region disappears (Johnstone & Bayliss 1995). The functional significance of differences in degree of aggregation and of PG size is not yet understood. It has been suggested that the aggregation helps to keep the PGs in the tissue since there is no evidence that they are held there by any form of binding.

Versican. Versican is a large proteoglycan of similar domain structure to aggrecan and also is able to form aggregates. However, it has far fewer GAG chains attached to its protein core. Versican is found mainly in tissues such as ligaments and tendons. It is present in the annulus but not the nucleus of the disc (Hayes et al 2001, Melrose et al 2001).

Small proteoglycans. The disc also contains several members of the family of small leucine-rich proteoglycans. These consist of a short protein core with only one or two GAG chains attached to it. To date, decorin, biglycan, fibromodulin and lumican have been identified in the disc, all at higher concentrations in the annulus than in the nucleus apart from lumican. Decorin and fibromodulin bind to the outside of collagen fibrils and thus have roles in regulating collagen fibril diameter. Biglycan is known to bind growth factors (Johnstone et al 1993, Sztrolovics et al 1999).

Fixed-charge density (FCD)

One important property of the GAGs, especially in relation to the disc's mechanical function, is that they are charged. Both CS and KS contain anionic groups (SO_3^- and COO^-), which impart a net negative charge to the matrix. The FCD confers important properties on the disc since it controls the distribution of charged solutes and hence osmotic pressure, as discussed later.

Collagen

Collagen is the main structural protein in the body, making up about 80% of the total body protein. It is not one single substance, but a family of proteins of which there are approximately 21 members identified so far, with varying chemical composition and tertiary structure. There are at least 29 genes controlling the production of all these types of collagen. All members of the collagen family have three amino acid chains with at least some part of their molecule having these three chains coiled together forming a super helix. Chemical bonds, or cross-links, form both within the collagen molecule and between adjacent molecules. The physical and mechanical properties depend on the amino acid composition since this defines the tertiary structure and conformation of the protein and also its interactions with other collagen and matrix molecules.

The collagen types can be classified into subgroups depending on their structure or organization. One example of such a classification is shown in Figure 5.3. Fibrillar collagens (types I, II, III, V and XI), as their name suggests, form fibrils. The extensive helical structure of fibrillar collagen and cross-links which form render these collagens very stable. They are highly insoluble, resistant to enzymatic breakdown, and are mechanically strong. Two of them, types I and II, are the most common collagen throughout the body, making up more than 80% of the total collagen. Type I collagen is found in tissues such as tendon, ligament and the outer region of intervertebral disc but is also the major collagen of skin and bone. Type II collagen is mainly found in tissues with a high degree of compressive loading, such as cartilage and the eardrum. Exactly how the mechanical properties of these different types relate to their chemistry remains unclear.

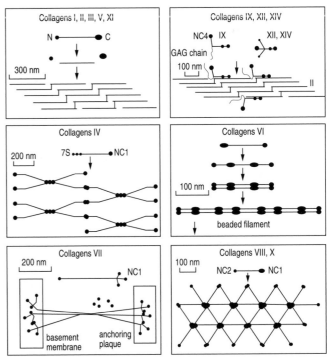

Figure 5.3 Schematic showing the organization of the different collagen types.

Collagen types in disc

There are 10 types of collagen identified to date in the disc. Types I and II are complementary, approximately 80% of the outer annulus being type I collagen, the amount decreasing centrally and vice versa for type II collagen. The other types present in the disc include fibrillar collagens V and XI, other minor collagens including types III and VI, which are mostly cell associated, the basement membrane collagen, type IV, and the fibril-associated collagens with an interrupted triple helix (FACIT) collagen, types IX, XII and XIV. The FACIT collagens bind to the surface of type I and II collagen and may control their fibril diameter. Hence, some of these collagens, while only making up a small percentage of the total, may be a potent influence on the mechanical properties of the tissue.

Collagen organization in the disc

The organization of collagen fibrils in the disc is highly specialized. The three-dimensional collagen framework of the disc has been shown in scanning electron micrographs (Takeda 1975). In the nucleus the collagen fibrils are much finer than in the annulus, mostly about 0.05 μm in diameter, and are arranged in a loose irregular meshwork. In the annulus, collagen is arranged in 15–25 concentric lamellae made of parallel bundles of fine fibrils 0.1–0.2 μm in diameter. These lamellae are visible to the naked eye and vary from 100 to 500 μm in width, the outer lamellae being thickest. Their width varies with age and location, with the posterior lamellae not as wide as those in the rest of the disc (Marchand & Ahmed 1990). The fibre bundles of each lamella run obliquely between the adjacent vertebral bodies and are firmly anchored to them or to the cartilaginous endplate. The resulting angle formed between the fibre bundles of the lamellae and the vertebral bodies varies between 40 and 70 degrees, the direction of the fibres alternating in the neighbouring lamellae.

The arrangement of the collagen network in the disc has an important influence on how load is distributed. The angle between the fibre bundles of the adjacent lamellae is able to change since the lamellae are loosely interconnected. Even though collagen is only slightly extensible, the fact that the lamellae can move separately gives the structure itself considerable extensibility, especially in the vertical direction. The arrangement of the collagen network is shown schematically in Figure 5.4.

Other matrix constituents

In addition to collagen and PG the disc contains a considerable fraction of non-collagenous proteins. These include structural glycoproteins, such as elastin (Mikawa et al 1986) and other less well-characterized constituents. Some may be associated with the cell as has been found in other cartilages, where they are strongly implicated in the interaction of the cell with the extracellular matrix. Amyloid, extravascular plasma proteins and endogenous proteinase inhibitors are

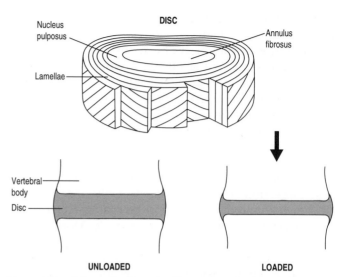

Figure 5.4 Schematic view of collagen organization of the disc showing the direction of the collagen bundles in adjacent annulus lamellae and possible changes in the network on loading.

also found in disc tissue and may be involved in ageing and degenerative processes. The proportion of these components changes with development and ageing and also varies with position (Nerlich et al 1997, Hayes et al 2001). The concentration of some proteins such as fibronectin increases markedly in degenerate discs (Oegema et al 2000).

Proteinases

The disc, like all other tissues, has to have the capability to remodel itself, which entails both breaking down or degrading the original matrix and synthesizing new components. Proteinase enzymes, which can break down collagen, proteoglycans and other matrix macromolecules have been identified in the disc (Sedowofia et al 1982). Some proteinases, such as cathepsins B and D, are more active at acid pH, while others, including matrix metalloproteinases and aggrecanase, are more active at neutral pH. Matrix metalloproteinases (MMPs), a family of enzymes each able to degrade specific macromolecules and together able to break down all matrix components, have been found in the disc. Only members of the subgroup collagenases (MMPs 1, 8 and 13) can disrupt the triple helix of collagen, but the degraded collagen fragments can be further broken down by other MMPs, the gelatinases (MMPs 2 and 9). The proteoglycan core protein is broken down from both ends by many MMPs but particularly the stromelysins (MMPs 3, 10 and 11). However, the most common degradation site is near the HA-binding region, leaving a stub of aggrecan attached to HA together with non-aggregated aggrecan fragments. The activity of MMPs is complex. MMPs are produced by the cells as inactive precursors which require activation before they can degrade matrix molecules. They also have naturally occurring inhibitors (tissue inhibitors of MMPs or TIMPs).

In degenerate discs MMP concentrations increase (Crean et al 1997), as shown in Figure 5.5A, and turnover, which is normally slow (>2 years for PGs; > 10 years for collagen), is more rapid in degeneration (Antoniou et al 1996a). The increased proteoglycan degradation and MMP activity seen in disc disease could result not only from an increased synthesis of MMPs, but also from greater activation of those present or from decreased levels of TIMPs (Roberts et al 2000).

Cells

The disc has a low cellularity; the mean cell density of the adult human disc is about 5500 cells mm^{-3} (Maroudas et al 1975). The cell density is not uniform throughout the tissue, being highest near the end-plate and at the periphery of the annulus, i.e. in the regions nearest the blood supply. The primary function of these cells is the manufacture and maintenance of the matrix.

There are distinct differences between cells in the annulus and nucleus, possibly reflecting their different developmental origin. In the infant human disc, the cells of the nucleus are notochordal. These notochordal cells disappear by 4–10 years in humans and are replaced by rounded chondrocyte-like cells surrounded by a capsule with long processes extending into the matrix. The cells of the inner annulus are also rounded, but those in the outer regions of the annulus are long and thin and extend along the collagen fibrils of the lamellae (Errington et al 1998). While disc cells have not yet been fully characterized, it is now clear that there are different cell types, which remain distinct in culture and produce different sets of extracellular matrix proteins.

Water

Water containing dissolved solutes is the main constituent of the disc. It occupies 65–90% of the tissue volume, depending on age and region. Since the cell density is low, most of the water is extracellular. Some of it is associated with the collagen fibrils, the intrafibrillar fraction. This fraction, which is about 1.0 g water/1.0 g dry collagen, may be considerable in old or degenerate discs, which have low PG concentrations. This intrafibrillar water is freely exchangeable and is accessible to small solutes such as glucose, but large molecules, such as the PGs themselves, are excluded from this fraction. The effective concentration of PGs is then often underestimated (Maroudas 1990).

Nerves and blood vessels

Compared to other sites in the body, the intervertebral discs have few blood vessels or nerves in the healthy adult. In contrast, in utero and in young discs, there are blood vessels in the annulus fibrosus and large vascular channels in the thick cartilage end-plate. These diminish during development. The cartilage end-plate decreases to become a thin layer, approximately 1.5 mm thick, of totally avascular hyaline cartilage. Few, if any, vessels remain present in the outer annulus. The adult disc is almost avascular; it is the largest avascular structure in the body. However, with increasing age and/or degeneration, the vascularity of the annulus increases again (Kauppila 1995) (Figure 5.5B).

Innervation in healthy and diseased discs follows a similar pattern to blood vessels. The normal adult disc has nerve fibres in the outer few millimetres of the annulus fibrosus. They originate from the sinuvertebral nerve and paravertebral sympathetic trunk, their distribution apparently being non-segmental, with reports of pain relief at the L4–S1 disc levels when anaesthetic is applied to the L2 nerve root. The nerves lie predominantly parallel to the collagen bundles in the annulus and particularly between the annular lamellae, although sometimes nerve fibres can be seen to cross them. Innervation is both autonomic and sensory, the former commonly co-distributing with blood vessels in the disc, presumably when the nerve facilitates vascular control. The

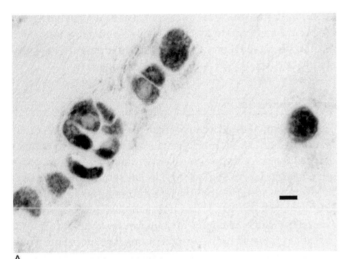

A

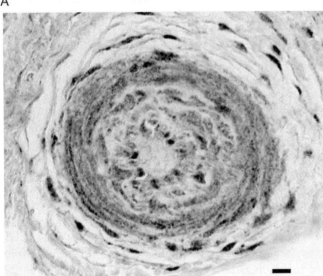

B

Figure 5.5 A MMPs produced by cells in degenerate discs. B Blood vessels in annulus of degenerate discs.

sensory innervation may be involved in both nociception and proprioception, since it is known that mechanoreceptors occur in the outer 2–3 lamellae of human discs and the longitudinal ligaments (Roberts et al 1995). Golgi tendon organ receptors (GTO) appear to be the most common proprioreceptors, although pacinian corpuscles and Ruffini endings have also been observed. The relative frequency of these mechanoreceptors may reflect the level and rate of change of stress seen in the disc, since GTOs are high threshold, slow adapting receptors which only become active at the extremes of movement in other localities. The mechanoreceptors in the disc may be important in influencing the activity of spinal muscles. Electrical stimulation of the disc innervation elicits reaction in the lumbar multifidus and longissimus paraspinal muscles (Indahl et al 1997).

In degenerate intervertebral discs removed from patients with back pain the innervation seen is more extensive than in normal controls, with both number and size of nerves increasing. Both thick myelinated nerve bundles (diameter 15–25 μm) and thin (diameter 0.25–2.5 μm) nerves are found in degenerate discs and nerves also penetrate more centrally in degenerate than in normal discs (Freemont et al 1997).

DISC DISEASES

Disorders of the intervertebral disc include spinal deformities such as scoliosis (when the spine is bent laterally), kyphosis (when it is abnormally humped), disc herniation or disc degeneration. These will each be discussed in turn.

Spinal deformities

In both scoliosis and kyphosis the intervertebral discs are wedged, as can be the vertebral bodies. There are many congenital, neuromuscular or other disorders which result in scoliosis, but in the majority of affected individuals there is no known cause (idiopathic). As far as is known the compositional and structural changes in the scoliotic disc are the same whatever the initiating factor.

Several properties such as the type of collagen, its cross-linking pattern and turnover and glycosaminoglycan contents have all been shown to vary across the disc from the concave to the convex side of the curve (Crean et al 1997, Duance et al 1998). The scoliotic disc also shows marked calcification, particularly in the end-plate (Roberts et al 1993). More recently, techniques used to study nutrient pathways have demonstrated that these are affected in scoliosis with those at the apex of the curve being most compromised (Urban et al 2001a). This may be directly responsible for the diminished cell numbers seen in these discs (Urban et al 2001b).

Disc herniation

Disc herniation or 'slipped' or prolapsed discs are the most common disc disorder leading to spinal surgery, with 12 000 operations for it being carried out annually in England.

The cause of disc herniation is not clear. It could arise from purely mechanical overload or because the matrix is weaker than normal. Poorly synthesized or structured matrix or matrix which has been partially degraded (e.g. via MMPs) could lead to a mechanically inferior matrix, which might predispose to rupture under normal loading conditions.

The posterolateral disc bulges (protrusion) or ruptures either partially (extrusion) or totally (sequestration). Clinical symptoms result from pressure on the spinal nerves, depending at what level the prolapse occurs. L4–5 and L5–S1 discs are most commonly involved affecting the sciatic nerve, resulting in sciatica. However, since more than 70% of individuals with disc prolapses identifiable on MRI are asymptomatic (Boos et al 1995) there must be other factor(s) involved in addition to mechanical factors. Possible suggestions include sensitization of the nerve roots via inflammatory mediators which might be released from the herniated discs (Brisby et al 2000).

The natural history of symptomatic herniated discs, if left unoperated, is often to resorb. They become vascularized and have high levels of cytokines and proteases, such as matrix metalloproteinases, which can degrade the extracellular matrix.

Disc degeneration

The disc shows degenerative changes relatively early in its life with about 10% of individuals aged 10–20 years having degenerate discs and with degeneration increasing steeply with ageing (Miller et al 1988). The causes are unknown but twin studies indicate that there is a strong genetic influence (Sambrook et al 1999). When twins discordant for the major risk factors such as heavy physical work or smoking were examined (i.e. one twin smoked but not the other) the influence of the environment was insignificant compared to that of the genes (Battie et al 1995). Disc degeneration appears to be a complex polygenetic disorder; associations between disc degeneration and polymorphisms of several genes such as aggrecan, collagen IX and vitamin D receptors have already been reported (Videman et al 1998, Annunen et al 1999, Kawaguchi et al 1999, Paassilta et al 2001).

Disc degeneration is thought to lead to back pain, either directly or indirectly. One of the main compositional changes in degenerate discs is loss of proteoglycan and hence water and actual disc height. The associated loss of stiffness leads to increased disc bulging on loading. These changes can in turn alter the loading on adjacent spinal structures such as muscles, ligaments, facet capsules and bone, all of which are highly innervated. It can contribute to the symptoms associated with spinal stenosis. In this condition, which occurs later in life, the spinal canal becomes narrowed due to increased ossification of the vertebral bodies bordering on the spinal canal and/or the thickening and sometimes calcification of ligamentum flavum. Slight bulging of the disc in such a narrowed canal will therefore cause symptoms.

In addition to the loss of proteoglycan and water, other biochemical changes which can occur in degenerate discs include a shift in the types of collagen produced, altered collagen cross-linking and increased proteinase content. Morphologically, the disc becomes cracked and fissured, perhaps due to loss of glycosaminoglycan and water, with more irregular, disrupted collagen organization and annular lamellae. In addition degenerate discs have more blood vessels and innervation than 'normal' discs (Freemont et al 1997). The degeneration-induced changes in disc composition and structure can be visualized to some extent by MRI (Thompson et al 1990, Antoniou et al 1998).

FUNCTION OF THE CONSTITUENTS OF THE DISC

The major functions of the discs are mechanical as the discs serve both to transmit load and to act as joints. These mechanical functions are directly related to the concentration and arrangement of the two major structural components of the tissue, collagen and PG.

A structural model

The functions of the macromolecular constituents of the matrix are demonstrated in a physical model (Broom & Marra 1985). This model consists of a network of string enclosing balloons, which inflate the network and prevent it from collapsing. The resulting structure is able to support compressive loads though neither the string nor the balloons could do so alone, as the string would collapse and the balloons would fly apart. In the disc, collagen forms a structural framework which, like the string network of the model, is strong in tension but collapses under a compressive load if unsupported. PGs are held in the matrix by the collagen network as the balloons are held in the string network. PGs imbibe water, as discussed later, and inflate the collagen network, as the balloons inflate the string network; in so doing, they enable the tissue to support compressive loads without collapsing.

The biophysical function of proteoglycans and collagen

The osmotic pressure of proteoglycan solutions

The high osmotic pressure of PG solutions arises mainly from the polyelectrolyte nature of the PGs. Because of the fixed negative charges on the GAGs, the total number of ions in the disc is always greater than in the plasma and the excess number of ions in the disc leads to the high osmotic pressure in the tissue. PG size or degree of aggregation has little influence on osmotic pressure compared to charge density (Comper & Preston 1974). In the nucleus of the resting adult disc the FCD lies between 0.2 and 0.4 mEq ml^{-1} depending on age, giving an osmotic pressure of 0.1–0.3 MPa (1–3 atmospheres). The FCD of the annulus, and hence its osmotic pressure, is somewhat lower, but is still considerable in comparison with that of non-weight-bearing tissues. It should be noted that the osmotic pressure rises steeply with an increase in FCD or PG content arising, for instance, as the result of fluid expression under load.

Swelling pressure of the disc

The disc contains PGs at concentrations which lead to an osmotic pressure, π, of several atmospheres. PGs at such concentrations in contact with saline solutions would tend to imbibe water and hence cause the tissue to swell. In vivo this tendency to swell is opposed by: (i) the combined effects of body weight and muscle tension, Pa; and (ii) the net restraining force of the collagen network of the disc, Pc. At equilibrium these effective pressures are balanced. Thus we can say:

$$Pa = (\pi - Pc) = Ps \qquad \text{(equation 1)}$$

where Ps is called the net swelling pressure of the tissue. Ps varies with the composition and hence with region of the disc and will be affected by factors such as age and degeneration which affect tissue organization and composition and also with load-induced changes in hydration, since both π and Pc vary with hydration.

Swelling pressure and tissue fluid content

Fluid content depends on the applied load, on the loading history and on tissue composition.

If the load on the disc at equilibrium is increased, the equilibrium is disturbed by the increase in Pa since now Pa>Ps; fluid is thus expressed to restore equilibrium. As fluid is expressed the PG concentration, and hence the osmotic pressure, increases but the volume of the tissue, and hence the collagen network tension, decreases. The net effect is an increase in the swelling pressure Ps (equation 1). If the load is maintained, fluid will continue to be expressed from the tissue until the swelling pressure increases sufficiently to balance the applied pressure.

Conversely, if the load on the tissue is reduced Pa<Ps and the disc swells. During swelling, the PGs are diluted and their osmotic pressure, π, decreases; as the volume increases, the tension in the collagen network also increases and Pc rises. The swelling pressure is consequently reduced. If the load on the disc is completely removed, for instance when the disc is placed in saline solution in vitro, swelling will finally cease when the reduced osmotic pressure is balanced by the increased collagen tension.

Figure 5.6 shows the increase in volume of a bovine tail disc after incubation in saline for 5 hours. Swelling was considerable, especially in the nucleus where the collagen network is weakest; here the fluid content of similarly swollen discs may increase 200–300% (Urban & Maroudas 1981). Swelling in the annulus was directional and dictated by the collagen organization. It should be noted that following disc herniation, sequestrated disc fragments are in effect unloaded fragments of disc, which can swell considerably.

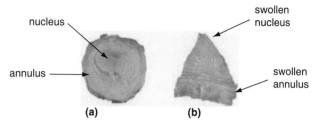

Figure 5.6   Swelling of the unloaded disc. A An intact bovine tail disc after removal of adjacent tissues. B the same disc after immersing for 5 hours in saline at 4°C. The nucleus pulposus in particular has swollen considerably; swelling has increased the height of the annulus fibrosus more than the width.

Hydraulic permeability

In the schematic view of the disc matrix shown in Figure 5.2 the matrix can be seen to consist of PGs densely packed between collagen fibrils. The collagen fibrils are spaced at 20–60 nanometres whereas, because of their close packing, the distance between the GAG chains is only 2–4 nanometres (Byers et al 1983). The fine pore structure of the matrix is thus determined by the PG concentration rather than by the collagen network; the higher the PG concentration, the more closely packed are the GAGs and the smaller the effective 'pores' formed by the entangled GAG chains. A change in the water content of the disc alters PG concentration and thus pore size; if the tissue swells, the PG concentration is diluted and the effective pore size increases. Conversely, if the disc loses fluid, the pore size decreases as the same number of PG chains pack into a smaller volume of tissue.

Pore size relates directly to hydraulic permeability and thus the rate at which fluid moves in and out of the disc; small pores impart a low hydraulic permeability and thus restrict fluid flow.

Solute partitions and transport

Proteoglycans, because they are charged and divide the extracellular spaces into small pores, control the concentration of dissolved solutes in the disc. The imbalance of charge in the matrix leads to the concentration of positive ions, such as calcium and sodium, being higher in the disc than in the external plasma (Maroudas 1980). The distribution of ions is important because it governs the osmotic pressure of the disc as discussed. Charge also affects the concentration of other molecules which enter the disc, such as antibiotics; positively charged antibiotics such as aminoglycosides will reach higher concentrations in the disc than negatively charged antibiotics such as penicillin (Thomas et al 1995).

The concentration of large uncharged molecules in the disc is governed by the pore size distribution and this also depends on PG concentration. Many of the larger serum proteins have diameters which are greater than the 2–4 nanometre diameter of the 'pores' formed between the interdigitating GAG chains and are thus virtually excluded

from the normal disc matrix on account of their size. Even glucose (mol wt <200) is sterically excluded from about 10% of the pores in a normal disc (Urban et al 1979). In disc degeneration, as PG concentration falls, pore size increases and some of the pores become accessible to these large molecules. This process has not been investigated in the disc, but loss of PGs allows large molecules such as growth factor complexes to penetrate into osteoarthritic articular cartilage, possibly influencing the development and progression of arthritis (Schneiderman et al 1995).

Proteoglycans also govern the movement of solutes through the tissue. Solutes can move by diffusion under concentration gradients or through convective flow, i.e. with fluid moving in and out of the disc in response to changes in mechanical load. In both cases, their movement is restricted by the GAG network. Whether a solute moves by diffusion or whether transport is aided by convection depends on solute size. Small solutes such as glucose, oxygen and lactate, which can diffuse rapidly, move almost entirely by diffusion; larger solutes such as enzymes or proteases, which diffuse more slowly, are affected by fluid movement (Thornton et al 1987, O'Hara et al 1990).

MECHANICAL BEHAVIOUR OF THE DISC IN RELATION TO ITS COMPOSITION

The disc's behaviour under load depends both on the load and on the organization of its extracellular matrix.

Loads on the lumbar spine

In vivo the disc is always under load as a result of the combined effects of body weight and muscle activity. Loads applied to the disc lead to a rise in pressure. Nachemson (1960) found that even in a relaxed supine subject the pressure on the lower lumbar discs was 0.1–0.2 MPa, whereas in unsupported sitting it rose to about 0.6–0.7 MPa. Peak pressures during strenuous activity may rise considerably above these values. Recent in vivo measurements have monitored changes in intradiscal pressure over 24 hours and confirmed these early results for the most part (Wilke et al 1999), with the pressure lower in degenerate than in normal discs (Sato et al 1999). Because of the relationship between disc pressure and posture, the intradiscal pressure tends to follow a cyclic pattern: it is at its lowest during sleep, and then increases 5- to 6-fold during the day's activities.

The deformation of the disc under load

Disc height alters with changes in load by two mechanisms. When the load on the disc is increased the disc deforms initially through a rearrangement of the collagen network (see Fig. 5.4). The extent of this deformation varies from disc to disc, but the factors which govern this are not understood. No consistent pattern with age, sex or degree of degeneration has been found (Shirazi-Adl et al 1984). For changes in load of short duration this deformation is virtually constant volume. However, if the load is maintained the disc loses height or creeps, and a large part of the creep deformation results from fluid loss (Keller & Nathan 1999). Thus, for each applied load, the extent of the initial deformation will depend largely on the structure and integrity of the collagen network (Iatridis et al 1999). In contrast, the rate and magnitude of the creep deformation is related more to the PG content. Degenerate discs of low PG content will be much less able to retain fluid in the face of applied pressure than normal discs (Fig. 5.7A).

The amount of water exchanged between disc and surroundings with changes in load is quite considerable. In vivo MRI studies which imaged discs of normal office worker volunteers immediately after rising and then after a day's work estimated that, on average, discs lose around 25% of their fluid content during the day and that this fluid is reimbibed at night during rest (Boos et al 1993).

A schematic view of the diurnal fluid cycle and its relationship to swelling pressure is shown in Figure 5.7B. Initially the disc is assumed to be at equilibrium at point (1) (after a night's rest - 7 a.m.). The pressure on the disc is suddenly increased to (2) (on rising, for example). The disc is no longer in equilibrium. Thus there is a driving force expressing fluid from the tissue which depends on the difference between (2) and the swelling pressure curve. While the pressure on the disc is maintained, fluid is expressed from the tissue. The rate of fluid loss depends partly on the driving force (it is fastest when the driving force is greatest) and partly on the hydraulic permeability of the tissue at point (2). Fluid loss is thus fastest initially. As fluid is expressed the PG concentration rises and the hydraulic permeability falls; also, the driving force diminishes as the equilibrium curve is approached. All these mechanisms help to limit the amount of fluid lost from the disc. When the pressure on the disc is released (points 3 to 4 – on retiring to rest at night, for example), the disc now lies under the swelling pressure curve and thus will have a tendency to imbibe fluid in order to dilute the PGs. During swelling (during rest at night – points 4 to 1) the hydraulic permeability increases; thus, the rate of fluid flow does not decrease drastically as equilibrium is approached. Swelling thus tends to be faster than fluid loss and hence the disc is able to replace the fluid lost in 16 hours of activity with 8 hours of rest.

Changes in height during the day are thought in part to arise from loss of fluid from the disc. Eklund & Corlett (1984) measured 6 mm height loss on average during the day, and found that the rate of shrinkage depended on the load on the spine. MRI measurements have correlated this loss in height with fluid loss (Paajanen et al 1994). In contrast, Thornton et al (1987) found that the Skylab astronauts, who were weightless for 85 days, grew about 5 cm in height, in part probably through swelling of their discs under low external loads.

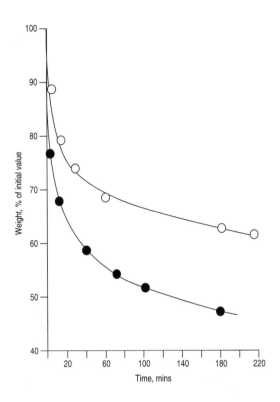

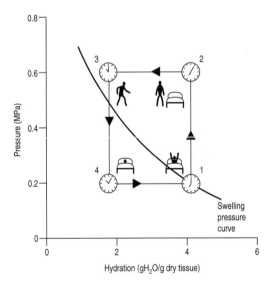

Figure 5.7 Disc fluid content depends on disc composition and on load. A Rates of fluid expression from disc slices in vitro in relation to disc proteoglycan content (open circle: high initial PG content; solid circles: low initial PG content). B Schematic of the diurnal fluid cycle in relation to the disc swelling pressure curve. (1) 7 a.m.: at rest; (2) 7.05 a.m.: pressure increase on rising; (3) 11 p.m.: before retiring; (4) pressure drop on retiring.

CELL ENERGY METABOLISM AND DISC NUTRITION

Although the disc has a low cell density, the continuing activity of the cells is vital to the health of the disc since the cells are responsible for turning over and renewing matrix constituents.

Energy metabolism

Disc cells produce the energy necessary for their survival and function mainly from glucose, which is broken down by glycolysis, even in the presence of oxygen, to produce lactic acid. Through this pathway one molecule of glucose produces two molecules of lactic acid and two molecules of ATP, the cellular energy source. ATP can be produced more efficiently by oxidative phosphorylation since this pathway, which requires oxygen as well as glucose, produces up to 36 molecules of ATP from one molecule of glucose. However, it seems that only around 15% of the disc's ATP is produced by oxidative phosphorylation (Holm et al 1981) and that disc cells do not need oxygen to survive (Horner & Urban 2001). Without oxygen, however, cell functional activity falls steeply.

Disc nutrition

The disc is avascular. Nutrients such as oxygen and glucose, essential for cell survival and activity, reach the cells by diffusion through the matrix of the disc from the blood vessels in contact with the annulus periphery and with the cartilaginous end-plate, as shown schematically in Figure 5.8A.

Waste products produced by the cells are removed from the tissue by the same blood vessels. The route through the endplate may disappear if a calcified layer forms, as happens in scoliosis (Roberts et al 1996) or disc degeneration (Nachemson et al 1970); the nucleus cells may then be at risk.

Because of its size and avascularity, steep gradients in the concentration of nutrients exist in the disc. Holm et al (1981) have shown that while the outer annulus is in equilibrium with the blood oxygen, in the disc interior oxygen concentrations are very low and lactic acid concentrations high so that the deep regions are acidic. The disc thus appears to be in a precarious metabolic state with any loss of nutrient supply leading to cell death and disc degeneration. Indeed, factors affecting the blood supply to the vertebral body, such as atherosclerosis (Kauppila 1997, Kauppila et al 1997), sickle cell anaemia, caisson disease and Gaucher's disease (Jones 1997), all appear to lead to a significant increase in disc degeneration.

In experimental tests, factors which affect the microcirculation, such as vibration or smoking, were seen to lead to a rapid fall in oxygen concentrations in the disc nucleus and a rise in lactate concentration (Holm & Nachemson 1988; see Figure 5.8B). Long-term exercise – or lack of it – appears to have a permanent effect on movement of nutrients into

Figure 5.8 A Schematic view of the nutritional pathways into the disc and of the blood vessels at the vertebral body–disc interface. Adapted from Holm et al 1981. B Effect of exposure to smoke on the time course of (i) oxygen tensions and (ii) lactate concentrations measured in vivo in the centre of the nucleus pulposus (open squares: exposed to smoke; closed circles: no smoke control). Adapted from Holm & Nachemson 1988.

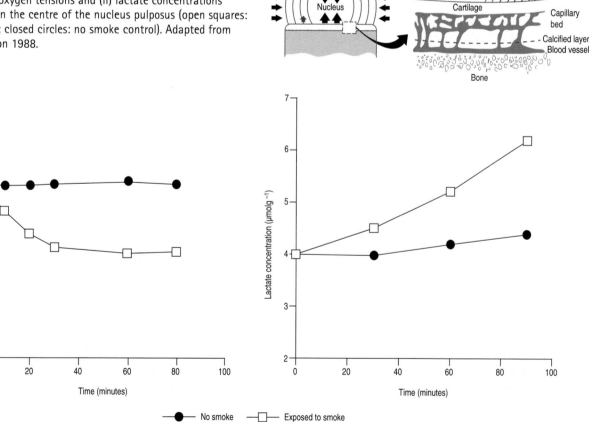

the disc and thus on their concentration in the tissue. The mechanism is not known but it has been suggested that exercise affects the external capillary bed at the disc–bone interface (Holm & Nachemson 1983). Holm & Nachemson (1982) examined dogs' discs which had been fused. After 3 months a fall in cellular activity could be observed, PGs were lost and the fluid content of the discs fell. The reverse occurred in dogs which were vigorously trained over several months; this resulted in increased cellular activity and PG content. It is, however, not clear whether the effect of load or exercise was entirely due to change in nutrient supply; as will be discussed below, cell metabolism is also very sensitive to mechanical stress.

CELL METABOLISM AND MATRIX TURNOVER

In vivo measurements

Relatively little is known about matrix synthesis and turnover in the disc. In vivo studies in animals using radioactive labelling demonstrated that PGs are synthesized in vivo in both adult and young animals. Turnover time (i.e. the average time to replace all PGs) was only a few weeks in 6-week-old guinea pigs, but was over 2 years in adult dogs (Lohmander et al 1973, Urban et al 1979).

Recently, new techniques have been used to examine turnover in discs obtained from human surgical and autopsy material. These rely on examining tissue-specific markers of breakdown or synthesis using newly developed antibodies. Breakdown can be measured by antibodies to neo-epitopes, produced when molecules such as aggrecan or collagen are cleaved by proteinases (Hughes et al 1998). Also, tissues can be examined for molecules produced only during synthesis. For instance, after the collagen molecule is exported from the cell but before it can be assembled into the matrix, a protein domain, the propeptide, is removed enzymically. These propeptides are relatively small and diffuse from the tissue within days. Their presence in the tissue thus indicates that there is active collagen synthesis.

Antoniou et al (1996a, 1996b) have used these markers to examine discs over a range of degenerative grades and ages. Although results varied from region to region of the disc, in general they were able to identify three matrix turnover phases. Phase I (growth) was characterized by both active synthesis and active degradation of matrix molecules. Phase II (maturation and ageing) was distinguished by a progressive drop in both synthetic activity and denaturation of type II collagen. Phase III (degeneration) showed a fall in aggrecan and collagen II synthesis but an increase in collagen II degradation and in collagen I synthesis. Tracer measurements on human discs removed at surgery are in agreement, finding that PG synthesis varies across the disc and was low in degenerate discs (Johnstone & Bayliss 1995).

Since disc cells are active throughout life, potentially they might be able to repair the disc after injury or damage.

Animal models do indeed suggest that PG replacement is possible. When dog discs were treated with chymopapain and PGs were lost from the disc and end-plate, it was observed that the undamaged disc cells were able to synthesize PGs, and expansion of the disc was observed after several months (Garvin & Jennings 1973, Oegema et al 1983). There is no evidence, however, that PGs can be replaced after chymopapain treatment in humans (Leivseth et al 1999), probably because in damaged human discs many disc cells are lost before treatment is started.

Extracellular influences on disc cell metabolism

Over the last 10 years development of methods for studying matrix metabolism (Bayliss et al 1986, Maldonado & Oegema 1992) has increased understanding of the factors influencing cellular activity. Disc cells appear to make a variety of matrix macromolecules but rates of synthesis vary depending on the cell origin; nucleus cells, for instance, produce aggrecan at much higher rates than outer annulus cells. Matrix synthesis also varies with age; rates of biosynthesis are fastest in cells taken from immature discs.

Using these culture methods, it has become apparent that disc cells respond to a variety of extracellular stimuli and that the matrix produced depends not only on cell origin, but that the extracellular environment also has a powerful influence on cell metabolism.

Growth factors and cytokines

Disc cells respond to growth factors, such as IGF-1, which are responsible for stimulating matrix production (Thompson et al 1991, Osada et al 1996). They also respond to cytokines such as IL-1 and TNF-α, which both stimulate activity of MMPs and other agents involved in matrix breakdown and repress synthesis of matrix macromolecules. The concentration of cytokines increases in herniated tissue (Kang et al 1996), possibly because inflammatory cells invade and populate the protruding disc. These cytokines may have a positive role to play in stimulating resorption of the protrusion; however, they may also set off a degenerative cascade in the disc itself and possibly also stimulate pain in the nerve fibres in the outer regions of the disc.

Nutrient levels

Several studies have now shown that if nutrient supply to the disc is impeded, concentrations of oxygen and glucose in the centre of the disc fall and concentrations of lactic acid rise so that the disc becomes acidic (Diamant et al 1968). In acidic pH or low oxygen, even if the cells survive, the amount of PG produced falls significantly (Ishihara & Urban 1999). Even though PG turnover is slow, a decrease in rate of production will eventually lead to a fall in PG concentration in the tissue with consequent changes in disc biomechanics; loss of PG appears to be one of the first signs of disc degeneration.

Mechanical stress

The disc is under constantly varying mechanical forces. With every movement or change in posture, the load on the disc alters as can be seen in recent continuous in vivo pressure measurements (Wilke et al 1999). Cells of most tissues are very responsive to mechanical forces and recent work has shown that this is also true for disc cells.

In vivo responses to load

Most of the information in vivo comes from experimental studies where animals or joints have been subjected to abnormal mechanical loads for days to months. Little is known about the effects of exercise as such, though heavy exercise (40 km running per day) appeared to stimulate matrix synthesis marginally in dog discs (Puustjarvi et al 1993). However, abnormal loads appear to have detrimental effects. Spinal fusion, for instance, appears to lead to degenerative changes in adjacent discs. Degenerative changes and cell death have also been seen after discs have been subjected to high continuous compressive loading (Higuchi et al 1983, Lotz et al 1998). Long-term wedging can also produce disc abnormalities (Pazzaglia et al 1997). These studies all indicate that degenerative changes can be induced by abnormal forces on an otherwise healthy disc and that these changes result from alterations in cellular activity rather than from matrix damage as such. While some of the effects of load in vivo might arise from alterations in the blood supply to the disc, in vitro tests have shown that disc cells themselves respond to load-induced changes in their environment.

In vitro studies

While in vivo studies have demonstrated an overall response of the disc cells to mechanical signals, understanding of the precise mechanical signals which stimulate the cells can only be obtained from in vitro experiments where specific responses to controlled mechanical signals can be investigated. Few studies on disc cells have so far been reported. However, results have shown that disc cells are very sensitive to mechanical stress and responses depend both on the cell type and on the precise nature of the mechanical signal.

The type of mechanical signals seen by the cell depends on how the disc is loaded. When the matrix is loaded, hydrostatic pressure rises, the cell and matrix deform and fluid is expressed. Fluid moves along the cell boundary and, as a consequence of fluid expression, the extracellular concentration of macromolecules increases. The change in pressure or extent of fluid loss depends on the magnitude and duration of the load and on the disc composition. The signals seen by the cells on each change of load are thus very complex, as indicated in Figure 5.9.

In vitro tests have shown that disc cells, as those of other cartilages, are sensitive to the magnitude of the load and

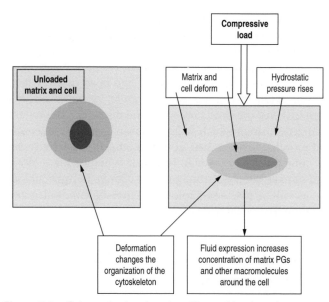

Figure 5.9 Schematic showing the effects of load on the environment of the cell. On loading the disc matrix and cell deform, hydrostatic pressure rises, fluid is expressed, thus changing the composition of the matrix arou.nd the cell.

respond to each of these signals via different pathways. Nucleus cells, for instance, are very responsive to hydrostatic pressure; pressure in the low physiological range (0.3 MPa) stimulates PG synthesis significantly, whereas high pressure (3 MPa) inhibits PG synthesis but stimulates production of MMPs. The effect of hydrostatic pressure appears to be mediated in part by nitric oxide (Liu et al 2001). Disc cells are also very sensitive to changes in hydration, with synthesis rates showing a bimodal response to load (Fig. 5.10); rates fall if fluid is expressed or if the disc

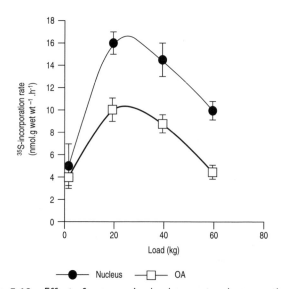

Figure 5.10 Effect of compressive load on proteoglycan synthesis by cells of the bovine nucleus pulposus and annulus fibrosus. The whole disc was incubated at 37°C in vitro under load and rates of synthesis measured over 8 hours (solid circles: nucleus; open squares: outer annulus). Adapted from Ohshima et al 1995.

swells (Ohshima et al 1995). Here the signal appears mediated by the change in cell volume. Responses to fluid movement and to stretch, however, appear to be regulated by cell–matrix interactions.

The complexity is increased because the response varies with cell type. Annulus and nucleus cells have been shown to respond differently to the same mechanical signal in several studies. For example, only nucleus and inner annulus cells are affected by a rise in hydrostatic pressure; outer annulus cells show no response to even high levels of pressure (Ishihara et al 1996). Figure 5.10 shows that annulus cells produce less PG than nucleus cells and are less influenced by compressive load.

These in vitro tests demonstrate the sensitivity of disc cells to different mechanical signals. Load-induced changes in the extracellular environment of the cell alter production of matrix macromolecules and of proteases and hence can affect the overall composition of the disc in the long term. However, while in vitro tests are able to examine cellular responses to simple signals such as controlled stretch or fluid movement or pressure rise, in vivo the cell will be exposed to simultaneous changes in all these signals. Each signal will vary in duration and magnitude depending on the loading regime and nature of the matrix. The overall response of the cell to load thus depends on how it integrates these different signals to produce extracellular matrix. At present we understand little of this process. Thus, although it is apparent that mechanical loading can affect the disc matrix in the long term, at present we are far from being able to predict the net response of the disc cells to any mechanical intervention.

CONCLUSION

In order to function adequately, the disc must retain a well-ordered extracellular matrix throughout life. Disc cells make and maintain this matrix; any loss of cellular function will eventually lead to loss of matrix components and disc degeneration. At present, we understand little of the behaviour of these cells. We need to understand more about their behaviour in health and disease in order to preserve their activity, prevent disc degeneration and even possibly promote disc repair.

KEYWORDS	
nucleus pulposus	collagen
cartilage end-plate	proteinases
proteoglycans	disc nutrition

Acknowledgements

We thank the Arthritis Research Campaign (U0511) and the EU Consortium EURODISC(QLK6-CT-2002-02582) for support.

References

Annunen S, Paassilta P, Lohiniva J et al 1999 An allele of COL9A2 associated with intervertebral disc disease. Science 285: 409–412

Antoniou J, Steffen T, Nelson F et al 1996a The human lumbar intervertebral disc: evidence for changes in the biosynthesis and denaturation of the extracellular matrix with growth, maturation, ageing, and degeneration. Journal of Clinical Investigation 98: 996–1003

Antoniou J, Goudsouzian N M, Heathfield T F et al 1996b The human lumbar endplate: evidence of changes in biosynthesis and denaturation of the extracellular matrix with growth, maturation, ageing, and degeneration. Spine 21: 1153–1161

Antoniou J, Pike G B, Steffen T, Baramki H, Poole A R, Aebi M, Alini M 1998 Quantitative magnetic resonance imaging in the assessment of degenerative disc disease. Magnetic Resonance in Medicine 40: 900–907

Battie M C, Videman T, Gibbons L E, Fisher L D, Manninen H, Gill K 1995 1995 Volvo Award in clinical sciences. Determinants of lumbar disc degeneration: a study relating lifetime exposures and magnetic resonance imaging findings in identical twins. Spine 20: 2601–2612

Bayliss M T, Urban J P G, Johnstone B, Holm S 1986 In vitro method for measuring synthesis rates in the intervertebral disc. Journal of Orthopaedic Research 4: 10–17

Boos N, Wallin A, Gbedegbegnon T, Aebi M, Boesch C 1993 Quantitative MR imaging of lumbar intervertebral disks and vertebral bodies: influence of diurnal water content variations. Radiology 188: 351–354

Boos N, Rieder R, Schade V, Spratt K F, Semmer N, Aebi M 1995 Volvo Award in clinical sciences. The diagnostic accuracy of magnetic resonance imaging, work perception, and psychosocial factors in identifying symptomatic disc herniations. Spine 20: 2613–2625

Brisby H, Byrod G, Olmarker K, Miller V M, Aoki Y, Rydevik B 2000 Nitric oxide as a mediator of nucleus pulposus-induced effects on spinal nerve roots. Journal of Orthopaedic Research 18: 815–820

Broom N D, Marra D L 1985 New structural concepts of articular cartilage demonstrated with a physical model. Connective Tissue Research 14: 1–8

Buckwalter J A 1995 Ageing and degeneration of the human intervertebral disc. Spine 20: 1307–1314

Byers P D, Bayliss M T, Maroudas A, Urban J, Weightman B 1983 Hypothesizing about joints. In: Maroudas A, Holbrow E J (eds) Studies in joint disease 2. Pitman, London, pp 241–276

Comper W D, Preston B N 1974 Model connective tissue systems: a study of polyion-mobile ion and of excluded-volume interactions of proteoglycans. Biochemical Journal 143: 1–9

Coventry M B, Ghormley R K, Kernohan J W 1945 The intervertebral disc: its microscopic anatomy and pathology; changes in the intervertebral disc concomitant with age. Journal of Bone and Joint Surgery 27: 233–247

Crean J K, Roberts S, Jaffray D C, Eisenstein S M, Duance V C 1997 Matrix metalloproteinases in the human intervertebral disc: role in disc degeneration and scoliosis. Spine 22: 2877–2884

Diamant B, Karlsson J, Nachemson A 1968 Correlation between lactate levels and pH in discs of patients with lumbar rhizopathies. Experientia 24: 1195–1196

Duance V C, Crean J K, Sims T J et al 1998 Changes in collagen cross-linking in degenerative disc disease and scoliosis. Spine 23: 2545–2551

Eklund J A, Corlett E N 1984 Shrinkage as a measure of the effect of load on the spine. Spine 9: 189–194

Errington R J, Puustjarvi K, White I F, Roberts S, Urban J G 1998 Characterisation of cytoplasm-filled processes in cells of the intervertebral disc. Journal of Anatomy 192: 369–378

Freemont A J, Peacock T E, Goupille P, Hoyland J A, O'Brien J, Jayson M-I V 1997 Nerve ingrowth into diseased intervertebral disc in chronic back pain. Lancet 350: 178–181

Garvin P, Jennings R B 1973 Long term effects of chymopapain on intervertebral discs of dogs. Clinical Orthopaedics 921: 281–295

Hayes A J, Benjamin M, Ralphs J R 2001 Extracellular matrix in development of the intervertebral disc. Matrix Biology 20: 107–121

Higuchi M, Abe K, Kaneda K 1983 Changes in the nucleus pulposus of the intervertebral disc in bipedal mice: a light and electron microscopic study. Clinical Orthopaedics 175: 251–257

Holm S, Nachemson A 1982 Nutritional changes in the canine intervertebral disc after spinal fusion. Clinical Orthopaedics 169: 243–258

Holm S, Nachemson A 1983 Variation in the nutrition of the canine intervertebral disc induced by motion. Spine 8: 866–874.

Holm S, Nachemson A 1988 Nutrition of the intervertebral disc: acute effects of cigarette smoking: an experimental animal study. Upsala Journal of Medical Sciences 93: 91–99

Holm S, Maroudas A, Urban J P, Selstam G, Nachemson A 1981 Nutrition of the intervertebral disc: solute transport and metabolism. Connective Tissue Research 8: 101–119

Horner H A, Urban J P 2001 2001 Volvo Award winner in basic science studies. Effect of nutrient supply on the viability of cells from the nucleus pulposus of the intervertebral disc. Spine 26: 2543–2549

Hughes C E, Little C B, Buttner F H, Bartnik E, Caterson B 1998 Differential expression of aggrecanase and matrix metalloproteinase activity in chondrocytes isolated from bovine and porcine articular cartilage. Journal of Biological Chemistry 273: 30576–30582

Iatridis J C, Kumar S, Foster R J, Weidenbaum M, Mow V C 1999 Shear mechanical properties of human lumbar annulus fibrosus. Journal of Orthopaedic Research 17: 732–737

Indahl A, Kaigle A M, Reikeras O, Holm S H 1997 Interaction between the porcine lumbar intervertebral disc, zygapophysial joints, and paraspinal muscles. Spine 22: 2834–2840

Iozzo R V, Murdoch A D 1996 Proteoglycans of the extracellular environment: clues from the gene and protein side offer novel perspectives in molecular diversity and function. FASEB Journal 10: 598–614

Ishihara H, Urban J P 1999 Effects of low oxygen concentrations and metabolic inhibitors on proteoglycan and protein synthesis rates in the intervertebral disc. Journal of Orthopaedic Research 17: 829–835

Ishihara H, McNally D S, Urban J G, Hall A C 1996 Effects of hydrostatic pressure on matrix synthesis in different regions of the intervertebral disk. Journal of Applied Physiology 80: 839–846

Johnstone B, Bayliss M T 1995 The large proteoglycans of the human intervertebral disc: changes in their biosynthesis and structure with age, topography, and pathology. Spine 20: 674–684

Johnstone B, Markopolous M, Neame P, Caterson B 1993 Identification and characterization of glycanated and non-glycanated forms of biglycan and decorin in the human intervertebral disc. Biochemical Journal 292: 661–666

Jones J P 1997 Subchondral osteonecrosis can conceivably cause disk degeneration and 'primary'osteoarthritis. In: Urbaniak J R, Jones J P (eds) Osteonecrosis. American Academy of Orthopaedic Surgery, Park Ridge, Illinois, pp 135–142

Kang J D, Georgescu H I, McIntyre-Larkin L, Stefanovic-Racic M, Donaldson W F, Evans C H 1996 Herniated lumbar intervertebral discs spontaneously produced matrix metalloproteinases, nitric oxide, interleukin-6, and prostaglandin E2. Spine 21: 271–277

Kauppila L I 1995 Ingrowth of blood vessels in disc degeneration: angiographic and histological studies of cadaveric spines. Journal of Bone and Joint Surgery (American volume) 77: 26–31

Kauppila L I 1997 Prevalence of stenotic changes in arteries supplying the lumbar spine: a post-mortem angiographic study on 140 subjects. Annals of the Rheumatic Diseases 56: 591–595

Kauppila L I, McAlindon T, Evans S, Wilson P W, Kiel D, Felson D T 1997 Disc degeneration/back pain and calcification of the abdominal aorta: a 25-year follow-up study in Framingham. Spine 22: 1642–1647

Kawaguchi Y, Osada R, Kanamori M et al 1999 Association between an aggrecan gene polymorphism and lumbar disc degeneration. Spine 24: 2456–2460.

Keller T S, Nathan M 1999 Height change caused by creep in intervertebral discs: a sagittal plane model. Journal of Spinal Disorders 12: 313–324

Leivseth G, Salvesen R, Hemminghytt S, Brinckmann P, Frobin W 1999 Do human lumbar discs reconstitute after chemonucleolysis? A 7-year follow-up study. Spine 24: 342–347

Liu G Z, Ishihara H, Osada R, Kimura T, Tsuji H 2001 Nitric oxide mediates the change of proteoglycan synthesis in the human lumbar intervertebral disc in response to hydrostatic pressure. Spine 26: 134–141

Lohmander S, Antonopolous C, Friberg U 1973 Chemical and metabolic heterogeneity of chondroitin sulfate and keratan sulfate in guinea pig cartilage and nucleus pulposus. Biochimica et Biophysica Acta 304: 430–448

Lotz J C, Colliou O K, Chin J R, Duncan N A, Liebenberg E 1998 1998 Volvo Award winner in biomechanical studies. Compression-induced degeneration of the intervertebral disc: an in vivo mouse model and finite-element study. Spine 23: 2493–2506

Maldonado B A, Oegema-TR J 1992 Initial characterization of the metabolism of intervertebral disc cells encapsulated in microspheres. Journal of Orthopaedic Research 10: 677–690

Marchand F, Ahmed A M 1990 Investigation of the laminate structure of lumbar disc annulus fibrosus. Spine 15: 402–410

Maroudas A 1980 Physical chemistry of articular cartilage and the intervertebral disc. In: Sokoloff L (ed) The joints and synovial fluid II. Academic Press, New York, pp 240–293

Maroudas A 1990 Different ways of expressing concentration of cartilage constituents with special reference to the tissue's organization and functional properties. In: Maroudas A, Keuttner K (eds) Methods in cartilage research. Academic Press, London, pp 219

Maroudas A, Stockwell R A, Nachemson A, Urban J 1975 Factors involved in the nutrition of the human lumbar intervertebral disc: cellularity and diffusion of glucose in vitro. Journal of Anatomy 120: 113–130

Melrose J, Ghosh P, Taylor T K 2001 A comparative analysis of the differential spatial and temporal distributions of the large (aggrecan, versican) and small (decorin, biglycan, fibromodulin) proteoglycans of the intervertebral disc. Journal of Anatomy 198: 3–15

Mikawa Y, Hamagami H, Shikata J, Yamamuro T 1986 Elastin in the human intervertebral disk: a histological and biochemical study comparing it with elastin in the human yellow ligament. Archives of Orthopaedic and Trauma Surgery 105: 343–349

Miller J, Schmatz C, Schultz A 1988 Lumbar disc degeneration: correlation with age, sex, and spine level in 600 autopsy specimens. Spine 13: 173–178

Nachemson A 1960 Lumbar intradiscal pressure. Acta Orthopaedica Scandinavica 43 (Suppl.): 1–104

Nachemson A, Lewin T, Maroudas A, Freeman M A F 1970 In vitro diffusion of dye through the end-plates and annulus fibrosus of human lumbar intervertebral discs. Acta Orthopaedica Scandinavica 41: 589–607

Nerlich A G, Schleicher E D, Boos N 1997 1997 Volvo Award winner in basic science studies. Immunohistologic markers for age-related changes of human lumbar intervertebral discs. Spine 22: 2781–2795

Oegema T R J, Bradford D S, Cooper K M, Hunter R E 1983 Comparison of the biochemistry of proteoglycans isolated from normal, idiopathic scoliotic and cerebral palsy spines. Spine 8: 378–384

Oegema T R, Johnson S L, Aguiar D J, Ogilvie J W 2000 Fibronectin and its fragments increase with degeneration in the human intervertebral disc. Spine 25: 2742–2747

O'Hara B P, Urban J P G, Maroudas A 1990 Influence of cyclic loading on the nutrition of articular cartilage. Annals of the Rheumatic Diseases 49: 536–539

Ohshima H, Urban J P G, Bergel D H 1995 The effect of static load on matrix synthesis rates in the intervertebral disc measured in vitro by a new perfusion technique. Journal of Orthopaedic Research 13: 22–29

Osada R, Ohshima H, Ishihara H et al 1996 Autocrine/paracrine mechanism of insulin-like growth factor-1 secretion, and the effect of insulin-like growth factor-1 on proteoglycan synthesis in bovine intervertebral discs. Journal of Orthopaedic Research 14: 690–699

Paajanen H, Lehto I, Alanen A, Erkintalo M, Komu M 1994 Diurnal fluid changes of lumbar discs measured indirectly by magnetic resonance imaging. Journal of Orthopaedic Research 12: 509–514

Paassilta P, Lohiniva J, Goring H H et al 2001 Identification of a novel common genetic risk factor for lumbar disk disease. JAMA 285: 1843–1849

Pazzaglia U E, Andrini L, Di Nucci A 1997 The effects of mechanical forces on bones and joints: experimental study on the rat tail. Journal of Bone and Joint Surgery (British volume) 79: 1024–1030

Peacock A 1951 Observations on the postnatal development of the intervertebral disc in man. Journal of Anatomy 86: 162–179

Puustjarvi K, Lammi M, Kiviranta I, Helminen H J, Tammi M 1993 Proteoglycan synthesis in canine intervertebral discs after long distance running training. Journal of Orthopaedic Research 11: 738–746

Roberts S, Menage J, Urban J P G 1989 Biochemical and structural properties of the cartilage end-plate and its relation to the intervertebral disc. Spine 14: 166–174

Roberts S, Menage J, Eisenstein S M 1993 The cartilage end-plate and intervertebral disc in scoliosis: calcification and other sequelae. Journal of Orthopaedic Research 11: 747–757

Roberts S, Eisenstein S M, Menage J, Evans E H, Ashton I K 1995 Mechanoreceptors in intervertebral discs: morphology, distribution, and neuropeptides [see comments]. Spine 20: 2645–2651

Roberts S, Urban J P G, Evans H, Eisenstein S M 1996 Transport properties of the human cartilage endplate in relation to its composition and calcification. Spine 21: 415–420

Roberts S, Caterson B, Menage J, Evans E H, Jaffray D C, Eisenstein S M 2000 Matrix metalloproteinases and aggrecanase: their role in disorders of the human intervertebral disc. Spine 25: 3005–3013

Sambrook P N, MacGregor A J, Spector T D 1999 Genetic influences on cervical and lumbar disc degeneration: a magnetic resonance imaging study in twins. Arthritis and Rheumatism 42: 366–372

Sato K, Kikuchi S, Yonezawa T 1999 In vivo intradiscal pressure measurement in healthy individuals and in patients with ongoing back problems. Spine 24: 2468–2474

Schneiderman R, Rosenberg N, Hiss J et al 1995 Concentration and size distribution of insulin-like growth factor-I in human normal and osteoarthritic synovial fluid and cartilage. Archives of Biochemistry and Biophysics 324: 173–188

Sedowofia K A, Tomlinson I W, Weiss J B 1982 Collagenlytic enzyme systems in human intervertebral discs: their control mechanism, and their possible roles in the initiation of biomechanical failure. Spine 7: 213–222

Shirazi-Adl S A, Shrivastava S C, Ahmed A M 1984 Stress analysis of the lumbar disc-body unit in compression: a three-dimensional non-linear finite element study. Spine 9: 120–134

Sztrolovics R, Alini M, Mort J S, Roughley P J 1999 Age-related changes in fibromodulin and lumican in human intervertebral discs. Spine 24: 1765–1771

Takeda T 1975 Three-dimensional observations of collagen framework of human lumbar discs. Journal of the Japanese Orthopedic Association 49: 45–57

Thomas R D M, Batten J J, Want S, McCarthy I D, Brown M, Hughes S P F 1995 A new in-vitro model to investigate antibiotic penetration of the intervertebral disc. Journal of Bone and Joint Surgery 77B: 967–970

Thompson J P, Pearce R H, Schechter M T, Adams M E, Tsang I K Y, Bishop P B 1990 Preliminary evaluation of a scheme for grading the gross morphology of the human intervertebral disc. Spine 15: 411–415

Thompson J P, Oegema T R, Bradford D S 1991 Stimulation of mature canine intervertebral disc by growth factors. Spine 16: 253–260

Thornton W E, Moore T P, Pool S L 1987 Fluid shifts in weightlessness. Aviation, Space and Environmental Medicine 58: A86–A90

Urban J P, Maroudas A 1981 Swelling of the intervertebral disc in vitro. Connective Tissue Research 9: 1–10

Urban J P G, Roberts S 1995 Development and degeneration of the intervertebral discs. Molecular Medicine Today 1: 329–335

Urban J P G, Holm S, Maroudas A 1979 Diffusion of small solutes into the intervertebral disc: an in vivo study. Biorheology 15: 203–223

Urban M R, Fairbank J C, Etherington P J, Loh F L, Winlove C P, Urban J P 2001a Electrochemical measurement of transport into scoliotic intervertebral discs in vivo using nitrous oxide as a tracer. Spine 26: 984–990

Urban M R, Fairbank J C, Bibby S R, Urban J P 2001b Intervertebral disc composition in neuromuscular scoliosis: changes in cell density and glycosaminoglycan concentration at the curve apex. Spine 26: 610–617

Videman T, Leppavuori J, Kaprio J 1998 Iatragenic polymorphisms of the vitamin D receptor gene associated with intervertebral disc degeneration. Proceedings of the International Society for the Study of the Lumbar Spine, Brussels, 59 [abstract]

Wilke H J, Neef P, Caimi M, Hoogland T, Claes L E 1999 New in vivo measurements of pressures in the intervertebral disc in daily life. Spine 24: 755–762

Woods A, Couchman J R 2001 Syndecan-4 and focal adhesion function. Current Opinion in Cell Biology 13: 578–583

Chapter **6**

Clinical biomechanics of the thoracic spine including the ribcage

S. J. Edmondston

INTRODUCTION

An understanding of the biomechanics of the thoracic spine and ribcage is important in the practice of manual therapy as it provides a basis for the interpretation of patterns of clinical presentation in patients with 'mechanical' pain disorders of the thoracic region. Surprisingly, the thoracic spine has been a relatively limited focus of biomechanical research which may explain why this region of the spine has been considered an enigma relative to the cervical and lumbar regions (Singer & Edmondston 2000). The perception that thoracic musculoskeletal pain disorders are less common is supported by the limited epidemiological data which suggests that these account for less than 15% of spinal pain presentations in the general population and in manual therapy practice (Hinkley & Drysdale 1995, Linton et al 1998). Despite this, the severity of symptoms and associated level of disability can be equal to those of patients with lumbar spine disorders (Occhipiniti et al 1993), which may explain the resurgent interest in this region of the spine from a clinical and biomechanical perspective.

The presence of the ribcage and the complex mechanical interaction between the spine and ribcage present significant methodological problems for biomechanical studies of the thoracic spine. Finite element models and animal laboratory studies provide much of the data on movement patterns and stability of the thoracic spine/ribcage complex. Many of the ex vivo studies of human thoracic mechanics have been conducted on specimens without an intact ribcage which may limit the applicability of the findings to clinical practice as thoracic spine mobility and loadbearing are significantly influenced by the ribcage (Andriacchi et al 1974, Berg 1993). Clinical studies of thoracic posture mechanics have used radiological imaging techniques (Goh et al 2000) but these techniques have limited value in kinematic studies. However, a clearer understanding of thoracic spine mechanics has been achieved though the combined results of motion analysis studies of asymptomatic subjects in conjunction with clinical observation (Gregerson & Lucas 1967, Lee 1994, Willems et al 1996).

Although the thoracic spine is anatomically well defined, the functional boundaries of this region of the spine are less distinct. In this review, emphasis is given to regional differences in the mechanics of the thoracic spine, which are reflected in the skeletal and articular anatomy. The upper thoracic spine may be considered as being functionally part of the cervical spine, while the low thoracic motion segment anatomy results in movement patterns more closely resembling those of the lumbar spine. The 'functional' thoracic spine therefore seems to consist of the motion segments between T3 and T9 (Lee 1993). This arbitrary division of the thoracic spine into functional regions seems consistent with the patterns of clinical presentation of mechanical pain disorders which have been described in this region (Lee 1994, Singer & Edmondston 2000).

The biomechanics of the thoracic spine will be considered in this review in relation to the two common patterns of clinical presentation. The first is the disorders where pain is predominantly associated with spinal loading and load attenuation. The biomechanics of thoracic loadbearing are reviewed with reference to loadsharing in the motion segment, influences on spinal curvature and the muscular and postural responses to loadbearing. The second issue relates to situations where symptoms relate more to movement activities or restriction of movement. The interaction between mechanical stability and mobility requirements is reviewed, with reference to the variability in the range and patterns of movement in the different regions of the thoracic spine. The primary objective is to summarize the current knowledge of thoracic spine and ribcage biomechanics which have particular relevance to the practice of manual therapy.

LOADBEARING BIOMECHANICS OF THE THORACIC SPINE

The compressive load on the thoracic spine increases caudally from about 9% of body weight at T1 to 47% of body weight at T12 (White 1969). The ability to sustain the increasing loading demands is achieved through a progressive increase in vertebral body size, end-plate cross-sectional area and bone content, particularly in the lower six vertebral segments (Edmondston et al 1994a, Singer et al 1995). Cancellous bone density and architecture is relatively constant between T2 and T12 which suggests that the skeletal adaptation to increasing load is that of an increase in bone mass rather than of cancellous bone density (Edmondston et al 1994b). The loadbearing capacity of the thoracic spine may be up to three times greater when the ribcage is intact (Andriacchi et al 1974). According to Pal & Routal (1986), 76% of compressive load in the upper thoracic spine is transferred through the vertebral body/intervertebral disc complex. This loadsharing ratio is likely to be similar in the mid-thoracic region, due to the anterior location of the line of gravity relative to the spine. The preferential loading of the anterior spinal structures in the

mid-thoracic region is reflected in the higher incidence of disc degeneration and vertebral body deformity in these segments (Singer 1997, Goh et al 1999). In the low thoracic spine, a greater proportion of the compressive load may be transferred through the posterior column formed by the interlocking laminae and articular facets, as well as the lower costovertebral joints (Pal & Routal 1987). The medial taper of the articular facets and 'wrap-around' configuration of the mortice joints at the thoracolumbar junction would act to provide a stable platform for compressive loadbearing in this region of the spine, while restricting torsional mobility (Singer & Malmivaara 2000).

The intervertebral disc has an important role in attenuating the static and impact compressive loads applied to the thoracic spine during functional and recreational activities. Although the response of the lumbar disc to compressive loading has been investigated in radiological and laboratory studies, there are few comparative studies of the mechanical properties of thoracic discs in compression (Martinez et al 1997, Wisleder et al 2001). Regional variations in the mechanical properties of thoracic intervertebral discs in response to compressive loading have been reported in ex vivo studies. When normalized for differences in height, the upper and mid-thoracic discs undergo greater deformation and creep in response to a specific load than do the discs in the low thoracic and upper lumbar regions (Koeller et al 1984). Differences in water content do not appear to account for the more viscous mechanical behaviour of the upper and mid-thoracic discs in response to compressive load (Koeller et al 1984). Instead this may be due to differences in disc morphology and biochemistry, and the structural arrangement of the annular lamellae (Pooni et al 1986, Scott et al 1994, Putz & Müller-Gerbl 2000). In the lumbar spine, compressive load is evenly distributed across the surface of the vertebral end-plate, independent of the position of the motion segment. In the thoracic spine, the uniform load distribution across the end-plate becomes asymmetric when loaded outside the neutral position (Horst & Brinckmann 1981).

Since the thoracic discs are a potential source of pain, these observations in relation to the biomechanical response to compressive loading may explain the common clinical presentation of mid-thoracic pain associated with sustained loading activities such as word processing and driving. Indeed, a higher prevalence of thoracic pain has been reported in an occupational survey comparing spinal pain symptoms in bus drivers (28%) compared to employees in the same company with non-driving occupations (10%) (Anderson 1992).

BIOMECHANICS OF THE THORACIC KYPHOSIS

The thoracic kyphosis is the primary curve of the spinal axis, persisting from embryological development. In standing postures the form of the thoracic spine is maintained by the tensile forces in the posterior ligaments and spinal extensor muscles, and the balanced compressive loads transferred through the vertebral bodies and discs (White et al 1977). The thoracic curvature in standing is largely influenced by the location of the line of gravity and the shape of the vertebral bodies and intervertebral discs (Pearsall & Reid 1992, Manns et al 1996, Goh et al 1999). In a comparison of clinical and post mortem radiographs, Singer et al (1994) found little difference in the resting form of the kyphosis confirming the importance of ligamentous tension and skeletal and disc morphology in determining thoracic curvature.

The resting length of antagonistic muscle groups and the level of recruitment of trunk musculature have been hypothesized to influence the sagittal plane curvatures of the spine (White & Sahrmann 1994). However, Toppenberg & Bullock (1986) were unable to demonstrate an association between the length of trunk and lower limb muscles and the thoracic kyphosis. In relaxed standing, relatively low levels of phasic muscle activity are required to maintain the upright posture and correct for postural sway (Ortengren & Andersson 1977). This low-level muscle activity would seem unlikely to have much influence on thoracic curvature. Similarly, trunk muscle strength is unlikely to influence neutral spinal curvature, a hypothesis confirmed by Walker et al (1987). Incremental spinal loading studies have examined the influence of trunk muscle recruitment on thoracic curvature. Klausen (1965) observed no change in thoracic curvature when external loads of up to 40 kg were applied using a backpack. Similarly, Edmondston et al (2000) reported no change in the thoracic kyphosis, despite a linear increase in EMG activity of the erector spinae muscles, when the subjects held loads of up to 20% of body weight. A non-linear increase in abdominal muscle recruitment was also noted during this loading study. Hence the optimal response to loading in the thoracic spine appears to be one in which the neutral curvature is maintained through an increase in the balanced trunk muscle activation associated with unloaded standing.

MECHANICAL STABILITY OF THE THORACIC SPINE

Normal mechanical function of the thoracic spine is dependent on an appropriate interaction between mobility and stability in the motion segments. The ribcage and sternum provide additional stability for the thoracic spine during loadbearing and movement, and thoracic stiffness is significantly reduced when the integrity of the ribcage is compromised (Berg 1993, Shea et al 1996). Stability during dynamic loading tasks is further enhanced by an increase in intrathoracic pressure, which is achieved through coordinated contraction of the diaphragm, together with the deep abdominal and intercostal muscles (Morris et al 1961, Hodges & Gandevia 2000).

In response to an applied force, the motion segment displays non-linear behaviour, with minimal resistance to movement initially (neutral zone), followed by an elastic zone in which movement (displacement) is proportional to load (Panjabi et al 1989). Control of segmental movement in the neutral zone is dependent on muscle contraction while in the elastic range motion control is provided by ligamentous tension and the intervertebral disc (Panjabi 1992). In the lumbar spine, the range of the neutral zone is greatest in the sagittal plane while in the thoracic spine the sagittal plane neutral zone is smaller than in the coronal and horizontal planes (Oda et al 1996) (Table 6.1).

It is evident from experimental studies that considerable anatomical disruption is required to produce mechanical instability in the thoracic spine. Transection of all posterior ligaments and destabilization of the costovertebral joint is required to cause flexion instability of the motion segment (Shea et al 1996). Similarly, extension stability in the motion segment is compromised following complete transection of the intervertebral disc and rib head resection (Panjabi et al 1981, Feiertag et al 1995). Stability of the thoracic spine in the coronal plane is dependent more on the costotransverse ligament complex than the midline ligaments. The strain in the lateral ligaments of the thoracic spine may be up to 5.6% with only 1 degree of lateral flexion while the strain in the midline ligaments, for the equivalent movement, has been shown to be only 1% (Panjabi & Goel 1982, Jiang et al 1994). The influence of the posterior ligaments and rib joints on the mobility and neutral zone of the thoracic motion segments was examined by Oda and co-workers (1996) using a canine model. Following removal of these structures, the neutral zone increased by less than 2 degrees and 4 degrees in the sagittal and axial planes respectively. The greatest increase in neutral zone was in the frontal plane where the change was 7.3 degrees.

The changes in the neutral zone of the motion segment may result from injury or degeneration of the motion segment, particularly of the intervertebral disc. In the lumbar spine, changes in neutral zone, which may relate to clinical instability, are greater in the sagittal plane (Wilke et al 1995). Similarly, radiological and clinical patterns of lumbar segmental instability are observed more commonly with sagittal plane movements (Boden & Wiesel 1990, O'Sullivan 2000). In contrast, the sagittal plane neutral zone in the thoracic spine is very small due to the narrow disc height and coronal orientation of the zygapophysial joints, which

Table 6.1 Comparison of neutral zone ranges for thoracic and lumbar spine motion segments

	Sagittal plane	Coronal plane	Axial plane
Thoracic*	0.6	3.5	2.1
Lumbar†	1.7	2.9	0.2

All numbers are in degrees.
Data from *Oda et al 1996, †Wilke et al 1995.

strongly constrain sagittal movement. The higher range of unconstrained movement (neutral zone) in axial rotation and lateral flexion is consistent with the description of rotational instability as a pattern of patient presentation in the mid-thoracic spine (Lee 1994). While motion palpation tests for examining the stability of the thoracic motion segments have been proposed (Lowcock 1991), it is not possible to examine the range or patterns of segmental motion in the thoracic spine using radiological imaging techniques.

REGIONAL MOBILITY OF THE THORACIC SPINE

Normal movement of the thoracic spine is required to facilitate functional tasks and recreational activities. An understanding of the kinematics of the thoracic spine, including regional variations and the anatomical influences on movement, is required in the interpretation of any movement examination of patients with thoracic pain disorders. Unfortunately, the unique anatomy of the thoracic spine, particularly the presence of the ribcage, presents significant difficulties for in vivo investigations of thoracic movement. Much of the reported data come from cadaveric studies which are limited by the requirement to dissect the ribcage and related muscles prior to analysis. Stereo-radiography techniques cannot be used in the thoracic spine due to poor vertebral definition and superimposition of the ribs, although rotational mobility has been measured using CT (Singer et al 1989). Given the ethical constraints associated with invasive measurement techniques, surface measurements using electromagnetic motion analysis systems are increasingly being employed (Willems et al 1996). However, the extent to which surface measurements reflect the movement patterns of the underlying joints remains questionable (Stokes 2000). Despite these difficulties, data derived from studies using each of these analysis techniques provide a more complete understanding of the kinematics of the thoracic spine and support the development of biomechanical models.

Upper thoracic region

Descriptions of the ranges of movement in the thoracic spine highlight the regional differences in motion segment anatomy. Upper thoracic mobility contributes to normal cervical spine function and to functional movements of the thorax. Sagittal movements are accompanied by little movement in the other planes, possibly due to the symmetrical anterior rotation of the upper ribs which may act to constrain coupled movements (Willems et al 1996). A range of upper thoracic sagittal movement of about 5 degrees per segment has been reported in both in vivo and cadaveric studies (White 1969, Willems et al 1996). The proportion of this range which is extension is reported as being between 30 and 50% which may reflect differences in the reference point for measurement in these studies. Symmetrical posterior rotation of the ribs, such that the posterior part of the

rib moves inferiorly, occurs during extension of the upper thoracic spine (Lee 1993).

The kinematics of upper thoracic rotation and lateral flexion are more complex due to the asymmetrical movement patterns in the spinal motion segments and ribs. The constraining influence of the ribs on these movements is confirmed by the overall lower ranges of segmental motion reported in ex vivo studies compared to measurements from human subjects. Lateral flexion occurs around an axis located within the disc space between the mid-disc and ipsilateral margin of the vertebra (White 1969). The bilateral range of upper thoracic lateral flexion reported in ex vivo studies is 6–8 degrees per segment compared to about 4 degrees per segment from clinical studies (White 1969, Willems et al 1996). Axial rotation in the upper thoracic spine occurs around an axis located forward of the anterior margin of the vertebral body (Davis 1959). The in vivo range of upper thoracic rotation is about 8 degrees per segment compared to about 12 degrees per segment from the ex vivo studies (White 1969, Willems et al 1996). Movement coupling between rotation and lateral flexion in this region of the spine may be inconsistent within and between individuals due to the influence of the muscles which span the cervicothoracic junction, and the associated effect on spinal and rib movement (Willems et al 1996). Descriptions of rib movement associated with coronal and axial plane spinal movement are based on clinical observation (Lee 1994). Lateral flexion of the upper thoracic spine is associated with ipsilateral anterior rotation and contralateral posterior rotation of the upper ribs. Rib movement is more pronounced during cervicothoracic rotation where posterior rotation of the right ribs and anterior rotation of the left ribs accompanies right rotation and vice versa.

Mid-thoracic region

The mid-thoracic spine (T3–9) is most mobile in axial rotation with the range of movement achievable in sitting being the same as that in standing (Gregersen & Lucas 1967). The axis of rotation for this movement lies within the vertebral body, which, together with the coronal plane orientation of the zygapophysial joints, promotes lateral translation of the articular facets. This is accompanied by ipsilateral translation and tilt of the vertebral body. However, these coupled movements would be limited due to the thin intervertebral discs and tension in the costal ligaments (Davis 1959). Tension developed in the costal ligaments causes posterior rotation of the ipsilateral rib and anterior rotation of the contralateral rib during axial rotation in the mid-thoracic spine (Lee 1993) (Fig. 6.1). The range of axial rotation in the mid-thoracic spine has been reported as being about 10 degrees per segment, based on cadaveric and in vivo surface measurements (White 1969, Willems et al 1996). In contrast, Gregersen & Lucas (1967) were able to obtain more direct measurement from human subjects by recording movements from Steinmann pins inserted into the spinous

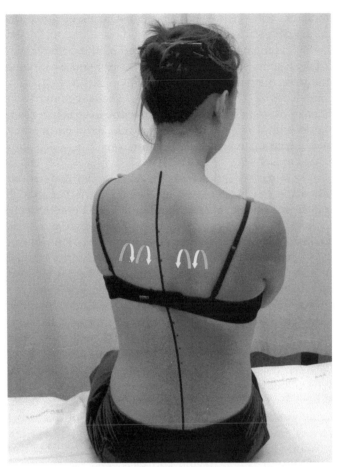

Figure 6.1 Response of the mid-thoracic spine to rotation. Right rotation of the trunk is associated with ipsilateral lateral flexion of the thoracic spine. Right rotation of the thorax is associated with posterior rotation of the ipsilateral ribs and anterior rotation of the contralateral ribs (white arrows).

processes. These investigators reported a segmental range of axial rotation of about 5 degrees per segment. During normal gait, axial rotation is greatest in the mid-thoracic segments (up to 2.5 degrees per segment) (Gregersen & Lucas 1967). The greater rotational mobility of the mid-thoracic spine, and the associated torsion and shear forces transferred to the intervertebral discs, may contribute to the higher prevalence of disc degeneration in these segments (Singer 1997).

Approximation of the ribcage during lateral flexion of the mid-thoracic spine limits mobility in the coronal plane. A segmental range of lateral flexion of 4 degrees per segment has been reported in clinical studies compared to 6 degrees per segment in the cadaveric experiments where the ribcage was removed (White 1969, Willems et al 1996). Lateral flexion of the mid-thoracic spine produces concurrent anterior rotation of the ipsilateral ribs and posterior rotation of the contralateral ribs. This asymmetrical rib movement may contribute the contralateral rotation of the thorax which is observed clinically during trunk lateral flexion (Lee 1993).

Sagittal plane movement is relatively limited in the mid-thoracic spine. The axis of rotation for sagittal rotation is located in the disc space of the caudad motion segment. However, the exact location is different for flexion and extension (Panjabi et al 1984). Anterior sagittal rotation (flexion) and the associated anterior translation are constrained by the vertical articular facets of the zygapophysial joints (Panjabi et al 1984). Flexion is limited by tension in the posterior spinal ligaments and approximation of the ribs, which rotate anteriorly during this movement (Lee 1993). Mid-thoracic extension is associated with posterior translation of the superior vertebra, which is less constrained by the articular facets of the zygapophysial joints. In contrast, vertebral motion in extension is guided by the contact of the inferior articular facet or the spinous process on the vertebra below resulting in a constrained axis of rotation (Panjabi et al 1984). The posterior vertebral translation during extension induces posterior rotation of the ribs (Lee 1993). The range of sagittal movement has been determined as being about 5 degrees per segment in cadaveric and in vivo studies (White 1969, Willems et al 1996). The consistency between cadaveric and clinical studies is possibly due to the greater influence of the zygapophysial joints, rather than the ribcage, in determining the range of sagittal movement.

Low thoracic region

Movement in the low thoracic spine is influenced by the variability in posterior element morphology and the anatomy of the lower two ribs, which articulate with one vertebral body and have no anterior attachment. Zygapophysial joint asymmetry (tropism) and different patterns of transition from coronal to sagittal orientation result in considerable variability between individuals in the ranges of motion and patterns of coupled motion in this region (Gregersen & Lucas 1967, Singer et al 1989). The greater disc height and more sagittal orientation of the zygapophysial joints in the low thoracic region facilitate mobility in the sagittal plane (White 1969, Pooni et al 1986). Evidence for these anatomical influences on movement in the low thoracic spine comes from the cadaveric study of White (1969) who reported 8 degrees of sagittal movement at T9/10 compared with 20 degrees at T11/12. This compares with 5 degrees per segment between T8 and T12 determined using a surface measurement technique in an in vivo study (Willems et al 1996). Mobility in the coronal plane in the low thoracic region is similar to that in the upper and mid-thoracic segments. A range of 6 degrees per segment between T8 and T12 was reported in the clinical study of Willems and co-workers (1996). In contrast, cadaveric measurements of low thoracic lateral flexion show an increase in range from 6 degrees at T9/10 to 12 degrees at T11/12 (White 1969). These results highlight the influence of zygapophysial joint orientation on mobility in the thoracolumbar junction region (T11–L1) compared to the adjacent cephalad segments (Malmivaara et al 1987, Singer et al 1989).

The low thoracic spine (T8–12) has a more limited range of axial rotation compared to the upper and mid-thoracic regions. In vivo studies have reported ranges of motion of between 5 and 7 degrees per segment (Gregersen & Lucas 1967, Willems et al 1996). As with movement in the other planes, variability in the segmental range of axial rotation within this region is due to the changing orientation of the zygapophysial joints. Based on measurements from CT scans, unilateral segmental rotation was found to decrease from 2.8 degrees per segment at T10/11 to 1.8 degrees per segment at T12/L1 (Singer et al 1989). These investigators found no significant difference in segmental rotation between subjects with an abrupt change in zygapophysial joint orientation compared to those in which it was more gradual. However, a 'mortice'-type configuration of the zygapophysial joints observed in some individuals in this region may further constrain axial rotation due to the medial taper of the joint surfaces and the extended mamillary process of the superior articular facet (Singer et al 1989).

Movement coupling in rotation/lateral flexion

Movement of the thoracic spine rarely occurs in a single plane. Due to various structural and anatomical influences, spinal movement in one plane is inevitably accompanied by one or more coupled movements (Harrison et al 1998). Movement coupling principles provide the foundation for the interpretation of patterns of movement impairment and technique selection in some methods of manual therapy practice (Evjenth & Hamberg 1984, Gibbons & Tehan 1998). In particular, patterns of movement coupling in the frontal

and horizontal planes have been the focus of numerous cadaveric and in vivo studies for almost 100 years (Lovett 1905). It is apparent that the primary direction of movement influences the range and direction of coupled movements and that regional differences in coupled motion exist in the thoracic spine (Willems et al 1996). These regional variations in movement coupling may be due to vertebral orientation within the kyphosis, zygapophysial joint anatomy and the costal articulations (Veldhuizen & Scholten 1987, Singer et al 1989).

A summary of studies examining coupled rotation and lateral flexion is presented in Table 6.2. The variation in movement coupling between rotation and lateral flexion is likely to be due to differences in study design and measurement techniques (Gregersen & Lucas 1967, Panjabi et al 1976, Willems et al 1996). Furthermore, analysis of coupled movement is difficult owing to the small ranges of movement which are subject to significant measurement error (Panjabi et al 1976). In these studies, measurements have been derived from the spine rather than from analysis of movement of the thorax (spine and ribcage) as a whole complex. This seems important considering the interaction between spinal and rib movement as previously described. From clinical observation it does appear that rotation is associated with coupled ipsilateral lateral flexion of the spine (see Fig. 6.1). However, consideration of the associated rib movement leads to the (untested) hypothesis that rotation of the thorax (spine and ribcage) is associated with contralateral lateral flexion and vice versa. Movement of the thorax into right rotation is associated with posterior rotation of the ipsilateral ribs (Lee 1993). In contrast, right lateral flexion is associated with anterior rotation of the ipsilateral ribs. Therefore, it seems likely that right rotation of the thorax would be accompanied by coupled left lateral

Table 6.2 Summary of studies which have examined patterns of coupled movement in the thoracic spine

Author	Method	Region	Primary movement	Coupled movement
Gregersen & Lucas 1967	Normal volunteers	Upper and middle	LF	Ipsilateral rot.
		Lower	LF	Variable pattern
White 1969	Cadaver	Upper	LF	Ipsilateral rot.
		Middle and lower	LF	Ipsilateral rot. (variable)
Panjabi et al 1976	Cadaver	Middle	Rot.	Contralateral LF
		Middle	LF	Contralateral rot.
Lee 1993	Biomechanical model	Middle	Rot.	Ipsilateral LF
			LF	Contralateral rot.
Willems et al 1996	Surface measurement (3-Space Fastrak system)	Upper	LF	Contralateral rot. (53%)
			Rot.	Contralateral LF (82%)
		Middle	LF	Ipsilateral rot. (83%)
			Rot.	Ipsilateral LF (99%)
		Lower	LF	Ipsilateral rot. (68%)
			Rot.	Ipsilateral LF (93%)

LF = lateral flexion; rot. = rotation.

flexion as in both cases the right-sided ribs would rotate posteriorly. This functional approach to the interpretation of movement coupling in the thoracic spine/ribcage complex appears to have greater relevance to the practice of manual therapy than consideration of coupled motion of the spine in isolation.

Movement of the thoracic spine and ribcage during respiration

Movement of the ribcage during inspiration is initiated by the diaphragm, which elevates the lower ribs as the contraction causes depression of the central tendon (DeTroyer & Estenne 1988). Rib movement occurs around a mediolateral axis, which extends from the costovertebral joint towards the rib tubercle (Rickenbacher et al 1985, Saumarez 1986). In the upper ribs this axis is located at about 35 degrees to the coronal plane whereas in the lower ribs the axis is oriented closer to the sagittal plane. Consequently, movement of the upper ribs elevates the sternum and increases the anteroposterior diameter of the ribcage ('pump-handle') while movement of the lower ribs has a greater influence on the lateral dimensions of the ribcage ('bucket-handle') (Harris & Holmes 1996). Although both actions of the ribs occur simultaneously, the proportion of 'pump-handle' movement is greater in the upper ribs while the 'bucket-handle' action is more dominant in the lower ribs (Mitchell & Mitchell 1995). The lower two ribs have no anterior attachment and have a 'caliper'-type action (Mitchell & Mitchell 1995).

During quiet respiration there is relatively little movement of the upper ribs. However, on exertion, upper ribcage movement increases due to the action of the accessory respiratory muscles (scalenii, sternomastoid and pectoralis minor) (DeTroyer & Estenne 1988). The role of the intercostal muscles in respiration remains contentious but these muscles could have an inspiratory or expiratory function dependent on their level of activity in different costal segments (Loring & Woodbridge 1991). Deep inspiration in sitting is associated with extension of the lumbar and thoracic spine, possibly to accommodate the concurrent posterior (pump-handle) rotation of the ribs (Leong et al 1999).

MUSCLE ACTIONS ON THE THORACIC SPINE AND RIBCAGE

Movement of the thoracic spine and ribcage is dependent on coordinated contraction of the associated musculature. Sagittal movements of the thorax are achieved through the activation of the thoracic fibres of iliocostalis and longissimus, which act around the thoracic kyphosis (Macintosh & Bogduk 1994). Generation of extension moments during functional tasks is associated with synergistic activation of the diaphragm and abdominal muscles, which elevate intra-abdominal pressure (IAP) (Morris et al 1961, Stokes 2000). The increase in IAP in particular contributes to the extensor moment, reducing the tension generated in the extensor muscles and the associated compressive forces transferred to the thoracolumbar spine (Morris et al 1961, Daggfeldt & Thorstensson 1997).

Generation of axial torque provides trunk rotation during locomotion, and for sporting activities such as golf and racquet sports. The oblique abdominal muscles generate the forces required for thoracic spine rotation. Due to the anterior location of these muscles, contraction is associated with combined flexion and rotation of the trunk (Bogduk 1986). The flexion movement is resisted by simultaneous contraction of the ipsilateral thoracic fibres of iliocostalis and longissumus (Rickenbacher et al 1985). More specific control of thoracic rotation may be achieved through unilateral contraction of the contralateral thoracic multifidus and rotatores muscles. The oblique orientation of these fibres promotes movement in the horizontal plane rather than the extension movement generated by the lumbar multifidus (Bojadsen et al 2000). The relative role of the oblique abdominal and thoracic erector spinae in generating axial torque in the thoracic spine remains uncertain. Lateral flexion of the thorax is controlled by the eccentric action of iliocostalis and longissumus, with a lesser contribution from the medial intersegmental muscles. The contralateral medial tract muscles (semispinalis, multifidus and rotatores) control the associated rotation produced by the long fibres of iliocostalis. (Rickenbacher et al 1985).

BIOMECHANICAL CONSIDERATIONS IN MANUAL THERAPY PRACTICE

Knowledge of the regional biomechanics of the thoracic spine and ribcage assists the clinician in the interpretation of active movement and motion palpation examination in relation to the patient's symptoms. Normal mechanics of the cervical spine and shoulder are dependent on normal mobility in the upper thoracic spine. A habitual flexed upper thoracic posture may reduce the capacity of the muscles, which provide cervicothoracic retraction to work in the functional range. Further, the upper ribs will be drawn into anterior rotation due to the flexed position of the upper thoracic spine. Restriction of cervical extension and rotation movements is inevitable due to the restriction of upper rib mobility and the requirement for movement out of the neutral spinal alignment. Consequently, restricted upper thoracic mobility may increase the movement demands on the more mobile lower cervical segments, with the potential for symptom development or exacerbation.

Upper thoracic extension is required to accommodate the later range of bilateral flexion of the shoulders, while ipsilateral flexion of the upper thoracic spine is observed during unilateral shoulder elevation (Culham & Peat 1993, Sobel et al 1996). Consequently, changes in upper thoracic posture and mobility may lead to subacromial pathology due to the effects on scapula and glenohumeral mechanics (Sobel et al 1996). Similarly, restriction of upper rib mobility may produce symptoms and physical signs consistent with those of subacromial impingement or thoracic outlet syndrome (Lindgren & Leino 1988, Boyle 1999). Based on these observations, examination of upper thoracic and rib mobility would be important in patients with shoulder pain related to overhead activities.

Due to their location in the apex of the kyphosis, the anterior elements of the mid-thoracic spine are subjected to high compressive loads (White et al 1977). Progressive wedge deformity of the vertebral bodies and disc space narrowing are common, even in relatively young individuals (Wood et al 1995). These anatomical changes can reduce the mobility of the mid-thoracic motion segments and ribs, particularly in axial rotation and extension. This pattern of movement restriction is commonly seen in patients with chronic postural pain associated with sustained loading activities. In older patients, mid-thoracic mobility may be further reduced due to the preferential development of anterior vertebral osteophytes in this region (Nathan 1962). On physical examination, a region of relatively limited mid-thoracic motion may be observed during trunk rotation, which is more evident when rotation is performed with the arms elevated (Fig. 6.2). This is often associated with compensatory contralateral lateral flexion of the lumbar spine and cramp-like discomfort in the lower thorax due to the increased torsional loading transferred to this region. In extension, a physical barrier to movement may occur due to the reduced disc height, which would promote early approximation of the bony posterior elements. The influence of these anatomical changes on mid-thoracic extension should be considered in clinical tests which involve passive physiological movement and overpressure. This physical barrier to extension should also be considered when prescribing mobility and posture correction exercises for the thoracic spine.

Anatomical variation in the low thoracic spine, particularly the thoracolumbar junction, should be considered in the examination of movement in this region. The transition from a coronal to sagittal zygapophysial joint orientation may be gradual or abrupt resulting in individual differences in patterns of segmental mobility. The application of motion palpation and mobilization techniques should account for the relatively limited potential for extension and rotation, particularly under weight-bearing conditions.

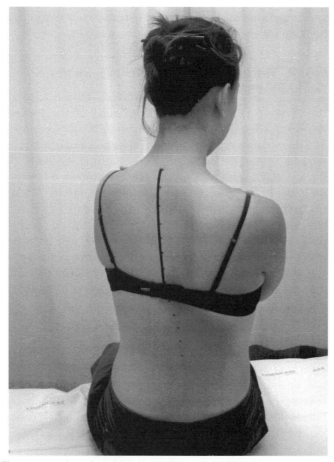
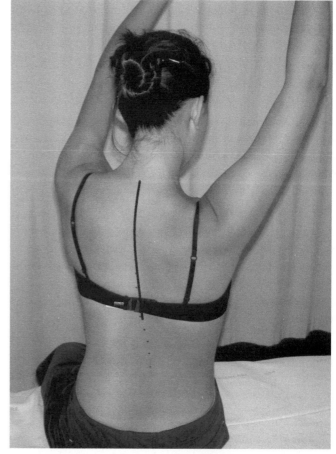

Figure 6.2 A patient with restricted mid-thoracic rotation demonstrates reduced movement of the mid-thoracic region on movement testing (A). This limitation of movement is more evident when tested in relative thoracic extension (arms elevated) (B), and is associated with compensatory contralateral flexion of the lumbar spine.

Manipulative techniques applied to this region which involve end-range extension or rotation have the potential to produce discomfort or even injury to the joint surfaces or related peri-articular tissues (Singer & Giles 1990).

Accessory motion palpation techniques have been advocated for the assessment of range and quality of segmental motion in patients with thoracic spine pain (Magarey 1994). In particular, changes in the through-range resistance to movement (stiffness) in response to posteroanterior (PA) forces applied to the spinous processes may assist in the identification of a symptomatic segment. In asymptomatic subjects, the PA stiffness of the thoracic vertebral segments increases from an average of 9.1 N/mm at T4 to 11.4 N/mm at T10 (Edmondston et al 1999). Departure from this segmental increase in PA stiffness may be indicative of abnormal motion segment function if associated with a relevant symptom response. The thoracic spine is supported by the compressible ribcage such that assessment of PA stiffness may be strongly influenced by ribcage stiffness. However, ribcage stiffness, measured via sternal loading, is significantly lower than the PA stiffness of the thoracic spine and accounts for only 33% of the variation between individuals (Edmondston et al 1999). This suggests that factors other than ribcage stiffness determine the movement response to PA motion palpation tests in the thoracic spine.

Posteroanterior load applied to the thoracic spine therefore results in a global movement of the spine and ribcage and a more specific movement of the loaded segment. One possible influence on the response to PA loading in the thoracic spine is the orientation of the applied force. The application of PA force to the spinous process induces anterior translation and posterior rotation (extension) of the related vertebral segment. When a movement force of 200 N is directed anteriorly or perpendicular to the spinal curvature, a resultant anterior translation of equivalent force is accompanied by an extension moment of up to 5.5 Nm (Lee 1989). In contrast, an equivalent force directed towards the vertebral body eliminates the extension moment but induces a longitudinal force of up to half the applied load (Lee 1989). Therefore, the movement response to PA accessory motion palpation in the thoracic spine may be influenced by the method in which the test is applied. Consistency in the method of application is required to achieve comparable responses on subsequent testing occasions.

CONCLUSION

The thoracic spine and ribcage complex has been a relatively limited focus for biomechanical research. This can be attributed to the complex interaction between the spine and ribcage during movement, and technical difficulties, which limit the potential for direct measurement of vertebral and rib motion. Despite this, a better understanding of the biomechanics of the thoracic spine is beginning to emerge. This review provides a summary of the response to load-bearing and the adaptations to the dual requirement for stability and mobility. Regional variations in thoracic spine kinematics reflect the influence of the anatomical diversity of this region of the spine, and recognition of this is important in the application and interpretation of clinical tests and treatment techniques in manual therapy practice.

KEYWORDS	
thoracic spine	biomechanics
ribcage	coupled motion

References

Anderson R 1992 The back pain of bus drivers. Spine 17: 1481–1488

Andriacchi T, Schultz A, Belytschko T, Galante J 1974 A model for studies of mechanical interactions between the human spine and rib cage. Journal of Biomechanics 7: 497–507

Berg E E 1993 The sternal-rib complex: a possible fourth column in thoracic spinal fractures. Spine 18: 1916–1919

Boden S D, Wiesel S W 1990 Lumbosacral segmental motion in normal individuals. Have we been measuring instability properly? Spine 15: 751–757

Bogduk N 1986 The anatomy and function of the lumbar back muscles. In: Grieve G P (ed) Modern Manual Therapy. Churchill Livingstone, Edinburgh, Ch 13, pp 138–145

Bojadsen T W, Silva E S, Rodrigues A J, Amadio A C 2000 Comparative study of Mm. multifidi in lumbar and thoracic spine. Journal of Electromyography and Kinesiology 10: 143–149

Boyle J J W 1999 Is the pain and dysfunction of shoulder impingement lesion really second rib syndrome in disguise? Two case reports. Manual Therapy 4: 44–48

Culham E, Peat M 1993 Functional anatomy of the shoulder complex. Journal of Orthopaedic and Sports Physical Therapy 18: 342–350

Daggfeldt K, Thorstensson A 1997 The role of intra-abdominal pressure in spinal loading. Journal of Biomechanics 30: 1149–1155

Davis P R 1959 The medial inclination of the human thoracic intervertebral articular facets. Journal of Anatomy 93: 68–74

DeTroyer A, Estenne M 1988 Functional anatomy of the respiratory muscles. In: Belman M J (ed) Respiratory muscles: function in health and disease. Saunders, Philadelphia

Edmondston S J, Singer K P, Day R E, Breidahl P D, Price R I 1994a In-vitro relationships between vertebral body density, size and compressive strength in the elderly thoracolumbar spine. Clinical Biomechanics 9: 180–186

Edmondston S J, Breidahl W H, Singer K P, Day R E, Price R I 1994b Segmental trends in cancellous bone structure in the thoracolumbar spine: histological and radiological comparisons. Australasian Radiology 38: 272–277

Edmondston S J, Allison G T, Althorpe B M, McConnell D R, Samuel K K 1999 Comparison of ribcage and posteroanterior thoracic spine stiffness: an investigation of the normal response. Manual Therapy 4: 157–162

Edmondston S J, Allison G T, Dahl B-R, Look D, Poirier D, Wapnah M 2000 Trunk muscle and postural responses to incremented spinal loading. International Federation of Orthopaedic Manipulative Therapists 7th Scientific Conference, Perth, Australia

Evjenth O, Hamberg J 1984 Muscle stretching in manual therapy: a clinical manual. Alfta Rehab, Sweden

Feiertag M A, Horton W C, Norman J T, Proctor F C, Hutton W C 1995 The effect of different surgical releases on thoracic spinal motion. Spine 20: 1604–1611

Gibbons P, Tehan P 1998 Muscle energy concepts and coupled motion of the spine. Manual Therapy 3: 95–101

Goh S, Price R I, Leedman P J, Singer K P 1999 The relative influence of vertebral body and intervertebral disk shape on the thoracic kyphosis. Clinical Biomechanics 14: 439–448

Goh S, Price R I, Leedman P J, Singer K P 2000 A comparison of three methods for measuring thoracic kyphosis: implications for clinical studies. Rheumatology 39: 310–315

Gregersen G G, Lucas D B 1967 An in vivo study of the axial rotation of the human thoracolumbar spine. Journal of Bone and Joint Surgery 49A: 247–262

Harris J D, Holmes T G 1996 Ribcage and thoracic spine. Physical Medicine and Rehabilitation Clinics of North America 7: 761–771

Harrison D E, Harrison D D, Troyanovich S J 1998 Three-dimensional spinal coupling mechanics. I: A review of the literature. Journal of Manipulative and Physiological Therapeutics 21: 101–113

Hinkley H J, Drysdale I P 1995 Audit of 1000 patients attending the clinic of the British College of Naturopathy and Osteopathy. British Osteopathic Journal 16: 17–22

Hodges P W, Gandevia S C 2000 Changes in intra-abdominal pressure during postural and respiratory activation of the human diaphragm. Journal of Applied Physiology 89: 967–976

Horst M, Brinckmann P 1981 Measurement of the distribution of axial stress on the end-plate of the vertebral body. Spine 6: 217–232

Jiang H, Raso J V, Moreau M J, Russell G, Hill D L, Bagnall K M 1994 Quantitative morphology of the lateral ligaments of the spine: assessment of their importance in maintaining lateral stability. Spine 19: 2676–2982

Klausen K 1965 The form and function of the loaded human spine. Acta Physiologica Scandinavica 65: 176–190

Koeller W, Meier W, Hartmann M 1984 Biomechanical properties of the human intervertebral discs subjected to axial compression: a comparison of lumbar and thoracic discs. Spine 9: 725–733

Lee M 1989 Mechanics of spinal joint manipulation in the thoracic and lumbar spine: a theoretical study of posteroanterior force techniques. Clinical Biomechanics 4: 249–251

Lee D 1993 Biomechanics of the thorax: a clinical model of in vivo function. Journal of Manual and Manipulative Therapy 1: 13–21

Lee D 1994 Manual therapy for the thorax: DOPC, British Columbia

Leong J C Y, Lu W W, Luk K K D, Karlberg E M 1999 Kinematics of the chest cage and spine during breathing in healthy individuals and in patients with adolescent idiopathic scoliosis. Spine 24: 1310–1315

Lindgren K A, Leino E 1988 Subluxation of the first rib: a possible thoracic outlet syndrome mechanism. Archives of Physical Medicine and Rehabilitation 69: 692–695

Linton S J, Hellsing A-L, Hallden K 1998 A population-based study of spinal pain among 35–45-year-old individuals. Spine 23: 1457–1463

Loring S H, Woodbridge J A 1991 Intercostal muscle action inferred from finite-element analysis. Journal of Applied Physiology 70: 2712–2718

Lovett R W 1905 The mechanism of the normal spine and its relation to scoliosis. Boston Medical and Surgical Journal 13: 349–358

Lowcock J 1991 Thoracic joint stability and clinical stress tests. Orthopaedic Division of the Canadian Physiotherapy Association Newsletter (Nov/Dec)

Macintosh J E, Bogduk N 1994 The anatomy and function of the lumbar back muscles. In: Boyling J D, Palastanga N (eds) Grieve's Modern Manual Therapy. Churchill Livingstone, Edinburgh, pp 189–209

Magarey M E 1994 Examination of the cervical and thoracic spine. In: Grant R (ed) Physical therapy for the cervical and thoracic spine, 2nd edn. Churchill Livingstone, Edinburgh

Malmivaara A, Videman T, Kuosma E, Troup J D G 1987 Facet joint orientation, facet and costovertebral joint osteoarthritis, disc degeneration, vertebral body osteophytosis, and Schmorl's nodes in the thoracolumbar junctional region of cadaveric spines. Spine 12: 458–463

Manns R A, Haddaway M J, McCall I W, Pullicino V C, Davie M W J 1996 The relative contribution of disc and vertebral morphometry to the angle of kyphosis in asymptomatic subjects. Clinical Radiology 51: 258–262

Martinez J B, Oloyede V O, Broom N D 1997 Biomechanics of load-bearing of the intervertebral disc: an experimental and finite element model. Medical Engineering and Physics 19: 145–156

Mitchell F L, Mitchell P K G 1995 The muscle energy manual. MET Press, East Lansing, Michigan

Morris J M, Lucas B D, Bresler B 1961 Role of the trunk in stability of the spine. Journal of Bone and Joint Surgery 43A: 327–351

Nathan H 1962 Osteophytes of the vertebral column. Journal of Bone and Joint Surgery 44A: 243–268

Occhipiniti E, Colombini D, Grieco A 1993 Study of distribution and characteristics of spinal disorders using a validated questionnaire in a group of male subjects not exposed to occupational spinal risk factors. Spine 18: 1150–1159

Oda I, Abumi K, Duosai L, Shono Y, Kaneda K 1996 Biomechanical role of the posterior elements, costovertebral joints, and rib cage in the stability of the thoracic spine. Spine 21: 1423–1429

Ortengren R, Andersson G B J 1977 Electromyographic studies of trunk muscles with special reference to the functional anatomy of the lumbar spine. Spine 2: 44–52

O'Sullivan P B 2000 Lumbar segmental 'instability': clinical presentation and specific stabilizing exercise management. Manual Therapy 5: 2–12

Pal G P, Routal R V 1986 A study of weight transmission through the cervical and upper thoracic regions of the vertebral column in man. Journal of Anatomy 148: 245–261

Pal G P, Routal R V 1987 Transmission of weight through the lower thoracic and lumbar regions of the vertebral column in man. Journal of Anatomy 152: 93–105

Panjabi M M 1992 The stabilising system of the spine. II: Neutral zone and instability hypothesis. Journal of Spinal Disorders 5: 390–397

Panjabi M M, Goel V K 1982 Physiologic strains in the lumbar spinal ligaments. Spine 7: 192–203

Panjabi M M, Brand R A, White A A 1976 Mechanical properties of the human thoracic spine. Journal of Bone and Joint Surgery 58A: 642–652

Panjabi M M, Hausfeld J N, White A A 1981 A biomechanical study of the ligamentous stability of the thoracic spine in man. Acta Orthopaedica Scandinavica 52: 315–326

Panjabi M M, Krag M H, Dimnet J C, Walter S D, Brand R A 1984 Thoracic spine centres of rotation in the sagittal plane. Journal of Orthopaedic Research 1: 387–394

Panjabi M M, Abumi K, Daranceau J 1989 Spinal stability and intersegmental muscle forces. Spine 14: 194–200

Pearsall D J, Reid J G 1992 Line of gravity relative to the upright vertebral posture. Clinical Biomechanics 7: 80–86

Pooni J S, Hukins D W, Harris P F, Hilton R C, Davies K E 1986 Comparison of the structure of human intervertebral discs in the cervical, thoracic and lumbar regions of the spine. Surgical and Radiological Anatomy 8: 175–182

Putz V R, Muller-Gerbl M 2000 Ligaments of the human vertebral column. In: Giles L G F, Singer K P (eds) Clinical anatomy and management of thoracic spine pain. Butterworth Heinemann, Oxford

Rickenbacher J, Landolt A M, Theiler K 1985 Applied anatomy of the back. Springer-Verlag, Berlin

Saumarez R C 1986 An analysis of possible movements of the upper rib cage. Journal of Applied Physiology 60: 678–689

Scott J E, Bosworth T R, Cribb A M, Taylor J R 1994 The chemical morphology of age-related changes in human intervertebral disc glycosaminoglycans from cervical, thoracic and lumbar nucleus pulposus and annulus fibrosis. Journal of Anatomy 184: 73–82

Shea K G, Schlegel J D, Bachus K N, Dunn H K, West J R 1996 The contribution of the rib cage to thoracic spine stability. In: Proceedings of the International Society for the Study of the Lumbar Spine, Vermont

Singer K P 1997 Pathomechanics of the aging thoracic spine. In: Lawrence D (ed) Advances in chiropractic. Mosby Yearbook, Chicago

Singer K P, Edmondston S J 2000 The enigma of the thoracic spine. In: Giles L G F, Singer K P (eds) Clinical anatomy and management of thoracic spine pain. Butterworth Heinemann, Oxford

Singer K P, Giles L G F 1990 Manual therapy considerations at the thoracolumbar junction: an anatomical and functional perspective. Journal of Manipulative and Physiological Therapeutics 13: 83–88

Singer K P, Malmivaara A 2000 Pathoanatomical characteristics of the thoracolumbar junctional region. In: Giles L G F, Singer K P (eds) Clinical anatomy and management of thoracic spine pain. Butterworth Heinemann, Oxford

Singer K P, Day R E, Breidahl P D 1989 In vivo axial rotation at the thoracolumbar junction: an investigation using low dose CT in healthy male volunteers. Clinical Biomechanics 4: 145–150

Singer K P, Edmondston S J, Day R E, Breidahl W H 1994 Computer-assisted and Cobb angle determination of the thoracic kyphosis: an in-vivo and in-vitro comparison. Spine 19: 1381–1384

Singer K P, Edmondston S J, Day R E, Breidahl P D, Price R I 1995 Prediction of thoracic and lumbar vertebral body compressive strength: correlations with bone mineral density and vertebral region. Bone 17: 167–174

Sobel J S, Kremert I, Winters J C, Arendzen J H, de Jong B M 1996 The influence of the mobility in the cervicothoracic spine and the upper ribs (shoulder girdle) on the mobility of the scapulohumeral joint. Journal of Manipulative and Physiological Therapeutics 19: 469–474

Stokes I A F 2000 Biomechanics of the thoracic spine and ribcage. In: Giles L G F, Singer K P (eds) Clinical anatomy and management of thoracic spine pain. Butterworth Heinemann, Oxford

Toppenberg R M, Bullock M I 1986 The interrelationship of spinal curves, pelvic tilt and muscle lengths in the adolescent female. Australian Journal of Physiotherapy 32: 6–12

Veldhuizen A G, Scholten P J M 1987 Kinematics of the scoliotic spine as related to the normal spine. Spine 12: 852–858

Walker M L, Rothstein J M, Finucane S D, Lamb R L 1987 Relationships between lumbar lordosis, pelvic tilt, and abdominal muscle performance. Physical Therapy 67: 512–516

White A A 1969 An analysis of the mechanics of the thoracic spine in man. Acta Orthopaedica Scandinavica 127(Suppl.): 8–92

White S G, Sahrmann S A 1994 A movement system balance approach to management of musculoskeletal pain. In: Grant R (ed) Physical therapy for the cervical and thoracic spine, 2nd edn. Churchill Livingstone, Edinburgh

White A A, Panjabi M M, Thomas C L 1977 The clinical biomechanics of kyphotic deformities. Clinical Orthopaedics and Related Research 128: 8–17

Wilke H-J, Wolf S, Claes L E, Arand M, Wiesend A 1995 Stability increase of the lumbar spine with different muscle groups. Spine 20: 192–198

Willems J M, Jull G A, Ng J K-F 1996 An in-vivo study of the primary and coupled rotations of the thoracic spine. Clinical Biomechanics 11: 311–316

Wisleder D, Smith M B, Mosher T J, Zatsiorsky V 2001 Lumbar spine mechanical response to axial compression load in vivo. Spine 26(18): E403–409

Wood K B, Garvey T A, Gundry C, Heithoff K B 1995 Magnetic resonance imaging of the thoracic spine. Journal of Bone and Joint Surgery 77A: 1631–1638

Chapter **7**

Clinical biomechanics of the lumbar spine

J. Cholewicki, S. P. Silfies

INTRODUCTION

There are three basic mechanical functions for the lumbar spine: protection of the spinal cord and nerve roots, permitting motion between the pelvis and thorax, and transmission of loads between the pelvis and thorax. Failure in any one of these three mechanical functions could result immediately in, or lead to, a clinical problem. The topic of spinal kinematics has been covered in a number of biomechanics texts and the discussion of spinal cord and nerve root protection is probably better suited by an anatomical approach. However, the biomechanics of spinal load transmission in the context of mechanical equilibrium, stability and injury mechanisms has considerable implications for clinical evaluation and treatment strategies and it will be the focus of this chapter.

The support of loads that arise from interaction between external and muscular forces is probably the single most important mechanical function of the spine. Because the muscles act through a relatively small moment arm in relation to the moment arm of external forces, the spine sustains extremely high loads. Not surprisingly, mechanical factors are often identified as the primary cause in a large percentage of low back disorders (Cherkin et al 1992, Deyo & Weinstein 2001, Kerr et al 2001, Marras et al 1995, McCowin et al 1991). While other psychosocial and pathophysiological factors leading to low back pain (LBP) have also been identified, this chapter will focus solely on the mechanical factors. Therefore, when referring to LBP or injury throughout this chapter we are implicitly considering only the mechanical causes.

Currently, the assessment of spine loads and subsequently the elucidation of the mechanisms of injury are possible only through biomechanical modelling. Other methods of in vivo load measurement exist, such as instrumented implants (Rohlmann et al 2000), but they are very limited owing to their invasiveness, patient population and technological constraints. Therefore, much of this chapter is devoted to the discussion of biomechanical equilibrium and stability models and conceptual models of lumbar spine injury. We will summarize the current research and discuss the application of an instability/motor control injury model to the clinical evaluation and treatment of patients with mechanical low back dysfunction.

THEORETICAL BASIS OF STRUCTURAL ANALYSES OF EQUILIBRIUM AND STABILITY

For the safe support of loads by any mechanical structure, its material must withstand the load and the structure itself must be stable. This leads to a two-step approach in the structural analysis of mechanical systems. The first level analysis relies on the force and moment equilibrium conditions for the computation of loads arising at various locations of interest in the structure. Depending on the system, this analysis can be static or dynamic. In the latter case, the inertial forces are included in the equations of equilibrium. The standard approach is to draw a free body diagram, which is a representation of an isolated part of a system with all of the forces and moments acting on it. For example, to estimate the loads acting at the L3–4 intervertebral joint during lifting, a free body diagram is drawn (Fig. 7.1). The sum of forces and moments arising from the upper body mass, muscle action, weight held in hands and the joint reaction forces must be zero to satisfy the static equilibrium condition. The unknown muscle and joint reaction

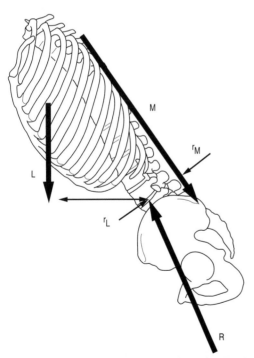

Figure 7.1 A free body diagram of the lumbar spine for the calculation of the reaction forces (R) acting on the L3–4 intervertebral joint. Because the moment arm (r_L) of the load (L) is usually much greater than the moment arm (r_M) of the combined erector spine muscles, their force (M) must be much greater to balance the moment equilibrium equation. From the force equilibrium equation, it follows that the joint reaction force is the sum of load and muscle force (R = L + M).

forces can be computed by solving the moment and force equations simultaneously. One should note that the large resultant joint compression force stems mainly from the muscle action and can be several times greater than the combined upper body weight and the weight held in hands.

The second level analysis examines whether the equilibrium state defined in the first level analysis is stable. The terms 'stability' and 'instability' referring to given joints or systems of joints are often misused in biomechanics literature. Within spine biomechanics, the stability concept is complicated by several clinical definitions of segmental instability consisting of a variety of diagnostic findings (White & Panjabi 1990). Several attempts to clarify and standardize the terms 'stability' and 'instability' have been made. Pope & Panjabi (1985) proposed that 'stability' (or 'instability') is a mechanical entity and should be treated as such. Definitions should not be based on suspected injury mechanism or 'clinical history'. Similarly, Ashton-Miller & Schultz (1991) called for a standard use of these terms in biomechanics. However, both 'clinical instability' and 'mechanical stability/instability' may be used concurrently if a clear understanding of the distinctions between them exists.

From a mechanical point of view, stability analysis refers to the study of an unperturbed state of a system. A perturbation is applied and certain quantities, which characterize the state of the system at any time, are measured. If, as the system goes from the unperturbed to perturbed state, the changes in those quantities do not exceed their earlier established measures, the unperturbed state is called stable. If these quantities exceed their earlier established measures, the unperturbed state is unstable (Leipholz 1987). An example of a clinical application of this definition is testing of patients' static standing or seated balance. A clinician provides perturbation to a patient to ascertain his ability to maintain balance and to return to equilibrium or a stable state. If the patient fails to maintain balance or his sway exceeds some normative distance, his stance will be classified as unstable.

The state of a dynamic system is generally characterized with parameters describing its motion. Therefore, the stability of the dynamic system will refer to the stability of its unperturbed motion. A control mechanism(s), if present, becomes an integral part of such a system and will also affect its stability. For example, a constant velocity and intended trajectory can describe unperturbed motion of a car on cruise control. A multitude of system parameters will affect this car's stability when it encounters a perturbation such as a bump on a road or a gust of wind: stiffness of the suspension, friction between the tyres and the road or the quality of the cruise control, to mention only a few. Similarly, in the most general terms, spine stability refers to the capability of maintaining and controlling physiological spine movements and it includes a motor control system. Hypermobility, for example, is one of the spine characteristics. It does not necessarily imply instability of the entire spine system, especially if it can be adequately compensated for and controlled resulting in coordinated and physiological spine movement. Unfortunately, current biomechanical models are still limited to static analyses of stability, although the mathematical theory is available to study fully dynamic systems (Leipholz 1987). These models focus on muscle and joint stiffness and various muscle recruitment patterns. However, some inferences about motor control and the dynamic stability of the spine can be made by comparing static spine stability obtained from these models and patients' responses to various perturbations (see p. 78). For example, the dynamic response of a patient to sudden trunk loading depends on the static stability of the spine exhibited prior to sudden loading and the muscle reflex response (motor control) after sudden loading (Cholewicki et al 2000).

In a static example, let us examine stability of the equilibrium states of the four mechanical systems represented by balls on different surfaces in Figure 7.2. Each system is in a static equilibrium. Upon perturbation, only the balls in the last two examples will return to their original equilibrium positions. These two systems are therefore stable. The balls in the first two examples will be displaced away from their original equilibrium positions following the perturbations, indicating unstable equilibrium states of these systems.

The mathematical formulation of the stability problem in elastostatic systems such as one considered above relies on the minimum potential energy principle. A mechanical system is stable only if its total potential energy is at a relative mini-

mum. In other words, any mechanical perturbation would cause the potential energy of a stable system to rise and it would then tend to return to its relative equilibrium. It can easily be seen in Figure 7.2 that the potential energies of stable systems are at their respective minima. It should also be noted that static equilibrium is a necessary but not a sufficient condition for stability. If a system is not in equilibrium, it is not stable by definition. Furthermore, the stability state can be quantified with the measure of the curvature of the potential energy. The larger the curvature (depth) of the potential energy in the vicinity of its minimum, the more stable the system is. For example, the system represented in Figure 7.2D is more stable than the system represented in Figure 7.2C.

In a more realistic example of an inverted pendulum resembling a spine model, the change in potential energy in various forms must be considered (Fig. 7.3). The total potential energy (V) of such a system after the perturbation is the difference between the elastic energy (U) stored in springs and the work (W) performed by the external load:

$$V = U - W \qquad \text{(equation 1)}$$

Furthermore, the elastic energy stored in springs is proportional to their stiffness (k)

$$U = \tfrac{1}{2} k\, x_1^2 + \tfrac{1}{2} k\, x_2^2 \qquad \text{(equation 2)}$$

where x_1 and x_2 are the changes in the springs' length. The work performed by the external load (L) is given by:

$$W = L\, e \qquad \text{(equation 3)}$$

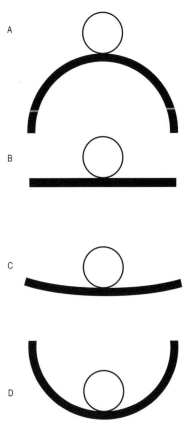

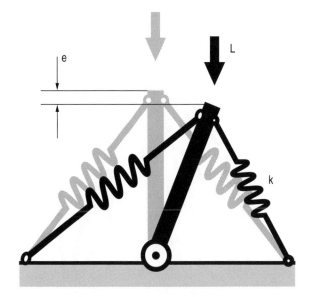

Figure 7.2 A simple mechanical system illustrating the principle of the minimum potential energy. In all four cases (A, B, C, and D) the system satisfies static equilibrium conditions. However, only the C and D cases are stable, because each of these systems' potential energy is at its respective minimum.

Figure 7.3 A simplified spine model illustrating the energy approach to analysis of stability. The total potential energy of such a system after the perturbation is the potential energy stored in springs (muscles) minus the work performed by the external load (L). Stiffer springs (k) store more potential energy and create a more stable system.

Now it remains to examine the total potential energy for its behaviour around the equilibrium state. Mathematically, the first derivative of the potential energy must be equal to zero to satisfy the static equilibrium requirement and the second derivative must be greater than zero for stability (equations 4 and 5). The second derivative also quantifies the curvature of the potential energy ($V'' > 0$ implies the concave surface) and hence the stability of the system.

$V' = 0$ static equilibrium (equation 4)

$V'' > 0$ stability (equation 5)

Equations 1 and 5 can be interpreted in the following way. If upon the perturbation, the amount of stored elastic energy is greater than the work performed by the external forces, the overall energy of the system will rise. Such a system is stable and it will return to its original equilibrium configuration. In contrast, if the elastic potential energy stored in springs is less than the external work, the system is unstable and it will continue to deform seeking the minimum potential energy – it will buckle. It can be seen by combining equations 1, 2 and 3 that the stiffer the springs are, the more stable the system is. This is because more elastic potential energy is stored upon the perturbation. Similarly, the larger the external load is, the less stable the system. The final observation is that an elastostatic system, or the forces acting upon it, need not be symmetrical for it to be stable, as long as the static equilibrium is satisfied.

The minimum potential energy principle is one classical approach used to determine the stability criteria of an elastic system with multiple degrees of freedom (Fig. 7.4). The only difference from the previous examples is that now the potential energy forms a multidimensional surface around the equilibrium state (number of dimensions equals the number of degrees of freedom). Therefore, partial, second order derivatives of the potential energy with respect to each coordinate must now be greater than zero to satisfy stability criteria. In other words, the potential energy surface must be concave in every direction at the point of equilibrium to form the minimum and for the entire system to be stable. If this surface is convex in the direction of any one degree of freedom, the entire system will be unstable. The average curvature of the potential energy surface – termed the stability index (SI) by Cholewicki & McGill (1996) – can be used to quantify the relative stability of a multi-degree of freedom system.

In the lumbar spine, muscles, along with ligaments and other passive tissues, play the stabilizing role by momentarily storing the elastic potential energy in response to mechanical perturbations. The muscles act as variable stiffness springs whose stiffness is proportional to the muscle force. If the spine is sufficiently stable it will resist external perturbations without the need for active feedback control. In other words, the spine will return to its equilibrium state after the perturbation even if no change in muscle activation had occurred. Due to inherent delays in feedback loops, active control of relatively small and transient perturbations may not be efficient and/or effective. Several issues pertaining to the stability of the lumbar spine will be discussed in more detail later in the chapter.

In summary, a complete biomechanical assessment of spine injury potential, injury mechanisms or the biomechanical evaluation of the effectiveness of various prevention and rehabilitation approaches should encompass the two analytical steps outlined above. The estimation of tissue loads is necessary to assess the risk of tissue failure under various spine-loading scenarios. However, tissue integrity alone does not assure the structural stability of the spine. Therefore, the assessment of spine stability is also necessary to further elucidate the potential or effects of structural failure due to buckling.

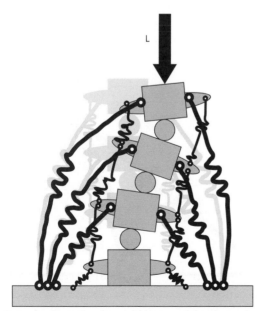

Figure 7.4 A schematic of a multidegree-of-freedom spine model. If one of the degrees of freedom becomes unstable, the entire structure is unstable and it will buckle under the load (L). Muscle and ligaments must provide stability with a coordinated muscle recruitment pattern.

Estimating spine loads

The biomechanical analysis of spinal loads begins with a free body diagram and the equations for static or dynamic equilibrium of forces and moments. Models containing even minimal anatomical detail result in a mathematically indeterminate problem caused by existence of multiple tissues that can generate or support forces and moments about a given joint. There are two basic methods for solving the problem of mathematical indeterminacy in a biomechanical spine model: optimization and EMG-assisted approaches. Each of these methods offers a number of distinctive assets and liabilities.

Optimization methods

An optimization method relies on formulating an objective function that serves as a criterion for selecting a unique solution of force partitioning among various tissues out of the infinitely large set of viable solutions. This criterion may consist of minimizing the sum of muscle forces (Yettram & Jackman 1980), the sum of muscle stress, disc compression, joint shear force, or some combination of these (e.g. Bean et al 1988, Schultz et al 1983). Because the optimization solution converges on a singular set of muscle forces to meet the moment constraints, it is insensitive to the transient changes in load sharing among agonist muscles during the exertion. Current objective functions are not able to respond to the many different ways in which muscles are recruited to perform similar tasks even when the kinematics or resultant moment patterns are the same. A popular objective function in many low back optimization models, minimization of muscle stress and disc compression, predicts no antagonist muscle co-activation (co-contraction), defined as the contraction of muscles above the minimum stress necessary to satisfy the moment equilibrium about a given joint (Hughes et al 2001). In turn, this optimization scheme underestimates the joint compression forces during isometric exertions by 23–43% when compared with an EMG-assisted approach (Cholewicki et al 1995, Hughes et al 1995). The antagonistic co-activation of trunk muscles is often demonstrated with EMG during many activities (Granata & Orishimo 2001, Lavender et al 1993, 1992b). Among other hypotheses, the antagonist muscle co-activation is explained as necessary for providing mechanical stability to the spinal column (Bergmark 1989, Cholewicki & McGill 1996, Crisco & Panjabi 1991, Gardner-Morse et al 1995, Granata & Marras 2000).

EMG-assisted methods

An EMG-assisted method partitions the forces among the muscles according to their normalized EMG activity, cross-sectional areas and assumptions regarding their maximum force-generating potential (Granata & Marras 1995, McGill 1992a). In the dynamic version of this method, predicted muscle forces are further modulated with coefficients accounting for instantaneous muscle length, velocity of contraction and passive elastic contributions. EMG-assisted partitioning of muscle forces is inherently consistent with physiologically observed muscle activation patterns. However, due to imperfections in EMG recording and processing and anatomical modelling, the simultaneous moment equations in three dimensions are not satisfied very well in complex tasks (Granata & Marras 1995, McGill 1992a).

To remedy the equilibrium problem, a hybrid approach, termed EMG-assisted optimization (EMGAO), was developed (Cholewicki & McGill 1994). In this method, an optimization algorithm is used to satisfy the equilibrium equations in a way that provides the best possible match between the predicted muscle forces and their myoelectric profiles. Minimal adjustments are applied to the individual muscle forces estimated initially from EMG, to balance all moment and force equations. The EMGAO combines some principal advantages of the optimization and EMG-assisted methods. It preserves the physiologically observed (through EMG) muscle activation patterns while satisfying the equilibrium constraint equations exactly (Cholewicki et al 1995).

Despite the obvious advantage of better physiological accuracy of the EMG and EMGAO spine models, they require complex data acquisition and processing methodologies. For the applications that require only rough estimates of spinal loading, optimization or even single muscle equivalent models may suffice (Kingma et al 1998, McGill et al 1996, van Dieën & de Looze 1999b). However, simulations with such models will always produce identical results for the same loading (input) conditions. It is not possible to detect differences in neuromuscular control between the subjects or the different features among the 'normal' and 'abnormal' muscle activation patterns or their effects on spine forces. The EMG-assisted models are better suited for this purpose because their input is biologically sensitive to the various patterns of muscle recruitment.

Stability of the lumbar spine

In vitro estimates of the critical loads of isolated osteoligamentous spine segments highlight the importance of the mechanical stability of the spine. In a classic experiment Lucas & Bresler (1961) determined the critical load for a thoracolumbar spine to be approximately 20 N (4.5 lb). This indicates that the spine is unable to sustain compressive loads and will buckle under very low loads. A later replication of this study established the critical load for a lumbar spine to be approximately 90 N (20 lb) (Crisco et al 1992). The lumbar spine must support an upper body weight four to five times greater than its buckling threshold load. If any additional external forces are acting on the torso, spine stability surfaces as the most important issue in supporting and transmitting such loads. It becomes clear that the static or dynamic equilibrium analysis in a spine model is not enough to study the above phenomena. It is now necessary to incorporate structural stability analysis tools into the biomechanical models.

Trunk muscles as variable stiffness springs

Stability analysis has been applied to spine modelling only relatively recently (Bergmark 1989, Cholewicki & McGill 1996, Crisco & Panjabi 1991, Gardner-Morse et al 1995, Granata & Marras 2000). To our knowledge, Bergmark (1989) was the first to incorporate a spring-like short-range muscle stiffness into the calculations of stability in a multiple degrees of freedom spine model. Short-range muscle stiffness, also called high frequency stiffness, relates small changes in the muscle length and force, such that they will not result in the change of cross-bridge attachment distribution. The mechanical properties of the whole muscle/tendon unit within this short range are essentially elastic (conservative) (Rack & Westbury 1973, 1974) and can be modelled with a mechanical spring (Hogan 1990). The short-range stiffness of the muscle has been shown to be linearly related to the muscle force (Morgan 1977, Zahalak & Heyman 1979), although some researchers have reported a non-linear relationship (Hatta et al 1988, Stein & Gordon 1986). Beyond this short range the muscle stiffness is modulated by spinal reflexes and eventually by voluntary responses (Diener et al 1983, Nashner & Cordo 1981, Winters et al 1988, Zajac & Winters 1990).

The short-range muscle stiffness (k) can be roughly estimated as being proportional to the muscle force (F) and inversely proportional to its length (L) (Rack & Westbury 1974):

$$k = q\frac{F}{L} \qquad \text{(equation 6)}$$

The proportionality constant q varies anywhere between 5 and 100 depending on muscle excitation and tendon-to-muscle length ratio (Cholewicki & McGill 1995, Crisco & Panjabi 1991). For more accurate estimates of muscle stiffness, especially in dynamic simulations, a distribution–moment model of the muscle activation dynamics (calcium release and diffusion) (Cholewicki & McGill 1995, 1996, Zahalak 1986, Zahalak & Ma 1990) or a model with an enhanced spring-like muscle performance through an improved muscle reflex loop (Gielen & Houk 1987, Ramos et al 1990, Stein & Oguztoreli 1984, Winters 1995) is better suited.

The ligaments, intervertebral disc and other passive structures also contribute to the stability of the lumbar spine by acting as non-linear springs. Their contribution to spine stability may have been overlooked in the past. The passive stiffness of the osteoligamentous lumbar spine increases significantly with a compressive load placed on the spine. In fact, the osteoligamentous lumbar spine can carry up to 1200 N (270 lb) if this load is distributed to follow the spine curvature (follower load) (Patwardhan et al 1999), which may be the likely in vivo scenario. Nevertheless, more research is necessary to establish the extent of relative sharing of the stabilizing roles between the passive and active (muscles) tissues in the spine.

Spine stabilizing role of trunk muscles

The effects of different trunk muscle activation patterns on spine stability have been studied through experimentation with stability models of various complexities using both optimization and EMG-assisted methods. Optimization models were shown to be able to predict antagonistic muscle co-activation if the stability criteria were incorporated into their objective functions (Cholewicki et al 1997, Granata & Marras 2000, Stokes & Gardner-Morse 1999). These studies demonstrated that the antagonistic muscle co-contraction increases spine stability in exchange for a

greater spine compression force penalty. In fact, a low level of trunk muscle co-contraction, in the range of 1–2% of a maximum voluntary exertion, is necessary to maintain the spine in a stable equilibrium around its neutral posture (Cholewicki et al 1997).

It is easy to see from the earlier discussion that increased muscle force increases muscle stiffness, which causes more of the elastic potential energy to be stored in the muscles upon the transient perturbations, which in turn leads to greater spine stability. Therefore, there appears to be an ample stability safety margin in tasks that require a lot of muscular effort (Cholewicki & McGill 1996). In contrast, tasks that demand very little muscle activity, such as upright standing with no load, are characterized by low spine stability. The tasks that challenge spine stability the most are those in which spine posture is maintained within its neutral zone, where ligaments are relatively slack, and there are very few muscles activated to stabilize it. It seems reasonable for the neuromuscular system to maintain the most stability during heavy lifting or other high intensity exertion tasks, when the spine buckling would have deleterious effects. On the other hand, low energy expenditure may be an objective of the motor control system during standing, sitting or walking tasks that must be sustained over longer periods. Figure 7.5 conceptually compares injury risks due to tissue overload and spine instability as functions of task demand.

In addition to the overall intensity of muscle co-activation, the stability of the spinal column depends on muscle architecture (Crisco & Panjabi 1991). Large muscles with greater moment arms are more effective in stabilizing the spine than smaller intervertebral muscles. However, each vertebral body must have at least one muscle fascicle attached and activated, otherwise the spine will always be unstable (Crisco & Panjabi 1991). In addition, for any given activation

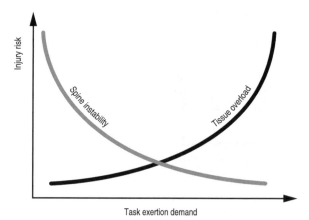

Figure 7.5 Conceptual view of the musculoskeletal injury risks as a function of task exertion demand. Likelihood of tissue overload and failure increases with increased task exertion. However, spine structural failure due to buckling (and in turn some tissue overstraining due to the buckling event) is more likely to occur when the muscle forces are low. Adapted from Cholewicki & McGill (1996).

level of the muscles that attach to each lumbar vertebra, there exists an upper limit for the activation of the large muscles that attach only to the pelvis and ribcage (Bergmark 1989). Beyond this limit, the spine becomes unstable. It is analogous to holding a stack of tennis balls by grasping only the top and bottom ones. Each joint must be stabilized prior to activating large trunk muscles, which apply compressive forces between the ribcage and pelvis (Fig. 7.6).

Based on the above functional dichotomy and on whether the muscles cross a single intervertebral joint or span across all joints from the ribcage to pelvis, Bergmark (1989) divided the trunk muscles into 'local' and 'global' systems. The transversus abdominis, portions of the internal oblique and lumbar multifidus have been labelled as local trunk muscles, whereas the rectus abdominis, external oblique and lumbar erector spinae muscle groups belong to the global muscle system. Unfortunately, the above classification and Bergmark's work are often misinterpreted as identifying the muscles that are spine stabilizers and the muscles that are moment generators. While there may be some trunk muscles that are clinically more important than others, this notion is not supported by mechanical stability analyses. All trunk muscles contribute to spine stability and all muscles that cross a given joint contribute to the joint moment. The overall stability of the spine depends on the individual forces, and hence stiffness, of all trunk muscles as well as their relative force magnitudes. The total joint moment is the sum of products of all muscle forces and their respective moment arms.

The stability of the lumbar spine is a highly non-linear function of the trunk muscle forces. First, as discussed above, stability depends on both absolute and relative muscle forces. Second, the relative contribution of a muscle to

spinal stability depends on the magnitude and direction of external trunk loading (Cholewicki & VanVliet 2002). Simulations with muscle 'knock out' in a spine stability model showed that no single muscle group contributed more than 30% to the overall stability of the lumbar spine (Cholewicki & VanVliet 2002). No single muscle group could be identified as the most important spine stabilizer and no clear distinction was found between the local and global muscles as related to stability. Finally, increased spine stiffness due to spine compression force and the ligament forces that are dependent on spine posture must be also considered among the factors determining the overall stability of the spine.

Role of intra-abdominal pressure in spine stability

Much controversy surrounds the mechanical role of increased intra-abdominal pressure (IAP) in preparation for or during physical exertions. Very high pressures, commonly observed during strenuous activities, were originally hypothesized to reduce the compressive forces on the lumbar spine (Bartelink 1957, Keith 1923, Morris et al 1961). The pressure produced within the abdominal cavity exerts a hydrostatic force down on the pelvic floor and up on the diaphragm. This force adds tensile load to the spine and produces trunk extension moment and was therefore assumed to reduce spine compression force. Later, however, researchers observed that the forceful contraction of abdominal muscles that appears to be necessary to generate IAP would cancel out the tensile force and extensor moment obtained from IAP (McGill & Norman 1987). In fact, in vivo intradiscal pressure measurements would suggest that the lumbar spine compression force increases, rather than decreases, with voluntary increase in IAP (Valsalva manoeuvre) (Nachemson et al 1986) (Fig. 7.7).

If the transversus abdominis and/or oblique muscles were recruited preferentially to create IAP without the activation of rectus abdominis, then perhaps a net spinal unloading effect could be achieved with IAP (Daggfeldt & Thorstensson 1997, Nachemson et al 1986). Additionally, a small trunk extension moment can be produced with contraction of the diaphragm alone (Hodges et al 2001). The question then arises as to whether people can generate IAP with such a preferential muscle recruitment pattern and without the penalty of additional compressive forces from other longitudinally oriented muscles. Indeed among all abdominal wall muscles, activation of transversus abdominis correlates the best with IAP (Cresswell & Thorstensson 1989; Cresswell et al 1992, 1994) and it is recruited first in preparation for rapid limb movements (Hodges & Richardson 1996, 1998, 1999). However, an overall pattern of trunk muscle co-contraction associated with increased IAP was observed by other researchers who hypothesized that it enhances spine stability with a resultant increase in spine compressive load (Cholewicki et al 1999a, Cresswell et al 1994, Marras & Mirka 1996, McGill & Norman 1987, McGill & Sharratt 1990).

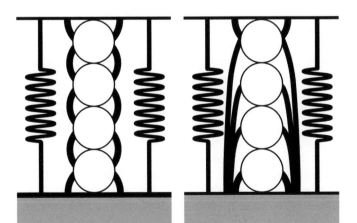

Figure 7.6 A schematic illustration of the relationship between the multisegmental muscles (muscles that span the pelvis and ribcage), intersegmental muscles (muscles that span individual intervertebral joints) and spine stability. Each intervertebral joint must have a muscle fascicle attached and activated according to one or both of the two depicted architectures (Crisco & Panjabi 1991). Furthermore, for any given activation of the intersegmental muscles, there exists a limit for the activation of the multisegmental muscles beyond which buckling will occur.

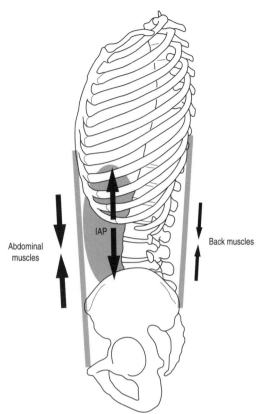

Figure 7.7 Intra-abdominal pressure (IAP) mechanics. The tensile force and the trunk extensor moment achieved through the action of IAP on the pelvic floor and the diaphragm is offset or even exceeded by the concomitant increase in the abdominal and back muscle co-contraction necessary to generate IAP.

Further support for the spine-stabilizing role of IAP came from a report of increased trunk stiffness stemming from voluntarily generated IAP (Cholewicki et al 1999b). In this study, a significant increase in EMG activity of all major abdominal, lumbar and thoracic muscles was documented when subjects elevated their IAP from its resting value to 40% and 80% of the maximum voluntarily generated pressure. Along with this increase in muscle co-contraction, trunk stiffness rose significantly by 12% and 32%, respectively, indicating enhanced stability of the lumbar spine (Cholewicki et al 1999b). Undeniably, this enhancement of spine stability via IAP and trunk muscle co-contraction came about with the price of increased spine compression force (Gardner-Morse & Stokes 1998, Granata & Marras 2000).

Generally, individuals are unable to decouple an increase in IAP from trunk muscle co-contraction during steady-state exertions (Cholewicki et al 2002a). IAP, intrathoracic pressure (ITP) and trunk muscle co-contraction are highly correlated regardless of whether subjects attempt to increase IAP without trunk muscle co-contraction or to co-contract their muscles without elevating their IAP. These entities may dissociate temporarily during transient states such as exhaling (Cholewicki et al 2002a) or in preparation for a rapid arm movement (Hodges & Richardson 1996,

1998, 1999), but they appear to be tightly coupled under steady-state exertions.

The concurrent rise in intrathoracic pressure, IAP and muscle co-contraction during physical exertions can easily be explained, based on stability requirements. A high-level physical exertion, such as a lift, throw or jump, requires a rapid contraction of limb and other muscles that originate on the thorax. To execute an effective lift or throw, not only must the 'mechanical slack' be taken up from the muscles prior to the exertion, but a rigid base from which these muscles originate must also be created. Co-contraction of the latissimus dorsi, thoracic erector spinae and intercostal muscles against the ITP increases the rigidity of the ribcage while the co-contraction of the abdominal wall and lumbar erector spinae muscles against the IAP increases stability of the lumbar spine (Cholewicki et al 1999a). Furthermore, ITP helps the contracting diaphragm to increase IAP by reducing the transdiaphragmatic pressure (Cholewicki et al 2002a). Therefore, the co-contraction of all trunk muscles, including the abdominal wall, erector spinae and latissimus dorsi, along with the increase in IAP and ITP, stiffens both the lumbar spine and the thoracic cage, with a net effect of increased spine compression force.

There are other possible mechanical and physiological effects of increased IAP during physical exertion. Abdominal wall muscles, especially oblique and transversus abdominis, can gain greater mechanical advantage if they contract around the pressurized abdomen than if they collapse inward along their straight lines of action (Cresswell & Thorstensson 1989). A concomitant increase in the cerebrospinal fluid pressure may act as a safety mechanism by opposing a rise in arterial blood pressure (Porth et al 1984). Although it has been suggested that exhaling during such exertions may reduce blood pressure and minimize the risk of a stroke (Narloch & Brandstater 1995), this strategy would also reduce IAP, ITP and the level of trunk muscle co-contraction. As a result, reduced spine stability and rigidity of the thorax would compromise the intended physical performance.

In summary, the extremely high IAP levels generated by competitive weightlifters (McGill et al 1990) do not reduce the spine compression force, but rather prevent the collapse of the ribcage and the buckling of the lumbar spine. Likewise, the increased IAP observed in individuals preparing for sudden trunk loading (Cresswell et al 1994) or in patients with non-specific LBP (Fairbank et al 1980, Hemborg & Moritz 1985), likely serves to enhance spine stability prior to any movement.

Role of abdominal belts and lumbar supports in spine stability

The notion of the beneficial role of abdominal belts and lumbar supports was inspired by the early theories of intra-abdominal pressure (IAP) reducing spine compression forces. Because wearing a belt helps in generating higher IAP (Harman et al 1989, McGill et al 1990), it was assumed that the belt was helpful in protecting the lumbar spine from excessive forces (Harman et al 1989, Lander et al 1990, 1992). However, the literature to date does not support this notion. A very thorough and systematic literature review on lumbar supports by van Poppel et al (2000) demonstrated that many contradictory results and findings of 'no effect' rule out most of the benefits with which the belts are often credited. For example, some studies found that abdominal belts marginally increase trunk strength; decrease spine compression force, spinal shrinkage and muscle EMG (Bourne & Reilly 1991, Granata et al 1997, Lee & Kang 2002, Smith et al 1996, Sullivan & Mayhew 1995, Warren et al 2001, Woldstad & Sherman 1998). Others found no such effects (Ciriello & Snook 1995, Ivancic et al 2002, Lantz & Schultz 1986a, Majkowski et al 1998, Marras et al 2000, McGill & Norman 1987, Rabinowitz et al 1998, Reyna et al 1995). The positive findings are often related to the altered kinematics of task execution imposed by the belt and lower trunk moments, which in turn result in misleadingly smaller spine compression forces (Granata et al 1997, Woldstad & Sherman 1998).

The only consistent finding across various studies is that belts reduce trunk range of motion and increase trunk stiffness (Axelsson et al 1992, Buchalter et al 1988, Cholewicki et al 1999b, Fidler & Plasmans 1983, Lantz & Schultz 1986b, McGill et al 1994, Tuong et al 1998). Again, it has been shown mathematically that this increase in trunk stiffness translates directly into enhanced stability of the lumbar spine, even around its neutral posture (Ivancic et al 2002). Thus, an abdominal belt and IAP can each individually or additively increase spine stability. Specifically, the estimates of these effects are as high as a 40% increase in spine stability due to wearing a belt and another 40% due to generating large IAP for a combined effect from both mechanisms of more than an 80% increase in spine stability (Cholewicki et al 1999b, Ivancic et al 2002). However, the difference between the two mechanisms is that the increase in spine stability due to high IAP is actively gained from muscle co-contraction associated with IAP. In contrast, the stabilizing effect of the belt is a passive mechanism stemming from the interaction of the wide and stiff belt placed between the ribcage and pelvis.

Even though the spine stabilizing function of lumbar supports is relatively well documented, no objective clinically relevant benefits have been found. A prescription of abdominal belts to manual load-handling workers does not reduce the incidence of low back injuries (Jellema et al 2001, Reddell et al 1992, Wassell et al 2000). The efficacy of lumbosacral orthoses in the treatment of spine fractures or following a fusion surgery has not been completely proven (Axelsson et al 1995, Ohana et al 2000). Even the concern of muscle weakening following long-term belt wearing appears to be unsupported in the literature (Holmström & Moritz 1992, Walsh & Schwartz 1990). However, many studies report that people perceive a sense of security and/or pain relief from wearing lumbar supports (Ahlgren & Hansen 1978, Alaranta & Hurri 1988, Million et al 1981). Perhaps such mechanical effects are too small to be detected objectively.

If we consider that only 1–2% of the maximum voluntary contraction (MVC) is required from trunk muscles to maintain the spine in a stable upright posture (Cholewicki et al 1997) (see p. 72), the estimated belt effects might indeed be very small. An abdominal belt can enhance spine stability around its neutral posture by 40% at the most (Cholewicki et al 1999a, Ivancic et al 2002). Even if we assume full adaptation to this additional stability, the expected reduction in trunk muscle co-contraction will not exceed 0.8% MVC (40% × 2% MVC). Clearly, such small differences in muscle activation are beyond the detection accuracy of our current EMG recording techniques. Furthermore, based on a simple but realistic model of trunk flexors and extensors (Cholewicki et al 1997), we can estimate the difference in spine compression force that corresponds to the 0.8% MVC reduction in muscle co-contraction to be roughly 35 N. Again, such a small reduction in the spine load appears neither statistically significant nor clinically relevant. Where then does the subjective perception of the benefits of wearing an abdominal belt or a lumbar support come from?

Let us examine a similar analogy to the one above. The addition of a 32 kg mass to the trunk requires an increase in trunk muscle co-contraction of approximately 1–2% MVC above the 1–2% MVC already required to maintain a stable upright posture of the spine without additional load (Cholewicki et al 1997). Could, then, a reduction of 0.8% MVC be perceived as a relief equivalent to the removal of 12.8–25.6 kg from the upper body? Furthermore, sustained muscular contractions of 5% MVC or greater will eventually result in pain while the less intense contraction can be sustained indefinitely (Jonsson 1978). Could it be that patients with low back pain, who exhibit more muscle co-contraction during the activities of daily living (Lariviere et al 2000, Marras et al 2001, van Dieën et al 2003), benefit from the reduction of muscle co-contraction below the 5% MVC threshold with the help of lumbosacral orthoses? Suggestions of improved trunk proprioception with lumbosacral orthoses have also been made (McNair & Heine 1999, Newcomer et al 2001). Perhaps enhanced proprioception in the lumbar spine may reduce the likelihood of low back injury and pain due to motor control error (see section on stability based concept of musculoskeletal injury). Therefore, the perceived muscle weakening following long-term belt wearing might instead be motor control deconditioning. There are currently no data to help answer the above questions. For now, the identification of exact mechanisms underlying the sensation of the protective function of lumbar supports and back pain relief from wearing lumbosacral orthoses must await results from more theoretical and experimental studies.

BIOMECHANICS OF SPINE INJURY AND PAIN

Low back pain (LBP) is a multifactorial problem. Numerous risk factors associated with acute low back injury and/or chronic disability have been identified. These risk factors fall into one of three major categories: demographic, such as an individual's strength and age; psychosocial, such as psychological stress and job satisfaction; and biomechanical, such as posture and the load handled (Frank et al 1996). While their reported relative importance depends on the quality of the measurement tools used, it appears that the worst-case scenario is a combination of factors from all three categories (Kerr et al 2001). A well-designed prevention or rehabilitation programme must take into account all three factors. The following sections will focus only on the biomechanical aspects of LBP and injury.

Equilibrium based concept of musculoskeletal injury

The conventional model of musculoskeletal injury is based on the concept of tissue overload during physical exertion. Tissue load tolerance is compared to the estimated loads in vivo. The injury is likely to occur if the tissue loads approach or exceed the tissue tolerance levels at any given time. This model encompasses several aspects of tissue failure such as the accumulation of microtrauma during repetitive exertions, tissue creep, fatigue and/or unbalanced tissue loading (Kumar 2001).

The in vivo estimates of the compressive loads sustained by the lumbar spine during moderate physical exertions range between 2000 and 6000 N (450–1350 lb) (Davis et al 1998, Potvin 1997, van Dieën et al 2001). In the extreme case of competitive weightlifting, spine compression can reach 18 500 N (4150 lb) (Cholewicki et al 1991). On the other hand, the highest reported compressive load that a spinal motion segment withstood to failure during in vitro tests was just under 16 000 N (2900 lb) (Hutton et al 1979). On average, specimens fail under loads of approximately 6000 N (1350 lb) (Brinckmann et al 1989, Granhed et al 1989, Porter et al 1989). This apparent paradox of incompatibility between in vivo spine loads and in vitro tolerance levels motivated the formulation of several spine-unloading theories. The mechanisms involving intra-abdominal pressure (discussed in the section on the role of intra-abdominal pressure in spine stability), lumbodorsal fascia as the hydraulic amplifier, and the posterior ligamentous system have been proposed (Gracovetsky et al 1985, 1989, 1990). These hypotheses found very little support from the studies that followed (Adams & Hutton 1986, Cholewicki & McGill 1992, McGill & Norman 1988), but unfortunately many of the recommendations derived from these theories are still being perpetuated.

Direct comparisons between in vivo and in vitro failure loads are ill-advised because the cadaveric specimens are generally harvested from individuals older than the populations used in in vivo studies (Brinckmann et al 1989, Granhed et al 1989, Porter et al 1989). The specimens are frequently degenerated and have less bone mineral content, related often to prolonged bed rest or illness. On the other hand, sub-failure injuries can occur much earlier, before the ultimate load is reached (Oxland & Panjabi 1992). Accumulation of end-plate fractures, which are often missed on conventional roentgenograms, and internal disc disruption have been proposed as the mechanisms leading to LBP and intervertebral disc degeneration (Schwarzer et al 1995, van Dieën et al 1999). Consistent with this model, exposure to both high cumulative and large peak spinal loads can lead to LBP (Norman et al 1998).

In addition to joint compression, the load borne by the spine includes shear forces and bending moments. Facets and the intervertebral disc support anterior joint shear force, which results mostly from the upper body weight and lifted load. Unless a spondylolysis or spondylolysthesis is present, anterior shear force does not appear to be a threat to the integrity of the lumbar spine (Cyron et al 1979). In vivo estimates of anterior shear of approximately 200 N (Potvin 1991) are well below the ultimate strength of the motion segments reported to be between 620 and 980 N (140-220 lb) (Miller et al 1986, Osvalder et al 1993).

Posterior ligamentous structures fail under relatively low loads when the lumbar spine is subjected to flexion moments (Adams et al 1980, Osvalder et al 1990). Thus, ruptured supraspinous and interspinous ligaments are commonly seen in adult spines (Grenier et al 1989, Rissanen 1960). Posterior disc herniation is also associated with flexion moments applied in the presence of a large spine compression force (Adams & Hutton 1982a, 1982b). In addition, the ligaments and disc exhibit viscoelastic behaviour and creep when loaded during prolonged spine flexion. Peak lumbar flexion increased by 5.5 degrees after sitting for 20 minutes with fully flexed posture (McGill 1992b). Full recovery of spine mechanical properties took 30 minutes (McGill 1992b). However, the neurophysiological response pathways between lumbar ligaments and muscles may not fully recover even after 7 hours (Jackson et al 2001, Solomonow et al 2002). Therefore, repetitive tasks performed in flexed postures constitute a significant risk factor for overloading posterior ligaments and may lead to LBP.

Despite the many identified biomechanical risk factors, the conventional model of musculoskeletal injury possesses several limitations that make it inconsistent with some documented circumstances of low back injury and LBP. Reported low back injuries in an occupational setting rarely involve near-maximum exertions (McGill 1997). An injury sustained during sub-maximal tasks is difficult to explain with the overload model when the same individual or others performed the same task repeatedly in the past without any adverse effects. Sudden spine loading, trips and slips are also identified as causes of LBP (Bigos et al 1986, Frymoyer et al 1983, Manning et al 1984, Omino & Hayashi 1992, Troup et al 1981), but these scenarios may not necessarily produce tissue loads that are above their physiological limits. Finally, there is no consensus in the literature on the most detrimental biomechanical factors associated with LBP. Some researchers have identified peak loads while others have identified cumulative spine compression forces as the pertinent risk factors (Kerr et al 2001, Norman et al 1998, van Dieën et al 2001). Shear forces, excessive bending and twisting, the frequency of movement and whole body vibration have also been proposed as risk factors (Damkot et al 1984, Kelsey et al 1984, Kerr et al 2001, Manning et al 1984, Marras et al 1995, Pope et al 1998). It appears that any activity requiring physical exertion constitutes a risk factor for sustaining low back injury. Therefore, not all of these data are consistent with the model of tissue overload presented above. However, an injury model based on spine instability may better explain the above findings.

Stability based concept of musculoskeletal injury

A stability based model of spine injury was first proposed by Panjabi (1992a). He identified three subsystems: the passive subsystem consisting of ligamentous structures and disc; the active subsystem consisting of muscles; and the motor control coordinating the fulfilment of stability demands between the other two subsystems. A variety of mechanoreceptors, including but not limited to muscle spindles, Golgi tendon organs, joint receptors and cutaneous receptors, provide continuous feedback to the motor control system. A dysfunction in any of these subsystems may result in or lead to a clinical problem and/or it must be compensated by the remaining subsystems (Fig. 7.8). Cholewicki & McGill (1996) extended this model further and quantified the stability of the lumbar spine given its posture, external loads and trunk muscle activation (EMG). They demonstrated that spine instability or buckling could occur if the level of muscle co-contraction is low or their activation pattern is erroneous. Furthermore, Cholewicki & McGill (1992) observed a minor injury via fluoroscopy of a power lifter executing an extremely heavy lift. A hyperflexion at only one intervertebral level (L4–5) occurred during the lift suggesting a buckling phenomenon of the lumbar spine. Thus, the above studies highlighted motor control error as a possible factor precipitating low back injury and pain.

The motor control of spine stability is extremely complex. If we assume 5 degrees of freedom at each intervertebral joint (three axes of rotation and anteroposterior and lateral translations), the entire lumbar spine will comprise 30 degrees of freedom (5×6 joints). With a multitude of muscles and redundant lines of action, there exists an infinite number of possible muscle activation patterns that will satisfy equilibrium constraints, but an adequate stability level may not necessarily be achieved.

Problems of motor control and stability of the lumbar spine constitute an extension of the traditional equilibrium based approach to musculoskeletal injury. To date, very few spine stability studies have been published and they are limited to static conditions (Bergmark 1989, Cholewicki & McGill 1996, Gardner-Morse et al 1995, Granata & Marras 2000). Nevertheless, these recent efforts have opened new horizons for understanding spine disability and LBP. Based on stability analyses, it is now possible to explain several phenomena that traditional approaches have been unable to adequately elucidate. New hypotheses regarding spine injury mechanisms were formulated and tested. The following sections explore certain features of this model in more detail and in this context review the research related to muscle recruitment pattern and motor control in healthy individuals and in patients with mechanical LBP.

Explanation for injury occurrence under very low loads

Situations when individuals 'throw out their back' when picking up small objects from the floor or tying their shoelaces are common. Traditional equilibrium modelling does not provide an adequate explanation for such phenomena. Stability, on the other hand, offers much insight into possible injury mechanisms. Light tasks requiring little muscular effort create a scenario in which the spine is most vulnerable to buckling (Cholewicki & McGill 1996). In these situations, muscular fatigue or a motor control error may lead to spine instability. To prevent spine buckling, small intervertebral muscles that bridge an unstable lumbar level must be activated. Independent recruitment of large muscles that span several lumbar levels may not be a suitable response, as these muscles increase the compressive load on the spinal column. Their activation would increase the buckling effect, if unaccompanied by activation of small intervertebral muscles. Consequently, small muscles and passive supporting structures may be overloaded and injured or joint instability may result in abnormal motions which would irritate soft tissues, nerve roots or nociceptors.

As discussed on p. 72, co-activation of 1–2% MVC of trunk flexors and extensors is present and necessary to assure the mechanical stability of the spine in an upright posture (Cholewicki et al 1997). This level of muscle co-activation must be maintained throughout the duration of an entire day when individuals are walking or sitting. A two-fold increase in trunk muscle co-contraction was necessary to maintain spine stability when stiffness of

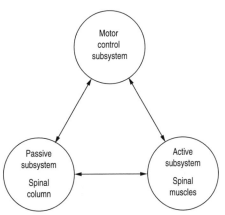

Figure 7.8 Panjabi's model of spinal stability and its motor control. Adapted with permission from Panjabi (1992).

contribution of the passive subsystem was reduced in a biomechanical model (Cholewicki et al 1997). This decrease in passive subsystem stiffness can be the result of mechanical trauma or a sub-failure injury (Oxland & Panjabi 1992). Because sustained muscular contractions at the level of 5% MVC or greater lead to muscular fatigue and pain (Jonsson 1978), the co-activation of trunk muscles during upright standing should be well below the 5% MVC value. Consequently, if decreased passive stiffness or motor control dysfunction exists, these muscles may increase activation and become fatigued, resulting in an inability to provide the adequate degree of spine stability when attempting certain physical tasks. These events may lead to a vicious cycle in which the spine becomes repeatedly re-injured because of muscle fatigue. Clinically, increased levels of muscle co-activation may indicate dysfunction of the passive stabilizing system of the lumbar spine. A similar hypothesis was first proposed by Panjabi (1992a, 1992b). This serves as a plausible explanation for chronic mechanical LBP.

There is also evidence of poor position sense, diminished postural control and slow reaction times in patients with mechanical LBP (Oddsson et al 1999, Taimela et al 1999, Wilder et al 1996). Certainly, if trunk stability is compromised by abnormal patterns of muscle activation or poor postural control it leaves the spine vulnerable to injury, especially under sudden loading conditions. A motor control problem fits with an instability/motor control model of low back injury, which overcomes many limitations of the conventional model. Using the instability/motor control model, injuries that occur at low effort levels such as a bending movement, twisting or reaching for an object can finally be explained.

Muscle recruitment patterns and low back pain

Biomechanical modelling of lumbar spine stability clearly identifies antagonist muscle co-activation as a mechanism by which the entire spinal column becomes stiffer, hence more stable (see p. 72). It has been suggested that 25% MVC of the trunk musculature provides maximal trunk stiffness (Cresswell & Thorstensson 1994). Even larger levels of trunk muscle co-activation may be necessary to stabilize the lumbar spine during more complex and dynamic tasks (Lavender et al 1992a, Marras & Mirka 1996). Antagonist muscle co-activation functions to increase spinal stability by increasing muscle stiffness (Cholewicki et al 1999a, Cresswell et al 1994, Gardner-Morse & Stokes 1998, Gracovetsky et al 1985) and by providing compressive loads to the spinal column (Janevic et al 1991, Stokes et al 2002). It is not surprising, then, that a number of studies have reported more antagonistic muscle co-contraction during various activities in patients with LBP (Lariviere et al 2000, Marras et al 2001, van Dieën et al 2003).

In general, inconsistent differences in trunk muscle recruitment patterns in patients with mechanical LBP have been reported and thus, no particular pattern of muscle

dysfunction can be identified (Cresswell & Thorstensson 1994, Edgerton et al 1996, Hodges & Richardson 1996, Mannion & Dolan 1994, O'Sullivan et al 1997a, Paquet et al 1994, Peach et al 1998, Sihvonen et al 1991). Patients with a clinical diagnosis of lumbar instability appear to preferentially activate the rectus abdominis and/or external oblique muscle groups (O'Sullivan et al 1997a, 1998, Silfies 2002). These patterns of muscle activation were interpreted as a dysfunction of the transversus abdominis and lumbar multifidus muscle groups in providing adequate compensation for a mechanically compromised osteo-ligamentous spine or passive subsystem. However, others did not find such a pattern in LBP patients (van Dieën et al 2003).

Two models have been proposed in the past to explain different muscle recruitment patterns in patients with LBP. The pain–spasm–pain model postulates that pain results in increased muscle activity, which in turn will cause pain (Roland 1986). The pain–adaptation model states that pain decreases the activation of muscles when active as agonists and increases it when the muscle is active as antagonist (Lund et al 1991). The effects of such a control strategy would be that movement velocity is reduced and movement excursions are limited. Both theories yield conflicting predictions on how LBP patients would alter trunk muscle recruitment in response to their pain, yet both find some supportive evidence in the literature.

Recent work by van Dieën et al (2003) demonstrated a higher lumbar to thoracic erector spinae activation ratio and a greater level of trunk muscle co-contraction in a LBP group compared to asymptomatic controls. These EMG data were then fed into a biomechanical model (Cholewicki & McGill 1996), which indicated that this change in recruitment pattern enhanced spinal stability (van Dieën et al 2003). These authors suggested that patients might be utilizing many different muscle recruitment patterns with a common goal of enhancing spinal stability.

Motor control of spine stability and low back pain

Due to the multisegmental structure of the human body, any voluntary movement is associated with postural adjustments. Thus, control of balance and lumbar stability are essential requirements for pain-free function of the spine. Motor control operates through the integration of several different pathways. Spinal pathways use proprioceptive input from sensory organs, muscles and joint structures to assist in postural control and trunk stability. The peripheral sensory system (spinal reflex pathways) also functions in conjunction with brain stem and cognitive programming. The brain stem coordinates visual, vestibular and joint receptor information, while cognitive programming is based upon repeated or stored central commands.

The functional assessment of trunk motor control related to the maintenance of spinal stability is difficult owing to the complexity of this system and the continually changing demands for stability and movement. Motor control research related to spine stability has been accomplished predominantly through monitoring of EMG activation patterns (synergist and antagonist), postural control parameters and muscle onset and offset timing. Several models of testing muscle response to a controlled challenge have been established:

1. use of anticipated self-perturbation of the extremities (Hodges & Richardson 1996, 1997b, Zattara & Bouisset 1988)
2. use of expected or unexpected external loading or loading of the trunk (Radebold et al 2000, van Dieën & de Looze 1999a, Wilder et al 1996)
3. standing or seated balance control (Mientjes & Frank 1999, Radebold et al 2001, Takala et al 1997)
4. use of forced or altered breathing patterns (Hamaoui et al 2002, McGill et al 1995)
5. use of expected or unexpected perturbation of a support surface (Huang et al 2001).

Postural adjustments triggered prior to the onset of voluntary movements appear variable and task specific in asymptomatic individuals (Andersson et al 1995, Oddsson et al 1999). It has been demonstrated that combinations of planned tasks with unexpected perturbation could cause some conflict between the two commands that may increase the risk of injury or motor control errors (Oddsson et al 1999). In addition, pain or prior injury to musculoskeletal tissues containing mechanoreceptors may also provide inaccurate information to the motor control system creating a mechanism for motor control errors and further injury to musculoskeletal tissue (De Luca 1993, Hodges & Richardson 1998, Mientjes & Frank 1999, Radebold et al 2000, Solomonow et al 2001, Takala et al 1997).

Through analysis of asymptomatic individuals during self-perturbation of an extremity, the transversus abdominis (TrA) and internal oblique (IO) have been identified as acting in a feed-forward or preparatory manner (Hodges & Richardson 1996, 1997b, 1999, Hodges et al 1999). It also appears that activation of the TrA and IO may be a general response to disturbance of the centre of mass, as their activation was not direction or movement specific (Aruin & Latash 1995, Hodges & Richardson 1997a). This preparatory activation of the TrA may contribute to control of spinal segmental motion, which theoretically is necessary to prepare the spine for contraction of other musculature. It follows from this discussion that the trunk musculature would require appropriate recruitment and timing to maintain stability of the spine during static posturing and movement (Cholewicki et al 1997, Gardner-Morse & Stokes 1998, Hodges & Richardson 1996). In turn, this would require accurate and timely information from the mechanoreceptors in the spine to allow for appropriate adjustments of the trunk musculature via the motor control system to maintain spinal stability.

A number of studies compared postural control of asymptomatic individuals to patients with LBP. Results of studies employing unilateral self-perturbation of the limbs suggest that there is a dysfunction in the motor control system related to delayed activation of the transverse abdominis muscle group in chronic LBP subjects. This delayed activation of the TrA could be a contributing factor to the inability to stabilize the spine (Hodges 2001, Hodges & Richardson 1996, 1997b). In a sudden trunk loading paradigm, patients with LBP demonstrated delayed onset latencies of trunk muscles. In addition, LBP subjects responded with a pattern of trunk muscle co-contraction instead of the selected directional response utilized by healthy subjects (Magnusson et al 1996, Radebold et al 2000, 2001, Wilder et al 1996). These prolonged latencies and co-contraction patterns may represent a motor control adaptation for enhancing lumbar stability or an impairment making it difficult for patients to cope safely with sudden and unexpected loading.

Impairments in standing postural control have been reported in patients with LBP (Mientjes & Frank 1999, Takala et al 1997). Increased body sway has been related to dysfunction in proprioception stemming from damage or injury to lumbar spine tissue containing mechanoreceptors. Similar findings were reported for sitting balance, with LBP patients performing significantly poorer especially with increased seat instability and lack of visual feedback (Radebold et al 2001). This finding appears to support the notion that proprioceptive input is somehow altered in patients with LBP, as absence of visual feedback increases the challenge to postural control. Significant correlations between poor sitting balance with eyes closed and longer trunk muscle response latencies to a sudden load release (Radebold et al 2001) support the hypothesis that altered gross motor control stems from nociceptive stimuli or poor proprioception. This hypothesis is further supported by studies that have documented poor lumbar position sense (Gill & Callaghan 1998, Parkhurst & Burnett 1994, Taimela et al 1999) and longer psychomotor reaction speed (Luoto et al 1996, 1999, Taimela et al 1993) in patients with mechanical LBP. Thus, studies testing spinal reflexes and brain stem pathways of the motor control system reveal alterations of both the feed-forward and feedback neuromotor strategies in patients with LBP.

Cause or effect?

While it is well documented that differences in motor control parameters do exist in individuals with mechanical LBP, it is not known at this time whether these differences are the cause or effect of LBP. Longitudinal prospective studies are necessary to answer this question, but to date none have been published.

Impaired proprioception in the lumbar spine, delayed trunk muscle reflex response and poor postural control may represent predisposing factors to the development of LBP by hindering proper responses to dynamic loading and failure to provide adequate stability to the spine. Individuals susceptible to LBP could inherently possess those risk factors or acquire them after the first episode of back injury (Fig. 7.9). For example, the subjects used in a majority of the studies were classified as having chronic LBP and may

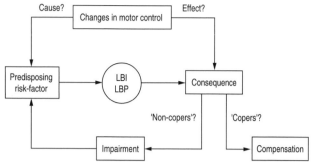

Figure 7.9 A diagram of the relationship between low back pain (LBP) or injury (LBI) and motor control changes documented in literature. It is currently not known whether the differences in motor control in LBP patients are the cause or effect of LBP. Furthermore, one of the most important clinical questions is which changes constitute functional adaptation and which are impairment ('copers' vs 'non-copers')

represent those who are unable to develop appropriate mechanisms via the active and motor control subsystems to allow for pain-free function of the spine ('non-copers'). On the other hand, one study that reported similar motor control changes in first-time injured athletes in spite of their clinical and functional recovery raised the possibility of a chronic condition being a series of acute events (Cholewicki et al 2002b). The recovery of damaged mechanoreceptors and in turn motor control may take longer than functional recovery and subsidence of pain. This impairment, in turn, can further predispose an individual to sustain recurrent low back injuries. In fact, previous back trouble appears to be the best predictor of future LBP (Bigos et al 1991, Feyer et al 2000, Greene et al 2001, Schneider et al 2000).

The changes in motor control observed in LBP patients could also result from LBP. They could function as a compensation mechanism designed to stabilize the lumbar spine following injury or may be an impairment caused by LBP (Fig. 7.9). Damage or inflammation in tissues containing mechanoreceptors could alter their feedback and in turn impair motor control. Finally, changes in muscle recruitment pattern could also result from inhibition or hyperactivity of specific muscles due to pain (Edgerton et al 1996) or be caused by pain itself (Arendt-Nielsen et al 1996, Cobb et al 1975, Sterling et al 2001, Zedka et al 1999).

To our knowledge, only one prospective study addressed the causality issue of ankle joint instability and postural control (Tropp et al 1984). These authors found that poor performance in a postural control task resulted in a significantly higher risk of sustaining ankle sprain injury among professional soccer players. Thus, these results would suggest that impaired motor control is the cause of injuries, although extrapolation from the ankle joint to the spine is uncertain. In either case, intervention based upon restoring a functional and adequate motor control strategy may be beneficial to individuals demonstrating alterations

within this subsystem. Therefore, the next question arises, as to which motor control alterations constitute beneficial adaptation and which are a detrimental impairment.

Impairment or adaptation?

The differences in muscle recruitment or neuromuscular control seen between patients with LBP and asymptomatic individuals have been hypothesized to be either (a) a compensation for underlying spinal instability, passive structure damage or proprioceptive dysfunction (Lariviere et al 2000, Radebold et al 2000, van Dieën et al 2003), or (b) some impairment predisposing these patients to sustain recurrent injuries (Cholewicki et al 2002b, Hodges & Richardson 1996, O'Sullivan et al 1997a, 1998, Radebold et al 2000, Sihvonen et al 1997). Correct classification of patients based on the above possibilities is a critical step for the selection of effective therapy (Fig. 7.9). Perhaps interpretation of the changes in motor control depends on many individual factors in a particular patient. For example, in someone with acute LBP this altered pattern may display hyperactivity or inhibition secondary to pain, while in a chronic (non-inflammatory) LBP, such an alteration may suggest an inadequate adaptive response in an attempt to enhance stability over a multitude of tasks ('non-coper'). Answering this question would require follow-up studies of acute LBP patients and monitoring muscle activation patterns of chronic LBP patients across a large number of tasks and conditions.

What changes constitute an impairment and which are an adaptation? From a biomechanical perspective, this piece of the puzzle is currently missing and is difficult to define without a 'standard motor control pattern' or an in vivo measurement of spine stability. Methods that allow quantification of stability or stiffness of the trunk in relation to the trunk motor control pattern are in the early stages of development. Once this quantification is achieved, the interpretation is still difficult. If trunk stiffness or stability in LBP patients is higher than in asymptomatic individuals, does that mean they are co-contracting too much and creating excessive spine compression forces? If this is the case, perhaps assisting them to decrease muscle activity or achieve skilled co-contraction strategies that can provide increased trunk stability without the excessive compression penalty is the right course of action. However, if LBP patients actually require that much co-contraction to maintain spine stability, this may indicate significant tissue damage and adequate adaptation ('copers'). In this case, altering the co-contraction strategy may not be the best intervention.

From a clinical perspective, the answer may be as follows: if an alteration in muscle activation or motor control allows the individual to function in daily activities, at work or at play, we might label this alteration as an adaptation. However, if this individual is demonstrating functional limitations and/or disability, we may label this pattern as an impairment. In clinical practice, we are inclined to lean towards the impairment label, as most patients are seeking assistance because of pain, functional limitation and/or disability. We therefore assume that they are protecting injured structures, avoiding nociceptive stimulation or are unable to adequately compensate for their dysfunction using their present motor control strategies and are thus impaired. Clinically, acuity of symptoms along with other clinical measurements of physical impairments and function guide our decision related to intervention with a particular patient. Thus, lumping all altered muscle activation patterns or motor control changes into either an adaptation or an impairment may be a gross misinterpretation of both clinical and research findings.

CLINICAL RELEVANCE OF TRUNK STABILITY AND MOTOR CONTROL

Review of the current research related to trunk motor control reveals considerable variability in co-contraction strategies, activation patterns and timing of muscle activation in the asymptomatic population. In part, this has created some difficulties in the research arena related to determining 'standard' motor control strategies. In some ways, this variability should be expected because of the redundancy of the trunk musculature and complexity of the motor control system (Latash et al 2002). If we take skilled golfers for example, and compare their swings, we would find they generally adhered to a pattern of motion, but with slight variations in joint range, trajectory, segment coordination and timing. Yet these individuals still accomplish the same task with relatively equal skill. In much the same way, more than one co-contraction, activation or timing pattern may be capable of achieving adequate spinal stabilization. Similar findings are reported in the literature related to knee instability, where no single 'good compensation' strategy was adopted by patients with anterior cruciate ligament injury (Rudolph et al 1998).

Clinical assessment of trunk stability and motor control

One clinical problem is identifying those patients with mechanical low back pain who would most benefit from a motor control training approach, as LBP results from a combination of factors. Our current inability to determine which impairments are contributing to an individual's mechanical LBP has been an obstacle within the clinical community. Since most LBP patients present with multiple impairments, we have acquiesced in treating them with a multifaceted approach. The routine rehabilitation programme for a patient diagnosed with mechanical LBP may consist of bracing, lower extremity muscle stretching, trunk muscle strengthening and endurance exercises, postural exercises, dynamic stabilization exercises, general conditioning exercises, modalities for reduction of pain and inflammation and education in proper lifting techniques. At present, treatment is essentially global because it is unclear which particular interventions help improve individual patient outcomes.

Ideally, during the evaluation of a patient with LBP, the clinician attempts to determine the presence or absence of potential factors that may be contributing to mechanical low back dysfunction. These factors are then used to establish a diagnosis and treatment plan. The present limitation to this clinical decision making process as it relates to the spinal instability/motor control model of LBP is that clinical tests for the evaluation of trunk motor control (muscle recruitment patterns, proprioception and postural control) are in their infancy. Evaluation of muscle activation patterns has recently achieved some attention based primarily on the work of O'Sullivan, Richardson, Jull and colleagues (Jull & Richardson 2000, Jull et al 1993, O'Sullivan 2000, O'Sullivan et al 1997a, Richardson & Jull 2000). Assessment of trunk stability during self-perturbation of the extremities has been proposed by Van Dillen and co-workers (Van Dillen et al 2001, 1998). This assessment technique uses observation of spine kinematics, muscle palpation and symptom reproduction in several different trunk positions (sitting, lying and standing). If patients are unable to maintain a neutral lumbar position while performing self-perturbation, the clinician hypothesizes that a motor control deficit exists. A review of the literature would also suggest that assessment of trunk proprioception or sitting balance, particularly without visual feedback, might provide evidence of motor control dysfunction (Radebold et al 2001).

To our knowledge, these types of clinical assessment techniques are at the forefront of current LBP research and have yet to be systematically developed and tested for validity and reliability in diagnosing motor control dysfunction. To date, our ability in most cases to make a clear clinical diagnosis of a motor control dysfunction in LBP patients is limited to many assumptions. For further discussion of clinical examination techniques, we refer you to the current research and chapters 10, 22 and 31 in this text on lumbar spine motor control.

Implications for rehabilitation strategies

Despite our inability to determine whether motor control differences are a risk factor for the development of LBP or the effect of injury and pain, a treatment approach for mechanical LBP has been developed based on Panjabi's model (Panjabi 1992a). According to this model, the muscular and motor control subsystems are trained to 'appropriately' control and stabilize the spine (Fritz et al 1998, Norris 1995, O'Sullivan et al 1997b, Richardson & Jull 2000, Saal & Saal 1989). Several studies have demonstrated the benefits of addressing motor control in the treatment of LBP. Patients receiving treatment programmes directed toward enhancing motor control demonstrated significantly less pain, a faster return to function, and had fewer reoccurrences of LBP at follow-up (Hides et al 2001, O'Sullivan et al 1997b, 1998, Sihvonen et al 1997). Thus, it may be possible to train the motor control system to provide sufficient dynamic stability to a mechanically compromised lumbar spine (Hides et al 2001). What remains inconclusive is whether such treatment truly improves the parameters of motor control such as muscle reaction times or patterns of activation. Improvements with these protocols may be due to other effects of training such as increased muscle strength or endurance, mood elevation, biochemical changes or modulation of pain. Only one study to date has demonstrated improved reaction times to match those of healthy control subjects during unexpected perturbation following a specialized rehabilitation programme (Wilder et al 1996).

According to the spine stability/motor control model and given the fact that all trunk muscles contribute to spinal stability (Cholewicki & VanVliet 2002), it would appear that training of the entire neuromotor apparatus might be more beneficial than focusing on individual muscle training. Given the variability of the motor control system (Latash et al 2002) and the redundancy in the trunk musculature, there may be more than one effective muscle activation pattern with which spine stability can be achieved. Recently, several rehabilitation strategies based on 'stabilization training' have been introduced (Norris 1995, O'Sullivan 2000, Richardson & Jull 2000, Saal & Saal 1989, Saal et al 1990). The aim of these strategies is to help individuals to develop better control of the trunk muscles so that they can be adequately recruited during physical activities. The lack of a 'gold standard' compensatory muscle activation strategy creates complications for designing treatment programmes to improve lumbar spine stability. As such, successful training strategies have to provide the opportunity for development of individualized compensatory patterns of the trunk musculature. This raises some questions regarding the effectiveness of programmes that emphasize one specific motor control training pattern.

Another aspect of a rehabilitation programme is the intensity of exercise. The research suggests that trunk muscle co-contractions at 1–2% MVC for a healthy spine, 2–5% MVC for a compromised spine or at most 10–25% MVC (Cholewicki & McGill 1996, Cholewicki et al 1997, Cresswell & Thorstensson 1994) are sufficient to stabilize the spine. Thus, traditional strengthening protocols (high load, low repetitions) may not be necessary to achieve adequate spine stabilization over the course of daily activities. Because large muscle forces are not typically required for daily function, it would appear that effective spine stabilization requires the ability to co-contract trunk muscles at low levels over long periods of time and under a variety of postures and tasks. In addition, we argued earlier that circumstances involving sudden spine motion and lower loads leave more room for motor control errors. Thus, the exercise prescription should lean toward the parameters of muscle endurance (low load, high repetitions), with emphasis on dynamic not static endurance activities.

Muscle timing and postural control are also important factors to maintaining appropriate spine stability particularly in the event of support surface unsteadiness and sudden or unexpected loading. Thus, dynamic exercises that challenge these particular parameters would be an important component of motor control rehabilitation. Again, we believe that these exercises should be completed in a way that allows the patient to develop their own stabilization strategies. This follows the line of intervention being proposed and tested regarding the rehabilitation of individuals with ankle, knee and shoulder instabilities (Beard et al 1994, Davies & Dickoff-Hoffman 1993, Eils & Rosenbaum 2001, Fitzgerald 1998, Maitland et al 1999, Rozzi et al 1999, Wilk et al 2002).

One would also expect that a learning process exists that may start with patients responding to these dynamic situations with gross co-contraction of the trunk musculature and eventually progressing to more skilled co-contraction patterns to achieve the desired control and stability. The motor learning theory of Bernstien hypothesizes that initial solutions to motor control problems result in 'freezing out' a portion of the degrees of freedom (Vereijken et al 1992a, 1992b). This 'freezing out' could be accomplished by keeping the joints or segments rigidly fixed, allowing little to no motion, or by coupling of several degrees of freedom to form a joint complex. Improvement in skill would then be characterized by gradually reducing gross co-contraction or freeing degrees of freedom and moving towards compensatory synergistic muscle patterns during dynamic activities (Vereijken et al 1992a, 1992b). Evidence of a gross co-contraction strategy in mechanical LBP subjects has been reported by several investigators (Lariviere et al 2000, Marras et al 2001, Radebold et al 2000, van Dieën et al 2003).

Further discussion of stabilization exercises, motor control training programmes and recommended progression is contained in chapters 22 and 31 in this text. Concerns related to spine compressive and shear forces arising with muscle co-contraction exercises were addressed in the recent research by several authors (Allison et al 1998, Arokoski et al 1999, 2001, 2002, Axler & McGill 1997, Callaghan et al 1998, McGill 1998, Vera-Garcia et al 2000).

The motor control assessment and treatment techniques described in this chapter are in their relative infancy. Further controlled studies are required to determine their diagnostic and prognostic value and the treatment efficacy they afford. Only recently, research tools have been developed to test the model of low back injury and pain based on motor control of lumbar spine stability. However, the hypotheses spawned from this model have already charted new directions in the prevention, diagnosis and rehabilitation of low back pain.

KEYWORDS	
lumbar spine	motor control
biomechanics	low back pain
stability	

Acknowledgment

The authors would like to acknowledge their financial support from the National Institutes of Health, grant 1R01 AR 46844-01A1.

References

Adams M A, Hutton W C 1982a The mechanics of prolapsed intervertebral disc. International Orthopaedics 6: 249–253

Adams M A, Hutton W C 1982b Prolapsed intervertebral disc: a hyper-flexion injury. 1981 Volvo Award in basic science. Spine 7: 184–191

Adams M A, Hutton W C 1986 Has the lumbar spine a margin of safety in forward bending? Clinical Biomechanics 1: 3–6

Adams M A, Hutton W C, Stott J R 1980 The resistance to flexion of the lumbar intervertebral joint. Spine 5: 245–253

Ahlgren S A, Hansen T 1978 The use of lumbosacral corsets prescribed for low back pain. Prosthetics and Orthotics International 2: 101–104

Alaranta H, Hurri H 1988 Compliance and subjective relief by corset treatment in chronic low back pain. Scandinavian Journal of Rehabilitation Medicine 20: 133–136

Allison G T, Godfrey P, Robinson G 1998 EMG signal amplitude assessment during abdominal bracing and hollowing. Journal of Electromyography and Kinesiology 8: 51–57

Andersson E, Oddsson L, Grundstrom H, Thorstensson A 1995 The role of the psoas and iliacus muscles for stability and movement of the lumbar spine, pelvis and hip. Scandinavian Journal of Medicine and Science in Sports 5: 10–16

Arendt-Nielsen L, Graven-Nielsen T, Svarrer H, Svensson P 1996 The influence of low back pain on muscle activity and coordination during gait: a clinical and experimental study. Pain 64: 231–240

Arokoski J P, Kankaanpaa M, Valta T et al 1999 Back and hip extensor muscle function during therapeutic exercises. Archives of Physical Medicine and Rehabilitation 80: 842–850

Arokoski J P, Valta T, Airaksinen O, Kankaanpaa M 2001 Back and abdominal muscle function during stabilization exercises. Archives of Physical Medicine and Rehabilitation 82: 1089–1098

Arokoski J P, Valta T, Kankaanpaa M, Airaksinen O 2002 Activation of paraspinal and abdominal muscles during manually assisted and non-assisted therapeutic exercise. American Journal of Physical Medicine and Rehabilitation 81: 326–335

Aruin A S, Latash M L 1995 Directional specificity of postural muscles in feed-forward postural reactions during fast voluntary arm movements. Experimental Brain Research 103: 323–332

Ashton-Miller J A, Schultz A B 1991 Spine instability and segmental hypermobility biomechanics: a call for the definition and standard use of terms. Seminars in Spine Surgery 3: 136–148

Axelsson P, Johnsson R, Stromqvist B 1992 Effect of lumbar orthosis on intervertebral mobility: a roentgen stereophotogrammetric analysis. Spine 17: 678–681

Axelsson P, Johnsson R, Stromqvist B, Nilsson L T, Akesson M 1995 Orthosis as prognostic instrument in lumbar fusion: no predictive value in 50 cases followed prospectively. Journal of Spinal Disorders 8: 284–288

Axler C T, McGill S M 1997 Low back loads over a variety of abdominal exercises: searching for the safest abdominal challenge. Medicine and Science in Sports and Exercise 29: 804–811

Bartelink D L 1957 The role of abdominal pressure in relieving the pressure on the lumbar intervertebral discs. Journal of Bone and Joint Surgery (British volume) 39: 718–725

Bean J C, Chaffin D B, Schultz A B 1988 Biomechanical model calculation of muscle contraction forces: a double linear programming method. Journal of Biomechanics 21: 59–66

Beard D J, Dodd C A, Trundle H R, Simpson A H 1994 Proprioception enhancement for anterior cruciate ligament deficiency: a prospective randomised trial of two physiotherapy regimes. Journal of Bone and Joint Surgery (British volume) 76: 654–659

Bergmark A 1989 Stability of the lumbar spine: a study in mechanical engineering. Acta Orthopaedica Scandinavica 230(Suppl.): 1–54

Bigos S J, Spengler D M, Martin N A et al 1986 Back injuries in industry: a retrospective study. II: Injury factors. Spine 11: 246–251

Bigos S J, Battie M C, Spengler D M et al 1991 A prospective study of work perceptions and psychosocial factors affecting the report of back injury [published erratum appears in Spine 1991 16(6): 688]. Spine 16: 1–6

Bourne N D, Reilly T 1991 Effect of a weightlifting belt on spinal shrinkage. British Journal of Sports Medicine 25: 209–212

Brinckmann P, Biggemann M, Hilweg D 1989 Prediction of the compressive strength of human lumbar vertebrae. Spine. 14: 606–610

Buchalter D, Kahanovitz N, Viola K, Dorsky S, Nordin M 1988 Three-dimensional spinal motion measurements. 2: A noninvasive assessment of lumbar brace immobilization of the spine. Journal of Spinal Disorders 1: 284–286

Callaghan J P, Gunning J L, McGill S M 1998 The relationship between lumbar spine load and muscle activity during extensor exercises. Physical Therapy 78: 8–18

Cherkin D C, Deyo R A, Volinn E, Loeser J D 1992 Use of the International Classification of Diseases (ICD-9-CM) to identify hospitalizations for mechanical low back problems in administrative databases. Spine 17: 817–825

Cholewicki J, McGill S M 1992 Lumbar posterior ligament involvement during extremely heavy lifts estimated from fluoroscopic measurements. Journal of Biomechanics 25: 17–28

Cholewicki J, McGill S M 1994 EMG assisted optimization: a hybrid approach for estimating muscle forces in an indeterminate biomechanical model. Journal of Biomechanics 27: 1287–1289

Cholewicki J, McGill S M 1995 Relationship between muscle force and stiffness in the whole mammalian muscle: a simulation study. Journal of Biomechanical Engineering 117: 339–342

Cholewicki J, McGill S M 1996 Mechanical stability of the in vivo lumbar spine: implications for injury and chronic low back pain. Clinical Biomechanics 11: 1–15

Cholewicki J, VanVliet J Jr 2002 Relative contribution of trunk muscles to the stability of the lumbar spine during isometric exertions. Clinical Biomechanics 17: 99–105

Cholewicki J, McGill S M, Norman R W 1991 Lumbar spine loads during the lifting of extremely heavy weights. Medicine and Science in Sports and Exercise 23: 1179–1186

Cholewicki J, McGill S M, Norman R W 1995 Comparison of muscle forces and joint load from an optimization and EMG assisted lumbar spine model: towards development of a hybrid approach. Journal of Biomechanics 28: 321–331

Cholewicki J, Panjabi M M, Khachatryan A 1997 Stabilizing function of trunk flexor-extensor muscles around a neutral spine posture. Spine 22: 2207–2212

Cholewicki J, Juluru K, McGill S M 1999a Intra-abdominal pressure mechanism for stabilizing the lumbar spine. Journal of Biomechanics 32: 13–17

Cholewicki J, Juluru K, Radebold A, Panjabi M M, McGill S M 1999b Lumbar spine stability can be augmented with an abdominal belt and/or increased intra-abdominal pressure. European Spine Journal 8: 388–395

Cholewicki J, Simons A P D, Radebold A 2000 Effects of external trunk loads on lumbar spine stability. Journal of Biomechanics 33: 1377–1385

Cholewicki J, Ivancic P C, Radebold A 2002a Can increased intra-abdominal pressure in humans be decoupled from trunk muscle co-contraction during steady state isometric exertions? European Journal of Applied Physiology 87: 127–133

Cholewicki J, Polzhofer G K, Galloway M T, Greene H S, Shah R A, Radebold A 2002b Neuromuscular function in athletes following recovery from an acute low back injury. Journal of Orthopaedic and Sports Physical Therapy 32: 569–576

Ciriello V M, Snook S H 1995 The effect of back belts on lumbar muscle fatigue. Spine 20: 1271–1278

Cobb C R, deVries H A, Urban R T, Luekens C A, Bagg R J 1975 Electrical activity in muscle pain. American Journal of Physical Medicine 54: 80–87

Cresswell A G, Thorstensson A 1989 The role of the abdominal musculature in the elevation of the intra-abdominal pressure during specified tasks. Ergonomics 32: 1237–1246

Cresswell A G, Thorstensson A 1994 Changes in intra-abdominal pressure, trunk muscle activation and force during isokinetic lifting and lowering. European Journal of Applied Physiology and Occupational Physiology 68: 315–321

Cresswell A G, Grundstrom H, Thorstensson A 1992 Observations on intra-abdominal pressure and patterns of abdominal intra-muscular activity in man. Acta Physiologica Scandinavica 144: 409–418

Cresswell A G, Oddsson L, Thorstensson A 1994 The influence of sudden perturbations on trunk muscle activity and intra-abdominal pressure while standing. Experimental Brain Research 98: 336–341

Crisco J J 3rd, Panjabi M M 1991 The intersegmental and multisegmental muscles of the lumbar spine: a biomechanical model comparing lateral stabilizing potential. Spine 16: 793–799

Crisco J J, Panjabi M M, Yamamoto I, Oxland T R 1992 Euler stability of the human ligamentous lumbar spine. II: Experiment. Clinical Biomechanics 7: 27–32

Cyron B M, Hutton W C, Stott J R 1979 Spondylolysis: the shearing stiffness of the lumbar intervertebral joint. Acta Orthopaedica Belgica 45: 459–469

Daggfeldt K, Thorstensson A 1997 The role of intra-abdominal pressure in spinal unloading. Journal of Biomechanics 30: 1149–1155

Damkot D K, Pope M H, Lord J, Frymoyer J W 1984 The relationship between work history, work environment and low-back pain in men. Spine 9: 395–399

Davies G J, Dickoff-Hoffman S 1993 Neuromuscular testing and rehabilitation of the shoulder complex. Journal of Orthopaedic and Sports Physical Therapy 18: 449–458

Davis K G, Marras W S, Walters T R 1998 Evaluation of spinal loading during lowering and lifting. Clinical Biomechanics 13: 141–152

De Luca D J 1993 Use of the surface EMG signal for performance evaluation of back muscles. Nerve Muscle 16: 210–216

Deyo R A, Weinstein J N 2001 Primary care: low back pain. New England Journal of Medicine 344: 363–370

Diener H C, Bootz F, Dichgans J, Bruzek W 1983 Variability of postural 'reflexes' in humans. Experimental Brain Research 52: 423–428

Edgerton V R, Wolf S L, Levendowski D J, Roy R R 1996 Theoretical basis for patterning EMG amplitudes to assess muscle dysfunction. Medicine and Science in Sports and Exercise 28: 744–751

Eils E, Rosenbaum D 2001 A multi-station proprioceptive exercise program in patients with ankle instability. Medicine and Science in Sports and Exercise 33: 1991–1998

Fairbank J C, O'Brien J P, Davis P R 1980 Intraabdominal pressure rise during weight lifting as an objective measure of low-back pain. Spine 5: 179–184

Feyer A M, Herbison P, Williamson A M et al 2000 The role of physical and psychological factors in occupational low back pain: a prospective cohort study. Occupational and Environmental Medicine 57: 116–120

Fidler M W, Plasmans C M 1983 The effect of four types of support on the segmental mobility of the lumbosacral spine. Journal of Bone and Joint Surgery (American volume) 65: 943–947

Fitzgerald G 1998 Non-operative anterior cruciate ligament rehabilitation for individuals participating in high level physical activity. Rehabilitation Sciences 165. Allegheny University of the Health Sciences, Philadelphia

Frank J W, Kerr M S, Brooker A S et al 1996 Disability resulting from occupational low back pain. I: What do we know about primary prevention? A review of the scientific evidence on prevention before disability begins. Spine 21: 2908–2917

Fritz J M, Erhard R E, Hagen B F 1998 Segmental instability of the lumbar spine. Physical Therapy 78: 889–896

Frymoyer J W, Pope M H, Clements J H, Wilder D G, MacPherson B, Ashikaga T 1983 Risk factors in low-back pain: an epidemiological survey. Journal of Bone and Joint Surgery (American volume) 65: 213–218

Gardner-Morse M G, Stokes I A 1998 The effects of abdominal muscle co-activation on lumbar spine stability. Spine 23: 86–91

Gardner-Morse M, Stokes I A, Laible J P 1995 Role of muscles in lumbar spine stability in maximum extension efforts. Journal of Orthopaedic Research 13: 802–808

Gielen C C, Houk J C 1987 A model of the motor servo: incorporating nonlinear spindle receptor and muscle mechanical properties. Biological Cybernetics 57: 217–231

Gill K P, Callaghan M J 1998 The measurement of lumbar proprioception in individuals with and without low back pain. Spine 23: 371–377

Gracovetsky S, Farfan H, Helleur C 1985 The abdominal mechanism. Spine 10: 317–324

Gracovetsky S, Kary M, Pitchen I, Levy S, Ben Said R 1989 The importance of pelvic tilt in reducing compressive stress in the spine during flexion–extension exercises. Spine 14: 412–416

Gracovetsky S, Kary M, Levy S, Ben Said R, Pitchen I, Helie J 1990 Analysis of spinal and muscular activity during flexion/extension and free lifts. Spine 15: 1333–1339

Granata K P, Marras W S 1995 An EMG-assisted model of trunk loading during free-dynamic lifting. Journal of Biomechanics 28: 1309–1317

Granata K P, Marras W S 2000 Cost–benefit of muscle cocontraction in protecting against spinal instability. Spine 25: 1398–1404

Granata K P, Orishimo K F 2001 Response of trunk muscle co-activation to changes in spinal stability. Journal of Biomechanics 34: 1117–1123

Granata K P, Marras W S, Davis K G 1997 Biomechanical assessment of lifting dynamics, muscle activity and spinal loads while using three different styles of lifting belt. Clinical Biomechanics 12: 107–115

Granhed H, Jonson R, Hansson T 1989 Mineral content and strength of lumbar vertebrae: a cadaver study. Acta Orthopaedica Scandinavica 60: 105–109

Greene H S, Cholewicki J, Galloway M T, Nguyen C V, Radebold A 2001 A history of low back injury is a risk factor for recurrent back injuries in varsity athletes. American Journal of Sports Medicine 29: 795–800

Grenier N, Greselle J F, Vital J M et al 1989 Normal and disrupted lumbar longitudinal ligaments: correlative MR and anatomic study. Radiology 171: 197–205

Hamaoui A, Do M, Poupard L, Bouisset S 2002 Does respiration perturb body balance more in chronic low back pain subjects than in healthy subjects? Clinical Biomechanics (Bristol, Avon) 17: 548

Harman E A, Rosenstein R M, Frykman P N, Nigro G A 1989 Effects of a belt on intra-abdominal pressure during weight lifting. Medicine and Science in Sports and Exercise 21: 186–190

Hatta I, Sugi H, Tamura Y 1988 Stiffness changes in frog skeletal muscle during contraction recorded using ultrasonic waves. Journal of Physiology 403: 193–209

Hemborg B, Moritz U 1985 Intra-abdominal pressure and trunk muscle activity during lifting. II: Chronic low-back patients. Scandinavian Journal of Rehabilitation Medicine 17: 5–13

Hides J A, Jull G A, Richardson C A 2001 Long-term effects of specific stabilizing exercises for first-episode low back pain. Spine 26: E243–248

Hodges P W 2001 Changes in motor planning of feed-forward postural responses of the trunk muscles in low back pain. Experimental Brain Research 141: 261–266

Hodges P W, Richardson C A 1996 Inefficient muscular stabilization of the lumbar spine associated with low back pain: a motor control evaluation of transversus abdominis. Spine 21: 2640–2650

Hodges P W, Richardson C A 1997a Feed-forward contraction of transversus abdominis is not influenced by the direction of arm movement. Experimental Brain Research 114: 362–370

Hodges P W, Richardson C A 1997b Contraction of the abdominal muscles associated with movement of the lower limb. Physical Therapy 77: 132–142; discussion 142–134

Hodges P W, Richardson C A 1998 Delayed postural contraction of transversus abdominis in low back pain associated with movement of the lower limb. Journal of Spinal Disorders 11: 46–56

Hodges P W, Richardson C A 1999 Altered trunk muscle recruitment in people with low back pain with upper limb movement at different speeds. Archives of Physical Medicine and Rehabilitation 80: 1005–1012

Hodges P, Cresswell A, Thorstensson A 1999 Preparatory trunk motion accompanies rapid upper limb movement. Experimental Brain Research 124: 69–79

Hodges P W, Cresswell A G, Daggfeldt K, Thorstensson A 2001 In vivo measurement of the effect of intra-abdominal pressure on the human spine. Journal of Biomechanics 34: 347–353

Hogan N 1990 Mechanical impedance of single- and multi-articular systems. In: Winters J M, Woo S L (eds) Multiple muscle systems: biomechanics and movement organization. Springer-Verlag, New York, pp 149–164.

Holmström E, Moritz U 1992 Effects of lumbar belts on trunk muscle strength and endurance: a follow-up study of construction workers. Journal of Spinal Disorders 5: 260–266

Huang Q M, Hodges P W, Thorstensson A 2001 Postural control of the trunk in response to lateral support surface translations during trunk movement and loading. Experimental Brain Research 141: 552–559

Hughes R E, Bean J C, Chaffin D B 1995 Evaluating the effect of co-contraction in optimization models. Journal of Biomechanics 28: 875–878

Hughes R E, Bean J C, Chaffin D B 2001 A method for classifying co-contraction of lumbar muscle activity. Journal of Applied Biomechanics 17: 253–258

Hutton W C, Cyron B M, Stott J R 1979 The compressive strength of lumbar vertebrae. Journal of Anatomy 129: 753–758

Ivancic P C, Cholewicki J, Radebold A 2002 Effects of the abdominal belt on muscle-generated spinal stability and L4/L5 joint compression force. Ergonomics 45: 501–513

Jackson M, Solomonow M, Zhou B, Baratta R V, Harris M 2001 Multifidus EMG and tension–relaxation recovery after prolonged static lumbar flexion. Spine 26: 715–723

Janevic J, Ashton-Miller J A, Schultz A B 1991 Large compressive preloads decrease lumbar motion segment flexibility. Journal of Orthopaedic Research 9: 228–236

Jellema P, van Tulder M W, van Poppel M N, Nachemson A L, Bouter L M 2001 Lumbar supports for prevention and treatment of low back pain: a systematic review within the framework of the Cochrane Back Review Group. Spine 26: 377–386

Jonsson B 1978 Kinesiology: with special reference to electromyographic kinesiology. Electroencephalography and Clinical Neurophysiology 34 (Suppl.): 417–428

Jull G A, Richardson C A 2000 Motor control problems in patients with spinal pain: a new direction for therapeutic exercise. Journal of Manipulative and Physiological Therapeutics 23: 115–117

Jull G, Richardson, C A, Toppenberg R, Comerford M, Bui B 1993 Towards a measurement of active muscle control for lumbar stabilisation. Australian Physiotherapy 39: 187–193

Keith A 1923 Man's posture: its evolution and disorders. Lecture IV: The adaptations of the abdomen and its viscera to the orthograde posture. British Medical Journal I: 587–590

Kelsey J L, Githens P B, White A A D et al 1984 An epidemiologic study of lifting and twisting on the job and risk for acute prolapsed lumbar intervertebral disc. Journal of Orthopaedic Research 2: 61–66

Kerr M S, Frank J W, Shannon H S et al 2001 Biomechanical and psychosocial risk factors for low back pain at work. American Journal of Public Health 91: 1069–1075

Kingma I, de Looze M P, van Dieën J H, Toussaint H M, Adams M A, Baten C T 1998 When is a lifting movement too asymmetric to identify low-back loading by 2-D analysis? Ergonomics 41: 1453–1461

Kumar S 2001 Theories of musculoskeletal injury causation. Ergonomics 44: 17–47

Lander J E, Simonton R L, Giacobbe J K 1990 The effectiveness of weight-belts during the squat exercise. Medicine and Science in Sports and Exercise 22: 117–126

Lander J E, Hundley J R, Simonton R L 1992 The effectiveness of weight-belts during multiple repetitions of the squat exercise. Medicine and Science in Sports and Exercise 24: 603–609

Lantz S A, Schultz A B 1986a Lumbar spine orthosis wearing. II: Effect on trunk muscle myoelectric activity. Spine 11: 838–842

Lantz S A, Schultz A B 1986b Lumbar spine orthosis wearing. I: Restriction of gross body motions. Spine 11: 834–837

Lariviere C, Gagnon D, Loisel P 2000 The comparison of trunk muscles EMG activation between subjects with and without chronic low back pain during flexion–extension and lateral bending tasks. Journal of Electromyography and Kinesiology 10: 79–91

Latash M L, Scholz J P, Schoner G 2002 Motor control strategies revealed in the structure of motor variability. Exercise and Sport Sciences Reviews 30: 26–31

Lavender S A, Tsuang Y H, Andersson G B, Hafezi A, Shin C C 1992a Trunk muscle cocontraction: the effects of moment direction and moment magnitude. Journal of Orthopaedic Research 10: 691–700

Lavender S A, Tsuang Y H, Hafezi A, Andersson G B, Chaffin D B, Hughes R E 1992b Co-activation of the trunk muscles during asymmetric loading of the torso. Human Factors 34: 239–247

Lavender S A, Tsuang Y H, Andersson G B 1993 Trunk muscle activation and cocontraction while resisting applied moments in a twisted posture. Ergonomics 36: 1145–1157

Lee Y H, Kang S M 2002 Effect of belt pressure and breath held on trunk electromyography. Spine 27: 282–290

Leipholz H H E 1987 Stability theory: an introduction to the stability of dynamic systems and rigid bodies. John Wiley, Stuttgart

Lucas D B, Bresler B 1961 Stability of the ligamentous spine. Biomechanics Laboratory, University of California, San Francisco

Lund J P, Donga R, Widmer C G, Stohler C S 1991 The pain-adaptation model: a discussion of the relationship between chronic musculoskeletal pain and motor activity. Canadian Journal of Physiology and Pharmacology 69: 683–694

Luoto S, Taimela S, Hurri H, Aalto H, Pyykko I, Alaranta H 1996 Psychomotor speed and postural control in chronic low back pain patients: a controlled follow-up study. Spine 21: 2621–2627

Luoto S, Taimela S, Hurri H, Alaranta H 1999 Mechanisms explaining the association between low back trouble and deficits in information processing: a controlled study with follow-up. Spine 24: 255–261

McCowin P R, Borenstein D, Wiesel S W 1991 The current approach to the medical diagnosis of low back pain. Orthopedic Clinics of North America 22: 315–325

McGill S M 1992a A myoelectrically based dynamic three-dimensional model to predict loads on lumbar spine tissues during lateral bending. Journal of Biomechanics 25: 395–414

McGill S M B S 1992b Creep response of the lumbar spine to prolonged full flexion. Clinical Biomechanics 7: 43–48

McGill S M 1998 Low back exercises: evidence for improving exercise regimens. Physical Therapy 78: 754–765

McGill S M 1997 The biomechanics of low back injury: implications on current practice in industry and the clinic. Journal of Biomechanics 30: 465–475

McGill S M, Norman R W 1987 Reassessment of the role of intra-abdominal pressure in spinal compression. Ergonomics 30: 1565–1588

McGill S M, Norman R W 1988 Potential of lumbodorsal fascia forces to generate back extension moments during squat lifts [see comments]. Journal of Biomedical Engineering 10: 312–318

McGill S M, Sharratt M T 1990 Relationship between intra-abdominal pressure and trunk EMG. Clinical Biomechanics 5: 59–67

McGill S M, Norman R W, Sharratt M T 1990 The effect of an abdominal belt on trunk muscle activity and intra-abdominal pressure during squat lifts. Ergonomics 33: 147–160

McGill S, Seguin J, Bennett G 1994 Passive stiffness of the lumbar torso in flexion, extension, lateral bending, and axial rotation: effect of belt wearing and breath holding. Spine 19: 696–704

McGill S M, Sharratt M T, Seguin J P 1995 Loads on spinal tissues during simultaneous lifting and ventilatory challenge. Ergonomics 38: 1772–1792

McGill S M, Norman R W, Cholewicki J 1996 A simple polynomial that predicts low-back compression during complex 3-D tasks. Ergonomics 39: 1107–1118

McNair P J, Heine P J 1999 Trunk proprioception: enhancement through lumbar bracing. Archives of Physical Medicine and Rehabilitation 80: 96–99

Magnusson M L, Aleksiev A, Wilder D G et al 1996 Unexpected load and asymmetric posture as etiologic factors in low back pain. European Spine Journal 5: 23–35

Maitland M E, Ajemian S V, Suter E 1999 Quadriceps femoris and hamstring muscle function in a person with an unstable knee. Physical Therapy 79: 66–75

Majkowski G R, Jovag B W, Taylor B T et al 1998 The effect of back belt use on isometric lifting force and fatigue of the lumbar paraspinal muscles. Spine 23: 2104–2109

Manning D P, Mitchell R G, Blanchfield L P 1984 Body movements and events contributing to accidental and nonaccidental back injuries. Spine 9: 734–739

Mannion A F, Dolan P 1994 Electromyographic median frequency changes during isometric contraction of the back extensors to fatigue. Spine 19: 1223–1229

Marras W S, Mirka G A 1996 Intra-abdominal pressure during trunk extension motions. Clinical Biomechanics 11: 267–274

Marras W S, Lavender S A, Leurgans S E et al 1995 Biomechanical risk factors for occupationally related low back disorders. Ergonomics 38: 377–410

Marras W S, Jorgensen M J, Davis K G 2000 Effect of foot movement and an elastic lumbar back support on spinal loading during free-dynamic symmetric and asymmetric lifting exertions. Ergonomics 43: 653–668

Marras W S, Davis K G, Ferguson S A, Lucas B R, Gupta P 2001 Spine loading characteristics of patients with low back pain compared with asymptomatic individuals. Spine 26: 2566–2574

Mientjes M I, Frank J S 1999 Balance in chronic low back pain patients compared to healthy people under various conditions in upright standing. Clinical Biomechanics (Bristol, Avon) 14: 710–716

Miller J A, Schultz A B, Warwick D N, Spencer D L 1986 Mechanical properties of lumbar spine motion segments under large loads. Journal of Biomechanics 19: 79–84

Million R, Nilsen K H, Jayson M I, Baker R D 1981 Evaluation of low back pain and assessment of lumbar corsets with and without back supports. Annals of the Rheumatic Diseases 40: 449–454

Morgan D L 1977 Separation of active and passive components of short-range stiffness of muscle. American Journal of Physiology 232: C45–49

Morris J M, Lucas D B, Bresler B 1961 The role of trunk in stability of the spine. Journal of Bone and Joint Surgery (American volume) 43: 327–351

Nachemson A L, Andersson B J, Schultz A B 1986 Valsalva maneuver biomechanics: effects on lumbar trunk loads of elevated intraabdominal pressures. Spine 11: 476–479

Narloch J A, Brandstater M E 1995 Influence of breathing technique on arterial blood pressure during heavy weight lifting. Archives of Physical Medicine and Rehabilitation 76: 457–462

Nashner L M, Cordo P J 1981 Relation of automatic postural responses and reaction-time voluntary movements of human leg muscles. Experimental Brain Research 43: 395–405

Newcomer K, Laskowski E R, Yu B, Johnson J C, An K N 2001 The effects of a lumbar support on repositioning error in subjects with low back pain. Archives of Physical Medicine and Rehabilitation 82: 906–910

Norman R, Wells R, Neumann P et al 1998 A comparison of peak vs cumulative physical work exposure risk factors for the reporting of low back pain in the automotive industry. Clinical Biomechanics 13: 561–573

Norris C 1995 Spinal stabilization. 5: An exercise programme to enhance lumbar stabilization. Physiotherapy 81: 138–146

Oddsson L I, Persson T, Cresswell A G, Thorstensson A 1999 Interaction between voluntary and postural motor commands during perturbed lifting. Spine 24: 545–552

Ohana N, Sheinis D, Rath E, Sasson A, Atar D 2000 Is there a need for lumbar orthosis in mild compression fractures of the thoracolumbar spine? A retrospective study comparing the radiographic results between early ambulation with and without lumbar orthosis. Journal of Spinal Disorders 13: 305–308

Omino K, Hayashi Y 1992 Preparation of dynamic posture and occurrence of low back pain. Ergonomics 35: 693–707

O'Sullivan P B 2000 Lumbar segmental 'instability': clinical presentation and specific stabilizing exercise management. Manual Therapy 5: 2–12

O'Sullivan P, Twomey L, Allison G, Sinclair J, Miller K 1997a Altered patterns of abdominal muscle activation in patients with chronic low back pain. Australian Journal of Physiotherapy 43: 91–98

O'Sullivan P B, Twomey L T, Allison G T 1997b Evaluation of specific stabilizing exercise in the treatment of chronic low back pain with radiologic diagnosis of spondylolysis or spondylolisthesis. Spine 22: 2959–2967

O'Sullivan P B, Twomey L, Allison G T 1998 Altered abdominal muscle recruitment in patients with chronic back pain following a specific exercise intervention. Journal of Orthopaedic and Sports Physical Therapy 27: 114–124

Osvalder A L, Neumann P, Lövsund P, Nordwall A 1990 Ultimate strength of the lumbar spine in flexion – an in vitro study. Journal of Biomechanics 23: 453–460

Osvalder A L, Neumann P, Lövsund P, Nordwall A 1993 A method for studying the biomechanical load response of the (in vitro) lumbar spine under dynamic flexion–shear loads. Journal of Biomechanics 26: 1227–1236

Oxland T R, Panjabi M M 1992 The onset and progression of spinal injury: a demonstration of neutral zone sensitivity. Journal of Biomechanics 25: 1165–1172

Panjabi M M 1992a The stabilizing system of the spine. I: Function, dysfunction, adaptation, and enhancement. Journal of Spinal Disorders 5: 383–389

Panjabi M M 1992b The stabilizing system of the spine. II: Neutral zone and instability hypothesis. Journal of Spinal Disorders 5: 390–396

Paquet N, Malouin F, Richards C L 1994 Hip–spine movement interaction and muscle activation patterns during sagittal trunk movements in low back pain patients. Spine 19: 596–603

Parkhurst T M, Burnett C N 1994 Injury and proprioception in the lower back. Journal of Orthopaedic and Sports Physical Therapy 19: 282–295

Patwardhan A G, Havey R M, Meade K P, Lee B, Dunlap B 1999 A follower load increases the load-carrying capacity of the lumbar spine in compression. Spine 24: 1003–1009

Peach J P, Sutarno C G, McGill S M 1998 Three-dimensional kinematics and trunk muscle myoelectric activity in the young lumbar spine: a database. Archives of Physical Medicine and Rehabilitation 79: 663–669

Pope M H, Panjabi M 1985 Biomechanical definitions of spinal instability. Spine 10: 255–256

Pope M H, Magnusson M, Wilder D G 1998 Low back pain and whole body vibration. Clinical Orthopaedics and Related Research 354: 241–248

Porter R W, Adams M A, Hutton W C 1989 Physical activity and the strength of the lumbar spine. Spine 14: 201–203

Porth C J, Bamrah V S, Tristani F E, Smith J J 1984 The Valsalva maneuver: mechanisms and clinical implications. Heart and Lung 13: 507–518

Potvin J R 1997 Use of NIOSH equation inputs to calculate lumbosacral compression forces. Ergonomics 40: 691–707

Potvin J R, Norman R W, McGill S M 1991 Reduction in anterior shear forces on the L4/L5 disc by the lumbar musculature. Clinical Biomechanics 6: 88–96

Rabinowitz D, Bridger R S, Lambert M I 1998 Lifting technique and abdominal belt usage: a biomechanical, physiological and subjective investigation. Safety Science 28: 155–164

Rack P M, Westbury D R 1973 The short range stiffness of active mammalian muscle and its effect on mechanical properties. Journal of Physiology 229: 16P–17P

Rack P M, Westbury D R 1974 The short range stiffness of active mammalian muscle and its effect on mechanical properties. Journal of Physiology 240: 331–350

Radebold A, Cholewicki J, Panjabi M M, Patel T C 2000 Muscle response pattern to sudden trunk loading in healthy individuals and in patients with chronic low back pain. Spine 25: 947–954

Radebold A, Cholewicki J, Polzhofer G K, Greene H S 2001 Impaired postural control of the lumbar spine is associated with delayed muscle response times in patients with chronic idiopathic low back pain. Spine 26: 724–730

Ramos C F, Hacisalihzade S S, Stark L W 1990 Behaviour space of a stretch reflex model and its implications for the neural control of voluntary movement. Medical and Biological Engineering and Computing 28: 15–23

Reddell C R, Congleton J J, Huchingson R D, Montgomery J F 1992 An evaluation of a weightlifting belt and back injury prevention training class for airline baggage handlers. Applied Ergonomics 23: 319–329

Reyna J R J, Leggett S H, Kenney K, Holmes B, Mooney V 1995 The effect of lumbar belts on isolated lumbar muscle. Spine 20: 68–73

Richardson C A, Jull G A 2000 Muscle control–pain control: what exercises would you prescribe? Manual Therapy 1: 2–10

Rissanen P M 1960 The surgical anatomy and pathology of the supraspinous and interspinous ligaments of the lumbar spine, with special reference to ligament ruptures. Acta Orthopaedica Scandinavica 46(Suppl.): 1–100

Rohlmann A, Graichen F, Weber U, Bergmann G 2000 Monitoring in vivo implant loads with a telemeterized internal spinal fixation device. Spine 25: 2981–2986

Roland M O 1986 A critical review of the evidence for a pain–spasm–pain cycle in spinal disorders. Clinical Biomechanics 1: 102–109

Rozzi S L, Lephart S M, Sterner R, Kuligowski L 1999 Balance training for persons with functionally unstable ankles. Journal of Orthopaedic and Sports Physical Therapy 29: 478–486

Rudolph K S, Eastlack M E, Axe M J, Snyder-Mackler L 1998 Basmajian Student Award paper. Movement patterns after anterior cruciate

ligament injury: a comparison of patients who compensate well for the injury and those who require operative stabilization. Journal of Electromyography and Kinesiology 8: 349–362

Saal J A, Saal J S 1989 Nonoperative treatment of herniated lumbar intervertebral disc with radiculopathy: an outcome study. Spine 14: 431–437

Saal J A, Saal J S, Herzog R J 1990 The natural history of lumbar intervertebral disc extrusions treated nonoperatively. Spine 15: 683–686

Schneider G A, Bigelow C, Amoroso P J 2000 Evaluating risk of re-injury among 1214 army airborne soldiers using a stratified survival model. American Journal of Preventive Medicine 18: 156–163

Schultz A, Haderspeck K, Warwick D, Portillo D 1983 Use of lumbar trunk muscles in isometric performance of mechanically complex standing tasks. Journal of Orthopaedic Research 1: 77–91

Schwarzer A C, Aprill C N, Derby R, Fortin J, Kine G, Bogduk N 1995 The prevalence and clinical features of internal disc disruption in patients with chronic low back pain. Spine 20: 1878–1883

Sihvonen T, Partanen J, Hanninen O, Soimakallio S 1991 Electric behavior of low back muscles during lumbar pelvic rhythm in low back pain patients and healthy controls. Archives of Physical Medicine and Rehabilitation 72: 1080–1087

Sihvonen T, Lindgren K A, Airaksinen O, Manninen H 1997 Movement disturbances of the lumbar spine and abnormal back muscle electromyographic findings in recurrent low back pain. Spine 22: 289–295

Silfies S 2002 Trunk muscle and motor control impairments in patients with lumbar instability. Department of Rehabilitation Sciences 184. Drexel University, Philadelphia

Smith E B, Rasmussen A A, Lechner D E, Gossman M R, Quintana J B, Grubbs B L 1996 The effects of lumbosacral support belts and abdominal muscle strength on functional lifting ability in healthy women. Spine 21: 356–366

Solomonow M, Eversull E, He Zhou B, Baratta R V, Zhu M P 2001 Neuromuscular neutral zones associated with viscoelastic hysteresis during cyclic lumbar flexion. Spine 26: E314–324

Solomonow M, Zhou B, Baratta R V, Zhu M, Lu Y 2002 Neuromuscular disorders associated with static lumbar flexion: a feline model. Journal of Electromyography and Kinesiology 12: 81–90

Stein R B, Gordon T 1986 Nonlinear stiffness – force relationships in whole mammalian skeletal muscles. Canadian Journal of Physiology and Pharmacology 64: 1236–1244

Stein R B, Oguztoreli M N 1984 Modification of muscle responses by spinal circuitry. Neuroscience 11: 231–240

Sterling M, Jull G, Wright A 2001 The effect of musculoskeletal pain on motor activity and control. Journal of Pain 2: 135–145

Stokes I, Gardner-Morse M 1999 Lumbar spinal muscle activation synergies predicted by multi-criteria cost function. Proceedings of 45th Annual Meeting, Orthopaedic Research Society, Anaheim, California

Stokes I A, Gardner-Morse M, Churchill D, Laible J P 2002 Measurement of a spinal motion segment stiffness matrix. Journal of Biomechanics 35: 517–521

Sullivan M S, Mayhew T P 1995 The effect of lumbar support belts on isometric force production during a simulated lift. Journal of Occupational Rehabilitation 5: 131–143

Taimela S, Osterman K, Alaranta H, Soukka A, Kujala U M 1993 Long psychomotor reaction time in patients with chronic low-back pain: preliminary report. Archives of Physical Medicine and Rehabilitation 74: 1161–1164

Taimela S, Kankaanpaa M, Luoto S 1999 The effect of lumbar fatigue on the ability to sense a change in lumbar position: a controlled study. Spine 24: 1322–1327

Takala E-P, Korhonen I, Viikari-Juntura E 1997 Postural sway and stepping response among working population: reproducibility, long-term stability, and associations with symptoms of the low back. Clinical Biomechanics 12: 429–437

Tropp H, Ekstrand J, Gillquist J 1984 Stabilometry in functional instability of the ankle and its value in predicting injury. Medicine and Science in Sports and Exercise 16: 64–66

Troup J D, Martin J W, Lloyd D C 1981 Back pain in industry: a prospective survey. Spine 6: 61–69

Tuong N H, Dansereau J, Maurais G, Herrera R 1998 Three-dimensional evaluation of lumbar orthosis effects on spinal behavior. Journal of Rehabilitation Research and Development 35: 34–42

van Dieën J H, de Looze M P 1999a Directionality of anticipatory activation of trunk muscles in a lifting task depends on load knowledge. Experimental Brain Research 128: 397–404

van Dieën J H, de Looze M P 1999b Sensitivity of single-equivalent trunk extensor muscle models to anatomical and functional assumptions. Journal of Biomechanics 32: 195–198

van Dieën J H, Weinans H, Toussaint H M 1999 Fractures of the lumbar vertebral endplate in the etiology of low back pain: a hypothesis on the causative role of spinal compression in a specific low back pain. Medical Hypotheses 53: 246–252

van Dieën J H, Dekkers J J, Groen V, Toussaint H M, Meijer O G 2001 Within-subject variability in low back load in a repetitively performed, mildly constrained lifting task. Spine 26: 1799–1804

van Dieën J H, Cholewicki J, Radebold A 2003 Trunk muscle recruitment patterns in low back pain patients enhance the stability of the lumbar spine. Spine 28: 834–841

Van Dillen L R, Sahrmann S A, Norton B J et al 1998 Reliability of physical examination items used for classification of patients with low back pain. Physical Therapy 78: 979–988

Van Dillen L R, Sahrmann S A, Norton B J et al 2001 Effect of active limb movements on symptoms in patients with low back pain. Journal of Orthopaedic and Sports Physical Therapy 31: 402–413; discussion 414–408

van Poppel M N, de Looze M P, Koes B W, Smid T, Bouter L M 2000 Mechanisms of action of lumbar supports: a systematic review. Spine 25: 2103–2113

Vera-Garcia F J, Grenier S G, McGill S M 2000 Abdominal muscle response during curl-ups on both stable and labile surfaces. Physical Therapy 80: 564–569

Vereijken B, van Emmerik R, Whiting H, Newell K 1992a Free(z)ing degrees of freedom in skill acquisition. Journal of Motor Behavior 24: 133–142

Vereijken B, Whiting H T, Beek W J 1992b A dynamical systems approach to skill acquisition. Quarterly Journal of Experimental Psychology 45 A: 323–344

Walsh N E, Schwartz R K 1990 The influence of prophylactic orthoses on abdominal strength and low back injury in the workplace. American Journal of Physical Medicine and Rehabilitation 69: 245–250

Warren L P, Appling S, Oladehin A, Griffin J 2001 Effect of soft lumbar support belt on abdominal oblique muscle activity in nonimpaired adults during squat lifting. Journal of Orthopaedic and Sports Physical Therapy 31: 316–323

Wassell J T, Gardner L I, Landsittel D P, Johnston J J, Johnston J M 2000 A prospective study of back belts for prevention of back pain and injury. JAMA 284: 2727–2732

White III A, Panjabi M 1990 Clinical instability. In: White III A, Panjabi M (eds) Clinical biomechanics of the spine. Lippincott, Philadelphia, pp 342–360

Wilder D G, Aleksiev A R, Magnusson M L, Pope M H, Spratt K F, Goel V K 1996 Muscular response to sudden load: a tool to evaluate fatigue and rehabilitation. Spine 21: 2628–2639

Wilk K E, Meister K, Andrews J R 2002 Current concepts in the rehabilitation of the overhead throwing athlete. American Journal of Sports Medicine 30: 136–151

Winters J M 1995 An improved muscle-reflex actuator for use in large-scale neuro-musculoskeletal models. Annals of Biomedical Engineering 23: 359–374

Winters J, Stark L, Seif-Naraghi A H 1988 An analysis of the sources of musculoskeletal system impedance. Journal of Biomechanics 21: 1011–1025

Woldstad J C, Sherman B R 1998 The effects of a back belt on posture, strength, and spinal compressive force during static lift exertions. International Journal of Industrial Ergonomics 22: 409–416

Yettram A L, Jackman M J 1980 Equilibrium analysis for the forces in the human spinal column and its musculature. Spine 5: 402–411

Zahalak G I 1986 A comparison of the mechanical behavior of the cat soleus muscle with a distribution-moment model. Journal of Biomechanical Engineering 108: 131–140

Zahalak G I, Heyman S J 1979 A quantitative evaluation of frequency response characteristics of active human skeletal muscle in vivo. Journal of Biomechanical Engineering 101: 28–37

Zahalak G I, Ma S P 1990 Muscle activation and contraction: constitutive relations based directly on cross-bridge kinetics. Journal of Biomechanical Engineering 112: 52–62

Zajac F E, Winters J M 1990 Modeling musculoskeletal movement systems: joint and body segmental dynamics, musculoskeletal actuation, and neuromuscular control. In: Winters J M, Woo S L-Y (eds) Multiple muscle systems: biomechanics and movement organization: Springer-Verlag, New York, pp 121–148.

Zattara M, Bouisset S 1988 Posturo-kinetic organisation during the early phase of voluntary upper limb movement. 1: Normal subjects. Journal of Neurology, Neurosurgery and Psychiatry 51: 956–965

Zedka M, Prochazka A, Knight B, Gillard D, Gauthier M 1999 Voluntary and reflex control of human back muscles during induced pain. Journal of Physiology 520 (2): 591–604

Chapter 8

Clinical biomechanics of lifting

S. Milanese

INTRODUCTION

Despite the increasing use of risk management programmes in industry, musculoskeletal injuries attributed to manual handling remain a major burden to the community in terms of financial costs and human suffering (Waters & Putz Anderson 1996, Chaffin et al 1999). Mechanical low back pain in particular remains a major health and safety issue for both the clinic based and the industrial physiotherapist alike. The use of mechanization and ergonomic re-engineering in the production process and the popularity of manual handling training programmes for workers appears to have done little to reduce the prevalence of low back pain. Given the increasing role of physiotherapists in the design and implementation of manual handling risk management programmes, it is pertinent for us to revisit the scientific basis underpinning our understanding of the risks involved in manual handling.

A review of the epidemiological literature on low back pain (Hildebrandt 1987) found 24 work-related factors reported by at least one published source as being associated with low back pain. These factors reflected those of an earlier landmark review that identified that heavy physical loading, manual handling, including lifting, bending, twisting, sitting, sustained non-neutral postures and vehicular driving, were associated with an increased risk of low back pain (Magora 1973). Chaffin & Park reported that workers involved in heavy lifting were at least eight times more likely to report suffering back injuries as those workers performing sedentary work tasks (Chaffin & Park 1973).

Despite the published evidence, the role of occupational risk factors in the development of disc degeneration and low back pain remains controversial. It has been reported that familial aggregation, age and other unexplained factors might play a more important role in disc degeneration than occupational loading factors (Videman & Battie 1999). It would appear to be prudent to conclude at this stage, in the absence of conclusive evidence, that the causes for low back pain are multifactorial, as indeed are the optimal management approaches.

CHARACTERISTICS OF LIFTING TASKS

There are very few tasks performed in the work, home or recreational environments that do not involve manual handling of some description, whether involving relatively low weights (pens, television remote controls, etc.) or the larger loads handled in the heavy industries such as the mining and foundry industries. Manual handling is a term used to describe any activity that involves the generation of physical force by the person to complete the task – pushing, pulling, carrying, lifting, etc. This review will limit itself to the manual handling task of lifting.

All lifting tasks share common characteristics. Lifting involves the movement of an object from one location to another location, generally traversing both vertical and horizontal distances, and can be subdivided into three stages:

1. *Access*. The initial stage involves the lifter getting the hand(s) in a position on the load to allow control of the load during lifting. The need to access the load is the key driver for the posture that the body adopts at the commencement of the lift. Confined or cramped workspaces, for example aircraft luggage holds, will also affect the posture assumed in this stage.
2. *Movement*. Pure lifting – i.e. pure vertical movement of a load during lifting – is rare, with most lifting involving a dimension of horizontal movement. The direction of the horizontal movement should also be considered, as movements of the load in directions away from the sagittal plane will involve twisting and/or asymmetrical loading of the spine. Successful completion of this stage will depend on generation of sufficient force by the musculoskeletal system and results in the development of increased stress on the spine.
3. *Placement*. At the completion of the lift the lifter must control the load to a set destination. Factors affecting this stage of the lift include the speed of lifting, the location of the destination, the nature of the load and the precision required in placing the load.

APPROACHES USED TO STUDY THE EFFECT OF LIFTING

There are three approaches traditionally used to study the effect of lifting on the human body:

Physiological approach

This approach examines the physiological demands (heart rate, O_2 consumption, ventilatory rate, EMG and blood lactate levels) of lifting on the human body. The determinants of safe lifting in this approach include the minimization of the energy demands on the lifter, reducing the accumulation of physical fatigue that may contribute to musculoskeletal injury (Waters & Putz Anderson 1996).

Psychophysical approach

Psychophysics examines the relationship between the perception of human sensations and physical stimuli (Waters & Putz Anderson 1996). Proponents of this approach believe that the worker's actual level of workload can be assessed by his/her subjective judgement or perception of physical stress (Waters & Putz Anderson 1996). Typical studies involve the measurement of maximal acceptable weight limits (MAWL) for specific task conditions and for various workers. The results of such measures allow the generation of tables of acceptable weight limits for various segments of the population (Snook & Ciriello 1991). Jorgensen et al (1999) examined subjects performing sagittal lifting activities and correlated the psychophysical limits with both calculated biomechanical and measured physiological values. They observed that the decisions made by subjects when increasing and lowering weights towards a MAWL appeared to correlate with both the biomechanical and physiological parameters. They felt that the psychophysical approach allowed lifters to address more of the risks associated with all parts of the body rather than those specific to the low back as seen in the traditional biomechanics approach.

Biomechanical approach

Ethical and methodological constraints limit the capacity to measure internal loads on the body during manual handling activities by direct measurement methods (Langrana et al 1990). The biomechanical loads on the lumbar spine are one of the contributing factors to the occurrence of low back pain (Langrana et al 1990). The biomechanical approach involves 'the systematic application of engineering concepts to the functioning of the human body to predict the distribution of internal musculoskeletal forces resulting from the interaction with externally applied forces of the task' (Waters & Putz Anderson 1996). The human body is considered to be a system of mechanical links, each of a known physical size and form and these dimensions are used to construct biomechanical models, which reduce the complexity of the system to enhance understanding (Chaffin et al 1999). The complexity of the mathematical formulation and ease of use of the biomechanical models vary significantly between the different models. Important considerations when using or interpreting the findings from a biomechanical model are (Waters & Putz Anderson 1996):

- the mechanical nature of the model (static vs dynamic)
- dimensionality of the model (two- or three-dimensional)
- accuracy of the representation (single or multiple muscles, IAP (intra-abdominal pressure), muscle co-contraction, active and passive elements)
- complexity of the input needed to use the model (mechanical parameters, physiological measures of muscle function, musculoskeletal geometry).

From an engineering mechanics perspective, in a three-dimensional modelling system the complexity of the input data which can be accepted by the system will often be limited by its mathematical capacity (Langrana et al 1990). Early models used simple vector moments, incorporating simple lines of pull to represent the muscular elements in the model. Given the cross-sectional dimensions of the muscles and the dynamic nature of their recruitment this limited the accuracy of the models in predicting internal spinal loads (Davis & Mirka 2000). The use of more complex modelling systems has improved the accuracy of the model outputs; however, this remains an area of concern when defining the validity of any modelling system.

In general, for clinical purposes, a biomechanical model need only be as complex as is necessary to accurately and reasonably describe the nature of the loads occurring in the lumbar spine due to a particular work task, and often involves a trade-off between criteria of accuracy and realism versus simplicity and ease of use (Granata & Marras 1996).

Decisions on safe lifting limits are made by comparing the internal stresses calculated using biomechanical models, with the experimentally induced failure loads of specific spinal tissue. If the computed internal stresses that result from the application of a known external load fall under the experimentally induced failure load of the spinal tissue, then the lift is considered to be 'safe'. When the calculated internal stresses exceed the capacity of the tissue then it is hypothesized that injury will occur. Biomechanical models can then be used to develop or support risk control strategies that minimize the calculated stresses, allowing a safety zone during manual handling activities.

Integrated approaches

It is not surprising, given the different approaches used, that calculated safe lifting limits may conflict between the approaches (Dempsey 1998, Ayoub & Woldstad 1999). This

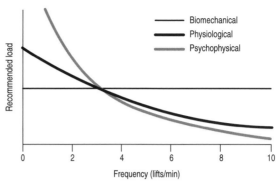

Figure 8.1 Example of conflicts among biomechanical, psychophysical and physiological criteria. Reproduced with permission from Ayoub & Woldstad 1999.

makes it difficult for the clinical practitioner to make a decision on proper safety limits for manual handling, as demonstrated in Figure 8.1. An attempt has been made to circumvent this problem with the development of integrated models. These models involve a unique approach that considers all three of the primary stress measures – biomechanical, physiological and psychophysical. A prime example of this approach is the revised National Institute for Occupational Safety and Health (NIOSH) lifting equation (Tables 8.1, 8.2, 8.3) (Waters et al 1994). The NIOSH lifting equation used population norms from the three approaches to develop the lifting model. The norms include:

1. *Biomechanical*: predicted maximum compressive forces on the L5/S1 should not exceed 3.4 kN.
2. *Physiological*: metabolic energy expenditure rates should not exceed safe limits (Table 8.4).
3. *Psychophysical*: safe limits should comply with the maximal acceptable weight limits of 75% of women and 99% of men.

Table 8.1 The revised NIOSH lifting equation (adapted from Waters et al 1994)

Revised NIOSH lifting equation RWL = LC × HM × VM × DM × AM × FM × CM	
Key to revised NIOSH lifting equation	
Lifting task descriptor	**Source**
Recommended weight limit (RWL)	
Load constant (LC): the maximum value for RWL	23 kg, 226 N
Horizontal multiplier (HM): related to horizontal distance from hand grip to body	25/H
Vertical multiplier (VM): related to height of load from ground level	1 − (0.003[V − 75])
Distance multiplier (DM): related to distance load moves vertically	0.82 + (4.5/D)
Asymmetry multiplier (AM): related to the angle of asymmetry from the mid-sagittal plane	1 − (0.0032 A)
Frequency multiplier (FM): related to the number of lifts per minute	See Table 8.2
Coupling multiplier (CM): related to the quality of the persons coupling with the load	See Table 8.3

Table 8.2 Frequency multiplier table for revised NIOSH lifting equation (reproduced with permission from Chaffin et al 1999)

Frequency Lifts/min (F)	Work duration					
	<1 hour		>1 but <2 hours		>2 but <8 hours	
	V<0.75	V>0.75	V<0.75	V>0.75	V<0.75	V>0.75
<0.2	1.00	1.00	0.95	0.95	0.85	0.85
0.5	0.97	0.97	0.92	0.92	0.81	0.81
1	0.94	0.94	0.88	0.88	0.75	0.75
2	0.91	0.91	0.84	0.84	0.65	0.65
3	0.88	0.88	0.79	0.79	0.55	0.55
4	0.84	0.84	0.72	0.72	0.45	0.45
5	0.8	0.8	0.60	0.60	0.35	0.35
6	0.75	0.75	0.50	0.50	0.27	0.27
7	0.70	0.70	0.42	0.42	0.22	0.22
8	0.60	0.60	0.35	0.35	0.18	0.18
9	0.52	0.52	0.30	0.30	0.00	0.15
10	0.45	0.45	0.26	0.26	0.00	0.13
11	0.41	0.41	0.00	0.23	0.00	0.00
12	0.37	0.37	0.00	0.21	0.00	0.00
13	0.00	0.34	0.00	0.00	0.00	0.00
14	0.00	0.31	0.00	0.00	0.00	0.00
15	0.00	0.28	0.00	0.00	0.00	0.00
>15	0.00	0.00	0.00	0.00	0.00	0.00

V = values in metres

BIOMECHANICS OF LIFTING

Biomechanical criteria for determining safe lifting

In developing criteria for safe levels of lifting the NIOSH lifting equation used three biomechanical criteria based on a review of the literature. These criteria were:

1. The joint between L5 and S1 is the level of greatest lumbar stress during lifting.
2. Compressive force at this level is the critical stress vector.
3. The compressive force criterion that defines increased risk is 3.4 kN (Waters et al 1994).

It has been proposed that at a compressive force of 3.4 kN on the lumbar spine, vertebral end-plate microfractures begin to occur in less than 1% of the male worker population and less than 25% of female workers during occasional lifting tasks, while compression levels above 6.4 kN are hazardous to the majority of workers (Chaffin et al 1999).

The mechanism for spinal injury under compressive load has been reported as occurring through failure of the endplates of the vertebral bodies and underlying trabeculae as the nucleus pulposus bulges upwards and downwards (Adams et al 2000). The magnitude of the compressive forces during a single lift is unlikely to cause end-plate failure, and it has been proposed that injury of this type is most likely to be cumulative (Fig. 8.2) (Adams & Dolan 1995). Lotz et al (1998) studied the effects of sustained compression on the intervertebral disc structure of mice and identified that compression resulted in disorganization of

Table 8.3 Coupling multiplier table for revised NIOSH lifting equation (reproduced with permission from Chaffin et al 1999)

Coupling type	Coupling multiplier	
	V < 0.75 m	V > 0.75 m
Good	1.00	1.00
Fair	0.95	1.00
Poor	0.90	0.90

Table 8.4 Metabolic energy expenditure limits (Kcal/min) for lifting, as used in the revised NIOSH lifting equation (adapted from Rodgers et al 1991)

Duration of lifting (during a work day)	Lift location (V) mm	
	V < 750	V > 750
< 1 hour	4.7	3.3
Between 1 and 2 hours	3.7	2.7
Between 2 and 8 hours	3.1	2.2

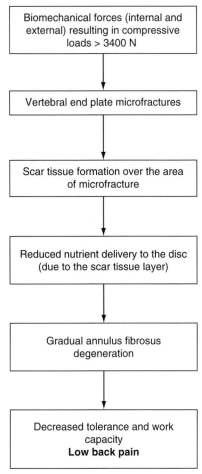

Figure 8.2 Proposed sequence of events for spinal degeneration following application of compressive forces. Adapted with permission from Marras 2001.

annular architecture, increased biomechanical instability (i.e. increased neutral zone), altered type 2 collagen and diminished cellularity. They reported that sustained compression resulted in cell death in the nucleus and inner annulus, possibly due to the mechanical stress or the adverse biochemical environment from the resultant water loss. Their observed annular morphological changes and increased biomechanical instability are consistent with those reported for degenerative human intervertebral discs. It was proposed that the effects of sustained or repeated compressive loading of the discs will hasten the disc degenerative process through cellular and biomechanical mechanisms (Adams et al 2000), even though they may fall below 'safe' biomechanical compressive levels.

Critical reviews of the criteria for the determination of safe lifting limits by Leamann (1994) and Dempsey (1998) identified that the use of compressive forces as the biomechanical 'safety' criterion may be flawed and both authors concluded that further research was needed. Other biomechanical criteria that may be used include the external hip moment, the anteroposterior (AP) shear force, lateral shear forces and the kinematic parameters of the torso (Marras

et al 1995, Ayoub & Woldstad 1999, Fathallah et al 1999). Shear forces in particular have been identified as potentially contributing to the risk of low back injury. However, safe limits for shear force exposure have not been as well established as those for compressive loads (Karwowski et al 1991, Davis & Marras 1998). Davis & Marras (1998) proposed a shear tolerance limit of 1 kN at which point there was an increased risk of tears of the annulus fibrosus; however, extensive work is still required in this area before shear tolerance values can be used as the biomechanical criterion for determining safe lifting limits.

Style of lifting

Lifting from below waist height is characterized by ankle dorsiflexion, knee, hip and lumbar flexion during the 'access' part of the lift, followed by ankle plantarflexion, knee, hip, and lumbar extension to perform the lift (Burgess-Limerick 2001). There are three main lifting techniques described in the literature, which involve different relative movements between the joints of the trunk and lower limbs (Fig. 8.3). The technique description pertains to the posture adopted at the start of the lift (Burgess-Limerick et al 1995, Burgess-Limerick 2001).

Squat lifting

At the commencement of the lift the body starts with a posture of ankle dorsiflexion, full knee flexion and hip flexion with the trunk maintained close to upright. Squat lifting can be further divided on biomechanical grounds into lifting with a small-sized load, which can be lifted between the knees, and lifting a larger load, which must be lifted in front of the knees in the squatting position (Chow 2001). Changes in load dimensions, and hence capacity to lift between the knees during squat lifting, will affect the distance of the load from the body, a powerful influence on the resultant stresses on the spine during lifting.

Stoop lifting

This describes the other extreme of lifting where the knees are minimally flexed, the ankles maintained in plantargrade and the trunk near maximal flexion. It is also termed the 'derrick' lift due to its similarity to the actions of the derrick crane (Oborne 1995). This lifting style is characterized by maximum lumbar flexion at commencement of the lift.

Semi-squat lifting

The posture involved lies between the stoop and squat lift with moderate trunk and knee flexion. Semi-squat lifting has been reported as the most common type of lift adopted when free dynamic lifting, with either of the two extremes of lifting styles rarely used when asked to perform free dynamic lifting, particularly over an extended period of time (Gagnon & Smyth 1992, Burgess-Limerick et al 1995, Burgess-Limerick & Abernethy 1997).

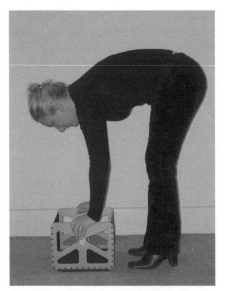 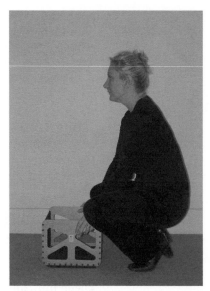 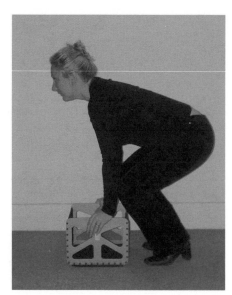

Figure 8.3 Three different lifting styles. A: Stoop lifting. B: Squat lifting. C: Semi-squat lifting.

A problem with defining the lifting styles by the posture demonstrated at the initiation of the lift is that it does not control for the movement pattern that the person uses when lifting (Burgess-Limerick et al 1995, Hsaing & McGorry 1997). When a person uses different lifting strategies there are changes in the coordination of the body and limb movements and in the motion pattern of the external load (Hsaing & McGorry 1997). During squat lifting, the lifter has a number of different strategies available to lift the load. They may pull the load closer to the body during the prelifting phase, use the body to jerk up the load during the lifting phase and then slide the load forward midway through the lift, or pull the load close to the body and develop a combined upward and forward momentum of the load before guiding it to touchdown (Hsaing & McGorry 1997) (Fig. 8.4). When teaching correct lifting we need to consider the motion patterns used in the lift as well as the initial posture. Hsaing & McGorry (1997) demonstrated that manipulation of the motion patterns of the load could be used to 'control' the estimated compressive forces on the lumbosacral joint, with the latter combined style

motion pattern demonstrating the lowest increase in compressive values.

The pros and cons of each lifting style will depend on the biomechanical stresses that the lifting style places on the lifter's trunk. In biomechanical terms, the main effect of different lifting styles will be on the magnitude and orientation of the moment of the load through affecting factors such as the object's centre of gravity, weight distribution (Oborne 1995) and the posture of the spine during the lift. Trunk postures during lifting have been shown to be associated with the risk of low back pain (Granata & Wilson 2001).

Spinal motion segment

It has been reported that 85–95% of all disc herniations related to manual handling occur at the L4/5 and L5/S1 spinal levels and the L5/S1 level sustains the largest amount of force (Chaffin et al 1999). Tichauer (1971) proposed that the load moment around the L5/S1 joint form the basis for setting safe limits for lifting and carrying. As described, the compressive force at this level has been used in setting biomechanical criteria. A range of other forces also act on the lumbar motion segment during lifting and these are shown in Figure 8.5. Lifting, with the concomitant development of flexor and extensor moments on the spine, results in development of both compression and shear forces over the motion segment (Burgess-Limerick 1999).

In full trunk flexion, as occurs in stoop lifting, 70% of the resistance to further lumbar flexion is provided by the intervertebral ligaments (in particular the short ligaments of the apophyseal joints) while the disc resists only 30% of the flexion torque. Once we move past the elastic limits of the ligaments, the interspinous and supraspinous liga-

Figure 8.4 Different lifting motion patterns. Reproduced with permission from Hsiang & McGorry 1997.

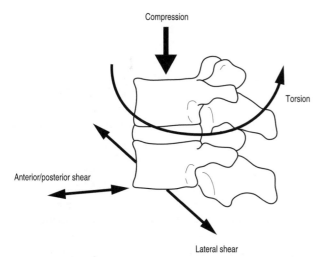

Figure 8.5 Forces acting on the spinal motion segment during lifting. Reproduced with permission from Marras 2001.

ments are damaged first (Adams et al 2000). Increased intradiscal pressure in this posture occurs due to tension in the posterior intervertebral ligaments and the posterior annulus.

When we lift there is an increase in the compressive forces on the lumbar motion segments through an increase in the magnitude of the load moment acting on the spine and an increase in muscle activity used to raise the load. As the vertical spacing of adjacent vertebrae is small compared to their length and width, small changes in the angle of motion segment flexion can lead to large changes in the distribution of stress in the motion segment, with this effect being exaggerated with pathological changes and creep loading (Adams et al 2000). When a cadaveric disc is loaded to reduce disc height by 20% (to simulate normal diurnal variation seen in vivo), the pressure in the nucleus falls by 36% while peaks of compressive stress rise in the annulus. Full lumbar flexion significantly increases the compressive pressure in the anterior annulus, while mid-flexion tends to equalize the compressive force across the whole disc (Adams et al 2000). Young, well-hydrated discs are less sensitive to changes in posture, and stress concentrations are only evident at the end of range (Dolan & Adams 2001). The apophyseal joints show similar changes secondary to narrowed disc spaces with peak compressive forces in the apophyseal joints changing from middle to upper regions in the flexed posture to the inferior margins in lordotic postures (Dolan & Adams 2001).

With the application of compressive force on the motion segment in a neutral position, the intervertebral disc provides the majority of the resistance. The facet joints provide little stiffness to compression in the neutral posture due to their vertical alignment; however, in the lordotic posture, such as in squat lifting, the facet joints can resist from 15 to 25% of the applied compressive load (Yang & King 1984),

which increases further in the presence of facet degeneration and/or disc narrowing (Dunlop et al 1984, Yang & King 1984). Three factors can increase the amount of compression force borne by the neural arch: pathological disc narrowing, prior long-term creep loading; and lordotic postures. When all factors are in place, the neural arch can resist up to 70% of the compressive stresses in the lordotic posture (Adams et al 2000).

Biomechanically the properties of the intervertebral disc are influenced by its geometric parameters, such as height and area. The height and area of the disc vary between disc levels, between different people and within the same disc itself. There is a decrease in disc height from the fifth decade of life while the disc area increases with age (Natarajan & Andersson 1999). Within the same person, the disc varies during the day due to diurnal variations, with a loss of height, particularly in the first few hours of the day and related to severity of loading of the spine. This diurnal change of disc height results in changing of the load-sharing capacity of the spinal elements during the day (Natarajan & Andersson 1999), with the disc taking more of the stress during flexion earlier in the day. Adams et al (1990) reported an increase in compression stiffness and more flexibility in flexion with diurnal changes.

During the application of anterior shear forces to the motion segment, as occurs with trunk flexion, the apophyseal joints provide the majority of the resistance to further anterior shear through the development of compressive stresses between the overlapping articular surfaces (Langrana et al 1990). In the general population there is wide variation between the anatomical orientation of the apophyseal joints of the lumbar spine (Bogduk 1997). In flexed lumbar postures, the apophyseal joints provide resistance to further flexion through passive stretching of the capsular fibres, but the capacity of the joints to resist anterior shear forces will depend on the orientation of the articular surfaces. Apophyseal joint articular surfaces parallel to the sagittal plane are less likely to be able effectively to resist significant increases in anterior shear forces that may develop from lifting in a flexed posture (Bogduk 1997). This may place greater anterior shear stress on the intervertebral disc, a plane that it is not well designed to resist, increasing the potential for injury to this structure.

A factor not always considered in biomechanical modelling, but one that has significance clinically, is the effect of creep on the motion segment. Human biological tissue has a viscoelastic nature and when subject to static or repeated postures undergoes creep, with a reduction in stiffness of the passive tissues of the motion segment (Best et al 1994). Viscoelastic creep has been demonstrated following cyclic and prolonged loading in flexion and has been shown to increase the laxity of the intervertebral joint, leading to high rates of instability, injury and low back pain in individuals involved in lifting (Gedalia et al 1999). Injuries associated with spinal instability can reportedly occur at compressive forces approaching 88 N (Granata & Wilson 2001).

It has been reported that the risk of low back injury is increased when lifting is performed many times during the day (Mundt et al 1993). The two mechanisms proposed include the altered muscle activation patterns found during fatiguing work activities, which may result in increased spinal compression, or the resultant muscle insufficiency, which may shift the loading to the passive tissue of the body. Sparto & Parnianpour (1998) used EMG-assisted biomechanical modelling to demonstrate minimal increase in spinal compression as a result of the changing muscle recruitment patterns and suggested that the injury mechanisms that result from repetitive or sustained posturing may be due to the change in the viscoelastic passive tissue responses or muscular insufficiency.

This raises the potential for reduced capacity of the passive structures of the spine to resist extra stresses, potentially resulting in temporary instability of the motion segment in that posture, increasing the risk of injury. The motion segment therefore relies more heavily on the dynamic components of motion segment stability, the abdominals and erector spinae to overcome the stress of any imposed loads (Solomonow et al 1999). Deficiencies in this dynamic stabilizing system may result in risk of injury below 'normal' biomechanical failure criteria.

The deformation and reduced thickness of the disc are thought to increase the laxity of the joints, increasing the range of IV movement as well as instability and injury (Solomonow et al 1999). Creep loading causes the annulus to resist a lower proportion of the bending moment applied to the spine and the ligaments to resist more. This implies that the annulus resists bending most strongly in the early morning when the disc is hydrated (Dolan & Adams 2001) and less during the day as the spine is subject to creep.

Intradiscal pressure

The pressures increase within the intervertebral disc during all manual handling activities (Kroemer & Grandjean 1997). Nachemson & Elfstrom (1970), in a review of intradiscal pressures during different lifting postures, identified that there was a sharp rise in intradiscal pressure at the level of L3/4 during stoop lifting compared with squat lifting when lifting a 20 kg load. When a load is held at a distance from the body, as in lifting a load in a squat lift around the knees, there is a significant increase in compressive forces at the lower lumbar levels, further increasing intradiscal pressure (Kroemer & Grandjean 1997). This increase in intradiscal pressure results from the increased muscular activity and lumbar flexion used in the lift posture.

Muscle activity

The erector spinae act to produce the extensor moment required to overcome the weight of the load and extend the trunk to the upright posture during lifting. For biomechanical modelling purposes, the action of the erector spinae muscles can be represented as a force moment acting on the spinal motion segment. Generally, this force moment has been represented as acting with a moment arm of 50 mm, a value resulting from the early work of Bartelink et al (1957). This value has been questioned with more recent work indicating that the moment arm of the erector spinae will vary between different lumbar postures. Tveit et al (1994) reported that the moment arm of the erector spinae increased by approximately 15% when the lordosis was increased, increasing the mechanical efficiency of the erector spinae. It was also reported that the upper lumbar and lower thoracic erector spinae portions of the erector spinae may contribute to the resultant extensor moment through their action on the erector spinae aponeurosis (or superficial dorsal tendon). This mechanism could theoretically increase the moment arm of the erector spinae to a maximum value of 85 mm, although this will depend on the specific anthropometric characteristics of the lifter and the posture assumed.

Extreme lumbar flexion postures are characterized by the absence of EMG activity in the lumbar erector spinae (McGill & Kippers 1994, McGorry et al 2001), termed the flexion–relaxation response (FRR). A similar reaction has also been demonstrated in the hamstring muscles (McGorry et al 2001). Lifting with a lordosis, such as in squat lifting, was shown to result in earlier peak EMG readings in the erector spinae than lifting with the lumbar spine in kyphosis. During stoop lifting, the FRR was evident and the peak EMG response was delayed towards the middle of the lift (Holmes et al 1992). While the torque values around the spinal motion segments were similar between the two lifts, the orientation of the motion segment and its capacity to resist the imposed forces were different. The lack of erector spinae activity which occurred early in the stoop lift (i.e. FRR) results in the flexed spinal motion segment resisting the flexor moment by the posteriorly placed passive structures, including the paravertebral ligaments, interspinous ligaments, posterior fibres of annulus fibrosus, and the passive elements of the muscular system.

Segmental muscle recruitment in the erector spinae muscles progresses in the caudad–cephalad direction during trunk extension from full flexion, independent of the speed of lifting (McGorry et al 2001). Solomonow et al (1998) identified a primary reflex arc between the mechanoreceptors in the spinal ligaments and facet joint capsules to the multifidus muscle. This reflex arc was triggered following the application of tensile loads to the spinal ligaments and resulted in contraction of the multifidus muscle at the level of ligament deformation and at one level above and/or below. This activity reached a peak when the stress in the ligament approached moderate levels that could potentially cause damage to the ligament tissue (Solomonow et al 1998). This reflex arc appears to be present to protect the passive tissue constraints of the spine towards the end range of lumbar flexion, although the presence of the FRR would suggest that this reflex arc is overridden at the extremes of range.

Experimentally based research, primarily on feline spines, has shown that this reflexive muscular activity decreased during cyclic activity because of desensitization of the mechanoreceptors in the viscoelastic structures as they become subject to laxity (Solomonow et al 1999). This was observed to occur even before fatigue of the erector spinae muscles set in. Gedalia et al (1999) observed that after 50 minutes of cyclic loading on the feline spine, recovery of this reflex arc did not appear to occur after 2 hours of rest. Taimela et al (1999) identified that there was a decrease in the capacity of human subjects to sense a change in lumbar position (proprioception) following lumbar fatigue activities in both control and low back pain patients, although this was significantly worse in LBP patients. The desensitization of the mechanoreceptors in the passive spinal tissues following repeated loading, as seen in feline spines, is an attractive mechanism to help explain the increased risk of low back pain following repeated manual handling. It could be hypothesized that following the cyclic loading of the passive intervertebral tissue resulting from repeated manual handling the human spine is more vulnerable to injury due to reduced neuromuscular control. This remains an exciting area for further research.

Contraction of the erector spinae muscles (in particular the pars lumborum fibres of the longissimus thoracis and iliocostalis lumborum) results in the development of a posterior shear force on the superior vertebrae. This has the potential effect of reducing the effect of anterior shear forces generated by the weight of the upper trunk and load (Burgess-Limerick 2001), but this capacity to resist anterior shear forces will depend on the lumbar posture used. The erector spinae (longissimus thoracis and iliocostalis lumborum) in the flexed posture have changed lines of action relative to the motion segment (by changing the cosine of the orientation of the line of action) and are therefore less able to resist the anterior shear forces seen to cause damage to the spine in full flexion (McGill et al 2000). Other muscles (multifidus, quadratus lumborum, psoas) also resist anterior shear and would appear to be less affected by the angle of trunk.

Despite the well-developed extensor muscles of the lumbar spine, biomechanical modelling indicated that the calculated extensor moments to be overcome at the lumbar spine when lifting heavy loads exceeded the demonstrable capacity of the erector spinae (Gedalia et al 1999). This suggested that other mechanisms must assist the activity of the erector spinae muscles in generating sufficient extensor moment to overcome the applied load. Gedalia et al (1999) provided an excellent review of the various perspectives put forward to explain the discrepancy between calculated and actual forces generated. Theories include the arch theory, where the lumbar spine is viewed as an arch braced by the intra-abdominal pressure (IAP), the hydraulic amplifier

theory, where the thoracolumbar fasciae surrounding the muscles act to brace the erector spinae muscles, increasing their power, or the passive posterior musculoligamentous system. In this latter system the passive ligamentous system and the passive tension generated in the erector spinae muscles was used to overcome the load early in the lift, until the moment arm of the load was sufficiently reduced as the trunk approached the erect posture for the active tension of the erector spinae muscles to take over.

Marras et al (2001) identified that patients with low back pain had higher resultant spinal compressive loads during free dynamic lifting despite reducing their effective trunk flexion moments by restricting their flexion range of motion and speed of movement. This increased spinal compressive load resulted from the increased levels of muscle coactivation demonstrated in this group, particularly when lifting below waist height. Another important factor was the influence of body weight, which Marras et al (2001) reported had a significant effect on increasing the spinal compressive load.

Intra-abdominal pressure

The concept that pressures within the trunk may assist with the mechanical efficiency of the trunk during lifting was first proposed in the 1920s. The original hypothesis was that the flexion moment created by the application of a load anterior to the axis of rotation of the motion segments would be counteracted by development of pressure in the trunk cavities (Chaffin et al 1999). It was hypothesized that this would reduce the activity required of the erector spinae muscles, reducing the stress on the vertebral column. Early work by Bartelink (1957) and Morris et al (1961) concluded that there would be a 30% reduction in stresses over the lumbosacral joint with the development of intra-abdominal pressure (IAP). Recently this hypothesis has been brought into question as a result of extensive laboratory based work in this area. Intra-abdominal pressure responses appear to be divided into an initial peak response at the commencement of the lift, a lower sustained pressure while the load was being raised and a further peak associated with the placement of the load. Interestingly, Hamberg et al (1978) used systematic strengthening exercises for the abdominal muscles and reported that while there were measurable increases in strength of the abdominal and back muscles these did not equate into increases in IAP while the subjects were lifting loads.

How the IAP was generated may also affect the biomechanical influence on the spine. When developed as a result of the Valsalva manoeuvre, the increase in IAP was accompanied with an increase in back extensor muscle activity which resulted in increases in spinal compression forces, as measured by disc pressure measurements and from biomechanical modelling (McGill & Norman 1987).

The role of IAP in lifting requires further clarification (Chaffin et al 1999). McGill & Norman (1987) and Marras et al

(2001) concluded that the co-contraction of several abdominal muscles (in particular the transversus abdominis and the oblique abdominals) acts to stiffen the torso, reducing the neutral zone, but also increasing IAP. It has been suggested that the muscle tensions involved would cancel any major unloading of the spinal disc due to increases in IAP (McGill & Norman 1987), hence the IAP has been depicted as a by-product of antagonistic co-contraction of the torso muscles to stabilize the spine during the act of lifting (Cholewicki et al 1999). Hodges et al (2001) have raised some questions about this proposal, suggesting that increases in IAP may in fact facilitate an extensor torque if the IAP is generated through selective muscle recruitment, in particular of the diaphragm, pelvic floor muscles and transversus abdominis (Hodges et al 2001).

Other joints

Biomechanical modelling of dynamic lifting has shown that the forces over the hip joint can be quite large, particularly when the load cannot be held close to the body. The capacity of the hip muscles to generate sufficient force to overcome the flexor moment generated by lifting loads is well documented (Farfan 1978, Bogduk 1997). Unfortunately the strong hip extensor muscles are only able to rotate the hip and pelvis backward on the femurs, leading to increased flexor moments acting on the lumbar spine (Bogduk 1997). The strong one-joint hip flexor muscles are less likely to be affected by lifting posture than the longer multijoint muscles. During lifting from the semi-squat posture the interaction between knee and hip extension allows the hamstrings and quadriceps to work together to maintain an adequate length–tension relationship facilitating their effectiveness, a situation that is less likely to occur during stoop lifting (Burgess-Limerick 1999).

In the squat lift position, the knees are in a 'close-packed' position, and the heels are generally off the ground. This places the body in an unstable position and places greater stress through the knees during the early part of the lift. Perturbations of the load during the lift may be less able to be withstood due to the relative instability of the body, increasing the potential for asymmetrical stresses through the lumbar spine. Postures of full knee flexion are generally discouraged in patients to avoid the significant patellofemoral joint compression that results from this posture, further exacerbated when a load is lifted. The patellofemoral joint is an area commonly involved in osteoarthritic changes in the ageing population. Stoop lifting and semi-squat lifting place less stress through the knee joints, allowing these joints to avoid the close-packed positions.

van Dieen et al (1999) presented an excellent review of the biomechanical evidence in support of advocating the squat lift compared to the stoop lift as a control measure to prevent low back pain. They concluded that the biomechanical literature did not provide substantial support for advocating the squat technique to prevent low back pain. They reported that the positive effects for squat lifting with respect to estimated spinal force moments and compression values were found only when the squat lift allowed lifting from a position between the feet, reducing the load on the low back by up to 30%. Issues with squat lifting include the higher ground reaction forces due to the greater vertical excursion of the body centre of mass, which are often ignored in static biomechanical modelling. They reported that in lifting tasks where the load was not lifted from a position between the feet, the net moment and compressive load through the lumbar spine were lower in stoop lifting. In contrast the shear and bending moments were higher in stoop lifting. Straker & Duncan (2000) found that subjects reported more discomfort and lower MAWL during squat lifting a medium-sized box from floor to knuckle height than with the stoop lift. It appears therefore that there is no clear-cut advantage offered by one extreme lifting style over the other. This is reflected in the clinical observation that subjects choose the semi-squat lifting style during free dynamic lifting rather than squat or stoop lifting.

RISK FACTORS

In considering the biomechanical effects on the spine of the different lifting styles, we need to consider the range of other factors that may influence the effect on the spine. These factors can be divided into three main categories and are listed in Table 8.5.

Personal risk factors

These are the characteristics of the worker that may affect the probability that an injury may occur.

Both age and gender have been shown to affect the biomechanical characteristics of the spine (Jager & Luttmann 1992). Age will affect the mechanical behaviour of the spinal motion segments, secondary to degenerative changes, as well as reducing the strength of the trunk muscle forces available to resist the internal pressures when lifting (Stubbs 1985). Gender differences are based on differences in anthropometric characteristics between male and female population groups which will affect trunk weight, centre of mass and muscle moment arms. It has also been suggested that differences in lumbar lordosis angles between genders will affect spinal stability during lifting (Granata & Orishimo 2001).

In the clinical application of risk management strategies to address risks associated with lifting, it is often difficult to address the personal risk factors. The basic tenet of ergonomics to 'fit the task to the person' is the safest guide when undertaking risk management programmes. Behavioural health programmes aiming to improve musculoskeletal and cardiovascular health and fitness, facilitate smoking cessation and improve workplace morale may be useful in reducing the risks associated with lifting activities.

Table 8.5 Risk factors associated with manual handling (adapted from Stubbs 1985 and Waters & Putz Anderson 1996)

Personal factors	Environmental factors	Job related factors	
		Task	Load
• Sex	• Humidity	• Location of load relative to worker. Reach and height	• Weight of object or force required to move the object
• Anthropometry (body weight and height)	• Light	• Distance object is to be moved	• Stability of load
• Physical fitness and training	• Noise	• Frequency and duration of handling activity	• Depth of load
• Lumbar mobility	• Vibration	• Bending and twisting	• Centre of gravity
• Strength	• Foot traction	• Postural requirements, preceding and during lift	• Breadth
• Medical history	• Space available		• Height of load
• Years of employment			• Height of load
• Smoking			
• Psychosocial factors			
• Anatomical abnormalities			
• Skill levels			
• Clothing worn			

However, they should only form a part of a total risk management strategy.

Environmental risk factors

These are conditions or characteristics of the external surroundings that may affect the probability of an injury. Issues such as the quality of the floor surface upon which the lift is to be performed, the ambient environment and the space available in which to perform the lift will all affect the risks associated with lifting activities.

Job related risk factors

These are the characteristics of the task that may affect the likelihood of an injury and are usually considered the most important in biomechanics as they directly affect the magnitude of the physical hazard to the worker (Waters & Putz Anderson 1996). They are also the easiest to measure and change in the occupational arena. However, consideration of just one of these factors – i.e. load mass – may underestimate the effect of the lift on the lumbar spine (Davis & Marras 2000). Changes in load weight may lead to changes in trunk dynamics, which may offset any of the benefits of the reduced load weights. It is therefore more important to consider how the person interacts with the load rather than the actual weight of the load itself.

Marras et al (1993, 1995) studied the contribution of various biomechanical workplace factors to the risk of low back injury in over 400 manual handling jobs in 48 different industries. They identified that the combination of five trunk motion and workplace factors were best associated with the risk of low back injury using multiple logistic regression modelling. These included lifting frequency, load moment, trunk lateral velocity, trunk twisting velocity and trunk sagittal angle. Other authors have identified factors such as asymmetry, speed of lift and horizontal and vertical position of load and load mass (van Dieen et al 1999).

As described, the NIOSH lifting equation has identified a number of different physical parameters that need to be considered when analysing a lift. The effects of job related risk factors are briefly described.

Horizontal position of the load

The horizontal position of the load relates to the position of the centre of mass of the load relative to the axis of rotation of the motion segment in the horizontal plane. The NIOSH lifting formula has defined the minimal distance that the centre of mass can be held from axis of rotation of the spine as 250 mm, which takes into account the abdominal cavity. Changes in the horizontal position of the load will have a dramatic effect on the moment of the load, significantly affecting spinal compression values. The increase in moment magnitude is non-linearly related to the increases in horizontal position of the load with an increasing rate of increase in moment magnitude as the load moves further away from the body (Schipplein et al 1995).

As the load moves away from the body, the lever arm of the load acting at the spinal level increases, magnifying the flexor torque produced at the spinal level. The spinal extensor muscles, working at a relatively fixed lever arm, must work significantly harder to balance the load. The increased activity of the extensor muscles result in increased compressive loads over the underlying motion segments. Chaffin et al (1999) have recommended that the minimization of the horizontal distance of the load is the most important control mechanism when considering the biomechanical effect of lifting on the body. Figure 8.6 describes the predicted L5/S1

Figure 8.6 Predicted L5/S1 compression forces for varying loads and different postures. Reproduced with permission from Chaffin et al 1999.

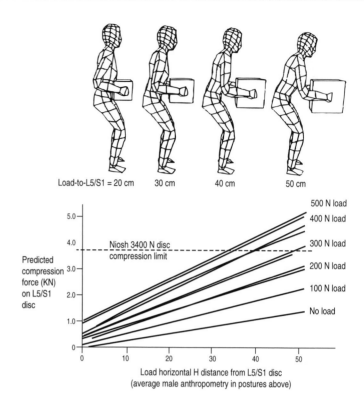

compressive forces for specific loads under different horizontal distances from the spine.

Increases in the horizontal distance of the load will not only increase the spinal compressive forces but it will also reduce the strength capacity of the subject (Kumar & Garand 1992), increasing the potential for injury in these postures (Kumar 1996). Furthermore, in a study of the effect of changes in horizontal distances of the load during peak exertions in stoop and squat lifting, Kumar (1996) found that reaching between full, three-quarters and half horizontal reach distances had significant effects on the strength capacity of the lifter.

Vertical position of the load

The height of the load relative to the lifter is a major driver behind the posture assumed when lifting, and hence the stresses through the body. Higher placed loads, such as with handles or on a raised stand, will reduce the degree of general flexion required to access the load. The less the degree of flexion required to access the load, the more likely the subject is to assume a neutral spine posture during lifting, reducing the biomechanical stresses through the spine, and facilitating trunk muscle activity (Tveit et al 1994, McGill et al 2000). The higher the load is placed vertically at the commencement of the lift, the shorter the vertical distance to be traversed during lifting, reducing the body's centre of mass vertical excursion, further reducing the biomechanical stresses on the spine (van Dieen et al 1999).

Lifting frequency

Increasing the frequency of the lift has been shown to have effects on safe lifting levels in both the physiological and psychophysical approaches. Mirka & Kelaher (1995) studied the effects of different lifting frequencies (between three and nine lifts per minute) on the kinematics of the trunk when free dynamic lifting. They reported that the higher frequencies of lifting resulted in higher levels of sagittal trunk acceleration, particularly between three and six lifts per minute. This occurred despite the fact that the frequencies used did not result in a state of continuous lifting, i.e. even at nine lifts per minute the subject had time between lifts to rest (Fig. 8.7). This was supported by Nussbaum et al (1997) who reported significant increases in spinal compression values, using an EMG-assisted biomechanical model, when lifting rates were increased 20% from preferred 'comfort' rates.

Increases in lifting frequencies are biomechanically problematic for the spine when they increase the speed of the lift. This has been shown to increase the load moment acting on the spine (Lavender et al 1999), increasing the spinal compression values (Mirka & Kelaher 1995) and placing the spine at greater risk of injury (Marras et al 1995).

An interesting observation from Mirka & Kelaher's study was that, as the lifts continued over the 20 minute time span, the lifters demonstrated significant increases in trunk sagittal acceleration, although the time at which this occurred varied between subjects (Mirka & Kelaher 1995). The timing of this change in trunk acceleration corre-

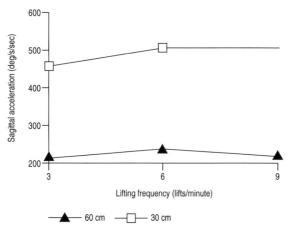

Figure 8.7 Saggital trunk acceleration values with different levels of lifting frequency. Reproduced with permission from Mirka & Kelaher 1995.

sponded to change of subject lifting styles from squat type lifting to a stoop lift (Mirka & Kelaher 1995). This change in lifting style corresponds to the findings from the physiological approach, which identified that the stoop lift was the most energy-efficient form of lifting.

Use of handles

The psychophysical approach has demonstrated that MAWLs were significantly higher for loads with handles compared to those without handles (Morrissey & Liou 1988, Drury et al 1989). Davis et al (1998) used an EMG-assisted biomechanical model to calculate the internal forces on the spine when lifting crates with and without handles from a conveyor to a pallet. They found that the presence of handles reduced the anteroposterior shear and compression forces on the lumbar spine for loading all levels of the pallet. They reported that this was due to the combination of several factors including kinematic variables, muscle co-activity, and increased vertical heights resulting from the use of the handles. Lifting without handles resulted in greater activity in the antagonistic trunk muscles, i.e. rectus abdominis, and greater maximum sagittal flexion of the trunk. This reflected the earlier findings of Kromodihardjo & Mital (1987) which reported that lifting loads with handles resulted in less biomechanical stress through the lumbar spine of the lifter.

Weight of the load

The weight of the load will have obvious effects on the load moment acting on the lumbar spine during lifting. Increases in load mass generally result in increased muscle activity, spinal loading and ultimately an increased risk of injury. Scholz (1993) reported that the load mass significantly affected the delay after the start of the lift before lumbar extension occurred. Increases in load mass increased

the time delay between the onset of knee extension and lumbar extension, implying that the passive constraints to further flexion in the lumbar spine were used to overcome the load moment for longer with heavier weights, before active lumbar extension occurred.

Davis & Marras (1998) found that several kinematic variables were significantly affected by changes in load weight when lifting loads over 20 kg but that overall postures were not. They reported that small changes in load weights during free dynamic lifting had a limited effect on spinal loads due to changes in trunk kinematics. Subjects tended to lift with an increased velocity and tended to hold the load further away from their body when lifting lower weights resulting in increased spinal loading. Davis & Marras (1998, 2000) expressed the ratio of computed dynamic compression values with the static compression values, calculated using static and dynamic biomechanical models (Fig. 8.8). They found that as the weight increased the ratio of dynamic to static compression values dropped, indicating that the dynamic factors had a greater influence over the lower loads. Unfortunately this study limited itself to loads over 9 kg and further work is required to investigate the effect of lower loads on trunk kinematics.

This study reinforced the need to consider the range of factors, not just the weight but also dynamic factors such as trunk kinematics and muscle recruitment patterns, when assessing the risks involved in lifting activities.

Asymmetry of the lift

Asymmetry during lifting has been identified as a risk factor for the development of low back pain (Marras et al 1995, Lavender et al 1999) and complex combined dynamic motions of the trunk commonly occur during many of the industrial activities that predispose workers to low back pain (Straker et al 1997). Asymmetrical lifting generates complex patterns of spinal loading, placing increased stresses on the lumbar spine, increasing intradiscal pressure and the stress on capsular ligaments (van Dieen & Kingma 1999, Chow 2001). Other proposed mechanisms for this increased risk from

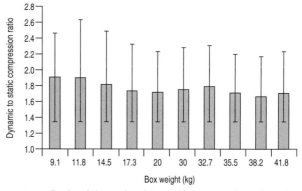

Figure 8.8 Ratio of dynamic with static compressive values during lifting. Reproduced with permission from Davis & Marras 2000.

asymmetrical lifting include the increased muscle force used during asymmetrical lifting either to generate sufficient torque to perform the lift or secondary to the lifter's perception of increased difficulty with asymmetrical lifting resulting in increased antagonistic muscle activation (van Dieen & Kingma 1999). This increase in muscle activation will result in higher spinal compression values.

Investigating only one component of the net resultant spinal forces (i.e. compression) and ignoring the other components, as occurs in traditional biomechanical modelling, may lead to erroneous judgements regarding the biomechanical risk involved (Straker et al 1997). This may result in underestimation of the spinal loading factors by up to 40% (Fathallah et al 1999). The combination of lateral shear and compression loading patterns appear to be the key to distinguishing the risk involved, particularly during asymmetrical lifting tasks. There is a need to further develop tolerance of spinal tissue to dynamic complex loading conditions (Fathallah et al 1999).

Asymmetrical lifting has also been shown to reduce the lifter's trunk extensor capability (Chow 2001) and increase the levels of antagonistic co-contraction of trunk muscles (Marras & Mirka 1992). This increase in muscle co-activation occurred in muscles other than the erector spinae or latissimus dorsi, which appeared to be consistently active in all asymmetrical movements. The increase in co-activation also occurred with increases in trunk torque and trunk velocity (Marras & Mirka 1992), resulting in increased spinal compression values.

Sudden and unexpected loading during lifting has been shown to increase the spinal compressive loading via muscular activation by up to 70% (Mannion et al 2000). It has been reported that the muscle activity demonstrated during sudden and unexpected lifting exceeded that which was required to overcome the load, dramatically increasing the compressive stresses on the spine. The increased weight of the load, due to inertial properties was shown to increase the compressive effect on the spine minimally compared to the effect of this increased muscle activity (Mannion et al 2000). Interestingly when subjects lifted an underestimated weight (up to 10 kg) at a self-selected, low velocity this increased muscle activity was not seen, and maximum compression values and lumbar angles were no different than when expected lifting of the same mass occurred (van der Burg & van Dieen 2001). This difference may be secondary to the timing of the perturbation, with the low rate of application of the perturbation during lifting an unexpected load allowing compensation to occur. Sudden increases in load mass during the lift may not allow compensatory mechanisms requiring sudden increases in muscle activity to occur with the resultant increase in compression values.

CONCLUSION

Lifting remains a significant risk factor for the development of low back pain in the community. When considering risk management strategies for the minimization of risks associated with lifting it is important to consider the range of parameters that affect the stresses on the lifter. It is no longer appropriate to consider manual handling training as a sufficient risk management strategy without assessing the whole person–task–environment system. The biomechanical approach, while not able to provide all the answers we need in the clinical environment, allows us to develop a better understanding of the influence of these parameters, and ultimately how we can change them to make the task of lifting safer.

KEYWORDS	
biomechanics lifting	lumbar spine

References

Adams M A, Dolan P 1995 Recent advances in lumbar spinal mechanics and their clinical significance. Clinical Biomechanics 10: 3–19

Adams M A, Dolan P, Hutton W C et al 1990 Diurnal changes in spinal mechanics and their clinical significance. Journal of Bone and Joint Surgery 72: 266–270

Adams M A, Freeman B J C, Morrison H P et al 2000a Mechanical initiation of intervertebral disc degeneration. Spine 25(13): 1625–1636

Adams M A, May S, Freeman B J C et al 2000b The effects of backward bending on lumbar intervertebral discs: relevance to physical therapy treatments for low back pain. Spine 25(4): 431–437

Ayoub M M, Woldstad J C 1999 Models in manual materials handling. In: Kumar S (ed) Biomechanics in ergonomics. Taylor and Francis, Philadelphia

Bartelink D L 1957 The role of abdominal pressure in relieving the pressure on the intervertebral discs. The Journal of Bone and Joint Surgery 39B(4): 718–725

Best T M, McElhaney J, Garrett W E et al 1994 Characterisation of the passive responses of live skeletal muscle tissue using the quasi-linear theory of visco-elasticity. Journal of Biomechanics 27: 413–419

Bogduk N 1997 Clinical anatomy of the lumbar spine and sacrum, 3rd edn. Churchill Livingstone, Sydney

Burgess-Limerick R 1999 Squat, stoop, or something in between? In: Straker L, Pollock C (eds) Proceedings of Cyberg 1999. Second International Cyberspace Conference on Ergonomics. International Ergonomics Association Press, Curtin University of Technology, Perth, Australia

Burgess-Limerick R 2001 Lifting techniques. In: Kumar W (ed) International encyclopaedia of ergonomics and human factors. Taylor and Francis, London

Burgess-Limerick R, Abernethy B, Neal R J et al 1995 Self selected manual lifting technique: functional consequences of interjoint coordination. Human Factors 37: 395–411

Burgess-Limerick R, Abernethy B 1997 Toward a quantitative definition of manual lifting postures. Human Factors 39(1): 141–148

Chaffin D B, Park K S 1973 A longitudinal study of low back pain as associated with occupational weight lifting factors. American Industrial Hygiene Journal 34: 513–525

Chaffin D B, Andersson G B J, Martin B J 1999 Occupational biomechanics, 3rd edn. John Wiley and Sons, New York

Cholewicki J, Juluru K, McGill S 1999 Intra-abdominal pressure mechanism for stabilising the lumbar spine. Journal of Biomechanics 32: 13–17

Chow D H K 2001 Lifting strategies. In: Karwowski W (ed) International encyclopaedia of ergonomics and human factors. Taylor and Francis, London

Davis K G, Marras W S 1998 Is changing the box weight an effective ergonomic control? In: Proceedings of the Human Factors and Ergonomics Society, 42nd Annual Conference, Chicago, IL, Oct 5–9, Human Factors and Ergonomics Society

Davis K G, Marras W S 2000 Assessment of the relationship between box weight and trunk kinematics: does a reduction in box weight necessarily correspond to a decrease in spinal loading. Human Factors 42(2): 195–208

Davis J R, Mirka G A 2000 Transverse contour modelling of trunk muscle distributed forces and spinal loads during lifting and twisting. Spine 25(2): 180–189

Davis K G, Marras W S, Waters T R 1998 Reduction of spinal loading through the use of handles. Ergonomics 41(8): 1155–1168

Dempsey P G 1998 A critical review of biomechanical, epidemiological, physiological and psychophysical criteria for designing manual materials handling tasks. Ergonomics 41(1): 73–88

Dolan P, Adams M A 2001 Recent advances in lumbar spinal mechanics and their significance for modelling. Clinical Biomechanics 16(Suppl. 1): S8–S16

Drury C G, Deeb J M, Hartman B et al 1989 Symmetric and asymmetric manual material handling. 1: Physiology and psychophysics. Ergonomics 32: 467–489

Dunlop R B, Adams M A, Hutton W C 1984 Disc space narrowing and the lumbar facet joints. Journal of Bone and Joint Surgery 66B: 706–710

Farfan H F 1978 The biomechanical advantage of lordosis and hip extension for upright activity: man as compared with other anthropoids. Spine 3: 336–342

Fathallah F A, Marras W S, Parnianpour M 1998 An assessment of complex spinal loading during dynamic lifting tasks. Spine 23(6): 706–716

Fathallah F A, Marras W S, Parnianpour M 1999 Regression models for predicting peak and continuous three dimensional spinal loads during symmetric and asymmetric lifting tasks. Human Factors 41(3): 373–388

Gagnon M, Smyth G 1992 Biomechanical exploration on dynamic modes of lifting. Ergonomics 35: 329–345

Gedalia U, Solomonow M, Zhou B et al 1999 Biomechanics of increased exposure to lumbar injury caused by cyclic loading. 2: Recovery of reflexive muscular stability with rest. Spine 24(23): 2461–2467

Granata K P, Marras W S 1996 Biomechanical models in ergonomics. In: Bhattacharya A, McGlothin J D (eds) Occupational ergonomics. Marcel Dekker, New York, pp 115–136

Granata K P, Orishimo K F 2001 Response of trunk muscle coactivation to changes in spinal stability. Journal of Biomechanics 34: 1117–1123

Granata K P, Sanford A H 2000 Lumbar-pelvic coordination is influenced by lifting task parameters. Spine 25(11): 1413–1418

Granata K P, Wilson S E 2001 Trunk posture and spinal stability. Clinical Biomechanics 16: 650–659

Hamberg J, Hemborg B, Holmström E, Löwing H, Moritz U, Nilsson M K, Åkesson I 1978 Abdominal muscular activity and intra-abdominal pressure at different lifting techniques, before and after training of the abdominal muscles In: Proceedings of the XIX International Congress on Occupational Health, Dubrovnik, Yugoslavia, Sept 25–30. International Commission on Occupational Health.

Hansson T, Keller T, Spengler D M 1987 Mechanical behaviour of the human lumbar spine II: fatigue strength during dynamic compressive loading. Journal of Orthopedic Research 5: 479–487

Hildebrandt V J 1987 A review of epidemiological research on risk factors of low back pain. In: Buckle P W (ed). Musculoskeletal disorders at work. Taylor and Francis, London

Hodges P W, Cresswell A G, Daggfeldt K et al 2001 In vivo measurement of the effect of intra-abdominal pressure on the human spine. Journal of Biomechanics 34: 347–353

Holmes J A, Damaser M S, Lehman S L 1992 Erector spinae activation and movement dynamics about the lumbar spine in lordotic and kyphotic squat lifting. Spine 17(3): 327–334

Hsaing S M, McGorry R W 1997 Three different lifting strategies for controlling the motion patterns of the external load. Ergonomics 40(9): 928–939

Jager M, Luttmann A 1992 The load on the lumbar spine during asymmetrical bi-manual materials handling. Ergonomics 35: 783–805

Jorgensen M J, Davis K G, Kirking B C et al 1999 Significance of biomechanical and physiological variables during the determination of maximum acceptable weight of lift. Ergonomics 42(9): 1216–1232

Karwowski W, Hancock P, Zurada J M et al 1991 Risk of low back overexertion injury due to manual load lifting in view of the catastrophe theory. In: Queinnec Y, Daniellou F (eds) Designing for everyone. Proceedings of the 11th Congress of the International Ergonomics Association, Taylor and Francis, London

Kroemer K H E, Grandjean E 1997 Fitting the task to the human: a textbook of occupational ergonomics, 5th edn. Taylor and Francis, London

Kromodihardjo S, Mital A 1987 Biomechanical analysis of manual lifting tasks. Journal of Biomedical Engineering 109: 132–137

Kumar S 1996 Spinal compression at peak isometric and isokinetic exertions in simulated lifting in symmetric and asymmetric planes. Clinical Biomechanics 11(5): 281–289

Kumar S, Garand D 1992 Static and dynamic lifting strength at different reach distances in symmetrical and asymmetrical planes. Ergonomics 35(7/8): 861–880

Langrana N A, Edwards W T, Sharma M 1990 Biomechanical analysis of loads on the lumbar spine. In: Weisel S W, Weinstein J N, Herkowitz H et al (eds) The lumbar spine: the International Society for the Study of the Lumbar Spine, 2nd edn. W B Saunders, Philadelphia

Lavender S A, Li Y C, Andersson G B J et al 1999 The effects of lifting speed on the peak external forward bending, lateral bending and twisting spine moments. Ergonomics 42(1): 111–125

Leamann T B 1994 Research to reality: a critical review of the validity of various criteria for the prevention of occupationally induced low back pain. Ergonomics 37(12): 1959–1974

Lotz J C, Colliou O K, Chin J R et al 1998 Compression induced degeneration of the intervertebral disc: an invivo mouse model and finite element study. Spine 23(23): 2493–2506

McGill S M, Kippers V 1994 Transfer of loads between lumbar tissues during flexion relaxation phenomen. Spine 19(19): 2190

McGill S M, Norman R W 1987 Effects of an anatomically detailed erector spinae model on L4/L5 disc compression and shear. Journal of Biomechanics 20(6): 591–600

McGill S, Hughson R L, Parks K 2000 Changes in lumbar lordosis modify the role of the extensor muscles. Clinical Biomechanics 15: 777–780

McGorry R W, Hsiang S M, Fathallah F A et al 2001 Timing of activation of the erector spinae and hamstrings during a trunk flexion and extension task. Spine 26(4): 418–425

Magora A 1973 Investigation of the relation between low back pain and occupation. IV: Physical requirements: bending, rotation, reaching and sudden maximal effort. Scandinavian Journal of Rehabilitative Medicine 5: 186–190

Mannion A F, Adams M A, Dolan P 2000 Sudden and unexpected loading generates high forces on the lumbar spine. Spine 25(7): 842–852

Marras W S 2001 Loads on the lumbar spine during dynamic work. In: Karwowski W (ed) International encyclopaedia of ergonomics and human factors. Taylor and Francis, London

Marras W S, Mirka G S 1992 A comprehensive evaluation of trunk response to asymmetric trunk motion. Spine 17(3): 318–326

Marras W S, Lavender S A, Leurgans S E et al 1993 The role of dynamic three dimensional trunk motion in occupationally related low back disorders: the effects of workplace factors, trunk position and trunk motion characteristics on the risk of injury. Spine 18: 617–628

Marras W S, Lavender S A, Leurgans S E et al 1995 Biomechanical risk factors for occupationally related low back disorders. Ergonomics 28: 377–410

Marras W S, Davis K G, Ferguson S A et al 2001 Spine loading characteristics of patients with low back pain compared with asymptomatic individuals. Spine 26(23): 2566–2574

Mirka G A, Kelaher D P 1995 The effects of lifting frequency on the dynamics of lifting. In: Proceedings of the Human Factors and Ergonomics Society, 39th Annual Conference, San Diego, CA, Oct 9–13, Human Factors and Ergonomics Society

Morris J M, Lucas D B, Bresler B 1961 Role of the trunk in stability of the spine. The Journal of Bone and Joint Surgery 43A(3): 327–351

Morrissey S J, Liou Y H 1988 Maximal acceptable weights in load carriage. Ergonomics 31: 217–226

Mundt D J, Kelsey J L, Golden A L 1993 An epidemiologic study of non-occupational lifting as a risk factor for herniated lumbar intervertebral disc. Spine 18: 595–602

Nachemson A, Elfstrom G 1970 Intravital dynamic pressure measurements in lumbar discs. Scandinavian Journal of Rehabilitation Medicine 1(Suppl. 1): 1–40

Natarajan R N, Andersson G B J 1999 The influence of disc height and cross sectional area on the mechanical response of the disc to physiologic loading. Spine 24(28): 1873–1881

Nussbaum M A, Caffin D B, Baker G 1997 Effects of pacing on spinal loads when using material handling systems. In: Proceedings of the Human Factors and Ergonomics Society, 41st Annual Conference, Albuquerque, NM, Sept 22–26, Human Factors and Ergonomics Society

Oborne D J 1995 Ergonomics at work. John Wiley, Chichester

Rodgers S H J, Yates J W, Garg A 1991 The physiological basis for manual guidelines. National Technical Information Service, report no. 91-227-330

Schipplein O D, Reinsel T E, Andersson G B J et al 1995 The influence of initial horizontal weight placement on the loads at the lumbar spine while lifting. Spine 20(17): 1895–1898

Scholz J P 1993 Organisational principles for the coordination of lifting. Human Movement Science 12: 427–459

Snook S H, Ciriello V M 1991 The design of manual handling tasks: revised tables of maximum acceptable weights and forces. Ergonomics 34(9): 1197–1213

Solomonow M, Zhou B, Harris M, et al 1998 The ligamento-muscular stabilising system of the spine. Spine 23(23): 2552–2562

Solomonow M, Zhou B, Baratta R V et al 1999 Biomechanics of increased exposure to lumbar injury caused by cyclic loading. 1: Loss of reflexive muscular stabilization Spine 24(23): 2426–2434

Sparto P J, Parnianpour M 1998 Estimation of trunk muscle forces and spinal loads during fatiguing repetitive trunk exertions. Spine 23(23): 2563–2573

Straker L M, Stevenson M G, Twomey L T, Smith L M 1997 A comparison of single and combination manual handling tasks risk assessment: Part 3 Biomechanical measures. Ergonomics 40: 708–728

Straker L, Duncan P 2000 Psychophysical and psychosocial comparison of squat and stoop lifting by young females. Australian Journal of Physiotherapy 46(1): 27–32

Stubbs D A 1985 Human constraints on manual working capacity: effects of age on intratruncal pressures. Ergonomics 28: 107–114

Taimela S, Kankaanpaa M, Luoto S 1999 The effect of lumbar fatigue on the ability to sense a change in lumbar position, a controlled study. Spine 24(13): 1322–1327

Tichauer E R 1971 A pilot study of the biomechanics of sitting in simulated industrial work situations. Journal of Safety Research 3(3): 98–115.

Tveit P, Daggfelt K, Hetland S, Thorstensson A 1994 Erector spinae lever arm length variations with changes in spinal curvature. Spine 19(2): 199–204

van der Burg J C E, van Dieen J H 2001 Underestimation of object mass in lifting does not increase the load on the low back. Journal of Biomechanics 34: 1447–1453

van Dieen J H, Kingma I 1999 Total trunk muscle force and spinal compression are lower in asymmetric moments as compared to pure extension moments. Journal of Biomechanics 32: 681–687

van Dieen J H, Hoozemans M J M, Tousaaint H M 1999 Stoop or squat: a review of biomechanical studies on lifting techniques. Clinical Biomechanics 14(10): 685–696

Videman T, Battie M C 1999 The influence of occupation on lumbar degeneration. Spine 124(11): 1164–1168

Waters T R, Putz-Andersson V, Garg A 1994 Applications manual for the revised NIOSH lifting equation. Department of Health and Human Services (NIOSH) publication no. 94–110, National Institute for Occupational Safety and Health, Washington DC

Waters T R, Putz Anderson V 1996 Manual materials handling. In: Bhattacharya A, McGlothin J D (eds) Occupational ergonomics. Marcel Dekker, New York, pp 329–350

Yang K H, King A L 1984 Mechanism of facet load transmission as a hypothesis for low back pain. Spine 9: 557–565

Chapter 9

Motor control of the cervical spine

E. A. Keshner

THE HEAD–NECK SYSTEM

Action of the cervical spine cannot be considered as the sum of isolated movements about several joints. It is a dynamic structure which acts to support the head on the trunk, orient the head in space and transmit forces arising from the trunk that will influence the position of the head. Thus, although neural control of the spine operates through the biomechanical structures, the control operations are very much dependent upon the goal of the movement. The musculoskeletal anatomy of the cervical spine has been studied in detail (see, for example, Kamibayashi & Richmond 1998, Sherk & Parke 1983, Worth 1994), but the neurophysiological control of that anatomy by the central nervous system (CNS) has been less focused upon. It is particularly difficult to identify sources of CNS control in the cervical spine of intact individuals because the presence of vital contents such as the carotid and vertebral arteries, spinal cord and larynx makes invasive recording procedures undesirable. Another reason is that the cervical spine is not analogous to the rest of the vertebral column. The neck is designed for enormous degrees of mobility and the vertebrae are smaller and more anatomically complicated (Bland & Boushey 1988). Finally, any control of the cervical spine must be considered in the context of the redundancies inherent in both its musculoskeletal and sensorimotor components.

THE PROBLEM OF MOTOR CONTROL IN THE CERVICAL SPINE

The cervical spine is a complex biomechanical linkage composed of multiple degrees of freedom of movement about each of its joints and at least 20 pairs of muscles, many of which are capable of performing similar actions. In fact, there appear to be more muscles than are necessary to perform the repertoire of head movements that humans make (Peterson et al 1989). This would increase the degrees of freedom for each task by increasing the choice of potential motor patterns available to the CNS. Thus the ultimate motor control problem in the cervical spine is how to simplify or reduce the degrees of freedom for efficient and timely production of an optimal movement pattern (Bernstein 1967). The purpose of this chapter is to report what is currently known about sensorimotor control of the musculoskeletal and neurophysiological components of the cervical spine in order to examine how the CNS solves the problem of redundancy.

Musculoskeletal redundancy

Complex multiple muscle systems have the potential for producing single movements with variable muscle activation patterns. Neural and mechanical redundancies in the head–neck complex potentially provide great flexibility for producing head and neck movements. Longer neck muscles cross many cervical vertebrae and can generate moments about both lower and upper cervical joints. Overall, the number of independently controlled muscle elements (including subdivisions of compartmentalized muscles) exceeds the number of degrees of freedom of neck motion. Because of their multiple insertions, many of the neck muscles have multiple functions or change their function depending on the initial position of each vertebral joint and the degree to which the joints are free to move in each of the planes of motion (Richmond et al 1991, 1992, Wickland et al 1991). The extent of functional variability in the neck muscles appears to depend upon the task being studied. Thus a great deal is known about the static organization of the human cervical spine, but the dynamic organization is less easily characterized and data from other species must be relied upon to draw conclusions about control of the cervical spine.

Vertebral column

The neurally controlled actions of the large number of muscles of the head and neck must be matched to and interact with the mechanics of the spine. All mammalian species examined hold the cervical vertebral column nearly vertical at rest (Graf et al 1995, Vidal et al 1986). In the cervical spine there are eight joints between the skull and the thoracic vertebrae, each having six degrees of freedom: three rotational (flexion/extension, axial rotation, and lateral bending) and three translational (up–down, side to side, anterior–posterior). But when analysed descriptively with videofluoroscopy, head–neck biomechanics appear much simpler than expected. Videofluoroscopy studies of the cervical spine performed on quadrupedal mammals in a resting position (de Waele et al 1989, Graf et al 1995, Vidal et al 1986) suggest that there are only two primary axes of motion in the cervical spine: the atlanto-occipital joint (C1–skull) and the cervciothoracic joint (C7–T1). In human cadavers (Panjabi et al 2001), the greatest degree of flexion occurred at CI–C2 and the greatest degree of extension was observed at skull–C1. Axial rotation was largest at C1–2 and with lateral bending moments the motion occurred across all vertebral levels.

Qualitative analyses in alert animals demonstrate that most active head movements are made about a restricted set of joint axes (Choi et al 2000, Keshner 1994). Horizontal plane motions occur about C1–2, sagittal plane actions about either C1–skull or C7–T1 and lateral plane motions by combined lateral flexion of C2–5. Fore–aft translation of the head is effected by combining pitch flexion about C7–T1 with pitch extension about C1–skull to keep the head level. However, all the cervical joints are actually involved to some extent in the final head movement, and the relative amount and pattern of motion at each cervical joint during head movement appears to depend upon the posture that the animal assumes. For example, vertebrae in a standing cat were observed to travel in a vertical, arcing motion, whereas in a prone cat those same vertebrae travelled more diagonally (Keshner 1994). It was determined that the prone cat moved primarily at C1 and C7 with additional motion at C4. Standing cats, however, tended to use all of the vertebrae to accomplish the full excursion of the head (Table 9.1). Similarly, a rhesus monkey used all of the cervical vertebrae when tracking a target in the upright position, but moved primarily at C1-skull when tracking in quadruped. Different muscles were activated to accomplish the same head movements depending upon the position of the animal. The moment arms of the muscles were not significantly different in the altered body positions (Keshner et al 1999), therefore different muscles were probably selected by each animal because the trajectory of the spinal column varied for the two body positions.

Muscles of the head and neck

Although the head represents only 7% of the body's total weight (Gowitzke & Milner 1980), more than 20 different muscles directly link the skull on either side of midline to the vertebral skeleton (Sherk & Parke 1983). Thus, a voluntary motor task in the head and neck could be accomplished through a variety of combinations of kinematic and muscle actions. The multiple choices might not be so surprising if

Table 9.1 Mean (± S.D.) angular excursion of each vertebra with respect to T, during ±20° head tracking movements in the sagittal plane in two body postures

	Monkey		Cat	
	Upright	Quadraped	Standing	Prone
Skull	32° ± 4°	26° ± 5°	*	*
C1	27° ± 3°	15° ± 6°	14° ± 2°	25° ± 9°
C2	25° ± 5°	11° ± 3°	15° ± 2°	30° ± 9°
C3	22° ± 4°	11° ± 3°	15° ± 3°	*
C4	24° ± 17°	12° ± 4°	17° ± 3°	42° ± 10°
C5	17° ± 2°	8° ± 3°	20° ± 4°	*
C6	16° ± 4°	7° ± 2°	24° ± 5°	*
C7	8° ± 5°	8° ± 1°	35° ± 7°	69° ± 33°

*Data not available.

the head were involved in the fine motor control and variety of motions found in the hand and fingers. Motions of the head relative to the trunk, however, are primarily directed towards orienting and stabilizing the position of the eyes and head in space (Goldberg & Peterson 1986, Outerbridge & Melvill Jones 1971), even during fine motor activities such as eating and scanning the environment. Despite this opportunity for response variability, our previous work in both humans (Keshner et al 1989) and cats (Keshner et al 1992, 1997) suggests that, within an animal, the CNS programmes neck muscles to respond in specific directions rather than generating an infinite variety of muscle patterns.

Neck muscle organization

Neck muscles are characteristically grouped in layers. The outer layer consists of long muscles that connect the skull and shoulder girdle. A deeper layer links the skull and vertebral column. The deepest layers consist of muscles that link the cervical and thoracic vertebrae. The outermost layer of muscles, connecting the skull with the shoulder girdle, consists of sternocleidomastoid and trapezius. Sternocleidomastoid is activated during flexion, contralateral rotation and lateral bending movements of the head. Trapezius has three segments and is classically described as a scapular muscle. Trapezius has been implicated in head extension because the superior fibres of that muscle originate on the external occipital protuberance (Lockhart et al 1972), although anatomical examination reveals that the muscle fibres become very sparse and essentially disappear around the level of the fourth cervical vertebra. Physiological studies of trapezius do not support its participation in pure head extension movements (Keshner et al 1989, Vasavada 1999, Vasavada et al 1998).

The next layer of muscles links the skull with the vertebral column. This group includes long dorsal (splenius capitis, semispinalis capitis and longissimus capitis) and a long ventral (longus capitis) muscles. Splenius capitis and longissimus capitis act as extensors and lateral flexors of the head. Semispinalis capitis is a head extensor muscle that participates minimally during ipsilateral lateral flexion. Longus capitis lies close to the vertebral bodies, thus it has little mechanical advantage for flexion. Rather it may be activated during ipsilateral rotation of the head. Slightly deeper to these muscles lie splenius cervicis, semispinalis cervicis, longissimus cervicis and longus colli which link the vertebrae to one another. The functions of these muscles should be similar to those of the capitis segments, but they have smaller moment arms because they lie closer to the vertebrae. The deepest layers of muscles are the suboccipital muscles, which include rectus capitis posterior major and minor, obliquus capitis superior and obliquus capitis inferior. All four muscles produce extension at the atlanto-occipital joint.

Neck muscle morphometry

From their anatomical descriptions, it would appear that many of the neck muscles perform overlapping actions.

However, an examination of muscle morphometry reveals considerable heterogeneity that could influence the moment generating capacity and, therefore, the optimal performance of each muscle in each task. In cats, each muscle differs in its relative content of fast and slow fibres, its sites of origin and insertion and the mechanics of action across the individual joints of the cervical column (Richmond & Abrahams 1975, Richmond & Vidal 1988, Richmond et al 1991, Selbie et al 1993, Wickland et al 1991).

Kamibayashi & Richmond (1998) studied the neck muscle architecture and morphometry, measuring musculotendon, fascicle and sarcomere length as well as muscle mass and pennation angles in ten human cadavers. Just as in cats, human neck muscles were found to be architecturally complex. Many muscles crossed two or more joints and had multiple attachments to different vertebrae. The number of tendons and vertebral level of attachments varied across specimens. Unlike limb muscles that have distinct tendinous attachments to bone, many neck muscles had very little tendon at their ends. Instead of distinct tendons, many neck muscles were found to have a complex architecture of internal tendons and aponeuroses. All of these factors affect the biomechanical consequences of muscle action and could influence their selection by the CNS for performance of a task.

FUNCTIONAL SYNERGIES

The task for the head–neck controller is to select which of the many muscles and joints will be operative in any movement to meet apparently conflicting goals of stability and mobility. These include producing a stable base of support for the mass of the head and the head's special sensory receptors to keep them in line with a target while permitting full range of motion of the head on the trunk. The problem for the controller is that these two goals require a decrease in the active degrees of freedom to accomplish joint stability, yet rely on joint flexibility to accomplish the movement.

One solution to the degrees of freedom problem is to organize the muscles as functional synergies. A synergy implies a consistent grouping of a set of muscles to accomplish a defined task (Tuller et al 1982). Synergies are conceptualized as units of control incorporating the muscles around a joint that will act together in a functional fashion. Thus the CNS relies on synergic mechanisms that are composed of a group of muscles that can span several joints and are constrained to act as a single unit. Instead of controlling each individual muscle, the CNS need only trigger a synergic unit to produce the joint torques required for a movement (Buchanan et al 1989). In the neck, Richmond et al (1992) observed dissociation between deep and superficial neck muscles in freely moving cats that would suggest control by different neural substrates. This differential control might be indicative of independent muscle synergies, each acting at a different axis of joint motion to produce a different movement goal. Separate actions of two groups of muscles, one producing the forces necessary to move the vertebral column and the other to align the head with a terminal target, would assist the head–neck controller in meeting its multiple criteria or goals (Thomson et al 1994).

Directional patterns of activation

Originally, synergists referred to those muscles producing the same direction of force (Beevor 1977). Experiments on complex motor systems, including the oral–facial system (Abbs & Cole 1988), the upper arm (Buchanan et al 1989) and the head and neck (Keshner et al 1989), have demonstrated that a single action can be accomplished through a variety of muscle patterns consisting of both agonists and antagonists. The controlled parameter appears to be the required force vector rather than the specific force–lever arm of any one muscle (Macpherson 1988, 1991).

It is theoretically possible that each individual head movement is produced by a variety of muscle patterns, thus requiring many muscles to satisfy all possible combinations. In that case, the CNS could then choose from a number of possible combinations to produce the desired outcome (Crowninshield & Brand 1981). It has been seen in both decerebrate and alert cats that the maximal excitation of a muscle when participating in any particular task is strongly related to a specific direction of motion (Keshner et al 1992, 1997). Thus muscles may be selected on the basis of the required force vector rather than on the goal of the task.

Concomitant studies in humans have been impeded by the methodology required to isolate individual neck muscle responses. Experimenters have mostly relied upon the implantation of fine wire electrodes (Takebe et al 1974, Vitti et al 1973), believed to be the only method that could distinguish between the overlapping neck muscles. There is a reluctance on the part of human subjects, however, to undergo invasive procedures with needle or wire electrodes, and these studies have only been able to measure the response of one muscle at any given time.

Measurement of a single muscle during any given head movement limits the conclusions that can be drawn concerning the programming of synergistic patterns of action. For example, Zangemeister et al (1982) recorded from two pairs of neck muscles with surface electrodes during ballistic head rotations and found that initial head position strongly influenced their results on the functional interaction of the two muscles. Keshner et al (1989) simultaneously recorded the activation of four neck muscles using surface electrodes during an isometric head stabilization task. When amplitude of electromyographic (EMG) activation was plotted against direction of applied force, each muscle exhibited a preferred direction of activation, which could be represented as a three-dimensional maximal activation direction vector having components in the flexion/extension, lateral bending and axial rotation directions (Fig. 9.1). Increasing the force applied to the head linearly increased

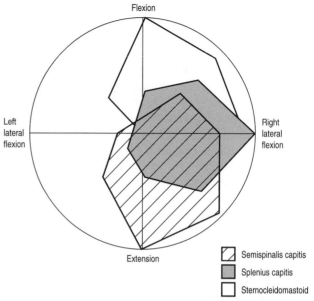

Figure 9.1 Mean percentage of maximum EMG activation in the frontal plane for three neck muscles in 15 subjects attempting to isometrically stabilize their heads against a 4.5 kg weight demonstrates overlapping activation but differing maximal activation directions. The point closest to the circumference is the direction of maximal activation for that muscle.

EMG output in preferred response directions and revealed a non-linear change in EMG activation in non-preferred directions, which changed from deactivation at low forces to activation at higher forces. These results demonstrate that describing the combined activation patterns of the muscles during each controlled head movement is necessary to reveal how the CNS programmes this complex motor system.

Directional tuning of neck muscles

Most studies of neck muscle activation examined moments about only one anatomical axis. However, most neck muscles have moment arms for more than one axis of rotation and their resultant moment arm direction is not aligned with an anatomical axis. Vasavada (1999) examined neck muscle EMG tuning curves while subjects generated three-dimensional isometric force moments against a stationary six-degrees-of-freedom rotational load cell attached to a head brace. Force moment output was displayed by a cursor on a computer screen to provide feedback to the subject. This task, where the head was rigidly stabilized, eliminated the need to protect the system against unwanted motion and resulted in more consistent patterns of muscle activation.

The neck muscles exhibited significant spatial tuning when subjects generated torques in the flexion, extension, lateral bending and intermediate directions. A test showed that each muscle's preferred direction was unique and consistent among subjects. Preferred activation directions were flexion for sternocleidomastoid, ipsilateral lateral flexion for splenius capitis and extension for semispinalis capitis. Trapezius was tuned toward lateral flexion but had the lowest activation levels and greatest variability. The maximal activation direction did not always correspond to the direction of the force moment produced by the muscle. For example, maximal activation of sternocleidomastoid was almost orthogonal to its moment arm direction, which was maximal in lateral flexion.

When axial rotation was included in the target moment, each muscle had a unique preferred direction which was consistent among subjects and usually dominated by a strong axial rotation component, shifting the maximal activation vectors even further from the moment arm direction. This behaviour can be explained by the fact that there are no muscles that produce powerful axial torques and therefore the CNS must activate the muscles that are available quite strongly to attain isometric torques equivalent to those in flexion/extension or lateral bending.

Thus, when the head–neck system is used in a situation with a single well-defined goal, neck muscles are activated in a consistent pattern over time and across subjects. When the task has multiple requirements such as maintaining head orientation and protecting the system from excessive forces, multiple strategies appear, each of which may use a different synergistic combination of muscles to produce the required net force moment (Peterson et al 2001).

Relationship between neck muscle activation and muscle mechanics

A likely control parameter for the CNS to employ in selecting the muscles that should participate in any given action would be the maximum moment arm of each muscle in order to maintain maximum mechanical advantage for each muscle. In one study (Keshner et al 1989) muscle tuning often corresponded to the direction of maximum mechanical advantage. Head position was not controlled in this study, and muscle activation patterns were found to differ across subjects, particularly in splenius capitis. When head position was controlled (Mayoux-Benhamou & Revel 1993, Vasavada 1999), directional tuning curves were consistent across subjects but did not correspond to the direction of the maximum moment arm. The EMG/moment relationship was non-linear and the maximum extension moment of the dorsal neck muscles occurred in the neutral head position.

The relationship between neck muscle activation patterns and maximum moment arm was also examined in cats during a head tracking task in the sagittal plane (Keshner et al 1997). A three-dimensional biomechanical model (Statler 2001) was developed to estimate how muscle moment arms and force generating capacities change during the head tracking movement. In some cases, modification of muscle activation patterns was consistent with changes in muscle moment arms or force generating poten-

tial. In other cases, however, changes in muscle activation patterns were observed without changes in muscle moment arms or force generating potential. Thus, the moment generating potential of the muscles appears to be just one of the variables that influence which muscles the CNS will select to participate in a movement.

Influence of posture on neck muscle activation patterns

Changes in cervical spine position

Muscle activation patterns have been found to differ between isometric (load control) and isoinertial (position control) tasks (Buchanan & Lloyd 1995, Tax et al 1990). In cats, spatial activation patterns and temporal relations between each muscle and a tracking device were affected by the plane of motion in which the head movement occurred. The plane of motion also affected the magnitude of muscle activation. It may be that a muscle's length and pulling direction, which can vary with cervical spine orientation, have a greater influence on its contribution to an action than mechanical efficiency (Mayoux-Benhamou & Revel 1993, Runciman & Richmond 1997).

Deep and superficial muscles in the cat neck were recorded during head turning movements (Thomson et al 1994). Some muscles varied their activity levels when the neck was horizontally or vertically positioned. Other muscles exhibited the same activity in either position, leading these investigators to purport the presence of both a varying and invariant synergy in the neck. The two groups of muscles seemed to be separated by those that were more superficial and attached to the lambdoidal crest (invariant) versus those that were lateral and caudal and attached intervertebrally or onto the scapula (variable). The variable synergy was assumed to reflect the changing lever arms of the muscles with changes in body position.

It is not clear whether postural effects are due to CNS selection of muscle activation patterns as a result of some fixed synergy, or whether the activation patterns are governed by the demands of the mechanical task including the mass of the system and the position of the thorax relative to the head (Richmond et al 1992). Orientation of the cervical spine (i.e. perpendicular or parallel to earth horizontal) was a significant variable in determining both the range of cervical joint motion and the amplitude and timing of the neck muscles (Statler & Keshner 2003). Changing the orientation of the neck did not lead to a large change in the moment arms of any of the muscles examined. Differences in muscle moment arms that did occur were too small to account for the different muscle activation patterns. It would appear that the functional capacity of the muscles was not compromised by the small changes in head–neck position required. Thus the mechanical properties of the muscles were not the relevant parameters generating the switch between muscle activation patterns. Differences in EMG activation with initial orientation could be due to a shift in the gravitational force vectors on the mechanical system requiring additional energy from the muscles to maintain a common output.

Changes in whole body posture

Neck muscle activation was also examined in a rhesus monkey (*Macaca mulatta*) in two body positions (Choi et al 2000, Peterson et al 2001). The animal produced sinusoidal (0.25 Hz) head tracking movements in the sagittal plane when seated with trunk and head vertical or while standing in the quadrupedal position. Vertebral motion was found to vary with body posture, occurring synchronously at all joints in upright, and primarily at skull-C1 in the quadrupedal position. EMG activation increased in the quadrupedal position and extensor muscles were concurrently activated when the neck was reaching peak extension. When upright, activation of muscles attaching to the upper cervical column (biventer cervicis, complexus, obliquus capitis inferior, rectus capitis posterior minor) peaked prior to full extension of the neck. Activation of muscles attaching to the lower vertebrae or scapula (rhomboideus capitis, semispinalis cervicis, splenius capitis, levator scapula anterior) peaked when the neck moved towards flexion. Only rectus capitis posterior major responded when the neck was fully extended. Thus, when upright, muscles are activated in functional groupings defined by their anatomical attachments. In the quadrupedal position, gravity acting on the horizontally oriented head produced greater activation and a collective response of the muscles. These results suggest a connection between central recruitment and the mechanical requirements of the task, which might include orientation of the spine relative to gravity and its interaction with muscle length–tension properties (Mayoux-Benhamou et al 1997).

Altering the system mechanics

Changing the inertial mass of the system has less impact on the selection of muscles and the behavioural response than does changing postural orientation (Fig. 9.2). In the cat, adding a weight to the head during a voluntary tracking task had little effect other than to increase the amplitude of each muscle's EMG response (Statler & Keshner 2003). Increased response amplitudes were observed in the sagittal plane when the head was weighted but not in the horizontal plane. In a study of human subjects attempting to stabilize a weighted head during whole body rotations in the horizontal and sagittal planes (Keshner et al 1999), the behaviour of the head was found to change relatively little with added inertia. As adding inertia to a passive mechanical system should cause substantial changes in dynamics, neural mechanisms must be invoked to maintain the constant response dynamics. The principal effect on muscle EMG responses was to increase the delay in the response at high frequencies. Opposing neck muscles continued to be reciprocally activated even with an increased inertial mass.

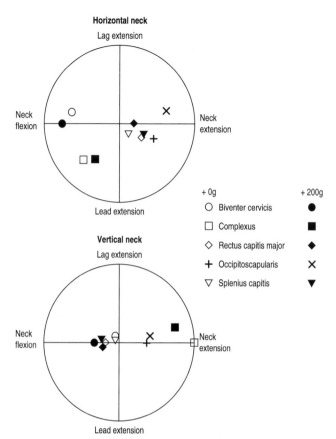

Figure 9.2 Polar plots of the amplitude (distance from the origin) and phase (location on axis) of the muscle EMG response in the cat during ±20° voluntary head tracking in the sagittal plane at 0.25 Hz. The cervical spine was parallel to the earth horizontal in the top plot and perpendicular to earth horizontal in the bottom plot. Open symbols are the response of the muscle with no weight added to the head. Filled symbols are the response of each muscle when a 200 g weight was placed on the head. Note the greater difference in muscle activation between the two neck postures rather than between the 0 g and 200 g responses.

A mathematical model of head–neck control (Peng et al 1996) has identified stiffness and the vestibulocollic reflex as the primary contributors to the control of head stabilization in space. It seems likely that the amount of both stiffness and reflex output are under central control and that these parameters were readjusted to maintain a consistent frequency response pattern of head movement when the head was weighted. Stiffness modulation should play a more significant role in the vertical than in the horizontal plane because of the greater influence of gravity on motions in the vertical plane that stimulates muscle receptors, thereby altering muscle preactivation levels and initial muscle stiffness.

NEURAL CONTROL OF THE CERVICAL SPINE

Several areas of the nervous system have been implicated in control of the cervical spine. These can be condensed into those that initiate the vestibular and cervical proprioceptive reflexes and those involved in voluntary head motions. Reflex responses of the neck, which include the vestibulocollic (VCR) and cervicocollic (CCR) reflexes, respond reactively to acceleratory and proprioceptive stimuli to maintain the orientation of the head in space (VCR) and the head on the trunk (CCR). Voluntary responses are those used for tracking and acquiring exteroceptive (visual, auditory, olfactory) information and can occur as either anticipatory or pursuit actions. The normal repertoire of head movement responses emerges from combinations of input and output signals.

Vestibulospinal pathways are considered to be the primary conveyor of descending inputs to the neck because of their monosynaptic and disynaptic connections with cervical motoneurons. Cervical proprioceptive inputs have a significant influence on the vestibulospinal signals (Gdowski & McCrea 2000) and a role in head stabilization as evidenced in studies of cervical proprioceptive disorders that have demonstrated distinct orientation and postural disturbances (Brandt 1996, Karlberg et al 1995). Other descending pathways, particularly those from the reticulospinal system (Peterson 1984, Peterson et al 1978), have been shown to be equally important for eliciting the VCR response.

Convergence of vestibular and somatosensory input onto the vestibulospinal and reticulospinal (Brink et al 1980) neurons is well documented and occurs at the level of the vestibular nuclear complex and adjacent reticular formation and upon spinal interneurons (Boyle & Pompeiano 1980, Kasper et al 1988, Peterson 1984, Wilson et al 1990). Convergence of afferent input may occur at the level of the motoneuron as well (Brink et al 1980). The combined signals initiate a series of interspinal reflexes that align the body segments (Roberts 1973, Wilson et al 1984).

Precise descriptions of the anatomy and neurophysiology of the pathways involved in these actions are comprehensively described elsewhere (Berthoz et al 1992, Wilson & Melvill Jones 1979). However, descriptions of isolated pathway locations and actions cannot convey how all of these control pathways operate through the biomechanics of the system to produce smooth, purposeful motions of the head and neck. This chapter will focus on the behavioural correlates that elucidate the motor control properties of the head and neck.

Characteristics of the cervical spine reflexes

The CCR and VCR reflexes appear perfectly suited through their dynamic and somatotopic characteristics to compensate for positional disturbances of the head and neck with respect to the trunk (Dutia & Price 1987, Peterson et al 1985, Schor et al 1988). The VCR produces a counter-rotation of the head on the trunk during transient postural reactions that is disturbed in patients with labyrinthine deficit (Horak et al 1994, Keshner et al 1987). The CCR stabilizes

the head on the body and can provide information about the rotation of the head on the trunk.

Angular vestibulocollic reflex

Specific influences of labyrinthine signals on head and limb movements have been studied in the cat and monkey. With head position fixed relative to the body, and the semicircular canals stimulated by either angular rotation in the horizontal plane or by electrical stimulation applied to individual canal nerves, a compensatory action of the neck and eye muscles away from the direction of stimulation was evoked (Suzuki & Cohen 1964). Electrical stimulation also results in reciprocal limb movements so that the body is pushed into a vertical position by extension of the opposite limb (Cohen et al 1966). Thus, when the restrained animal does not have to compensate for normal environmental forces, converging vestibular and spinal inputs either sum or cancel their effects so that the animal appears to attain a position of optimum stability and orientation in space.

It is probable that the disynaptic vestibular pathways contribute to the VCR. Nevertheless, the evidence that is available demonstrates that these pathways by themselves are not sufficient to produce the dynamics of the reflex (Wilson & Schor 1999). Other inputs to the VCR include the reticulospinal pathways, which have been shown to replace the short-latency connections when vestibulospinal pathways are interrupted (Peterson 1984, Peterson et al 1978). Furthermore, the VCR is not sufficient for purposeful head stabilization in a dynamic environment. The simple response pathways identified in reduced preparations, such as decerebrate cats, are not as readily elicited in alert animals (Banovetz et al 1995, Boyle et al 1996, Wilson & Schor 1999) and are not adequate to produce the forces necessary to counteract external disturbances.

Cervicocollic reflex

Recent findings (Gdowski & McCrea 2000) suggest that correct alignment of the head with the trunk and with the gravitoinertial vertical (Imai et al 2001) requires that the vestibular system receive ascending somatosensory inputs. Thus, to attain an appropriate postural response, a convergence of sensory information from the vestibular and somatosensory systems is needed to align the body with respect to earth vertical and to align various body parts with respect to each other.

The CCR arises from a stretch of the neck muscles (Ezure et al 1983, Peterson et al 1985) as would occur if the body were turning under a fixed head. Although there is an abundance of evidence that the neck proprioceptors provide information regarding the position and movement of the head with respect to the trunk, the actual receptors eliciting this response are not well delineated. The muscle spindle is the most obvious receptor to produce the CCR response, but the physiological evidence suggests this reaction is not a simple spindle reflex (Wilson 1992). The evidence suggests the presence of more signal processing between the receptors and motoneurons than expected from a monosynaptic pathway, and there is evidence for a contribution from presynaptic inhibition in the CCR response (Banovetz et al 1995, Wilson 1988).

Linear vestibulocollic reflex

Because of the difficulty in isolating outputs from the otoliths, little is known about the actions of this component of the vestibular system. The otoliths are stimulated by linear accelerations of the head and their inputs have been found to modify both eye and head stabilizing responses (Schor & Miller 1981, 1982, Schor et al 1985). Studies of neck reflex activation in alert cats (Banovetz et al 1995, Lacour et al 1987) and head stabilization in humans (Keshner et al 1995) found VCR responses to pitch or roll rotations that contain an added component from activation of otolith organs. Otolith contributions to compensatory eye and neck responses increased with stimulus frequency, but the otolith system alone was unable to produce perfect compensation (Borel & Lacour 1982). There is some suggestion that convergence of canal and otolith input on vestibulospinal neurons supplies combined angular and linear acceleration inputs to the vestibulospinal reflexes in the neck (Uchino et al 2000); however, the otoliths have been described as having a distinct functional effect during locomotion. In order to maintain a stable head fixation distance over the optimal range of walking velocities, it was proposed that compensatory head pitch movements were produced predominantly by the angular vestibulocollic reflex at low walking speeds and by the linear vestibulocollic reflex at higher speeds (Hirasaki et al 1999).

MULTIMODAL CONTROL OF THE HEAD AND NECK

Although the CCR and VCR appear to be all that is necessary to compensate for positional disturbances of the head and neck, most of the research indicates that more than one mechanism actually contributes to control of the cervical spine (Fig. 9.3). Multiple pathways contribute to stabilization of the head by the neck, and there is evidence that remaining pathways may compensate for the loss or injury of any one pathway, although it would not be a complete functional substitution (Keshner 2000, Keshner & Chen 1996).

In a series of studies in which seated subjects were rotated with predictive sinusoids, the natural mechanics of the head–neck system were found to be adequate to produce head stabilization (Barnes & Rance 1974, 1975, Bizzi et al 1978). Other studies that examined stabilization of the head when the trunk was fixed, however, demonstrated that the VCR and CCR also made a strong contribution to this response (Goldberg & Peterson 1986, Keshner & Peterson 1995, Viviani & Berthoz 1975). Voluntary motor commands and mechanical properties of the system also accounted for compensatory head motions in monkeys and

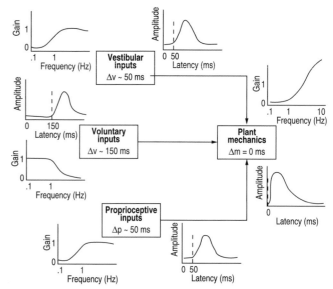

Figure 9.3 Flow diagram depicting the potential pathways participating in head stabilization. Graphs surrounding each control box illustrate the expected activation of each control mechanism in the time (latency) and frequency domains.

humans undergoing horizontal trunk rotations when the trunk was fixed (Bizzi et al 1976, Gresty 1987, Guitton et al 1986, Keshner & Peterson 1995) and in humans in the vertical plane (Keshner et al 1995).

Mechanisms controlling head stabilization

Differential frequency characteristics of the mechanisms potentially controlling head stability (Fig. 9.4) were revealed through a paradigm of fixing the trunk to the seat so that only the head was free to move. Subjects were randomly rotated in the dark in the vertical and horizontal planes (Keshner & Chen 1996, Keshner & Peterson 1995, Keshner et al 1995) with a range of sinusoidal frequencies. Voluntary control was manipulated by either distracting the subjects with a mental task or requiring that they stabilize to a visual image.

In the horizontal plane, responses of the neck with respect to the trunk were similar to responses that were predicted by an underdamped, second order linear system (see Fig. 9.4). Amplitudes of the neck with respect to trunk amplitudes rose at approximately 40 dB/decade and, when amplitudes were large enough to be meaningful, response phases shifted from 0 degrees to −180 degrees. A plateau in the response dynamics that appeared around 1.5–2.5 Hz (see arrow in Fig. 9.4) implies that an additional control mechanism was operating to damp the rising response. Resonant responses of the head (implying that stabilization was lost and the head moved more than the trunk) were observed above 2.5 Hz. These data suggest that the head was locked to the trunk at low frequencies, had a small area

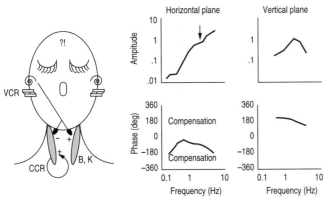

Figure 9.4 The cartoon on the left depicts the mechanisms contributing to stabilization of the head. Canal and otolith signals descend from the labyrinths to excite the contralateral and inhibit the ipsilateral neck muscles via the VCR. Proprioceptive inputs from the neck generate excitation of the ipsilateral neck muscles via the CCR. Descending voluntary signals (?!) and the intrinsic mechanics of the neck such as viscoelasticity (B) and stiffness (K) also influence the response. On the right are bode plots of the amplitude and phase of the average neck with respect to trunk response to horizontal and vertical plane pseudorandom sum-of-sine rotations during a mental distraction task. Phases of ±180° and amplitudes equal to 1 indicate that the head is perfectly compensating for motion of the trunk to stay stable in space. A phase of 0° indicates that the head is moving with the trunk. Amplitudes greater than 1 mean that the head is moving more than the trunk. The vertical arrow indicates the plateau in the horizontal plane dynamics that appeared around 1.5–2.5 Hz.

responses controlled by visual signals. Above 1 Hz, mechanical factors (e.g., inertia, stiffness and viscoelasticity) become important and act with little delay.

Linear translations of the subject when the trunk was free to move also reveal a significant somatosensory component of head stabilization as a result of motion of the trunk at the neck (Forssberg & Hirschfeld 1994, Gresty 1989, Vibert et al 2001). The relative importance of the VCR and CCR for head–neck stabilization is probably dependent upon the degrees of freedom and postural requirements of the task.

Influence of task on neck muscle activation patterns

In alert cats, movements generated in a particular direction during a voluntary head–tracking task used different muscle patterns than the same head movements generated by the neck reflexes (Keshner et al 1992). Correspondingly, the maximal response of individual muscles occurred at different orientations for the two tasks (Fig. 9.5). But each voluntary and reflex head movement in the cat was produced by an identifiable and repeatable pattern of neck muscle activation during orienting and stabilizing behaviours (Baker et al 1985, Keshner et al 1992, Roucoux & Crommelinck 1988). This was also true in head-fixed monkeys during pursuit eye movements (Lestienne et al 1984). This would imply that each head motion task is executed by a specific muscular pattern that is not repeated in any other direction.

Different patterns of muscle activation during reflex and voluntary head motions suggest that the sensorimotor transformation process is different for reflex and voluntary

of compensation for trunk motion, and then stabilization was lost as frequency increased. The simple second order response pattern would suggest that voluntary mechanisms act to stabilize the head to the trunk at low frequencies and that head inertia and other biomechanical factors predominate at high frequencies. In the mid-frequency range, reflexes may become active to dampen and delay control by the system mechanics. In the vertical plane, larger response amplitudes imply that head stabilization improves at low frequencies (< 1 Hz). The response is similar to the responses in the horizontal plane at the mid-frequencies but the high frequency resonance is not observed. Enhanced otolith contributions may have occurred at low frequencies in the vertical plane due to gravitational input, thereby smoothing the performance of the head stabilizing system throughout the frequency range.

Thus, the reflexes appear to be predominant in the frequency range of natural locomotion (1.5–2 Hz) (Hirasaki et al 1999) and their function is to damp oscillations of the head at higher frequencies or with altered system mechanics (Keshner et al 1999). Below 1 Hz, the head is primarily stabilized by longer latency (>100 ms) voluntary pathways and, perhaps, otolith signals. Voluntary responses are observed as anticipatory torques in the neck muscles or

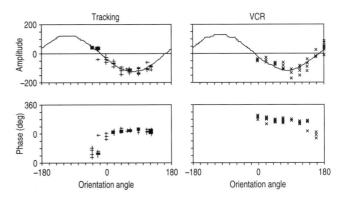

Figure 9.5 Plots of amplitudes and phases of the right complexus muscle EMG responses during ±20° voluntary head tracking and VCR trials at 0.25 Hz in different head orientations. Responses are derived from a least-squares fit to five days of data from one cat. A sinusoid fit to the amplitude data illustrates the sinusoidal pattern of EMG output with maximum and minimum responses shifted +22° in the VCR task. A 90° phase shift in the VCR relative to tracking indicates a response related to the velocity rather than the position of the head.

tasks, thereby modifying the directional results. Numerous sites have the potential to be a locus for the sensorimotor transformation of voluntary movements. Neurons of the pontomedullary reticular formation, many that monosynaptically excite motoneurons supplying neck and axial muscles (Peterson et al 1978, 1984), get inputs from head and trunk areas of motor cortex in the cat (Alstermark et al 1983, Peterson et al 1975). Convergent semicircular canal and neck proprioceptive inputs were recorded at cortical levels in alert cats during a passive rotation task (Mergner et al 1985). There are also widespread reciprocal projections between cerebellum and neck afferents (Chan et al 1982, Wilson et al 1976).

Transformation of vestibular inputs to neck motor output during the VCR occurs primarily in the brainstem nuclei. Head movements need to be constrained during the reflex task and may include only a few joints, thereby restricting the system to one pattern of muscle activation, whereas motor solutions for voluntary head tracking need constant adjustment. Multiple sensory input is also operative during voluntary movements, as are changing muscle lengths, multiarticular motions and a changing visual scene.

MODELS OF THE HEAD AND NECK

The head and neck serve as a strong correlate of the whole body during postural restabilization because of their multisegmental, multi-muscle arrangement (Graf et al 1997, Winters & Goldsmith 1983). A critical gap in our knowledge is at the output end where we know very little about the biomechanical action of neck muscles as a function of neck geometry. The complexity of the neck motor system poses a difficult challenge for creating useful predictive models. The most common approach to a dynamic model of the head and neck is the lumped parameter model where single parameters are used to represent the inertia, viscosity and elasticity of the system. Goldberg & Peterson (1986) have shown that the lumped parameter model provides an excellent fit to properties of a passive head–neck system. However, discrepancies between rigid models and physical data exist and suggest a need in the models for greater freedom of joint motion.

A biomechanical model first developed to study how surgical changes in musculoskeletal geometry and musculotendon parameters affect muscle force and its moment about the joints (Delp & Loan 1995) has been applied to the cat (Keshner et al 1997, Statler 2001, Statler & Keshner 2003) and to the human (Vasavada 1999, Vasavada et al 1998) neck. The model uses a graphical interface that allows visualization of the musculoskeletal geometry and permits manipulation of the model parameters. To create a model using this system, the geometry of the bones, the kinematics of the joints and the lines of action and force generating parameters (physiological cross-sectional area, muscle fibre length, tendon slack length and fibre pennation angle) of the muscles are specified. Once musculoskeletal geometry

is specified, muscle lengths and moment arms can be computed over a range of body positions. Given a set of muscle activation patterns from electromyographic recordings, the forces and moments generated by each modelled muscle can be estimated. Also, the moments developed by passive structures such as intervertebral ligaments can be incorporated. Moment arms of each muscle are computed from the mathematical descriptions of the muscle lines of action and the joint kinematics. The model can be used to predict the motor control consequences occurring as a result of cervical joint limitations.

A homeomorphic model of head and neck sensorimotor integration has been developed (Keshner et al 1999, Peng et al 1996) to interpret experimental data from human subjects. The model is 'lumped' parameter in type because of gaps in available data and to avoid unnecessary complexity. The model is based on the biomechanics, that is, the geometry and physics, of the joints and masses involved. Layered on top of the biomechanics are stiffness (position dependence), viscosity (velocity dependence) and extrinsic torques. The goal is to split out contributions of specific sensory loops and motor control pathways that are relevant to human health. The model (Fig. 9.6) simulating the response of the head to a horizontal trunk displacement incorporates head mechanics, the VCR and the CCR, with parameters drawn from numerous experimental studies (Peng et al 1996). A more complex two-joint model of pitch-plane head motion including VCR and CCR loops has also been developed and can simulate experimental results (Keshner et al 1999), but the addition of the second joint has increased the mechanical complexity. In the pitch plane the head is unstable without active control. In response to a step input, it

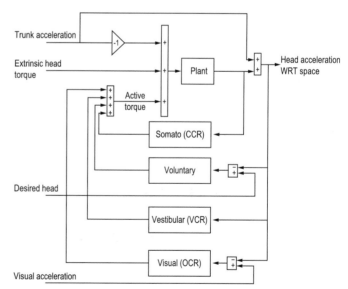

Figure 9.6 Control loops believed to participate in head stabilization and incorporated into the homeomorphic model of head stability. In addition to the inertial (I), cervicocollic (CCR), and vestibulocollic (VCR) inputs, somatosensory, visual (visuocollic reflex = OCR) and vestibular error signals (shown as ± control signals) are combined, delayed and coupled to the head.

'falls over' with a pronounced 'bounce' on the top trace of the time domain simulation when there is no compensation. The addition of static vestibular or proprioceptive inputs results in a head that still leans forwards but remains much closer to upright. The addition of dynamic compensation using the VCR and CCR improves stability.

CONCLUSION

Dynamic studies have indicated that visual and voluntary control of neck muscles and the dynamic and static VCR and CCR preferentially govern the head–neck system in different frequency domains. Thus neural control of the cervical system may be redundant but it is not excessive. Each component of the system is necessary to have a flexible and functional system. Redundant control allows the system to compensate for injury as well as creating a potential for substantial variability within and between subjects. Kinematic studies have indicated the existence of specific muscle activation patterns for voluntary force generation in the neck, of reflex and voluntary control strategies for stabilizing the head during body perturbations, and of several control strategies for voluntary head tracking that vary with posture. Each strategy appears to be executed by a specific muscle synergy that is presumably optimized to efficiently meet the demands of the task and the neural controllers must compensate for these task and posture dependent variations. Models need to be further developed to explain and delineate the multiple levels of control and response in the cervical spine.

KEYWORDS	
biomechanical model	neck muscles
cervical spine	neural control
cervicocollic	posture
CNS	redundancy
directional tuning	reflex
electromyography	reticulospinal
EMG	vertebrae
head tracking	vestibular
kinematics	vestibulocollic
mathematical model	vestibulospinal
moment arms	videofluoroscopy
muscle activation patterns	voluntary control

References

Abbs J H, Cole K J 1988 Neural mechanisms of motor equivalence and goal achievement. In: Wise S P (ed) Higher brain functions: recent explorations of the brain's emergent properties. Wiley, New York, pp 15–43

Alstermark B, Pinter M, Sasaki S 1983 Convergence on reticulospinal neurons mediating contralateral pyramidal disynaptic EPSPS to neck motoneurons. Brain Research 259: 151–154

Baker J, Goldberg J, Peterson B 1985 Spatial and temporal response properties of the vestibulocollic reflex in decerebrate cats. Journal of Neurophysiology 54: 735–756

Banovetz J, Baker J F, Peterson B W 1995 Spatial coordination by vestibular descending signals. I: Reflex excitation of neck muscles in alert and decerebrate cats. Experimental Brain Research 105: 345–362

Barnes G R, Rance B H 1974 Transmission of angular acceleration to the head in the seated human subject. Aerospace Medicine 45: 4121–4126

Barnes G R, Rance B H 1975 Head movement induced by angular oscillation of the body in the pitch and roll axes. Aviation Space Environmental Medicine 46: 987–993

Beevor C E 1977 The Croonian lectures on muscular movements and their representation in the central nervous system. In: Payton O D, Hirt S, Newton R A (eds) Scientific bases for neurophysiologic approaches to therapeutic exercise: an anthology. F A Davis, Philadelphia, pp 5–12

Bernstein N 1967 The problem of interrelation of co-ordination and localization. In: Bernstein N The coordination and regulation of movements. Pergamon Press, New York, pp 15–59

Berthoz A, Graf W, Vidal P P (eds) 1992 The head–neck sensory motor system. Oxford, New York

Bizzi E, Polit A, Morasso P 1976 Mechanisms underlying achievement of final head position. Journal of Neurophysiology 39: 435–444

Bizzi E, Dev P, Morasso P, Polit A 1978 Effect of load disturbances during centrally initiated movements. Journal of Neurophysiology 41: 542–556

Bland J H, Boushey D R 1988 The cervical spine, from anatomy and physiology to clinical care. In: Berthoz A, Graf W, Vidal P P (eds) The head–neck sensory motor system. Oxford, New York, pp 135–140

Borel L, Lacour M 1982 Functional coupling of the stabilizing eye and head reflexes during horizontal and vertical linear motion in the cat. Experimental Brain Research 91: 191–206

Boyle R, Pompeiano O 1980 Responses of vestibulospinal neurons to sinusoidal rotation of neck. Journal of Neurophysiology 44: 633–649

Boyle R, Belton T, McCrea R A 1996 Responses of identified vestibulospinal neurons to voluntary and reflex eye and head movements in the alert squirrel monkey. Annals of the New York Academy of Sciences 781: 244–263

Brandt T 1996 Cervical vertigo: reality or fiction? Audiology and Neuro-Otology 1: 187–196

Brink E E, Hirai N, Wilson V J 1980 Influence of neck afferents on vestibulospinal neurons. Experimental Brain Research 38: 285–292

Buchanan T S, Lloyd D G 1995 Muscle activity is different for humans performing static tasks, which require force control and position control. Neuroscience Letters 194: 61–64

Buchanan T S, Rovai G P, Rymer W Z 1989 Strategies for muscle activation during isometric torque generation at the human elbow. Journal of Neurophysiology 62: 1201–1212

Chan Y S, Manzoni D, Pompeiano O 1982 Response characteristics of cerebellar dentate and lateral cortex neurons to sinusoidal stimulation of neck and labyrinth receptors. Neuroscience 7: 2993–3011

Choi H, Keshner E A, Peterson B W 2000 Primate neck muscle activation patterns during head tracking in two postures. Society for Neuroscience Abstracts 26: 2212

Cohen B, Tokumasu K, Goto K 1966 Semicircular canal nerve eye and head movements: the effect of changes in initial eye and head position on the plane of the induced movement. Archives of Ophthalmology 76: 523–531

Crowninshield R D, Brand R A 1981 A physiologically based criteria of muscle force prediction in locomotion. Journal of Biomechanics 14: 793–801

de Waele C, Graf W, Josset P, Vidal P P 1989 A radiological analysis of the postural syndromes following hemilabyrinthectomy and selective canal and otolith lesions in the guinea pig. Experimental Brain Research 77: 166–182

Delp S L, Loan J P 1995 A graphics-based software system to develop and analyze models of musculoskeletal structures. Computers in Biology and Medicine 25: 21–34

Dutia M B, Price R F 1987 Interaction between the vestibulocollic reflex and the cervicocollic stretch reflex in the decerebrate cat. Journal of Physiology (London) 387: 19–30

Ezure K, Fukushima K, Schor R H, Wilson V J 1983 Compartmentalization of the cervicocollic reflex in cat splenius muscle. Experimental Brain Research 51: 397–404

Forssberg H, Hirschfeld H 1994 Postural adjustments in sitting humans following external perturbations: muscle activity and kinematics. Experimental Brain Research 97: 515–527

Gdowski G T, McCrea R A 2000 Neck proprioceptive inputs to primate vestibular nucleus neurons. Experimental Brain Research 135: 511–526

Goldberg J, Peterson B W 1986 Reflex and mechanical contributions to head stabilization in alert cats. Journal of Neurophysiology 56: 857–875

Gowitzke B A, Milner M 1980 Understanding the scientific basis of human movement. Williams and Wilkins, Baltimore

Graf W, De Waele C, Vidal P P 1995 Functional anatomy of the head–neck movement system of quadrupedal and bipedal mammals. Journal of Anatomy 186: 55–74

Graf W, Keshner E, Richmond F J, Shinoda Y, Statler K, Uchino Y 1997 How to construct and move a cat's neck. Journal of Vestibular Research 7: 219–237

Gresty M 1987 Stability of the head: studies in normal subjects and in patients with labyrinthine disease, head tremor, and dystonia. Movement Disorders 2: 165–185

Gresty M 1989 Stability of the head in pitch (neck flexion–extension): studies in normal subjects and patients with axial rigidity. Movement Disorders 4: 233–248

Guitton D, Kearney R E, Wereley N, Peterson B W 1986 Visual, vestibular and voluntary contributions to human head stabilization. Experimental Brain Research 64: 59–69

Hirasaki E, Moore S T, Raphan T, Cohen B 1999 Effects of walking velocity on vertical head and body movements during locomotion. Experimental Brain Research 127: 117–130

Horak F B, Shupert C L, Dietz V, Horstmann G 1994 Vestibular and somatosensory contributions to responses to head and body displacements in stance. Experimental Brain Research 100: 93–106

Imai T, Moore S T, Raphan T, Cohen B 2001 Interaction of the body, head, and eyes during walking and turning. Experimental Brain Research 136: 1–18

Kamibayashi L K, Richmond F J 1998 Morphometry of human neck muscles. Spine 23: 1314–1323

Karlberg M, Persson L, Magnusson M 1995 Impaired postural control in patients with cervico-brachial pain. Acta Oto-Laryngologica 520 (2) (Suppl.): 440–442

Kasper J, Schor R H, Wilson V J 1988 Response of vestibular neurons to head rotations in vertical planes. II: Response to neck stimulation and vestibular neck-interaction. Journal of Neurophysiology 60: 1765–1778

Keshner E A 1994 Vertebral orientations and muscle activation patterns during controlled head movements in cats. Experimental Brain Research 98: 546–550

Keshner E A 2000 Modulating active stiffness affects head stabilizing strategies in young and elderly adults during trunk rotations in the vertical plane. Gait and Posture 11: 1–11

Keshner E A, Chen K J 1996 Mechanisms controlling head stabilization in the elderly during random rotations in the vertical plane. Journal of Motor Behavior 28: 324–336

Keshner E A, Peterson B W 1995 Mechanisms controlling human head stability. I: Head–neck dynamics during random rotations in the horizontal plane. Journal of Neurophysiology 73: 2293–2301

Keshner E A, Allum J H J, Pfaltz C R 1987 Postural coactivation and adaptation in the sway stabilizing responses of normals and patients with bilateral peripheral vestibular deficit. Experimental Brain Research 69: 66–72

Keshner E A, Campbell D, Katz R, Peterson B W 1989 Neck muscle activation patterns in humans during isometric head stabilization. Experimental Brain Research 75: 335–364

Keshner E A, Baker J F, Banovetz J, Peterson B W 1992 Patterns of neck muscle activation in cats during reflex and voluntary head movements. Experimental Brain Research 88: 361–374

Keshner E A, Cromwell R, Peterson B W 1995 Mechanisms controlling human head stability. II: Head–neck characteristics during random rotations in the vertical plane. Journal of Neurophysiology 73: 2302–2312

Keshner E A, Statler K D, Delp S L 1997 Kinematics of the freely moving head and neck in the alert cat. Experimental Brain Research 115: 257–266

Keshner E A, Hain T C, Chen K J 1999 Predicting control mechanisms for human head stabilization by altering the passive mechanics. Journal of Vestibular Research 9: 423–434

Lacour M L, Borel J, Barthelemy J, Harlay S, Xerri C 1987 Dynamic properties of the vertical otolith-neck reflexes in the alert cat. Experimental Brain Research 65: 559–568

Lestienne F, Vidal P P, Berthoz A 1984 Gaze changing behaviour in head restrained monkey. Experimental Brain Research 53: 349–356

Lockhart R D, Hamilton G F, Fyfe F W 1972 Anatomy of the human body. J B Lippincott, New York

Macpherson J M 1988 Strategies that simplify the control of quadrupedal stance. I: Forces at the ground. Journal of Neurophysiology 60: 204–217

Macpherson J M 1991 How flexible are muscle synergies? In: Humphrey D R, Freund H J (eds) Motor control: concepts and issues. Wiley, New York, pp 33–47

Mayoux-Benhamou M A, Revel M 1993 Influence of head position on dorsal neck muscle efficiency. Electromyography and Clinical Neurophysiology 33: 161–166

Mayoux-Benhamou M A, Revel M A, Vallee C 1997 Selective electromyography of dorsal neck muscles in humans. Experimental Brain Research 113: 353–360

Mergner T, Becker W, Deecke L 1985 Canal–neck interaction in vestibular neurons of the cat's cerebral cortex. Experimental Brain Research 61: 94–108

Outerbridge J S, Melvill Jones G 1971 Reflex vestibular control of head movements in man. Aerospace Medicine 42: 935–940

Panjabi M M, Crisco J J, Vasavada A et al 2001 Mechanical properties of the human cervical spine as shown by three-dimensional load-displacement curves. Spine 26: 2692–2700

Peng G C, Hain T C, Peterson B W 1996 A dynamical model for reflex activated head movements in the horizontal plane. Biological Cybernetics 75: 309–319

Peterson B W 1984 The reticulospinal system and its role in the control of movement. In: Barnes C D (ed) Brainstem control of spinal cord function. Academic Press, New York, pp 27–86

Peterson B W, Maunz R A, Pitts N G, Mackel R G 1975 Patterns of projection and branching of reticulospinal neurons. Experimental Brain Research 23: 333–351

Peterson B W, Pitts N G, Fukushima K, Mackel R 1978 Reticulospinal excitation and inhibition of neck motoneurons. Experimental Brain Research 32: 471–489

Peterson B W, Goldberg J, Bilotto G, Fuller J H 1985 The cervicocollic reflex: its dynamic properties and interaction with vestibular reflexes. Journal of Neurophysiology 54: 90–109

Peterson B W, Pellionisz A J, Baker J F, Keshner E A 1989 Functional morphology and neural control of neck muscles in mammals. American Zoologist 29: 139–149

Peterson B W, Choi H, Hain T, Keshner E, Peng G C 2001 Dynamic and kinematic strategies for head movement control. Annals of the New York Academy of Sciences 942: 381–393

Richmond F J R, Abrahams V C 1975 Morphology and enzyme histochemistry of dorsal muscles of the cat neck. Journal of Neurophysiology 38: 1312–1321

Richmond F J R, Vidal P P 1988 The motor system: joints and muscles of the neck. In: Peterson B W, Richmond F J (eds) Control of head movement. Oxford University Press, New York, p 121

Richmond F J R, Gordon D C, Loeb G E 1991 Heterogeneous structure and function among intervertebral muscles. In: Berthoz A, Graf W, Vidal P P (eds) The head–neck sensory motor system: Oxford University Press, New York, pp 101–103

Richmond F J R, Thomson D B, Lob G E 1992 Electromyographic studies of neck muscles in the intact cat. I: Patterns of recruitment underlying posture and movement during natural behaviors. Experimental Brain Research 88: 41–58

Roberts T D M 1973 Reflex balance. Nature 244: 156–158

Roucoux A, Crommelinck M 1988 Control of head movement during visual orientation. In: Peterson B W, Richmond F J (eds) Control of head movement. Oxford University Press, New York, pp 208–223

Runciman R J, Richmond F J 1997 Shoulder and forelimb orientations and loading in sitting cats: implications for head and shoulder movement. Journal of Biomechanics 30: 911–919

Schor R H, Miller A D 1981 Vestibular reflexes in neck and forelimb muscles evoked by roll tilt. Journal of Neurophysiology 46: 167–178

Schor R H, Miller A D 1982 Relationship of cat vestibular neurons to otolith-spinal reflexes. Experimental Brain Research 47: 137–144

Schor R H, Miller A D, Timerick S J B, Tomko D L 1985 Responses to head tilt in cat central vestibular neurons. II: Frequency dependence of neural response vectors. Journal of Neurophysiology 53: 1444–1452

Schor R H, Kearney R E, Dieringer N 1988 Reflex stabilization of the head. In: Peterson B W, Richmond F J (eds) Control of head movement. Oxford University Press, New York, pp 141–166

Selbie W S, Thomson D B, Richmond F J R 1993 Suboccipital muscles in the cat neck: morphometry and histochemistry of the rectus capitis muscle complex. Journal of Morphology 216: 47–63

Sherk H H, Parke W W 1983 Normal adult anatomy. In: Cervical Spine Research Society (ed) The cervical spine. J B Lippincott, New York, pp 8–22

Statler K D 2001 A computer graphics based model of the cat head and neck used to examine joint movement, moment generating potential and EMG patterns in voluntary head and neck movements. PhD Thesis, Department of Biomedical Engineering, Northwestern University, Evanston, Illinois

Statler K D, Keshner E A 2003 Effects of inertial load and cervical-spine orientation on a head tracking task in the alert cat. Experimental Brain Research 148: 202–210.

Suzuki J-I, Cohen B 1964 Head, eye, body, and limb movements from semicircular canal nerves. Experimental Neurology 10: 393–406

Takebe K, Vitti M, Basmajian J V 1974 The functions of semispinalis capitis and splenius capitis muscles: an electromyographic study. Anatomical Records 179: 477–480

Tax A A M, Denier van der Gon J J, Erkelens C J 1990 Differences in central control of m. biceps brachii in movement tasks and force tasks. Experimental Brain Research 79: 138–142

Thomson D B, Loeb G E, Richmond F J R 1994 Effect of neck posture on the activation of feline neck muscles during voluntary head turns. Journal of Neurophysiology 72: 2004–2014

Tuller B, Turvey M T, Fitch H L 1982 The Bernstein perspective. II: The concept of muscle linkage or coordinative structure. In: Kelso J A S (ed) Human motor behavior: an introduction. Lawrence Erlbaum, New Jersey, pp 253–270

Uchino Y, Sato H, Kushiro K, Zakir M M, Isu N 2000 Canal and otolith inputs to single vestibular neurons in cats. Archives of Italian Biology 138: 3–13

Vasavada A N, Peterson B W, Delp S L 2002 Three-dimensional spatial tuning of neck muscle activation in humans. Experimental Brain Research 147: 437–448

Vasavada A N, Li S, Delp S L 1998 Influence of muscle morphometry and moment arms on the moment-generating capacity of human neck muscles. Spine 23: 412–422

Vibert N, MacDougall H G, de Waele C et al 2001 Variability in the control of head movements in seated humans: a link with whiplash injuries. Journal of Physiology 532: 851–868

Vidal P P, Graf W, Berthoz A 1986 The orientation of the cervical vertebral column in unrestrained awake animals. I: Resting position. Experimental Brain Research 61: 549–559

Vitti M, Fujiwara M, Basmajian J V, Iida M 1973 The integrated roles of longus colli and sternocleidomastoid muscles: an electromyographic study. Anatomical Records 177: 471–484

Viviani P, Berthoz A 1975 Dynamics of the head–neck system in response to small perturbations: analysis and modeling in the frequency domain. Biological Cybernetics 19: 19–37

Wickland C R, Baker J F, Peterson B W 1991 Torque vectors of neck muscles in the cat. Experimental Brain Research 84: 649–659

Wilson V J 1988 Convergence of neck and vestibular signals on spinal interneurons. Progress in Brain Research 76: 137–143

Wilson V J 1992 Physiologic properties and central actions of neck muscle spindles. In: Berthoz A, Graf W, Vidal P P (eds) The head–neck sensory motor system. Oxford University Press, New York, pp 175–178

Wilson V J, Melvill Jones G 1979 Mammalian vestibular physiology. Plenum Press, New York.

Wilson V J, Schor R H 1999 The neural substrate of the vestibulocollic reflex. What needs to be learned? Experimental Brain Research 129: 483–493

Wilson V J, Maeda M, Franck J I, Shimazu H 1976 Mossy fiber neck and second order labyrinthine projections to cat flocculus. Journal of Neurophysiology 39: 301–310

Wilson V J, Ezure K, Timerick S J B 1984 Tonic neck reflex of the decerebrate cat: response of spinal interneurons to natural stimulation of neck and vestibular receptors. Journal of Neurophysiology 51: 567–577

Wilson V J, Yamagata Y, Yates B J, Schor R H, Nonaka S 1990 Response of vestibular neurons to head rotations in vertical planes. III: Response of vestibulocollic neurons to vestibular and neck stimulation. Journal of Neurophysiology 164: 1695–1703

Winters J M, Goldsmith W 1983 Response of an advanced head–neck model to transient loading. Journal of Biomechanical Engineering 105: 63–70, 196–197

Worth D R 1994 Movements of the head and neck. In: Boyling J D, Palastanga N, Jull G A, Lee D G (eds) Grieve's Modern Manual Therapy, 2nd edn. Churchill Livingstone, Edinburgh, pp 53–68

Zangemeister W H, Stark L, Meienberg O, Waite T 1982 Neural control of head rotation: electromyographic evidence. Journal of Neurological Sciences 55: 1–14

Chapter 10

Motor control of the trunk

P. W. Hodges

INTRODUCTION

It is well accepted that the spine is inherently unstable and dependent on the contribution of muscles in addition to the passive elements of the spine to maintain stability and to control movement (Panjabi 1992b). Although trunk muscles must have sufficient strength and endurance to satisfy the demands of spinal control, the efficacy of the muscle system is dependent on its controller, the central nervous system (CNS) (Panjabi 1992b). The challenge for the CNS to move and control the spine is immense, despite constant changes in internal and external forces. The CNS must continually interpret the status of stability, plan mechanisms to overcome predictable challenges and rapidly initiate activity in response to unexpected challenges. It must interpret the afferent input from the peripheral mechanoreceptors, and other sensory systems, compare these requirements against an 'internal model of body dynamics' and then generate a coordinated response of the trunk muscles so that the muscle activity occurs at the right time, at the right amount, and so on. To further complicate this issue, muscle activity must be coordinated to maintain control of the spine within a hierarchy of interdependent levels: control of intervertebral translation and rotation, control of spinal posture/orientation, control of body with respect to the environment. Finally, unlike the muscles of the limb, trunk muscles perform a variety of homeostatic functions in addition to movement and control of the trunk, including respiration and continence. This chapter reviews the elements that contribute to the control and movement of the trunk, the strategies used by the CNS to undertake this control and factors that complicate or compromise this control owing to conflict between trunk muscle functions and pain.

BIOMECHANICAL DEMANDS FOR CONTROL OF MOVEMENT AND STABILITY

Optimal trunk function is a complex interplay between movement and control of the integrity of the spine and pelvis at the intersegmental level, at a global level involving the control of orientation (e.g. control of lordosis, control of pelvic rotation), and the contribution of the trunk to maintenance of equilibrium of the body with respect to gravity and other external forces (Fig. 10.1). All movements and postures are a complex interaction of movement and stability (Massion 1992). In reality, even static postures involve movement (for example small cyclical movements of the trunk and lower limbs compensate for disturbance to posture from respiration (Gurfinkel et al 1971, Hodges et al 2002a)), and movement occurs in conjunction with a subtle background of postural adjustments. Movement perturbs stability as a result of the interaction between internal and external forces (Massion 1992). These forces include the reactive moments from limb movements, changes in the influence of gravity on the body as a result of the modification of the position of the centre of mass with movement and the interaction with objects and the environment (for example catching a ball). Even a simple action such as a movement of a limb changes the position of the centre of mass and is associated with reactive moments that are equal in amplitude but opposite in direction to the forces producing the moment. There is considerable argument about which parts of a task are movement related and which are purely posture related. In fact movement is used by the CNS to maintain stability and minimize energy expenditure. Rather than making the spine rigid, the CNS uses coordinated movement to oppose and dissipate forces acting on the trunk. For instance, small movements of the trunk are initiated prior to limb movements that are opposed to the direction of reactive forces (Hodges et al 1999, 2000a), and rotation of the pelvis occurs around each orthogonal axis during gait (Perry 1992). Thus the control of movement and stability of the spine is complex. Moreover, the strategies used by the CNS and the muscles involved vary between the three levels of control (intersegmental control, orientation control and control of body equilibrium). However, the understanding of the demands of stability is complicated by disagreement regarding the definition of the term 'stability'.

Models of stability

The most common contemporary view of spinal stability is based on the Euler model which considers the control of buckling forces (see, for example, Crisco & Panjabi 1991, Gardner-Morse et al 1995, Cholewicki & McGill 1996). This is based on the understanding that buckling failure of the lumbar spine, devoid of muscle, occurs with compressive loading of as little as 90 N (Lucas & Bresler 1960). This model argues that activity and stiffness of antagonistic muscles is required to maintain the lumbar spine in a mechanically stable equilibrium (Crisco & Panjabi 1991, Gardner-Morse et al 1995, Cholewicki & McGill 1996). Due to the emphasis on buckling, this element relates particularly to the control of orientation and it has been argued that muscles act like guy wires to stiffen the intervertebral joints that they span (Crisco & Panjabi 1991). This definition is relatively static and suggests the maintenance of a set position of the spine. Few studies have considered this model in more dynamic terms (Cholewicki et al 1997).

While control of buckling is a critical element of stability, there are additional factors to consider. Firstly, in terms of spinal health, this should be broadened to include the control of spinal movement; it is important to consider the control of the progression of changes in curvature and intervertebral motion. Secondly, the definition must incorporate control of the other components of stability, namely

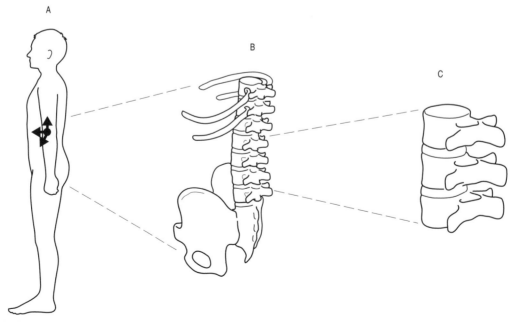

Figure 10.1 Multiple levels of trunk control. A: Control of equilibrium of the body. B: Control of trunk orientation. C: Intersegmental control.

the fine-tuning of intersegmental motion and the contribution of the trunk to postural equilibrium.

Control of intersegmental translation and rotation is important, but cannot be completely separated from the control of spinal orientation and buckling forces (Panjabi et al 1989). Buckling can occur at the intervertebral level, but separate attention must be paid to control of translations and rotations. For instance, during an arc of movement it is important to control the coordination between translation and rotation at the intervertebral levels (Bogduk et al 1995). It has been shown that if stability of the spine is modelled with muscles of varying lengths, but leaving one segment with no muscle attachment, the spine remains unstable with stability equivalent to that achieved with no muscle at all, thus highlighting the importance of segmental attachment of the spinal muscles (Crisco & Panjabi 1991); segmental control is an essential component for spinal stability.

At a more general level, as the trunk forms a large proportion of the mass of the body, trunk movement is important for the control of postural equilibrium with respect to external forces. If the equilibrium of the body is disturbed by external forces (such as an unexpected movement of the support surface) or internal forces (for example due to reactive forces from limb movement), movement of the trunk occurs to move the centre of mass over the base of support or alter the orientation of the body (see, for example, Horak & Nashner 1986, Keshner et al 1988). This stability function of the trunk is important to consider as it may influence the accuracy of control of spinal orientation or intervertebral motion. In particular, situations are likely to arise in which the requirement to move the trunk to restore balance may conflict with the demand to control the orientation of the spine.

The same principles of control of orientation and intersegmental motion also apply to the pelvis. At one level there is the need to control orientation of the pelvis around the three orthogonal axes; however, there is also the requirement to control the relationship between segments of the pelvis. In upright positions the sacroiliac joint (SIJ) is subjected to considerable shear force as the mass of the upper body must be transferred to the lower limbs via the ilia (Snijders et al 1993, 1995). The body has two mechanisms to overcome this shear force: one is dependent on the shape of the sacroiliac joint (form closure) and the frictional characteristics of the joint surface; the other mechanism involves generation of compressive forces across the SIJ via muscle contraction (force closure) (Snijders et al 1993, 1995). As with the spine, different muscles and recruitment strategies are likely to be involved in control of each aspect of stability of the pelvis.

Control in Neutral

The spine exhibits least stiffness around the neutral position (Panjabi 1992a). Panjabi described this region of low stiffness as the 'neutral zone'. This region is important to consider as its stability is dependent on the contribution of the trunk muscles and it has been argued that the region may increase (and thus the requirement for muscle activity) in situations of clinical instability (Panjabi 1992a).

CONTROL ELEMENTS

Motor control of spinal stability requires an integrated system that has sensors to detect the status of the body, a control system to interpret the requirements for stability and plan appropriate responses, and the muscles to execute the response. Consideration of these elements, in particular the architectural properties of the trunk muscles, is critical to understanding the mechanisms used by the nervous system to control trunk muscles to coordinate movement and stability of the trunk.

Muscles

A large number of muscles have a mechanical affect on the spine and pelvis and all muscles are *required* to maintain optimal control. An important consideration is the redundancy in the muscle system (i.e. many muscles cross the joints and may be capable of performing similar functions). However, there is considerable variation in the architectural properties of the trunk muscles, which has led to the proposal by several authors that there may be functional differentiation in the muscle system. This has implications for the potential contribution of these muscles to control and movement of the spine. In a general sense it is clear that the mechanical advantage of muscles to move and control the trunk varies due to factors such as the length of the moment arm and proximity to the joint, muscle attachments and the length and orientation of the muscle fascicles. Thus it has been argued variously that muscles are biomechanically more suited to either motion or stability (see, for example, Goff 1972, Janda 1978, Bergmark 1989, Richardson et al 1999, Sahrman 2002). In addition, as mentioned in the previous section, there are several elements to stability and there is likely to be some differentiation of contribution of muscles within this component. In reality there is likely to be a spectrum with muscles at the extremes that are ideally suited to control of intervertebral motion or spinal orientation and torque production; others in the middle of the spectrum make some contribution to both. Although simple division of muscles into groups is likely to oversimplify the complex control of lumbopelvic motion and stability, it provides a useful definition to consider as it contributes to our understanding of why the CNS uses different strategies to control the different muscle groups.

Bergmark (1989) presented a model for the trunk that considered differentiation in the contribution of muscle to stability. This model identified muscles as either 'local' or 'global', based on anatomical characteristics (Fig. 10.2). The local muscles are those that cross one/few segments and have a limited moment arm to move the joint, but an ideal anatomy to control intervertebral motion. Bergmark

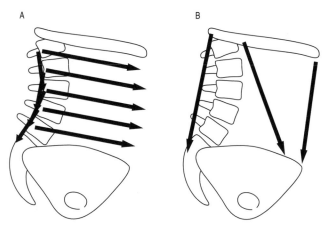

Figure 10.2 Local and global muscles of the trunk. A: Local muscles attach directly to the spine and control intervertebral motion. B: Global muscles transcend the spine and control spinal orientation.

included muscles such as the lumbar multifidus in this group; however, other muscles that satisfy these criteria are transversus abdominis (TrA) (Fig. 10.2A), intertransversarii and interspinales. In contrast, the global muscles have attachments to the pelvis and thorax and thus transcend multiple segments. These muscles have a larger moment arm and, thus, a larger torque generating capacity, and are suited to the control of orientation and balancing external forces. Examples of the global muscles include rectus abdominis, obliquus externus abdominis, obliquus internus abdominis and the thoracic erector spinae. Muscles such as the lateral fibres of quadratus lumborum and parts of psoas also meet these criteria. There is considerable overlap between these systems with some muscles sharing features of both, such as the lumbar portions of longissimus and iliocostalis, which have one attachment to the lumbar vertebrae and share some features of the local system.

Considering this model, it is clear that optimal function of both systems is required to maintain spinal function. The local system has only a limited ability to influence the control of orientation and, similarly, the global system has only a limited ability to control intervertebral motion. In fact, the contribution made by the global system to the control of intervertebral motion occurs as a result of compressive forces exerted by co-activation of antagonist global muscles. While compression can assist in the control of shear and rotation forces, this is associated with a cost: firstly, global co-activation increases the compressive load on lumbar segments (Gardner-Morse & Stokes 1998) resulting in increased intradiscal pressure and loading through the posterior elements; secondly, antagonist global muscle co-activation results in a restriction of spinal motion or rigidity of the spine and, as mentioned above, movement is an important component of optimal spinal control. In contrast, local muscles allow controlled spinal motion and have the ability to control individual segments rather than providing a general compressive force across the spine. Specific fea-

tures of the muscles that are intrinsic to the spine and those that lie superficially are presented in the following sections.

Intrinsic lumbopelvic muscles

Transversus abdominis (TrA) is a sheet-like muscle that attaches from the inguinal ligament, iliac crest, thoracolumbar fascia and the lower six ribs (Urquhart et al 2001). The attachment to the spine is via the three layers of the thoracolumbar fascia. The posterior layer of the fascia attaches to the spinous processes, the middle layer to the transverse processes and the anterior layer runs over quadratus lumborum (Williams et al 1989). The contribution of TrA to spinal control is complex. Its muscle fibres have a relatively horizontal orientation and therefore it has minimal ability to move the spine. However, it may contribute to rotation (Hemborg 1983, Cresswell et al 1992, Urquhart et al 2002). Its contribution to spinal control is likely to involve its role in modulation of intra-abdominal pressure (IAP) and tensioning the thoracolumbar fascia. TrA has been shown to be the abdominal muscle most closely associated with the control of IAP (Cresswell et al 1992, 1994) and recent data confirm that spinal stiffness is increased by IAP (Hodges et al 2001b, 2001d). Fascial tension may directly restrict intervertebral motion or provide gentle segmental compression via the posterior layer of the thoracolumbar fascia (Gracovetsky et al 1985). Recent porcine studies confirm that the combined effect of IAP and fascial tension is required for TrA to increase intervertebral stiffness and the mechanical effect of its contraction on the mid-lumbar regions is reduced if the fascial attachments are cut (Hodges et al 2002b). For sacroiliac support, TrA acts on the lever formed by the ilia to increase anterior compression of the SIJ (Snijders et al 1995); this has been confirmed in vivo (Richardson et al 2002).

Multifidus has five fascicles that arise from the spinous process and lamina of each lumbar vertebra and descend in a caudolateral direction (Macintosh & Bogduk 1986). The most superficial fibres of each fascicle cross up to five segments and attach caudally to the ilia and sacrum. In contrast, the deep fibres attach from the inferior border of a lamina and cross a minimum of two segments to attach on the mamillary process and facet joint capsule (Lewin et al 1962). The superficial fibres are distant from the centres of rotation of the lumbar vertebrae, have an extension moment arm and can control the lumbar lordosis (Macintosh & Bogduk 1986). In contrast, the deep fibres have a limited moment arm and have only a minor ability to extend the spine (Panjabi et al 1989). While many trunk muscles are suited architecturally to the control of spinal orientation, most have a limited ability to control intervertebral shear and torsion (Panjabi et al 1989, Bogduk 1997). The deep fibres of multifidus are ideally placed to control these motions. Multifidus can control intervertebral motion by generation of intervertebral compression (Wilke et al 1995). The proximity of deep multifidus to the centre of rotation results in compression with minimal extension moment to be overcome by antagonistic muscle activity. In addition, multifidus may contribute to the control of intervertebral motion by control of anterior rotation and translation of the vertebrae (Macintosh & Bogduk 1986), or via tensioning the thoracolumbar fascia as it expands on contraction (Gracovetsky et al 1977). Several studies have provided in vitro and in vivo evidence of the ability of multifidus to control intervertebral motion (Kaigle et al 1995, Wilke et al 1995).

Other muscles that share features with the intrinsic muscles are the interspinales, intertransversarii, posterior fibres of psoas, medial fibres of quadratus lumborum and the lumbar portions of longissimus and iliocostalis. The interspinales and intertransversarii are small muscles that have a high density of muscle spindles (see below) and have been argued to have an important sensory rather than motor function (Nitz & Peck 1986b). The posterior fibres of psoas that attach to the transverse processes of the lumbar vertebrae have a minimal moment arm for spinal movement and have been argued to provide primarily an intersegmental compressive force (Bogduk et al 1992), and may have a primary function in intersegmental stability (Gibbons 2001). However, this requires clarification with EMG studies of this portion of the muscle. The medial fibres of quadratus lumborum, along with the lumbar erector spinae, have one attachment to the transverse processes of the lumbar spine and thus have a segmental attachment such that these muscles may contribute to both elements of spinal control and have been implicated in spinal stability (McGill et al 1996). Of the other abdominal muscles, obliquus internus has an attachment to the thoracolumbar fascia in a small proportion of people, thus providing a segmental attachment to the spine (Bogduk 1997). Anteriorly this muscle has fibres that are parallel to those of TrA and may contribute to the force closure of the SIJ (Snijders et al 1995). However, despite the similarities to TrA there are distinct differences in control of these two muscles.

Superficial lumbopelvic muscles

The contribution of the superficial muscles to lumbopelvic movement and stability is generally predictable based on the moment arm and direction of force provided by the muscles; that is, flexors generate flexion torque and oppose extension. Thus, in standing, the extensor muscles may be active to overcome trunk flexion due to gravity. However, it has been generally considered that antagonist trunk muscles are co-activated to stiffen the spine and prevent buckling (Gardner-Morse & Stokes 1998, McGill 2002). Muscles that provide this control include the oblique abdominal muscles, rectus abdominis, lateral fibres of quadratus lumborum, thoracic portions of the longissimus and iliocostalis. Furthermore, a contribution may also be provided by the lumbar erector spinae, superficial fibres of multifidus, medial fibres of quadratus lumborum, anterior fibres of psoas and latissimus dorsi. Recent studies using a Euler model have highlighted the important contribution of the

obliquus externus and long erector spinae in this role (McGill 2002). Several authors argue that muscles such as the gluteus maximus may also contribute to the general control of the spine and generation of segmental compression (Vleeming et al 1995).

Sensors

Multiple sensors contribute to the sensation of movement and position of the spine and pelvis. These include free nerve endings and receptors in the muscles, ligaments, annulus fibrosus, joint capsules and skin, with contributions from other senses such as vision and the vestibular and auditory systems. Muscle spindles are the most complex of the mechanoreceptors and consist of sensory and contractile components that lie in parallel with muscle fibres so that they are stretched with the muscle (Gandevia et al 1992). The sensory component has two main types of sensory endings, bag and chain fibres. These endings are sensitive to length and/or velocity of lengthening. The contractile component of the muscle spindle provides a mechanism for the CNS to control the sensitivity of the muscle spindle and to adapt the spindle to changes in muscle length. The contractile component of the muscle spindle is innervated by a special class of motor neurons, called gamma motoneurons. It is considered that alpha and gamma motoneurons are co-activated during muscle contraction. Many studies have confirmed that the input from muscle spindles is critical for the perception of movement (Gandevia & McCloskey 1976), yet stimulation of single muscle afferents does not result in conscious perception (Macefield et al 1990). Spinal muscles have varying densities of muscle spindles; notably, the deep segmental muscles have a high density of muscle spindles (Nitz & Peck 1986b) which is consistent with the proposal that these muscles have a critical role in sensation of intervertebral motion.

Golgi tendon organs are located in series with the muscle fibres in the tendon. These receptors provide an inhibitory input to the alpha motoneurons and were originally proposed to contribute only to strong contractions to prevent damage to the muscles. However, each receptor is attached to a small population of muscle fibres and is sensitive to small forces to provide discrete detection of tension in different parts of the muscle (Houk & Simon 1967). Thus, these receptors are likely to provide an important contribution to feedback during movement.

Joint receptors are encapsulated receptors (Ruffini endings and pacinian corpuscles) situated in the joint capsule. The contribution of these receptors to perception of movement and movement control has often been considered to be limited (Gandevia & McCloskey 1976). While some receptors are activated at specific ranges of motion, the majority fire at the end of range when the joint capsule is stretched (Nade et al 1987). Other joint structures such as the ligaments also contain receptors which may contribute to proprioception. Mechanoreceptors are also present in the annulus of the disc (Roberts et al 1995). Electrical and mechanical stimulation of the mechanoreceptors in disc and other ligamentous structures modulates activity of muscles of the spine, including the multifidus muscle (see, for example, Indahl et al 1995, Solomonow et al 1998) (Fig. 10.3).

There are several types of tactile receptors distributed in the layers of the skin. These receptors include pacinican corpuscles, Meissner corpuscles, Merkel cells and Ruffini endings and provide important tactile information. While input from the cutaneous receptors is important for the perception of movement of large (e.g. knee, Edin 2001) and small joints (e.g. hand, Collins et al 2000) and is critical for the coordination of grip force (see Johansson & Westling 1988), it is not known whether this input contributes to control of the spine.

The vestibular apparatus involves the saccule and utricle, which detect the position of the head with respect to gravity, and the semicircular canals, which provide information of acceleration of the head around the three major axes. The major function of the vestibular apparatus is to provide information about movements of the head. Integration of vestibular information and proprioceptive

information from the neck and trunk allow the interpretation of the position of the body relative to gravity. Interestingly, it has been argued that data from the control of the trunk are consistent with the presence of a gravity receptor in the trunk, in the region of the kidney, although the neural substrate of this mechanism is unclear (Mittelstaedt 1996).

The visual and auditory systems provide information regarding the interaction between the body and the environment or objects (Schmidt & Lee 1999). As such, vision provides an important contribution to control of movement and, although hearing does not play a major role in movement control, auditory information may provide useful feedback from environmental factors and issues such as success of performance (Jenison 1997), for instance for feedback of the accuracy of movements involved in tasks such as foot contact during running.

Although input from all sensory elements may provide information of disturbances to spinal stability, it is also critical to consider that sensory input is also required to provide input regarding the instantaneous status of the body and the internal and external forces acting on it, as well as development of an 'internal model' of the body and its dynamics so that the effect of movements and forces can be

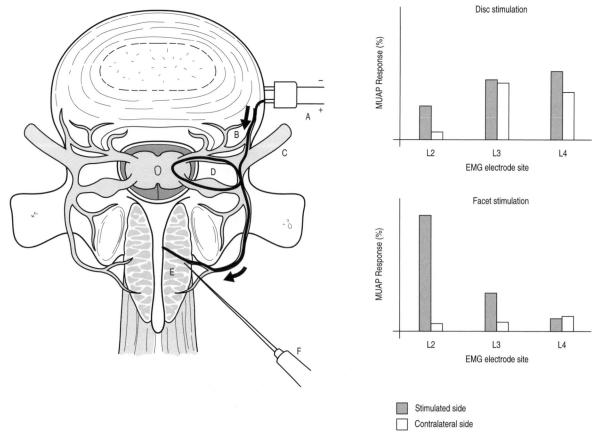

Figure 10.3 Muscle response to electrical stimulation of the intervertebral disc and facet joint. Electrical stimulation (A) of mechanoreceptors is associated with a short latency response of the multifidus muscles (E). Adapted from Indahl et al 1995.

predicted (Gahery & Massion 1981, Gurfinkel 1994). Input from all sources, including vestibular and proprioceptive, is required for the development, upkeep and interpretation of this model.

Controller

It is beyond the scope of this chapter to provide a detailed description of the organization of the control system. However, several important issues require consideration. Firstly, trunk muscles receive inputs from various parts of the CNS including corticospinal inputs (Plassman & Gandevia 1989), which to some extent, unlike the limb muscles, course the spinal cord bilaterally or send collaterals to both sides (Kuypers 1981, Mori et al 1995). However, it is generally considered that there is more significant control of the trunk muscles by the brain stem and spinal structures (Kuypers 1981), for example the vestibulospinal and reticulospinal systems. This is consistent with the relatively small size of the representation on the motor and sensory homunculi. The following section will consider the mechanisms of control of the trunk muscles from a behavioural perspective, that is, consideration of the organization of muscle recruitment rather than consideration of the specific neural structure and events involved in their production.

CONTROL MODELS

The CNS has two primary strategies for the control of the movement and stability of the body, including the trunk: feedforward or 'open'-loop strategies for situations in which the outcome of a perturbation is predictable and the CNS can plan strategies in advance; and feedback or 'closed'-loop strategies in which responses are generated in reaction to sensory input (visual, vestibular, proprioceptive input, etc.) from unpredictable perturbations (Schmidt & Lee 1999) (Fig. 10.4). In addition, due to time taken to initiate a response to sensory input, the CNS may also generate an underlying level of tonic activity to increase the muscle

stiffness and act as the first line of defence against an unexpected perturbation (Johansson et al 1991). This latter control strategy includes components of both feedforward and feedback mediated control. In general, normal function involves a complex combination of these strategies. As mentioned above, there is considerable redundancy in the motor system and multiple strategies could be used by the CNS in any given situation. The following sections outline evidence which argues that the CNS draws on the architectural properties of trunk muscles in a specific manner to concurrently meet the demands of movement and control of stability (i.e. control of intervertebral motion, orientation and body equilibrium).

Open-loop control of the trunk

Open-loop control implies that all aspects of the movement performance are pre-planned by the CNS and the movement occurs without modification by sensory feedback (Fig. 10.4). Movements that are likely to fit into this category are predictable ballistic and repetitive movements and predictable challenges to spinal control such as voluntary limb movements. Basic evidence that this type of control exists comes from studies of humans and animals with deafferented limbs. In these cases, limb movement can occur that is almost indistinguishable from that of a limb with a full complement of sensory input except for fine controlled movements of the fingers, which appear slightly clumsy (Taub & Berman 1968). To reconcile these observations, theories have been developed of mechanisms of generation of movement patterns. In animals the presence of central pattern generators (CPG) has been confirmed (Grillner 1981). Basically, a CPG is a collection of neurons that may control a repetitive function such as locomotion or respiration. These neuron groups can control the alternating contraction of muscles to perform the movement and while they can be modified by afferent feedback they can function independently of feedback. The existence of CPGs has not been confirmed in humans. Another organizational theory to explain the central control of movement is the concept of the motor programme.

The motor programme theory involves a memory based mechanism whereby a generalized motor programme is stored as an abstract representation of a group of movements that are retrieved when a movement is performed (Schmidt & Lee 1999). This theory argues that the CNS stores details of invariant features of a movement (for example order of events, relative timing, relative force). This information is accessed, with selected task duration and muscles, when the movement is performed. There are several problems to consider: for instance, a large amount of information would need to be stored to cover the full complement of movement possibilities and there are a large number of degrees of freedom. This issue was highlighted by Bernstein (1967), who argued that there are too many components that need to be controlled concurrently. For

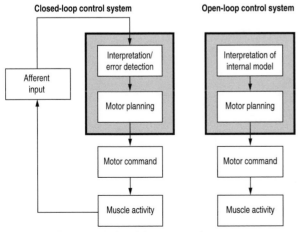

Figure 10.4   Open- and closed-loop control systems.

even the simplest movements of the hand, motion of each joint between the fingertip and the floor requires consideration. This is compounded when considering all of the muscles that are available to control each joint and the motor units within each muscle. As suggested by Bernstein, this is an enormous problem for the CNS in view of the resources required to individually control the large number of muscles and joints. A system is needed that can reduce processing demands, for instance by grouping degrees of freedom together.

Another model of movement control, the dynamic pattern theory (Kelso 1984), has been presented to reconcile some of these difficulties in movement control. The dynamic pattern theory argues that there is no central representation of all components of the movement, but instead the organization of the muscle contractions and joint movement is coordinated by environmental invariants and limb dynamics. Central to this theory is the idea that movements are attracted to steady-state behaviours and movements follow the principles of non-linear dynamics. In other words, if a particular variable is changed systematically the system may move between separate stable states. A familiar example to illustrate this point is the transition from walking to running. In the dynamic pattern theory it is argued that at slower speeds the movements of the arm and legs are 'attracted' to a coordinated pattern that is walking, yet at faster speeds the pattern changes, in part for reasons

of efficiency. Thus, coordinated movement is self-organized according to the characteristics of limb behaviour and environmental constraints. Currently the debate continues regarding these two theories. In reality movement may be coordinated by a hybrid of both possibilities.

Lumbopelvic stability is controlled in a feedforward or open-loop manner when the perturbation to the trunk is predictable. For instance, activity of the trunk muscles occurs in advance of the muscle responsible for movement of the upper (Belenkii et al 1967, Bouisset & Zattara 1981, Aruin & Latash 1995, Hodges & Richardson 1997b) and lower limbs (Hodges & Richardson 1997a) and prior to loading when a mass is added to the trunk in a predictable manner (Cresswell et al 1994) (Fig. 10.5). In this type of task the CNS predicts the effect that this movement will have on the body and plans a sequence of muscle activity to overcome this perturbation. This prediction involves an 'internal system of body dynamics' which is an abstract construct built up over a lifetime of movement experience and holds information of the interaction between internal and external forces (Gurfinkel 1994). Several possibilities could explain the organization of the movement and postural parts of the task. In general the postural activity could exist as a part of the motor command for movement or the postural part could be organized separately, but in parallel with the movement command. Several studies have investigated this question and are generally in support of the

Figure 10.5 Feedforward control of trunk stability. Rapid arm movement is associated with a sequence of trunk muscle activity that varies between directions of limb movement. Onsets of activity of deltoid and the trunk muscles are shown. The deep muscle, transversus abdominis, is controlled separately and does not vary with movement direction. Adapted from Hodges & Richardson 1996. Key: TrA = transversus abdominis, OI = obliquus internus abdominis, OE = obliquus externus abdominis, RA = rectus abdominis, ES = erector spinae.

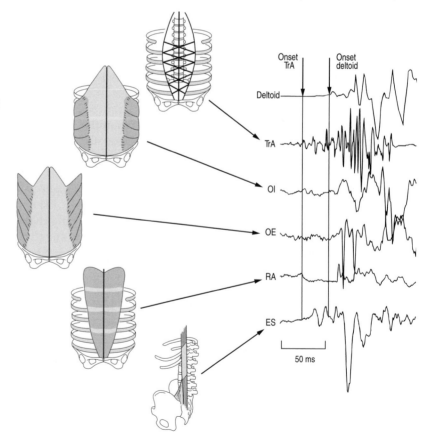

parallel process model (Massion 1992). An important feature of this feedforward control of the spine is that it provides insight into the differential strategies used by the CNS to control each of the elements of stability and how these may be integrated. Consistent with the architectural properties of the trunk muscles described above (pp. 121–123), the temporal and spatial parameters of activity of the superficial trunk muscles are linked to the direction of forces acting on the spine (i.e. superficial trunk muscle activity is earlier and larger in amplitude when their activity opposes the direction of reactive forces), and thus consistent with the control of orientation of the spine (Aruin & Latash 1995, Hodges & Richardson 1997b, Hodges et al 1999). In association with limb movements, this activity has also been shown to be consistent with the control of the disturbance to equilibrium and to move the COM (centre of mass) in a manner consistent with the maintenance of upright stance (Aruin & Latash 1995, Hodges et al 1999). In contrast, activity of the deep intrinsic muscles (both TrA and multifidus) is independent of the direction of reactive forces (Hodges & Richardson 1997b, Moseley et al 2000). This is consistent with the architectural properties of these muscles to provide a general increase in intervertebral control. Thus, the data suggest that the CNS uses feedforward non-direction-specific activity of the intrinsic muscles to control intervertebral motion and tuned direction-specific responses of the superficial muscles to control spinal orientation (Hodges & Richardson 1997b). Recent data suggest that the CNS uses discrete strategies to control each factor. When the preparation for movement is manipulated or subjects perform an attention demanding task, the latency for limb movement and the postural activity of the superficial muscles is delayed but there is no change in the latency of the deep muscle response (TrA, Hodges & Richardson 1999; deep fibres of multifidus, Moseley et al 2001a). This suggests that the deep muscle response is more rudimentary and may be controlled by a more basic mechanism by the CNS. Importantly, these responses have been shown to be linked to the speed of limb movement (Hodges & Richardson 1997c) and the mass of the limb (Zattara & Bouisset 1986, Hodges & Richardson 1997a), suggesting that the CNS predicts the amplitude of the reactive forces and adjusts the feedforward responses accordingly.

Repetitive limb movements may also provide an example of open-loop control. However, as the movement is ongoing it is not possible to exclude the contribution of afferent input to the organization of the trunk muscle activity, and studies have argued that spinal mechanisms dependent on afferent feedback may be important for this control (Zedka & Prochazka 1997). Although the mechanism for control of repetitive movement is not completely understood, there is evidence of differential activity of the deep and superficial muscles that is consistent with the different roles of these muscles. For instance, tonic activity of the intrinsic spinal muscles occurs in association with repetitive upper limb movement (TrA, Hodges & Gandevia

2000b; multifidus, Moseley et al 2002), repetitive lower limb movement during gait (Saunders et al 2002) and repetitive trunk movement (Cresswell et al 1992). In contrast, superficial muscle activity occurs in a phasic manner linked to the direction of limb movement.

Closed-loop control of the trunk

In a closed-loop system the command to move may be generated in a similar manner to an open-loop system; however, the intended movement is compared against feedback regarding the status of the body and its relationship to the environment (see Fig. 10.4). If the feedback differs from the intended movement an error command is generated to correct the movement performance. In this way sensory feedback is used to mould and correct movement performance (Schmidt & Lee 1999).

Clearly this type of control requires effective systems for detecting the state of the environment and the position and movements of the body segments. These sensors were outlined above (see section on sensors, pp. 123–125). Although the concept of closed-loop control may be considered in terms of higher information processing and consciousness, this system may operate at a variety of levels from simple monosynaptic reflexes to complex fine motor tasks involving coordinated finger movements. It is important to consider these different levels of control.

At the more basic end of the spectrum, closed-loop control may operate at the reflex level. This may include monosynaptic stretch reflexes, which involve stretch of a muscle spindle generating afferent impulse from the receptor region of the spindles that excite the alpha motoneurons in the same muscle, resulting in contraction. Short-latency reflexes have been identified in the paraspinal muscles when subjects catch an unexpected mass in their hands (Wilder et al 1996, Leinonen et al 2001, Moseley et al 2001b) and responses have been recorded in paraspinal (Dimitrijevic et al 1980) and abdominal muscles (Kondo et al 1986, Myriknas et al 2000) in response to a mechanical tap to the muscle. These reflex responses activate the paraspinal muscles en masse with no differentiation between deep and superficial components (Moseley et al 2001b). Simple responses are inflexible and represent a basic mechanism for the motor system to correct an error, for example to resist an imposed stretch. However, there appears to be some integration. For instance, reflex changes may occur in other related muscles, including contralateral muscles (Beith & Harrison 2001), and activity of TrA occurs prior to that of the paraspinal muscles when the trunk is unexpectedly flexed by addition of a mass to the front of the trunk (Cresswell et al 1994). Furthermore, activity of TrA and the paraspinal muscles occurs at the same time as the trunk is perturbed when a mass is added to the upper limbs during arm movement (Hodges et al 2001c). This latter finding suggests that afferent input from distant segments may be involved in initiation of the trunk muscle response. When the predictability of the perturbation is increased and higher centre input may influence the response, the paraspinal muscles are differentially active, with earlier activity of deep multifidus (Moseley et al 2001b) (Fig. 10.6). This also occurs when paraspinal muscle activity is reduced when load is removed from the trunk, by removal of a load from the upper limbs (Hodges et al 2002b). This unloading response is commonly argued to be due to removal of the support for muscle contraction from spindle afferent input (Angel et al 1965, Nitz & Peck 1986a).

Other basic responses have been identified in response to electrical and/or mechanical stimulation of afferents in the ligaments, annulus, facet joint capsule and SIJ in pigs (see Fig. 10.3), cats and humans (Indahl et al 1995, 1997, 1999; Solomonow et al 1998, 1999). In general, activity of multifidus was initiated with short latency on both sides and over multiple spinal segments in response to the stimulus. The nature of the response was affected by the site of stimulation on the annulus (Holm et al 2000) and SIJ (Indahl et al 1999), and could be modified by injection of analgesic or saline into the facet joint capsule. These reflexes provide a strategy for mechanical stimulation of the spinal structures to influence trunk muscle activity in a reflex manner. Alternatively the response may modulate descending drive to the muscles.

More complex than simple stretch reflexes are the long-loop reflexes that involve information processing at higher levels of the CNS, including transcortical mechanisms. These responses have a longer latency than the simple stretch reflex, are more flexible and can be modified voluntarily (Marsden et al 1977). Due to their flexibility these responses are thought to have a greater role in error correction. Another response group are the triggered responses (Schmidt & Lee 1999). These responses are faster than a voluntary reaction

time but involve a more complex and widespread response than is initiated via simple reflex mechanisms. For instance, when the support surface on which a person is standing is rapidly moved, a complex interplay of several body segments, including response of trunk muscles, is initiated in order to maintain the equilibrium of the body (Horak & Nashner 1986, Keshner & Allum 1990). Two main strategies have been identified that involve either ankle movement (ankle strategy) or hip movement (hip strategy), depending on the context and the support surface characteristics (Horak & Nashner 1986). Trunk movement, and thus activation of the superficial trunk muscles, is a critical component of these strategies, particularly the hip strategy.

The most complex level of closed-loop control is the fine control of long duration tasks that require accuracy. In these tasks, the sensory information may be used consciously to provide feedback of performance and continually modulate movement performance. However, even during these conscious goal-directed tasks, sensory information may be used at a subconscious level to modulate muscle activity.

Control of muscle stiffness

A third type of control strategy is related to both feedback and feedforward control and involves modulation of the 'tone' in specific muscles to provide an underlying degree of stability to the joints. This activity increases the stiffness of muscles that surround the joints (Bergmark 1989, Gardner-Morse et al 1995). Muscle stiffness is the property of muscles to act as springs (i.e. the ratio of length change to force change) and has viscoelastic and activity related components. Muscle stiffness provides control of forces applied to a joint and contributes to control before even the shortest reflex response could be initiated (Johansson et al

Figure 10.6 Feedback mediated response of the back muscles to loading of the trunk. When a load is dropped into the bucket held in the hands (A), activity of the deep, superficial and lateral components of the multifidus (onset indicated by arrows) occurs with short latency after the perturbation to the trunk. When the perturbation is expected, the deep and superficial fibres of multifidus are controlled differentially. Reproduced from Moseley et al 2003. Key: Deep MF = deep fibres of multifidus, Sup MF = superficial fibres of multifidus, Lat MF = lateral fibres of multifidus, ES T7 = erector spinae at T7

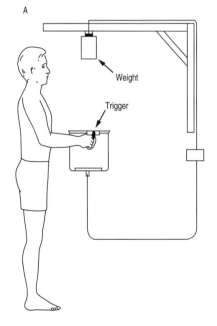
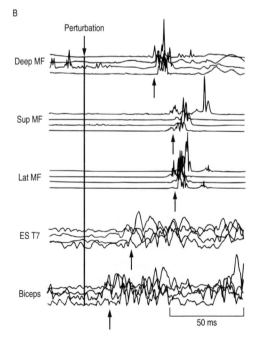

1991) and it has been argued that postural stability may be controlled by modulation of stiffness of the ankle muscles (Winter et al 1998). Similarly, stability of the trunk may be controlled by stiffness of the spinal muscles. Importantly, the activity related component of muscle stiffness is modulated by feedback from spindle and ligament afferents (Johansson et al 1991). It is the stretch reflex and the control of the gamma motoneurons, which control the sensitivity of the sensory component of the muscle spindles, that control this system. In addition, the reflex activity of multifidus muscle in response to stimulation of mechanoreceptors in the lumbar disc and ligaments (Indahl et al 1995, 1997, 1999) and supraspinous ligament in humans (Solomonow et al 1998) may contribute to stiffness control.

Integrated control of stability and movement of the trunk

It is important to consider that all the processes defined above may act concurrently and the outcome of feedforward processes may be moulded by later feedback mediated processes. In general, feedforward and feedback mediated responses closely match the demands of the task and are scaled to the amplitude of the perturbing forces and the context of the perturbation. As such, muscle activity directed to the control of stability represents a finely tuned component of human movement.

FACTORS THAT COMPLICATE MOTOR CONTROL OF THE TRUNK

The delicate balance of motor control of the trunk may be compromised by a number of factors including pain and conflict between the multiple functions of the trunk muscles. These factors present challenges to the motor control of the trunk muscles and may impair the control and stability of the lumbopelvic region.

The effect of pain and injury on motor control

Many studies have investigated changes in trunk muscle activity with acute and chronic pain. While most have evaluated the strength and endurance of the trunk muscles, this has led to variable results. For instance, some show reduced strength and endurance (see, for example, Suzuki et al 1977), while others do not (see, for example, Thorstensson & Arvidson 1982). It has been suggested that these changes may be more related to inactivity than pain (Thorstensson & Arvidson 1982). Furthermore, the importance of changes in strength and endurance is unclear as maximum strength and endurance are infrequently required in function and these parameters indicate little of how the muscles are used. Alternatively, studies have evaluated the control of the trunk muscles. It has been argued that impaired control of the trunk muscles may lead to inadequate support for the spine and pelvis, leading to injury and pain (Panjabi 1992b, Cholewicki et al 1997). This section considers this

issue in terms of the models of motor control of the trunk muscles presented in the previous section.

Changes in open–loop control mechanisms

The major factor that has implicated changes in the open-loop control of movement is changes in feedforward strategies. As mentioned above, these strategies are pre-planned by the nervous system and represent the pattern of muscle activity initiated by the CNS in advance of movement. Several studies have investigated the onset of muscle activity in association with rapid limb movements (Hodges & Richardson 1996, 1998). These studies investigated people with chronic recurrent low back pain (LBP) when their pain was in remission. The most consistent finding was delayed activity of TrA with arm and leg movements in all directions (Fig. 10.7). Thus, activity of TrA was absent in the period before movement. This is consistent with a compromise in the control of intervertebral motion (see section on models of stability). Activity of the superficial abdominal muscles was delayed only with specific movements. A major finding was that the change in TrA activity could not be explained by inhibition of the response or delayed transmission in the CNS, as the delay was different for each movement direction (i.e. there was a change in strategy, not a greater delay for the message to be transmitted to the motoneuron). Further studies have challenged the coordination of these responses, by manipulation of preparation for movement. These data suggest that the responses are a result of inappropriate motor planning rather than changes in excitability or transmission of the command in the CNS (Hodges, 2001a) (see Fig. 10.10).

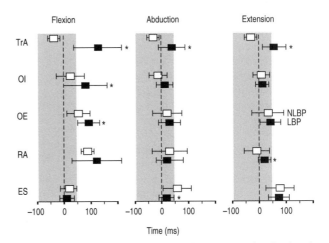

Figure 10.7 Group data for subjects with recurrent low back pain and matched control subjects showing the onset of EMG activity of the trunk muscles relative to that of deltoid with movement of the arm in three directions. Zero indicates the onset of deltoid EMG. The onset of TrA activity is delayed in low back pain subjects with movement in each direction thus failing to prepare the spine for the perturbation from limb movement. Adapted from Hodges & Richardson 1996. Key: TrA = transversus abdominis, OI = obliquus internus abdominis, OE = obliquus externus abdominis, RA = rectus abdominis, ES = erector spinae, NLBP = non low back pain, LBP = low back pain.

Changes in closed–loop control mechanisms

Changes in all elements of the closed-loop control system have been reported. However, as closed-loop control incorporates a complex interaction between input and output, in most studies it is difficult to determine the exact component or components of the system that are responsible for the change in motor control. For instance, if the amplitude of activity of a muscle is increased during a movement task it is difficult to determine whether the change results from inaccurate feedback from the periphery, inaccurate interpretation of normal feedback or inability to initiate an appropriate command. However, in specific instances the component can be identified.

The basis of closed-loop control is accurate feedback from movement. One of the most common of the motor control deficits that have been identified in association with lumbopelvic pain and injury is sensory deficit. This has been identified in two major ways, first by measurement of the acuity or smallest perceptible stimulation, such as the smallest movement that can be accurately detected, and secondly, the ability to accurately copy a position or return to a position of a limb after it has been demonstrated with the same or opposite limb. Using these methods studies have identified decreased acuity to spinal motion in low back pain (Taimela et al 1999) and impaired ability to accurately reposition with low back pain (Gill & Callaghan 1998, Brumagne et al 2000). Due to the importance of sensory information to closed-loop control of movement, deficits such as these may lead to impaired movement control at a number of levels. For instance, impaired acuity may lead to delayed reflex responses as a result of increased time to reach the threshold for movement detection. More complex changes are also possible, such as impaired coordination during voluntary movement due to inaccurate feedback from movement. This inaccurate feedback may lead to faulty error detection and correction. Another possibility is that inaccurate feedback may lead to development of a faulty 'internal model of body dynamics'. In this case the CNS may generate commands that are inaccurate for performance of the required movement. An additional possibility is that muscle spindle sensitivity may be altered by pain (see, for example, Pedersen et al 1997).

The mechanism for sensory feedback to change with injury and pain may be multifactorial. For instance, it may be due to injury to joint, muscle or cutaneous receptors. Alternatively it may be due to changes in interpretation of the afferent input such as the potential for afferent input to be misinterpreted as nociceptive in hyperalgesia. In addition, changes in muscle activity may affect sensory acuity. Muscle activity is known to augment acuity (Gandevia et al 1992); thus any change in activation may adversely affect movement sensation. Furthermore, many muscles, particularly the deep muscles close to the joints, have extensive attachments to joint structures and contraction is likely to affect sensation. Finally, several studies have argued that sensory acuity may be reduced by fatigue (Carpenter et al 1998); thus decreased muscle endurance with injury or pain may lead to impaired sensory acuity.

Changes in a variety of reflex responses have been identified in musculoskeletal pain syndromes. These changes include delayed onset of activity of the erector spinae to trunk loading (Magnusson et al 1996) and delayed offset of activity of the oblique abdominal and thoracolumbar erector spinae muscles of the trunk in response to unloading in chronic low back pain (Radebold et al 2000) (Fig. 10.8). However, others have failed to find changes in reflex

Figure 10.8 When a mass attached to the front (extension) or back (flexion) of the trunk and is suddenly removed the trunk muscles must reduce their activity to maintain the upright position of the trunk. When people have low back pain the offset of the external oblique abdominal and thoracic erector spinae muscles is delayed. Reproduced from Radebold et al 2000. Key: RA = rectus abdominis, EO = obliquus extensor abdominis, IO = obliquus internus abdominis, LD = latissimus dorsi, TE = thoracic erector spinae, LE = lumbar erector spinae.

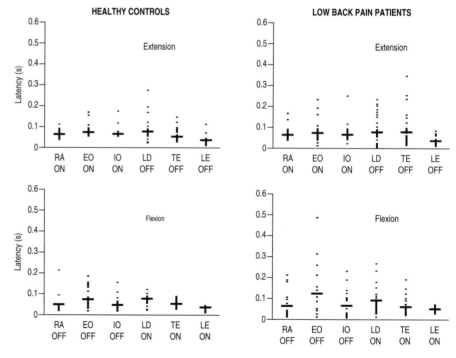

responses of the erector spinae, elicited by a muscle tap, with experimentally induced pain (Zedka et al 1999).

Changes in control of trunk muscle activity occur during ongoing functional movements (i.e. closed-loop control). For instance, reduced amplitude of activity of multifidus has been identified during functional tasks in people with low back pain (Lindgren et al 1993, Sihvonen et al 1997). In contrast, there has been considerable debate in the literature regarding the presence of augmented activity of the paraspinal muscles. In general these studies have had variable results with studies reporting increased (Wolf & Basmajian 1977, Arena et al 1989), decreased (Sihvonen et al 1997), asymmetrical (Cram & Steger 1983) and no change in activity (Collins et al 1982). A consistent finding has been sustained activity of the erector spinae muscles at the end of range of spinal flexion, a point at which the erector spinae muscles are normally inactive (the 'flexion–relaxation' phenomenon), in people with low back pain (Shirado et al 1995). This has been replicated by experimental pain (Zedka et al 1999) (Fig. 10.9) and has been shown to limit intervertebral motion (Kaigle et al 1998). During gait, periods of silence in the erector spinae are reduced activity between heel contacts during gait (Arendt-Nielsen et al 1996). Additional evidence of hyperactivity of the superficial trunk muscles comes from the study by Radebold and colleagues (2000) that indicates delayed reduction of EMG activity when a load is removed from the trunk.

Numerous studies have investigated parameters of ongoing closed-loop control of posture in people with low back pain. These studies have identified impairments of balance when standing on one (Luoto et al 1998) or two legs (Byl & Sinnott 1991) or sitting (Radebold et al 2001). Furthermore, an increased risk of low back pain or recurrence of pain has been identified for people with poor performance in a test of standing balance (Takala & Viikari-Juntura 2000). These changes indicate a general reduction of the accuracy of the postural control system in these patients. Other more complex elements of control have also been found to be altered in low back pain. For instance, people with low back pain have a slower reaction time (Luoto et al 1995), and slow reaction time has been associated with musculoskeletal injuries (including low back pain) in a variety of sports (Taimela & Kujala 1992).

Few studies have investigated the motor control of multifidus in LBP. However, changes in multifidus have been reported that may be indirectly associated with changes in control. For example, studies report changes in muscle fibre composition (Rantanen et al 1993), increased fatigability (Roy et al 1989, Biederman et al 1991), and reduced cross-sectional area of multifidus has been identified as little as 24 hours after the onset of acute, unilateral LBP (Hides et al 1994).

Thus, data appear to indicate that the deep local muscles and the superficial global muscles are commonly affected in an opposite manner by the presence of pain. Hypothetically, this may result in reduced efficiency of intervertebral control. As mentioned earlier, the superficial muscles are inefficient for providing control at the intervertebral level and can only do so at the cost of increased spinal loading and co-activation. As a result, a degree of the output of

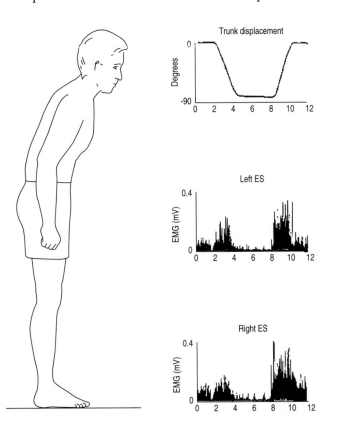
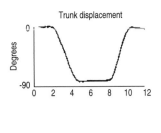
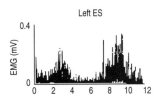
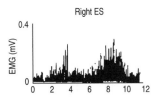

Figure 10.9 When back pain is induced experimentally by injection of hypertonic saline the normal relaxation of the paraspinal muscles at the end of trunk flexion (i.e. flexion relaxation) (middle panel) is lost and muscle activity is maintained although the range of motion is identical. Key: ES = erector spinae. Adapted from Zedka M, Prochazka A, Knight B, Gillard D and Gauthier M (1999).

these muscles must be diverted to intervertebral control. This is likely to compromise the ability of these muscles to deal with the control of orientation. This follows the hypothesis of Cholewicki et al (1997) who suggested that excessive activity in the superficial muscles might be a measurable compensation for poor passive or active segmental support.

Mechanism of changes in motor control

An important consideration is whether changes in motor control occur as a result of the pain (Fig. 10.10) or whether incompetent motor control strategies lead to inefficient spinal control, and thus microtrauma, nociceptor stimulation and pain as suggested by Janda (1978) and Farfan (1973). While neither possibility can be ruled out, injection of hypertonic saline into the lumbar longissimus muscle to produce transient pain induced changes in the feedforward responses of TrA that are similar to those identified in clinical pain (Hodges et al 2001a). Changes in global muscle activity differed between individuals. However, in all subjects, activity of at least one superficial trunk muscle was increased. This variability of the superficial muscles' response to pain is consistent with clinical observations. In separate studies, loss of relaxation of the erector spinae muscles has been replicated during trunk flexion (Zedka et al 1999) and gait (Arendt-Nielsen et al 1996) by experimentally induced pain. However, it is likely that the motor control changes may also precede LBP.

Several authors have argued that poor control may lead to microtrauma and eventual injury (Farfan 1973, Panjabi 1992b, Cholewicki et al 1997). Several studies have provided preliminary support for this hypothesis. For example, Janda (1978) identified that many people with chronic back pain also had minor neurological signs, and people

with slow reaction times have been shown to have an increased risk of injury (Taimela & Kujala 1992).

The mechanism for pain and nociceptor stimulation to affect motor control is poorly understood (see Fig. 10.10). Pain could affect motor output at any level of the motor system including the cortex, the motoneurons, reflex pathways and areas 'upstream' of the motor cortex involved in motor planning. Studies have identified changes in motoneuron excitability (Matre et al 1998), decreased cortical excitability (Valeriani et al 1999) and changes in sensitivity of muscle spindles (Pedersen et al 1997) in association with pain. However, the available data suggest that the change in motor control identified in LBP may be due to a change in motor planning, and not simple inhibition or transmission delays (Hodges 2001a). Consistent with this hypothesis, pain changes the activity of areas of the brain involved in motor planning (see Derbyshire et al 1997 for a review). While the exact mechanism is unknown, pain may have a direct affect on motor planning or may affect planning as a result of the attention-demanding nature of pain or stress associated with pain. In terms of attention, it has been argued that changes may arise due to an inability to ignore unnecessary information and the affect that this would have on limited attention resources (Luoto et al 1999). However, recent data indicate that the changes in control with rapid arm movements cannot be replicated by attention-demanding or stressful tasks (Moseley et al 2001a). However, fear of pain can replicate at least some features of the change in motor control identified with clinical and experimental pain (Moseley et al 2001a).

These changes in motor control may be at least partially explained by the 'pain–adaptation' model. This model hypothesizes that movement velocity and amplitude is reduced in the presence of pain (Lund et al 1991). In terms

Figure 10.10 Mechanism for pain to effect motor control.

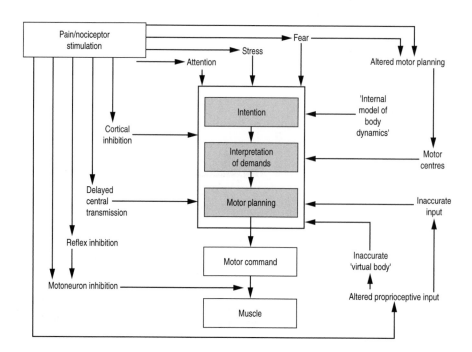

of limb and jaw movements, this is associated with reduced agonist activity and increased antagonist activity (Svensson et al 1995). In terms of the control of trunk stability, this model may suggest increased co-activation of the trunk muscles to increase trunk stiffness. This would be consistent with the prediction of Panjabi (1992b). As outlined above, one response of the nervous system to pain is augmented activity of the superficial global muscles. In a pain–adaptation model this would be interpreted as an attempt by the CNS to splint and restrict motion of a region of the spine to protect it from injury or reinjury. As a result, the deep muscle activity may be redundant and reduced but at the expense of fine-tuning of segmental control. This hypothesis requires further investigation.

Alternatively, pain may not affect motor control directly, but indirectly via the influence of pain on proprioception. In chronic pain, non-nociceptor mechanoreceptors may contribute to excitation of second order nociceptor neurons (Siddall & Cousins 1995) and pain may alter proprioceptive feedback (Capra & Ro 2000). Thus, pain may affect motor planning indirectly via inaccurate feedback and may influence feedforward responses as a result of development of an internal model of body dynamics that is built on faulty input.

A final factor to consider is that motoneuron excitability may be altered in the presence of pain and injury. One factor that may change motoneuron excitability is reflex inhibition. The mechanism for reflex inhibition is generally considered to involve inhibition of the alpha motoneuron as a result of afferent input from effusion (Stokes & Young 1984) or injury to joint structures (Ekholm et al 1960). For instance, when effusion is present in the knee the motoneuron excitability of quadriceps muscles is reduced (Spencer et al 1984). Furthermore, this affects certain muscles to different degrees, such as the oblique fibres of vastus medialis being inhibited with lower volumes of effusion than other vasti muscles. Reflex inhibition has also been argued to explain the rapid atrophy of multifidus in people with acute low back pain (Hides et al 1994), although this requires clarification.

Task conflict of the trunk muscles

Unlike limb muscles, the muscles of the trunk are involved in functions other than control and movement, such as respiration, continence and control of the abdominal contents. This introduces a challenge to the control system to coordinate these functions. As mentioned above (section on intrinsic lumbopelvic muscles), the contribution of TrA to lumbopelvic stability involves increased IAP and fascial tension. Changes in these parameters require co-activation of the diaphragm and pelvic floor muscles, which control displacement of the abdominal contents. Co-activation of these muscles has been termed the 'abdominal canister' (Hodges 1999) (Fig. 10.11). Studies have confirmed that activity of these muscles occurs in conjunction with TrA

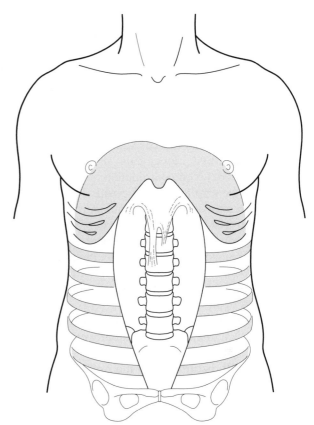

Figure 10.11   Abdominal canister. Activity of the muscles that surround the abdominal cavity are coordinated for control of lumbopelvic stability, respiration and continence.

during arm movements (Hodges et al 1997a, 2002d, Hodges & Gandevia 2000a, 2000b). However, their involvement in spinal control presents a challenge to the CNS to coordinate the respiratory and continence functions. To further complicate this system, respiration also presents a cyclical challenge to stability of the trunk and body equilibrium (Gurfinkel et al 1971).

Respiration

Normal quiet respiration involves cyclical activity of the diaphragm, parasternal intercostal and scalene muscles during inspiration, with expiration generated passively by the elastic recoil of the lung and chest wall (DeTroyer & Estenne 1988). However, when the demand for respiration is increased and the rate and depth of expiration are increased, abdominal muscles are phasically activated during the expiratory phase (Campbell 1952). If respiration is increased involuntarily (as in hypercapnoea) TrA is recruited at lower minute ventilation than the other abdominal muscles (DeTroyer et al 1990, Hodges et al 1997b). Recent data indicate that this may vary between regions of the abdominal wall, with activity of the mid-region of TrA recruited with lower respiratory demand (Urquhart and Hodges, unpublished observations). Recent studies of repetitive limb movements confirm that when the arm is moved repetitively to challenge the stability of the spine, tonic activity of the diaphragm and TrA is sustained, but is modulated with respiration to meet respiratory demands (Hodges & Gandevia 2000a, 2000b). In a mechanical sense, the diaphragm and TrA co-contract tonically, yet during inspiration diaphragm activity is increased and shortens (concentric), and TrA decreases its activity and lengthens (eccentric). The converse pattern occurs during expiration. Recent data confirm that this coordination also occurs during natural repetitive movements such as locomotion (Saunders et al 2002). This coordination occurs as if there is summation of the respiratory and postural drives to these muscles, which may occur at the motoneuron, providing a mechanism for the CNS to coordinate these functions. However, when respiratory drive is increased by respiratory disease (Hodges et al 2000b) or by breathing with an increased dead space to induce hypercapnoea (Hodges et al 2001e) this coordination is compromised and tonic activity of the diaphragm and TrA is reduced.

Respiratory movements of the ribcage and abdomen also generate a cyclical disturbance to stability of the trunk and body equilibrium. However, most studies have failed to identify a cyclical disturbance to the centre of pressure at the ground with respiration (Gurfinkel et al 1971, Bouisset & Duchene 1994). This is due to small amplitude cyclical movements of the lumbar spine, pelvis and lower limb that are time-locked to respiration that match and counteract the disturbance to postural stability (Gurfinkel et al 1971, Hodges et al 2002a). Importantly, this postural compensation does not occur when people have low back pain (Guillemot & Duplan 1995, Grimstone & Hodges 2003).

Continence

Similar to the challenge to respiration, the CNS must deal with the challenge to coordinate continence and spinal stability. Importantly, when intra-abdominal pressure is increased in association with contraction of the abdominal muscles, activity of the pelvic floor muscles is required to maintain continence. Numerous studies have confirmed that pelvic floor muscle activity occurs in conjunction with coughing (Deindl et al 1993) and lifting (Hemborg et al 1985) and recent data confirm that activity of the pelvic floor muscles precedes single limb movements in a non-direction-specific manner (similar to TrA and deep multifidus) and are tonically active during repetitive movements of the arm (Hodges et al 2002c). Other studies argue that voluntary activity of the pelvic floor muscles is associated with involuntary recruitment of TrA (Sapsford et al 2001, Critchley 2002) and, conversely, TrA activity is associated with pelvic floor muscle recruitment (Sapsford & Hodges 2001).

Other factors leading to task conflict

As mentioned above (section on models of stability), the trunk muscles contribute to control of intervertebral motion, trunk orientation and whole-body equilibrium as well as performing coordinated movement of the trunk. Theoretically, this coordination may also compromise the accuracy of stability. For instance, when body equilibrium is disturbed, movement of the trunk is required to maintain the position of the centre of mass over the base of support, and this demand may be inconsistent with the demand to maintain stability. Although in specific situations the trunk muscle activity has been found to be consistent with both tasks (Hodges et al 1999), this may not be the case in all situations. For instance, if the support surface is moved when a mass is being lifted, conflict between postural and movement tasks may arise. In this situation postural control has been shown to be compromised (Oddsson et al 1999, Huang et al 2001).

Implications of task conflict

Task conflict has important clinical implications for low back pain patients. It has been argued that respiratory and genitourinary problems are common in people with low back pain (Hurwitz & Morgenstern 1999, Finkelstein 2002) and this may compromise the normal coordination of postural, respiratory and continence functions of the trunk muscles. Thus, normal control of lumbopelvic stability and movement may be challenged by potential conflict between the multiple functions of the trunk muscles. This may lead to compromised accuracy of control.

Additional control issues

Several other factors present challenges to motor control of the trunk, namely the function of adjacent segments and the role of the trunk as a reference frame. Irrespective of the stability of the trunk, it has been argued from a largely clinical perspective that stability cannot be maintained in function if the motion of the adjacent joints is compromised, such that lumbar motion must compensate for reduced hip or thoracic flexibility. There is some evidence of this in the literature. For instance, hip range of motion has been shown to be reduced in people with low back pain (Ellison et al 1990).

The second additional factor that complicates the control of the trunk is that the CNS may use the trunk as a 'reference frame'. That is, the CNS may interpret the position of other regions with respect to the trunk. For instance, dancers have been shown to control the lower limb in relation to the trunk (Mouchnino et al 1990, 1993). If true, optimal control of the trunk has implications for coordination of regions other than the trunk. This requires further investigation.

CONCLUSION

In summary, multiple strategies are used by the CNS to coordinate movement and control of the lumbopelvic region. A major issue is the numerous factors that can lead to compromise of the efficiency of the control system, particularly of the deep local muscles of the region. It is activity of the deep muscles that is most commonly found to be impaired in the presence of pain and by conflict with other concurrent homeostatic functions. Although the deep muscles are not sufficient to provide control to the lumbar spine and pelvis, they provide a critical contribution, along with the superficial global muscles. Hypothetically, augmented activity of the superficial muscles (at the expense of the deep muscles) may compromise the quality of spinal control as these muscles have a limited ability to fine-tune intervertebral motion and their activity is associated with the cost of reduced flexibility of spinal motion due to co-contraction to counteract the torque output of these muscles. Furthermore, it may be argued that dependence on the superficial muscles may compromise other functions such as respiration due to the attachments to the thorax and ribcage. In contrast, normal control of the deep local muscles is likely to provide an efficient mechanism to control intervertebral motion without restricting spinal movement and without compromise to respiration. Thus, techniques to rehabilitate the coordination between these systems and motor control strategies can be justified.

KEYWORDS	
stability	sensor
open loop	controller
closed loop	task conflict

References

Angel R W, Eppler W, Iannone A 1965 Silent period produced by unloading of muscle during voluntary contraction. Journal of Physiology 180: 864–870

Arena J G, Sherman R A, Bruno G M, Young T R 1989 Electromyographic recordings of 5 types of low back pain subjects and non-pain controls in different positions. Pain 37: 57–65

Arendt-Nielsen L, Graven-Nielsen T, Svarrer H, Svensson P 1996 The influence of low back pain on muscle activity and coordination during gait: a clinical and experimental study. Pain 64: 231–240

Aruin A S, Latash M L 1995 Directional specificity of postural muscles in feed-forward postural reactions during fast voluntary arm movements. Experimental Brain Research 103: 323–332

Beith I D, Harrison P J 2001 Reflex control of the human internal oblique muscles. Abstracts - Society for Neuroscience 27: 930–933

Belenkii V, Gurfinkel V S, Paltsev Y 1967 Elements of control of voluntary movements. Biofizika 12: 135–141

Bergmark A 1989 Stability of the lumbar spine: a study in mechanical engineering. Acta Orthopaedica Scandinavica 60: 1–54

Bernstein N 1967 The co-ordination and regulation of movements. Pergamon Press, Oxford

Biederman H J, Shanks G L, Forrest W J, Inglis J 1991 Power spectrum analysis of electromyographic activity: discriminators in the differential assessment of patients with chronic low back pain. Spine 16: 1179–1184

Bogduk N 1997 Clinical anatomy of the lumbar spine and sacrum. Churchill Livingstone, London

Bogduk N, Pearcy M, Hadfeild G 1992 Anatomy and biomechanics of psoas major. Clinical Biomechanics 7: 109–119

Bogduk N, Amevo B, Pearcy M 1995 A biological basis for instantaneous centres of rotation of the vertebral column. Proceedings of the Institution of Mechanical Engineers Part H: 177–183

Bouisset S, Duchene J L 1994 Is body balance more perturbed by respiration in seating than in standing posture? Neuroreport 5: 957–960

Bouisset S, Zattara M 1981 A sequence of postural adjustments precedes voluntary movement. Neuroscience Letters 22: 263–270

Brumagne S, Cordo P, Lysens R, Verschueren S, Swinnen S 2000 The role of paraspinal muscle spindles in lumbosacral position sense in individuals with and without low back pain. Spine 25: 989–994

Byl N N, Sinnott P L 1991 Variations in balance and body sway in middle-aged adults: subjects with healthy backs compared with subjects with low back dysfunction. Spine 16: 325–330

Campbell E J M 1952 An electromyographic study of the role of the abdominal muscles in breathing. Journal of Physiology (London) 117: 222–233

Capra N F, Ro J Y 2000 Experimental muscle pain produces central modulation of proprioceptive signals arising from jaw muscle spindles. Pain 86: 151–162

Carpenter J E, Blasier R B, Pellizzon G G 1998 The effects of muscle fatigue on shoulder joint position sense. American Journal of Sports Medicine 26: 262–265

Cholewicki J, McGill S M 1996 Mechanical stability of the in vivo lumbar spine: implications for injury and chronic low back pain. Clinical Biomechanics 11: 1–15

Cholewicki J, Panjabi M M, Khachatryan A 1997 Stabilizing function of trunk flexor-extensor muscles around a neutral spine posture. Spine 22: 2207–2212

Collins G A, Cohen M J, Naliboff B D, Schandler S L 1982 Comparative analysis of paraspinal and frontalis EMG, heart rate and skin conductance in chronic low back pain patients and normals to various postures and stresses. Scandinavian Journal of Rehabilitation Medicine 14: 39–46

Collins D F, Refshauge K M, Gandevia S C 2000 Sensory integration in the perception of movements at the human metacarpophalangeal joint. Journal of Physiology 529(2): 505–515

Cram J R, Steger J C 1983 EMG scanning in the diagnosis of chronic pain. Biofeedback and Self-Regulation 8: 229–241

Cresswell A G, Grundstrom H, Thorstensson A 1992 Observations on intra-abdominal pressure and patterns of abdominal intra-muscular activity in man. Acta Physiologica Scandinavica 144: 409–418

Cresswell A G, Oddsson L, Thorstensson A 1994 The influence of sudden perturbations on trunk muscle activity and intra-abdominal pressure while standing. Experimental Brain Research 98: 336–341

Crisco J J, Panjabi M M 1991 The intersegmental and multisegmental muscles of the lumbar spine: a biomechanical model comparing lateral stabilising potential. Spine 7: 793–799

Critchley D 2002 Instructing pelvic floor contraction facilitates transversus abdominis thickness increase during low-abdominal hollowing. Physiotherapy Research International 7: 65–75

Deindl F, Vodusek D, Hesse U, Schussler B 1993 Activity patterns of pubococcygeal muscles in nulliparous continent women. British Journal of Urology 72: 46–51

Derbyshire S W, Jones A K, Gyulai F, Clark S, Townsend D, Firestone L L 1997 Pain processing during three levels of noxious stimulation produces differential patterns of central activity. Pain 73: 431–445

DeTroyer A, Estenne M 1988 Functional anatomy of the respiratory muscles. In: Belman M (ed) Respiratory muscles: Function in health and disease. W B Saunders, Philadelphia, Vol 9, pp 175–195

DeTroyer A, Estenne M, Ninane V, VanGansbeke D, Gorini M 1990 Transversus abdominis muscle function in humans. Journal of Applied Physiology 68: 1010–1016

Dimitrijevic M R, Gregoric M R, Sherwood A M, Spencer W A 1980 Reflex responses of paraspinal muscles to tapping. Journal of Neurology, Neurosurgery, and Psychiatry 43: 1112–1118

Edin B 2001 Cutaneous afferents provide information about knee joint movements in humans. Journal of Physiology 531: 289–297

Ekholm J, Eklund G, Skoglund S 1960 On reflex effects from knee joint of cats. Acta Physiologica Scandinavica 50: 167–174

Ellison J B, Rose S J, Sahrmann S A 1990 Patterns of hip rotation range of motion: a comparison between healthy subjects and patients with low back pain. Physical Therapy 70: 537–541

Farfan H F 1973 Mechanical disorders of the low back. Lea and Febiger, Philadelphia

Finkelstein M 2002 Medical conditions, medications, and urinary incontinence: analysis of a population-based survey. Canadian Family Physician 48: 96–101

Gahery Y, Massion J 1981 Co-ordination between posture and movement. Trends in Neuroscience 4: 199–202

Gandevia S C, McCloskey D I 1976 Joint sense, muscle sense, and their combination as position sense, measured at the dorsal interphalangeal joint of the middle finger. Journal of Physiology 260: 387–407

Gandevia S C, McCloskey D I, Burke D 1992 Kinaesthetic signals and muscle contraction. Trends in Neurosciences 15: 62–65

Gardner-Morse M G, Stokes I A 1998 The effects of abdominal muscle coactivation on lumbar spine stability. Spine 23: 86–91

Gardner-Morse M, Stokes I A F, Laible J P 1995 Role of muscles in lumbar spine stability in maximum extension efforts. Journal of Orthopaedic Research 13: 802–808

Gibbons S 2001 Biomechanics and stability mechanisms of psoas major. In: Vleeming A, Mooney V, Gracovetsky S A et al (eds) Fourth Interdisciplinary World Congress on Low Back Pain Pelvic Pain. European Conference Organisers, Montreal, Canada

Gill K P, Callaghan M J 1998 The measurement of lumbar proprioception in individuals with and without low back pain. Spine 23: 371–377

Goff B 1972 The application of recent advances in neurophysiology to Miss M. Rood's concept of neuromuscular facilitation. Physiotherapy 58: 409–415

Gracovetsky S, Farfan H F, Lamy C 1977 A mathematical model of the lumbar spine using an optimised system to control muscles and ligaments. Orthopedic Clinics of North America 8: 135–153

Gracovetsky S, Farfan H, Helleur C 1985 The abdominal mechanism. Spine 10: 317–324

Grillner S 1981 Control of locomotion in bipeds, tetrapods, and fish. In: Brookhart M, Mountcastle V B (eds) Handbook of physiology. The nervous system. Motor control. American Physiological Society, Washington D C, Vol 2, pt 2, pp 1179–1235

Grimstone S K, Hodges P W 2003 Impaired postural compensation for respiration in people with recurrent low back pain. Experimental Brain Research 151: 218–224

Guillemot A, Duplan B 1995 Étude de la prévalence des troubles posturaux au sein d'une cohorte de 106 lumbalgiques. In: Gagey P W B (ed) Entrées du système postural fin. Masson, Paris, pp 71–77

Gurfinkel V S 1994 The mechanisms of postural regulation in man. Soviet Scientific Reviews. Section F. Physiology and General Biology 7: 59–89

Gurfinkel V S, Kots Y M, Paltsev E I, Feldman A G 1971 The compensation of respiratory disturbances of erect posture of man as an example of the organisation of interarticular interaction. In: Gelfand I M, Gurfinkel V S, Formin S V, Tsetlin M L, (eds) Models of the structural functional organisation of certain biological systems. MIT Press, Cambridge, Massachusetts, pp 382–395

Hemborg B 1983 Intraabdominal pressure and trunk muscle activity during lifting. Department of Physical Therapy. University of Lund, Lund

Hemborg B, Moritz U, Löwing H 1985 Intra-abdominal pressure and trunk muscle activity during lifting. IV: The causal factors of the intra-abdominal pressure rise. Scandinavian Journal of Rehabilitation Medicine 17: 25–38

Hides J A, Stokes M J, Saide M, Jull G A, Cooper D H 1994 Evidence of lumbar multifidus muscle wasting ipsilateral to symptoms in patients with acute/subacute low back pain. Spine 19: 165–177

Hodges P W 1999 Is there a role for transversus abdominis in lumbo-pelvic stability? Manual Therapy 4: 74–86

Hodges P W 2001a Changes in motor planning of feedforward postural responses of the trunk muscles in low back pain. Experimental Brain Research 141: 261–266

Hodges P, Gandevia S 2000a Activation of the human diaphragm during a repetitive postural task. Journal of Physiology 522: 165–175

Hodges P, Gandevia S 2000b Changes in intra-abdominal pressure during postural and respiratory activation of the human diaphragm. Journal of Applied Physiology 89: 967–976

Hodges P W, Richardson C A 1996 Inefficient muscular stabilisation of the lumbar spine associated with low back pain: a motor control evaluation of transversus abdominis. Spine 21: 2640–2650

Hodges P W, Richardson C A 1997a Contraction of the abdominal muscles associated with movement of the lower limb. Physical Therapy 77: 132–144

Hodges P W, Richardson C A 1997b Feedforward contraction of transversus abdominis is not affected by the direction of arm movement. Experimental Brain Research 114: 362–370

Hodges P W, Richardson C A 1997c Relationship between limb movement speed and associated contraction of the trunk muscles. Ergonomics 40: 1220–1230

Hodges P W, Richardson C A 1998 Delayed postural contraction of transversus abdominis associated with movement of the lower limb in people with low back pain. Journal of Spinal Disorders 11: 46–56

Hodges P W, Richardson C A 1999 Transversus abdominis and the superficial abdominal muscles are controlled independently in a postural task. Neuroscience Letters 265: 91–94

Hodges P W, Butler J E, McKenzie D, Gandevia S C 1997a Contraction of the human diaphragm during postural adjustments. Journal of Physiology 505: 239–248

Hodges P W, Gandevia S C, Richardson C A 1997b Contractions of specific abdominal muscles in postural tasks are affected by respiratory maneuvers. Journal of Applied Physiology 83: 753–760

Hodges P W, Cresswell A G, Thorstensson A 1999 Preparatory trunk motion accompanies rapid upper limb movement. Experimental Brain Research 124: 69–79

Hodges P W, Cresswell A G, Daggfeldt K, Thorstensson A 2000a Three dimensional preparatory trunk motion precedes asymmetrical upper limb movement. Gait and Posture 11: 92–101

Hodges P W, McKenzie D K, Heijnen I, Gandevia S C 2000b Reduced contribution of the diaphragm to postural control in patients with severe chronic airflow limitation. Proceedings of the Annual Scientific Meeting of the Thoracic Society of Australia and New Zealand, Melbourne, Australia

Hodges P, Moseley G, Gabrielsson A, Gandevia S 2001a Acute experimental pain changes postural recruitment of the trunk muscles in pain-free humans. Abstracts - Society for Neuroscience 27: 304–311

Hodges P W, Cresswell A G, Daggfeldt K, Thorstensson A 2001b In vivo measurement of the effect of intra-abdominal pressure on the human spine. Journal of Biomechanics 34: 347–353

Hodges P W, Cresswell A G, Thorstensson A 2001c Perturbed arm movements cause short latency postural responses in trunk muscles. Experimental Brain Research 138: 243–250

Hodges P W, Eriksson A E M, Shirley D, Gandevia S C 2001d Lumbar spine stiffness is increased by elevation of intra-abdominal pressure.

Proceedings of the International Society for Biomechanics, Zurich, Switzerland

Hodges P W, Heijnen I, Gandevia S C 2001e Reduced postural activity of the diaphragm in humans when respiratory demand is increased. Journal of Physiology 537: 999–1008

Hodges P, Gurfinkel V S, Brumagne S, Smith T, Cordo P 2002a Coexistence of stability and mobility in postural control: evidence from postural compensation for respiration. Experimental Brain Research 144: 293–302

Hodges P, Moseley G, Gandevia S 2002b Differential control of the deep and superficial compartments of multifidus is dependent on input from higher centres. Seventh International Physiotherapy Congress, Sydney

Hodges P W, Sapsford R R, Pengel H M 2002c Feedforward activity of the pelvic floor muscles precedes rapid upper limb movements. Seventh International Physiotherapy Congress, Sydney, Australia

Hodges P, Kaigle-Holm A, Holm S, Erstrom L, Cresswell A, Hansson T, Thorstensson A 2003 Intervertebral stiffness of the spine is increased by evoked contraction of transversus abdominis and the diaphragm: in vivo porcine studies. Spine 28: 2594–2601

Holm S, Indahl A, Kaigle A, Gronblad M, Hansson T 2000 The neuromuscular role of mechanoreceptors in the porcine lumbar intervertebral disc. Proceedings of the International Society for the Study of the Lumbar Spine, Adelaide, Australia, p 263

Horak F, Nashner L M 1986 Central programming of postural movements: adaptation to altered support-surface configurations. Journal of Neurophysiology 55: 1369–1381

Houk J, Simon W 1967 Responses of Golgi tendon organs to forces applied to muscle tendon. Journal of Neurophysiology 30: 1466–1481

Huang Q M, Hodges P W, Thorstensson A 2001 Postural control of the trunk in response to lateral support surface translations during trunk movement and loading. Experimental Brain Research 141: 552–559

Hurwitz E, Morgenstern H 1999 Cross-sectional associations of asthma, hay fever, and other allergies with major depression and low-back pain among adults aged 20-39 years in the United States. American Journal of Epidemiology 150: 1107–1116

Indahl A, Kaigle A, Reikeras O, Holm S 1995 Electromyographic response of the porcine multifidus musculature after nerve stimulation. Spine 20: 2652–2658

Indahl A, Kaigle A M, Reikeras O, Holm S H 1997 Interaction between the porcine lumbar intervertebral disc, zygapophysial joints, and paraspinal muscles. Spine 22: 2834–2840

Indahl A, Kaigle A, Reikeras O, Holm S 1999 Sacroiliac joint involvement in activation of the porcine spinal and gluteal musculature. Journal of Spinal Disorders 12: 325–330

Janda V 1978 Muscles, central nervous motor regulation and back problems. In: Korr I M (ed) The neurobiologic mechanisms in manipulative therapy. Plenum Press, New York, pp 27–41

Jenison R 1997 On acoustic information for motion. Ecological Psychology 9: 131–151

Johansson R S, Westling G 1988 Programmed and triggered actions to rapid load changes during precision grip. Experimental Brain Research 71: 72–86

Johansson H, Sjolander P, Sojka P 1991 A sensory role for the cruciate ligaments. Clinical Orthopaedic and Related Research 268: 161–178

Kaigle A M, Holm S H, Hansson T H 1995 Experimental instability in the lumbar spine. Spine 20: 421–430

Kaigle A M, Wessberg P, Hansson T H 1998 Muscular and kinematic behavior of the lumbar spine during flexion-extension. Journal of Spinal Disorder 11: 163–174

Kelso J A S 1984 Phase transitions and critical behaviour in human bimanual coordination. American Journal of Physiology: Regulatory, Integrative, and Comparative Physiology 15: R1000–1004

Keshner E A, Allum J H J 1990 Muscle activation patterns coordinating postural stability from head to foot. In: Winters J M, Woo S L-Y (eds)

Multiple muscle systems: biomechanics and movement organization. Springer-Verlag, New York, pp 481–497

Keshner E A, Woollacott M H, Debu B 1988 Neck, trunk and limb muscle responses during postural perturbations in humans. Experimental Brain Research 71: 455–466

Kondo T, Bishop B, Shaw C F 1986 Phasic stretch reflex of the abdominal muscles. Experimental Neurology 94: 120–140

Kuypers H 1981 Anatomy of the descending pathways. In: Brookhart J, Mountcastle V (eds) Handbook of Physiology. The nervous system. Motor control. American Physiological Society, Bethesda, MD, vol 2, pt 1, pp 597–666

Leinonen V, Kankaanpaa M, Luukkonen M, Hanninen O, Airaksinen O, Taimela S 2001 Disc herniation-related back pain impairs feed-forward control of paraspinal muscles. Spine 26: E367–372

Lewin T, Moffett B, Viidik A 1962 The morphology of the lumbar synovial joints. Acta Morphologica Neerlanco Scandinavica 4: 299–319

Lindgren K-A, Sihvonen T, Leino E, Pitkänen M, Manninen H 1993 Exercise therapy effects on functional radiographic findings and segmental electromyographic activity in lumbar spine instability. Archives of Physical Medicine and Rehabilitation 74: 933–939

Lucas D B, Bresler B 1960 Stability of the ligamentous spine. Technical Report esr. 11, no. 40. Biomechanics Laboratory, University of California, Berkeley and San Francisco

Lund J P, Donga R, Widmer C G, Stohler C S 1991 The pain–adaptation model: a discussion of the relationship between chronic musculoskeletal pain and motor activity. Canadian Journal of Physiology and Pharmacology 69: 683–694

Luoto S, Heliövaara M, Hurri H, Alaranta H 1995 Static back endurance and the risk of low-back pain. Clinical Biomechanics 10: 323–324

Luoto S, Aalto H, Taimela S, Hurri H, Pyykko I, Alaranta H 1998 One-footed and externally disturbed two-footed postural control in patients with chronic low back pain and healthy control subjects: a controlled study with follow-up. Spine 23: 2081–2089

Luoto S, Taimela S, Hurri H, Alaranta H 1999 Mechanisms explaining the association between low back trouble and deficits in information processing: a controlled study with follow-up. Spine 24: 255–261

Macefield G, Gandevia S C, Burke D 1990 Perceptual responses to microstimulation of single afferents innervating joints, muscles and skin of the human hand. The Journal of Physiology 429: 113–129

McGill S 2002 Low back disorders: evidence based prevention and rehabilitation. Human Kinetics Publishers, Champaign, Illinois

McGill S, Juker D, Kropf P 1996 Quantitative intramuscular myoelectric activity of quadratus lumborum during a wide variety of tasks. Clinical Biomechanics (Bristol, Avon) 11: 170–172

Macintosh J E, Bogduk N 1986 The detailed biomechanics of the lumbar multifidus. Clinical Biomechanics 1: 205–231

Magnusson M, Aleksiev A, Wilder D, Pope M, Spratt K, Lee S 1996 Unexpected load and asymmetric posture as etiologic factors in low back pain. European Spine Journal 5: 23–35

Marsden C D, Merton P A, Morton H B 1977 Anticipatory postural responses in the human subject. Journal of Physiology (London) 275: 47P–48P

Massion J 1992 Movement, posture and equilibrium: interaction and coordination. Progress in Neurobiology 38: 35–56

Matre D A, Sinkjaer T, Svensson P, Arendt-Nielsen L 1998 Experimental muscle pain increases the human stretch reflex. Pain 75: 331–339

Mittelstaedt H 1996 Somatic graviception. Biological Psychology 42: 53–74

Mori S, Iwakiri H, Homma Y, Yokoyama T, Matsuyama K 1995 Neuroanatomical and neurophysiological bases of postural control. In: Fahn S, Hallet M, Leders H, Marsden C D (eds) Negative motoro phenomena. Lippincott-Raven, Philadelphia

Moseley G L, Hodges P W, Gandevia S C 2002 Deep and superficial fibres of multifidus are differentially active during voluntary arm movements. Spine 27: E29–36

Moseley G L, Hodges P W, Gandevia S C 2001a Attention demand, anxiety and acute pain cause differential effects on postural activation of the abdominal muscles in humans. Abstracts - Society for Neuroscience 304–312

Moseley G L, Hodges P W, Gandevia S C 2001b External perturbation to the trunk is associated with differential activity of the deep and superficial fibres of lumbar multifidus. In: Mooney A V, Gracovetsky V et al (eds) Fourth Interdisciplinary World Congress on Low Back and Pelvic Pain, Montreal, Canada, pp 241–242

Moseley G L, Hodges P W, Gandevia S C 2002 Deep and superficial fibers of lumbar multifidus are differentially active during voluntary arm movements. Spine 27: E29–36

Moseley G L, Hodges P W, Gandevia S C 2003 External perturbation of the trunk in standing humans results in differential activity of components of the medial back muscles. Journal of Physiology 547: 581–587

Mouchnino L, Aurenty R, Massion J, Pedotti A 1990 Coordinated control of posture and equilibrium during leg movement. In: Brandt T, Paulus W, Bles W, Dieterich M, Krafczyk S, Straube A (eds) Disorders of posture and gait. Georg Thieme, Stuttgart, pp 68–71

Mouchnino L, Aurenty R, Massion J, Pedotti A 1993 Is the trunk a reference frame for calculating leg position? Neuroreport 4: 125–127

Myriknas S E, Beith I D, Harrison P J 2000 Stretch reflexes in the rectus abdominis muscle in man. Experimental Physiology 85: 445–450

Nade S, Newbold P J, Straface S F 1987 The effects of direction and acceleration of movement of the knee joint of the dog on medial articular nerve discharge. Journal of Physiology 388: 505–519

Nitz A J, Peck D 1986a Comparison of muscle spindle concentrations in large and small human epaxial muscles acting in parallel combinations. American Surgeon 52: 273–277

Nitz A J, Peck D 1986b Comparison of muscle spindle concentrations in large and small human epaxial muscles acting in parallel combinations. American Surgeon 52: 273–277

Oddsson L I, Persson T, Cresswell A G, Thorstensson A 1999 Interaction between voluntary and postural motor commands during perturbed lifting. Spine 24: 545–552

Panjabi M M 1992a The stabilising system of the spine. II: Neutral zone and instability hypothesis. Journal of Spinal Disorders 5: 390–397

Panjabi M M 1992b The stabilizing system of the spine. I: Function, dysfunction, adaptation, and enhancement. Journal of Spinal Disorders 5: 383–389

Panjabi M M, Abumi K, Duranceau J, Oxland T 1989 Spinal stability and intersegmental muscle forces: a biomechanical model. Spine 14: 194–200

Pedersen J, Sjolander P, Wenngren B I, Johansson H 1997 Increased intramuscular concentration of bradykinin increases the static fusimotor drive to muscle spindles in neck muscles of the cat. Pain 70: 83–91

Perry J 1992 Gait analysis: normal and pathological function. SLACK Incorporated, Thorofare, New Jersey

Plassman B L, Gandevia S C 1989 Comparison of human motor cortical projections to abdominal muscles and intrinsic muscles of the hand. Experimental Brain Research 78: 301–308

Radebold A, Cholewicki J, Panjabi M M, Patel T C 2000 Muscle response pattern to sudden trunk loading in healthy individuals and in patients with chronic low back pain. Spine 25: 947–954

Radebold A, Cholewicki J, Polzhofer G K, Greene H S 2001 Impaired postural control of the lumbar spine is associated with delayed muscle response times in patients with chronic idiopathic low back pain. Spine 26: 724–730

Rantanen J, Hurme M, Falck B et al 1993 The lumbar multifidus muscle five years after surgery for a lumbar intervertebral disc herniation. Spine 18: 568–574

Richardson C A, Jull G A, Hodges P W, Hides J A 1999 Therapeutic exercise for spinal segmental stabilisation in low back pain: scientific basis and clinical approach. Churchill Livingstone, Edinburgh

Richardson C A, Snijders C J, Hides J A, Damen L, Pas M S, Storm J 2002 The relation between the transversus abdominis muscles, sacroiliac joint mechanics, and low back pain. Spine 27: 399–405

Roberts S, Eisenstein S M, Menage J, Evans E H, Ashton I K 1995 Mechanoreceptors in intervertebral discs: morphology, distribution, and neuropeptides. Spine 20: 2645–2651

Roy S H, DeLuca C J, Casavant D A 1989 Lumbar muscle fatigue and chronic low back pain. Spine 14: 992–1001

Sahrman S 2002 Diagnosis and treatment of movement impairment syndromes. Mosby, St Louis

Sapsford R R, Hodges P W 2001 Contraction of the pelvic floor muscles during abdominal maneuvers. Archives of Physical Medicine and Rehabilitation 82: 1081–1088

Sapsford R R, Hodges P W, Richardson C A, Cooper D H, Markwell S J, Jull G A 2001 Co-activation of the abdominal and pelvic floor muscles during voluntary exercises. Neurourology and Urodynamics 20: 31–42

Saunders S, Rath D, Hodges P W 2002 Respiratory and postural activation of the trunk muscles changes with mode and speed of locomotion. Gait and Posture, in press 2004

Schmidt R A, Lee T D 1999 Motor control and learning: a behavioural emphasis. Human Kinetics, Champaign, Illinois

Shirado O, Ito T, Kaneda K, Strax T E 1995 Flexion-relaxation phenomenon in the back muscles: a comparative study between healthy subjects and patients with chronic low back pain. American Journal of Physical Medicine Rehabilitation 74: 139–144

Siddall P J, Cousins M J 1995 Pain mechanisms and management: an update. Clinical and Experimental Pharmacology and Physiology 22: 679–688

Sihvonen T, Lindgren K A, Airaksinen O, Manninen H 1997 Movement disturbances of the lumbar spine and abnormal back muscle electromyographic findings in recurrent low back pain. Spine 22: 289–295

Snijders C J, Vleeming A, Stoeckart R 1993 Transfer of lumbosacral load to iliac bones and legs. 1: Biomechanics of self bracing of the sacroiliac joints and its significance for treatment and exercise. Clinical Biomechanics 8: 285–294

Snijders C J, Vleeming A, Stoeckart R, Mens J M A, Kleinrensink G J 1995 Biomechanical modelling of sacroiliac joint stability in different postures. Spine: State of the Art Reviews 9: 419–432

Solomonow M, Zhou B H, Harris M, Lu Y, Baratta R V 1998 The ligamento-muscular stabilizing system of the spine. Spine 23: 2552–2562

Solomonow M, Zhou B H, Baratta R V, Lu Y, Harris M 1999 Biomechanics of increased exposure to lumbar injury caused by cyclic loading: 1: Loss of reflexive muscular stabilization. Spine 24: 2426–2434

Spencer J D, Hayes K C, Alexander I J 1984 Knee joint effusion and quadriceps reflex inhibition in man. Archives of Physical Medicine and Rehabilitation 65: 171–177

Stokes M, Young A 1984 The contribution of reflex inhibition to arthrogenous muscle weakness. Clinical Science 67: 7–14

Suzuki N, Ohe K, Inoue H 1977 The strength of abdominal and back muscles in patients with low back pain. Central Japanese Journal of Orthopaedics and Traumatology 20: 332–334

Svensson P, Arendt-Nielsen L, Houe L 1995 Sensory-motor interactions of human experimental unilateral jaw muscle pain: a quantitative analysis. Pain 64: 241–249

Taimela S, Kujala U M 1992 Reaction times with reference to musculoskeletal complaints in adolescence. Perceptual and Motor Skills 75: 1075–1082

Taimela S, Kankaanpaa M, Luoto S 1999 The effect of lumbar fatigue on the ability to sense a change in lumbar position: a controlled study. Spine 24: 1322–1327

Takala E, Viikari-Juntura E 2000 Do functional tests predict low back pain? Spine 25: 2126–2132

Taub E, Berman A J 1968 Movement and learning in the absence of sensory feedback. In: Freedman S J (ed) The neurophysiology of spatially oriented behaviour. Dorsey Press, Homewood, Illinois

Thorstensson A, Arvidson Å 1982 Trunk muscle strength and low back pain. Scandinavian Journal of Rehabilitation Medicine 14: 69–75

Urquhart D M, Hodges P W, Story I, Barker P J, Briggs C A 2001 Regional morphology of transversus abdominis and obliquus internus abdominis. Proceedings of the Biennial Congress of Musculoskeletal Physiotherapists of Australia, Adelaide, Australia

Urquhart D, Story I, Hodges P 2002 Transversus abdominis recruitment in trunk rotation. International Physiotherapy Conference, Sydney, Australia

Valeriani M, Restuccia D, Di Lazzaro V et al 1999 Inhibition of the human primary motor area by painful heat stimulation of the skin. Clinical Neurophysiology 110: 1475–1480

Vleeming A, Pool-Goudzwaard A L, Stoeckart R, vanWingerden J-P, Snijders C J 1995 The posterior layer of the thoracolumbar fascia: its function in load transfer from spine to legs. Spine 20: 753–758

Wilder D G, Aleksiev A R, Magnusson M L, Pope M H, Spratt K F, Goel V K 1996 Muscular response to sudden load: a tool to evaluate fatigue and rehabilitation. Spine 21: 2628–2639

Wilke H J, Wolf S, Claes L E, Arand M, Wiesend A 1995 Stability increase of the lumbar spine with different muscle groups: a biomechanical in vitro study. Spine 20: 192–198

Williams P L, Warwick R, Dyson M, Bannister L H, (eds) 1989 Gray's Anatomy. Churchill Livingstone, London

Winter D A, Patla A E, Prince F, Ishac M, Gielo-Perczak K 1998 Stiffness control of balance in quiet standing. Journal of Neurophysiology 80: 1211–1221

Wolf S L, Basmajian J V 1977 Assessment of paraspinal electromyographic activity in normal subjects and chronic low back pain patients using a muscle biofeedback device. In: Asmussen E, Jorgensen K (eds) Biomechanics IV B. University Park Press, Baltimore, pp 319–324

Zattara M, Bouisset S 1986 Chronometric analysis of the posturo-kinetic programming of voluntary movement. Journal of Motor Behaviour 18: 215–223

Zedka M, Prochazka A 1997 Phasic activity in the human erector spinae during repetitive hand movements. Journal of Physiology 504: 727–734

Zedka M, Prochazka A, Knight B, Gillard D, Gauthier M 1999 Voluntary and reflex control of human back muscles during induced pain. Journal of Physiology 520: 591–604

Chapter **11**

The lumbar fasciae and segmental control

P. J. Barker, C. A. Briggs

OVERVIEW

The middle and posterior layers of lumbar fasciae encapsulate the paraspinal muscles and provide attachment for muscles converging from the back, limbs and abdominal wall. It has been proposed that these fasciae support the lumbar spine and sacroiliac joint via several mechanisms.

This chapter presents current evidence from anatomical, biomechanical, electromyographic (EMG) intra-abdominal (IAP) and intramuscular pressure studies. It incorporates these with proposed functions of fasciae and in particular with models of segmental control. The magnitude of forces involved and roles in different planes are discussed, with reference to directions for future research and low back pain management.

ANATOMY AND BIOMECHANICS

The lumbar fasciae are arranged in three layers. The anterior layer (ALF) is thin and membranous while the middle and posterior layers (MLF, PLF) are more fibrous. The latter two attach to lumbar transverse and spinous processes (respectively), collectively enclosing the paraspinal muscles. All three layers meet and fuse at the lateral raphe, between the twelfth rib and iliac crest (Farfan 1995). Attachments at this raphe include fascicles from transversus abdominis (TrA), internal oblique (IO) and external oblique (EO) as well as latissimus dorsi (LD) (Barker et al 2004, Bogduk & Macintosh 1984, Bogduk et al 1998, Tesh 1986, Vleeming et al 1995) (Fig. 11.1).

Lumbar fasciae are also termed 'thoracolumbar' fasciae, although only the posterior layer extends above the level of the twelfth rib and correctly deserves this name. Even 'fascia' may be an inappropriate classification for these tissues (Bogduk 1997, Gallaudet 1931), since the MLF and PLF blend medially with vertebral ligaments and form aponeurotic attachments for TrA and LD, so might also be considered ligamentous or tendinous (Bogduk 1997).

Anterior layer of lumbar fascia

The anterior layer of lumbar fascia (ALF) covers quadratus lumborum (QL), joins the MLF laterally at the lateral raphe

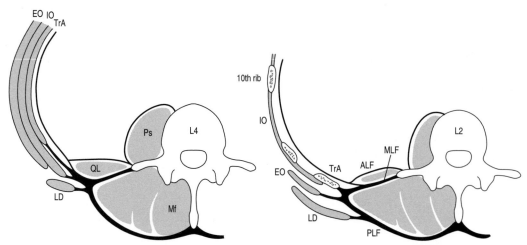

Figure 11.1 The lumbar fasciae in cross-section at L4 and L2. Note IO's attachment to the lateral raphe below L3 and EO's attachment to it above L3. Reproduced from Barker and Briggs 1999 Spine 24 (17): 1757–1764 with permission from Lippincott, Williams & Wilkins. Key: EO = external oblique; IO = internal oblique; TrA = transversus abdominis; LD = latissimus dorsi; QL = quadratus lumborum; Ps = psoas; Mf = multifidus; ALF = anterior lumbar fascia; MLF = middle lumbar fascia; PLF = posterior lumbar fascia.

and inserts medially on the anterior surface of each lumbar transverse process. It is thin (0.1 mm), membranous (Barker et al 2004b) and may blend with the fascia over psoas laterally.

The ALF displays thickenings superiorly and laterally. The lateral arcuate ligament is the superior thickening, providing attachment for the diaphragm and covering the upper part of QL. A second thickening passes vertically between the tip of the twelfth rib and the iliac crest. The remainder of the ALF lacks fibres and its capacity for tensile transmission appears to be minimal.

Middle layer of lumbar fascia

Bony and ligamentous attachments

The middle layer of lumbar fascia (MLF) arises from the iliac crest and posterior iliolumbar ligament, attaching superiorly to the medial part of the twelfth rib and lumbocostal ligament (Bogduk & Macintosh 1984, Williams et al 1995). Here, QL is tightly enclosed between the lumbocostal ligament and lateral arcuate ligament (Poirier 1901). Medially, the MLF attaches to the outer edge of each lumbar transverse process (Barker et al 2004b, Breathnach 1965, Sharpey et al 1867, Tesh et al 1987) and the intertransverse ligaments. Laterally, the MLF has only muscular attachments, of which the most extensive is to TrA (Fig. 11.2).

Fibre orientation

Fibres of the MLF radiate laterally from the tips of lumbar transverse processes. Superolateral fibres are short (~2 cm), angled up to 30 degrees above the horizontal before joining inferolateral fibres from the transverse process above, to form fibrous 'arches' between the processes (Barker et al 2004b, Tesh et al 1987, Testut & Latarjet 1948) (see Fig. 11.2). The majority of fibres are directed inferolaterally (approximately 10–25 degrees below horizontal) and are continuous with fascicles from the mid-region of TrA (Barker et al 2004b, Urquhart et al 2004). At the lateral raphe, a few fibres of the MLF may be reflected posteriorly to join the deep lamina of the PLF, encircling the lateral border of erector spinae (Tesh et al 1987). Since fibre orientation indicates the directional stiffness of a tissue (Hukins 1984, 1985; Minns et al 1973), the MLF is likely to be stiffer transversely.

Features and stiffness

The width of the MLF, from transverse processes to lateral raphe, is only 2–3 cm, the aponeurosis of TrA extending

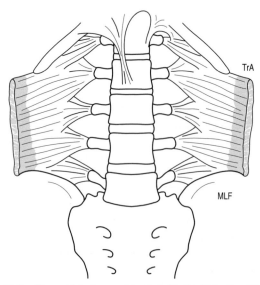

Figure 11.2 The middle layer of lumbar fascia. Note the thick attachments of the MLF to transverse processes, the extensive TrA aponeurosis and that MLF fibres are angled more towards horizontal inferiorly. Reproduced with permission from Barker et al 2004b. Key: TrA = transversus abdominis; MLF = middle lumbar fascia.

beyond this for 5–6 cm (Barker et al 2004a, 2004b) (see Fig. 11.2). The average thickness of the MLF varies greatly, being more than 50% thicker at its attachments to the transverse processes than between them (0.62:0.40 mm; Barker et al 2004b). These attachments are aligned primarily horizontally and may avulse the transverse process tips during contraction of TrA (Marshall 2001). Avulsion of the processes has been observed in dissections by traction on the MLF, confirming its capacity to transmit loads to the vertebral column (Barker et al 2004b). In unembalmed cadavers, transverse tensile loads of up to 50 N have been applied to TrA without the muscle or MLF tearing; however, their maximum capacity is likely to be greater than 50 N (Barker et al 2004a).

Although mechanical testing of the MLF on isolated segments is difficult (Tesh 1986), early anatomical texts referred to it as the strongest layer of lumbar fascia (Davies-Colley 1894, Sharpey et al 1867) and limited in vitro tests support this. In an unembalmed cadaver, Tesh (1986, 1987) inserted a balloon confined (by rigid horizontal dividers) to the lumbar region of the abdomen, then applied lateral flexion torques while varying the pressure in the balloon. Increasing the pressure (from 60 to 120 mmHg) was noted to right the trunk against applied lateral flexion force, requiring a proportional increase in restraining force necessary to retain lateral flexion. This force was up to 14.5 Nm or equivalent to 40% of the moment produced by body weight in extreme lateral flexion. If the position was sustained and both pressure and lateral flexion torque removed, then the pressure re-raised, the cadaver moved back to the neutral position. The force was attributed to tension generation in the MLF (Tesh 1986, Tesh et al 1987).

The MLF possesses thickenings via which it may transmit loads to the vertebral column. Although its stiffness has not been quantified, its tensile capacity is likely to be greater horizontally. The capacity of the MLF to resist loads in the coronal plane, at end of range lateral flexion, may be up to 14.5 Nm.

Muscle attachments

The MLF is attached to fascicles of TrA, LD (Bogduk & Macintosh 1984), EO and IO (Barker et al 2004a, Bogduk & Macintosh 1984, Vleeming et al 1995). EO attaches to it above the level of the transverse process of L3, IO below this level and TrA to the full length of the lateral raphe (Barker et al 2004a). The attachments of LD, IO and EO are relatively small and muscular (Gallaudet 1931) and fascicles of IO and LD oriented almost perpendicular to fibres of the MLF. Other muscles including QL, iliocostalis lumborum and the diaphragm have small attachments to the MLF. By contrast, the attachment of TrA is extensive and aponeurotic laterally (Testut & Latarjet 1948), with fascicles being directly continuous with fibres of the MLF (Barker et al 2004b).

Tensile effects of muscle attachments

Raster photography, a technique to indicate tensile transmission between muscles and fascia by comparing movement of fascial markers against a reference grid, was described by Vleeming et al (1995). Tension was applied to fascial attachments to simulate the effect of muscle contraction.

A similar technique was employed to determine the area of fascial movement following tensile loading of the lateral abdominal muscles and MLF in unembalmed cadavers (Barker et al 2004a). Tension on the attachment of TrA displaced more than double the area of fasciae than tension on IO or EO (Fig. 11.3) and resisted higher applied tension before failure. A strain gauge inserted into the MLF and PLF at their vertebral (L3) attachments indicated tension applied to TrA was transmitted more effectively to the MLF, its tensile force being almost twice that of the PLF and transmitted direct to vertebrae rather than across the midline (Barker et al 2004a) (see Fig. 11.3). Tesh's work (Tesh 1986) indicates the MLF is also most likely to transmit tensile forces generated from within TrA, since the intra-abdominal balloon pressure was sustained even when the PLF was incised. Mathematical calculations (Barker et al 2004a) indicate that during maximum contraction, the MLF may withstand a transverse hoop tension of 48 N per segment.

TrA therefore appears to be the only muscle that can transmit tension via the MLF to all lumbar vertebrae, its fascicles being attached and well aligned with fibres of the MLF throughout this region. TrA is the primary muscle attachment of the MLF, which in turn appears well structured to operate as this muscle's principal aponeurosis of origin.

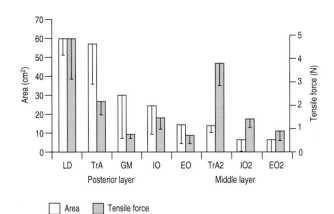

Figure 11.3 Fascial area and tensile forces. The areas of PLF and MLF displaced and tensile forces developed in fasciae with 10 N applied tension to attached muscles. 'Tensile force' indicates the transverse component of tensile force at L3. Reproduced from Barker and Briggs 1999 Spine 24 (17): 1757–1764 with permission from Lippincott, Williams & Wilkins. Key: PLF = posterior lumbar fascia; MLF = middle lumbar fascia; LD = latissimus dorsi; TrA = transversus abdominis; GM = gluteus maximus; IO = internal oblique; EO = external oblique.

Posterior layer of lumbar fascia

The posterior layer of lumbar fascia (PLF) surrounds the paraspinal muscles and consists of two laminae, which are progressively fused below T12 (Barker & Briggs 1999, Bogduk & Macintosh 1984). Figure 11.4 illustrates these two laminae with their fibre directions and attachments.

Bony and ligamentous attachments

The PLF attaches to lumbar and thoracic spinous processes, supraspinous and interspinous ligaments, the posterior superior iliac spine and posterior part of iliac crest as well as the ilium on the opposite side (Bogduk & Macintosh 1984, Tesh et al 1987). It is also reported to be continuous inferiorly with the long dorsal sacroiliac and sacrotuberous ligaments (Vleeming et al 1996, 1995), while its deep lamina attaches superolaterally at each rib angle (Barker & Briggs 1999). Fibres from the superficial lamina of the PLF cross the midline at all lumbar levels (Tesh et al 1987) although midline attachments become less evident below L3 (Bogduk & Macintosh 1984, Vleeming et al 1995).

Each interspinous ligament, via its sagittally oriented fibres, attaches the deep lamina of the PLF to the anterior upper border of the spinous process below. Its primary function has been proposed to anchor the PLF to the spine (Aspden et al 1987, Hukins et al 1990b) or to limit anterior shear forces on vertebrae (Farfan 1995, Tesh et al 1987). Lamellae within the spinous processes are also aligned in the sagittal plane (Gallios & Japiot 1925). However, the PLF itself approaches the spinous processes from a posterolateral angle, which varies with contraction of the paraspinal muscles (Tesh 1986).

The midline lumbar attachments of the PLF are variable and may require paraspinal muscle contraction for effective tensile transmission to the interspinous ligaments and spinous processes.

Fibre orientation

The superficial lamina of the PLF appears cross-hatched below T12. This has been attributed to fibres aligning superolaterally with LD and inferolaterally with the contralateral gluteus maximus (GM), (Vleeming et al 1995), although since the laminae are fused, exact origins are difficult to trace (Bogduk & Macintosh 1984). Serratus posterior inferior and TrA also have fascicles closely oriented with fibres of the PLF (see Fig. 11.4) so its fibre directions may be partly attributed to these muscles (Barker et al 2004a). Fibres in the deep lamina are predominantly superolateral (Bogduk & Macintosh 1984).

Fibre angles of the PLF are generally measured with the spine in extension and are cited here with reference to a horizontal axis. Barker & Briggs (1999) reported angles and/or presence of fascial fibres at alternate vertebral levels throughout the PLF in 20 cadavers. Superolateral fibres in the superficial lamina become more transverse in the upper lumbar spine, oriented almost 40 degrees above the

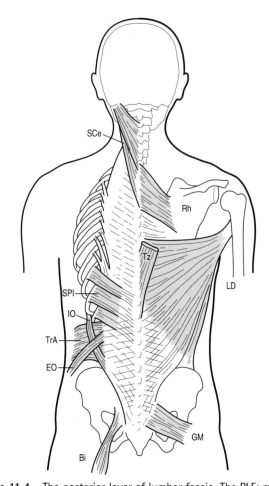

Figure 11.4 The posterior layer of lumbar fascia. The PLF: muscular attachments of deep (left) and superficial (right) laminae. Reproduced from Barker and Briggs 1999 Spine 24 (17): 1757–1764 with permission from Lippincott, Williams & Wilkins. Key: SCe = splenius cervicis; SPI = serratus posterior inferior; Bi = biceps femoris; Tz = trapezius; Rh = rhomboids; GM = gluteus maximus.

horizontal at L5 and 30 degrees at L1. At T9 they lie transversely, then are oriented increasingly inferolaterally to become continuous with the rhomboid muscles (see Fig. 11.4). In the lumbar region, inferolateral fibres (20 degrees below horizontal) cross the above fibres to create a hatched appearance (Barker & Briggs 1999).

The lattice formed by PLF fibres is thus more closely oriented towards a horizontal axis. Fibres in the deep lamina above T12 are consistently directed superolaterally at 20 degrees above the horizontal but decrease at T4, above which this lamina becomes more membranous (Barker & Briggs 1999).

Features and stiffness

The average thickness of the PLF (0.52 mm) is comparable with that of the middle layer (0.55 mm; Barker et al 2004b). Thickened fascial bands have been described in the PLF (Bogduk & Macintosh 1984) but regional differences are only minor (0.56 mm) at the spinous processes compared with between them (0.53 mm; Barker & Briggs 1999). The increase in thickness at vertebral attachments (6%) is slight compared with that observed in the middle layer (55%; Barker et al 2004b).

Both laminae of the PLF diminish in thickness and fibrosity in the thoracic region, yet the region of the superficial lamina between LD and rhomboid attachments can vary considerably (Barker & Briggs 1999). This lamina ends freely at the upper border of rhomboid minor while the deep lamina remains thin throughout the thoracic region, attaching superiorly to splenius cervicis (Barker & Briggs 1999) and fascia overlying the splenii (Bogduk & Macintosh 1984). The deep lamina thus forms an enclosed compartment that runs the length of the spine, surrounding the paraspinal and splenius muscles. Dye injection studies support this (Peck et al 1986).

The width of the PLF, from spinous processes to lateral raphe, is approximately 7 cm (Barker et al 2004a) per side. It lies approximately 7 cm behind the instantaneous axis of rotation for flexion, with almost double the moment arm of most posterior ligaments (Tesh 1986, Tesh et al 1987). Mechanical testing using samples of PLF indicates it may be up to four times stiffer transversely than longitudinally, and three times stiffer transversely than in an oblique (inferolateral) direction (Tesh 1986). Consistent with other connective tissues, stiffness of the PLF increases with deformation (Tesh 1986, Yahia et al 1993).

Transverse stiffness of samples of PLF has been reported at up to 113 MPa, which is relatively unimpressive compared with other fasciae (Tesh 1986). This, however, may be an underestimate, since isolated samples tend to be weaker than entire intact tissues with in situ attachments (Adams 1995, Adams & Green 1993). During maximal IAP and with contraction of the paraspinal muscles, the PLF has been estimated mathematically to withstand a maximum transverse ('hoop') tension of 90 N at each segment (Tesh 1986), although subsequent analysis indicates this tension is more correctly attributed to the MLF (Barker et al 2004a). Tests applying sub-failure tension to attached fascicles of TrA indicate the PLF is likely to withstand at least 50 N tension (Barker et al 2004a).

The numeric stiffness of the PLF is uncertain, but its transverse stiffness is up to four times greater than its longitudinal stiffness. Small tensile loads applied to muscle attachments are easily transmitted via the lumbar fasciae to vertebrae (Barker et al 2004a) and may play a role in influencing segmental movement around the neutral position.

Muscle attachments

The PLF receives the same attachments via the lateral raphe as the MLF (see Fig. 11.1A, B) as well as attachments from many extrinsic back muscles. These are illustrated (see Fig. 11.4) from superiorly to inferiorly, using combined findings of dissection and tensile studies (Barker & Briggs 1999, Bogduk & Macintosh 1984, Vleeming et al 1995).

In the thoracic region, the superficial lamina is attached to the rhomboids up to the level of T2 and to the lowest fascicles of trapezius at T11/12. The superficial lamina is also attached to LD, via an oblique aponeurotic junction above the iliac crest, and the contralateral GM, via fibres crossing the midline below L4. Inferiorly it is attached to ipsilateral fascicles of GM between the posterior superior iliac spine and the median sacral crest, at S2–4 levels.

The deep lamina is attached superiorly to the lower border of splenius cervicis. Here, serratus posterior superior (SPS) overlies the deep lamina without attaching to it and is, in turn, located deep to the rhomboids. SPS thus separates the two laminae of the PLF without attaching to either, while by contrast, at upper lumbar levels, serratus posterior inferior (SPI) is entirely continuous with the deep lamina. The deep lamina attaches laterally to the mid-region of TrA and to part of EO above L3 and part of IO below it. This lamina also has variable inferior attachments to the lumbar erector spinae aponeurosis (below L5; Hutchinson & Dall 1994) and the sacrotuberous ligament, which may provide indirect attachment to biceps femoris (Vleeming et al 1989).

Features of attached muscle regions

Most attachments to the PLF consist of groups of adjacent fascicles rather than entire muscle bellies, the exceptions being SPI and rhomboid muscles. All attachments have varying fascicle directions, lengths, moment arms and cross-sectional areas and consequently different vectors and capacities for stiffness or torque generation (Bergmark 1989).

Attaching fascicles of LD and GM are relatively long, directed superolaterally towards the axilla and inferolaterally towards the iliotibial tract, respectively. SPI has shorter fascicles, passing superolaterally toward the lower four ribs. Attaching fascicles of EO and TrA are relatively long and pass anteroinferiorly; those of EO almost vertically to the anterior iliac crest and those of TrA to the rectus sheath. IO's attached fascicles are comparatively short, passing superolaterally to the lower three to four ribs (Williams et al 1995) (see Fig. 11.4).

Cross-sectional areas of the muscle attachments vary considerably. LD, TrA, SPI, EO and IO are generally thin, broad muscles, with fascial attachments of LD and TrA being the most extensive. Bogduk et al (1998) reported fibres of LD had insufficient cross-sectional area to produce torque via the PLF at the sacroiliac joint (Bogduk et al 1998), but the attachment of GM appears to have a more substantial cross-sectional area (P. J. Barker, unpublished work, 2003).

Tensile effects of muscle attachments

Vleeming et al (1995) applied 50 N tension to attachments of the PLF in embalmed cadavers, reporting that both LD and GM transmitted tension to the posterior layer of lumbar fascia contralaterally, LD up to 2 cm and GM up to 4 cm past the midline. Traction to SPI and EO, biceps femoris and trapezius and gluteus medius produced variable, limited or no fascial displacement, respectively. Barker et al (2004a) performed a similar study in unembalmed cadavers using a lower (10 N) applied tension and found greatly increased tensile transmission, with every muscle tested (LD, GM, TrA, IO, EO) producing fascial movement and tensile force (see Fig. 11.3).

Most extensive PLF displacement resulted from tension on LD and TrA, bilaterally between T12 and S1, while tension on GM and IO caused fascial displacement below L3 and tension on EO above it. Tension on both obliques often produced only unilateral displacement (Barker et al 2004a). Transverse tensile force in the PLF was also found to be greatest when tension was applied to LD and TrA, with up to 50% of applied tensile force being transmitted to the fascia adjacent to the L3 spinous process (Barker et al 2004a) (see Fig. 11.3).

Two studies by Tesh (1986) concur that TrA transmits tension to the PLF. During inflation of a lumbar intra-abdominal balloon, markers on the PLF were noted to move laterally and if incised longitudinally, the edges of the incision sprang apart, indicating the PLF was transmitting tension. Tesh's concurrent CT study indicated that a Valsalva manoeuvre (performed in supine) drew the PLF anteriorly. Contraction of the paraspinal muscles has also been proposed to generate transverse tension in the PLF (Carr et al 1985, Farfan 1973, Gracovetsky et al 1977, Tesh et al 1987), with staining techniques indicating this mechanism may transmit tension to both supraspinous and interspinous ligaments (Tesh 1986).

A study of the PLF which perhaps has the greatest implications for segmental stability was also performed by Tesh (1986). The effects of applying lateral fascial tension on segmental sagittal rotation were investigated. Lateral tension of 20 N was applied direct to the PLF, via grips to simulate contraction of the lateral abdominal muscles, then segments were loaded in sagittal rotation via distracting their spinous processes. When lateral tension was applied, resistance to sagittal rotation increased from the onset of loading and throughout early range at all segments (Tesh 1986), so that additional sagittal force (e.g. 20 N) was required to achieve the same spinous process distraction (e.g. 1 mm; Fig. 11.5). Transverse loading of the PLF effectively stiffened the motion segment in the initial stage of flexion, without altering the final stiffness (Tesh 1986).

The PLF has extensive attachments to LD and TrA. Tensile and staining tests indicate that every muscle attachment is capable of generating some tension in the PLF and so via it may contribute to spinal stability (Bogduk & Macintosh 1984). Transverse tension in the PLF can increase segmental stiffness to sagittal plane rotation in early range (Tesh 1986).

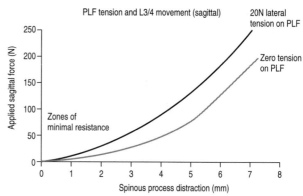

Figure 11.5 The effect of PLF tension on sagittal segmental movement. Typical load deformation curve taken from the L3–4 segment during sagittal rotation. Note that with 20 N applied lateral tension to the PLF, the curve moves to the left, its gradient indicating an increased stiffness in early sagittal displacement but no change at the end of the range. Adapted from Tesh 1986. Key: PLF = posterior lumbar fascia.

SEGMENTAL CONTROL

Comparative features of the middle and posterior layers of the lumbar fasciae

Both MLF and PLF are capable of transmitting tension from TrA to all lumbar vertebrae, with fibres of the middle layer being directly continuous with TrA fascicles laterally and thickened at their attachments to the transverse processes, medially. From the lateral raphe, the MLF provides a relatively short, direct route to vertebrae that generates almost double the transverse tension of the PLF when tension is applied to TrA. The MLF also appears to be the primary fascial restraint for tension generated within TrA (via an intra-abdominal balloon) and may resist substantial lateral flexion torques. It is, therefore, well structured to transmit a wide range of tensile loads from TrA, from one or both sides.

By contrast, the PLF's multiple fibre orientations indicate its suitability for tensile transmission from several attached muscles. Fibres in the PLF are not consistently oriented with fascicles of TrA and it forms a less direct route from TrA, which has been shown to transmit less tensile force (Barker et al 2004a) to vertebrae. Although the PLF is stiffest in the transverse direction, its vertebral attachments are relatively inconsistent, unthickened and mobile in the absence of paraspinal contraction. The MLF may consequently provide a more efficient route for TrA to influence segmental movement than the PLF.

Despite this, application of transverse tension to the PLF has been shown to increase resistance to inner range segmental movement in the sagittal plane (Tesh 1986).

Whether a similar stabilizing effect may be produced via the MLF remains to be demonstrated.

Related muscles

Attachments and classification
Functionally, spinal muscles may be classified as either 'global' or 'local' (Bergmark 1989). Global muscles attaching to the spine, including GM or LD, are generally superficial and responsible for generating large torques, whereas local muscles such as multifidus are deeper, with segmental attachments that generate small torques but are more important in influencing intersegmental movement. Although not originally classified (Bergmark 1989), TrA's anatomy (Barker et al 2004b, Urquhart et al 2004), and EMG activity (Hodges & Richardson 1997b) are consistent with a local function (Richardson et al 1999). The lumbar fasciae are related to muscles from both groups as well as some that are classified as part local and part global. These include QL, IO and certain regions of the erector spinae (Bergmark 1989).

IO was considered to be a partly local muscle due to its attachment to the lumbar fasciae (Bergmark 1989) and so EO might similarly be allocated to both categories. Both obliques are, however, primarily attached to the ribcage and pelvis, so better suited to act as global trunk rotators. Local and global muscles may respond differently to low back injury, with wasting and/or dysfunction documented in the former and excessive levels of co-contraction proposed to develop in the latter (Richardson et al 1999).

General EMG activity
In healthy subjects, collective EMG findings reveal that local muscles such as TrA and the deep fascicles of multifidus are active prior to the prime movers for limb movements, in all directions and at various speeds (Hodges & Richardson 1997a, 1997b, 1998, Moseley et al 2002). Their onset does not vary with the direction of limb movement, in contrast with onsets of adjacent muscles (Hodges & Richardson 1996, Moseley et al 2002) and their subsequent contraction is more tonic (sustained and submaximal) in nature (Hodges et al 1999, Richardson et al 1999).

From these findings, pre-contraction of TrA has been hypothesized to limit excess intersegmental movement occurring either via the lumbar fasciae or IAP generation (Hodges & Richardson 1997b). Tension from TrA may be transmitted via the MLF and PLF to the processes of lumbar vertebrae, 'anchoring' them during perturbations to the spine to help prevent excessive movement and potential segmental injury (Hodges & Richardson 1997b). Lumbar multifidus is relatively bulky (Macintosh et al 1986), so might also influence intersegmental movement by increasing tension in the overlying PLF. Only some of its fascicles, however, demonstrate an early onset of contraction, so its effect on vertebrae via the PLF is likely to be less efficient at limiting segmental movement than its direct compressive action (Hodges & Richardson 1996, Moseley et al 2002).

The MLF and PLF thus provide mechanisms via which (primarily) TrA may influence segmental control. Their efficiency depends on the effectiveness of contraction of TrA, which requires optimum motor control (Hodges & Richardson 1996, McGill & Norman 1993).

Local regional EMG activity
Regions of muscles that have different fascial attachments may also have different functions. To clarify the effect of each muscle, EMG activity within the relevant (attached or enclosed) muscle region must be considered.

The middle fascicles of TrA, which originate between the iliac crest and lower border of the costal margin, are those typically recorded from in EMG studies (Cresswell et al 1992, Hodges & Richardson 1997b, 1998, Hodges et al 1999). The contraction onset of TrA is noted to be delayed relative to the onset of the prime mover in subjects with low back pain (Hodges et al 2001) and the subsequent contraction becomes more phasic in nature (Hodges & Richardson 1996, Hodges et al 2001). TrA's contraction prior to limb movement has invariably been reported unilaterally, although studies performed on different sides and during bilateral limb movement consistently show this feature (Hodges & Richardson 1997b, Hodges et al 1999), indicating the contraction may occur bilaterally.

Additional activity in middle fascicles of TrA has been noted during trunk and pelvic rotation, with greater (unilateral) activity in ipsilateral trunk rotation and opposite pelvic rotation (Cresswell et al 1992). TrA's lowest fascicles may behave in a more tonic fashion than its middle fascicles throughout limb movements (Hodges et al 1999).

Only the posterior fascicles of IO and EO attach to vertebrae via the MLF and PLF. These fascicles are proposed to have the greatest capacity for stiffness generation (Bergmark 1989, Mirka et al 1997). However, electrode placement in most EMG studies of the obliques allows recording from fascicles either at or anterior to the mid-axillary line (Carman et al 1972, Davis & Mirka 2000, Hodges & Richardson 1997b, Mirka et al 1997), above the region where EO's fascicles attach to the fasciae and anterior to fascicles of IO with a fascial attachment. The proposed local function of these fascicles thus remains to be clarified.

The deep fascicles of lumbar multifidus have been shown to demonstrate an early onset of contraction prior to prime movers for limb movements and are thought to influence vertebral movement by their direct (compressive) action (Moseley et al 2002). In addition, multifidus may sometimes be active bilaterally during rotation (Donisch & Basmajian 1972).

Via both the MLF and PLF, an isolated, submaximal contraction of TrA may subtly increase stiffness of lumbar segments prior to trunk perturbations. Bilateral contraction of TrA is required for a symmetric fascial influence on segmental movement.

Global regional EMG activity

Anterior fascicles of EO and IO appear to behave predominantly in a global fashion. Each has an onset of contraction more specific to the direction of limb movement, with subsequent activity being more phasic (Hodges et al 1999, Richardson et al 1999). Subjects suffering low back pain may recruit fascicles of IO differently during drawing in of the abdominal wall (O'Sullivan et al 1997a). IO has also been noted to demonstrate an early onset of contraction prior to some limb movements, but not as early or as consistently as TrA (Hodges & Richardson 1997c, Richardson et al 1999). IO and EO are also recruited unilaterally as agonists for trunk rotation (Carman et al 1972) and bilaterally for flexion or to stabilize leg movements (Floyd & Silver 1950).

During gait and trunk rotation, fascicles of LD and GM that attach to the PLF are reported to contract contralaterally in an alternating phasic fashion (Mooney et al 2001) and may generate oblique tension across the PLF (Vleeming et al 1995). The paraspinal muscles may also generate tension in the PLF during contraction, for example during resisted extension or anti-gravity flexion (Donisch & Basmajian 1972, Floyd & Silver 1955).

While tension in the MLF is primarily influenced by contraction of TrA, the PLF may be more influenced by contraction of global, phasic muscles. This puts the MLF at an advantage for segmental stability.

Biomechanical roles of the lumbar fasciae

Longitudinal tension generation

The PLF has the largest moment arm of all extensor tissues (Tesh 1986) and has been proposed to oppose flexion moments in several ways. Although initially thought to generate passive longitudinal tension (Gracovetsky et al 1981), its fibres are not well oriented for this, possessing a relatively small vertical component (Barker & Briggs 1999, Bogduk & Macintosh 1984, McGill & Norman 1988, Tesh et al 1987, Vleeming et al 1995). Similar to a lattice, lateral tension generated by abdominal wall muscles might increase longitudinal tension in the PLF. This has been simulated in cadavers and a small amount of lumbar extension noted (Fairbank & O'Brien 1980). Initially the axial 'gain' was predicted mathematically to be up to 5:1 (Gracovetsky et al 1985), but subsequent studies indicate gains of less than 1:1, even if the effects of lumbar flexion on fibre angles are incorporated (Tesh et al 1987). Fasciae appear to contribute to spinal support more effectively by generating transverse than longitudinal tension.

Hydraulic amplifier effect

By enclosing paraspinal muscles and restricting radial expansion, the PLF may increase longitudinal tension in these muscles, enhancing their contraction and the extension moment generated by them. This is known as the hydraulic amplifier effect (Aspden 1992, Farfan 1973, Gracovetsky et al 1977). Intramuscular pressure recordings (Styf & Lysell 1987) support restriction by fascia, with mathematical analysis (based on behaviour of non-viscoelastic materials) indicating it may increase the effectiveness of the paraspinals by up to 30% (Hukins et al 1990a).

Lumbar segmental control

From the neutral position of the lumbar spine, each segment can move within a region of minimal resistance from surrounding tissues, known as the neutral zone (Panjabi 1992b). Control of this zone is thought to provide a better indication of spinal instability than physiologic range of movement (Panjabi 1992b, Panjabi et al 1989). Surrounding tissues can be classified into active, passive and neural control subsystems, and deficiency in any one has been proposed to permit excess movement, resulting in pain and disability (Panjabi 1992a).

The MLF and PLF may limit lumbar segmental movement by transmitting tension from contraction of TrA (Hodges & Richardson 1997b). Tesh's (1986) work (Tesh 1986) supports this theory, since applying lateral tension to the PLF effectively moved the segmental load deformation curve to the left, reducing the neutral zone (see Fig. 11.5). Although rarely performed, lumbar fasciectomy may result in a sensation of instability (S. N. Bell, personal communication, 2002) that is consistent with this proposal.

Lateral tension on the MLF was not tested but might be predicted to have a similar effect on segmental neutral zone movement and perhaps be more effective at transmitting tension from TrA in the transverse plane (Barker et al 2004a). The MLF and PLF are passive components in this mechanism, reliant on a relatively isolated bilateral, symmetrical contraction of TrA (and/or multifidus) to be effective. EMG findings collectively indicate that, in vivo, such a fascial mechanism is likely to precede trunk perturbations from the neutral position in the sagittal and coronal planes (Cresswell et al 1992, Hodges & Richardson 1997b, 1998, Moseley et al 2002).

Changes in onset of TrA observed with low back pain (Hodges & Richardson 1996, 1998, Hodges et al 2001) support this model of segmental stability, as do the results of rehabilitation aimed at retraining its motor control (Jull & Richardson 2000). Decreases in pain and functional disability have been noted in patients with spondylolysis and spondylolisthesis as well as reduced recurrence of injury in patients with first episode low back pain. Improvements following motor control retraining have been sustained for more than 2 years (Hides et al 2001, O'Sullivan et al 1997b). All of this provides considerable support for a role of TrA (and the MLF and/or PLF) in segmental control.

Load transfer across the midline

In noting that tension on LD and GM caused displacement of markers on the PLF bilaterally, Vleeming et al (1995) proposed that this layer may assist load transfer across the midline, particularly during activities involving contralateral limb extension or trunk rotation, such as swimming or walking.

Loose midline attachments of the PLF may enable some forces to be distributed across, rather than entirely to, the lumbar spine and sacroiliac joint. This proposal is supported by findings of tension studies (Barker et al 2004a, Vleeming et al 1995) and the co-contraction of contralateral GM and LD during gait and trunk rotation (Mooney et al 2001). Relatively low tensile loading has been noted to produce contralateral tension in the PLF (Barker et al 2004a, Vleeming et al 1995), indicating this layer has a greater capacity for contralateral tensile transmission tension, but potentially a reduced capacity for restraining movement of vertebrae, via the spinous processes.

Sacroiliac stability

The PLF lies directly behind the sacroiliac joint (SIJ), so tension in it can contribute to active force compression at the SIJ (Vleeming et al 1995). A functional relationship between the SIJ and PLF (with its attached muscles; particularly GM) is supported by several studies.

Biomechanical analysis of LD indicates that it may produce a limited effect (via the PLF) at the SIJ (Bogduk et al 1998). Tensile testing studies similarly indicate the effects of LD and TrA may only extend via the PLF to fascial markers at S1 (Barker et al 2004a, Vleeming et al 1995). By contrast, the fascial attachment of GM is thicker, more proximal to the SIJ and oriented perpendicular to its articular components (Dijkstra et al 1989), displacing markers as low as S3 (Barker et al 2004a).

Surface EMG studies indicate GM displays a greater signal amplitude than LD during gait and trunk rotation (Mooney et al 2001) and contraction of GM corresponds with a greater increase in SIJ stiffness (Wingerden et al 2001). The level of attachment of GM and the PLF also corresponds with the level at which pelvic belts are placed (Vleeming et al 1992) to brace the SIJ for effective relief of peripartum pain (Mens et al 1996). However, management regimes for sacroiliac dysfunction based on associations between GM and LD have given varied results (Mens et al 2000, Mooney et al 2001), while TrA is emerging to play a more important role in SIJ stiffness.

Richardson et al (2002) proposed that compression of the SIJ is produced by TrA's anterior iliac attachments, which are direct rather than via the lumbar fasciae. Pelvic belt placement, previously thought to simulate the effect of GM and the PLF posteriorly, might more correctly simulate the effect of TrA's fascicles anteriorly (Richardson et al 2002). The deep fascicles of multifidus also appear appropriate to contribute to stability of the SIJ via their anatomical features (Macintosh et al 1986) and EMG behaviour (Moseley et al 2002).

It is, therefore, increasingly evident that the lumbar fasciae and their attachments may be less important in sustaining SIJ stability than the anterior fibres of TrA. During certain activities, GM and LD may be recruited in a phasic fashion to provide additional posterior compression via the PLF.

Proprioception

The PLF and MLF may play a proprioceptive role in lumbar stability (Barker & Briggs 1999). Attached to ligaments and muscles as well as containing mechanoreceptors (Yahia et al 1992), they are closely related with each of Panjabi's passive, active and neural subsystems (Panjabi 1992a). The fasciae may form functional interfaces between these structures at a segmental level. Feedback from mechanoreceptors on the status of tension in related muscles and ligaments may be incorporated by the neural subsystem and tension in muscles modified to help prevent excess segmental movement (Panjabi 1992a).

If this mechanism is disrupted, proprioceptive feedback will be altered. A reduction in trunk proprioception and resultant sensation of instability following lumbar (PLF) fasciectomy (S. N. Bell, personal communication, 2002) is consistent with this. Histological studies report innervation of the PLF to be deficient in patients with chronic low back pain (Bednar et al 1995), which might similarly reduce proprioceptive feedback and segmental control. Proprioceptive deficiency is in keeping with reports of patients with low back pain having difficulty achieving preferential contraction of TrA (Richardson et al 1999) and highlights the importance of persisting with motor control retraining and incorporation into functional tasks (O'Sullivan et al 1997b) to avoid recurrence of injury.

Magnitude of segmental forces

Just two degrees of axial rotation has been reported to produce microtrauma of the intervertebral disc (Farfan et al 1970) and very small amounts (3%) of muscle contraction have been predicted capable of restoring segmental stability (Cholewicki & McGill 1996). Although limitation of neutral zone movement is now recognized as important in injury prevention (Cholewicki & McGill 1996, Panjabi 1992b), the stabilizing effects of TrA and/or lumbar fasciae have traditionally been discounted owing to their small capacity for force generation or transmission.

TrA's early onset of contraction enables it to act briefly and in relative isolation (together with MLF, PLF and deep multifidus) on the lumbar segments. Its small cross-sectional area (Richardson et al 1999) is well suited to generate small tensile loads and the fasciae are well structured to tolerate these. Fascial tensile forces are noted to increase with applied tension on TrA up to 10 N, but not proportionally above this (Barker et al 2004).

The low forces applied to fascia by Barker et al (2004a) and Tesh (1986) support the proposed capacity of fasciae to influence movement at all segments via an early onset, submaximal contraction of TrA. Although Tesh's study (Tesh 1986) simulated only about 20% of the maximum (90 N) lateral tension estimated by the author to be generated in the

PLF, this was sufficient to reduce neutral zone movement (see Fig. 11.5). The findings support the basis for exercises incorporating submaximal contraction of TrA (Richardson & Jull 1995, Richardson et al 1999) for management and prevention of low back pain.

Of interest, Tesh himself did not consider the effects of fascial tension to be adequate to influence segmental movement (Tesh 1986). In view of subsequent research recognizing the importance of limitation of the neutral zone (Panjabi 1992b) and the potential importance of an early onset of TrA contraction (Hodges & Richardson 1996), the effects, although relatively small, may still be significant.

Planar stability

Attachments to transverse and spinous processes (Farfan 1975), along with obliquely oriented fibres, permit the MLF and PLF to resist movement in all three movement planes. Vertebral processes maximize their leverage on segmental movement, providing the fasciae with approximately 7 cm moment arms (Tesh 1986) in the neutral position. Contraction of TrA prior to trunk perturbations has also been proposed to influence segmental neutral zone movement in multiple planes (Hodges & Richardson 1997b).

Coronal stability

From their intra-abdominal balloon experiments, Tesh and colleagues (Tesh 1986, Tesh et al 1987) proposed that if sufficient tension was generated (e.g. by TrA contraction) during lateral flexion, the MLF could contribute to segmental coronal plane stability by generating greater longitudinal tension

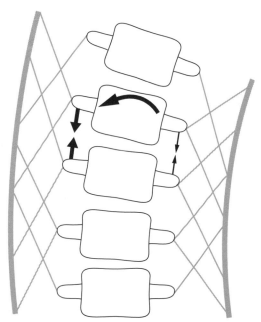

Figure 11.6 The MLF in lateral flexion. Asymmetry in MLF fibre angles during lateral flexion creates a corrective moment. Adapted from Tesh et al 1987.
Key: MLF = middle lumbar fascia.

on the convex side (Tesh et al 1987). The asymmetry was hypothesized to create a corrective moment that tended to approximate the transverse processes on that side (Fig. 11.6). It was therefore suggested that the MLF contributes increasingly to stability during trunk lateral flexion, while the PLF was able to be cut without affecting pressure (Tesh 1986).

The study indicated a tendency for tension from TrA and the MLF to return the spine to the neutral position (Tesh et al 1987), but did so using pressures associated with a strong contraction of TrA (120 mmHg) and from end of range lateral flexion rather than from the neutral position (in which fascial fibre angles would be symmetrical). Although indicative of a significant role for the MLF in the coronal plane, its application to segmental neutral zone motion is less clear than concurrent studies in the sagittal plane generating submaximal fascial tension (Tesh 1986) and requires further investigation. EMG studies do, however, indicate an onset of contraction of TrA prior to coronal trunk perturbations, so both MLF and PLF are likely to affect (inner range) coronal plane stability to some extent. Fibre angles dictate that this tensile effect will be more substantial in the transverse plane.

Sagittal stability

Since both spinous and transverse processes lie behind the instantaneous axis of rotation for flexion, the PLF and MLF may both contribute to sagittal plane stability, the PLF more so due to a longer moment arm. Tension on the PLF may be transmitted to vertebrae via the supraspinous and interspinous ligaments, helping to limit sagittal rotation and shear movements respectively (Farfan 1995).

Tesh's experiments (Tesh 1986) provide compelling evidence to support the role of the PLF in limiting segmental neutral zone movement in the sagittal plane (see Fig. 11.5). Fascial tension increased inner range stiffness during testing of all lumbar segments from four cadavers and the difference was reproducible if tension was detached then reapplied. The MLF has not been similarly tested, but has been shown to transmit lateral tension loads effectively (Barker et al 2004). EMG behaviour of TrA during sagittal trunk perturbations and with low back pain (Hodges & Richardson 1996) is consistent with such an (inner range) stabilizing role for both the MLF and PLF. Tensile transmission from TrA to the MLF may also help explain Kaigle et al's finding, in an in vivo porcine model, that removal of lumbar transverse processes (following facet joint injury) resulted in an increase in the neutral zone range for segmental sagittal rotation (Kaigle et al 1995).

Transverse stability

Very little axial rotation occurs in the lumbar spine owing to the orientation of facet joints (Bogduk 1997). Accurate testing of this movement is consequently difficult and no known studies have quantified the effects of fasciae on segmental rotation. However, minimal movement may be required to produce injury in this plane (Gracovetsky & Farfan 1986, Hickey & Hukins 1980) and twisting is commonly implicated in low back injury (Kelsey et al 1984, Marras et al 1993, 1995, Mundt et al 1993). Appropriately timed influences on the neutral zone may be particularly crucial for preventing injury in this plane.

Although EMG behaviour of TrA has not been reported in response to limb movements in the transverse plane, movements in sagittal and coronal planes are likely to generate alternating rotary demands in the transverse plane (Hodges & Richardson 1997b). On this basis, one might predict, TrA also demonstrates an early onset of contraction prior to transverse trunk peturbations.

Anatomical and transverse loading studies indicate TrA and the MLF and PLF are well structured to resist tension in the transverse plane (Barker et al 2004a, 2004b, Tesh 1986). Their effect on segmental movement might be expected, from fibre directions and the results of stiffness testing, to be several times the magnitude of those observed in the sagittal plane, and effected on a smaller range of motion.

Fascial disruption

The lumbar fasciae are frequently disrupted by injury or surgery. The MLF may be torn when its attachments are avulsed (Marshall 2001) and the PLF is routinely cut during lumbar spine surgery, lumbar fasciectomy or taking bone grafts from the iliac crest. The contribution of the relevant fascia(e) to segmental control is then compromised and one might expect the resultant deficiency to increase the individual's chance of low back injury. To date, however, this has not been reported, with management of the above conditions being largely symptomatic (Howarth & Petrie 1964).

It has been suggested that reattachment of the PLF to midline structures following surgery (Crock & Crock 1988) or the use of horizontal incisions (Aspden 1992) during spinal surgery may help to minimize rehabilitation time and impairment of spinal stability. During iliac crest bone grafts, an incision through the midline rather than iliac attachments of the PLF, followed by reattachment, has been reported to reduce postoperative pain over the harvest site (Hutchinson & Dall 1994). Further research into disruption of these mechanisms and the effects of surgical intervention is required.

CONCLUSION

The MLF and PLF are particularly well structured for transverse tension and capable of transmitting even small tensile loads from TrA to all lumbar vertebrae. Although the MLF may provide a more effective and isolated route, to date only the PLF has been demonstrated to limit segmental neutral zone movement (in the sagittal plane). EMG studies in healthy subjects indicate an early onset of contraction of TrA occurs prior to trunk perturbations in several directions, and under these circumstances both MLF and PLF are predicted to limit excess intersegmental movement occurring in all planes.

Disruption of the early contraction onset of TrA, as observed with low back pain, will eliminate this fascial influence on the neutral zone and is likely to increase predisposition to injury. The MLF and PLF also provide a mechanism for continuous proprioceptive feedback from each lumbar segment, with disruption of innervation possibly contributing to reduced segmental control in patients with chronic low back pain.

In addition to its segmental roles, the PLF has more global effects during activities that recruit its attached or enclosed global muscles and these may contribute to compression across the SIJ and lumbar spine as well as increase the effectiveness of paraspinal muscle contraction (respectively). Such global roles are effected on an underlying requirement for restriction of segmental movement, influenced by local muscle activity and transverse fascial tension from TrA. Further work elaborating the effects of MLF and PLF on segmental movement and the consequences of fascial disruption may provide greater insight into their roles in segmental control.

KEYWORDS	
anterior layer of lumbar fascia	hydraulic amplifier effect
middle layer of lumbar fascia	lumbar segmental stability
posterior layer of lumbar fascia	load transfer across the midline
lumbar fasciae	sacroiliac stability
muscle attachments	proprioception
local muscles	planar stability
global muscles	coronal stability
biomechanical roles	sagittal stability
longitudinal tension generation	transverse stability
	disruption
	segmental stability
	magnitude of forces

References

Adams M A 1995 Mechanical testing of the spine: an appraisal of methodology, results, and conclusions. Spine 20(19): 2151–2156

Adams M A, Green T P 1993 Tensile properties of the annulus fibrosus. I: The contribution of fibre-matrix interactions to tensile stiffness and strength. European Spine Journal 2: 203–208

Aspden R M 1992 Review of the functional anatomy of the spinal ligaments and the lumbar erector spinae muscles. Clinical Anatomy 5: 372–387

Aspden R M, Bornstein N H, Hukins D W 1987 Collagen organisation in the interspinous ligament and its relationship to tissue function. Journal of Anatomy 155: 141–151

Barker P J, Briggs C A 1999 Attachments of the posterior layer of lumbar fascia. Spine 24(17): 1757–1764

Barker P J, Briggs C A, Bogeski G 2004a Tensile transmission across the lumbar fasciae in unembalmed cadavers: effects of tension to various muscular attachments. Spine 29(2): 129–138

Barker P J, Urquhart D M, Briggs C A, Story I, Fahrer M 2004b The middle layer of lumbar fascia and muscle attachments to lumbar transverse processes: implications for fracture and segmental control. (submitted)

Bednar D A, Orr F W, Simon G T 1995 Observations on the pathomorphology of the thoracolumbar fascia in chronic mechanical back pain: a microscopic study. Spine 20(10): 1161–1164

Bergmark A 1989 Stability of the lumbar spine: a study in mechanical engineering. Acta Orthopaedica Scandinavica 230 (Suppl.): 1–54

Bogduk N 1997 Clinical anatomy of the lumbar spine and sacrum. Churchill Livingstone, New York, pp 115–117

Bogduk N, Macintosh J E 1984 The applied anatomy of the thoracolumbar fascia. Spine 9(2): 164–170

Bogduk N, Johnson G, Spalding D 1998 The morphology and biomechanics of latissimus dorsi. Clinical Biomechanics (Bristol, Avon) 13(6): 377–385

Breathnach A S 1965 Frazer's Anatomy of the human skeleton. J. & A. Churchill, London, pp 35–37

Carman B J, Blanton P L, Biggs N L 1972 Electromyographic study of the anterolateral abdominal musculature utilizing indwelling electrodes. American Journal of Physical Medicine 51(3): 113–129

Carr D, Gilbertson L, Frymoyer J, Krag M, Pope M 1985 Lumbar paraspinal compartment syndrome: a case report with physiologic and anatomic studies. Spine 10(9): 816–820

Cholewicki J, McGill S M 1996 Mechanical stability of the in vivo lumbar spine: implications for injury and chronic low back pain. Clinical Biomechanics (Bristol, Avon) 11(1): 1–15

Cresswell A G, Grundstrom H, Thorstensson A 1992 Observations on intra-abdominal pressure and patterns of abdominal intra-muscular activity in man. Acta Physiologica Scandinavica 144(4): 409–418

Crock H V, Crock M C 1988 A technique for decompression of the lumbar spinal canal. Neuro-Orthopedics 5: 96–99

Davies-Colley J N C 1894 The muscles. J & A Churchill, New York, pp 433–434

Davis J R, Mirka G A 2000 Transverse-contour modeling of trunk muscle-distributed forces and spinal loads during lifting and twisting. Spine 25(2): 180–189

Dijkstra P F, Vleeming A, Stoeckart R 1989 Complex motion tomography of the sacroiliac joint: an anatomical and roentgenological study. ROFO Fortschr Geb Rontgenstr Nuklearmed 150(6): 635–642

Donisch E W, Basmajian J V 1972 Electromyography of deep back muscles in man. American Journal of Anatomy 133(1): 25–36

Fairbank J C, O'Brien J P 1980 The abdominal cavity and thoraco-lumbar fascia as stabilisers of the lumbar spine in patients with low back pain. In: Engineering aspects of the spine. Mechanical Engineering Publications for the Institution of Mechanical Engineers, London, pp 83–88

Farfan H F 1973 Mechanical disorders of the low back. Lea & Febiger, Philadelphia, pp 1–39, 171–197

Farfan H F 1975 Muscular mechanism of the lumbar spine and the position of power and efficiency. Orthopedic Clinics of North America 6(1): 135–144

Farfan H F 1995 Form and function of the musculoskeletal system as revealed by mathematical analysis of the lumbar spine: an essay. Spine 20(13): 1462–1474

Farfan H F, Cossette J W, Robertson G H, Wells R V, Kraus H 1970 The effects of torsion on the lumbar intervertebral joints: the role of torsion in the production of disc degeneration. Journal of Bone and Joint Surgery (American volume) 52(3): 468–497

Floyd W F, Silver P H S 1950 Electromyographic study of patterns of activity of the anterior abdominal wall muscles in man. Journal of Anatomy 84: 132–145

Floyd W F, Silver P H S 1955 The function of the erectores spinae muscles in certain movements and postures in man. Journal of Physiology 129: 184–203

Gallaudet B B 1931 A description of the planes of fascia of the human body. Columbia University Press, New York, pp 2–59

Gallios M, Japiot M 1925 Architecture interieure des vertebres (statique et physiologie de la colonne vertebrale). Revue de Chirurgie 63: 687–708

Gracovetsky S, Farfan H 1986 The optimum spine. Spine 11(6): 543–573

Gracovetsky S, Farfan H F, Lamy C 1977 A mathematical model of the lumbar spine using an optimized system to control muscles and ligaments. Orthopedic Clinics of North America 8(1): 135–153

Gracovetsky S, Farfan H F, Lamy C 1981 The mechanism of the lumbar spine. Spine 6(3): 249–262

Gracovetsky S, Farfan H, Helleur C 1985 The abdominal mechanism. Spine 10(4): 317–324

Hickey D S, Hukins D W 1980 Relation between the structure of the annulus fibrosus and the function and failure of the intervertebral disc. Spine 5(2): 106–116

Hides J A, Jull G A, Richardson C A 2001 Long-term effects of specific stabilizing exercises for first-episode low back pain. Spine 26(11): E243–248

Hodges P W, Richardson C A 1996 Inefficient muscular stabilization of the lumbar spine associated with low back pain: a motor control evaluation of transversus abdominis. Spine 21(22): 2640–2650

Hodges P W, Richardson C A 1997a Relationship between limb movement speed and associated contraction of the trunk muscles. Ergonomics 40(11): 1220–1230

Hodges P W, Richardson C A 1997b Feedforward contraction of transversus abdominis is not influenced by the direction of arm movement. Experimental Brain Research 114(2): 362–370

Hodges P W, Richardson C A 1997c Contraction of the abdominal muscles associated with movement of the lower limb. Physical Therapy 77(2): 132–142

Hodges P W, Richardson C A 1998 Delayed postural contraction of transversus abdominis in low back pain associated with movement of the lower limb. Journal of Spinal Disorders 11(1): 46–56

Hodges P W, Cresswell A, Thorstensson A 1999 Preparatory trunk motion accompanies rapid upper limb movement. Experimental Brain Research 124(1): 69–79

Hodges P W, Moseley G L, Gabrielsson A, Gandevia S C 2001 Experimentally induced low back pain causes changes in motor control of the trunk muscles. Fourth Interdisciplinary World Congress on Low Back and Pelvic Pain, Montreal, European Conference Organizers, pp 184–185

Howarth M B, Petrie J G 1964 Injuries of the spine. Williams & Wilkins, Baltimore, p 265

Hukins D W L 1984 Connective tissue matrix: topics in molecular and structural biology. Macmillan, London, pp 211–240

Hukins D W L 1985 Composition and properties of connective tissues. Trends in Biochemical Science 10: 260–264

Hukins D W L, Aspden R M, Hickey D S 1990a Thoracolumbar fascia can increase the efficiency of the erector spinae muscles. Clinical Biomechanics 5: 30–34

Hukins D W L, Kirby M C, Sikoryn T A, Aspden R M, Cox A J 1990b Comparison of structure, mechanical properties, and functions of lumbar spinal ligaments. Spine 15(8): 787–795

Hutchinson M R, Dall B E 1994 Midline fascial splitting approach to the iliac crest for bone graft: a new approach. Spine 19(1): 62–66

Jull G A, Richardson C A 2000 Motor control problems in patients with spinal pain: a new direction for therapeutic exercise. Journal of Manipulative and Physiological Therapeutics 23(2): 115–117

Kaigle A M, Holm S H, Hansson T H 1995 Experimental instability in the lumbar spine. Spine 20: 421–430

Kelsey J L, Githens P B, White A A 3rd et al 1984 An epidemiologic study of lifting and twisting on the job and risk for acute prolapsed lumbar intervertebral disc. Journal of Orthopedic Research 2(1): 61–66

McGill S M, Norman R W 1988 Potential of lumbodorsal fascia forces to generate back extension moments during squat lifts. Journal of Biomedical Engineering 10(4): 312–318

McGill S M, Norman R W 1993 Low back biomechanics in industry: the prevention of injury through safer lifting. In: Grabiner M D (ed) Current issues in biomechanics. Human Kinetics Publishers, Champaign, Illinois, pp 69–121

Macintosh J E, Valencia F V, Bogduk N, Munro R R 1986 The morphology of the human lumbar multifidus. Clinical Biomechanics 1(4): 196–204

Marras W S, Lavender S A, Leurgans S E et al 1993 The role of dynamic three-dimensional trunk motion in occupationally-related low back disorders: the effects of workplace factors, trunk position, and trunk motion characteristics on risk of injury. Spine 18(5): 617–628

Marras W S, Lavender S A, Leurgans S E et al 1995 Biomechanical risk factors for occupationally related low back disorders. Ergonomics 38(2): 377–410

Marshall R 2001 Living anatomy: structure as the mirror of function. Melbourne University Press, Melbourne, Australia, pp 280–283

Mens J M, Vleeming A, Stoeckart R, Stam H J, Snijders C J 1996 Understanding peripartum pelvic pain: implications of a patient survey. Spine 21(11): 1363–1369; discussion 1369–1370

Mens J M, Snijders C J, Stam H J 2000 Diagonal trunk muscle exercises in peripartum pelvic pain: a randomized clinical trial. Physical Therapy 80(12): 1164–1173

Minns R J, Soden P D, Jackson D S 1973 The role of the fibrous components and ground substance in the mechanical properties of biological tissues: a preliminary investigation. Journal of Biomechanics 6(2): 153–165

Mirka G, Kelaher D, Baker A, Harrison A, Davis J 1997 Selective activation of the external oblique musculature during axial torque production. Clinical Biomechanics (Bristol, Avon) 12(3): 172–180

Mooney V, Pozos R, Vleeming A, Gulick J, Swenski D 2001 Exercise treatment for sacroiliac pain. Orthopedics 24(1): 29–32

Moseley G L, Hodges P W, Gandevia S C 2002 Deep and superficial fibers of the lumbar multifidus muscle are differentially active during voluntary arm movements. Spine 27(2): E29–36

Mundt D J, Kelsey J L, Golden A L et al 1993 An epidemiologic study of non-occupational lifting as a risk factor for herniated lumbar intervertebral disc. Northeast Collaborative Group on Low Back Pain. Spine 18(5): 595–602

O'Sullivan P, Twomey L, Allison G, Sinclair J, Miller K 1997a Altered patterns of abdominal muscle activation in patients with chronic low back pain. Australian Journal of Physiotherapy 43(2): 91–98

O'Sullivan P B, Twomey L T, Allison G T 1997b Evaluation of specific stabilizing exercise in the treatment of chronic low back pain with radiologic diagnosis of spondylolysis or spondylolisthesis. Spine 22(24): 2959–2967

Panjabi M M 1992a The stabilizing system of the spine. I: Function, dysfunction, adaptation, and enhancement. Journal of Spinal Disorders 5(4): 383–389

Panjabi M M 1992b The stabilizing system of the spine. II: Neutral zone and instability hypothesis. Journal of Spinal Disorders 5(4): 390–396

Panjabi M, Abumi K, Duranceau J, Oxland T 1989 Spinal stability and intersegmental muscle forces: a biomechanical model. Spine 14(2): 194–200

Peck D, Nicholls P J, Beard C, Allen J R 1986 Are there compartment syndromes in some patients with idiopathic back pain? Spine 11(5): 468–475

Poirier P 1901 Myologie. In: Poirer P, Charpy A (eds) Traité d'anatomie humaine. Masson et Compagnie, Paris, vol 2, pt 1, p 497

Richardson C A, Jull G A 1995 Muscle control-pain control. What exercises would you prescribe? Manual Therapy 1(1): 2–10

Richardson C A, Jull G A, Hodges P W, Hides J A 1999 Therapeutic exercise for spinal segmental stabilization in low back pain. Harcourt Brace, London, pp 4–59

Richardson C A, Snijders C J, Hides J A, Damen L, Pas M S, Storm J 2002 The relation between the transversus abdominis muscles, sacroiliac joint mechanics, and low back pain. Spine 27(4): 399–405

Sharpey W, Thomson A, Cleland J (eds) 1867 Quain's Elements of anatomy. James Walton Publishing, London, pp 248–253

Styf J, Lysell E 1987 Chronic compartment syndrome in the erector spinae muscle. Spine 12(7): 680–682

Tesh K M 1986 The abdominal muscles and vertebral stability. PhD thesis, Bioengineering Unit, University of Strathclyde, pp 166–349

Tesh K M, Dunn J S, Evans J H 1987 The abdominal muscles and vertebral stability. Spine 12(5): 501–508

Testut L, Latarjet A 1948 Traite d'anatomie humaine. G. Doin & Compagnie, Paris, pp 944–952

Urquhart D M, Barker P J, Hodges P W, Story I, Briggs C A 2004 Regional morphology of tranversus abdominis, obliquus internus and obliquus externus abdominis. (submitted)

Vleeming A, Stoeckart R, Snijders C J 1989 The sacrotuberous ligament: a conceptual approach to its dynamic role in stabilizing the sacroiliac joint. Clinical Biomechanics 4(4): 201–203

Vleeming A, Buyruk H M, Stoeckart R, Karamursel S, Snijders C J 1992 An integrated therapy for peripartum pelvic instability: a study of the biomechanical effects of pelvic belts. American Journal of Obstetrics and Gynecology 166(4): 1243–1247

Vleeming A, Pool-Goudzwaard A L, Stoeckart R, van Wingerden J P, Snijders C J 1995 The posterior layer of the thoracolumbar fascia: its function in load transfer from spine to legs. Spine 20(7): 753–758

Vleeming A, Pool-Goudzwaard A L, Hammudoghlu D, Stoeckart R, Snijders C J, Mens J M 1996 The function of the long dorsal sacroiliac ligament: its implication for understanding low back pain. Spine 21(5): 556–562

Williams P W, Bannister L H, Berry M M et al (eds) 1995 Gray's Anatomy. Churchill Livingstone, New York, pp 809–829

Wingerden J P V, Vleeming A, Buyruk H M, Raissadat K 2001 Muscular contribution to force closure: sacroiliac joint stabilisation in vivo. Fourth Interdisciplinary World Congress on Low Back and Pelvic Pain, Montreal, European Conference Organizers, pp 153–159

Yahia L, Rhalmi S, Newman N, Isler M 1992 Sensory innervation of human thoracolumbar fascia: an immunohistochemical study. Acta Orthopaedica Scandinavica 63(2): 195–197

Yahia L H, Pigeon P, DesRosiers E A 1993 Viscoelastic properties of the human lumbodorsal fascia. Journal of Biomedical Engineering 15(5): 425–429

Chapter 12

Neurophysiology of pain and pain modulation

A. Wright, M. Zusman

INTRODUCTION

In clinical practice manual therapists often see the impact of pain on an individual. Pain can change rapidly from no pain, or minimal levels of pain, to a situation where the pain experience is so severe and pervasive that it drives all of the person's behaviour. Whiplash injury, acute back injury, major fracture or other acute trauma can all provide an indication of the impact of pain on previously pain-free individuals. The propensity for pain and disability to persist in the absence of obvious ongoing primary peripheral pathology is both baffling and challenging. This chapter includes evidence for peripheral and central nervous system mechanisms that might contribute to the enhancement and maintenance of clinically observed symptoms and signs. It also describes forebrain mechanisms that could allow emotions and cognitions to effectively sensitize spinal cord pain pathway neurons, possibly providing a mechanism for psychosocial factors to enhance pain perception. Potential interactions between the nociceptive and motor systems are considered. The level of change that occurs in the behaviour of individuals who experience pain implies a very marked enhancement of nociceptive system function and, consequent upon this, enormous neuroplasticity and change in many aspects of central nervous system function. Mechanisms contributing to that neuroplasticity will be described.

HYPERALGESIA AND ALLODYNIA

A large body of research has developed describing the ways in which nociceptive system function can be enhanced and pointing to the effects of this on somatomotor function. The nociceptive system is normally a quiescent system requiring strong, intense, potentially damaging stimulation before it becomes activated. Yet once an individual is experiencing pain, relatively innocuous stimuli activate the system and trigger pain perception. This altered perceptual state is encompassed by the phenomena of hyperalgesia, an exaggerated or increased response to a noxious stimulus, and allodynia, the production of pain by a stimulus that would not normally be painful (Merskey & Bogduk 1994).

It is now clear that after injury there may be distinct differences between the mechanisms leading to hyperalgesia in injured and uninjured tissue. It is also apparent that the time course and extent of hyperalgesia is different for different forms of injury.

It is widely recognized that prolonged C fibre input evokes two distinct forms of cutaneous hyperalgesia; these have been termed primary and secondary hyperalgesia (Hardy et al 1950). It is suggested that primary hyperalgesia is predominantly due to peripheral sensitization of nociceptors whereas secondary hyperalgesia is dependent on the process of central sensitization in cells processing nociceptive information at the spinal cord level (Torebjork et al 1992).

PERIPHERAL REGULATORY MECHANISMS

There is now a large body of research investigating modulatory mechanisms in both the periphery and the central nervous system. It has become apparent that these processes are of great importance in altering nociceptive system function following injury.

Nociceptor activation and sensitization

Many early studies pointed to sensitization of peripheral nociceptors as a mechanism underlying the increased sensitivity to subsequent stimulation that takes place following tissue injury. It is apparent that many peripheral nociceptors are polymodal, in the sense that they respond to chemical as well as mechanical and thermal nociceptive stimulation (Kumazawa 1996). It is also apparent that chemical mediators released into the tissues because of tissue injury promote sensitization of peripheral nociceptors. Key mediators which have been identified include bradykinin, serotonin, histamine, potassium ions, adenosine triphosphate, protons, prostaglandins, nitric oxide, leukotrienes, cytokines and growth factors (Dray 1995). The effects of these mediators involve binding to specific receptors, activation of ion channels for depolarization, activation of intracellular second messenger systems, release of a range of neuropeptides to promote neurogenic inflammation and alteration of neuronal properties by modifying gene transcription (Bevan 1996, Dray 1995). Release of a range of inflammatory mediators triggers phosphorylation and activation of a number of receptors and second messenger systems (Mizamura & Kumazawa 1996).

The actions of chemical mediators normally fall into one of two categories: either direct activation of nociceptive afferents or sensitization so that subsequent stimulation leads to an enhanced response. While polymodal receptors respond to a range of stimuli, it is apparent that different molecular receptors and second messenger systems are involved in excitation and sensitization for different stimulation modalities (Mizamura & Kumazawa 1996). It is therefore important to note that nociceptors may become differentially sensitized to thermal, mechanical and chemical stimuli. An individual nociceptor can potentially exhibit sensitization to thermal stimuli, for example, while retaining normal sensitivity to mechanical or chemical stimuli.

'Inflammatory soup'

One of the most fundamental influences on nociceptor sensitivity is the pH of the surrounding tissue. High local proton concentrations are known to occur in many inflammatory states and the consequent reduction in pH can contribute to sensitization and activation of polymodal nociceptors (Handwerker & Reeh 1991, 1992, Reeh & Steen 1996). Altered pH of the local chemical environment of peripheral nociceptors is a particularly important factor in inducing mechanical sensitization and ischaemic pain (Dray 1995, Steen et al 1992). Combinations of inflammatory mediators and combination of chemical mediators with altered tissue pH appear to be more effective in inducing sensitization than individual chemical mediators alone (Handwerker & Reeh 1991). Thus in the natural situation it appears to be a blend of chemical mediators, termed 'inflammatory soup' by Handwerker & Reeh, that produces sensitization of peripheral nociceptors (Handwerker & Reeh 1991).

Multiple forms of peripheral sensitization

Endogenous chemicals act on a variety of receptors, activate three major intracellular second messenger systems and influence different ion channels (Dray 1995, Mizamura & Kumazawa 1996), resulting in distinctions between thermal, mechanical and chemical sensitization in specific populations of nociceptors (Mizamura & Kumazawa 1996). For example, prostaglandins may induce sensitization to chemical mediators at much lower concentrations than those required to induce sensitization to heat stimuli (Mizamura & Kumazawa 1996). The vanilloid receptor VR1 has been identified as a specific molecular mechanism for thermal hyperalgesia, as well as sensitization following capsaicin administration (Cesare et al 1999). The receptor will normally respond to temperatures in excess of 45°C. However, under low pH conditions there is a significant reduction in the activation threshold of the receptor such that VR1 may be activated at normal tissue temperatures (Harding 1999, Thacker 2002). This could potentially contribute to ongoing pain.

As noted above, nociceptor activation and sensitization can be produced through a number of different mechanisms. It can occur as a result of a direct influence of chemical mediators on membrane ion channels. It can also occur as a result of the action of chemical mediators on G-proteins and second messenger systems.

Membrane ion channels

One example is the fact that increased proton concentration results in increased membrane permeability to cations and sustained changes in neuronal activation. The mechanism of action of protons appears to be very similar to that of exogenously applied capsaicin (Dray 1995). Proton binding leads to phosphorylation of sodium channels resulting in a more sustained open state of the receptor and greater sodium influx to the cell (Kingsley 2000). Adenosine triphosphate, bradykinin, serotonin and prostaglandins may act on receptors that produce changes in potassium ion permeability (Dray 1995). The overall consequence is a significantly increased number of action potentials generated by peripheral nociceptors.

G-protein coupled intracellular cascades

One of the most effective mechanisms for sensitizing nociceptors is activation of G-protein coupled second messenger systems. These intracellular cascades result in very significant amplification of the neuronal signal. Binding of a chemical mediator to a G-protein receptor results in activation of that receptor and guanosine triphosphate (GTP) binding. The activated G-protein is released into the cytosol and may then bind to an appropriate enzyme such as adenylate cyclase causing it to catalyse a second messenger protein. In this case the second messenger will be cyclic adenosine monophosphate (cAMP), which in turn will activate protein kinase A (PKA). PKA is then responsible for phosphorylation of membrane ion channels and increased ion flux. Because binding to one G-protein receptor can lead to activation of not one but many ion channels, this process has the ability to greatly amplify the initial signal.

It is also apparent that kinins such as bradykinin may act on appropriate receptors causing phospholipase C activation among other effects. This leads to the release of intracellular calcium and diacylglycerol (DAG), which in turn activates protein kinase C (PKC). These pathways lead to activation of ion channels to increase membrane permeability, particularly for sodium and calcium ions (Dray 1995). Increased intracellular calcium ion concentration also leads to the release of neuropeptides such as substance P and stimulation of arachidonic acid production (Dray 1995).

Inhibition of hyperpolarization

Another mechanism by which peripheral sensitization can occur is inhibition of the hyperpolarization that occurs after impulse generation. This slow after-hyperpolarization limits the number of action potentials that can be generated following stimulation. Prostaglandins and bradykinin act to inhibit this phenomenon, allowing the neuron to fire repetitively (Dray 1995). This may also be one of the mechanisms activated by serotonin (Dray 1996).

Indirect mechanisms

Sensitization following the release of cytokines and leukotrienes appears to occur via indirect mechanisms whereby these agents stimulate other cells to release sensitizing agents. For example, leukotriene B4 stimulates the release of 8R,15SdiHETE from leucocytes, and this then acts to sensitize polymodal nociceptors (Levine et al 1993). Some of these agents may also act to induce receptors for other inflammatory mediators (Rang & Urban 1995).

In addition, Ca^{++} and calmodulin can activate nitric oxide synthase to trigger the production of nitric oxide. Nitric oxide functions as a messenger between neurons and surrounding tissues. As it diffuses widely through the tissues it can induce relaxation of vascular smooth muscle and it may contribute to the spread of sensitization in the peripheral tissues (Anbar and Gratt 1997).

Trophic factors

There is increasing evidence for the role of nerve growth factor (NGF) as a mediator of hyperalgesia (Anand 1995). Its actions include triggering mast cell degranulation, stimulating the release of neuropeptides and regulating other proteins such as proton activated ion channels (Anand 1995, Dray 1995, 1996, Shu & Mendell 1999). The induced hyperalgesia may be reduced by the administration of anti-nerve growth factor antibodies (Woolf et al 1994). It has been suggested that NGF may be particularly important for thermal sensitization and that it may condition the response of the VR1 receptor to capsaicin or thermal stimulation (Shu & Mendell 1999). Mechanical hyperalgesia appears to be induced over a much longer time period (Shu & Mendell 1999). Blockade of nerve growth factor function by the administration of the nerve growth factor specific tyrosine kinase receptor A coupled to human immunoglobulin-γ (trkA-IgG) prevents the development of thermal and mechanical hyperalgesia following joint inflammation (McMahon et al 1995). The trkA-IgG fusion molecule has the effect of binding nerve growth factor and reducing the amount of free NGF present in the tissues.

Other neurotrophins include brain-derived neurotrophic factor (BDNF) and glial cell line-derived neurotrophic factor (GDNF). Although expressed by peripheral afferents their primary effect appears to be related to modulation of central nervous system neurons. Activity induced phosphorylation of cAMP leads to activation of a gene transcription factor known as cyclic adenosine monophosphate response element binding protein (Woolf & Costigan 1999). This mediates transcription of BDNF within the dorsal root ganglion, which is then axoplasmically transported to presynaptic terminals in the dorsal horn. Subsequent peripheral stimulation will result in significantly increased release contributing to central sensitization.

The processes of peripheral sensitization are clearly one way in which nociceptive system activity can be increased in response to tissue injury. It is apparent that the sensitization process is relatively complex and that different forms of sensitization may develop depending on the nature of the injury or disease. Spontaneous discharge, reduced activation thresholds, inhibition of slow after-hyperpolarization and increased discharge rates in response to suprathreshold stimulation contribute to increasing the nociceptive afferent input to the central nervous system. These mechanisms are of considerable importance in the immediate period after tissue injury. Where pain persists beyond the time required for tissue healing it is likely that they will make a lesser contribution to ongoing pain and hyperalgesia.

Silent nociceptors

It is now well established that in some tissues there is a significant population of nociceptors that remain essentially inactive under normal conditions. These sleeping or silent nociceptors are activated because of tissue injury with consequent release of chemical mediators and increased tissue hypoxia (Schmidt 1996). Schmidt estimates that they may represent approximately one third of the total nociceptor population in joints (Schmidt 1996). They appear to be present in skin, joints and visceral tissue. At least 50% of visceral afferents may fall into this category (Mayer & Gebhart 1994). Once activated, these silent nociceptors exhibit marked sensitization with increased spontaneous discharge rates, reduced thresholds for evoked discharge and increased discharge rates in response to stimulation.

Phenotype change

A further mechanism contributing to enhanced activity of the nociceptive system is phenotype transformation (Woolf & Costigan 1999). It was proposed that in the situation where inflammation has been present for some time, transcriptional changes in gene expression might result in phenotypic changes in some myelinated Aβ afferents such that these fibres acquire the neurochemical properties of unmyelinated C fibres. Normally only C fibre (and a few Aδ) nociceptors contain the peptides necessary for clinically relevant central sensitization (e.g. substance P and calcitonin gene related peptide, CGRP) (Ma & Woolf 1995, 1996). However, it appears that the combination of inflammation, mechanical stimulation and release of growth factor molecules such as NGF bring about a genetically mediated phenotypic 'switch' (Woolf & Costigan 1999). Under these circumstances, myelinated afferents begin to express and release neuropeptides that are important for inducing long-term changes in neuronal sensitivity (Neumann et al 1996). Importantly, this means that these fibres can contribute to nociception by inducing sensitization in central nervous system neurons (Woolf & Costigan

1999). They may also contribute to the release of peptides and other chemical mediators responsible for peripheral sensitization and neurogenic inflammation. This conversion of myelinated Aβ afferents with low activation thresholds appears to be an additional mechanism for enhancing peripheral nociceptive input.

Activation of nociceptors, sensitization of currently responsive nociceptors, recruitment of mechanically insensitive or silent nociceptors and phenotype conversion of non-nociceptive afferents represent major mechanisms whereby tissue injury and inflammation can trigger both temporal and spatial summation of nociceptive afferent inputs to the central nervous system. Acting in concert, these mechanisms can contribute to substantial changes in peripheral nociceptive system function. Ultimately increased impulse activity in nociceptive neurons may be interpreted as pain at higher levels within the central nervous system. It is apparent, however, that there is not a constant link between the degree of tissue damage and the level of pain experienced. Modulatory influences will be discussed later in this chapter.

SPINAL CORD REGULATORY MECHANISMS

The existence of both wide dynamic range and nociceptive-specific neurons within the dorsal horn of the spinal cord is now widely recognized. Both cell types contribute to changes in nociceptive system function following injury (Fig. 12.1).

Wide dynamic range cells

Wide dynamic range cells are particularly prevalent in the deeper laminae of the dorsal horn. They receive input from both nociceptive and non-nociceptive afferent neurons and exhibit a graded response pattern related to the intensity of the afferent stimulus. If these neurons become sensitized and hyper-responsive they may discharge at a high rate following previously non-noxious stimulation (such as mild thermal or tactile stimulation) (Siddall & Cousins 1998). If the activity of the wide dynamic range neuron exceeds a threshold then the previously non-noxious stimulus will be perceived as painful. This phenomenon may, in part, provide the neurophysiological basis for the phenomenon of secondary hyperalgesia in which pain is perceived following stimulation of normal uninjured tissue.

Nociceptive-specific cells

Nociceptive-specific cells are located predominantly in the superficial laminae of the dorsal horn, where they receive inputs from unmyelinated C fibre afferents. Under normal conditions, their response characteristics include a lack of impulse generation in response to non-noxious stimulation and a relatively sluggish response to intense noxious stimulation of their peripheral receptive fields. However, fol-

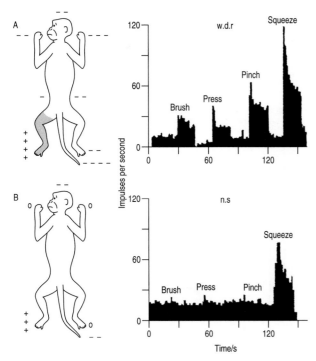

Figure 12.1 Response profiles of A: wide-dynamic range and B: nociceptive-specific neurons in the spinothalamic tract. The receptive fields of the cells are indicated on the figures to the left. Excitatory receptive fields are indicated by + signs and inhibitory receptive fields are indicated by − signs. Reproduced from Willis, 1985.

lowing stimulation of peripheral nociceptive afferents and the development of central sensitization, the response characteristics of nociceptive-specific neurons change (Cook et al 1987). Subliminal inputs from myelinated afferent neurons are enhanced and the cells begin to exhibit response characteristics that are similar to those of wide dynamic range neurons. Despite the fact that these cells can now be activated by non-noxious afferent inputs, it is likely that impulse activity generated by these neurons will contribute to pain perception at higher levels in the central nervous system. This may constitute another mechanism whereby normally non-nociceptive inputs from injured or uninjured tissues can contribute to pain perception.

The processes of central sensitization influence both wide dynamic range and nociceptive-specific cells in the dorsal horn of the spinal cord. Following tissue injury, the response characteristics of these cells change such that normally non-nociceptive afferent inputs via myelinated afferents can generate impulse activity that is likely to trigger pain perception.

Central sensitization

There is now considerable evidence that, as well as producing changes at their peripheral terminals, more than transient stimulation of unmyelinated C fibre (group IV) and

thinly myelinated Aδ (group III) primary afferents results in lasting increases in the excitability and responsiveness of both wide dynamic range and nociceptive-specific neurons in spinal cord pain pathways (Woolf & Salter 2000). The process of central sensitization (Woolf 1994) is an important aspect of neuroplasticity that contributes to enhanced activation of the nociceptive system in response to injury. This process may provide a link between the presence of pain and sensorimotor dysfunction in patients experiencing pain. Central sensitization describes the changes occurring at a cellular level to support the process of neuronal plasticity that occurs in nociceptive system neurons in spinal cord and supraspinal centres, because of activation of the nociceptive system (Woolf 1994).

The key to understanding the relevance of central sensitization to the production and interpretation of clinically observed symptoms and signs is to appreciate that spinal cord pain pathway neurons make more than routine hardwired connections with their prescribed receptive fields. As noted above, they also have a vast number of redundant, 'subliminal' connections with surrounding areas and structures. Under normal circumstances, the redundant inputs are too weak to be effective. Hence, normally the appropriate somatotopic map and sensory specificity are maintained. However, should the central neurons' usually high thresholds for excitation be significantly lowered for any reason, the potential exists for new connections to emerge. Under these circumstances, central pain pathway neurons display increased discharges to their normally effective inputs and discharges to previously ineffective inputs. As a consequence they respond to near and distant inputs that were formerly subliminal, normally inappropriate (e.g. along Aβ afferents) and non-somatotopic (Woolf & Doubell 1994). This contributes to some of the hallmarks of central sensitization in terms of expanded receptive fields and an exaggerated response to subsequent inputs.

This is the situation that prevails to varying degrees soon after dorsal horn pain pathway neurons receive a barrage of input along unmyelinated and thinly myelinated peripheral nociceptive afferents (Woolf & Doubell 1994). As a result, in addition to the production of excessive pain from local pathological tissue (peripheral sensitization), clinical manifestations of central sensitization include widespread spontaneously arising or non-noxiously provoked pain in distant normal tissue, mechanical allodynia, referred pain and referred tenderness. This process is initiated by activity in peripheral nociceptors, particularly those associated with unmyelinated afferent neurons but it appears that the process can also be sustained in the absence of peripheral nociceptor input (Coderre & Melzack 1987, Woolf 1983).

NMDA receptor activation

Activity in peripheral nociceptors releases the excitatory amino acid neurotransmitter glutamate. Glutamate then binds to two major ion channel receptor populations, α-amino-3-hydroxyl-5-methyl-isoxazoleproprionic acid (AMPA) and N-methyl-D-aspartate (NMDA). These receptors influence resting membrane potential and depolarization of dorsal horn nociceptive neurons. The NMDA receptor subtype in particular has been strongly implicated in the generation of central sensitization (Dickenson 1995, Mao et al 1995, Woolf 1994). Release of excitatory amino acids such as glutamate and concomitant release of excitatory neuropeptides such as substance P and neurokinin A from the presynaptic terminals of nociceptive afferents initiates a cascade of changes in postsynaptic spinal cord neurons (Duggan et al 1988, 1990; Wilcox 1991). These include activation of G-protein linked metabotrophic receptors such as the metabotrophic glutamate receptor (mGluR) and the neurokinin 1 receptor (NK1). G-protein mediated activation of phospholipase C leads to the release of Ca++ from intracellular compartments. G-protein binding also leads to activation of protein kinase C, which in turn modulates ion channel activity (Mao et al 1995, Woolf 1994). These changes up-regulate NMDA receptors and enhance the neuron's responsiveness to subsequent excitatory amino acid release (Woolf 1994). One outcome of this alteration in NMDA receptor function is an increased Ca++ influx into the cell. Increased intracellular Ca++ concentration reduces transmembrane potential and activates a number of enzymes such as PKA, tyrosine kinases, PKC and calcium calmodulin kinase. These kinases phosphorylate a range of receptors, ion channels and gene transcription factors, all of which contribute to relatively long lasting changes in the excitability of the dorsal horn neurons. These processes are summarized in Figure 12.2.

Nitric oxide production

One other effect of increased intracellular Ca++ concentration is to trigger the production of nitric oxide, which has important second messenger functions within the cell and is thought to be capable of diffusing out of the cell to bring about increased activation of and release of neurotransmitter from the primary afferent neuron (Meller & Gebhart 1993). Synthesis of nitric oxide is catalysed by the enzyme nitric oxide synthase, which is activated by binding of Ca++/calmodulin complexes (Gordh et al 1995). Nitric oxide in turn is thought to activate guanylate cyclase, triggering an intracellular cascade that eventually leads to release of stored intracellular Ca++. The capacity of nitric oxide to diffuse and influence adjacent neurons may be an important factor in the spread of sensitization that appears to occur in spinal cord neurons.

Long-term potentiation

Long-term potentiation (LTP) may be described as the increase in efficacy that occurs at a synapse following suitable prior activity. In other words, once primed by a barrage of nociceptive impulses, subsequent stimuli, including

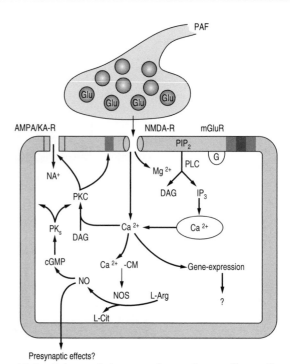

Figure 12.2 Release of glutamate from primary afferent fibres triggers many changes within spinal cord neurons. Activation of the NMDA receptor induces an influx of Ca++ through Ca++ channels, while activation of metabotrophic glutamate receptors mobilizes Ca++ from intracellular compartments. Reproduced from Mao et al 1995.
Key: PAF = primary afferent fibre; Glu = glutamate; AMPA/KA-R = RS-α-amino-3-hydroxy-5-methylisoxazole-4-propionic acid/kainic acid receptor; NMDA-R = N-methyl-D-aspartate receptor; mGluR = metabotrophic glutamate receptor; G = guanosine triphosphate (GTP) binding protein; PLC = phospholipase C; Ca++-CM = calcium-calmodulin complex; NOS = nitric oxide synthase; L-Arg = L-arginine; L-Cit = L-citrulline; cGMP = cyclic guanosine monophosphate; PK$_s$ = protein kinases.

those that are normally ineffective, elicit a much greater response from the postsynaptic neuron. At the first synapse in the dorsal horn this increase in excitability is expressed as excitatory postsynaptic action potentials that then travel to the brain.

LTP has been strongly linked with learning and memory at recognized centres in the brain, such as the hippocampus and cerebellum (Bear et al 2001). The physiological and structural changes necessary for learning and memory consolidation have profound implications for the production and maintenance of clinical pain. Evidence linking LTP and central sensitization is quite compelling. For instance, research to date has shown that the type and parameters of nociceptive afferent stimuli sufficient to induce LTP are similar to those that cause central sensitization and hyperalgesia. Moreover, demonstrable dorsal horn LTP and tissue insult-induced hyperalgesia possess the same signal transduction pathways, time course and pharmacological profile (Sandkühler 2000). This suggests that LTP at Aδ and C fibre synapses provides an attractive cellular model for injury-induced hyperalgesia (Sandkühler 2000).

The molecular changes currently thought to be responsible for expression of LTP are strongly linked to alterations in function of the AMPA receptor. However, the NMDA receptor, Ca++ influx and the activation of protein kinases are all involved since interruption of any one or all of these blocks the development of LTP. Nevertheless, at least two distinct changes that this cascade is capable of evoking in the AMPA receptor are of major importance. One is increased ionic conductance following AMPA receptor phosphorylation, the other is the insertion of entirely new AMPA receptors into the postsynaptic membrane. Notably, both of these events are mediated by protein kinases (PKC and calmodulin kinase, CaMK).

In the case of the former, synaptic efficacy is significantly increased by enhanced single channel conductance due to increased open channel time. This is the result of protein kinase mediated phosphorylation (Lin et al 2002). Acquisition by a synapse of additional receptor complexes, and with this greater transmitter binding to a given stimulus, involves a process known as exocytosis (Carroll et al 2001). Additional receptors in the postsynaptic membrane is one of several possible changes in nervous system structure, and therefore function, that is clearly important for learning and certain types of memory. Another is the discovery that following LTP postsynaptic structures form new synaptic connections with axons that contact them. A single axon can create multiple synapses on the same postsynaptic neuron. It is likely that within minutes, or at the most hours, following tissue insult, activity initiated biochemical events begin to bring about a change in nervous system anatomy as well as physiology. These mechanisms are likely to be initially responsible for clinically observed signs and symptoms but if maintained, they may also lay the foundation of long-term pain and disability (Carr & Goudas 1999).

In their final expression, the processes of learning and memory involve long-lasting protein phosphorylation due to the action of persistently active kinases. Such long-term physiological changes have the potential to become structurally permanent as a result of transcription mediated protein synthesis. In this way, learning is facilitated and memory consolidated by the construction of additional entirely new synapses (Bear et al 2001). In the present context this would constitute a specific basis for long-term pain. Experiments using fear-learning paradigms have demonstrated both AMPA receptor exocytosis and the synthesis of new protein contributing to the enhancement of LTP and long-term memory (Lin et al 2002, McKernan & Shinnick-Gallagher 1997, Scharf et al 2002). Experience with high 'emotional content' stimuli such as pain could consolidate 'laying down' of new synapses establishing a structural (as well as a physiological) basis for chronic pain.

Differential sensitization

There has been a very strong emphasis on the role of the NMDA receptor in the central sensitization process. However, as noted above, it has now become apparent that activation of the NMDA receptor may not be critical to the development of all forms of central sensitization; the AMPA receptor also appears to be of critical importance. It has been suggested that the NMDA receptor is particularly important in relation to thermal sensitization and that it plays a lesser role in mechanical sensitization (Meller et al 1996). Co-activation of spinal AMPA and mGluR receptors induces an acute mechanical sensitization (Meller et al 1996). This is mediated through activation of phospholipase A_2 leading to the production of arachidonic acid. It appears to be the products of the cyclooxygenase pathway for metabolism of arachidonic acid that are of most importance in generating mechanical sensitization (Meller et al 1996). Activation of NMDA receptors, phospholipase C, PKC and the production of nitric oxide appear to be less important factors in the development of mechanical sensitization and may be linked more to the development of thermal sensitization (Meller et al 1996).

Trophic factors

As noted previously, BDNF is released centrally from a subpopulation of peripheral nociceptive neurons and has an important role in enhancing phosphorylation of NMDA receptors to maintain central sensitization (Boucher et al 2000). It appears to be particularly important in facilitating the development of thermal hyperalgesia, since intrathecal administration of the fusion molecule, tyrosine kinase receptor B – human immunoglobulin-γ (trkB-IgG), significantly reduces thermal hyperalgesia induced by carageenan inflammation (Boucher et al 2000, Thompson et al 1999). It also appears likely that GDNF may play a role in the development of sensitization (Boucher et al 2000).

Neuroanatomical reorganization

Neuroanatomical reorganization of the laminar structure of the spinal cord is another important process that may contribute to alterations in nociceptive system function. This mechanism appears to be particularly important when nerve injury has occurred. Under these circumstances, myelinated axons that normally terminate in laminae III and IV of the dorsal horn have been shown to sprout into lamina II of the dorsal horn, potentially developing synaptic connections with intrinsic neurons involved in the transmission of nociceptive afferent inputs (Woolf et al 1992). It has been postulated that this may constitute a mechanism whereby normally innocuous afferent input could contribute to nociception (Woolf & Mannion 1999) and provide a neuroanatomical basis for the development of allodynia. Furthermore, it has been shown experimentally that in some cases dorsal horn inhibitory interneurons are lost ('dark cells'). It appears that the destruction of these neurons is a result of their susceptibility to a form of excitotoxicity (Sugimoto et al 1990, Woolf & Salter 2000). Were this additional alterations in anatomy to also occur, the result is likely to be intense intractable pain and varying degrees of chronic functional disability. It should be emphasized that such changes in neuroanatomy are likely to be mainly confined to situations in which the nervous system has been damaged and neuropathic pain has developed.

Enhanced activation of central nervous system neurons is dependent on a range of mechanisms. It is apparent that central sensitization and long-term potentiation in spinal cord neurons are relatively complex processes and that in common with peripheral processes, the nature of molecular changes underlying central sensitization may vary depending on the nature of the inducing stimulus. It is also apparent that other factors such as neuroanatomical reorganization may contribute to the changes that occur in central nervous system function post injury.

CENTRAL INTEGRATION OF NOCICEPTIVE INPUT

Pain and nociceptive inputs can exert a strong influence on motor function and emotional state. As well as interactions at spinal cord level, integration of nociception and other central nervous system functions must occur at higher centres. It is also clear that pain perception can be strongly modulated by descending systems originating in various parts of the brain (Cervero & Laird 1996, Stamford 1995).

This modulation can take the form of enhanced pain perception, as well as the reduced pain perception associated with analgesic effects (Cervero & Laird 1996). It is now becoming apparent that as well as being influenced by pain, motor activity and emotional state can in turn influence pain perception (Dubner & Ren 1999). Consequently, the central nervous system is better viewed as an integrated cyclical system rather than the simple cause and effect system enshrined in the distinction between afferent and efferent aspects of function.

Functional brain imaging

Functional brain imaging studies are increasingly providing a means of bridging the gap between psychological studies and basic neurophysiological studies, and allowing us to gain some basic understanding of the way in which nociception is intimately integrated with many other aspects of central nervous system function. This work is providing insights into the complex ways in which cognitive and emotional states can modulate pain perception. This is of considerable importance in understanding the influence of psychosocial factors on pain perception and pain report in the clinical situation.

Studies investigating both experimentally induced pain and clinical pain states provide substantial evidence for the involvement of a number of key brain sites in pain perception. Some notable regions include: the anterior cingulate cortex (ACC), anterior insular cortex (IC), primary somatosensory cortex (S1), secondary somatosensory cortex (S2), a number of regions in the thalamus and cerebellum, and interestingly, areas such as the premotor cortex that are normally linked to motor function (Casey 1999).

From this research there is abundant evidence of the distributed nature of the nociceptive system and the potential for close association between areas of the nervous system responding to pain and areas controlling motor function, and emotional state (Porro & Cavazzuti 1996). For example, it is clear that both the basal ganglia and the periaqueductal gray (PAG) region receive nociceptive inputs as well as coordinating important aspects of movement and motor control (Chudler & Dong 1995, Lovick 1991).

Attentional processes

Brain stem input from the ACC is particularly significant since the ACC has been invested with a pivotal role in integrating sensory and affective with attentional, cognitive and emotional aspects of pain (Casey 1999, Davis et al 2000, Hutchison et al 1999, Kwan et al 2000, Price 2000, Rainville et al 1997). This central role for the ACC has been demonstrated by using positron emission tomography (PET) as well as other imaging techniques (Fig. 12.3). PET is able to image changes in cerebral regional blood flow (rCBF) in response to a variety of noxious peripheral stimuli in awake human subjects (Casey 1999). Increases in rCBF responses during noxious stimulation are considered to reflect physiological changes in neuronal activity related to both nociceptive processing and the perception of pain. It is significant that, when methodological and analytical variations are taken into account, the same anatomical regions have been repeatedly highlighted across studies (Bushnell et al 1999, 2002, Casey 1999). Furthermore, the degree of rCBF response was found to correlate with reports of pain intensity in humans (Casey 1999, Hofbauer et al 2001).

In addition to the ACC and IC, the most consistently activated supraspinal regions, using a variety of noxious stimuli, were motor centres, namely the premotor cortex and cerebellar vermis (Casey 1999). Evidence suggests that complimentary activation of cortical and subcortical motor areas is related to instructions for movements or postures intended to escape painful stimulation (Hsieh et al 1994, Price 2000). Converging on the ACC is information from higher centres (S1, S2 via corticolimbic posterior parietal and insular cortices) that is considered to provide the organism with 'an overall sense of intrusion and threat to physical body and self' (Price 2000). This information is integrated with that from (pre)frontal cortical areas concerned with future implications of the pain and with establishing response priorities. These include decisions and strategies to escape pain and any pain-evoking situations.

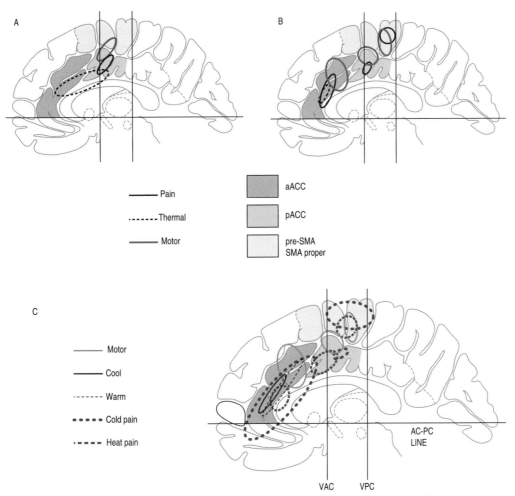

Figure 12.3 Spatial distribution of 95% confidence ellipses generated using the pooled activations of all subjects produced by: (A) the pain, thermal and motor tasks within the entire slice; (B) the pain, thermal and motor tasks within the aSCC, pACC and areas of the SMA; and (C) warm, cool, cold pain, heat pain and motor tasks situated within the aACC, pACC and SMA. Reproduced from Kwan et al 2000. Key: (aACC = anterior anterior cingulate cortex; pACC = posterior anterior cingulate cortex; SMA = supplementary motor area; VAC = vertical through anterior commissure; VPC = vertical through posterior commissure.

Movement and postural planning concerned with the avoidance of pain obviously require intimate anatomical cooperation with pre and supplementary motor centres as well as close connections with centres of emotion and motivation (Price 2000).

When imaging pain patients, it is frequently found that the same sensory and motor cortical and limbic centres could be activated by normally non-painful, as well as nociceptive stimuli (Bushnell et el 2002). This helps confirm the presence of supraspinal neuron sensitization. Various types of chronic pain are also associated with extensive reorganization of sites encoding peripheral stimuli in the somatosensory cortex. In patients with back pain, for example, in addition to a substantial increase in cortical activity to different intensities of peripheral cutaneous stimuli, there is a significant enlargement of the normal cortical representation of the back. The expansion occurs medially into the neighbouring area normally representative of the leg and foot (Flor et al 1997). The additional neuronal activity

associated with an enlarged cortical representation may serve to enhance and maintain the pain experience (Flor et al 1997). Such changes are an important example of the degree of neuroplasticity that is likely to occur in the presence of chronic pain.

Emotion

There is considerable overlap between the neuroanatomical and neurotransmitter systems modulating pain perception and those controlling emotional state (Chapman 1996). Bandler & Shipley (1994) describe a model of columnar organization that projects from regions of the frontal cortex, the hypothalamus, thalamus and amygdala to the PAG region of the mid-brain. These neuroanatomical connections may provide the basis for the interaction between cognitive and emotional states and pain perception, autonomic function and motor activity (Bandler & Shipley 1994).

Forebrain mediated modulatory systems

It is important to realise that central sensitization and long-term potentiation in spinal cord neurons can also be brought about by activity of pain modulatory systems that descend to the dorsal horn of the spinal cord from the brain and, moreover, that these descending brain stem pain facilitatory systems are heavily connected with, and strongly influenced by, activity in key forebrain structures. Neuronal activity in forebrain structures related to cognitions and emotions could lead to an imbalance of descending modulatory systems. If that imbalance leads to an increase in endogenous facilitation, normally innocuous stimuli could be perceived as painful. It is possible that for some individuals the diffuse nature and amplification of persistent pain may be in part the result of such an imbalance (see Fig. 12.4) (Dubner & Ren 1999).

The influence attention and focusing can have on the perception of pain in humans was noted by Miron et al (1989). This research showed that, with contrived changes in directed attention, human volunteers reported alterations in both the perceived intensity and unpleasantness, hence tolerance, of a transiently painful but non tissue damaging thermal stimulus. These and other findings prompted Dubner & Ren (1999) to contend that the addition of a behavioural variable such as attention to a potentially threatening stimulus results in sensitization of dorsal horn spinal cord neurons (see Fig. 12.5). In a series of behavioural studies incorporating electrophysiologically correlated data with a delayed-response task paradigm primates were rewarded for responding to a randomly delivered transient tissue threatening peripheral stimulus. It was found that expansion of receptive fields and increased responsiveness of second order trigeminal pain pathway neurons were directly related to the strength of engineered attention rather than stimulus intensity (Dubner & Ren 1999). Moreover, it was found that behavioural modulation

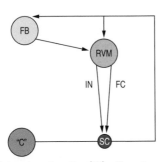

Figure 12.4 Peripheral nociceptive ('C') afferents sensitize spinal cord (SC) neurons as they ascend to supraspinal forebrain (FB) centres, on their way to giving excitatory collaterals to brain stem inhibitory (IN) and facilitatory (FC) nuclei. Pathways from these rostral ventromedial medullary (RVM) nuclei descend to modulate activity in the same SC neurons. The IN and FC nuclei are themselves contacted and may be influenced by activity occurring in the FB (cognitions, emotions, attention). In this way forebrain activity can diminish or enhance sensitization of SC neurons with or without ongoing 'C' afferent input.

associated with selective attention to a perceived threat utilizes the same forebrain and brain stem structures and mechanisms as are involved in the development, amplification and maintenance of persistent pain following actual tissue damage and inflammation (Dubner & Ren 1999). The critical implication is that because there is a shared central pain producing and sustaining mechanism, the clinical consequences of forebrain mediated selective attention are likely to be functionally indistinguishable from those initially triggered by the primary peripheral pathology (Dubner & Ren 1999, Moog et al 2002).

It is apparent that there is considerable overlap between mechanisms responsible for both inhibition and facilitation of nociceptive inputs from spinal cord neurons. Depending on stimulus intensity both inhibition and facilitation of dorsal horn pain pathway activity could be achieved from many of the same brain stem nuclei, especially those located in the rostral ventromedial medulla (RVM) (Urban & Gebhart 1999). Interestingly, despite this apparent anatomical overlap, the opposing neurophysiological consequences (inhibition, facilitation) have been shown to involve different spinal cord pathways and neurotransmitters, and to be dorsal horn lamina- and receptor-specific (Urban & Gebhart 1999). It has also been shown that simultaneously lesioning nominally inhibitory (nucleus raphe magnus, NRM) and facilitatory (nucleus reticularis gigantocellularis, NGC) sites completely reversed their customary (opposing) effects on spinal cord neurons (Wei et al 1999a).

The responses of wide dynamic range dorsal horn neurons (laminae I–VI) to mechanical peripheral stimuli can also be modulated by electrical and chemical (glutamate) stimulation applied at a range of sites in the rostral medial medulla (RMM) (Zhuo & Gebhart 2002). The often biphasic changes were specific for the site of RMM stimulation and not the particular neuron from which recordings were taken. Thus, individual dorsal horn neuron responses to noxious peripheral stimuli are enhanced by stimulation at some, and inhibited by stimulation at other, RMM sites. At some RMM sites, activity in the same neuron was facilitated with lower and inhibited with higher intensity stimulation in a similar manner to RVM nuclei.

Significantly, similar findings were obtained for responses evoked in dorsal horn neurons by both noxious and non-noxious mechanical peripheral stimulation. Together with other results, such findings led the authors to conclude that spinal transmission of noxious and non-noxious peripheral mechanical stimuli 'is subject to descending influences, including facilitatory influences that may contribute to exaggerated responses ... in some chronic pain states' (Zhuo & Gebhart 2002).

In this regard, certain brain stem nuclei have been identified as sources of potential tonic facilitation and persistent pain. These include the nucleus gigantocellularis, nucleus gigantocellularis pars alpha (Dubner & Ren 1999) and the dorsal reticular nucleus of the medulla (Lima & Almeida

2002). Descending facilitation is implicated in the development of centrally created secondary hyperalgesia associated with inflammatory and neuropathic pain (Porreca et al 2002). It is suggested that the reason for the existence of such a system is that descending facilitation initially has a discrete protective function, especially with inflammatory pain conditions (Porreca et al 2002).

By shifting the balance in favour of facilitation, forebrain activity related to attention and evaluation of threat could have a role in the initiation and maintenance of central sensitization in spinal cord neurons (Fig. 12.4). It might be anticipated that this would lead to clinically observed symptoms and signs that would be difficult to distinguish from symptoms and signs occurring as a result of peripheral injury. Understanding this is of considerable importance in clinical reasoning and the identification of patients where forebrain mediated central sensitization is strongly suspected of being the cause, or major component, of their prolonged pain and functional disability.

Certain cognitive styles have been associated with gross amplification of pain and its extension in the absence, or beyond the period for healing, of tissue damage (Aronoff 1998, Bacon et al 1994, Bass 2000, Crombez et al 1999, Ferrari & Schrader 2001, Jensen et al 1994, Keogh et al 2001, Linton 2000, Sullivan et al 2001, Vlaeyen & Linton 2000, Waddell et al 1993). These include somatization, catastrophizing, and hypervigilance. Figure 12.5 provides a model of the possible relationship between these factors and the development of chronic pain. Forebrain mediated central sensitization may provide a neuronal mechanism whereby such cognitive styles can contribute to up-regulation of the nociceptive system.

Loss of inhibition

On balance, the net effect of descending brain stem systems on spinal cord neurons, normally as well as under routine inflammatory conditions, seems to be inhibitory. However, it is possible for various factors to reduce this inhibition and shift the balance in favour of facilitation.

Experimental evidence for the importance of blockade of descending inhibitory pathways in inducing central sensitization include the observation that bilateral lesions of the dorsolateral funiculus in the rat led to a significant decrease in the latency for paw withdrawal to a noxious stimulus (Wei et al 1999b). Dorsolateral funiculi appear to be a preferred pathway for descending pain inhibitory systems (Dubner & Ren 1999, Urban & Gebhart 1999). Similarly, temporary spinal cord block (lidocaine (lignocaine)) caused dorsal horn nociceptive specific and wide dynamic range neurons to expand their receptive fields and increase their responsiveness to afferent input. These effects were further enhanced in experimentally 'inflamed' animals (hindpaw injection of complete Freund's Adjuvant or carrageenan) (Ren & Dubner 1996). Selective anaesthesia (lidocaine (lignocaine)) of the nucleus raphe magnus (NRM), in the RVM

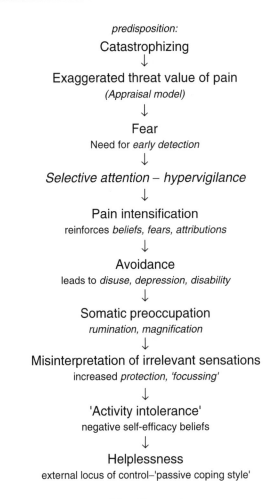

predisposition:
Catastrophizing
↓
Exaggerated threat value of pain
(Appraisal model)
↓
Fear
Need for *early detection*
↓
Selective attention – hypervigilance
↓
Pain intensification
reinforces *beliefs, fears, attributions*
↓
Avoidance
leads to *disuse, depression, disability*
↓
Somatic preoccupation
rumination, magnification
↓
Misinterpretation of irrelevant sensations
increased *protection, 'focussing'*
↓
'Activity intolerance'
negative self-efficacy beliefs
↓
Helplessness
external locus of control–'passive coping style'

You fix me!

Figure 12.5 Model of the relationship between some identified maladaptive cognitive processes and the development of chronic pain. Note the pivotal role of selective attention – hypervigilance.

caused nociceptive-specific neurons in the spinal cord to increase their background discharge, expand their receptive fields and respond in an exaggerated and abnormal manner to subsequent peripheral stimuli (Ren & Dubner 1996). In addition, selective chemical lesion of NRM 5HT-containing neurons in experimentally 'inflamed' animals resulted in demonstrable behavioural hypersensitivity. This was accompanied by the appearance of the Fos protein bilaterally in all laminae of the animals' spinal cord (Wei et al 1998). The Fos protein is a gene transcription by-product and recognized biological marker for enhanced neural activity (Menetrey et al 1989). Similar effects were observed in superficial laminae following lesions of an inhibitory noradrenergic locus coeruleus–dorsal horn pathway. The foregoing provides evidence for the importance of brain stem descending inhibitory systems in regulating the excitability of spinal cord pain pathway neurons (Wei et al 1998). Moreover, it suggests that disruption of one or more of the elements of this system can result in, among other things, the equivalent of central sensitization.

Facilitation

Among brain stem nuclei so far identified as the origin of descending (or locally acting) pain pathway facilitatory systems is the nucleus reticularis gigantocellularis (NGC). Low intensity stimulation in the RVM at or near the NGC has been shown to cause lingering excitation of some spinal cord spinothalamic tract neurons as well as a decrease in the latency of the tail-flick response (Haber et al 1980, Zhuo & Gebhart 1990). Stimulation of the NGC also enhanced the responses of primate spinothalamic tract neurons to transient noxious stimuli (Haber et al 1980). Selective lesions (ibotenic acid) of NGC in the 'inflamed' rat led to a significant increase in the latency for the paw withdrawal reflex and a marked reduction in the presence of Fos protein bilaterally in all laminae of the spinal cord. Such experiments provide evidence that NGC is capable of enhancing and/or maintaining central sensitization at the spinal cord level (Dubner & Ren 1999). Significantly, secondary hyperalgesia was completely blocked by ibotenic acid lesions of the medulla that included NGC (Urban et al 1996, 1999).

Almeida et al (1999) confirmed the presence of a nociceptively driven pathway from the dorsal reticular nucleus (DRt) of the medulla to superficial and deeper laminae of the dorsal horn of the spinal cord. Importantly, the findings were backed up by calculating the number of cells expressing noxiously induced c-fos in both superficial and deeper laminae of the spinal cord. The Fos protein is known to be a reliable marker of neuronal (hyper)activity (Menetrey et al 1989). Because it has every appearance of being reverberatory or self-sustaining, the DRt–dorsal horn circuit could be particularly significant, not only with respect to pain amplification but also in terms of chronicity.

Fields et al characterized specific groups of cells in RVM that may form the basis for bidirectional control (Fields et al 1983). They identified three distinct cell groups that show characteristically different responses during a thermal tail-flick test in the rat. The cells were described as off cells which show continuous ongoing activity and pause just before the tail-flick response occurs, on cells that are tonically inhibited but display a pronounced burst of activity just before the tail-flick response occurs and neutral cells whose activity is not specifically related to the pain response (Fields et al 1983).

This group hypothesized that off cells provide a tonic inhibition of nociceptive transmission cells in the spinal cord that is disinhibited and then facilitated by on cell activity when pain occurs.

Both types of neuron descend to appropriate laminae (I, II, IV) of the dorsal horn of the spinal cord and both may be influenced by stimulation of the PAG. Interestingly, Wei et al (1999a) recently demonstrated that the function of inhibitory 'off' cells may be suppressed (via inhibitory interneurons) by activity in nearby NGC neurons. Thus, NGC neurons probably exert their dorsal horn effects through several circuits. However, one mechanism for

endogenous descending facilitation, or sensitization, of spinal cord pain pathway neurons could be the local inhibition of a brain stem descending inhibitory system. The net effect of stimulation of NGC is facilitation of central sensitization at the spinal cord level (Ren et al 2000). It is possible that this facilitation may be initiated or controlled by the anterior cingulate cortex since electrical and chemical stimulation of ACC elicits marked facilitation of the tail-flick reflex to noxious thermal stimulation (Calejesan et al 2000). This effect is apparently mediated through relays in PAG and RVM.

There is now substantial evidence for pathways from acknowledged rostral 'pain relevant' cortical and subcortical centres to both the PAG and RVM. There is also compelling behavioural evidence that these forebrain centres are capable of exerting powerful clinically significant influences on various nuclei located within brain stem structures, including NGC. Together this anatomical, physiological and behavioural evidence helps confirm the long recognized, critical influence that such forebrain products as cognitions, emotions, attention and motivation have on the clinical pain experience. The evidence further endorses detrimental effects that recognized psychosocial factors have on motor control and adaptive function, both spontaneously and as a result of pain.

SOMATOMOTOR DYSFUNCTION

The major consequences of molecular changes in spinal cord neurons are increased synaptic efficacy and increased neuronal excitability. Neuronal plasticity leading to increased synaptic efficacy and increased neuronal excitability in spinal cord neurons conveying nociceptive information is also likely to influence activity in other neuronal pools with which the central nociceptive neurons make synaptic connections. This could account for changes in motor system function, which are clinical features of many pain states.

Enhanced withdrawal reflexes

It is clear that this hyperactive state of spinal cord neurons is associated with important changes in terms of sensorimotor function. In his seminal study, Woolf showed that the establishment of central sensitization is associated with facilitation of flexor withdrawal reflex responses (Woolf 1984). A prolonged increase in the response duration is maintained for several days and in some cases may still be present weeks later when tissue healing is presumed to have occurred (Woolf 1984).

Altered flexor withdrawal reflexes may be of clinical importance in tests such as the straight leg raise and the brachial plexus tension test. Increased muscle activity has been demonstrated in normal subjects when undergoing neural tissue provocation tests (Balster & Jull 1997). These studies support the proposal that muscle activity protects the nervous system from tensile forces. It has been suggested that this increase in muscle activity is due to activation of the flexor withdrawal reflex (Hall et al 1998, Wright et al 1994). Hall et al (1998) showed that flexor muscle activity is more easily elicited in chronic pain patients than in normal volunteers during the straight leg raise test (Hall et al 1998).

Vicious cycle model

In addition to increased muscle activation attributable to the influence of pain and tissue damage on alpha motoneuron function, it has been suggested that pain may influence the excitability of gamma motoneurons contributing to the development of increased muscle tension or spasm. The vicious cycle model is often alluded to in the literature. As outlined by Johansson & Sojka (1991), the basic concept is that stimulation of nociceptive afferents from muscles excites dynamic and static fusimotor neurons enhancing the sensitivity of primary and secondary muscle spindle afferents. Increased activity of primary muscle spindle afferents increases muscle stiffness. This increased muscle stiffness then leads to increased metabolite production and, following the vicious cycle formula, a further increase in muscle stiffness. In addition, increased activity in the secondary spindle afferents projects back onto the gamma system perpetuating enhanced muscle stiffness. These effects are thought to be important in generating muscle spasm and pain (Johansson & Sojka 1991).

There are several studies demonstrating enhanced activity in primary and secondary spindle afferents following the application of chemical mediators such as potassium chloride, lactic acid, bradykinin and serotonin (Djupsjobacka et al 1995, Johansson et al 1993). In addition to altered responses following local muscle injection, these researchers have also demonstrated modulation of secondary muscle spindle afferents following injection of bradykinin into the contralateral muscle (Djupsjobacka et al 1995). This model may provide some explanation of muscle spasm when it is a significant component of the clinical presentation. However, it provides very little explanation of situations in which we see muscle inhibition and wastage as a result of pain and a number of studies have failed to show an increase in resting EMG activity as might be postulated by this model.

Pain adaptation model

Lund and colleagues refuted the vicious cycle model and suggested that pain reduces the ability to contract muscles rather than making them hyperactive (Lund et al 1991). Their model, termed the pain adaptation theory, is strongly linked to the phenomenon of central sensitization. They propose that the effect of noxious stimulation is to alter the activity of type II spinal cord interneurons such that there is increased inhibition of agonist motor units and increased facilitation of antagonist motor units. This leads to an overall limitation of movement in any desired direction. The proposed alterations in neural function would be manifest as a reduction in the ability to activate the agonist muscle, a time delay in activating the agonist muscle and a reduction in the maximum force output from the agonist muscle. Increased activity in antagonist muscles and a delay in producing reciprocal inhibition of these muscles might also be anticipated. Movement becomes slower, muscles appear to be weaker and the overall range of movement accomplished may be reduced (Lund et al 1991). Deficits of this type have been demonstrated in patients with low back pain and in normal subjects following the injection of hypertonic saline into the lumbar paraspinal muscles (Arendt-Nielsen et al 1996) and the muscles of mastication (Svensson et al 1996). This model may represent a good explanation of the limitation of movement that occurs in the acute pain situation. It is apparent, however, that motor dysfunction in chronic pain states may be a somewhat more complex phenomenon.

Emerging models

Over the last decade researchers have begun to investigate the influence of pain on patterns of neuromuscular activation and control. It has been suggested that the presence of pain leads to inhibition or delayed activation of muscles or muscle groups that perform key synergistic functions to limit unwanted motion (Sterling et al 2002). This produces alterations in the patterns of motor activity and recruitment during functional movement. It has been suggested that this inhibition usually occurs in the deep muscles, local to the involved joint, that perform a synergistic function in order to control joint stability (Hides et al 1996, Hodges & Richardson 1996, Voight & Wieder 1991).

In both the lumbar and the cervical spine, the dysfunctional muscles appear to be the deep muscles that attach directly to the vertebrae. These muscles span the vertebrae and perform important synergistic functions to stabilize articular segments, rather than being primarily responsible for movement production (Cholewicki et al 1997). It appears that while changes in the control of these muscles may be initiated in the presence of pain and tissue injury, they are often sustained beyond the acute pain phase and may contribute to the chronicity of many musculoskeletal problems.

It is clear that pain can produce many changes in motor activity. Some of these changes can be explained by peripheral mechanisms in the muscles themselves and by mechanisms within the central nervous system. Certainly, pain has a potent effect on motor activity and control. The dysfunction that occurs in the neuromuscular system in the presence of pain is complex. In addition to the more obvious changes, such as increased muscle activity in some muscle groups and inhibition of others, more subtle anomalous patterns of neuromuscular activation appear to occur. Some elements of both the vicious cycle and pain adaptation models may be important in acute and chronic pain states. However, neither of these models can fully explain the prolonged changes in motor function that are seen after tissue injury. Loss of selective activation and inhibition of certain muscles that perform key synergistic functions, leading to altered patterns of neuromuscular activation, and the ensuing loss of joint stability and control are initiated with acute pain and tissue injury. However, these phenomena persist and could be one reason for chronic symptoms.

CONCLUSION

Recent advances in our knowledge of pain have provided a much greater insight into the many ways in which nociceptive system activity can be enhanced in response to tissue injury. It is clear that both peripheral and central mechanisms are important and that subtle variations in the mechanisms activated can result in different forms of altered sensitivity being induced. Mechanisms exist to sensitize nociceptors, to recruit previously inactive nociceptors and to utilize afferent inputs via myelinated neurons to contribute to nociception. These mechanisms contribute to substantial spatial and temporal summation of nociceptive inputs. Central mechanisms appear to be particularly important in controlling the spread of sensitivity to uninjured tissues surrounding the region of tissue damage.

Rapidly developing areas of research are also improving our knowledge of the interrelationship between pain, motor function and emotional state. We are beginning to move away from a largely peripheralist view of tissue injury to a much more integrated understanding of the influence of pain and injury on the central nervous system and the patient as a whole. This encompasses an emerging view of the nociceptive system as a highly distributed system that interacts with many other neuronal systems. The immense impact of pain and tissue injury on the central nervous system and the plasticity induced by the presence of pain are becoming increasingly apparent. It is now clear that the relative setting of descending facilitatory and inhibitory projections from brain to spinal cord may significantly affect the perceptions of nociceptive inputs. Cognitions, emotions and attentional state can all have important influences on the balance between descending inhibition and facilitation. Ultimately, improved understanding of these mechanisms should lead to the development of a more comprehensive approach to the management of patients with pain.

KEYWORDS

musculoskeletal pain	central sensitization
peripheral sensitization	pain inhibitory mechanisms

References

Almeida A, Storkson R, Lima D, Hole K, Tjolsen A 1999 The medullary dorsal reticular nucleus facilitates pain behaviour induced by formalin in the rat. European Journal of Neuroscience 11: 110–122

Anand P 1995 Nerve growth factor regulates nociception in human health and disease. British Journal of Anaesthesia 75: 201–208

Anbar M, Gratt B M 1997 Role of nitric oxide in the physiopathology of pain. Journal of Pain Symptom Management 14: 225–254

Arendt-Nielsen L, Graven-Nielsen T, Svarrer H, Svensson P 1996 The influence of low back pain on muscle activity and coordination during gait: a clinical and experimental study. Pain 64: 231–240

Aronoff G M 1998 Myofascial pain syndrome and fibromyalgia: a critical assessment and alternate view. Clinical Journal of Pain, 14: 74–85

Bacon N M, Bacon S F, Atkinson J H, et al 1994 Somatization symptoms in chronic low back pain patients. Psychosomatic Medicine 56: 118–127

Balster S M, Jull G A 1997 Upper trapezius muscle activity during the brachial plexus tension test in asymptomatic subjects. Manual Therapy 2: 144–149

Bandler R, Shipley M T 1994 Columnar organization in the midbrain periaqueductal gray: modules for emotional expression? Trends in Neurosciences 17: 379–389

Bass C 2000 Somatization. Medicine 28(5): 68–71

Bear M F, Connors B W, Paradiso M A 2001 Neuroscience: exploring the brain. Lippincott, Philadelphia, chs 23–24

Bevan S 1996 Signal transduction in nociceptive afferent neurons in inflammatory conditions. In: Kumazawa T, Kruger L, Mizumura K (eds) Progress in brain research. Elsevier Science BV, Amsterdam, vol 113, pp 201–213

Boucher T J, Kerr B J, Ramer M S, Thompson S W N, McMahon S B 2000 Neurotrophic factor effects on pain-signaling systems. In: Devor M, Rowbotham M C, Wiesenfeld-Hallin Z (eds) Proceedings of the 9th World Congress on Pain, Progress in Pain Research and Management. IASP Press, Seattle, vol 16, pp 175–189

Bushnell M C, Duncan G H, Hofbauer R K, Ha B, Chen J I, Carrier B 1999 Pain perception: is there a role for primary somatosensory cortex? Proceedings of the National Academy of Sciences of the United States of America 96: 7705–7709

Bushnell M K, Villemure C, Strigo I, Duncan G H 2002 Imaging pain in the brain: the role of the cerebral cortex in pain perception and modulation. Journal of Musculoskeletal Pain 10(1/2): 59–72

Calejesan A A, Kim S J, Zhuo M 2000: Descending facilitatory modulation of a behavioural nociceptive response by stimulation in the adult rat anterior cingulate cortex. European Journal of Pain 4: 83–96

Carr D B, Goudas L C 1999 Acute pain. Lancet 353: 2051–2058

Carroll R C, Beattie E C, von Zastrow M, Malenka R C 2001 Role of AMPA receptor endocytosis in synaptic plasticity. Nature Reviews Neuroscience 2: 315–324

Casey K L, 1999 Forebrain mechanisms of nociception and pain: analysis through imaging. Proceedings of the National Academy of Sciences of the United States of America 96: 7668–7674

Cervero F, Laird J M A 1996 From acute to chronic pain: mechanisms and hypotheses. In: Carli G, Zimmerman M (eds) Progress in brain research. Elsevier Science BV, Amsterdam, vol 110, pp 3–15

Cesare P, Moriondo A, Vellani V, McNaughton P A 1999 Ion channels gated by heat. Proceedings of the National Academy of Sciences of the United States of America 96: 7658–7663

Chapman C R 1996 Limbic processes and the affective dimension of pain. In: Carli G, Zimmerman M (eds) Progress in brain research. Elsevier Science BV, Amsterdam, vol 110, pp 63–81

Cholewicki J, Panjabi M M, Khachatryan A 1997 Stabilizing function of trunk flexor-extensor muscles around a neutral spine posture. Spine 22: 2207–2212.

Chudler E H, Dong W K 1995 The role of the basal ganglia in nociception and pain. Pain 64: 3–38

Coderre T J, Melzack R 1987 Cutaneous hyperalgesia: contributions of the peripheral and central nervous systems to the increase in pain sensitivity after injury. Brain Research 404: 95–106

Cook A J, Woolf C J, Wall P D, McMahon S B 1987 Dynamic receptive field plasticity in rat spinal cord dorsal horn following C primary afferent input. Nature 325: 151–153

Crombez G, Eccleston C, Baeyens F et al 1999 Attention to chronic pain is dependent upon pain-related fear. Journal of Psychosomatic Research 47(5): 403–410

Davis K D, Taub E, Duffner F et al 2000 Activation of the anterior cingulate cortex by thalamic stimulation in patients with chronic pain: a positron emission tomography study. Journal of Neurosurgery 92: 64–69

Dickenson A H 1995 Central acute pain mechanisms. Annals of Medicine 27: 223–227

Djupsjöbacka M, Johansson H, Bergenheim M, Wenngren B I 1995 Influences on the gamma-muscle spindle system from muscle afferents stimulated by increased intramuscular concentrations of bradykinin and 5-HT. Neuroscience Research 22: 325–353

Dray A 1995 Inflammatory mediators of pain. British Journal of Anaesthesia 75: 125–131

Dray A 1996 Neurogenic mechanisms and neuropeptides in chronic pain. In: Carli G, Zimmerman M (eds) Progress in brain research. Elsevier, Amsterdam, vol 110, pp 85–94

Dubner R, Ren K 1999 Endogenous mechanisms of sensory modulation. 6(Suppl.): S45–53

Duggan A W, Hendry I A, Morton C R, Hutchinson W D, Zhao Z Q 1988 Cutaneous stimuli releasing immunoreactive substance P in the dorsal horn of the cat. Brain Research 451: 261–273

Duggan A W, Hope P J, Jarrot B, Schaible H-G, Fleetwood-Walker S M 1990 Release, spread, and persistence of immunoreactive neurokinin A in the dorsal horn of the cat following noxious cutaneous stimulation: studies with antibody microprobes. Neuroscience 35: 195–202

Ferrari R, Schrader H 2001 The late whiplash syndrome: a biopsychosocial approach. Journal of Neurology, Neurosurgery and Psychiatry 70: 722–726

Fields H L, Bry J, Hentall I, Zorman G 1983 The activity of neurons in the rostral medulla of the rat during withdrawal from noxious heat. Journal of Neuroscience 3: 2545–2552

Flor H, Braun C, Elbert T, Birbaumer N 1997 Extensive reorganisation of primary somatosensory cortex in chronic back pain patients. Neuroscience Letters 224: 5–8

Gordh T, Karlsten R, Kristensen J 1995 Intervention with spinal NMDA, adenosine, and NO systems for pain modulation. Annals of Medicine, 27: 229–234

Haber L H, Martin R F, Chung J M, Willis W D 1980 Inhibition and excitation of primate spinothalamic tract neurons by stimulation in region of nucleus reticularis gigantocellularis. Journal of Neurophysiology 43: 1578–1593

Hall T, Zusman M, Elvey R 1998 Adverse mechanical tension in the nervous system? Analysis of straight leg raise. Manual Therapy 3: 140–146

Handwerker H O, Reeh P W 1991 Pain and inflammation. In: Bond M R, Charlton I E, Woolf C J (eds) Pain research and clinical management. Proceedings of the VIth World Congress on Pain. Elsevier, Amsterdam, pp 59–70

Handwerker H O, Reeh P W 1992 Nociceptors, chemosensitivity and sensitization by chemical agents. In: Willis W D (ed) Hyperalgesia and allodynia. Raven Press, New York, pp 107–115

Harding V 1999 The role of movement in acute pain. In: Max M (ed) Pain 1999 – an updated review. IASP Press, Seattle, pp 159–169

Hardy J D, Wolff H G, Goodell H 1950 Experimental evidence of the nature of cutaneous hyperalgesia. Journal of Clinical Investigation 29: 115–140

Hides J A, Richardson C A, Jull G A 1996 Multifidus muscle recovery is not automatic following resolution of acute first episode low back pain. Spine 21: 2763–2769

Hodges P W, Richardson C A 1996 Insufficient muscular stabilisation of the lumbar spine associated with low back pain: a motor control examination of transversus abdominus. Spine 21: 2640–2650

Hofbauer R K, Rainville P, Duncan G H, Bushnell M C 2001 Cortical representation of the sensory dimension of pain. Journal of Neurophysiology 86: 402–411

Hsieh J C, Hagermark O, Stahle-Backdahl M et al 1994 Urge to scratch represented in the human cerebral cortex during itch. Journal of Neurophysiology 72: 3004–3008

Hutchison W D, Davis K D, Lozano A M, Tasker R R, Dostrovsky J O 1999 Pain-related neurons in the human cingulate cortex. Nature Neuroscience 2: 403–405

Jensen M P, Turner J A, Romano J M, Lawler B K 1994 Relationship of pain-specific beliefs to chronic pain adjustment. Pain 57: 301–309

Johansson H, Sojka P 1991 Pathophysiological mechanisms involved in genesis and spread of muscular tension in occupational muscle pain and in chronic musculoskeletal pain syndromes: a hypothesis. Medical Hypotheses 35: 196–203

Johansson H, Djupsjobacka M, Sjolander P 1993 Influences of the gamma-muscle spindle system from muscle afferents stimulated by KCL and lactic acid. Neuroscience Research 16: 49–57

Keogh E, Ellery D, Hunt C, Hannent I 2001 Selective attentional bias for pain-related stimuli amongst pain fearful individuals. Pain 91(1/2): 91–100

Kingsley R E 2000 Concise text of neuroscience. Lippincott, Philadelphia, pp 102–103

Kumazawa T 1996 The polymodal nociceptor: bio-warning and defense system. Progress in Brain Research 113: 3–18

Kwan C L, Crawley A P, Mikulis D J, Davis K D 2000 An fMRI study of the anterior cingulate cortex and surrounding medial wall activations evoked by noxious cutaneous heat and cold stimuli. Pain 85: 359–374

Levine J D, Fields H L, Basbaum A I 1993 Peptides and the primary afferent nociceptor. Journal of Neuroscience 13: 2273–2286

Lima D, Almeida A 2002 The medullary dorsal reticular nucleus as a pronociceptive centre of the pain control system. Progress in Neurobiology 66: 81–108

Lin B, Brücher F A, Colgin L L, Lynch 2002 Long-term potentiation alters the modulator pharmacology of AMPA-type glutamate receptors. Journal of Neurophysiology 87: 2790–2800

Linton S J 2000 A review of psychological risk factors in back and neck pain. Spine 25: 1148–1156

Lovick T A 1991 Interactions between descending pathways from the dorsal and ventrolateral periaqueductal gray matter in the rat. In: Depaulis A, Bandlier R (eds) The midbrain periaqueductal gray matter. Plenum Press, New York, pp 101–120

Lund J P, Donga R, Widmar C G, Stohler C S 1991 The pain adaptation model: a discussion of the relationship between chronic musculoskeletal pain and motor activity. Canadian Journal of Physiology and Pharmacology 69: 683–694

Ma Q P, Woolf C J 1995 Noxious stimuli induce an N-methyl-D-aspartate receptor-dependent hypersensitivity of the flexion withdrawal reflex to touch: implications for the treatment of mechanical allodynia. Pain 61: 383–390

Ma Q-P, Woolf C J 1996 Progressive tactile hypersensitivity: an inflammation-induced incremental increase in the excitability of the spinal cord. Pain 67: 97–106

McKernan M G, Shinnick-Galagher P 1997 Fear conditioning induces a lasting potentiation of synaptic currents in vitro. Nature 390: 607–611

McMahon S B, Bennett D L, Priestley J V, Shelton D L 1995 The biological effects of endogenous nerve growth factor on adult sensory neurons revealed by a trkA-IgG fusion molecule. Nature Medicine 1: 774–780

Mao J, Price D D, Mayer D J 1995 Mechanisms of hyperalgesia and morphine tolerance: a current view of their possible interactions. Pain 62: 259–274

Mayer E A, Gebhart G F 1994 Basic and clinical aspects of visceral hyperalgesia. Gastroenterology 107: 271–293

Meller S T, Gebhart G F 1993 Nitric oxide (NO) and nociceptive processing in the spinal cord. Pain 52: 127–136

Meller S T, Dykstra C, Gebhart G F 1996 Acute mechanical hyperalgesia in the rat can be produced by coactivation of spinal ionotropic AMPA and metabotropic glutamate receptors, activation of phospholipase A2 and generation of cyclooxygenase products. In: Carli G, Zimmerman M (eds) Progress in brain research. Elsevier Science BV, Amsterdam, vol 110, pp 177–192

Menetrey D, Gannon A, Levine J D, Basbaum A I 1989 Expression of c-fos protein in interneurons and projection neurons of the rat spinal cord in response to noxious somatic, articular, and visceral stimulation. Journal of Comparative Neurology 285: 177–195

Merskey H, Bogduk N 1994 Classification of chronic pain: descriptions of chronic pain syndromes and definitions of pain terms. IASP Press, Seattle

Miron D, Duncan G H, Bushnell M K 1989 Effects of attention on the intensity and unpleasantness of thermal pain. Pain 39: 345–352

Mizamura K, Kumazawa T 1996 Modification of nociceptor response by inflammatory mediators and second messengers implicated in their action: a study in canine testicular polymodal receptors. In: Kumazawa T, Kruger L, Mizumura K (eds) Progress in brain research. Elsevier Science BV, Amsterdam, vol 113, pp 115–141

Moog M, Quintner J, Hall T, Zusman M 2002 The late whiplash syndrome: a psychophysical study. European Journal of Pain 6: 283–294

Neumann S, Doubell T P, Leslie T A et al 1996 Inflammatory pain hypersensitivity mediated by phenotypic switch in myelinated primary sensory neurones. Nature 384: 360–364

Porreca F, Ossipov M H, Gebhart G F 2002 Chronic pain and medullary descending facilitation. Trends in Neuroscience 25: 319–325

Porro C A, Cavazzuti M 1996 Functional imaging of the pain system in man and animals. In: Carli G, Zimmerman M (eds) Progress in brain research. Elsevier Science BV, Amsterdam, vol 110, pp 47–62

Price D D 2000 Psychological and neural mechanisms of the affective dimension of pain. Science 288: 1769–1772

Rainville P, Duncan G H, Price D D, Carrier B, Bushnell M C 1997 Pain affect encoded in human anterior cingulate but not somatosensory cortex. Science 277: 968–971

Rang H P, Urban L 1995 New molecules in analgesia. British Journal of Anaesthesia 75: 145–156

Reeh P W, Steen K H 1996 Tissue acidosis in nociception and pain. In: Kumazawa T, Kruger L, Mizumura K (eds) Progress in brain research. Elsevier Science BV, Amsterdam, vol 113, pp 143–151

Ren K, Dubner R 1996 Enhanced descending modulation of nociception in rats with persistent hindpaw inflammation. Journal of Neurophysiology 76: 3025–3037

Ren K, Wei F, Dubner R, Murphy A, Hoffman G E 2000 Progesterone attenuates persistent inflammatory hyperalgesia in female rats: involvement of spinal NMDA receptor mechanisms. Brain Research, 865: 272–277

Sandkühler J 2000 Learning and memory in pain pathways. Pain 88: 113–118

Scharf M T, Woo N H, Lattal K M et al 2002 Protein synthesis is required for the enhancement of long-term potentiation and long-term memory by spaced learning. Journal of Neurophysiology 87: 2770–2777

Schmidt R F 1996 The articular polymodal nociceptor in health and disease. In: Kumazawa T, Kruger L, Mizumura K. (eds) Progress in brain research. Elsevier Science BV, Amsterdam, vol 113, pp 53–81

Shu X Q, Mendell L M 1999 Neurotrophins and hyperalgesia. Proceedings of the National Academy of Sciences of the United States of America 96: 7693–7696

Siddall P J, Cousins M J 1998 Introduction to pain mechanisms: implications for neural blockade. In: Cousins M J, Bridenbaugh P O (eds) Neural blockade in clinical anesthesia and management of pain. Lippincott-Raven, Philadelphia

Stamford J A 1995 Descending control of pain. British Journal of Anaesthesia 75: 217–227

Steen K H, Reeh P W, Anton F, Handwerker H O 1992 Protons selectively induce lasting excitation and sensitisation to mechanical stimuli of nociceptors in rat skin, in vivo. Journal of Neuroscience 12: 86–95.

Sterling M, Jull G, Wright A 2001 The effect of musculoskeletal pain on motor activity and control. Journal of Pain 2: 135–145

Sugimoto T, Bennett G J, Kajander K C 1990 Transsynaptic degeneration in the superficial dorsal horn after sciatic nerve injury: effects of a chronic constriction injury, transection, and strychnine. Pain 42: 205–213

Sullivan M J, Thorn B, Haythornthwaite J A et al 2001 Theoretical perspectives on the relation between catastrophizing and pain. Clinical Journal of Pain 17: 52–64

Svensson P, Arendt-Nielson L, Houe L 1996 Sensory-motor interactions of human experimental jaw muscle pain: a quantitative analysis. Pain 64: 241–250

Thacker M, Gifford L 2002 A review of the physiotherapy management of complex regional pain syndrome. In: Gifford L (ed) Topical issues in pain 3. CNS Press, Falmouth, pp 119–141

Thompson S W, Bennett D L, Kerr B J, Bradbury E J, McMahon S B 1999 Brain-derived neurotrophic factor is an endogenous modulator of nociceptive responses in the spinal cord. Proceedings of the National Academy of Sciences of the United States of America 96: 7714–7718

Torebjork E, Lundberg L, La Motte R 1992 Central changes in the processing of mechanoreceptive input in capsaicin-induced secondary hyperalgesia in humans. Journal of Physiology (London) 448: 765–780

Urban M O, Gebhart G F 1999 Supraspinal contributions to hyperalgesia. Proceedings of the National Academy of Sciences of the United States of America 96: 7687–7692

Urban M O, Jiang M C, Gebhart G F 1996 Participation of central descending nociceptive facilitatory systems in secondary hyperalgesia produced by mustard oil. Brain Research 737: 83–91

Vlaeyen J W, Linton S J 2000 Fear-avoidance and its consequences in chronic musculoskeletal pain: a state of the art. Pain 85: 317–332

Voight M L, Wieder D L 1991 Comparative reflex response times of vastus medialis obliquus and vastus lateralis in normal subjects and subjects with extensor mechanism dysfunction: an electromyographic study. American Journal of Sports Medicine 19: 131–137

Waddell G, Newton M, Henderson I, Somerville D, Main C J 1993 A fear-avoidance beliefs questionnaire (FABQ) and the role of fear-avoidance beliefs in chronic low back pain and disability. Pain 52: 157–168

Wei F, Ren K, Dubner R 1998 Inflammation-induced Fos protein expression in the rat spinal cord is enhanced following dorsolateral or ventrolateral funiculus lesions. Brain Research 782: 136–141

Wei F, Dubner R, Ren K 1999a Nucleus reticularis gigantocellularis and nucleus raphe magnus in the brain stem exert opposite effects on behavioural hyperalgesia and spinal Fos protein expression after peripheral inflammation. Pain 80: 127–141

Wei F, Dubner R, Ren K 1999b Dorsolateral funiculus-lesions unmask inhibitory or disfacilitatory mechanisms which modulate the effects of innocuous mechanical stimulation on spinal Fos expression after inflammation. Brain Research 820: 112–116

Wilcox G L 1991 Excitatory neurotransmitters and pain. In: Bond M, Woolf C J, Charlton J E (eds) Pain research and clinical management. Proceedings of the VIth World Congress on Pain. Elsevier, Amsterdam, pp 97–117

Willis W D 1985 Anatomy and physiology of nociceptive ascending pathways. Philosophical Transactions of the Royal Society of London Series B 308: 253–268

Woolf C J 1983 Evidence for a central component of post-injury pain hypersensitivity. Nature 306: 686–688

Woolf C J 1984 Long term alteration in the excitability of the flexion reflex produced by peripheral tissue injury in the chronic decerebrate rat. Pain 18: 325–343

Woolf C J 1994 A new strategy for the treatment of inflammatory pain: prevention or elimination of central sensitisation. Drugs 47: 1–9

Woolf C J, Costigan M 1999 Transcriptional and posttranslational plasticity and the generation of inflammatory pain. Proceedings of the National Academy of Sciences of the United States of America 96: 7723–7730

Woolf C J, Doubell T P 1994 The pathophysiology of chronic pain: increased sensitivity to low threshold $A\beta$-fibre inputs. Current Opinion in Neurobiology 4: 525–534

Woolf C J, Mannion R J 1999 Neuropathic pain: aetiology, symptoms, mechanisms, and management: Lancet 353: 1959–1964

Woolf C J, Salter M W 2000 Neuronal plasticity: increasing the gain in pain. Science 288: 1765–1768

Woolf C J, Shortland P, Coggeshall R E 1992 Peripheral nerve injury triggers central sprouting of myelinated afferents. Nature 355: 75–78

Woolf C J, Safieh-Garabedian B, Ma Q-P, Crilly P, Winter J 1994 Nerve growth factor contributes to the generation of inflammatory sensory hypersensitivity. Neuroscience 62: 327–331

Wright A, Thurnwald P, O'Callaghan J, Smith J, Vixenzino B 1994 Hyperalgesia in tennis elbow patients. Journal of Musculoskeletal Pain 2: 83–97

Zhuo M, Gebhart G F 1990 Spinal cholinergic and monoaminergic receptors mediate descending inhibition from the nuclei reticularis gigantocellularis and gigantocellularis pars alpha in the rat. Brain Research 535: 67–78

Zhuo M, Gebhart G F 2002 Modulation of noxious and non-noxious spinal mechanical transmission from the rostral medial medulla in the rat. Journal of Neurophysiology 88: 2928–2941

Chapter 13

The effect of pain on motor control

M. Galea

INTRODUCTION

Pain involves a complex series of sensory and behavioural responses. Under normal circumstances, pain is the consequence of stimuli that either threaten or cause injury (Willis 1989). The responses to such stimuli include not only the perception of pain which may have a range of sensory qualities, but also responses such as arousal, distress, somatic and autonomic reflexes and endocrine changes. Such stimuli activate a sequence of events involving nociceptors, ascending somatosensory pathways, the thalamus and the cerebral cortex. Motivational–affective responses are triggered by another, related, system that operates in parallel with this sensory–discriminative system (Melzack & Casey 1968). Even the memory of pain can condition behaviour (fear avoidance). Musculoskeletal pain influences motor performance and because of this, the behaviour of a person in pain is an important element of an assessment by a health professional. Since the biological role of pain has been regarded as a protective one, the commonly observed lack of mobility, choice of posture and/or avoidance of movement of the person in pain have been interpreted as protective mechanisms that avoid further injury. While this is a logical response of the human system to acute pain, it does not serve a useful purpose in chronic pain situations and does not provide a framework for rehabilitation.

Despite the high prevalence of pain arising from deep structures such as muscle and articular tissues, much of our knowledge about mechanisms of acute and chronic pain has been derived from studies of the effects of nociceptive cutaneous stimuli in experimental animals, experimental subjects and people in pain. However, although it might appear reasonable to generalize these findings to pain produced by stimulation of deep tissues (muscle, joints and viscera), clinical studies suggest that there may be important differences between cutaneous and deep pain. This review will focus on the effects of deep pain on motor control. While there have been a large number of studies that have investigated changes in reflexes in response to a painful stimulus, more recent work has identified changes in the patterns of muscle activation in response to pain. These findings will be discussed with reference to motor control theories.

One of the problems in using painful stimuli in the experimental situation is stimulus control. Unlike stimuli used for the study of other sensory systems which can be well-defined and repeatedly applied, painful stimuli are difficult to control, and their repeated application can dramatically alter the behaviour of the sensory receptors (Willis 1989). There are also difficulties in interpretation of studies of motor behaviour of subjects with clinical pain disorders because of the variety of conditions and heterogeneity within these populations. In order to investigate the mechanisms underlying changes in motor performance, a number of experimental models in both animals and humans have been developed. Intramuscular injections of hypertonic (5%) saline, introduced in the 1930s by Kellgren (1938), are being used more commonly to induce pain in previously pain-free subjects. Muscle pain induced by hypertonic saline appears to have very similar characteristics to the subjectively perceived qualities and the motor performance effects of clinical musculoskeletal pain (Arendt-Nielsen et al 1996). The muscles selected for injection are those usually affected in clinical conditions. Thus, injections have been made into paraspinal muscles and muscles of the jaw, wrist and lower leg. Animal models have been developed for acute joint inflammation or arthritis involving the injection of kaolin (aluminium silicate) and carrageenan (a sulphated polysaccharide) into a joint. The injection of complete Freund's Adjuvant into a joint provides a model for a chronic inflammatory condition. In both models, joint swelling and increased temperature are observed, along with behavioural changes such as limping, guarding of the affected limb and hyperalgesia to heat and mechanical stimuli. Such experimental models of joint pain cannot be used in humans for obvious reasons, although some researchers have injected saline into the knee joint to cause an artificial effusion (Hopkins et al 2000). Investigations of the effects of joint pain in humans have focused on clinical subjects with acute joint sprains or chronic joint conditions.

DIFFERENCES BETWEEN CUTANEOUS AND DEEP PAIN

Sites of termination of nociceptive afferents in the dorsal horn

Cutaneous nociceptive afferents have well-circumscribed termination sites in the dorsal horn, typically up to 500 microns in the rostrocaudal direction. Deep nociceptive afferents, on the other hand, especially those innervating visceral tissues, have an extensive longitudinal distribution over several segments in the dorsal horn (Sugiura et al 1989). Dorsal horn neurons responsive to these inputs often have very large receptive fields and receive convergent somatic and visceral inputs. This multisegmental distribution may account for the diffuse and poorly localized nature of deep pain sensations. Cutaneous and deep afferents involved in nociception also differ in the laminar distribution of their terminals in the spinal cord. The superficial dorsal horn (laminae I and II) is the site of termination of myelinated and unmyelinated cutaneous nociceptive afferents, whereas deep afferents (from muscles and joints) involved in nociception terminate in lamina I and/or in laminae IV and V (Mense 1986, Craig et al 1988, Hoheisel et al 1989, Yu & Mense 1990). Nociceptive-specific neurons are predominantly in lamina I and the outer part of lamina II, whereas wide-dynamic range cells are more concentrated in lamina V. These differences in terminal projections imply that there are different intraspinal connections and therefore differential central processing of cutaneous and deep inputs occurs in the dorsal horn.

Referral of pain

Mechanosensitive receptive fields (RF) of muscle nociceptors extend over a small portion of the muscle (Mense & Meyer 1985). At the level of dorsal horn, RFs of neurons processing information from muscle nociceptors are also small, but many of the cells have multiple RFs from deep tissues and often additional input from the skin. The multiplicity of RFs and the convergence from skin and deep tissues provide support for the convergence–projection theory (Ruch 1946) and may explain the referral of deep pain to cutaneous regions as well as the diffuse nature of deep pain sensations. This is exemplified by the results of an experiment in which hypertonic saline was injected into masseter muscle. There was a loss of mechanosensitivity to threshold level monofilament stimuli applied to facial skin, not only at the site of pain but also on the contralateral side (Stohler et al 2001). This suggests that muscle nociceptors excite neurons in the trigeminal nucleus caudalis that suppress thalamic transmission from touch receptors on both sides of the face. The number of dorsal horn cells that receive information exclusively from muscle nociceptors appears to be relatively small. The more medially a cell is located in the dorsal horn the more distal is the site of its deep receptive field (Yu & Mense 1990). This somatotopic arrangement may be important for the control of local reflexes.

Muscle pain

Nociceptors are found throughout skeletal muscle, most densely in the region of tendons, fascia and aponeuroses (Stacey 1969). There is a view that muscle pain may become chronic through a series of vicious cycles. Lesions of muscle are likely to induce the release of endogenous sensitizing and pain-producing substances such as kinins and prostaglandins. These substances cause vasodilation and may cause local oedema in high concentrations. The increase in interstitial pressure may compress veins, leading to venous congestion and ischaemia. Ischaemia, in turn, is a powerful promoting factor for the release of nociceptive substances such as bradykinin or prostaglandin E_2. These have a sensitizing effect on nociceptors. Strong input from muscle nociceptors can lead to increases in the excitability of dorsal horn neurons and a contribution to central sensitization, forming a vicious circle (Mense 1991). Ischaemia may lead to failure of the calcium pump and local contracture, which may impair local circulation and enhance the ischaemia. Such a mechanism has been proposed for the development and maintenance of trigger points (Simons 1990).

Deep somatic pain has been associated with local increases of muscle tone (Travell & Simons 1983). The term 'vicious cycle' has also been given to a process whereby nociceptive afferent fibres stimulated by a painful lesion activate gamma motoneurons, which increases the discharge rate of the muscle spindles. This leads to activation of the muscle via monosynaptic connections with the alpha motoneuron and hypertonus in the affected muscles (Johansson & Sojka 1991). This in turn leads to ischaemia and the processes described above. This model is discussed further below.

Joint pain

Nociceptors in joints are located in the joint capsule and ligaments, bone, periosteum, articular fat pads and around blood vessels, but not in the joint cartilage (Wyke 1981). In conditions such as osteoarthritis, joint pain is the major symptom, with movement related pain the most common type of pain reported. The stimulus for pain in the chronic stages is most probably mechanical, since the anatomy of the joint is abnormal and leads to mechanical stresses on the capsule, ligaments and peri-articular tissues. Some inflammation may occur, leading to the release of chemical stimuli. Weakness has been observed in muscles surrounding a painful joint, although it is not clear that pain is the stimulus for this (Shakespeare et al 1985, Fahrer et al 1988, Fischer-Rasmussen et al 2001).

Increased background activity as well as increased responses to noxious and innocuous joint movement in Aβ, Aδ and C afferent fibres have been observed following acute inflammation. 'Silent nociceptors' are neurons that do not respond to peripheral mechanical stimuli in normal intact tissue, but begin to respond to innocuous and noxious stimuli, as well as to pressure and joint movement following joint inflammation (Schaible & Schmidt, 1988).

PAIN AND THE BRAIN

A matrix of structures in the nervous system has been identified as being variably activated during pain experience. The type, duration and location of stimulus differs considerably between clinical studies (neuropathic pain, idio-

pathic pain, cancer pain and post-stroke pain have all been studied). Experimental stimuli include ethanol injection, hot and cold probes, and each pain stimulus has varied with respect to intensity and quality.

The thalamus represents the final link in the transmission of impulses to the cerebral cortex, processing almost all sensory and motor information prior to its transfer to cortical areas. There is a differential pattern of connectivity of afferent information in the thalamus, with spinothalamic afferents mediating the sensory–discriminative aspects of pain terminating in the ventral posterolateral nucleus, and medial thalamic nuclei (the central lateral nucleus, the intralaminar complex and the mediodorsal nucleus), receiving additional information from the reticular formation, the cerebellum, and globus pallidus (see Galea 2002 for review). The diffuse projections of the intralaminar nuclei to many different areas of the cortex have been considered to be part of a non-specific arousal system, but it is also possible that their role is concerned with affective states induced by a painful stimulus (see Galea 2002 for review).

The basal ganglia are associated with planned action (Brooks et al 1993) and movement (Colebatch et al 1991). Their connections through the thalamus with the prefrontal cortex, supplementary motor cortex, motor cortex and anterior congulate cortex (Côte & Crutcher 1991) form a circuit associated with motor preparation or response selection. A number of brain stem structures, including the peri-aqueductal grey matter (Bernard & Bandler 1998) and the reticular formation, have extensive connections with all levels of the nervous system and are involved in the nociceptive, autonomic and motor systems as well as in pain modulation.

Multiple cortical areas are activated by painful stimuli, including the primary somatosensory cortex (Bushnell et al 1999), secondary somatosensory cortex, anterior cingulate cortex (Talbot et al 1991), insula, prefrontal cortex (Treede et al 1999) and supplementary motor area (Coghill et al 1994). These cortical regions also give rise to corticospinal projection (Galea & Darian-Smith 1994). This distributed activation of cerebral structures reflects the complex nature of pain, involving discriminative, affective, autonomic and motor components (Coghill et al 1994). Parietal areas are mainly concerned with the sensory–discriminative aspects whereas frontal–limbic connections subserve the affective dimension of pain experience.

Corticospinal projections are the only direct link between the sensorimotor cortex and the spinal cord and form a parallel, distributed system arising from cortical areas with complex cortical and thalamic interconnections, and converging on different parts of the spinal circuitry. There are projections to all laminae of the dorsal horn, mainly from postcentral cortical areas, including laminae containing spinothalamic neurons (Coulter & Jones 1977, Cheema et al 1984, Ralston & Ralston 1985). Precentral cortical areas project predominantly to laminae VII and VIII, with neurons from primary motor cortex projecting directly onto motoneurons in lamina IX (Galea & Darian-Smith 1997, Maier et al 1997). The dorsal caudal cingulate area projects to the dorsal portion of the intermediate zone of the spinal cord (Dum & Strick 1996). It must be emphasized that apart from the direct projections to motoneurons, the majority of these corticospinal projections terminate on interneurons that are also part of spinal circuits involved in movement. The 'state' of the interneurons is dependent on the combined influence on descending pathways, spinal interactions and afferent input and is related to the upcoming motor task.

It is well known that stimulation of corticospinal projections from primary and secondary somatosensory areas can result in primary afferent depolarization (PAD) in fibres of the dorsal root (Carpenter et al 1963, Andersen et al 1964). Stimulation of sensorimotor cortex can elicit both excitatory and inhibitory responses in dorsal horn neurons, particularly in laminae IV and V (Lundberg et al 1962, Wall 1967, Fetz 1968). Corticospinal projections to the superficial laminae from primary somatosensory cortex may directly modulate nociceptive-specific neurons (Cheema et al 1984). Posterior parietal cortex has connections with the primary somatosensory cortex and other polymodal association areas, including the limbic system (Cavada & Goldman-Rakic 1989) and is part of a general attentional system. The cingulate cortex is involved in affective and motor behaviour (Devinsky et al 1995). This region contains neurons that fire in anticipation of pain and could therefore be involved in avoidance behaviour (Koyama et al 1998). The insula receives converging information about all five sensory modalities and has extensive connections with the limbic system and the spinal cord (see Galea 2002 for review). The role of many of these areas in the control of movement is still under investigation. However all these regions, through the corticospinal tract, may exert a modulatory effect on both motor and sensory functions, including pain.

CHANGES IN REFLEX ACTIVITY IN RESPONSE TO PAIN

Measures of reflex activity (H reflex, nociceptive reflex and blink reflex) have been used in human subjects as an index of subjective pain, as they correlate with other physiological parameters and with verbal report (Gracely 1994). However, changes in reflex activity have been reported in relation to muscle or joint pain. Reflexes are important elements of motor activity, first identified and categorized in the 19th century by Marshall Hall (1790–1857), but described clearly as a structural and functional entity by Sherrington and co-workers in the early part of the 20th century. Sherrington's view of the reflex as an elementary unit of behaviour dominated the field of motor control until recently. A brief review of the best known reflexes mediated by the spinal cord, and categorized in terms of their main sensory input, provides a useful framework for later discussion of motor control theories.

Stretch reflex

The largest diameter sensory nerves, the Ia fibres from muscle spindles, make monosynaptic excitatory synapses on their own motoneurons and disynaptic inhibitory synapses onto antagonist motoneurons. This reflex is induced by stretching of muscle spindles and results in contraction of the stretched muscle and reciprocal inhibition of the antagonist. Muscle spindles themselves are innervated by gamma motoneurons, which regulate the sensitivity of the muscle spindle to stretch (Fig. 13.1A).

Tension feedback reflex

The large diameter group II fibres from the Golgi tendon organs (GTOs) make disynaptic inhibitory connections with motoneurons and excitatory connections with antagonist (inverse myotatic reflex). The effects on the motoneurons from a given muscle are the reverse of those in the stretch reflex. The GTOs are especially sensitive to tension arising from muscle contraction. The effect of a muscle contraction is to decrease the amount of contraction of that muscle but increase the excitation of opposing muscles. Combined with the stretch reflex, the inverse myotatic reflex contributes to overall muscle stiffness. The γ motor innervation of spindles keeps the muscle under resting tension and the GTO becomes exquisitely sensitive to tension changes due to active muscle contraction (Shepherd 1994) (Fig. 13.1B).

Group II reflexes

The group II afferents from muscle spindles arise from the group II (flower spray) endings in chain fibres and make disynaptic connections onto motoneurons. Excitatory connections are directed mainly to flexor muscles, and inhibitory connections to extensor muscles (Fig. 13.1C).

Flexor reflex

A noxious stimulus applied to skin or muscle characteristically produces withdrawal of the affected limb. This is termed the flexor reflex, and can be mediated by a wide range of receptors collectively referred to as the flexor reflex afferents (FRAs) (Eccles & Lundberg 1959). Where Sherrington (1910) described the flexion reflex as a mechanism for withdrawing a limb from noxious stimuli, Lundberg promoted the concept that the FRA systems are used during normal movements (Lundberg et al 1987) (Fig. 13.1D).

Reflex changes following painful stimuli

Withdrawal reflexes

Noxious stimulation of articular or muscle tissues can evoke activation of a limb flexion reflex (Gardner 1950,

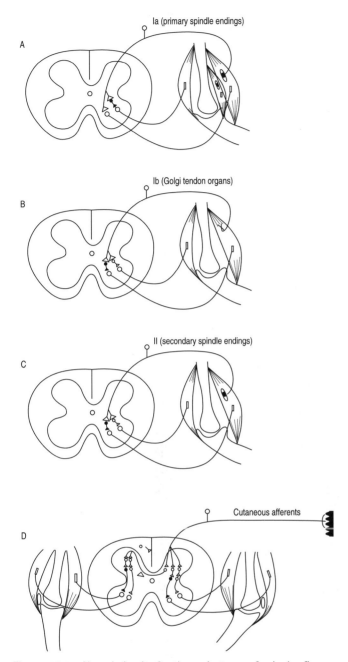

Figure 13.1 Neural circuits for the main types of spinal reflexes. Inhibitory terminals and interneurons are filled (black), while excitatory connections are unfilled (white). A: Stretch reflex – detects phasic stretch of muscle and contributes to the control of movement. B: Inverse myotatic reflex – detects tension and contributes to the control of muscle force and stiffness. C: Group II reflex – detects steady stretch of muscle and contributes to postural control. D: Flexor reflex – detects harmful stimuli and serves to withdraw a limb from harm.

Ia (primary spindle endings)

Ib (Golgi tendon organs)

II (secondary spindle endings)

Cutaneous afferents

Paintal 1961, Mense 1986, He et al 1988). Injection of algesic chemicals into the temporomandibular joint results in a sustained reflex increase in activity in tongue and jaw-opening muscles; weaker excitatory effects are observed in jaw-closing muscles (Broton & Sessle 1988). These effects

have been viewed as responses that serve to protect the limb from further noxious stimulation, and as mechanisms counteracting excessive movement so as to prevent further damage to the joint or muscle tissues (Schaible & Schmidt 1985, Mense 1986, He et al 1988). Although painful stimuli may evoke flexion, painful stimuli are not necessary for segmental activation of FRA pathways. Nociceptive afferent input presumably contacts spinal circuits involved both in flexion reflexes and perception of pain. Indeed, there is evidence for withdrawal reflexes in response to pain that are distinct from spinal motor pathways producing flexion (Schouenberg & Sjölund 1983, McCrea 1994). High intensity stimulation of limb muscle afferents can produce a prolonged facilitation of the flexor reflex (Wall & Woolf 1984) and this effect may be related to pathophysiological responses to injury or inflammation.

Stretch reflexes

There is conflicting evidence about the influence of pain on stretch reflexes. Activation of muscle nociceptors leads to increased fusimotor firing and increased sensitivity of the Ia muscle spindle afferents to stretch (Appelberg et al 1983, Johansson et al 1993, Pedersen et al 1997, Wang et al 2000). In contrast, Mense & Skeppar (1991) demonstrated inhibition of extensor gamma motoneurons following induced inflammatory muscle pain in the cat. There have been equivocal results in human experimental subjects. Matre et al (1998) demonstrated facilitation of the stretch reflex in the soleus and tibialis anterior muscles following injection of hypertonic saline, although without a corresponding increase in the amplitude of the H reflex, indicating that the excitability of the alpha motoneuron pool was unchanged. This increase in the stretch reflex disappeared with voluntary contraction of the muscle under investigation. On the other hand, Zedka et al (1999) found no increase in reflex activity in erector spinae muscles injected with hypertonic saline. These discrepancies could be partly due to differences in the techniques used to elicit reflex responses as well as differences in the function of the experimental muscle selected.

ABNORMAL MUSCLE ACTIVITY IN CHRONIC PAIN

Muscle hyperactivity

Observations of increased muscle tone associated with painful muscles (Travell & Simons 1983) led to attempts to explain these findings. One proposal is the facilitation of the gamma motor system by muscle pain (Johansson & Sojka 1991). The gamma motoneurons receive information from a wide variety of inputs, including the skin and joint ligaments, which contributes to the coordination of muscle tone, posture and movement. Group III and IV muscle afferents (comprising mechanoreceptors and nociceptors) are known to have a powerful influence on gamma motoneurons (Johansson et al 1989, Mense & Skeppar

1991). The hypothesis proposed by Johansson & Sojka involves stimulation of group III and IV nociceptors by chemical inflammatory mediators released by muscle contraction. Metabolites released during muscle contraction have been shown to activate group III and IV receptors (Rybicki et al 1985). These nociceptors synapse with and excite gamma motoneurons that stimulate muscle spindles, causing an increase in the output of the group Ia and II afferents. This stimulates alpha motoneurons, causing further muscle contractions that generate further metabolites and complete a positive feedback loop. Increased activity in the group II afferents excites the gamma motoneurons, which stimulate the muscle spindle. This constitutes a second positive feedback loop that can be maintained without group III or IV nociceptive input (Gladden et al 1998).

There is evidence that increased concentrations of metabolites from muscle contractions, including lactic acid, potassium chloride (Jovanovic et al 1990), arachidonic acid (Djupsjöbacka et al 1994), bradykinin (Djupsjöbacka et al 1995, Pedersen et al 1997) and 5-HT (Djupsjöbacka et al 1995), result in increases in gamma motoneuron activity and sensitivity of the muscle spindle afferents, thereby leading to increases in muscle stiffness. Increased gamma motoneuron activity has been induced by fatiguing contractions (Nelson & Hutton 1985, Ljubisavljevic & Anastasijevic 1994). Experimentally induced pain has been shown to be associated with changes in the fusimotor system (Thunberg et al 2002). Neck and paraspinal muscles are rich in muscle spindles (Richmond & Abrahams 1975, Amonoo-Kuofi 1982, Boyd-Clark et al 2002). These spindles, many of which lack a bag_1 fibre, are controlled by the static fusimotor system and concerned mainly with postural muscle activity (Price & Dutia 1989). Thus changes in muscle stiffness in these muscles are likely to cause disturbances in motor coordination and proprioception. Indeed, stimulation of fusimotor activity through application of muscle vibration to neck muscles has been shown to cause motor and balance disturbances (Lund 1980, Biguer et al 1988).

Muscle inhibition

Despite this experimental support for the Johansson–Sojka hypothesis, clinical observations suggest that there is inhibition of muscle activity during muscle pain. An alternative model, the pain–adaptation model, proposes that muscle dysfunction is a normal protective adaptation and is not one of the causes of pain (Lund et al 1993). Nociceptive input from painful muscle, joint and skin converge on interneurons at the segmental level and as a consequence motoneurons to the painful muscles are inhibited. In this way the amplitude of movement will be limited and potentially prevent further damage.

The relationship between muscle pain and muscle activity has been examined at rest, during static contractions and during dynamic tasks (Graven-Nielsen et al 1997). A review of this issue is complicated by different experimental paradigms and subject types. EMG activity has been shown to be higher at rest in some studies of subjects with induced muscle pain (Cobb et al 1975) but studies of patients in pain, for example low back pain (Nouwen & Bush 1984, Sherman 1985), myofascial pain (Durette et al 1991) or experimentally induced muscle pain (Stohler et al 1996), have shown no such increased activity.

The maximum voluntary contraction in painful muscles has been shown to be reduced in experimentally induced pain (Graven-Nielsen et al 1997) and in a number of disorders, including temporomandibular joint dysfunction (Molin 1972), fibromyalgia (Jacobsen & Danneskiold-Samsoe 1987, Bäckman et al 1988) and low back pain (Thorstensson & Arvidson 1982, Kankaanpää et al 1998).

Studies that have investigated the effect of pain on movement have shown that there is an inhibition of the painful muscle and facilitation of its antagonist. In activities such as walking there are changes in the coordination of muscle activity leading to reductions in movement amplitude and reduced stride time following experimentally induced muscle pain in muscles of the lower leg (Graven-Nielsen et al 1997, Madeleine et al 1999a). Zedka et al (1999) showed that injections of hypertonic saline into the erector spinae on one side resulted in a reduction in the velocity and range of voluntary trunk motion and a reduction in EMG amplitude in the affected muscle, consistent with the pain–adaptation model of Lund et al (1993). When subjects voluntarily overcame this guarding strategy and produced identical trunk movements before and during pain, the reduced amplitude in EMG activity persisted, indicating that the observed changes involve more than just a strategy to reduce movement. In contrast, no pain-induced changes in motor unit activity have been observed in cases of experimentally induced pain in extensor carpi ulnaris (Birch et al 2000). Changes in muscle activity and coordination during muscle pain therefore appear to be dependent on the functional role of the muscle and the level of muscle activity.

These experimental manipulations can only provide an indication of the effect of acute pain. Other investigations have identified specific deficits in the chronic pain situation. Patients with chronic low back pain fatigue faster (Kankaanpää et al 1998) and have poorer balance performance and delayed postural response times compared with healthy control subjects (Radebold et al 2000, 2001, Newcomer et al 2002). Investigations of patients with chronic low back pain have identified a deficit in the recruitment of the transversus abdominis during a postural perturbation produced by rapid arm movement (Hodges & Richardson 1996) or movement of the lower limb (Hodges & Richardson 1998), resulting in sub-optimal control of the lumbar spine in preparation for movement. A study in normal subjects has shown that trunk muscle fatigue is one factor that can alter anticipatory postural adjustments (Allison & Henry 2002) and there is individual variability in the preparatory strategies used to deal with sudden trunk loading (Lavender et al 1993). Such impairments of postural control could compromise the stability of the lumbar spine, making a person vulnerable to further injury. A similar phenomenon has been described in patients with chronic wrist pain. Such patients demonstrate a disturbance of fine motor control of the wrist on the unaffected side and it has been argued that this incoordination might result in additional overuse injury (Smeulders et al 2002).

Wasting of another muscle contributing to stability of the lumbar spine, multifidus, has been reported in patients with low back pain, with the site of wasting corresponding to the clinically determined level of symptoms (Hides et al 1994), suggesting a localized reflex inhibition. Reflex inhibition of the quadriceps has also been associated with knee joint pathology, especially effusion (Shakespeare et al 1985, Young et al 1987), and patients with patellofemoral pain are reported to have deficits in the timing of activation of the vastus medialis during a functional stepping task (Cowan et al 2001). While these findings are consistent with the pain–adaptation model, the resultant motor deficit not only limits the amount of movement, but also makes the affected region vulnerable to further damage. However, it is not known whether these motor deficits are compensatory mechanisms developed in response to pain or whether they are, in fact, predisposing factors to injury.

Wider effects

It also needs to be highlighted that nociceptive stimuli can have effects that extend beyond the local region. Nociceptive stimuli applied to extensor digitorum brevis in the foot produces a depression of Ia excitation and Ib inhibition of the soleus motoneurons through intercalated interneurons (Rossi et al 1999). Conversely, facilitation of soleus motoneurons has been observed following the induction of an artificial knee effusion, which usually inhibits the quadriceps (Hopkins et al 2000). Injection of hypertonic saline into the trapezius muscle on one side prior to the performance of a low-load, repetitive work task resulted not only in a reduction of muscle activity in the injected muscle but also a reduced working rhythm, a tendency to increase the amplitude of arm movements and a prolongation of the duration of the role of the non-affected arm in the task (Madeleine et al 1999b). Changes in rhythmic activity, such as chewing (Westberg et al 1997) or locomotion (Martin & Arendt-Nielsen 2000), following hypertonic saline into the masseter or soleus respectively, demonstrate that the performance of other muscle groups participating in the motor patterns is also affected, and possibly reflecting a change in the underlying motor programmes.

These studies have generated much data; however, there is still no clear consensus as to the effect of pain on motor control. This is perhaps partly because of the tendency of many of these studies to consider only local stimulus–response issues. An examination of motor control

theories provides a context for drawing together some of these findings.

MODELS OF MOTOR CONTROL

Motor control models and theories have generally been developed around the following questions:

1. What is the basic unit of nervous system organization in relation to the basic unit of motor function?
2. What principles apply to the organization of motor control?

Reflex model

The reflex model of motor control originated with Sherrington (1947) who found that specific stimuli such as stretch or pain induced distinct stereotyped movements called reflexes. An underlying assumption of this model is that afferent input is a prerequisite for motor output. The concept of feedback in relation to motor control was introduced much later with the view that the human motor system might be controlled in ways similar to the control of mechanical systems. One such system is a servomechanism that relies on feedback signals to maintain a constant output.

Building on Sherrington's (1947) original notion of reflexes as elementary units of motor behaviour (see Fig. 13.1), successive researchers have described the circuitry by which reflex pathways were coordinated. Lundberg (1979) showed that different reflex pathways may share common interneurons. One of the best examples of this principle is the Ia interneuron. This neuron not only mediates inhibition of antagonistic muscles in the stretch reflex, but is also part of an inhibitory pathway from flexor reflex afferents onto motoneurons, and a nodal point for control of spinal neurons by descending pathways such as the corticospinal, rubrospinal and vestibulospinal tracts which are important for skilled movement and postural tasks (Fig. 13.2).

Hierarchical model

The concept of the nervous system being organized as a hierarchy has a long history in clinical neurology. For example, we distinguish between the lower motoneuron in the spinal cord and the upper motoneuron in the brain stem or cerebral cortex. The neurologist Hughlings Jackson (1835–1911) formulated the idea that there were successive levels of motor control in the nervous system, with the control of automatic or reflexive movements by lower levels and purposive movements by higher levels (Fig. 13.3). It is now realized that motor control in mammals is not strictly hierarchical and the historical distinction between voluntary and reflex control is becoming increasingly blurred. For example, every voluntary movement is associated with automatic postural adjustments that occur unconsciously.

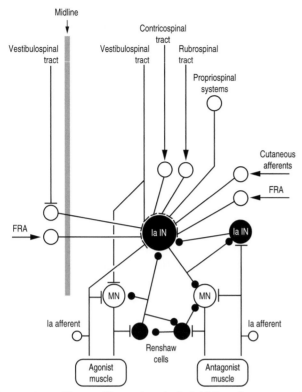

Figure 13.2 Diagram illustrating the Ia inhibitory interneuron (Ia IN) as an integrating node in a number of spinal circuits. Excitatory neurons and synaptic terminals are unfilled (white), inhibitory connections are filled (black). Reproduced from Shepherd 1998 with permission of Oxford University Press Inc.
Key: FRA = flexor reflex afferents; MN = motoneuron; Ia afferent, sensory nerve from muscle spindle.

Many volitional actions are often adjusted automatically by sensory feedback.

There are two basic systems for control of movement: feedback or closed-loop systems and feedforward or open-loop systems. Feedback control is usually required for slow movements or those requiring accuracy and this type of

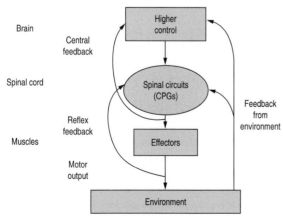

Figure 13.3 Connections of spinal circuits.
Key: CPG = central pattern generator.

control is typical during the early phases of skill acquisition. The control of movement fluctuates between feedback and feedforward modes of control. Rapid movements and well-learned movements are performed with feedforward control. Sensory information cannot be used during rapid movements because the movement occurs faster than the nervous system can process the sensory information.

The motor programme concept is based on an open-loop system of control and assumes that all movements are pre-planned and stored in memory until required for action. Motor programmes have been defined as sets of muscle commands that are structured before a movement sequence begins, and that allow the entire movement sequence to be performed without the influence of peripheral feedback. Such programmes contain details of the order and timing of events and the relative force to be exerted. An example of such programmes is the ability of the spinal cord to generate intrinsic rhythms or repeating patterns of muscle activity. Studies of both vertebrates and invertebrates have demonstrated that this property lies within neural circuits forming central pattern generators. Central pattern generators are recognized as key organizing principles for understanding the mechanisms of locomotion, and other rhythmical activities such as respiration. These circuits generate essential rhythmical features of the motor pattern and receive sensory feedback signals (see Fig. 13.3). However, the linear view that underlies the idea of a closed loop system, inputs, outputs, stimuli and responses, with feedback closing the loop, is only useful for simple systems. In a more complex system, the concept of feedback is inadequate.

Feedforward control models involve the delivery of information to other parts of the system to 'prepare' it for upcoming motor commands. Postural adjustments are an example of feedforward mechanisms and have been shown to precede self-initiated arm, leg and trunk movements to minimize postural instability that would otherwise have resulted (Lee 1980, Massion et al 1982, Frank & Earl, 1990). This type of control is dependent on the nervous system having an accurate internal model of the body and the external environment. An inappropriate internal model can lead to poor predictions about the sensory consequences of situations and actions, resulting in anticipatory movements that are ineffective or destabilizing (Horak 1991).

Systems model

It is not reasonable to assume that each individual neural and muscular component of the human body is controlled separately by the nervous system, as this would be a major computational task. Bernstein (1967) proposed a solution that the multiple degrees of freedom for movement are constrained to act as synergies or coordinative structures (i.e. functional groups of muscles and joints that are constrained to act as a unit). Examples of these synergies are the postural movement strategies described by Horak & Nashner

(1986), which are used to recover stability in response to brief perturbations of the supporting surface (Fig. 13.4). In this view, control is exerted not over muscles or sensory receptors (reflex model) nor over muscle activation patterns (hierarchical model) but over abstract aspects of motor behaviour, such as the relations between kinematic variables and the accomplishment of task goals.

The dynamical action theory, an elaboration of systems theory, proposes that movement emerges naturally out of the complex interactions among many interconnected elements (physical, environmental and neural), without specific commands or motor programmes in the central nervous system.

At the core of the dynamical action theory is the notion that human behaviour is governed by a generic process of self-organization, which refers to the spontaneous formation of patterns and pattern change. This idea takes into account the coordinative relations of various parts of a system, as well as the environment in which the interaction between the parts takes place. The coordinative structures are the units of action and are functionally linked, but not necessarily mechanically linked (Kelso & Tuller 1984). This view of motor control, that is that musculoskeletal variables are not controlled individually but are partitioned into a smaller number of coordinative structures, has led to hypotheses about how these coordinative structures operate using the framework of task dynamics (Saltzman & Kelso, 1987). The critical issues are that the coordinative structures are constrained by the particular tasks that are being performed, and that the units of action are specified in dynamic terms rather than kinematic or muscular variables. Thus the task will determine many features of the action, such as movement trajectory for example. This might explain the conflicting observations on the effect of pain in different muscle groups that have different functional roles.

Nervous system changes

It needs to be recognized that neural representations of body parts and movements are labile throughout life, changing according to the amount they are activated by peripheral inputs. This phenomenon has been most graphically demonstrated by the experiments of Merzenich and colleagues (1983, 1984) in which the reorganized cortical representations of the hand in the primary somatosensory cortex were mapped in the monkey following peripheral nerve lesions or digit amputation (Fig. 13.5A). These findings, and others illustrating similar reorganization in other brain regions, indicate that topographic maps in the adult brain are not hard-wired, but can vary depending on spatial shifts in the collective activity of neurons with experience, a reorganization which is not haphazard but context-dependent. The brain itself, therefore, can be viewed as a dynamical system (Kelso 1995). Byl et al (1996) showed in monkeys that rapid, repetitive, highly stereotypic movements can actively degrade the cortical representations of sensory information guiding fine motor hand movements. This 'dedifferentiation' of sensory feedback information from the hand led to focal dystonia and subsequent lack of use of the hand (Fig. 13.5B). Similarly, altered use of a part of the body will change the cortical representation of that part in sensorimotor cortical areas, and may therefore lead to prolonged movement dysfunction.

A dynamical view of pain and motor control

Studying individual elements of movement has increased our knowledge of the component parts of movement, but it has not contributed a great deal to our understanding of the function of individual elements related to behaviour as a whole. There is still a lack of understanding about how these elements function together or change with altered input, such as a painful stimulus. What is clear from this review is that:

- groups of cells rather than single cells are the main units of activity in the nervous system
- functional synergies of muscles rather than single muscles are the main units of motor control and coordination of action
- there is distributed control of these systems.

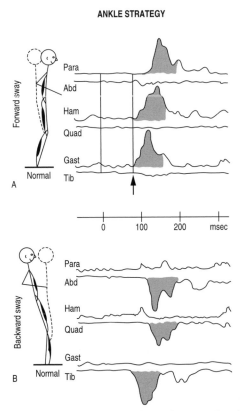

ANKLE STRATEGY

Figure 13.4 Muscle synergy and body motion associated with the ankle strategy for controlling forward sway (A) and backward sway (B). Reproduced from Horak & Nashner 1986 with permission of the American Physiological Society.

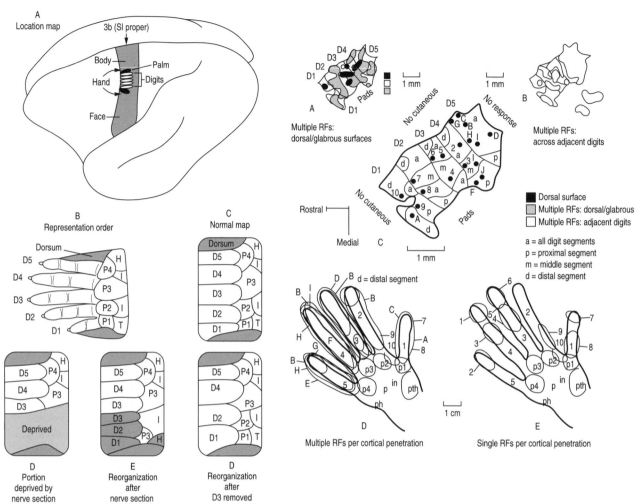

Figure 13.5   Left-hand panel: Reorganization of primary somatosensory cortex (area 3b) in owl monkeys. A: Dorsolateral view of an owl monkey brain showing the location of the hand representation within area 3b. B: Ventral surface of the hand split along the palm to reflect the somatotopic pattern of hand representation. C: Pattern of hand representation in area 3b. D: Portion of the hand representation deprived of normal activation by section of the median nerve. E: Somatotopic pattern of the reorganized cortex months after median nerve section. Most of the activation is from receptors on the dorsum of the digits 1–3. F: Reorganization after D3 removal. Digits and pads of the hand are traditionally numbered. Insular (I), hypothenar (H), and thenar (T) pads are indicated. Reproduced from Kaas 1992 with permission of MIT Press. Right-hand panel: Diagram illustrating an experience induced degradation of the hand representation in somatosensory cortex of a monkey following training on a hand-squeezing strategy. A, B, and C: Receptive fields on the hand and reconstruction of the topographic representations of the hand surface on the somatosensory cortex (area 3b) with penetration sites correlated with receptive fields on digits D and E, illustrating an abnormal 'map' of the hand. The magnitude of area 3b with multiple receptive fields was so extensive that separate drawings were necessary to clearly represent this (illustration A representing the overlap extending from the dorsal to the glabrous surface and illustration B representing the overlap to adjacent digits). D and E: Outlines of territories over which neurons were driven with receptive fields, larger than normal size, on broad hand surfaces, with abbreviations of the cortical penetration sites matched to the topographical drawing in illustration C. Reproduced from Byl et al 1997 with permission of the American Physical Therapy Association.

A reductionist approach investigating individual circuits is therefore unlikely to provide an indication of how the whole system operates, particularly with a multidimensional phenomenon such as pain.

Kelso (1995) has provided an example illustrating the key concepts of pattern formation that is useful for understanding how different elements may work together to bring about a coordinated whole. The Rayleigh–Bénard experiment involves heating a fluid from below and cooling it from above. This is an open system, activated by the appli-

cation of a temperature gradient. The fluid contains many molecules and as temperature increases slightly, the heat is dissipated among them in a random fashion, and there is no visible motion of the fluid. As temperature increases, the fluid now begins to move as a coordinated whole in an orderly rolling motion called convection rolls (Fig. 13.6A). The temperature gradient is the driving influence behind the motion, a so-called control parameter. However, this control parameter does not prescribe or contain the code for the emerging pattern. As Kelso (1995) states, rolling motions

Actions are modulated according to changing environmental circumstances, but there are 'rules', also known as constraints, that preserve qualitative aspects of a movement's structure. One of these is that timing of activity in components of a functional unit is generally independent of the amplitude of the activity. Constancy in timing relationships in muscle activity has been most clearly demonstrated in studies of locomotion, for example the duration of the step cycle decreases when speed of locomotion increases, and also in other rhythmical activities such as mastication (Grillner 1975). Since pain appears to disrupt qualitative aspects of movement such as timing of muscle activity in certain tasks (see, for example, Hodges & Richardson 1999, Martin & Arendt-Nielsen 2000), it is almost certainly a critical control parameter that can lead to radical alterations in the organization of motor activity and lead to dysfunctional movement patterns. Examples of this are the altered patterns of activity of the abdominal musculature in low back pain (Hodges & Richardson 1996, O'Sullivan et al 1997). Because of the adaptability of the nervous system, such patterns are likely to persist. This view of the motor control system provides a framework for understanding the effect of pain on motor activity, and a basis for the development of specific rehabilitation strategies to reverse the dysfunction.

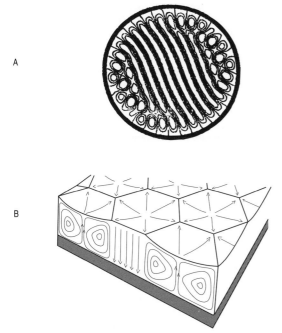

Figure 13.6 Convection patterns in fluid that is heated (refer to text for description). A reproduced from Kelso 1995 with permission of MIT Press. B reproduced from Velarde & Normand 1980 with permission of Alan D. Iselin.

are not the only possibilities. In an open container surface tension may also affect the flow, and its net effect is tesselation of the surface and the formation of hexagonal cells (Fig. 13.6B). Two quite distinct mechanisms can give rise to the same dynamic pattern, and conversely the same mechanism can give rise to different patterns, i.e. the mechanism—pattern relationship is not fixed.

KEYWORDS	
muscle pain	abnormal muscle activity
joint pain	motor control models
reflex activity	dynamical systems

References

Allison G T, Henry S M 2002 The influence of fatigue on trunk muscle response to sudden arm movements: a pilot study. Clinical Biomechanics 17: 414–417

Amonoo-Kuofi H S 1982 The number and distribution of muscle spindles in human intrinsic postvertebral muscles. Journal of Anatomy 135: 585–599

Andersen P, Eccles J C, Sears T A 1964 Cortically evoked depolarization of primary afferent fibers in the spinal cord. Journal of Neurophysiology 27: 63–77

Appelberg B, Hulliger M, Johansson H, Sojka P 1983 Actions on gamma-motoneurons elicited by electrical stimulation of group III muscle afferent fibres in the hind limb of the cat. Journal of Physiology 335: 275–292

Arendt-Neilsen L, Graven-Nielsen T, Svarrer H, Svensson P 1996 The influence of low back pain on muscle activity and coordination during gait: a clinical and experimental study. Pain 64: 231–240

Bäckman E, Bengtsson A, Bengtsoon M, Lennmarken C 1988 Skeletal muscle function in fibromyalgia: effect of regional sympathetic blockade with guanethidine. Acta Neurologica Scandinavica 77: 187–191

Bernard J F, Bandler R 1998 Parallel circuits for emotional coping behaviour: new pieces in the puzzle. Journal of Comparative Neurology 401: 429–436

Bernstein N A 1967 The coordination and regulation of movements. Pergamon Press, Elmsford, New York

Biguer B, Donaldson M L, Hein A, Jeannerod M 1988 Neck muscle vibration modifies the representation of visual motion and direction in man. Brain 111: 1405–1424

Birch L, Christensen H, Arendt-Nielsen L, Graven-Nielsen T, Søgaard K 2000 The influence of experimental muscle pain on motor unit activity during low-level contraction. European Journal of Applied Physiology 83: 200–206

Boyd-Clark L C, Briggs C A, Galea M P 2002 Muscle spindle distribution, morphology, and density in longus colli and multifidus muscles of the cervical spine. Spine 27: 694–701

Brooks D J 1993 Functional imaging in relation to parkinsonian syndromes. Journal of Neurological Sciences 115: 1–17

Broton J G, Sessle B J 1988 Reflex excitation of masticatory muscles induced by algesic chemicals applied to the temporomandibular joint of the cat. Archives of Oral Biology 33: 741–747

Bushnell M C, Duncan G H, Hofbauer R K, Ha B, Chen J-I, Carrier B 1999 Pain perception: is there a role for primary somatosensory cortex? Proceedings of the National Academy of Sciences USA 96: 7705–7709

Bly N N, Merzenich M M, Jenkins W M 1996 A primate genesis model of focal dystonia and repetitive strain injury.

I: Learning-induced dedifferentiation of the representation of the hand in the primary somatosensory cortex in adult monkeys. Neurology 76: 508–520

Bly N N, Merzenich M M, Cheung S, Bedenbaugh P, Nagarajan S S, Jenkins W M 1997 A primate model for studying focal dystonia and repetitive strain injury: effects on primary somatosensory cortex. Physical Therapy 77(3): 269–284

Carpenter D, Lundberg A, Norrsell U 1963 Primary afferent depolarization evoked from the sensorimotor cortex. Acta Physiologica Scandinavica 59: 126–142

Cavada C, Goldman-Rakic P S 1989 Posterior parietal cortex in rhesus monkey. II: Evidence for segregated corticocortical networks linking sensory and limbic areas with the frontal lobe. Journal of Comparative Neurology 287: 422–445

Cheema S S, Rustioni A, Whitsel B L 1984 Light and electron microscopic evidence for a direct corticospinal projection to superficial laminae of the dorsal horn in cats and monkeys. Journal of Comparative Neurology 225: 276–290

Cobb C R, de Vries H A, Urban R T, Luekens C A, Bagg R J 1975 Electrical activity in muscle pain. American Journal of Physical Medicine 54: 80–87

Coghill R C, Talbot J D, Evans A C, et al 1994 Distributed processing of pain and vibration by the human brain. Journal of Neuroscience 14: 4095–4108

Colebatch J G, Deiber M-P, Passingham R E, Friston K J, Frackowiak R S J 1991 Regional cerebral blood flow during voluntary arm and hand movements in human subjects. Journal of Neurophysiology 65: 1392–1401

Côté L, Crutcher M D 1991 The basal ganglia. In: Kandel E R, Schwartz J H, Jessell T M (eds) Principles of neural science, 3rd edn. Elsevier, New York, pp 647–659

Coulter J D, Jones E G 1977 Differential distribution of corticospinal projections from individual cytoarchitectonic fields in the monkey. Brain Research 129: 335–340

Cowan S M, Bennell K L, Hodges P W, Crossley K M, McConnell J 2001 Delayed onset of electromyographic activity of vastus medialis obliquus relative to vastus lateralis in subjects with patellofemoral pain syndrome. Archives of Physical Medicine and Rehabilitation 82: 183–189

Craig A D, Hepplemann B, Schaible H G 1988 The projection of the medial and posterior articular nerves of the cat's knee to the spinal cord. Journal of Comparative Neurology 276: 279–288

Devinsky O, Morrell M J, Vogt B A 1995 Contributions of anterior cingulate cortex to behaviour. Brain 118: 279–306

Djupsjöbacka M, Johansson H, Bergenheim M 1994 Influences on the γ-muscle spindle system from muscle afferents stimulated by increased intramuscular concentrations of arachidonic acid. Brain Research 663: 293–302

Djupsjöbacka M, Johansson H, Bergenheim M, Wenngren B I 1995 Influences on the γ-muscle spindle system from muscle afferents stimulated by increased intramuscular concentrations of bradykinin and 5-HT. Neuroscience Research 22: 325–333

Dum R P, Strick P L 1996 Spinal cord terminations of the medial wall motor areas in macaque monkeys. Journal of Neuroscience 16: 6513–6525

Durette M R, Rodriguez A A, Agre J C, Silverman J L 1991 Needle electromyographic evaluation of patients with myofascial or fibromyalgic pain. American Journal of Physical Medicine 70: 154–156

Eccles J C, Lundberg A 1959 Synaptic action in motoneurones by afferents which may evoke the flexion reflex. Archives Italiennes de Biologie 97: 199–221

Fahrer H, Rentsch H U, Gerber N J, Beyeler C, Hess C W, Grunig B 1988 Knee effusion and reflex inhibition of the quadriceps: a bar to effective retraining. Journal of Bone and Joint Surgery 70: 635–638

Fetz E E 1968 Pyramidal tract effects on interneurons in the cat lumbar dorsal horn. Journal of Neurophysiology 31: 69–80

Fischer-Rasmussen T, Krogsgaard M, Jensen D B, Dyhre-Poulsen P 2001 Inhibition of dynamic thigh muscle contraction by electrical stimulation of the posterior cruciate ligament in humans. Muscle Nerve 24: 1482–1488

Fox J L 1984 The brain's way of keeping touch. Science 225: 820–821

Frank J S, Earl M 1990 Coordination of posture and movement. Physical Therapy 70: 855–863

Galea M P 2002 The neuroanatomy of pain. In: Strong J, Unruh A, Wright A, Baxter G D (eds) Pain: a textbook for therapists. Churchill Livingstone, Edinburgh

Galea M P, Darian-Smith I 1994 Multiple corticospinal neuron populations in the macaque monkey are specified by their unique cortical origins, spinal terminations and connections. Cerebral Cortex 4: 166–194

Galea M P, Darian-Smith I 1997 Corticospinal projection patterns following unilateral cervical spinal cord section in the newborn and juvenile macaque monkey. Journal of Comparative Neurology 381: 282–306

Gardner E 1950 Reflex muscular responses to stimulation of articular nerves in the cat. American Journal of Physiology 161: 133–141

Gladden M H, Jankowska E, Czarkowska-Bauch J 1998 New observations on coupling between group II muscle afferents and feline γ motoneurons. Journal of Physiology 512: 507–520

Gracely R H 1994 Studies of pain in normal man. In: Wall P D, Melzack R (eds) Textbook of pain. Churchill-Livingstone, Edinburgh, pp 315–355

Graven-Nielsen T, Svensson P, Arendt-Nielsen L 1997 Effects of experimental muscle pain on muscle activity and co-ordination during static and dynamic motor function. Electroencephalography and Clinical Neurophysiology 105: 156–164

Grillner S 1975 Locomotion in vertebrates. Physiological Reviews 55: 247–304

He X, Proske U, Schaible H-G, Schmidt R F 1988 Acute inflammation of the knee joint in the cat alters responses of flexor motoneurons to leg movements. Journal of Neurophysiology 59: 326–340

Hides J A, Stokes M J, Saide M, Jull G A, Cooper D H 1994 Evidence of lumbar multifidus muscle wasting ipsilateral to symptoms in patients with acute/subacute low back pain. Spine 19: 165–172

Hodges P W, Richardson C A 1996 Inefficient muscular stabilization of the lumbar spine associated with low back pain. Spine 21: 2640–2650

Hodges P W, Richardson C A 1998 Delayed postural contraction of transversus abdominis in low back pain associated with movement of the lower limb. Journal of Spinal Disorders 11: 46–56

Hodges P W, Richardson C A 1999 Altered trunk muscles recruitment in people with low back pain with upper limb movement at different speeds. Archives of Physical Medicine and Rehabilitation 80: 1005–1012

Hoheisel U, Lehmann-Willenbrock E, Mense 1989 Termination patterns of identified group II and III afferent fibres from deep tissues in the spinal cord of the cat. Neuroscience 28: 495–507

Hopkins J T, Ingersoll C D, Edwards J E, Cordova M L 2000 Changes in soleus motoneuron pool excitability after artificial knee joint effusion. Archives of Physical Medicine and Rehabilitation 81: 1199–1203

Horak F 1991 Assumptions underlying motor control for neurologic rehabilitation. In: Lister M (ed) Contemporary management of motor control problems. Proceedings of the II Step Conference. Foundation for Physical Therapy USA, Alexandria, Virginia, pp 11–27

Horak F, Nashner L 1986 Central programming of postural movements: adaptation to altered support surface configurations. Journal of Neurophysiology 55: 1369–1381

Jacobsen S, Danneskiold-Samsoe B 1987 Isometric and isokinetic muscle strength in patients with fibrositis syndrome: new characteristics for a difficult definable category of patient. Scandinavian Journal of Rheumatology 16: 61–65

Johansson H, Sojka P 1991 Pathological mechanisms involved in genesis and spread of muscular tension in occupational muscle pain and in chronic musculoskeletal pain syndromes: a hypothesis. Medical Hypotheses 35(3): 196–203

Johansson H, Sjölander P, Sojka P, Wadell I 1989 Different fusimotor reflexes from the ipsi- and contralateral hindlimbs of the cat assessed in the same primary muscle spindle afferents. Journal of Physiology (Paris) 83: 1–12

Johansson H, Djupsjöbacka M, Sjölander P 1993 Influences on the gamma-muscle spindle system from muscle afferents stimulated by KCl and lactic acid. Neuroscience Research 16: 49–57

Jovanovic K, Anastasijevic R, Vuco J 1990 Reflex effects on γ fusimotor neurones of chemically induced discharges in small-diameter muscle afferents in decerebrate cats. Brain Research 521: 89–94

Kaas J H 1992 The reorganization of sensory and motor maps in adult mammals. In: Gazzaniga M (ed) The cognitive neurosciences. MIT Press, Cambridge, Massachusetts

Kankaanpää M, Taimela S, Laaksonen D, Hanninen O, Airaksinen O 1998 Back and hip extensor fatigability in chronic low back pain patients and controls. Archives of Physical Medicine and Rehabilitation 79(4): 412–417

Kellgren J H 1938 Observations on referred pain arising from muscle. Clinical Sciences 3: 175–190

Kelso J A S 1995 Dynamic patterns: the self-organization of brain and behaviour. MIT Press, Cambridge, Massachusetts

Kelso J A S, Tuller B 1984 A dynamical basis for action systems. In: Gazzaniga M (ed) Handbook of cognitive neuroscience. Plenum Press, New York, pp 321–356

Koyama T, Tanaka Y Z, Mikami A 1998 Nociceptive neurons in macaque anterior cingulate activate during anticipation of pain. NeuroReport 9: 2663–2667.

Lavender S A, Marras W S, Miller R A 1993 The development of response strategies in preparation for sudden loading to the torso. Spine 18: 2097–2105

Lee W 1980 Anticipatory control of postural and task muscles during rapid arm flexion. Journal of Motor Behaviour 12: 185–196

Ljubisavljevic M, Anastasijevic R 1994 Fusimotor-induced changes in muscle spindle outflow and responsiveness in muscle fatigue in decerebrate cats. Neuroscience 63: 339–348

Lund S 1980 Postural effects of neck muscle vibration in man. Experientia 36: 1398

Lund J P, Stohler C S, Widmer C G 1993 The relationship between pain and muscle activity in fibromyalgia and similar conditions. In: Vaeroy H, Merskey H (eds) Progress in fibromyalgia and myofascial pain. Elsevier, Amsterdam, pp 311–327

Lundberg A 1979 Integration in a propriospinal motor centre controlling the forelimb in the cat. In: Asanuma H, Wilson V J (eds) Integration in the nervous system. Igaku-Shoin, Tokyo, pp 47–64

Lundberg A, Norrsell U, Voorhoeve P 1962 Pyramidal effects on lumbosacral interneurons activated by somatic afferents. Acta Physiologica Scandinavica 56: 220–229

Lundberg A, Malmgren K, Schomburg E D 1987 Reflex pathways from group II muscle afferents. 2: Functional characteristics of reflex pathways to alpha-motoneurons. Experimental Brain Research 65: 282–293

McCrea D A 1994 Can sense be made of spinal interneuron circuits? In: Cordo P, Harnad S (eds) Movement control. Cambridge University Press, New York, pp 31–41

Madeleine P, Voigt M, Arendt-Nielsen L 1999a Reorganisation of human step initiation during acute experimental muscle pain. Gait and Posture 10: 240–247

Madeleine P, Lundager B, Voigt M, Arendt-Nielsen L 1999b Shoulder muscle co-ordination during chronic and acute experimental neck-shoulder pain: an occupational pain study. European Journal of Applied Physiology and Occupational Physiology 79: 127–140

Maier M A, Davis J N, Armand J et al 1997 Comparison of cortico-motoneuronal (CM) connections from macaque motor cortex and supplementary motor area. Society for Neuroscience Abstracts 23: 1274

Martin H A, Arendt-Nielsen L 2000 Effect of muscle pain and intrathecal AP-5 on electromyographic patterns during treadmill walking in the rat. Progress in Neuro-Psychopharmacology and Biological Psychiatry 24: 1151–1175

Massion J, Hugon M, Wiesendanger M 1982 Anticipatory postural changes induced by active unloading and comparison with passive unloading in man. Pflügers Archives 393: 292–296

Matre D A, Sinkjaer T, Svensson P, Arendt-Nielsen L 1998 Experimental muscle pain increases the human stretch reflex. Pain 75: 331–339

Melzack R, Casey K L 1968 Sensory, motivational and central control determinants of pain. In: Kenshalo D R (ed) The skin senses. C C Thomas, Springfield, Illinois, pp 423–443

Mense S 1986 Slowly conducting fibres from deep tissues: neurological properties and central nervous action. Progress in Sensory Physiology 6: 139–219

Mense S 1991 Considerations concerning the neurobiological basis of muscle pain. Canadian Journal of Physiological Pharmacology 69: 610–616

Mense S, Meyer H 1985 Different types of slowly conducting afferent units in cat skeletal muscle and tendon. Journal of Physiology 363: 403–417

Mense S, Skeppar P 1991 Discharge behaviour of feline gamma-motorneurons following induction of an artificial myositis. Pain 46: 201–210

Merzenich M M, Kaas J H, Wall J T, Nelson R J, Sur M, Felleman D J 1983 Topographic reorganization of somatosensory cortical areas 3b and 1 in adult monkeys following restricted deafferentation. Neuroscience 8: 33–55

Merzenich M M, Nelson R J, Stryker M P, Cynader M S, Shoppmann A, Zook J M 1984 Somatosensory cortical map changes following digit amputation in adult monkeys. Journal of Comparative Neurology 224: 591–605

Molin C 1972 Vertical isometric forces of the mandible. Acta Odontologia Scandinavica 30: 485–499

Nelson D L, Hutton R S 1985 Dynamic and static stretch responses in muscle spindle receptors in fatigued muscle. Medicine and Science in Sport and Exercise 17: 445–450

Newcomer K L, Jacobson T D, Gabriel D A, Larson D R, Brey R H, An K N 2002 Muscle activation patterns in subjects with and without low back pain. Archives of Physical Medicine and Rehabilitation 83: 816–821

Nouwen A, Bush C 1984 The relationship between paraspinal EMG and chronic low back pain. Pain 20: 109–123

O'Sullivan P, Twomey L, Allison G, Sinclair J, Miller K 1997 Altered patterns of abdominal muscle activation in patients with chronic low back pain. Australian Journal of Physiotherapy 43: 91–98

Paintal A S 1961 Participation by pressure-pain receptors of mammalian spindles in the flexion reflex. Journal of Physiology (London) 156: 498–514

Pedersen J, Sjölander P, Wenngren B I, Johansson H 1997 Increased intramuscular concentration of bradykinin increases the static fusimotor drive to muscle spindles in neck muscles of the cat. Pain 70: 83–91

Price R F, Dutia M B 1989 Physiological properties of tandem muscle spindles in neck and hind-limb muscles. Progress in Brain Research 80: 47–57

Radebold A, Cholewicki J, Panjabi M M, Patel T C 2000 Muscle response pattern to sudden trunk loading in healthy individuals and in patients with chronic low back pain. Spine 25: 947–954

Radebold A, Cholewicki J, Polzhofer G K, Greene H S 2001 Impaired postural control of the lumbar spine is associated with delayed muscle response times in patients with chronic idiopathic low back pain. Spine 26(7): 724–730

Ralston D D, Ralston H J 1985 The terminations of corticospinal tract axons in the macaque monkey. Journal of Comparative Neurology 242: 325–337

Richmond F J, Abrahams V C 1975 Morphology and distribution of muscle spindles in dorsal muscles of the cat neck. Journal of Neurophysiology 38: 1322–1339

Rossi A, Decchi B, Ginanneschi F 1999 Presynaptic excitability changes of group Ia fibres to muscle nociceptive stimulation in humans. Brain Research 818: 12–22

Ruch T C 1946 Visceral sensation and referred pain. In: Fulton J F (ed) Howell's Textbook of physiology, 15th edn. Saunders, Philadelphia, pp 385–401

Rybicki K J, Waldrop T G, Kaufman M P 1985 Increasing gracilis muscle interstitial potassium concentrations stimulate group III and IV afferents. Journal of Applied Physiology 58: 936–941

Saltzman E, Kelso J A S 1987 Skilled actions: a task-dynamic approach. Psychological Review 94: 84–106

Schaible H G, Schmidt R F 1985 Effects of an experimental arthritis on the sensory properties of fine articular afferent units. Journal of Neurophysiology 54: 1109–1122

Schaible H-G, Schmidt R F 1988 Time course of mechanosensitivity changes in articular afferents during a developing experimental arthritis. Journal of Neurophysiology 60: 180–195

Schouenborg J, Sjölund B H 1983 Activity evoked by A- and C-afferent fibres in rat dorsal horn neurons and its relation to a flexion reflex. Journal of Neurophysiology 50: 1108–1121

Shakespeare D T, Stokes M, Sherman K P, Young A 1985 Reflex inhibition of the quadriceps after meniscectomy: lack of association with pain. Clinical Physiology 5: 137–144

Shepherd G M 1994 Neurobiology, 3rd edn. Oxford University Press, New York

Shepherd G 1998 The synaptic organization of the brain, 4th edn. Oxford University Press, New York

Sherman R A 1985 Relationships between strength of low back muscle contraction and reported intensity of chronic low back pain. American Journal of Physical Medicine 64: 190–200

Sherrington C S 1910 Flexion reflex of the limb, crossed extension reflex, and reflex stepping and standing. Journal of Physiology 47: 196–214

Sherrington C S 1947 The integrative action of the nervous system, 2nd edn. Cambridge University Press, Cambridge

Simons D G 1990 Muscular pain syndromes. In: Fricton J R, Awad E (eds) Advances in pain research and therapy. Raven Press, New York, vol 17, pp 1–41

Smeulders M J, Kreulen M, Hage J J, Ritt M J, Mulder T 2002 Motor control impairment of the contralateral wrist in patients with unilateral chronic wrist pain. American Journal of Physical Medicine and Rehabilitation 81(3): 177–181

Stacey M J 1969 Free nerve endings in skeletal muscle of the cat. Journal of Anatomy 105: 231–254

Stohler C S, Zhang X, Lund J P 1996 The effect of experimental jaw muscle pain on postural muscle activity. Pain 66: 215–221

Stohler C S, Kowalski C J, Lund J P 2001 Muscle pain inhibits cutaneous touch perception. Pain 92: 327–333

Sugiura Y, Terui N, Hosoya K 1989 Distribution of unmyelinated primary afferent fibres in the dorsal horn. In: Cervero F, Bennett G J, Headley P M (eds) Processing of sensory information in superficial dorsal horn of the spinal cord. Plenum Press, New York, pp 15–27

Talbot J D, Marrett S, Evans A C, Meyer E, Bushnell M C, Duncan G H 1991 Multiple representations of pain in human cerebral cortex. Science 251: 1355–1358.

Thorstensson A, Arvidson A 1982 Trunk muscle strength and low back pain. Scandinavian Journal of Rehabilitation Medicine 14: 69–75

Thunberg J, Ljubisavljevic M, Djupsjöbäcka M, Johansson H 2002 Effects on the fusimotor-muscle spindle system induced by intramuscular injections of hypertonic saline. Experimental Brain Research 143: 319–326

Travell J G, Simons D G 1983 Myofascial pain and dysfunction: the trigger point manual. Williams and Wilkins, Baltimore

Treede R-D, Kenshalo D R, Gracely R H, Jones A K P 1999 The cortical representation of pain. Pain 79: 105–111

Velarde M G, Normand C 1980 Convection. Scientific American 243: 78–93

Wall P D 1967 The laminar organization of dorsal horn and effects of descending impulses. Journal of Physiology 188: 403–423

Wall P D, Woolf C J 1984 Muscle but not cutaneous C-afferent input produces prolonged increases in the excitability of the flexion reflex in the rat. Journal of Physiology 356: 443–458

Wang K, Svensson P, Arendt-Nielsen L 2000 Effect of tonic muscle pain on short-latency jaw-stretch reflexes in humans. Pain 88: 189–197

Westberg K-G, Clavelou P, Schwartz G, Lund J P 1997 Effects of chemical stimulation of masseter muscle nociceptors on trigeminal motoneuron and interneuron activities during fictive mastication in the rabbit. Pain 73: 295–308

Willis W D 1989 Neural mechanisms of pain discrimination. In: Lund J (ed) Sensory processing in the mammalian brain. Oxford University Press, New York, pp 130–143

Wyke B 1981 The neurology of joints: a review of general principles. Clinics in Rheumatic Diseases 7: 233–239

Young A, Stokes M, Iles J F 1987 Effects of joint pathology on muscle. Clinical Orthopaedics 219: 21–27

Yu X-M, Mense S 1990 Somatotopical arrangement of rat spinal dorsal horn cells processing input from deep tissues. Neuroscience Letters 108: 43–47

Zedka M, Prochazka A, Knight B, Gillard D, Gauthier M 1999 Voluntary and reflex control of human back muscles during induced pain. Journal of Physiology 520(2): 591–604

Chapter 14

The spine and the effect of ageing

K. P. Singer

CHAPTER CONTENTS

INTRODUCTION

In the absence of overt pathology, it is often difficult to distinguish between the effects of age per se and spinal degenerative changes, as both often overlap within the same relative grey scale. There are also different opinions as to whether many individuals achieve old age without some evidence of frank degenerative or pathological changes in spinal joints. Most published reviews on the health of the spine are written from a clinical perspective – pathology, radiology, surgery, biochemistry, clinical anatomy and so on – with an absence of large-scale epidemiological surveys to clarify the issue. The major post mortem survey of the vertebral column conducted over the lifetime of the German pathologist Georg Schmorl (Schmorl 1929, Schmorl & Junghanns 1971) and the large population based radiological studies of Dodge et al (1970) and Lawrence (1977) all indicate that spinal degenerative changes have an extremely high prevalence in adult populations. However, although all elements of the spine undergo degenerative changes with age, only some features of this process are associated with spinal pathology and pain (Andersson 1998).

It is clear that age and degenerative changes both function to constrain the system against further injury or damage. In the case of the spine, which serves three prime objectives of mobility, stability and protection of neural elements, excessive static or dynamic loading stress can induce local or regional degenerative change. Consequently, this chapter draws upon literature which presents both age and degeneration models and their influences upon the spine. There are relatively few reports which document the patterns of age-related degenerative change occurring throughout a single vertebral column; most focus on either the lumbar or the cervical region. Of clinical interest is the well recognized tendency for stress to accumulate at the transitional zones between regions with resultant symptoms arising from dysfunction or trauma and their degenerative sequelae. As the literature on normal ageing and disease of the human spine is extensive, this summary draws upon selected reviews and a general model of the vertebral column upon which regional patterns of degeneration may be viewed. Reference is made to literature to illustrate degenerative conditions which are represented in specific areas of the spine.

A GENERAL MODEL OF THE SPINE AND PHYSIO-LOGICAL RESPONSES TO AGEING

Normal physiological strains are well accommodated by each functional mobile segment; this comprises an intervertebral disc (IVD) with an annulus fibrosus and nucleus pulposus and the vertebral end-plates (VEP) which include the bony epiphyseal rim at the periphery of the vertebral bodies to regulate their circumferential and vertical growth (O'Rahilly et al 1980). The thin superior and inferior cartilaginous end-plates connect with the subchondral bony lamella which supports the cancellous trabecular structure within the vertebral body. Paired synovial zygapophysial joints link both vertebrae posteriorly and articulate closely to regulate both load and movement of the segment. Applied moments from muscle actions and axial compressive loads may be coupled with shear, bending (rotations) and torsion about the long axis of the spine, which are in turn moderated by the unique geometry of the segment's zygapophysial and ligamentous anatomy (Fig. 14.1). Inertial strains from dynamic loading, even several times the individual's body weight, may also be tolerated by the spine given its unique capacity to attenuate energy (Adams et al 2002).

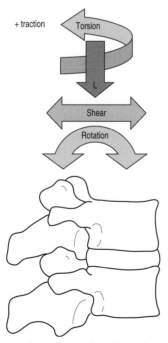

Figure 14.1 The motion segment is subjected to applied moments from muscle actions and axial loading, which may be coupled with shear, bending and torsion about the long axis of the spine. These forces are in turn moderated by the segment's zygapophysial joints and disposition of the ligamentous anatomy.

The configuration of the nucleus pulposus comprises amorphous mucopolysaccharides, from the fetal period, which continuously differentiate peripherally with the transverse growth of the annulus fibrosus. Formed through multiple fibrous concentric laminar layers, the annulus layers are orientated 40–90 degrees relative to each other. This arrangement provides considerable resistance to strains from external force moments and from the internal hydraulic pressures exerted by the nucleus as it deforms in response to load. At the superior and inferior surfaces of the disc, fibres penetrate the VEP and also fuse with the anterior and posterior longitudinal ligaments. Throughout life there is a progressive loss of differentiation between the nucleus and the annulus which on T2-weighted MRI scans is seen as a reduction in the high signal from the central disc region. In the younger individual, the nucleus is more gelatinous but this is gradually replaced by fibrocartilage to become more dehydrated and desiccated in the elderly (Prescher 1998). By the third decade of life, it becomes more difficult to distinguish boundaries between these two principal IVD elements. The outermost layers of the annulus comprise mostly type I collagen whereas type II collagen is represented to a higher extent in the innermost layers and within the nucleus. The IVD is designed to attenuate dynamic and static loads through hydraulic mechanisms related to its capacity to bind or express water. The proteoglycan gel, principally within the nucleus, maintains fluid content under load in turn sustained by the collagen weave of the surrounding disc matrix which permits deformations in response to physiological motions. With ageing there is a reduction in the nucleus capacity to bind water which is demonstrated through imaging studies as an apparent reduction in vertical disc height, with 'fissures' in the region of the nucleus. This trend has also been demonstrated mechanically from ex vivo assessments of axial load distributions using disc profilometry, whereby greater loading occurs preferentially through the region of the annulus with a relative decompression in the region of the dehydrated nucleus (Adams et al 2002, McNally et al 1992). The reduction in elasticity of the disc can contribute to an increase in the transfer of compressive loads to the VEP, leading to subchondral trabecular microfractures (Hahn et al 1994), a process which may contribute to sclerosis of the end-plate. Radiological demonstration of such changes may be seen in MRI investigations of the spine as the increased signal from T2-weighted image sequences described by Modic et al (1988).

The disc is essentially aneural apart from the peripheral superficial outer third, although with injury to the disc, vascular ingrowth associated with repair may contribute vasomotor nerves (Coppes et al 1997). The disc is also avascular, apart from the peripheral annulus, with a reliance upon nutritional substances transported via diffusion across the VEPs (Roberts et al 1997) or through vessels which communicate directly with the outer annular layers. Consequently, disruption to either system, occurring through normal ageing, surgical intervention, spinal deformity or trauma, can disrupt and lengthen the pathways of nutritional support to the disc and is presumed to contribute to subsequent disc degeneration (Buckwalter 1995, Urban & Roberts 1995). In the case of the VEP, sclerosis associated with end-plate lesions or coincident with ageing would likely contribute to this degenerative sequelae of the disc.

The consequence of either ageing or injury to the functional mobile segment may be degeneration of its elements with initial progressive increase in strain tolerance beyond the normal, which may progress to increased segmental mobility. One mechanical response to such changes, particularly affecting the stability and function of the IVD, is spondylosis, initiated through osteogenic stimulation in the junctional region between the VEP periphery and the annulus, resulting in the early formation of osteophytes (Vernon-Roberts & Pirie 1977). Experimentally induced osteoarthrosis of the paired zygapophysial joints, arising from annular rim lesions of the IVD, which has been produced in the sheep model (Moore et al 1999) confirms earlier post mortem observations (Oegema & Bradford 1991, Osti et al 1992).

The posterior paired zygapophysial, costotransverse and costovertebral joints are true synovial joints invested with hyaline articular cartilage, a capsule and synovium. These joint pairings contribute stability of the respective segment(s), and facilitate respiratory excursions of the thorax and regional mobility within the vertebral column. Each may respond to undue strain with typical degenerative patterns of synovial joints characterized by mechanical changes of the articular cartilage. Subchondral bone sclerosis, fissuring and detachment of the cartilage and marginal joint osteophytosis may follow changes in the IVD, particularly a loss of vertical height which in turn alters the mechanical alignment of the respective superior and inferior articular processes of the posterior joints, contributing to subluxation (Oegema & Bradford 1991). Bumper cartilage formations are associated with evidence of articular cartilage degeneration and fissuring, ossification of the ligamentum flavum and reactive hyperplasia at the posterior joint margins (see Ch. 3, Fig. 3.3). A further consequence of degenerative changes leading to altered morphology of the IVD and vertebral bodies is the response by the spinal ligaments. With progressive deformation of the segment, ligaments may demonstrate buckling and, in response to exaggerated segmental motion strains, subsequent hypertrophic changes may contribute to stenotic change within the vertebral and intervertebral canals (Benini 1990, Weinstein et al 1977). Considerable ossification within the ligamentum flavum may occur as part of degeneration of the articular triad, although this tends to predominate in the region of the lower thoracic and upper lumbar segments (Maigne et al 1992, Malmivaara 1988).

Against this background, it is possible to examine specific patterns of degeneration and age changes as they are represented from reported surveys. Indeed, when spinal degenerative patterns are merged onto a common spinal model, the most mobile cervical and lumbar segments and their respective stiffer transitional junctions can be clearly and differentially identified. For the entire spine, there is a tendency for large segmental mobility to induce local strains and ultimately degenerative sequelae. In the case of the bony thorax, high levels of degenerative change are seen at the respective costovertebral joint articulations of the first and last ribs as a consequence of the muscle attachments and the transfer of large torques from this musculature of the neck and trunk, respectively. When one considers the complete vertebral column as a multisegmented curved rod, with physiological inflexions that cross the neutral axis line, the literature presents evidence of stress accumulations at points of both maximum and minimum change in curve. The transitional junctions, having less relative motion, are designed more for stability. They represent locations where axial compressive load is greater, the change in spinal curvature is least and the trend is for arthrosis of their synovial joints. In contrast, where the curvature away from the neutral axis line is maximum, as in the middle region of the lordosis and kyphosis, and where bending, torsion and shear stresses are relatively higher, the trend is for greater disc degeneration (Fig. 14.2). A mixed pattern of degenerative change within a mobile segment emerges where an advanced level of either arthrosis or IVD degeneration has developed.

PATTERNS OF AGE CHANGES IN THE SPINE

The major degenerative conditions reviewed in this chapter are listed in Box 14.1 and include osteoporosis and anomalies of spinal curvature, and changes which arise secondary to trauma. Inflammatory disease of the spine is excluded from this discussion; the interested reader is directed to the compilation by Klippel & Dieppe (1998) for a thorough review. Degenerative conditions which principally have a spinal manifestation may involve various elements of the functional mobile segment, either singularly as in the case of early IVD degeneration or across this joint complex, exemplified by late zygapophysial joint arthrosis coincident with IVD degeneration (Fujiwara et al 2000).

Disc degeneration

Literature describing the incidence of disc degeneration (DD) throughout the vertebral column concentrates predominantly on the lumbar and cervical regions of the spine (Kramer 1981). An active debate has existed on the aetiology of DD, from which two main models emerge. Mechanical strains of the annulus fibrosus may result in a rim lesion which initiates this degenerative sequence (Osti et al 1990, 1992), or a lesion to the VEP may affect the discs' nutrition. The latter pathology has been confirmed experimentally (Ariga et al 2001) and demonstrated clinically and

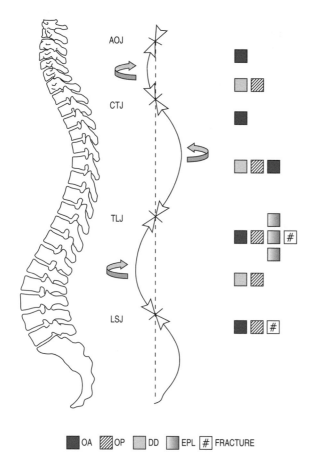

OA ░░**OP** **DD** **EPL** #**FRACTURE**

Figure 14.2 The human vertebral column comprises a balanced 'S'-shaped multisegmented curved rod with physiological inflexions that cross the neutral axis line. Evidence of stress accumulations is seen at points of both maximum and minimum change along this curve. The transitional junctions are constrained against motion, sustain higher axial compressive loads and show high levels of arthrosis of their synovial joints. Where the spinal segments depart from the neutral axis line in the middle lordoses and kyphosis, and where bending, torsion and shear stresses are relatively higher, the tendency is for higher levels of disc degeneration.
Key: AOJ = atlanto-axial junction; CTJ = cervicothoracic junction; TLJ = thoracolumbar junction; LSJ = lumbosacral junction; OA = osteoarthritis; OP = osteophytes; DD = disc degeneration; EPL = end-plate lesions.

at post mortem (Pfirrmann & Resnick 2001). From post mortem studies, discs with altered vascularity during the second decade of life show precursor changes to early degeneration (Boos et al 2002). The pathway of age-related degeneration change has been described by Buckwalter as compromised nutrition, loss of viable cells, cell senescence, post-translational modification of matrix proteins, accumulation of degraded matrix molecules, a reduction in pH levels that may impede cell function and ultimately induce cell death, and finally, fatigue failure of the matrix (Buckwalter 1995). Radiological reviews of large populations undertaken by Dodge et al (1970) and Lawrence (1977) have indicated that the highest prevalence of DD is in the

Box 14.1   Major types of degenerative and ageing effects in the human spine including those related to metabolic disease or arising in response to trauma

Degenerative conditions
  Degenerative disc disease, osteophytosis and ossification
  Diffuse idiopathic skeletal hyperostosis
  Vertebral end-plate lesions and Schmorl's nodes
  Scheuermann's disease
  Zygapophysial and costovertebral joint osteoarthritis

Spinal alignment anomalies
  Degenerative scoliosis and kyphosis, spondylolisthesis
Osteoporosis and osteoporotic fracture
Trauma
  Spinal fractures including the transitional junctions
  Intervertebral disc injury and prolapse

mid-cervical, mid-thoracic and mid-lumbar discs. These regions show a marked degree of reactive changes of the vertebral bodies with marginal osteophyte formation (Fig. 14.3). The incidence of DD was commonly linked to occupation and gender; with a greater frequency in males. In the survey by Bobko et al, it was noted that manual labourers were susceptible to DD within the cervicothoracic junction (CTJ) region in contrast to white collar workers where DD was more common within the C4–5 and C5–6 discs (Bobko et al 1966). Early post mortem studies of von Lushka (1850, 1858) demonstrated a large proportion of cervical discs with fissures and clefts. This was considered to be a normal characteristic of the region, an observation which was subsequently confirmed by Töndury (1959) and other workers (Bland 1987, Penning 1988). Complete transverse clefts which extend across and into the region of the uncovertebral joints may be found in the middle of healthy cervical discs on coronal inspection (Ten Have & Eulderink 1980). The high frequency of degenerative findings in the mid-cervical spine is well documented (Fletcher et al 1990, Milne 1991) and appears to relate to the combination of disc facet and interfacet angles seen in the mid-cervical vertebrae. Large anteroposterior translation during sagittal motion and combined lateral flexion and axial rotation (Milne 1991, 1993) is thought to result in greater shear forces in the intervertebral discs. The variations in orientation of the zygapophysial joints through the cervicothoracic transition may in part account for the discal degeneration in the upper thoracic spine.

Significant trends in degenerative changes in the cervicothoracic transition with respect to age have been identified (Boyle et al 1998b). The frequency of osteophytic lipping decreases from the mid-cervical mobile segments with the lowest incidence of marginal vertebral osteophyte formation occurring at the C7–T1 vertebral segment (Nathan 1962). From post mortem reviews of the thoracic

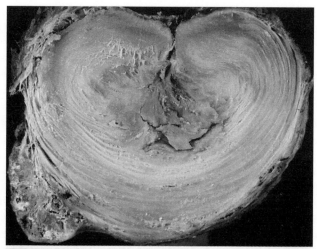

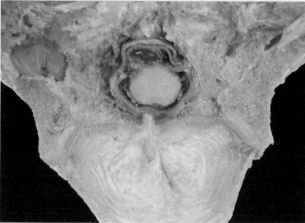

Figure 14.3 Macro-histology of the T10–11 and L2–3 discs sectioned in the horizontal plane at the mid-height of the disc of two elderly cases. The thoracic example (upper) depicts a central disc prolapse deforming the anterior dural sac. Note that the posterolateral disc is prevented from prolapse due to the location of the costovertebral joints in a manner analogous to the uncovertebral joints in the cervical spine. In the lower illustration age-related changes are demonstrated in the form of the large right-sided anterolateral osteophyte and central disintegration of the nucleus. A central fissure is evident through the posterior annulus.

spine, the most severely affected discs were located predominantly within the middle segments, peaking between T6 and T7, with a greater incidence in males (Singer 2000). Given the higher amplitude of axial plane segmental motion in the mid-thoracic spine, reported from in vivo investigations (Gregersen & Lucas 1967), these degenerative changes may relate to rotation strains imposed upon these segments. Investigation into the effects of torsion on lumbar IVDs has concluded that relatively small rotation strains induced potential injury in the annulus fibrosus (Farfan et al 1970). Similarly a torsion induced strain response from the relatively large axial plane motions possible in the mid-thoracic segments may be a major factor contributing to the DD seen in these segments (Lawrence 1977, Singer 2000).

The pattern of age-related decline in anterior disc height in men typifies the disc ageing process associated with senile kyphosis, as described by Schmorl & Junghanns (1971). Hence in older males without marked spinal osteopenia it is speculated that the cumulative effects of axial loading and torsional stresses result in degeneration of the anterior annulus and osteophytosis (Schmorl & Junghanns 1971). This early observation has been confirmed in recent series (Goh et al 1999, Manns et al 1996, Resnick 1985). In older women, however, loading through the anterior aspect of the kyphotic curve is more likely to produce progressive change of the vertebral bodies, causing the wedge deformity commonly associated with spinal osteoporosis. Mechanically, the middle vertebral segments appear predisposed to greater axial compressive and bending moments, due to their position within the apex of the thoracic kyphosis (Singer et al 1995).

Osteophytosis

A review by Nathan (1962) saw osteophyte formation and its associated IVD degeneration as an attempt to distribute force more uniformly across the VEPs and to achieve stress reduction on the segment. In his study of 346 skeletal spinal columns, Nathan (1962) reported a higher incidence of vertebral body osteophytes, including complete fusion between adjoining vertebrae, in the lower thoracic levels. Where thoracolumbar disc degeneration is present, marginal osteophyte formation of the vertebral body is frequently seen (Lawrence 1977, Vernon-Roberts 1992). This pattern of excess bone formation is commonly referred to as spondylosis deformans (Resnick 1985) and is seen in approximately 60% of women and 80% of men (Schmorl & Junghanns 1971). In an advanced stage, with complete ossification of the ligaments from several adjacent vertebrae, this presentation may form part of diffuse idiopathic skeletal hyperostosis (DISH) (Belanger & Rowe 2001). The degree of intervertebral space narrowing and subsequent tilting of the vertebral bodies, resulting from disc degeneration, often determines the extent and the type of marginal osteophytes (Malmivaara 1987, Nathan, 1994). In summary, the segments that appear susceptible to osteophytes are often the most mobile regions with the higher levels of DD, or where local stress may be accumulated.

Ossification within spinal ligaments

Ossification of the attachments of the ligamentum flavum, which is considered to be a response to stress, has been reported from several surveys of skeletal vertebral columns (Davis 1955, Maigne et al 1992, Nathan 1959). The high frequency of laminar projections of bone localized in the region of the lower thoracic and thoracolumbar junction (TLJ) levels suggests that this is a normal feature of the region, from the third decade of life. Maigne et al (1992) suggested that the size and frequency of these processes projecting into the ligamentum flavum acted to regulate the segmental response to torsion of the vertebral column, whereas Prescher (1998) considered this to be a reaction to flexion strain. Maigne et al noted that immediately above the TLJ, where the zygapophysial joints were configured to facilitate rotation, the spicules were more developed (Maigne et al 1992) (Fig. 14.4).

Diffuse idiopathic skeletal hyperostosis

Ankylosing hyperostosis of the spine may result in ossification of spinal ligaments without evident disc disease. Typically this condition affects older men, being uncommon in men younger than 40 years, and does not usually result in severe disability (Weinfeld et al 1997). According to surveys by Resnick & Niwayama (1976, 1995) radiographic evidence of DISH may be found in 12% of the population. In the majority of these cases, the thoracic spine is involved (Malone et al 1998), particularly on the right side of the

T5–12 vertebral bodies due to the influence of the descending abdominal aorta (Resnick & Niwayama 1976). There are few published large-scale studies of the prevalence of DISH; however, a recent investigation of 2364 patients identified 25% of males and 15% of females over the age of 50 years with radiographic features of this disease (Weinfeld et al 1997). The pathology of DISH also involves bone spur formation (enthesophytes) within peri-articular ligaments of other large joints.

The condition may be largely asymptomatic; however, when symptoms are present they commonly consist of spinal stiffness, particularly in the morning, and thoracic back pain, with spinal tenderness reported to be present in up to 90% of cases (Utsinger 1985). Loss of spinal mobility and associated diminished thoracic cage motion has been described (Resnick & Niwayama 1976). The principal features consist of multiple consecutive flowing osteophytes along the course of the anterior longitudinal ligament, involving at least four adjacent vertebrae, relatively pre-

Figure 14.4 Photomicrographs of 100 μm-thick horizontal histological sections at T11–12, to highlight ossification within the ligamentum flavum (arrows). A, B: The ligament is bounded by attachments to the superior articular process and laminae as it helps forms the dorsal wall of the vertebral canal between the paired zygapophysial joints laterally and adjacent laminae. In both, there is an expansion of the ligamentum flavum towards the vertebral canal which, in some cases, contributes to central stenosis. From macerated vertebrae at the thoracolumbar junction. Black arrows depict the location of ossicles between T11 and T12 which project into the ligamentum flavum. C, D: Hypertrophic enlargement of the superior aspect of the sap is evident on the left zygapophysial joint (Z) in D. Adapted from Singer 2000.
Key: sap = superior articular process; iap = inferior articular process; LF = ligamentum flavum; MP = mammillary process; Z = zygapophysial joint.

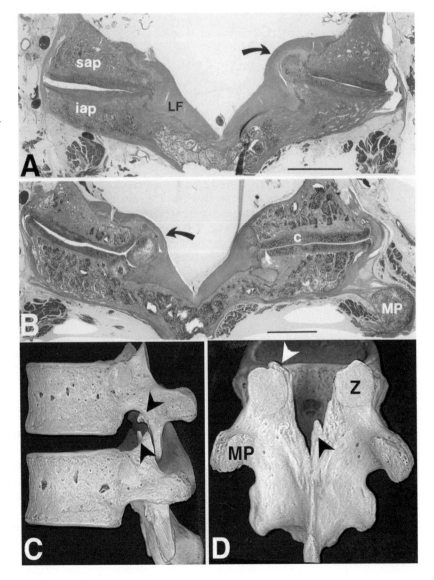

served disc spaces and VEPs (Fig. 14.5), and the absence of sacroiliac or zygapophysial joint sclerosis or ankylosis.

The coexistence of multiple pathologies with DISH was a feature of the post mortem investigation by Vernon-Roberts et al (1974). In their study, osteoporosis, Schmorl's nodes and lateral projection of disc tissues were found to be associated with DISH. The thickened syndesmophytes acted to bridge the disc space and maintain disc height, in contrast to other forms of spinal degenerative condition.

Vertebral end-plate lesions and Schmorl's nodes

The vertebral end-plate is a membrane of tissue comprising hyaline cartilage and a thin trabecular layer at the discovertebral junction (Grignon et al 2000). Its role is to mediate axial compressive load applied to the IVD and permit transfer of this energy within the subchondral and cancellous bone of the vertebral body. Cyclic physiological axial loading, as occurs with gait, acts as pump mechanism to assist diffusion of nutrients within the vascular vertebral body across the VEP to the disc. Abrupt or fatigue axial loading of the spine may cause localized failure of the VEP resulting in either a frank sharply demarcated vertebral intra-osseous prolapse, often termed a Schmorl's node (SN), or marked irregularity of the end-plate. The repair process for both lesions often results in bony sclerosis which can significantly impair the normal nutrient exchange to the IVD by extending this diffusion pathway.

Several authors have suggested that SNs appear most frequently in areas of VEP weakness, possibly resulting from congenital deficiency of the cartilage end-plate at the site of the remnant notochord. Another theory suggests that scarring of degenerated blood vessels supplying the juvenile disc, whereby the end-plate thickness is reduced,

increases susceptibility to nuclear extrusion (Begg 1954, Resnick & Niwayama 1978, Schmorl & Junghanns 1971).

Schmorl's nodes have been reported to occur during the late teens (Fisk et al 1984), with lesions as frequent in the young as in the older individual (Hilton et al 1976, Schmorl & Junghanns 1971). Cadaveric studies of lumbar spines have indicated that SNs develop at an early age and can exhibit advanced degenerative changes (Vernon-Roberts & Pirie 1977). Previous literature investigating the incidence of SNs and VEP lesions has focused on lower thoracic and upper lumbar segments. The reported incidence of SNs for these investigations have ranged between 38 and 79%, with the variation related to age, sex and racial characteristics of the study sample and geographical issues. Schmorl's nodes are found most commonly in males and are considered to be related to a genetic disposition, strenuous occupations (Schmorl & Junghanns 1971) or sports involving dynamic and violent axial loading as might occur with a heavy landing in flexion (Fisk et al 1984). Using cadaver spines containing T9–12 vertebral bodies, Hilton et al found most SNs located within the T10–11 and T11–12 segments with no age-related variation (Hilton et al 1976). These authors reported a 60% incidence of SNs in spines of those under the age of 20, with the youngest 13 years of age (Hilton et al 1976). A higher incidence was found by Malmivaara et al who reported SNs in 29 of 37 male cadaveric specimens (T10–L1) aged 21–69 years (Malmivaara et al 1987b).

In a post mortem radiographic survey, 64 of 90 spines had evidence of SNs (Singer 1997). Both male and female spines displayed SNs throughout the spine, the majority located within the T10–L2 segments. All authors agree that the inferior end-plate is more susceptible to infraction (Hilton et al 1976, Malmivaara 1987, Yasuma et al 1988) which implies that the VEP fails under compression.

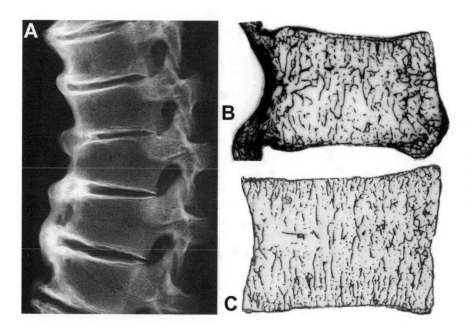

Figure 14.5 Marked osteophytic development is shown in this lower thoracic sample with diffuse idiopathic skeletal hyperostosis (DISH). From the anterior aspect (A), extensive bridging osteophytes are seen spanning multiple adjacent levels. The internal disc height is preserved and the kyphotic angulation contributed to by vertebral body wedging. Inspection of the median sagittal view from one cleared vertebral body stained with von Kossa (B) shows the extent of the thickened cortical nature of the osteophytes. In contrast a normal vertebral body without marked focal degeneration shows regular end-plates and a predominance of vertical trabecular bone (C).

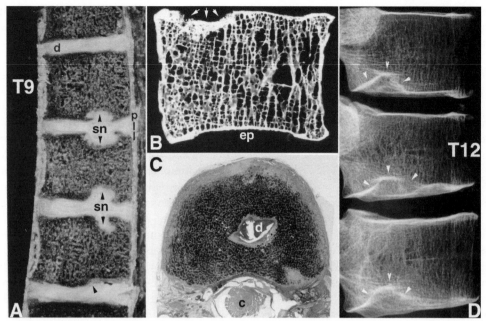

Figure 14.6 Intravertebral protrusions, or Schmorl's nodes, are depicted from several views to highlight their location and extent (A). They may project cranially and/or caudally through the vertebral end-plate (arrows). End-plate irregularities are typically in the lower thoracic spine, as represented by the inferior end-plate of T11 (arrow). A depression on the superior end-plate of a 2 mm-thick bone section from T11 is shown at B with slight sclerosing of the end-plate compared with the regular thin inferior end-plate. A central Schmorl's node at T12 (C), in a 100 μm-thick horizontal histological section shows disc material surrounded by sclerotic bony margins. Multiple Schmorl's nodes are shown at the thoracolumbar junction (D), all approximately in the same location and affecting the inferior vertebral end-plate, a characteristic of Scheuermann's disease. Adapted from Singer 2000.
Key: c = spinal cord; d = disc; ep = end-plate; pll = posterior longitudinal ligament; sn = Schmorl's nodes.

Pfirrmann et al made the observation from their post mortem study that SNs were not necessarily associated with evident DD; however, their series of 100 cases were from an elderly post mortem sample (Pfirrmann & Resnick 2001). Figure 14.6 depicts the typical location and presence of multiple SNs in the lower thoracic segments.

Zygapophysial and costovertebral joint degeneration

There appear to be specific sites within the spine where preferential degeneration of the synovial joints occur. The upper and lower segments of the thoracic region show a tendency for zygapophysial and costovertebral joint degeneration according to the skeletal surveys of Shore (1935a, 1935b) and Nathan et al (1964). Similar trends for osteophytic remodelling of the zygapophysial joints of the lumbosacral junction have been reported (Cihak 1970, Inman & Saunders 1942, Resnick 1985). This may be due to the design of these elements which provide stability and protection in contrast the adjacent mobile segments which show a correspondingly higher frequency of discal disease (Resnick 1985) (see Fig. 14.1). The development of osteophytes and eventual bony fusion of costovertebral and costotransverse joints in aged vertebral columns was also noted by Schmorl

& Junghans (1971) in their extensive survey of spinal pathology (compare Fig. 3.5, in Ch. 3, Zygapophysial joints).

Shore believed that maintaining an erect head posture on a changing thoracic kyphosis induced localized stress on the CTJ (Shore 1935a). The increasing thoracic kyphosis, which is particularly evident in the aged female population (Fon et al 1980, Singer et al 1990), and the resulting alteration in cervical spine curvature (Boyle et al 2002) may dispose the CTJ to degenerative changes. The CTJ and TLJ represent transitional areas between mobile and relatively immobile regions of the spine. At the CTJ, Boyle et al found evident IVD and VEP changes, along with osteophytic formation, which were more pronounced in the mobile segments immediately above the transition (Boyle et al 1998a, 1998b). This observation was consistent with the patterns of osteophytic formation noted by Nathan (1962). It was considered that the upper thoracic region and thoracic cage acted to impede intersegmental motion and thus safeguard these levels from marked degeneration (Boyle et al 1998a, 1998b). At the TLJ, Malmivaara and co-workers (Malmivaara 1987, Malmivaara et al 1987a) demonstrated that particular pathologies tended to be concentrated at each segment. The T10–11 segment was characterized by disc degeneration, vertebral body osteophytosis and SNs; the T11–12 segment tended to show both anterior and posterior degeneration involving zygapophysial and costovertebral joints, while the T12–L1 joint was characterized primarily by posterior joint degeneration. A comparison of zygapophysial joint orientation with degenerative findings suggested that the posterior elements play a significant role in resisting torsional loads. Asymmetry in the zygapophysial joint orientation tended to result in degenerative changes occurring mostly on the sagittal facing facet (Malmivaara 1987), an observation also made by Farfan et al at the lumbosacral junction (Farfan et al 1972).

Scheuermann's disease

Scheuermann's disease (SD) is a common problem that affects the adolescent spine although late manifestations may also be seen. Major signs are SNs and several wedged vertebral bodies which may contribute to an accentuated thoracic kyphosis. Although the reported incidence varies widely, SD is found in approximately 10% of the population, with males and females affected equally (Bradford & McBride 1987). Age of onset is typically before puberty and a key diagnostic feature is the inability of the individual to correct the thoracic deformity. A genetic link is proposed in the aetiology of SD; however, this is yet to be conclusively defined (Aufdermaur 1981).

Pathological areas of growth cartilage within VEPs, reported by Ascani & La Rosa, have been implicated in disordered endochondral ossification (Ascani & Rosa 1994). The extent of vertebral wedging has been related to growth disturbance and mechanical loading, which together produce the deformity. Shortening of the hamstring and pectoral muscles is a common presenting feature. There may be compensatory changes in the lumbar and cervical lordoses. Back extensor muscle function has been found to be reduced in patients with SD compared with controls (Murray et al 1993).

Pain in the interscapular region and at the CTJ is a common presenting symptom in younger patients with SD, while older individuals report more backache, with a distribution which implicates the TLJ segments (Ascani & Rosa 1994). Symptoms tend to decline with progressive ossification. A careful follow-up study involving 61 patients reported that the natural history of the disease was benign despite the cosmetic and structural disturbances which produce a characteristic hyperkyphosis (Murray et al 1993).

Heithoff et al (1994) described patients with thoracolumbar SD who had associated degenerative DD, suggesting that this was a manifestation of an intrinsic defect in the cartilagenous end-plate, resulting in inadequate nutrition and structural weakness, which initiated early disc degeneration. Associated co-morbidities may be osteomalacia, Paget's disease, infection and trauma. In the case of trauma, 10% of cases seen at post mortem showed acute rupture of the VEP (Fahey et al 1998).

DEGENERATIVE SPINAL CURVATURE ANOMALIES

Scoliosis

Idiopathic scoliosis involves a lateral curvature of the spine which is introduced through a disturbance in the longitudinal growth of the spine. It may occur early in the growth of the child and particularly during the early adolescent years (Weinstein 1994). Four main curve patterns have been identified: thoracic, lumbar, thoracolumbar and double major curves. Each of these curvature patterns has its own characteristics and predictable end-point (Weinstein 1994). Management of this disorder is based on the skeletal maturity of the patient at the time of assessment in relation to projected curve progression and its association with mechanical compromise, disability, back pain and possibly respiratory complications. The key concerns are skeletal immaturity, particularly related to curves of larger magnitude. It is well accepted that the severity of the scoliosis can continue to progress through the life span (Ascani et al 1986, Gillespy et al 1985). Disc degeneration is known to develop due to the often extreme compression and ipsilateral tension strains experienced within wedged scoliotic IVDs. In scoliosis, markedly higher levels of the reducible collagen cross-links have been reported on the convex side of the scoliotic disc (Duance et al 1998). This finding appears to parallel changes observed in IVD in degenerative disease to suggest that these reflect increased matrix remodelling. A cascade of degenerative changes occurs in advanced scoliosis due to the attempt to stabilize against the asymmetric mechanical loads induced by this deformity (Fig. 14.7).

A less common form, congenital scoliosis, occurs through defects in formation or segmentation of the vertebral column. These vertebral anomalies include: hemivertebrae, wedge vertebrae and unilateral bar formations (McMaster 1994). The progression of congenital scoliosis depends upon the location of the vertebral anomaly, its type, the extent of growth imbalance it introduces to the spinal column and the age of the individual at the time of diagnosis.

Kyphosis

Reference ranges for thoracic kyphosis include a wide spectrum across the age span (Fon et al 1980), in part due to a lack of standard assessment system (Singer et al 1990). Alteration in mechanics of the thoracic spine, secondary to an increased kyphosis, can have clinical implications in terms of respiratory function compromise, pain and long-term deformity. Postural subsidence with ageing is represented by a loss of vertical height, anterior deformation of the vertebral body and disc (Goh et al 1999) and an increase in thoracic kyphosis (Fig. 14.8), which can in turn contribute to secondary changes within the axial skeleton in terms of structure, mechanics and function. A progressive increase in kyphotic angulation becomes most marked in

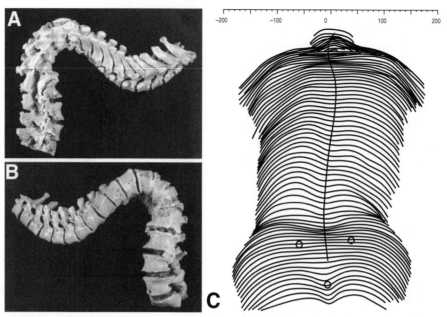

Figure 14.7 An elderly macerated spinal column depicting severe kyphoscoliosis and marked osteophytic fusion across several segments within the region of the thoracolumbar transition, depicted from a posterior (A) and anterior aspect (B). Note the remarkable osseous degeneration and remodelling. C: A surface contour image of a marked scoliosis in an elderly woman, showing the typical rib hump appearance and asymmetry of the thoracic cage.

postmenopausal women (Fig. 14.9), whereas in males the kyphos is less susceptible to change, unless influenced by trauma or metabolic disease (Seeman 1995).

Osteoporosis and osteoporotic fracture

Osteoporosis is an endocrine disease characterized by decreased bone mass and micro-architectural deterioration of bone, which may lead to bone fragility and subsequently to an increased rate of fracture. Although resorption of bone follows the normal process of ageing, it may be induced through disordered metabolism of bone and is accelerated following menopause in women (Kanis 1996). The concern by health economists regarding the full impact of this disease in Western societies is mounting, given the rapidly increasing proportion of older individuals who will require various forms of management of this 'silent' epidemic. More recently, osteoporosis in men has become recognized as having a potentially significant bearing on healthcare costs although the impact may be delayed in onset compared with women (Seeman 2001b).

Osteoporotic fractures are uncommon in young adults of either sex as their bone mass, as assessed by dual energy X-ray absorptiometry (DXA), is within normal ranges and bone loading stress is well within acceptable limits. With ageing, a gender difference in bone fragility emerges due to the dynamic change in relationship between the mechanics of load transfer and the margins of safety. Men accumulate more periosteal bone than women with a corresponding

increase in vertebral cross-sectional area which confers a relatively higher loadbearing capability such that reductions in bone strength are less dramatic than those seen in women. During ageing, this ratio is disturbed and fracture risk increases as the stress on bone begins to approximate its strength. About 20% of postmenopausal women have a stress to strength ratio imbalance, whereas only 2–3% of men are at risk of fracture due to the greater preservation of strength (Seeman 2001a).

The epidemiology of osteoporosis is well known whereby the risk factors of age, sex and racial contributors to bone loss and corresponding fracture risk increase exponentially with age (Matkovic et al 1995). For the thoracic spine, one in four women over the age of 60 years will show at least one vertebral body fracture on radiographic examination, while the incidence increases to 100% in women over 80 years of age (Melton 1995).

The mid-thoracic segments are the most vulnerable to osteoporotic collapse or progressive wedge deformity due to the mechanical disadvantage of these segments situated within the apex of the thoracic kyphosis (Edmondston et al 1997). The second peak for thoracic osteoporotic fracture is at the thoracolumbar junction (De Smet et al 1988), where more rapid loading of the thoracic spine can induce a pivot of the stiffened thorax on the TLJ. These more dynamic loads may be sufficient to cause marked collapse fractures under compression. Degenerative change to the IVD is not common in osteoporosis, suggesting a sparing of the IVD despite the vertebral body collapse (Fig. 14.10).

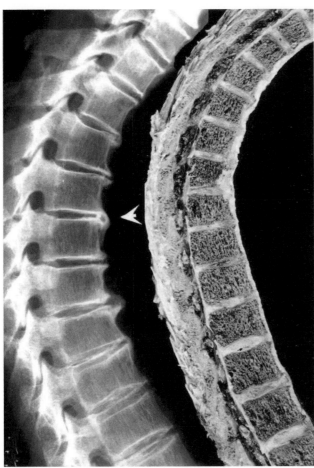

Figure 14.8   Radiographic and macroscopic illustrations of the thoracic kyphotic deformity. Marginal osteophytosis is evident at several levels with fusion across the anterior discovertebral junctions (arrow). Slight anterior wedging of multiple vertebral bodies is noted, particularly in the middle segments.

Spinal trauma

Trauma to the spine may act to initiate degenerative changes through inadequate attempt at remodelling and subsequent strains applied to the injured site, or where the effects of ageing further compound the response to injury. The most common mechanisms of spinal fracture of any region involve dynamic flexion and axial loads (Meyer 1992), commonly mediated through falls or motor vehicle injuries (Daffner 1990). Transitional regions of the human spinal column are considered to be particularly vulnerable to injury due to the abrupt changes in vertebral morphology which alter spinal mechanics and load transmission (Kazarian 1981, Singer et al 1989). In a study of 2461 spinal fractures, 54% occurred between T11 and L2 (Rehn 1968). The most commonly reported injury at the thoracolumbar junction is the wedge compression fracture (Harkönen et al 1979, Willén et al 1990). While the cervicothoracic junction is not affected by trauma to the same extent, the injuries can be severe when forces are localized to these segments (Evans 1991).

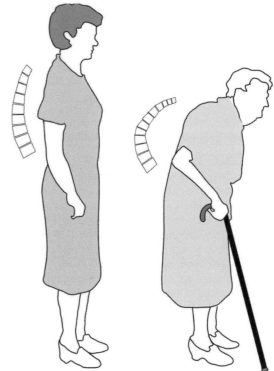

Figure 14.9   Schematic illustration of the sequential adjustment in cervicothoracic spinal posture over the lifespan. The accentuated thoracic kyphosis tends to reduce the cervical lordosis as a compensation to preserve forward gaze. Reproduced from Boyle et al 2002.

Rapid loading in flexion can induce traumatic VEP ruptures. In a recent post mortem study of 70 spinal trauma cases most acute SNs were identified in spines from individuals aged between 11 and 30 years (Fahey 1998). The male to female ratio was 9:1, and SNs were predominantly confined to the T8–L1 segments. Of clinical interest was the absence of radiological detection of these acute SN injuries. The coexistence of other spine pathologies, particularly DISH and ankylosing spondylitis, can complicate the management of patients with spinal fracture (Bernini et al 1981). Traumatic spinal injury, particularly discal lesions, can initiate subsequent degenerative change through rim lesions (Osti et al 1990) to more subtle disruptions to nutritional pathways via VEP damage.

Intervertebral disc prolapse

The entity of disc prolapse was first described in a classic report of paraplegia (Key 1838). Clinically, the regions susceptible to this injury and the resulting disc degeneration typically are those with higher levels of mobility within the cervical and lumbar regions (Kramer 1981, Kramer et al 1991). What is not often appreciated is the high frequency of macroscopic discal prolapse within the thoracic region (Andrae 1929, Singer 2000) (see Fig. 14.3). Many of the pro-

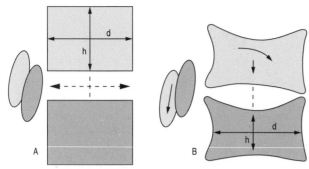

Figure 14.10 Schematic model to illustrate the effect of normal motion segment alignment between paired vertebral bodies, their paired zygapophysial joints posteriorly and a normal intervertebral disc (A). With advancing years and effect of osteoporosis, the vertebral bodies may demonstrate a reduced vertical height (h), most evident anteriorly, loss of disc height and subluxation of the zygapophysial joints and a slight anterior tilt of the superior vertebrae on the subjacent due to anterior disc wedging (B). An expansion in depth (d) of the vertebral body may be accounted for by endosteal bone deposition and osteophytic formation. The cumulative effect is accentuation of regional spinal curvature and focal deformity where isolated vertebral bodies are wedged through incident fracture.

lapses tend to be small and flat in appearance, an observation confirmed by Schmorl & Junghanns in their large post mortem series (Schmorl & Junghanns 1971).

From a review of seven clinical studies involving 221 cases of surgically confirmed thoracic prolapse, the level within the thoracic spine that showed most frequent protrusion was the T11–12 (see Fig. 14.3). This may be attributed to the relatively greater disc height and volume at this region, coupled with localization of torsional forces which can occur immediately above the level of TLJ transition. Indeed, Markolf (1972) proposed that the eleventh and twelfth thoracic vertebrae represented a site of structural weakness for stresses in the vertebral column, due to the reduced constraint of the ribcage and the change in zygapophysial joint morphology which facilitated rotation above the transitional levels and impeded it below. The implication of disc prolapse is decompression of the nucleus, fissuring of the annulus and the cascade of changes which follow this injury (Buckwalter 1995, Singer & Fazey 2004).

CONCLUSION

The human spine contributes a large proportion of the musculoskeletal presentations seen in manual therapy

practice. This chapter has reviewed the effect of age on the human spine including those degenerative processes which are secondary to metabolic disease, spinal deformity or trauma. Given the projections for an aged population and the prevalence of spinal degenerative conditions, it must be emphasized that patients presenting with any ankylosis and advanced degenerative condition of the spinal column are vulnerable to stress concentration at points of force application. A careful history and appropriate imaging, where indicated, will complement the assessment and assist in determining the appropriateness of manual therapy. Ageing of the spine is not merely a chronological process, as remodelling and repair follow such insults as disease, deformity, trauma or surgery. While the spines of some older individuals exhibit relatively few degenerative changes, those that do reflect a fundamental biological strategy to stabilize the segment(s) against further damage from imposed loads (Kirkaldy-Willis & Farfan 1982). When the spine is seen as a single system with regions of either high stress localization at the transitional junctions or torsion-related strains in regions of mobility, the typical patterns of degenerative responses can be recognized. Age-related physiological responses to abnormal development, trauma and disease can then be superimposed upon this mechanical framework to extend the explanation of how some insults are attenuated better than others.

Efforts to disclose further the natural history of disc cell function, to manipulate disc cells and improve disc nutrition, study vertebral end-plate structure and function will assist management of discal disease. Beyond these issues, refinements in tissue engineering, gene therapy and the potential of stem cells in disc therapy will contribute to moderating some of the ageing changes of this critical spinal element (Gruber & Hanley 2003).

KEYWORDS	
spine	osteoporosis
ageing	fracture
pathology	trauma
degeneration	Schmorl's nodes
intervertebral disc	Scheuermann's disease
vertebral end-plate	scoliosis
zygapophysial joint	kyphosis
osteoarthritis	disc prolapse

References

Adams M, Bogduk N, Burton A K, Dolan P 2002 Biomechanics of back pain. Churchill Livingstone, Edinburgh

Andersson G B 1998 What are the age-related changes in the spine? Baillières Clinical Rheumatology 12: 161–173

Andrae R 1929 Über Knorpelknötchen am hinteren Ende der Wirbelbandscheiben im Bereich des Spinalkanals. Beitrage zur Pathologischen Anatomie und zur Allemeinen Pathologischen 82: 464–474

Ariga K, Miyamoto S, Nakase T et al 2001 The relationship between apoptosis of endplate chondrocytes and ageing and degeneration of the intervertebral disc. Spine 26: 2414–2420

Ascani E, Rosa G L 1994 Scheuermann's kyphosis. In: Weinstein S L (ed) The pediatric spine: principles and practice. Raven Press, New York, pp 557–584

Ascani E, Bartolozzi P, Logroscino C A et al 1986 The natural history of untreated idiopathic scoliosis after skeletal maturity. Spine 11: 784–789

Aufdermaur M, 1981 Juvenile kyphosis (Scheuermann's disease): radiography, histology, and pathogenesis. Clincial Orthopaedics and Related Research 154: 167–174

Begg A C 1954 Nuclear herniations of the intervertebral disc. Journal of Bone and Joint Surgery 36B: 180–193

Belanger T A, Rowe D E 2001 Diffuse idiopathic skeletal hyperostosis: musculoskeletal manifestations. Journal of the American Academy of Orthopaedic Surgery 9: 258–267

Benini A 1990 Segmental instability and lumbar spinal canal stenosis. Neurochirurgia 33: 146–157

Bernini P M, Floman Y, Marvel J P, Rothman R H 1981 Multiple thoracic spine fractures complicating ankylosing hyperostosis of the spine. Journal of Trauma 21: 811–814

Bland J 1987 Disorders of the cervical spine. Saunders, Philadelphia

Bobko G, Rabai K, Zsadon B 1966 Contribution to the clinical picture of cervical spondylosis. Zeitschrift für Rheumaforsch 25: 181–186

Boos N, Weissbach S, Rohrbach H, Weiler C, Spratt K F, Nerlich A G 2002 2002 Volvo Award in basic science. Classification of age-related changes in lumbar intervertebral discs. Spine 27: 2631–2644

Boyle J J W, Singer K P, Milne N 1998a Pathoanatomy of the intervertebral discs at the cervicothoracic junction. Manual Therapy 3: 72–77

Boyle J W W, Milne N, Singer K P 1998b Clinical anatomy of the cervicothoracic junction. In: Giles L, Singer K P (eds) Clinical anatomy and management of cervical spine pain. Butterworth Heinemann, Oxford, pp 40–52

Boyle J W W, Milne N, Singer K P, 2002 Influence of age on cervicothoracic spinal curvature: postural implications. Clinical Biomechanics 17: 361–367

Bradford D, McBride G 1987 Surgical management of thoracolumbar spine fractures with incomplete neurologic deficts. Clinical Orthopaedics and Related Research 218: 201–216

Buckwalter J A 1995 Aging and degeneration of the human intervertebral disc. Spine 20: 1307–1314

Cihak R 1970 Variations of lumbosacral joints and their morphogenesis. Acta Universitatis Carolinae Medica 16: 145–165

Coppes M H, Marani E, Thomeer R T, Groen G J 1997 Innervation of 'painful' lumbar discs. Spine 22: 2342–2349

Daffner R H 1990 Thoracic and lumbar vertebral trauma. Orthopaedic Clinics of North America 21: 463–482

Davis P 1955 Observations on the movements of the human lower thoracic and lumbar vertebrae. Journal of Anatomy 89: 565

De Smet A A, Robinson R G, Johnson B E, Lukert B P 1988 Spinal compression fractures in osteoporotic women: patterns and relationship to hyperkyphosis. Radiology 166: 497–500

Dodge H J, Mikkelsen W M, Duff I F 1970 Age–sex specific prevalence of radiographic abnormalities of the joints of the hands, wrists and cervical spine of adult residents of the Tecumseh, Michigan, Community Health Study area, 1962–1965. Journal of Chronic Diseases 23: 151–159

Duance V C, Crean J K, Sims T J et al 1998 Changes in collagen cross-linking in degenerative disc disease and scoliosis. Spine 23: 2545–2451

Edmondston S J, Singer K, Day R, Price R E, Breidahl W H 1997 Ex-vivo estimation of thoracolumbar vertebral body compressive strength: the relative contributions of bone densitometry and vertebral morphometry. Osteoporosis International 7: 142–148

Evans D K 1991 Dislocations at the cervicothoracic junction. Journal of Bone and Joint Surgery 65B: 124–127

Fahey V, Opeskin K, Silberstein M, Anderson R, Briggs C 1998 The pathogenesis of Schmorl's nodes in relation to acute trauma: an autopsy study. Spine 23: 2272–2275

Farfan H F, Cossette J W, Robertson G H, Wells R V, Kraus H 1970 The effects of torsion on the lumbar intervertebral joints: the role of torsion in the production of disc degeneration. Journal of Bone and Joint Surgery 52A: 468–497

Farfan H, Huberdeau R, Dubow H 1972 Lumbar intervertebral disc degeneration: the influence of geometrical features on the pattern of disc degeneration – a post mortem study. Journal of Bone and Joint Surgery 54B: 492–510

Fisk J W, Baigent M L, Hill P D 1984 Scheuermann's disease: clinical and radiological survey of 17 and 18 year olds. American Journal of Physical Medicine 63: 18–30

Fletcher G, Haughton V, Ho K, Yu S 1990 Age-related changes in the cervical facet joints: studies with cryomicrotomy, MR and CT. American Journal of Roentgenology 154: 817–820

Fon G, Pitt M, Thies A 1980 Thoracic kyphosis: range in normal subjects. American Journal of Roentgenology 134: 979–983

Fujiwara A, Lim T H, An H S et al 2000 The effect of disc degeneration and facet joint osteoarthritis on the segmental flexibility of the lumbar spine. Spine 25: 3036–3044

Gillespy T, Gillespy T, Revak C 1985 Progressive senile scoliosis: seven cases of increasing spinal curves in elderly patients. Skeletal Radiology 13: 280–286

Goh S, Price R I, Leedman P J, Singer K P 1999 The relative influence of thoracic vertebral and disc morphometry on thoracic kyphosis. Clinical Biomechanics 14: 439–448

Gregersen G, Lucas D 1967 An in vivo study of the axial rotation of the human thoraco-lumbar spine. Journal of Bone and Joint Surgery 49A: 247–262

Grignon B, Grignon Y, Mainard D, Braun M, Netter P, Roland J 2000 The structure of the cartilaginous end-plates in elder people. Surgical and Radiologic Anatomy 22: 13–19

Gruber H E, Hanley E N J 2003 Recent advances in disc cell biology. Spine 28: 186–193

Hahn M, Vogel M, Amling M et al 1994 Mikrokallusformationen der spongiosa. Pathologe 15: 297–302

Harkönen M, Kataja M, Keski-Nisula T et al 1979 Injuries of the thoracolumbar junction. Archives of Orthopaedic and Traumatic Surgery 94: 35–41

Heithoff K B, Gundry C R, Burton C V, Winter R B 1994 Juvenile discogenic disease. Spine 19: 335–340

Hilton R, Ball J, Benn R 1976 Vertebral end-plate lesions (Schmorl's nodes) in the dorsolumbar spine. Annals of the Rheumatic Diseases 35: 127–132

Inman V, Saunders J D 1942 The clinico-anatomical aspects of the lumbosacral region. Radiology 38: 669–678

Kanis J A 1996 Textbook of osteoporosis. Blackwell Science, Oxford

Kazarian L 1981 Injuries to the human spinal column: biomechanics and injury classification. Exercise and Sport Sciences Reviews 9: 297–352

Key C 1838 On paraplegic depending on disease of the ligaments of the spine. Guy's Hospital Report 3: 17–34

Kirkaldy-Willis W H, Farfan H F 1982 Instability of the lumbar spine. Clinical Orthopaedics and Related Research 165: 110–123

Klippel J H, Dieppe P A 1998 Rheumatology. Mosby, London

Kramer J 1981 Intervertebral disk diseases: causes, diagnosis, treatment and prophylaxis. Georg Thieme Verlag, Stuttgart

Kramer J, Rivera C A, Kleefield J 1991 Degenerative disorders of the cervical spine. Rheumatic Disease Clinics of North America 17: 741–755

Lawrence J S 1977 Rheumatism in populations. Heinemann, London

McMaster M J 1994 Congenital scoliosis. In: Weinstein S L (ed) The pediatric spine: principles and practice. Raven, New York, pp 227–244

McNally D S, Adams M A, Goodship A E 1992 Measurement of stress distribution within intact loaded intervertebral discs. In: Little E G (ed) Technology transfer between high tech engineering and biomechanics. Elsevier Amsterdam, pp 139–159

Maigne J Y, Ayral X, Guèrin-Surville H 1992 Frequency and size of ossifications in the caudal attachments of the ligamentum flavum of the thoracic spine: role of rotatory strains in their development. Surgical and Radiologic Anatomy 14: 119–124

Malmivaara A 1987 Disc degeneration in the thoracolumbar junctional region: evaluation by radiography and discography in autopsy. Acta Radiologica 28: 755–760

Malmivaara A 1988 Thoracolumbar junctional region of the spine: an anatomical, pathological and radiological study [Abstract]. Acta Radiologica 29: 621

Malmivaara A, Videman T, Kuosma E, Troup J D G 1987a Facet joint orientation, facet and costovertebral joint osteoarthrosis, disc degeneration, vertebral body osteophytosis and Schmorl's nodes in the thoracolumbar junctional region of cadaveric spines. Spine 12: 458–463

Malmivaara A, Videman T, Kuosma E, Troup J D G 1987b Plain radiographic, discographic, and direct observations of Schmorl's nodes in the thoracolumbar junctional region of the cadaveric spine. Spine 12: 453–457

Malone D G, Caruso J R, Baldwin N G 1998 Degenerative and non-infectious inflammatory diseases. In: Benzel E C, Stillerman C B (eds) Thoracic spine. Quality Medical Publishing, St Louis, pp 597–606

Manns R A, Haddaway M J, McCall I W, Cassar Pullicino V, Davie M W J 1996 The relative contribution of disc and vertebral morphometry to the angle of kyphosis in asymptomatic subjects. Clinical Radiology 51: 258–262

Markolf K L 1972 Deformation of the thoracolumbar intervertebral joints in response to external loads. Journal of Bone and Joint Surgery 54A: 511–533

Matkovic V, Klisovic D, Ilich J Z 1995 Epidemiology of fractures during growth and aging. Physical Medicine and Rehabilitation Clinics of North America 6: 415–439

Melton J L 1995 Epidemiology of fractures. In: Riggs L B, Melton J L (eds) Osteoporosis: etiology, diagnosis, and management, 2nd edn. Lippincott-Raven, Philadelphia, pp 225–247

Meyer S 1992 Thoracic spine trauma. Seminars in Roentgenology 27: 254–261

Milne N 1991 The role of zygapophysial joint orientation and uncinate processes in controlling motion in the cervical spine. Journal of Anatomy 178: 189–201

Milne N 1993 Composite motion in cervical disc segments. Clinical Biomechanics 8: 193–202

Modic M, Masaryk T, Ross J, Carter J 1988 Imaging of degenerative disk disease. Radiology 168: 177–186

Moore R J, Crotti T N, Osti O L, Fraser R D, Vernon-Roberts B 1999 Osteoarthrosis of the facet joints resulting from anular rim lesions in sheep lumbar discs. Spine 24: 519–525

Murray P M, Weinstein S L, Spratt K F 1993 The natural history and long-term follow-up of Scheuermann's kyphosis. Journal of Bone and Joint Surgery 75A: 236–248

Nathan H 1959 The para-articular processes of the thoracic vertebrae. Anatomical Record 133: 605–618

Nathan H 1962 Osteophytes of the vertebral column: an anatomical study of their development according to age, race and sex with considerations as to their etiology and significance. Journal of Bone and Joint Surgery 44A: 243–268

Nathan H, Weinberg H, Robin G C, Aviad I 1964 The costovertebral joints: anatomico-clinical observations in arthritis. Arthritis and Rheumatology 7: 228–240

O'Rahilly R, Muller F, Meyer D B 1980 The human vertebral column at the end of the embryonic period proper. 1: The column as a whole. Journal of Anatomy 131: 565–575

Oegema T R, Bradford D S 1991 The inter-relationship of facet joint osteoarthritis and degenerative disc disease. British Journal of Rheumatology 30: 16–20

Osti O L, Vernon-Roberts B, Fraser R D 1990 Annulus tears and intervertebral disc degeneration: an experimental study using an animal model. Spine 15: 762–767

Osti O L, Vernon-Roberts B, Moore R, Fraser R D 1992 Annular tears and disc degeneration in the lumbar spine: a post-mortem study of 135 discs. Journal of Bone and Joint Surgery 74B: 678–682

Penning L 1988 Differences in anatomy, motion, development and aging of the upper and lower cervical disk segments. Clinical Biomechanics 3: 37–47

Pfirrmann C W A, Resnick D 2001 Schmorl nodes of the thoracic and lumbar spine: radiologic-pathologic study of prevalence, characterization, and correlation with degenerative changes of 1650 spinal levels in 100 cadavers. Radiology 219: 368–374

Prescher A 1998 Anatomy and pathology of the aging spine. European Journal of Radiology 27: 181–195

Rehn J 1968 Die knöcheren Verletzungen der Wirbelsäule, Bedeutung des Erstbefundes für die spätere Begutachtung. Die Wirbelsäule in Forschung und Praxis 40: 131–138

Resnick D 1985 Degenerative diseases of the vertebral column. Radiology 156: 3–14

Resnick D, Niwayama G 1976 Radiographic and pathologic features of spinal involvement in diffuse idiopathic skeletal hyperostosis (DISH). Radiology 119: 559–563

Resnick D, Niwayama G 1978 Intravertebral disk herniations: cartilaginous (Schmorl's) nodes. Radiology 126: 57–65

Resnick D, Niwayama G 1995 Diffuse idiopathic skeletal hyperostosis (DISH): ankylosing hyperostosis of Forestier and Rotes-Querol. In: Resnick D (eds) Diagnosis of bone and joint disorders. Saunders, Philadelphia, pp 1463–1508

Roberts S, McCall I W, Menage J, Haddaway M J, Eisenstein S M 1997 Does the thickness of the vertebral subchondral bone reflect the composition of the intervertebral disc? European Spine Journal 6: 385–389

Schmorl G 1929 Zur pathologische Anatomie der Wirbelsäule. Klinik Wochenscrift 8: 1243–1249

Schmorl G, Junghanns H 1971 The human spine in health and disease. Grune and Stratton, New York

Seeman E 1995 The dilemma of osteoporosis in men. American Journal of Medicine 98(Suppl. 2A): 76–88S

Seeman E 2001a During aging, men lose less bone than women because they gain more periosteal bone, not because they resorb less endosteal bone. Calcified Tissue International 69: 205–208

Seeman E 2001b Unresolved issues in osteoporosis in men. Reviews of Endocrinology and Metabolic Disorders 2: 45–64

Shore L 1935a On osteo-arthritis in the dorsal intervertebral joints: a study in morbid anatomy. British Journal of Surgery 22: 833–849

Shore L R 1935b Some examples of disease of the vertebral column found in skeletons of ancient Egypt: a contribution to paleopathology. British Journal of Surgery 22: 256–271

Singer K P 1997 Pathomechanics of the aging thoracic spine. In: Lawrence D (eds) Advances in chiropractic. Mosby, St Louis, pp 129–153

Singer K P 2000 Pathology of the thoracic spine. In: Giles L, Singer K P (eds) Clinical anatomy and management of thoracic spine pain. Butterworth Heinemann, Oxford, pp 63–82

Singer K P, Fazey P J 2004 Disc herniation – non-operative treatment. In: Herkowitz H K et al (eds) The lumbar spine, 3 edn. Raven-Lippincott, Philadelphia, in press

Singer K P, Willén J, Breidahl P D, Day R E 1989 The influence of zygapophyseal joint orientation on spinal injuries at the thoracolumbar junction. Surgical and Radiologic Anatomy 11: 233–239

Singer K P, Jones T J, Breidahl P D 1990 A comparison of radiographic and computer-assisted measurements of thoracic and thoracolumbar sagittal curvature. Skeletal Radiology 19: 21–26

Singer K P, Edmondston S J, Day R E, Price E, Breidahl P B 1995 Prediction of compressive strength of isolated lumbar and thoracic vertebral bodies: relationships to age, geometry, bone density and spinal curvature. Bone 17: 167–174

Ten Have H A M J, Eulderink F 1980 Degenerative changes in the cervical spine and their relationship to its mobility. Journal of Pathology 132: 133–159

Töndury G 1959 La colonne cervicale, son développement et ses modifications durant la vie. Acta Orthopedica Belgica 25: 602–627

Urban J P, Roberts S 1995 Development and degeneration of the intervertebral discs. Molecular Medicine Today 1: 329–335

Utsinger P 1985 Diffuse idiopathic skeletal hyperostosis. Clinics in Rheumatic Diseases 11: 325–351

Vernon-Roberts B 1992 Age-related and degenerative pathology of the intervertebral discs and apophyseal joints. In: Jayson M I V (ed) The lumbar spine and back pain. Churchill Livingstone, Edinburgh, pp 17–42

Vernon-Roberts B, Pirie C J 1977 Degenerative changes in the intervertebral discs of the lumbar spine and their sequelae. Rheumatology and Rehabilitation 16: 13–21

Vernon-Roberts B, Pirie C J, Trenwith V 1974 Pathology of the dorsal spine in ankylosing hyperostosis. Annals of the Rheumatic Diseases 33: 281–288

von Luschka H 1850 Die nerven des menschlichen wirbelkanales. Laupp and Siebeck, Tubingen

von Luschka H 1858 Die Halbbgelenke des Menschlichen Körpers. Druck und Verlag von Georg Reimer, Berlin, p 144

Weinfeld R M, Olson P N, Maki D D, Griffiths H J 1997 The prevalence of diffuse idiopathic skeletal hyperostosis (DISH) in two large American Midwest metropolitan hospital populations. Skeletal Radiology 26: 222–225

Weinstein S L 1994 Adolescent idiopathic scoliosis: prevalence and natural history. In: Weinstein S L (ed) The pediatric spine. Raven, New York, pp 463–478

Weinstein P, Ehni G, Wilson C 1977 Clinical features of lumbar spondylosis and stenosis. In: Weinstein P R, Ehni G, Wilson C B (eds) Lumbar spondylosis, diagnosis, management and surgical treatment. Year Book Medical Publisher, Chicago

Willén J, Anderson J, Tomooka K, Singer K 1990 The natural history of burst fractures in the thoracolumbar spine (T12 & L1). Journal of Spinal Disorders 3: 39–46

Yasuma T, Saito S, Kihara K 1988 Schmorl's nodes: correlation of X-ray and histological findings in postmortem specimens. Acta Pathological Japonica 38(6): 723–733

SECTION 3

Clinical sciences for manual therapy of the spine

Chapter **15**

How inflammation and minor nerve injury contribute to pain in nerve root and peripheral neuropathies

J. Greening

INTRODUCTION

Spinal and peripheral nerve injury involving axonal degeneration is known to cause neuropathic symptoms associated with sensory and motor fibre changes. These conditions are easy to diagnose when associated with objective loss of nerve conduction velocity (NCV) or muscle weakness. However, many patients present without objective signs of nerve dysfunction but with symptoms suggestive of neuropathy (paraesthesia, spontaneous pain, lancinating, burning pain). Examples are non-specific back pain, chronic whiplash disorders and non-specific arm pain. Patients may complain of pain that is not in a dermatomal, myotomal or single peripheral nerve distribution and symptoms may be associated with hyperalgesic or allodynic sensory changes. Over the past decade neurophysiologists and clinicians have made considerable progress towards understanding how minor nerve injury or inflammation without major axonal degeneration can cause changes similar to frank nerve injury with altered sensory thresholds and neuropathic symptoms.

This chapter will review the evidence for altered nerve function, morphology and neuropathic symptoms following minor peripheral nerve and nerve root injury. The effects of inflammatory mediators and mechanical compression on these structures will be examined and related to clinical studies where possible. While most of this work has been carried out in animals using large peripheral nerves, usually the sciatic, some of the neuropathological mechanisms involved are similar to experimental models of nerve root injury. Clinical studies confirm that these animal models of nerve injury may be relevant to the many patients musculoskeletal physiotherapists see with these chronic pain problems. Table 15.1 gives characteristics of sensory nerve fibre types.

MINOR PERIPHERAL NERVE INJURY

Animal models used to investigate the consequences of minor peripheral nerve injury include chronic constriction injury (CCI) where four loose ligatures are applied to the

Table 15.1 Characteristics of sensory nerve fibre types

Classification	Morphological fibre type	Respond to
Aβ	Large myelinated fibres	Different types of mechanoreceptor responding to innocuous stimuli, e.g.: • Pacinian corpuscle – vibration • Meissner's corpuscle – light touch
Aδ	Small myelinated fibres	• Mechanoreceptors • Cold-sensitive thermoreceptors • Nociceptors responding to noxious pressure and heat
C	Non-myelinated fibres	• Warmth-sensitive thermoreceptors • Nociceptor responding to noxious pressure, heat and irritant chemicals

sciatic nerve in the thigh (Bennett & Xie 1988) and a neuritis model where inflammatory materials are applied to the nerve sheath (Eliav et al 1999, 2001). In both models, the animal develops significant pain behaviours and sensory testing over the paw reveals marked mechanical allodynia and thermal hyperalgesia. In the CCI model the nerve swells either side of the ligatures and increased endoneurial fluid pressure probably causes venous stasis with subsequent axonal ischaemia and degeneration. In this injury model, nerve fibre loss is not apparent across all fascicles and where it occurs is most pronounced in the large myelinated Aβ fibres (Bennett & Xie 1988, Coggeshall et al 1993). Damage to Aδ and C fibres does occur but to a much lesser extent (Basbaum et al 1991). Recordings from nerve fibres demonstrate changed firing patterns. Normally transduction of sensory signals in response to different stimuli only occurs at the sensory terminal of afferent neurons. The rest of the axon length is not able to generate electrical activity. Following both the CCI and neuritis injury, electrophysiological recording of nerve fibres indicates changed firing patterns and ectopic activity at different sites along the nerve length. Spontaneous and abnormal mechanically evoked firing has been demonstrated arising from the associated dorsal root ganglion (DRG), the lesion site and the peripheral nociceptor terminals (Kajander & Bennett 1992, Koltzenburg et al 1994, Tal & Eliav 1996). Spontaneous Aβ firing occurs that is correlated with the presence of mechanical hyperalgesia in animal models (Tal & Eliav 1996). Centrally mediated mechanical hyperalgesia due to Aβ fibre stimulation has also been demonstrated in a human experimental model (Torebjork et al 1992), which may be maintained by sustained peripheral nociceptor activity (Anderson et al 1995). Using the CCI model, Koltzenburg et al (1994) reported that more than 10% of the C fibres showed spontaneous activity. Since most of these C fibres are nociceptors, this finding may be very relevant to pain symptoms. Many of these C fibres developed novel chemical sensitivity; for example, some developed an increased firing rate to noradrenaline (norepinephrine). This response may help explain some of the pathophysiology of sympathetic maintained pain states. Ectopic firing patterns of C fibres both in the periphery, at the dorsal root ganglion and at

sites of inflammation along the nerve trunk trigger a cascade of events within the central nervous system. These include increased central excitability, leading to chronic pain (Devor 1988, McMahon et al 1993; for review see Greening & Lynn 1998).

PERIPHERAL NEURITIS

Chromic gut, the suture material used for CCI studies, is an inflammatory material. Maves et al (1993) investigated the effects of using both chromic gut and silk ligatures. Heat hyperalgesia was only observed when the chromic gut was used. Interestingly heat hyperalgesia occurred even when the chromic gut sutures were laid alongside the nerve, with no ligation at all. Eliav et al (1999) investigated the consequences of inducing an inflammatory reaction of the sciatic nerve sheath. It appears that this very minor nerve injury, in which axonal loss is not apparent, leads to pain related behaviours and hyperalgesia and allodynia on sensory testing. Later studies using this animal model demonstrated increased mechanosensitivity of the Aβ fibres (Eliav et al 2001) and of deep nociceptor axons (Wallas & Bove 2001) at the lesion site. This has considerable clinical importance. In this situation nerve conduction studies will be normal. The increased sensitivity of the Aβ fibres and deep nociceptors to muscle means that limb movement is likely to provoke painful symptoms. In addition, nerve inflammation will involve C fibres present in the nerve sheath (nervi nervorum) (Bove & Light 1995, Zochodne 1993, Zochodne & Ho 1993). Local elevation of neurotrophin and other inflammatory mediators such as bradykinin and serotonin may sensitize these nociceptors (Koltzenburg et al 1999). The relative contributions that the nervi nervorum on the one hand, and the axons within the nerve trunk itself on the other, make to pain behaviour and dorsal horn neuronal excitability under conditions of local neuritis excitability remains to be evaluated (Bove & Light 1997).

A chronic or acute neuritis along a nerve trunk due to infection, mechanical irritation or vascular dysfunction will produce ectopic discharge and may therefore result in neuropathic pain in the absence of any detectable neural degeneration. Such an explanation may be of importance to complex regional pain syndrome I (reflex sympathetic dystrophy) where there is pain without evidence of structural nerve damage (Eliav et al 2001). Patients with arm pain where work practices such as repetitive hand and arm use seem to precede symptoms have been diagnosed as having non-specific arm pain (NSAP) (Harrington et al 1998). Patients present without evidence of major nerve or tissue damage but do have subtle change to Aβ and C fibre function and altered sympathetic reflexes (Greening et al 2003). Tests of nerve mechanosensitivity, such as the upper limb tension tests, frequently produce painful symptoms with restricted ranges of arm movement in patients with NSAP (Byng 1997, Greening et al 2001). These patients also report marked tenderness and referred pain on palpation over discrete areas of the median and ulnar nerves (Greening et al 2003), signs that may indicate sites of nerve inflammation or constriction. The sustained muscle activity and limb postures associated with keyboard use have been suggested to alter the nerve environment sufficiently to cause symptoms in NSAP (Greening & Lynn 1999)

In the nerve trunk, axons are packed within endoneurial connective tissue and organized into fascicles by the perineurium. While the perineurium confers considerable tensile strength to the nerve trunk it also acts as a diffusion barrier, protecting the interior of the fascicles by maintaining their chemical environment. A second major component to the maintenance of the chemical environment of the nerve fibres is the blood–nerve barrier. An early indication of nerve injury in both animal and human studies is disruption to this barrier with proliferation of endothelial cells and loss of tight cell junctions (Eliav et al 1999, Mackinnon et al 1986). These changes would allow cytokines access to the nerve fibre environment and induce C fibre activity (Sorkin et al 1997). The next section reviews the role of cytokines and neurotrophic factors in the production of neuropathic symptoms. Figure 15.1 depicts areas of ectopic firing and sensitization following nerve inflammation.

THE ROLE OF CYTOKINES AND NEUROTROPHINS IN NEUROPATHIC PAIN

Cytokines

Following nerve damage or inflammation, neuronal and non-neuronal cells such as macrophages and Schwann cells secrete cytokines and nerve growth factor (NGF) as part of the inflammatory response (Ebadi et al 1997, Murphy et al 1999). If nerve fibres are damaged cytokines play a part in wallerian degeneration in a number of ways:

- mediation of inflammatory events, e.g. they activate macrophages and Schwann cells
- regulation of the production of cytokines such as interleukin (IL-1), IL-6 and tumour necrosis factor alpha (TNFα)
- by inducing the production of nerve growth factor (Tal 1999).

Cytokines produce effects by their interactions with neuronal and non-neuronal cells. They have the potential to modify synaptic transmission and nociception (Ebadi et al 1997, Watkins et al 1995a, 1995b), and have been shown to be involved in the production of peripheral sensitization, ectopic nerve firing and central sensitization. Following minor nerve manipulation without axon degeneration, changes to the blood–nerve barrier allow cytokines access to the nerve fibres. Many of these cytokines have a pro-inflammatory action and have been associated with mechanical allodynia (IL-β, IL-6 and TNFα) (DeLeo et al 1996). Not all cytokines have the same pro-inflammatory action – IL-10, for example, inhibits the production of pro-inflammatory cytokines (Wagner et al 1998)

The pro-inflammatory cytokine TNFα, released by many cells closely associated with nerves, has been found to induce mechanical hyperalgesia following injection into the paw (Cunha et al 1992), exerting its action directly on terminal C fibre endings. Interestingly, endoneurial injection

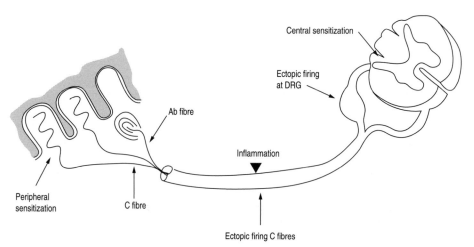

Figure 15.1 Areas of ectopic firing and sensitization following nerve inflammation. Key: DRG = dorsal root ganglion.

Central sensitization

Ectopic firing at DRG

Ab fibre

Inflammation

Peripheral sensitization

C fibre

Ectopic firing C fibres

of TNFα has also been shown to produce relatively long term (3 days) thermal hyperalgesia and mechanical allodynia (Wagner & Myers 1996). Just applying TNFα to the epineurium resulted in acute mechanical hyperalgesia (Sorkin & Doom 2000). Sorkin et al (1997) have shown a direct action of TNFα on intact axons by induction of ectopic activity in C fibres. Blocking the action of TNFα receptor following CCI in rats significantly attenuated the duration of mechanical and heat hyperalgesia (Sommer et al 1998). Nerve biopsies from patients with painful and non-painful peripheral neuropathies have revealed higher levels of TNFα in Schwann cells in the painful conditions and serum soluble TNFα receptor 1 levels higher in patients with a centrally mediated mechanical allodynia (Empl et al 2001).

Neurotrophins

Neurotrophins, for example nerve growth factor (NGF), are large peptides produced by a number of cell types including muscle cells, skin keratinocytes and Schwann cells in peripheral nerves. After the developmental period, sensory neurons are not dependent on NGF for survival and NGF is not significantly expressed in peripheral nerves. However, neurotrophins do play a part in regulating function in the adult nervous system. Following nerve injury or tissue inflammation, there is an up-regulation of NGF in the periphery. Elevated levels of NGF appear to sensitize C fibres directly or indirectly via immunocompetent cells, for example by the degranulation of mast cells, resulting in the release of prostoglandins and bradykinin (Andreev et al 1995, Koltzenburg et al 1999, Tal & Liberman 1997). Elevated levels of NGF can increase the synthesis, axonal transport and neuronal content, both peripherally and centrally, of the algesic neuropeptides substance P and calcitonin gene related peptide (CGRP). In contrast, a reduction in the uptake and transport of NGF following nerve constriction or axonal degeneration exposes the nerve cell body to decreased levels of NGF. This will have several effects on sensory nerve function including a complex change in neuronal peptide expression (e.g. substance P, CGRP falling and levels of galanin rising (McMahon et al 1997, Xu et al 1996)). Therefore, elevated or decreased levels of NGF will alter synaptic function in the dorsal horn and may be involved in increasing the receptive field size of central neurones, a factor that could lead to the spread of symptoms beyond single peripheral or dermatomal nerve boundaries. Supplying exogenous NGF to damaged peripheral nerves within the first 3 weeks following CCI injury can reduce the resulting hyperalgesia (Ren et al 1995). However, NGF antibodies can also reduce the effects of CCI (Herzberg et al 1997), so the consequences of CCI cannot just be the result of reduced NGF availability. Human studies of levels of NGF following nerve injury (Anand et al 1997) found reduced levels of NGF in injured nerves and dorsal root ganglion (DRG), but found normal levels of NGF distal to the injury, with areas of high concentration at neuroma formation. This suggests that early NGF administration may help prevent neuronal degeneration while in the more chronic stage anti-NGF treatment may help relieve chronic pain.

The main points regarding the role of cytokines and NGF are summarized in Box 15.1. Having established mechanisms of minor peripheral nerve injury, the effect of such injuries at the level of the nerve root and dorsal root ganglion is now considered.

INFLAMMATION AND COMPRESSION OF NERVE ROOTS AND DORSAL ROOT GANGLION

Non-specific low back pain, with or without radiculopathy, is a growing problem. An approach to its management has been one that relates pain to discrete structural abnormalities of the spine. However, structural and morphological changes do not necessarily predict pain and disability. Furthermore, the wide variations in treatment and treatment outcomes indicate that the pathophysiology of low back pain and radiculopathy is likely to be complex. For example, the relationship between sciatica and disc herniation was first demonstrated by Mixter & Barr in 1934. They attributed sciatica to compression of spinal nerve roots by herniated disc material. However, although inflamed nerve roots are very sensitive to manipulation during lumbar surgery producing leg and back pain, investigations have not

---

Box 15.1 Cytokines and nerve growth factor

- Cytokines and nerve growth factor (NGF) are peptides produced by neuronal and non-neuronal cells, e.g. macrophages, Schwann cells
- Cytokines mediate inflammatory events, e.g. activate macrophages and Schwann cells
- Following nerve inflammation or minor trauma, changes in the blood/nerve barrier allow cytokine access to nerve fibres
- The pro-inflammatory cytokine TNFα induces ectopic activity in C fibres
- Patients with painful neuropathies have Schwann cells with high levels of TNFα
- Following inflammation, elevated levels of NGF sensitize C fibres directly or indirectly via immunocompetent cells
- Increased availability of NGF elevates the neuronal content of the algesic neuropeptides substance P and calcitonin gene related peptide
- In acute nerve injuries, supplying NGF to damaged nerves reduces hyperalgesia by preventing neuronal degeneration; in chronic injuries NGF antibodies may relieve chronic pain

shown a correlation between compression of normal nerve roots and such pain (Boden et al 1990, Kuslich et al 1991). Isolated acute compression of uninflamed nerves, whether peripheral or central, leads to paraesthesia, sensory loss and reflex abnormalities without painful symptoms (Rydevik et al 1984).

DISC HERNIATION: EFFECTS ON NERVE ROOTS

Current concepts regarding radiculopathy following disc herniation indicate that this condition is not merely the result of nerve compression. Instead it appears that the nerve is sensitized (inflamed) by the herniated nucleus pulposus having gained access to the nerve via the epidural space. Animal studies have shown that the application of autologous nucleus pulposus material applied epidurally (without nerve compression) can induce significant histological and functional change in nerve roots (Olmarker et al 1993). These changes were significantly attenuated by the early intravenous administration of methylprednisolone (a glucocorticosteriod), supporting the hypothesis that inflammatory mechanisms may be related to the induced nerve root injury. Further studies have revealed leukotaxis and increase in vascular permeability (Olmarker et al 1995), axonal oedema and structural changes to Schwann cells (Olmarker et al 1996), and periradicular fibrosis (Cooper et al 1995). In vivo studies have shown spontaneous axonal firing, spontaneous activity and increased mechanosensitivity of the DRG, with decreased mechanical threshold over receptive fields in the foot (Takebayashi et al 2001). Yabuki et al (1998, 2000) reported decreased blood flow to the corresponding DRG and corresponding hind paw, an effect significantly reduced by the infiltration of lidocaine (lignocaine) to the affected nerve roots (Onda et al 2001). While an inflammatory reaction around the spinal nerve without compression clearly produces marked functional and histological changes, these effects are even more marked when nerve traction and inflammation occur together. Omarker & Myers (1998) demonstrated that displacement of the fourth lumbar root combined with disc puncture produced a greater degree of thermal hyperalgesia than when the two procedures were applied separately.

Incision of the annulus fibrosus with leakage of disc material produced similar changes to those described above with a reduction in nerve conduction velocity (NCV) to 20% less than the velocity of the non-incision group (Kayama et al 1996). However, a histological study of the affected nerve roots demonstrated no difference between the two groups. In this instance the reduction in conduction velocity may have been due to the vascular changes observed in the annular incision group. Here the axonal capillaries were increased in number, enlarged, with many showing thrombus formations. Thrombus formation would result in stasis of capillary blood flow, the reduction in NCV being related to nerve root ischaemia. This discrepancy between functional and structural changes has been

reported in other studies (Olmarker et al 1993, 1996). In the clinical situation, leakage of nucleus pulposus material could account for back pain and sciatica in patients without visible disc herniation on imaging studies.

Inflammatory reactions clearly play a part in the radiculopathy associated with disc herniation. The cytokine TNFα has been suggested to play a significant role in mediating the inflammatory response of spinal nerve roots. Effects of TNFα on nerve roots include the induction of pain behaviours, mechanical allodynia, neural oedema formation, intravascular thrombosis, blood flow reduction and myelin splitting (Igarashi et al 2000, Olmarker & Larsson 1998). It has also been shown that local application of TNFα to spinal nerve roots reduces nerve conduction velocity similar to that observed following application of nucleus pulposus material (Aoki et al 2002). TNFα is known to be produced and released from chondrocyte-like cells of the nucleus pulposus (Olmarker & Larsson 1998). Selective inhibition of TNFα effectively blocked these nucleus pulposus induced changes (Olmarker & Rydevik 2001). However, treatment was initiated at the same time as the injury, a scenario never possible in the clinical setting. The inherent ability of the nucleus pulposus to produce TNFα may explain the thrombus formation and other vascular changes in the absence of significant numbers of inflammatory cells found in a clinical histological study of herniated disc and associated soft tissues (Cooper et al 1995).

Prostaglandins are also important mediators of inflammatory reactions. They are generated from the breakdown products of damaged cell membranes. It has been reported that prostaglandin E2 (PGE2) plays a role in radiculopathy (Ozaktay et al 1998). PGE2 synthesis is regulated by phospholipase A_2 and cyclo-oxygenase (COX). COX exists in two forms, COX-1 and COX-2. The glucocorticosteriods interrupt the entire process of prostoglandin induction, while non-steroidal anti-inflammatory drugs (NSAIDs) act by interrupting the COX-1 pathway. COX-2 is induced in many cells following stimulation by inflammatory mediators including IL-1β and TNFα. Immunohistological studies have demonstrated COX-2, IL-1β, and TNFα in cultured herniated human disc material (Miyamoto et al 2000). PGE2 was produced by these disc cells following stimulation with cytokines. This suggests that COX-2 and inflammatory cytokines play a role in the production of back pain and radiculopathy. Clinical and immunohistological studies (O'Donnell & O'Donnell 1996, Virri et al 2001) have found a correlation between restriction of straight leg raising, the PGE2 content of extruded disc material and the presence of inflammatory cells. In contrast, an assay of phospholipase A_2 (an activator of arachidonic acid metabolites) from tissue taken from herniated and normal discs failed to show any significant elevation (Gronblad et al 1996). Cornefjord et al (2001) exposed compressed spinal nerve roots to either diclofenac or ketoprofen (non-steroidal anti-inflammatory drugs, NSAIDs) for 7 days following the experimental procedure. Although none of the animals appeared to exhibit gross signs of neurological defect, conduction velocity was significantly higher in the treated animals. Early pharmacological intervention with these strong anti-inflammatory agents appears to have a 'neuroprotective' effect on spinal nerve roots. In a double blind comparative trial with ibuprofen, nimesulide, a cyclo-oxygenase (COX)-2-selective anti-inflammatory agent, appeared more effective for treating acute low back pain (Pohjolainen et al 2000).

Clearly, one mechanism through which a herniated disc may initiate symptoms in low back pain or sciatica is as a result of inflammation induced by the release of pro-inflammatory chemicals from the nucleus pulposus. Both prostaglandins and cytokines appear to have a role and an effective drug therapy may be a combination of selective COX-2 inhibitors and inhibition of specific cytokines. The TNFα targeting drugs thalidomide and infliximab have given promising results in the treatment of ankylosing spondylitis, a systemic inflammatory rheumatic disease (Toussirot & Wendling 2001). However, these are potent drugs and their use in patients with discrete inflammatory conditions remains to be evaluated.

The mechanism of this neuropathological pain state is more complicated than simply chemical irritation of nerve roots and the dorsal root ganglion (DRG). Nerve pain due to damage from neural tissue oedema or mechanical injury from direct compression of nerve tissue by herniated disc material or spinal stenosis is also possible. Zhang et al (1999) demonstrated changed behavioural response, thermal hyperalgesia and mechanical allodynia with spontaneous firing of the DRG following a DRG compression injury. In these animals there were no motor deficits and little evidence of DRG cell degeneration. Although signs of inflammation were not looked for, the authors concluded that an inflammatory reaction was in part responsible for the observed changes. Rydvick et al (1989) found endoneurial oedema in their studies of DRG compression; Howe et al (1997) evoked DRG firing with the application of mechanical stimuli.

COMPARISONS BETWEEN INJURY PROXIMAL OR DISTAL TO THE DORSAL ROOT GANGLION

Comparisons with the peripheral CCI model using both chromic gut and silk ligatures applied to nerve roots have been performed. As noted above, chromic gut sutures produce an inflammatory reaction as well as a mild compressive effect to the nerve while silk would produce only mild compression. Kawakami et al (1994a), found heat hyperalgesia only in the chromic gut treated nerve roots, not those where silk ligatures were used. Similarly, the peripheral CCI model morphological changes (loss of Aβ fibres) found in both the chromic gut and silk ligature groups did not correlate with the sensory hyperalgesia. This demonstrates that mechanical compression alone was insufficient to produce the hyperalgesia. Changes in neuropeptide content of the

spinal nerve and DRG similar to those observed in the peripheral CCI model have also been found (Cornefjord et al 1995, Kawakami et al 1994b). Unlike peripheral nerve injury studies, the involvement of NGF in nerve root injuries does not appear to have been evaluated. Presumably if the peripheral neural connections are not compromised then levels of NGF in the DRG are unaffected, although spinal cord neurotrophin levels may change.

To examine whether the effects of nerve root injury are more severe than those of peripheral nerve injury, Winkelstein et al (2001) compared the effect of CCI to the L5 nerve root and transection of the spinal nerve (i.e. injury proximal or distal to the DRG). They assessed the severity of the behavioural response to mechanical and thermal tests, the induction of a spinal neuroimmune reaction and the response to using cytokine antagonists (for IL-1 and TNFα). The overall cytokine expression and degree of astrocyte and glia activation at the spinal cord were the same in both injuries. However, the pharmacological treatments were more effective at alleviating the mechanical hyperalgesia in the spinal nerve injury than the nerve root injury. This suggests that the nerve root injury produces a stronger centrally mediated response than the peripheral injury.

Are there specific anatomical points regarding nerve roots that make them more or less vulnerable to the effects of disc herniation and inflammatory mediators? The dorsal and ventral roots of the spinal nerves transverse the subarachnoid space separately, fusing in or close to their intervertebral foramen to form the mixed spinal nerve. Anatomically, nerve roots differ significantly from peripheral nerves. Nerve roots are bathed in cerebral spinal fluid and have a dural covering compared to the epineurium surrounding peripheral nerves. The spinal nerve has only a thin layer of epineurium near to the dorsal root ganglion (DRG) whereas the peripheral nerve has a thick epineurium (Garfin et al 1995). Byrod et al (1995) reported a rapid transport pathway between the epidural space and the intraneural capillaries of the nerve roots making the potential protective properties of the dura and arachnoid around the nerve roots appear less important. Thus, herniated disc contents have a rapid route to the axons of the spinal nerves. Smith et al (1993), observed that the L4/5 nerve roots moved linearly 2–5 mm within the intervertebral foramen with straight leg raising. Periradicular fibrosis would limit movement exposing the nerve roots to traction and irritation. This group also observed lateral movement towards the pedicle, effectively causing the nerve root to move into a posterolaterally herniated disc. Box 15.2 summarizes the effects of inflammation on nerve roots.

NERVE ROOTS AND TRAUMA: WHIPLASH INJURIES

Nerve root injury is a potential source of pain following traumatic injuries to the spine. Patients with chronic

---

Box 15.2 Inflammation and nerve roots

- Chondrocyte-like cells in the nucleus pulposus produce and release TNFα
- Rapid transport route between epidural space and intraneural capillaries allows herniated disc materials access to nerve fibres
- Periradicular fibrosis following inflammation exposes nerve roots to traction and irritation
- Nerve root injury produces a stronger centrally mediated response than peripheral nerve injury making pharmacological intervention less effective

Box 15.3 Conclusion

- Nerve inflammation without sign of frank axon degeneration can produce neuropathic symptoms
- Nerve conduction studies will be normal, but there may be changed sensory thresholds and neural provocation tests will be positive
- Management should include the early administration of anti-inflammatory medication
- COX-2 inhibitors are effective for low back pain
- Clinically, cytokine inhibitors remain unevaluated for these injuries

---

whiplash associated disorders (WAD), without signs of nerve conduction abnormalities, complain of neck and arm pain. The mechanisms underlying chronic pain following cervical whiplash injuries are unclear. Significant soft tissue injury following cervical whiplash injury has been demonstrated (Yoganandan et al 2001). This traumatic injury may expose DRG and spinal nerve roots to traction and inflammatory mediators. In a pig study, Svensson et al (1998) investigated the effects of pressure changes within the inner volume of the spinal canal during neck extension/flexion injuries. These injuries produced dysfunction and damage to DRG cell membrane. This effect was not apparent when the neck was only exposed to static loading. Kivioja et al (2001) assayed blood levels of TNFα, IL-6 pro-inflammatory cytokines and IL-10 anti-inflammatory cytokine in patients with WAD, ankle sprain, multiple sclerosis and control subjects. Significantly high levels of these cytokines were found in the WAD group at 3 days post injury but not at 14 days. Curatolo et al (2001) found increased sensitivity to neck and leg intramuscular and cutaneous electrical stimulation in WAD patients. Local anaesthetic infiltration of muscle tender points affected neither intensity of neck pain nor pain thresholds. Centrally mediated hyperalgesia therefore appeared to be independent of nociceptive input arising from the painful muscles. It is possible, in the acute stage, that cervical nerve roots and ganglia, having undergone minor trauma, may be exposed to proinflammatory cytokines, becoming a potent source of nociceptive input. The stage could then be set for central sensitization and chronic pain. A peripheral neuropathic component to the symptoms associated with chronic WAD should also be considered. Elevated plasma levels of the algesic neuropeptides calcitonin gene related peptide (CGRP) and substance P (Sub P) have been found in WAD patients (Alpar et al 2002). All patients had normal nerve conduction studies for the median nerve, yet chronic arm pain and levels of CGRP and Sub P decreased significantly in the patient group who received surgery to decompress the carpal tunnel.

Improvement in the operated group was maintained at a 2-year follow-up.

CONCLUSION

Nerves that have sustained minor injury or inflammation are capable of producing neuropathic symptoms. Clinically these types of injuries may occur where nerves are subject to inflammation and/or compression from herniated disc material, annular fissures, spinal stenosis, acceleration/deceleration injuries or mechanical irritation from limb posture and sustained muscle activity. In these minor nerve injuries, particularly neuritis, clinical nerve conduction studies are likely to be normal. The clinician should be aware that in such circumstances, the only other indication of nerve injury, apart from symptom characteristics, would be changed sensory thresholds and positive neural provocation tests.

Management of these conditions should include the early administration of anti-inflammatory medication. The effectiveness of COX-2 inhibitors has been demonstrated for low back pain and they may be useful in the treatment of minor peripheral neuropathies. Novel therapies such as cytokine inhibition remain unevaluated in these patients. The sequelae of nerve root injury may be more resistant to pharmacological intervention than peripheral nerve injury. Understanding the role of inflammation in neuropathic pain improves understanding of the complex pathophysiological mechanisms of low back pain and some non-specific limb pains. Box 15.3 summarizes the main points of this chapter.

KEYWORDS	
neuritis	neuropathic pain
inflammation	whiplash
cytokines	non-specific arm pain
neurotrophins	

Acknowledgements

I would like to thank Dr B. Lynn (University College, London) for his helpful comments during the preparation of this chapter and E. Greening for Fig. 15.1.

References

Alpar E K, Onvoha G, Killampalli V, Waters R 2002 Management of chronic pain in whiplash injury. Journal of Bone and Joint Surgery 84B(6): 807–811

Anand P, Terenghi G, Birch R et al 1997 Endogenous NGF and CNTF levels in human peripheral nerve injury. Neuroreport 8(8): 1935–1938

Anderson O K, Gracely R H, Arendt-Neilsen L 1995 Facilitation of the human nociceptive reflex by stimulation of A beta fibres in a secondary hyperalgesic area sustained by nociceptive input from the primary hyperalgesic area. Acta Physiologica Scandinavica 155(1): 87–89

Andreev N Y, Dimitrieva N, Koltzenburg M, McMahon S B 1995 Peripheral administration of nerve growth factor in the adult rat produces a thermal hyperalgesia that requires the presence of sympathetic post-ganglionic neurones. Pain 63(1): 109–115

Aoki Y, Rydevik B, Kikuchi S, Olmarker K 2002 Local application of disc-related cytokines on spinal nerve roots. Spine 27(15): 1614–1617

Basbaum A, Gautron M, Jazat F, Mayes M, Guilbaud G 1991 The spectrum of fibre loss in a model of neuropathic pain in the rat; an electron microscopic study. Pain 47: 359–367

Bennett G J, Xie Y K 1988 A peripheral mononeuropathy in rat that produces disorders of pain sensation like those seen in man. Pain 33(1): 87–107

Boden S D, Davis D O, Dina T S, Patronas N J, Wiesel S W 1990 Abnormal magnetic-resonance scans of the lumbar spine in asymptomatic subjects: a prospective investigation. Journal of Bone and Joint Surgery (American volume) 72(3): 403–408

Bove G M, Light A R 1995 Calcitonin gene-related peptide and peripherin immunoreactivity in nerve sheaths. Somatosensory and Motor Research 12(1): 49–57

Bove G M, Light A R 1997 The nervi nervorum: missing link for neuropathic pain? Pain Forum 6: 181–190

Byng J 1997 Overuse syndromes of the upper limb and the upper limb tension test: a comparison between patients, asymptomatic keyboard workers and asymptomatic non-keyboard workers. Manual Therapy 2: 157–164

Byrod G, Olmarker K, Konno S, Larsson K, Takahashi K, Rydevik B 1995 A rapid transport route between the epidural space and the intraneural capillaries of the nerve roots. Spine 20(2): 138–143

Coggeshall R E, Dougherty P M, Pover C M, Carlton S M 1993 Is large myelinated fiber loss associated with hyperalgesia in a model of experimental peripheral neuropathy in the rat? Pain 52(2): 233–242

Cooper R G, Freemont A J, Hoyland J A et al 1995 Herniated intervertebral disc-associated periradicular fibrosis and vascular abnormalities occur without inflammatory cell infiltration. Spine 20(5): 591–598

Cornefjord M, Olmarker K, Farley D B, Weinstein J N, Rydevik B 1995 Neuropeptide changes in compressed spinal nerve roots. Spine 20(6): 670–673

Cornefjord M, Olmarker K, Otani K, Rydevik B 2001 Effects of diclofenac and ketoprofen on nerve conduction velocity in experimental nerve root compression. Spine 26(20): 2193–2197

Cunha F Q, Poole S, Lorenzetti B B, Ferreira S H 1992 The pivotal role of tumour necrosis factor alpha in the development of inflammatory hyperalgesia. British Journal of Pharmacology 107(3): 660–664

Curatolo M, Petersen-Felix S, Arendt-Nielsen L, Giani C, Zbinden A M, Radanov B P 2001 Central hypersensitivity in chronic pain after whiplash injury. Clinical Journal of Pain 17(14): 306–315

DeLeo J A, Colburn R W, Nichols M, Malhotra A 1996 Interleukin-6-mediated hyperalgesia/allodynia and increased spinal IL-6 expression in a rat mononeuropathy model. Journal of Interferon and Cytokine Research 16(9): 695–700

Devor M 1988 Central changes mediating neuropathic pain. In: Dubner G, Gebhart G F, Bond M R (eds) Proceedings of the Fifth World Congress on Pain. Elsevier Science, Amsterdam

Ebadi M, Bashir R M, Heidrick M L et al 1997 Neurotrophins and their receptors in nerve injury and repair. Neurochemistry International 30(4–5): 347–374

Eliav E, Herzberg U, Ruda M A, Bennett G J 1999 Neuropathic pain from an experimental neuritis of the rat sciatic nerve. Pain 83(2): 169–182

Eliav E, Benoliel R, Tal M 2001 Inflammation with no axonal damage of the rat saphenous nerve trunk induces ectopic discharge and mechanosensitivity in myelinated axons. Neuroscience Letters 311(1): 49–52

Empl M, Renaud S, Erne B et al 2001 TNF-alpha expression in painful and nonpainful neuropathies. Neurology 56(10): 1371–1377

Garfin S R, Rydevik B, Lind B, Massie J 1995 Spinal nerve root compression. Spine 20(16): 1810–1820

Greening J, Lynn B 1998 Minor peripheral nerve injuries: an underestimated source of pain? Manual Therapy 3(4): 187–194

Greening J, Lynn B 1999 Possible causes of pain in repetitive strain injury. In: Devor M, Rowbotham M C, Wiesenfeld-Hallin Z (eds) 1999 Progress in pain research and management. IASP Press, Seattle, vol 16, pp 697–710

Greening J, Lynn B, Leary R, Warren L, O'Higgins P, Hall-Craggs M 2001 The use of ultrasound imaging to demonstrate reduced movement of the median nerve during wrist flexion in patients with non-specific arm pain. Journal of Hand Surgery 26: 5

Greening J, Lynn B, Leary R 2003 Sensory and autonomic function and ultrasound nerve imaging in RSI patients and keyboard workers. Pain 104: 275–281

Gronblad M, Virri J, Ronkko S et al 1996 A controlled biochemical and immunohistochemical study of human synovial-type (group II) phospholipase A2 and inflammatory cells in macroscopically normal, degenerated, and herniated human lumbar disc tissues. Spine 21(22): 2531–2538

Harrington J M, Carter J T, Birrell L, Gompertz D 1998 Surveillance case definitions for work related upper limb pain syndromes. Occupational and Environmental Medicine 55(4): 264–271

Herzberg U, Eliav E, Dorsey J M, Gracely R H, Kopin I J 1997 NGF involvement in pain induced by chronic constriction injury of the rat sciatic nerve. Neuroreport 8(7): 1613–1618

Howe J F, Loeser J D, Calvin W H 1997 Mechanosensitivity of dorsal root ganglia and chronically injured axons: a physiological basis for the radicular pain of nerve compression. Pain 3: 25–41

Igarashi T, Kikuchi S, Shubayev V, Myers R R 2000 Volvo Award winner in basic science studies. Exogenous tumor necrosis factor-alpha mimics nucleus pulposus-induced neuropathology: molecular, histologic, and behavioral comparisons in rats. Spine 25(23): 2975–2980

Kajander K C, Bennett G J 1992 Onset of a painful peripheral neuropathy in rat: a partial and differential deafferentation and spontaneous discharge in A beta and A delta primary afferent neurons. Journal of Neurophysiology 68(3): 734–744

Kawakami M, Weinstein J N, Chatani K, Spratt K F, Meller S T, Gebhart G F 1994a Experimental lumbar radiculopathy: behavioral and histologic changes in a model of radicular pain after spinal nerve root irritation with chromic gut ligatures in the rat. Spine 19(16): 1795–1802

Kawakami M, Weinstein J N, Spratt K F et al 1994b Experimental lumbar radiculopathy: immunohistochemical and quantitative demonstrations of pain induced by lumbar nerve root irritation of the rat. Spine 19(16): 1780–1794

Kayama, S, Konno S, Olmarker K, Yabuki S, Kikuchi S 1996 Incision of the annulus fibrosus induces nerve root morphologic, vascular, and functional changes: an experimental study. Spine 21(22): 2539–2543

Kivioja J, Ozenci V, Rinaldi L, Kouwenhoven M, Lindgren U, Link H 2001 Systemic immune response in whiplash injury and ankle sprain: elevated IL-6 and IL-10. Clinical Immunology 101(1): 106–112

Koltzenburg M, Torebjork H E, Wahren L K 1994 Nociceptor modulated central sensitization causes mechanical hyperalgesia in acute chemogenic and chronic neuropathic pain. Brain 117(3): 579–591

Koltzenburg M, Bennett D L, Shelton D L, McMahon S B 1999 Neutralization of endogenous NGF prevents the sensitization of nociceptors supplying inflamed skin. European Journal of Neuroscience 11(5): 1698–1704

Kuslich S D, Ulstrom C L, Michael C J 1991 The tissue origin of low back pain and sciatica: a report of pain response to tissue stimulation during operations on the lumbar spine using local anesthesia. Orthopedic Clinics of North America 22(2): 181–187

Mackinnon S E, Dellon A, Hudson A R, Hunter D A 1986 Chronic human nerve compression – a histological assessment. Neuropathology and Applied Neurobiology 12(6): 547–565

McMahon S B, Lewin G R, Wall P D 1993 Central hyperexcitability triggered by noxious inputs. Current Opinion in Neurobiology 3(4): 602–610

McMahon S B, Bennett D L, Michael G J, Priestly J V 1997 Neurotrophic factors and pain. In: Jensen T S, Turner J A, Wiesenfield-Hallin Z (eds). Proceedings of the Eighth World Congress on Pain. Progress in pain research and management. IASP Press, Seattle, vol 8, pp 353–379

Maves T J, Pechman P S, Gebhart G F, Meller S T 1993 Possible chemical contribution from chromic gut sutures produces disorders of pain sensation like those seen in man. Pain 54(1): 57–69

Mixter W J, Barr J S 1934 Rupture of the intervertebral disc with involvement of the spinal canal. New England Medical Journal 211: 210–215

Miyamoto H, Saura R, Harada T, Doita M, Mizuno K 2000 The role of cyclooxygenase-2 and inflammatory cytokines in pain induction of herniated lumbar intervertebral disc. Kobe Journal of Medical Sciences 46(1–2): 13–28

Murphy P G, Borthwick L S, Johnston R S, Kuchel G, Richardson P M 1999 Nature of the retrograde signal from injured nerves that induces interleukin-6 mRNA in neurons. Journal of Neuroscience 19(10): 3791–3800

O'Donnell J L, O'Donnell A L 1996 Prostaglandin E2 content in herniated lumbar disc disease. Spine 21(14): 1653–1655

Olmarker K, Larsson K 1998 Tumor necrosis factor alpha and nucleus-pulposus-induced nerve root injury. Spine 23(23): 2538–2544

Olmarker K, Rydevik B 2001 Selective inhibition of tumor necrosis factor-alpha prevents nucleus pulposus-induced thrombus formation, intraneural edema, and reduction of nerve conduction velocity: possible implications for future pharmacologic treatment strategies of sciatica. Spine 26(8): 863–869

Olmarker K, Rydevik B, Nordborg C 1993 Autologous nucleus pulposus induces neurophysiologic and histologic changes in porcine cauda equina nerve roots. Spine 18(11): 1425–1432

Olmarker K, Blomquist J, Stromberg J, Nannmark U, Thomsen P, Rydevik B 1995 Inflammatogenic properties of nucleus pulposus. Spine 20(6): 665–669

Olmarker K, Nordborg C, Larsson K, Rydevik B 1996 Ultrastructural changes in spinal nerve roots induced by autologous nucleus pulposus. Spine 21(4): 411–414

Omarker K, Myers R R 1998 Pathogenesis of sciatic pain: role of herniated nucleus pulposus and deformation of spinal nerve root and dorsal root ganglion. Pain 78(2): 99–105

Onda A, Yabuki S, Kikuchi S, Satoh K, Myers R R 2001 Effects of lidocaine on blood flow and endoneurial fluid pressure in a rat model of herniated nucleus pulposus. Spine 26(20): 2186–2191

Ozaktay A C, Kallakuri S, Cavanaugh J M 1998 Phospholipase A2 sensitivity of the dorsal root and dorsal root ganglion. Spine 23(12): 1297–1306

Pohjolainen T, Jekunen A, Autio L, Vuorela H 2000 Treatment of acute low back pain with the COX-2-selective anti-inflammatory drug nimesulide: results of a randomized, double-blind comparative trial versus ibuprofen. Spine 25(12): 1579–1585

Ren K, Thomas D A, Dubner R 1995 Nerve growth factor alleviates a painful peripheral neuropathy in rats. Brain Research 699(2): 286–292

Rydevik B, Brown M D, Lundborg G 1984 Pathoanatomy and pathophysiology of nerve root compression. Spine 9(1): 7–15

Rydevik B L, Myers R R, Powell H C 1989 Pressure increase in the dorsal root ganglion following mechanical compression: closed compartment syndrome in nerve roots. Spine 14(6): 574–576

Smith S A, Massie J B, Chesnut R, Garfin S R 1993 Straight leg raising: anatomical effects on the spinal nerve root without and with fusion. Spine 18(8): 992–999

Sommer C, Schmidt C, George A 1998 Hyperalgesia in experimental neuropathy is dependent on the TNF receptor 1. Experimental Neurology 151(1): 138–142

Sorkin L S, Doom C M 2000 Epineurial application of TNF elicits an acute mechanical hyperalgesia in the awake rat. Journal of the Peripheral Nervous System 5(2): 96–100

Sorkin L S, Xiao W H, Wagner R, Myers R R 1997 Tumour necrosis factor-alpha induces ectopic activity in nociceptive primary afferent fibres. Neuroscience 81(1): 255–262

Svensson M Y, Aldman B, Bostrom O et al 1998 Nerve cell damages in whiplash injuries; animal experimental studies. Orthopade 27(12): 820–826

Takebayashi T, Cavanaugh J M, Cuneyt O A, Kallakuri S, Chen C 2001 Effect of nucleus pulposus on the neural activity of dorsal root ganglion. Spine 26(8): 940–945

Tal M 1999 A role for inflammation in chronic pain. Current Review of Pain 3(6): 440–446

Tal M, Eliav E 1996 Abnormal discharge originates at the site of nerve injury in experimental constriction neuropathy (CCI) in the rat. Pain 64(3): 511–518

Tal M, Liberman R 1997 Local injection of nerve growth factor (NGF) triggers degranulation of mast cells in rat paw. Neuroscience Letters 221(2–3): 129–132

Torebjork H E, Lundberg L E, LaMotte R H 1992 Central changes in processing of mechanoreceptive input in capsaicin-induced secondary hyperalgesia in humans. Journal of Physiology 448: 765–780

Toussirot E, Wendling D 2001 Therapeutic advances in ankylosing spondylitis. Expert Opinion on Investigational Drugs 10(1): 21–29

Virri J, Gronblad M, Seitsalo S, Habtemariam A, Kaapa E, Karaharju E 2001 Comparison of the prevalence of inflammatory cells in subtypes of disc herniations and associations with straight leg raising. Spine 26(21): 2311–2315

Wagner R, Myers R R 1996 Endoneurial injection of TNF-alpha produces neuropathic pain behaviors. Neuroreport 7(18): 2897–2901

Wagner R, Janjigian M, Myers R R 1998 Anti-inflammatory interleukin-10 therapy in CCI neuropathy decreases thermal hyperalgesia, macrophage recruitment, and endoneurial TNF-alpha expression. Pain 74(1): 35–42

Wallas T R, Bove G M 2001 Pain-related responses following nerve inflammation and injury. Abstracts-Society for Neuroscience

Watkins L R, Goehler L E, Relton J, Brewer M T, Maier S F 1995a Mechanisms of tumor necrosis factor-alpha (TNF-alpha) hyperalgesia. Brain Research 692(1–2): 244–250

Watkins L R, Maier S F, Goehler L E 1995b Cytokine-to-brain communication: a review and analysis of alternative mechanisms. Life Sciences 57(11): 1011–1026

Winkelstein B A, Rutkowski M D, Sweitzer S M, Pahl J L, DeLeo J A 2001 Nerve injury proximal or distal to the DRG induces similar spinal glial activation and selective cytokine expression but differential behavioral responses to pharmacologic treatment. Journal of Comparative Neurology 439(2): 127–139

Xu J, Pollock C H, Kajander K C 1996 Chromic gut suture reduces calcitonin-gene-related peptide and substance P levels in the spinal cord following chronic constriction injury in the rat. Pain 64(3): 503–509

Yabuki S, Kikuchi S, Olmarker K, Myers R R 1998 Acute effects of nucleus pulposus on blood flow and endoneurial fluid pressure in rat dorsal root ganglia. Spine 23(23): 2517–2523

Yabuki S, Igarashi T, Kikuchi S 2000 Application of nucleus pulposus to the nerve root simultaneously reduces blood flow in dorsal root ganglion and corresponding hindpaw in the rat. Spine 25(12): 1471–1476

Yoganandan N, Cusick J F, Pintar F A, Rao R D 2001 Whiplash injury determination with conventional spine imaging and cryomicrotomy. Spine 26(22): 2443–2448

Zhang J M, Song X J, LaMotte R H 1999 Enhanced excitability of sensory neurons in rats with cutaneous hyperalgesia produced by chronic compression of the dorsal root ganglion. Journal of Neurophysiology 6: 3359–3366

Zochodne D W 1993 Epineurial peptides: a role in neuropathic pain? Canadian Journal of Neurological Sciences 20(1): 69–72

Zochodne D W, Ho L T 1993 Evidence that capsaicin hyperaemia of rat sciatic vasa nervorum is local, opiate-sensitive and involves mast cells. Journal of Physiology 468: 325–333

Chapter 16

Chronic pain and motor control

G. L. Moseley, P. W. Hodges

INTRODUCTION

Pain is essentially motoric, that is, the basic biological function of pain is to escape or prevent danger and promote survival (Melzack 1996, Wall & Melzack 1999). Not surprisingly then, people who have had pain usually develop 'abnormal' movement patterns. Abnormal movement patterns can be compensatory to pain, causative of pain, both compensatory and causative, or neither. In chronic pain the relationship between pain and movement is particularly complex. This is probably because chronic pain is clinically and physiologically distinct from acute pain. As such, it presents distinct aetiological and therapeutic challenges.

Aside from the ambiguity concerning what definitively constitutes chronic pain, there seem to be two factors that make the relationship between chronic pain and motor control difficult to understand: the first is a limited understanding of the physiological complexities of chronic pain and the second is the potent effects of cognitive and emotional factors often characteristic of chronic pain on motor control and motor learning. This chapter attempts to provide an overview of the challenges associated with chronic pain as they relate to its physiological complexities (see Doubell et al 1999 and Butler 2000 for a more detailed review) and cognitive and emotional complexities, and the impact of these complexities on motor control. It is important to note that much of the material presented here is of particular relevance to a portion of patients, namely those with chronic unremitting pain, particularly those in whom conventional strategies are of limited effect. This chapter presents a conceptual model for understanding the relationship between pain and motor control in these patients. Finally, the chapter discusses clinical implications for the assessment, management and progression of motor control training in what is a difficult patient group.

CHALLENGES IN CHRONIC PAIN: PHYSIOLOGICAL COMPLEXITIES

According to the International Association for the Study of Pain (IASP), chronic pain is pain of more than 3 months duration (Merskey & Bogduk 1994). However, this definition is only partially helpful because it does not give any details as to the mechanism or aetiology of the pain, details which are often more important than its duration. For example, even if the duration of the pain is identical, there are fundamental differences in both aetiology and management response between chronic pain due to a peripheral nerve injury or a malignant cancer or pain of no known pathology.

One proposal that accounts in part for such ambiguity suggests that chronic pain be regarded according to the underlying physiological mechanisms (Woolf et al 1998). This approach has benefits and limitations. Categorizing pain in this manner may distinguish between the examples mentioned above and provide sufficient information to enable optimal management responses, including pharmaceutical and interventionist strategies. However, it may also lead to an overestimation of the contribution of physiological mechanisms, such that structural or primary nociceptive mechanisms are overlooked. Suffice it to acknowledge that specific neural mechanisms contribute to some extent to any chronic pain situation and necessarily have an effect on sensorimotor performance. These neural mechanisms can occur rapidly and act within both the peripheral and the central nervous system.

Peripheral mechanisms of chronic pain

When cells are damaged, inflammatory mediators are released into the extracellular fluid. Inflammation causes an elevation of the resting membrane potential of nociceptors which, in effect, reduces their activation threshold (Raja et al 1999). This altered state is a normal product of injury and is called peripheral sensitization, by virtue of the altered response and stimulus modality properties of the peripheral nociceptor.

Clinically, peripheral sensitization manifests as both primary hyperalgesia and allodynia. Although these terms are used interchangeably, they represent distinct clinical presentations. Hyperalgesia means that a stimulus that normally results in pain now results in more pain. Allodynia means that a stimulus that does not normally result in pain now does result in pain. Allodynia in particular has implications for patients because it means that even subtle motor control deficits may be sufficient to maintain nociceptive input, which in turn may maintain inflammation, and so on.

Damage to the peripheral nerve induces more robust changes in the properties and function of the primary nociceptor. These changes increase nociceptive input at the dorsal horn (Devor & Seltzer 1999). When a nerve is cut, fine processes start to grow out of the proximal side of the cut within days of the injury. Ideally, the regenerating sprouts reach the target tissue on the other side of the cut thereby restoring normal function. However, if the sprouts fail to reach their target, or are prevented from doing so, they can turn back on themselves or form small tangles (Devor &

Seltzer 1999). When this happens, the newly formed neural structure begins to spontaneously generate action potentials in the proximal (and possibly peripheral (Raminsky 1978)) nerve section (Wall & Gutnick 1974, Weisenfeld & Lindblom 1980). Such sites have been called ectopic impulse generators or abnormal impulse generating sites (AIGS) (Butler 2000).

Animal studies have identified AIGS at sites of nerve compression and minor nerve damage (Amir & Devor 1993, Xie et al 1993, Pinault 1995, Chen & Devor 1998). AIGS are generally sensitive to mechanical input and can be further augmented by exposure to thermal (Matzner & Devor 1987, Blenk et al 1996) and chemical stimuli such as anoxia, inflammatory mediators (Tracey & Walker 1995, Michaelis et al 1998) and noradrenaline (norepinephrine) (Wall & Gutnick 1974, Janig et al 1996) (although see Michaelis et al 1997).

The dorsal root ganglion (DRG) can also function as an AIGS when the peripheral nerve becomes damaged or stressed (Devor & Seltzer 1999). Like other AIGS, dorsal root ganglion AIGS also display sensitivity to mechanical input, and consequently they have been proposed as a source of chronic spinal pain exacerbated by movement (Wall & Gutnick 1974, Howe et al 1977). In fact, the DRG and nerve root may be subject to considerable tensile stress during manoeuvres such as the straight leg raise (Nowicki et al 1996) and it is not unreasonable that this stress could be translated into the generation of both efferent and afferent action potentials (Nordin et al 1984). Efferent impulses generated by a sensitized DRG will cause neurogenic inflammation at the peripheral terminals of sensory neurons associated with the DRG, which means that radiation of symptoms, and potentially signs, can be mediated at the DRG. Generally, this mechanism is acknowledged in clinical texts (see, for example, Brieg 1978, Butler 2000).

Dorsal root ganglion AIGS may also be particularly sensitive to chemical and humoral factors, such as prostaglandins and noradrenaline (norepinephrine), because, unlike the rest of the peripheral nervous system, the DRG is readily permeable to vascular circuits (Wadhwani & Rapoport 1987, Allen & Kiernan 1994). This has particular ramifications in people with chronic pain because those people are often characterized by elevated levels of such hormones by virtue of the long-term stress associated with chronic pain (Melzack 1999).

Alterations in neural structure and behaviour at a peripheral and spinal level probably have a direct impact on the activity (and possibly the neural properties) of alpha and gamma motoneurons. Early theories proposed that sensitization of the primary nociceptor caused facilitation of gamma motoneuron loops (Travell et al 1942), which caused spasm of discrete groups of sarcomeres, which in turn led to anoxia and build-up of algesic chemicals and nociception (the so-called 'vicious cycle'). This proposal has been shown to be simplistic: sensorimotor loops are facilitated or inhibited according to the task at hand (Graven-Nielsen et al 1997). Although supraspinal mechanisms are almost certainly more important in this regard (Zedka et al 1999), sensitization of primary nociceptors will magnify the role of spinal sensorimotor mechanisms, at least at lower levels of muscle activity (Matre et al 1999).

Collectively, the available findings suggest that peripheral mechanisms that enhance nociceptive sensitivity are associated with changes in motor and endocrine function. Caution should be exercised, however, because the relationship between nociception and pain is complex. In fact, the body of evidence suggests that central rather than peripheral processes may be more important in the development and maintenance of chronic pain.

Central mechanisms of chronic pain

Primary nociceptors terminate in the dorsal horn at synaptic connections with second order nociceptors. There are two types of second order nociceptor: nociceptor-specific (NS) and polymodal or wide dynamic range (WDR). As their names suggest, in normal state NS neurons are activated by peripheral nociceptive input while WDR neurons can be activated by nociceptive and non-nociceptive input (i.e. synaptic input from Aβ as well as Aδ and C fibres) (Doubell et al 1999). WDR neurons are thought to be particularly important in chronic pain and therefore they have been the focus of most of the research. Because WDR neurons can be activated by non-nociceptive input, they are also of particular relevance to motor control and training.

Experimental pain models usually utilize peripheral nerve injury to investigate WDR neuron changes in chronic pain, partly because of the relative ease of this paradigm, but primarily because it allows quantification of the nociceptive stimulus. Reduction of normal inhibitory inputs ('disinhibition') caused by removal of supraspinal projections to the WDR neuron can cause sensitization (Doubell et al 1999). These and other findings suggest that sensitization mechanisms are probably activated in the absence of peripheral damage when descending projections are intact and facilitatory supraspinal input predominates. This situation has potent implications for chronic pain patients in whom demonstrable structural pathology is absent. These patients are often characterized by catastrophic interpretations of their pain and the conviction that their body is vulnerable. Such factors are likely to promote descending facilitatory mechanisms.

Regardless of whether it is mediated by peripheral input, disinhibition or increased descending facilitation, if second order nociceptors remain active they undergo rapid and substantial sensitization (see Doubell et al 1999, Mannion & Woolf 2000 for review). The changes that occur are collectively termed central sensitization and manifest clinically as secondary hyperalgesia and allodynia: potentiation (elevated resting membrane potential), which reduces the activation threshold of the second order nociceptor; altered gene expression; sprouting at the receptive (and possibly terminal) synapses.

Sustained activity of second order nociceptors results in changes in its gene expression (Ji & Rupp 1997). The genetic changes are thought to regulate the synthesis of neurotransmitter and receptor molecules, thus effecting greater synaptic efficacy as well as new synaptic connections (Dubner & Ruda 1992). The changes effect increased receptor fields within the dorsal horn, manifesting clinically as spreading pain and potentially incurring autonomic involvement.

Cortical structures are known to undergo structural reorganization in patients in whom no peripheral neuropathy is demonstrable. Flor and colleagues (1997) measured the extent of somatosensory cortex activated by noxious cutaneous stimulation to the finger and back of chronic low back pain (LBP) patients. The area activated by noxious back stimulation was elevated in the patients compared to age matched controls, and the area activated increased as a function of the duration of their pain (R = 0.71). The authors posited that cortical changes play a role in maintaining pain in the absence of tissue pathology.

Although alterations in the somatosensory cortex may be involved in some chronic pain states, the importance of these alterations is unclear. Most likely, the available findings reflect the relative accessibility for measurement of the somatosensory cortex compared to deeper cortical structures. In fact, across pain studies, the somatosensory cortex is infrequently active and although it demonstrates more activity in some studies of chronic pain patients (e.g. Coghill et al 1998), other studies report no difference in activity (e.g. Derbyshire et al 1994) and still others report more or less activity depending on the individual (Di Piero et al 1994).

In fact, of all the cortical structures that have been studied during pain only the anterior cingulate cortex (ACC) consistently demonstrates increased activity across studies (Peyron et al 2000). Notably, the ACC is also active during non-nociceptive but biologically threatening events such as anticipated pain (Sawamoto et al 2000) and anxiety (Kimbrell et al 1999, Osuch et al 2000). In chronic pain patients, the ACC seems to be chronically active (Hsieh et al 1995) and abnormal ACC neurotransmitter release during nociceptive stimulation has been reported (Grachev et al 2000).

These findings are important because the ACC has long been thought to be important in motor responses. However, movement is not permitted in imaging studies and chronic pain patients are often characterized by immobility. Further, in experimental pain, ACC activity occurs before activity in other cortical areas and too early to represent a response mechanism. Thus it seems that the motor function of the ACC during pain is part of a mechanism by which the brain makes sense of the nociceptive information according to what it should do about it (see Wall 1999 for a review).

Evaluation of ACC function suggests that it plays a complex and pivotal role in both establishing an emotional valence to pain and coordinating the perception of bodily threat with other areas involved in selection and planning of an appropriate behavioural/motor response strategy (Price 2000). These functions are evidenced by the fact that the

ACC directly projects to motor and supplementary motor areas (Price 2000), and receives direct projections from reticular formation neurons, which in turn have demonstrated clear relevance to escape behaviour and fear responses, but not to sensory–discriminative aspects of pain, for example nucleus gigantocellularis (Willis 1985) and peri-aqueductal grey nucleus (Mayer & Price 1976). Overwhelmingly, the distal origins of these neural mechanisms are instigated by activity in WDR rather than nociceptor-specific second order neurons (Vogt et al 1993) and activity relates to affective/emotional–motivational functions (Bushnell 1995).

There are two main reasons why the central mechanisms involving the ACC are important for chronic pain and motor control. The first is that the mechanisms are central in, and probably common to, the emotional and motor dimensions of pain. That is, activity is modulated according to the perceived threat value associated with pain and the perceived vulnerability of the body. Interpretations that emphasize threat and somatic vulnerability are typically definitive of chronic pain patients, especially those in whom no demonstrable tissue pathology has been identified (e.g. 'non-specific' spinal pain) (Sullivan et al 1995, Crombez et al 1998a, 1998b). Thus, factors that impart threat or emotional valence to pain are thought to have a greater impact on motor control than factors that impart stimulus intensity or sensory qualities to pain. Further, as cognitive and emotional factors contribute more to pain, so too the impact of pain on motor control increases (Price 2000). This notion appears theoretically sound and initial data seem supportive (see below).

The second reason that mechanisms involving the ACC are considered important in chronic pain and motor control is that the majority of presynaptic projections from the dorsal horn are WDR, rather than NS, neurons (Bushnell & Duncan 1989). Thus, sensitization of the dorsal horn, which almost exclusively involves WDR neurons, will have a profound effect on the motor and emotional/motivational dimensions of pain. This means that the sensitization process promotes escape-type responses, makes the pain more unpleasant and motivates the individual to do something about it. Although such a response seems biologically prudent, it also means that in states of sensitization, the impact of pain on motor output is increased.

Implications of neural changes associated with chronic pain

From a biological perspective, the ability of the nervous system to rapidly augment the sensitivity of nociceptive and pain mechanisms serves to protect vulnerable tissue and promote survival of the organism. In this sense, changes can be considered normal neural adaptations to demand. However, humans are able to incorporate complex reasoning, learning and emotional mechanisms such that a myriad of psychological and social factors can have an effect on these neural adaptations. This means that much

of the neural adaptation associated with many chronic pain situations can be considered a normal response to an abnormal set of circumstances.

Regardless of the specific aetiology, and despite its obvious evolutionary benefits, nociceptive sensitization presents substantial barriers to rehabilitation. First, increased sensitivity of the peripheral nociceptor reduces the kinematic margin for error, such that even slight motor control abnormalities may be sufficient to drive nociceptive pathways. Second, tolerance of the nervous system to non-nociceptive stimulation is reduced because WDR neurons receive non-nociceptive input pre-synaptically. Thus, there is a fine line between doing enough to promote control, strength and endurance changes and doing too much so that the sensitized nociceptive system is activated. The latter situation manifests clinically as a 'flare-up', typically associated with severe pain, sometimes with paraesthesia and nausea. The third barrier to rehabilitation is that cortically mediated modulation of nociception and pain may be sufficient to increase and possibly maintain pain. Perceived threat and somatic vulnerability are central to this effect. Finally, structural reorganization of the CNS can result in inaccurate transmission of proprioceptive information, which may disrupt the internal spatial representation of the body, thereby further compromising motor control. These issues as they influence assessment, management and progression are discussed later.

CHALLENGES IN CHRONIC PAIN: PSYCHOSOCIAL FACTORS

Chronic pain is sometimes understood to represent a collection of psychosocial characteristics, all of which are conceptually attached to long-lasting pain. These characteristics, broadly categorized as 'psychosocial' factors, include social exclusion, disability, depression, cognitive disruption, fear of pain and (re)injury and catastrophic thought processes. The importance of psychosocial factors in the development of chronic spinal pain has been emphasized (Burton et al 1995, Burton 1997, Schade et al 1999) and there is mounting evidence that beliefs relating to pain, stress, somatic hypervigilance and fear disrupt motor control (Weinberg & Hunt 1976, Brown & Donnenwirth 1990, Ebersbach et al 1995, Jones & Cale 1997, Watson et al 1997, Marsh & Geel 2000, van Galen & van Huygevoort 2000, van Dieen et al 2003, Moseley et al 2004c). Such factors have been linked directly to motor control changes, but probably also disrupt motor control by virtue of their demand on CNS performance.

The effect of cognitive and emotional factors on CNS performance in chronic pain

People with chronic pain have reduced cognitive capacity and difficulties are dependent on emotional factors associated with pain, rather than pain itself (Dufton 1989). For example, during functional restoration, improvement in psychomotor performance is associated with reduction in distress rather than a reduction in pain (Luoto et al 1999). People who report catastrophic thought processes are particularly affected. Crombez et al (1997) divided 124 non-chronic pain subjects into catastrophizers and non-catastrophizers, using the Pain Catastrophizing Scale (Sullivan et al 1995), and measured task performance during a noxious stimulation. They found that attentional interference was significantly greater in the catastrophizing group although there was no difference in the reported intensity or unpleasantness of the stimulus between groups. A similar effect has been shown to be related to the threat value of a stimulus (Crombez et al 1998a). That study evaluated performance on a tone discrimination task that was combined with transient cutaneous stimulation. The subjects who were told that the stimulation would be painful demonstrated reduced performance on the tone discrimination task. The only difference between groups was the addition of impending threat. Based on these results, Eccleston & Crombez (1999) proposed that pain interrupts cognitive performance according to its threat value and the degree of emotional arousal with which it is associated.

The impact on CNS performance of the threat value of pain may be mediated via fear mechanisms (Crombez et al 1998a). Initial evidence appears supportive of this proposal. Crombez and colleagues (1999) compared fearful and non-fearful chronic low back pain patients on a numerical task and found that performance at the task was best predicted using the interaction between pain severity and pain related fear. In other work that measured how long it took subjects to detect a dot presented after pain relevant and neutral words, Asmundson et al (1997) found that fear of pain was a determinant of the latency of the response in a group of chronic pain patients but not in control subjects. While this is in contrast to later work by Keogh and colleagues (2001), which found an effect in a non-patient group, the weight of evidence indicates that fear of pain impacts on CNS performance.

Any demand on CNS resources may feasibly reduce motor control. Findings from studies in which motor and attention demanding tasks are co-presented include the disruption of normal standing balance (Marsh & Geel 2000), reduction in speed and stability of walking (Ebersbach et al 1995), and reduced speed and increased error rate in handwriting (Brown & Donnenwirth 1990). As such, it is possible that the impact of pain on motor control parameters is secondary to the substantial attention demand inherent in pain. It is also possible that the emotional and cognitive aspects of pain also have an impact on motor control, independent of the demand on attention.

The effect of cognitive and emotional factors on motor control in chronic pain

The effect of stress and fear on motor control relating to spinal control has been investigated using postural control of the trunk muscles (Moseley et al 2004a, 2004c) and back muscle activity during lifting (Marras et al 2000), bending (Watson et al 1997), and walking (Lamoth et al (in press)).

The impetus for most studies has come from findings in people with chronic spinal pain or non-patients given experimentally induced acute pain. Our group has used the model of postural control of the trunk during limb movement to investigate pain and motor control. In short, normally during limb movements the deepest trunk muscles, transversus abdominis (TrA) and deep multifidus (Deep MF), are controlled independently to the superficial trunk muscles (Hodges & Richardson 1999, Moseley et al 2002, 2003). The independent strategy for TrA is lost in chronic recurrent LBP patients (Hodges & Richardson 1996, Hodges 2001). Although postural control of deep multifidus has not been studied in patients, abnormalities of multifidus have been identified in EMG and morphological studies (Sihvonen et al 1991, Hides et al 1994, 1996, Arendt-Nielsen et al 1996).

According to biomechanics, dysfunction of the deep trunk muscles will compromise intersegmental control and result in nociceptive stimulation of spinal structures (Panjabi 1992). Abnormality of the TrA response has been observed during acute experimental LBP elicited by intramuscular injection of hypertonic saline (Fig. 16.1), which suggests that alteration of the response may also be consequent to pain (Hodges et al 2003). Similar abnormalities observed in patients while they were pain-free (Hodges & Richardson 1996, 1998) raises the possibility that changes caused by pain may not always return to normal. Alternatively, perhaps some people have motor control changes prior to pain. Finally, perhaps aspects of pain such

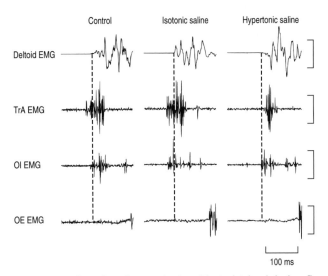

Figure 16.1 Raw data from a single subject obtained during flexion of the arm, showing delay in activation of transversus abdominis (TrA) obliquus internus (OI) and externus (OE) during low back pain induced by intramuscular injection of hypertonic saline. Vertical dashed line marks onset of anterior deltoid EMG.

as stress and fear, which are characteristic of chronic pain, are sufficient to interrupt normal function of the deep trunk muscles.

Stress

Stress, commonly inherent to pain, has previously been shown to alter motor control (Weinberg & Hunt 1976, Jones & Cale 1997, van Galen & van Huygevoort 2000). For example, during a throwing task, Weinberg & Hunt (1976) made subjects stressed by advising them that they were not performing well enough and that more was expected of them. Increased stress led to reduced performance at the task. Similar findings have been reported from a pen placement task (van Galen & van Huygevoort 2000), pinching and grasping tasks (Noteboom 2000) and during handwriting (Jones & Cale 1997).

The majority of work has investigated motor control during voluntary tasks. One aspect of voluntary tasks is that they are vulnerable to volitional alteration of the movement (e.g. guarding). In contrast, investigation of preparatory postural responses provides information about aspects of motor control that are not dependent on volitional control. In one study to investigate the effect of psychosocial stress subjects performed rapid arm movements while they also performed a Stroop task (Moseley et al 2004b), a recognized attention-demanding paradigm. Subjects were encouraged and were given positive feedback with regard to their performance. Thus, the Stroop test provided a non-stressful demand on CNS information processing resources. However, the Stroop test was then repeated but the subjects were given negative feedback about their performance ('you are not performing well enough') and the investigators appeared unhappy with the subject and with each other. Psychosocial stress has been elicited in this manner by others (Marras et al 2000) and subjective (reported distress) and physiological measures verified the efficacy of this strategy in effecting a stress response (Fig. 16.2).

During the non-stressful Stroop task, the reaction time of postural activation of the deep trunk muscles was not affected; however, those of the superficial trunk muscles and the prime mover were delayed. This finding demonstrated that the response of the deep trunk muscles does not require CNS processing resources that are limited by performance of the cognitive task. In contrast, the responses of the superficial trunk muscles and the prime mover were dependent on further processing because their reaction time was delayed by performance of the cognitive task. When subjects became stressed, the reaction time of postural activation of the deep trunk muscles was delayed in a similar fashion to that observed for the prime mover and superficial trunk muscles (Fig. 16.3).

Thus, psychosocial stress was sufficient to change motor control of the deep trunk muscles, although the effect was different to that observed during pain. This finding is consistent with a recent study that used an EMG based biomechanical model to evaluate the amount of spinal loading associated with a lifting task under different levels of stress (Marras et al 2000). That study found that when the researchers appeared unhappy with the performance and irritated by the subject there was an increase in trunk muscle activity. According to their model, this equated to increased spinal loads. A similar effect has been reported where activity of the shoulder muscles during keyboard work increased when the subjects became stressed (Ekberg et al 1995).

The mechanism(s) by which stress has an effect on motor control are not fully understood. Differential effects on distinct muscle fibre groups cannot be excluded but no clear data exist. At the spinal level, altered afferent input (Behrends et al 1983) has been reported to have an effect, but descending supraspinal modulation of the alpha motoneuron, both inhibitory (Willer et al 1981) and facilitatory (Willer et al 1979), probably has the most potent effect (Andersen 1996).

Apart from being consequent to preparations for an upcoming movement or postural task, descending input is also dependent on cognitive and emotional factors. Accordingly, supraspinal inputs can have an effect on the sensory neurons that access the alpha motoneuron

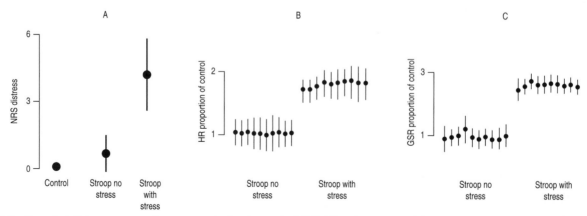

Figure 16.2 Reported distress measured on a numerical rating scale (NRS) (A) and heart rate (B) and galvanic skin response (GSR) (C) during control, non-stressful and stressful attention-demanding task. Each measure suggests an increase in stress in the final condition.

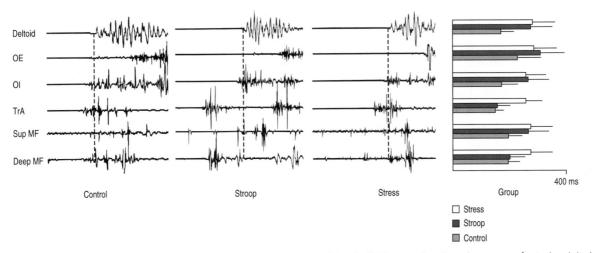

Figure 16.3 Raw data from a single subject and group data showing the delay in EMG onset for the prime mover (anterior deltoid) and superficial trunk muscles during the non-stressful attention-demanding task (Stroop) and a delay in the onset of the deep trunk muscles during the stressful attention-demanding task (stress). Obliquus internus (OI), externus (OE), transversus abdominis (TrA) superficial (Sup MF) and deep (Deep MF) multifidus are shown.

(i.e. within nociceptive components of the sensory system) or directly on the alpha motoneuron (Andersen 1996). The latter mechanism allows the CNS to 'prime' certain motor pathways in preparation for sensory input. Such mechanisms have implications for those patients who attempt a movement expecting it to be painful. It is feasible, then that in this type of situation motor patterns may appear to be associated with nociception when in fact they are not.

The majority of findings have been drawn from healthy subjects and are applicable to the current context by virtue of the importance allocated to psychosocial stressors in the development of chronicity. More insight is obtained from data from chronic pain patients. Studies in chronic LBP and orofacial pain patients report elevated EMG activity associated with stress, compared to non-patients, during static and dynamic tasks (Flor & Turk 1989, Flor et al 1992). The general pattern is consistent with a 'muscle tension model' of chronic pain, which has tenets in common with the so-called 'vicious cycle' proposed by Travell's group (1942). In effect, these models propose that psychophysical stressors increase muscle tension, which increases pain, which increases psychophysical stressors, and so on.

Based on this line, EMG biofeedback training was developed as a way to reduce muscle tension. Biofeedback training has generally been effective in reducing chronic low back pain and its psychosocial impact (Flor et al 1983, Stuckey et al 1986, Middaugh & Kee 1987, Biedermann et al 1989, Sherman & Arena 1992, Flor & Birbaumer 1993, Newton-John et al 1995, Arena & Blanchard 1996, Hasenbring et al 1999; although, see Bush et al 1985 for a contrary view). However, there is little support for its efficacy as a sole treatment (Sherman & Arena 1992). This is probably because the mechanism of effect appears to be unrelated to muscle tension. Holroyd's group (Holroyd et al 1984) demonstrated that the effect of biofeedback training was dependent on how well the patients perceived

themselves to be able to control muscle tension rather than their actual ability to do so. These results were replicated by others (Blanchard et al 1982), and Rokicki's group (1997) demonstrated a significant relationship between pain relief associated with biofeedback therapy and changes in self-efficacy measures. They argued that the treatment effect is mediated by cognitive factors directly, rather than via alterations in muscle activity.

An alternative explanation may lie in the effect of intensive sustained somatic awareness of the low back on cortical representations of the area and the so-called 'internal body dynamic'. Flor and colleagues (1997) demonstrated substantial cortical reorganization associated with chronic low back pain and found a strong link between the extent of reorganization and the duration of the pain. While too little is known about cortical reorganization in chronic low back pain to suggest a developed thesis, it may be that changes in cortical representation in response to training, regardless of the training objective, may contribute to its therapeutic effect.

Recent work suggests that the muscle tension model is too simplistic (see, for example, Matre et al 1998, Svensson et al 1998, Zedka et al 1999, Capra & Ro 2000) and offers support for the pain adaptation model (Lund et al 1991). This model stipulates that in the event of pain, the alteration in motor control serves to limit movement by imparting a general stiffness to the associated body segment(s). Movement limitation and 'guarding' often characterize chronic pain patients and have been implicated in the development of chronicity (see, for example, Main & Watson 1996). Most data highlight the import of cognitive factors and fear in this relationship.

Cognitive factors and fear

Innovative work identified cognitive factors and fear as important in altered motor control of the trunk muscles

(Watson et al 1997). In low back pain patients, the normal relaxation of the back muscles at end of flexion range the so-called flexion-relaxation phenomenon (FRP), is often, although not always, absent (Kippers & Parker 1984, Sihvonen et al 1991). In order to quantify this response, Ahern and colleagues (1988) devised the flexion-relaxation ratio (FRR), which provided a measure of the relationship between maximum muscle activity during bending and the muscle activity at end of range.

Watson et al (1997) determined the FRR using erector spinae (ES) surface EMG. Subjects also completed the Fear Avoidance Beliefs Questionnaire (FABQ) (Waddell et al 1993), the Pain Self-Efficacy Questionnaire (PSEQ) (Nicholas et al 1992), the Oswestry Disability Questionnaire (ODQ) (Fairbank et al 1980) and a visual analogue scale (VAS) of current pain intensity. The authors investigated the relationship between the FRR and each of the self-report variables. A relationship was identified between FRR and FABQ, while there was no relationship between FRR and VAS or ODQ. When Watson's group evaluated the effect of a cognitive-behavioural pain management programme, they reported strong correlations between the change in FRR and the change in PSEQ (r >0.45, P <0.03), and FABQ (r >–0.3, P <0.04). These findings imply that trunk muscle function during movement is affected in chronic low back pain according to fear of pain and (re)injury, and by the patient's perception of their ability to perform everyday tasks.

We investigated the effect of fear of low back pain on postural activation of the trunk muscles during arm movement (Moseley et al 2004c). Fear of LBP was elicited by random and unpredictable noxious shocks delivered to the back. Similar to the response observed during pain, when subjects were fearful of impending LBP, the simplistic and automatic response of the deep trunk muscles was delayed (Fig. 16.4). Interestingly, the effect was observed in deep multifidus and transversus abdominis, whereas, during acute experimental pain, an effect was only consistently observed in transversus abdominis.

Trials in which subjects were fearful of elbow pain (stimulation of the olecranon) were also conducted. In this condition, there was no effect on postural activation of the trunk muscles (Fig. 16.4). This demonstrated that the effect of fear of pain on motor control was dependent on the anatomical relevance of the impending pain. This finding is consistent with previous work during static tasks (Flor & Turk 1989, Flor et al 1992, Vlaeyen et al 1999).

Motor control of the postural activation of the trunk muscles was further assessed during repetitive arm movements. Previous investigation during experimentally induced acute LBP demonstrated that impairment of the postural response of transversus abdominis during repetitive arm movements was a consistent effect, and that there was a variable effect on the superficial trunk muscles (Hodges et al 2003). During fear of LBP, a similar though less marked effect was identified. In particular, transversus abdominis and deep multifidus demonstrated reduced

modulation, reduced mean amplitude and reduced coherence with arm movement. There was no effect of fear of LBP on the speed or range of arm movement or reaction time of the task. The causative mechanism of deep trunk muscle impairment during fear of LBP is not clear; however, it is important to note that a marked disruption of the postural activation of the trunk muscles during repetitive movement was observed.

Using a similar noxious stimulus paradigm, the effect of fear of low back pain on back muscle activity during gait has also been investigated (Lamoth et al 2004). Lamoth's group has previously identified robust alterations in the ratio of thoracic to lumbar ES activity in chronic low back pain patients (Lamoth et al 2001a, 2001b). Aspects of this effect were reproduced in normal subjects by experimental induction of acute pain (via hypertonic saline injection) and fear of pain (via noxious cutaneous shock) (Lamoth et al 2004). Those findings corroborate in a general way the results of postural adjustment studies and further support a guarding model of motor dysfunction associated with pain. Together, the findings that relate to fear of pain suggest that either the effect of pain on motor control is mediated by fear mechanisms, or both fear and pain have a common impact on motor control. Either way, fear of pain appears to be of importance from a clinical perspective.

It is notable that in normal subjects the induction of fear of pain seems to have a greater impact on motor strategy than the induction of acute pain. A potential explanation for this finding lies in a model proposed by Bolles & Fanselow (1980). Based on animal studies, they posited that fear and pain incorporate separate systems, such that when an animal is first stimulated nociceptively, the fear system is aroused and the pain system is inhibited. When fear has subsided, the pain system is able to organize recuperative and protective behaviour. This model presents a paradox to pain researchers. The ethical and practical constraints of eliciting pain experimentally are such that once the subject is exposed to a nociceptive stimulus, that stimulus is unlikely to cause fear because the subject knows that it will not get worse, will not last long and, importantly, is not indicative of damage. Therefore, it is likely that fear mechanisms are less involved in experimental pain than in clinical pain.

Aside from pain and self-efficacy, there is little work that investigates the effect of other pain related cognitions on motor control in chronic pain patients. This is probably because the complexity introduced by numerous variables that influence cognitive schema and motor task performance makes investigation difficult.

One attempt to investigate this issue evaluated change in simple motor tasks and pain-specific cognitions after a non-physical intervention (Moseley 2004). Measures were obtained before and after an intensive one-to-one education session in which there was no opportunity to be physically active. There was a significant relationship between cogni-

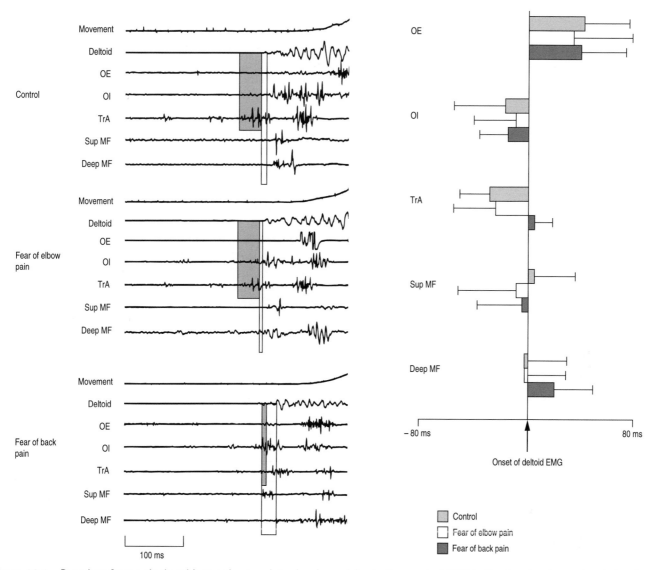

Figure 16.4   Raw data from a single subject and group data showing a delay in the onset of EMG in the deep trunk muscles during fear of back pain, but not fear of elbow pain. The short and long rectangles mark the latency between the onset of deltoid and transversus abdominis (TrA) EMG and deep multifidus (Deep MF) EMG, respectively. Note no delay in the deep trunk muscles, relative to deltoid, during fear of elbow pain. Obliquus internus (OI) and externus (OE) and superficial multifidus (Sup MF) are also shown.

tive and motor change (Fig. 16.5), which suggests a direct relationship between pain cognitions and motor control. Importantly, subjects did not perceive that they were attempting the task any differently. Thus, the findings suggest that in chronic low back pain patients, inappropriate pain cognitions may compromise motor control even when subjects are not consciously altering their movement response. Regardless of whether the mechanism of effect involves changes in pain threshold or tolerance and/or in motor response selection, the finding has direct implications for assessment and management.

In general, the available data suggest that psychosocial factors that commonly characterize chronic pain impact directly on motor control. It is proposed that fear of pain, a cognitive conviction that the body segment (i.e. spine) is

vulnerable and in cases of marked somatic hypervigilance or supraspinal reorganization, any threatening stimuli have an effect on motor control. For chronic pain patients, particularly those characterized by these factors, the magnitude and robustness of the impact may be sufficient to limit the utility of conventional motor control assessment and training strategies.

CLINICAL IMPLICATIONS

Schematic representation of the current thought in chronic pain and motor control

The available data on chronic pain and motor control can be summarized according to Figure 16.6. Physiologic complexities (Fig. 16.6A) caused by a myriad of adaptive

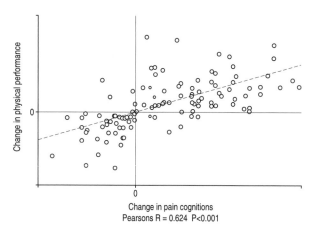

Figure 16.5 Plot and linear regression of the change in cognitive factors and motor performance during an education session on the neurophysiology of pain in which there was no opportunity to be physically active.

responses within (primarily but not exclusively) the CNS, will enhance nociception mediated protective spinal and supraspinal reflex mechanisms. The changes may lead to non-nociception initiated protective mechanisms, particularly in those patients who are hypervigilant to somatic information. Finally, and over time, supraspinal reorganization and altered somatic input will lead to disruption of the internal body dynamic (i.e. the body is not where the CNS perceives it to be) (Fig. 16.6A). Each of these physiological complexities alters motor output.

Cognitive and emotional factors that are characteristic of chronic pain disrupt motor control by three mechanisms (Fig. 16.6B). First, by enhancing the general disruptive effect of pain on CNS performance, stimulus processing is compromised. This may lead to impaired motor control although it may only be apparent in complex motor tasks. The second mechanism is by determining inappropriate motor–behavioural response strategies (e.g. guarding, bracing, avoidance). The third is by pro-

moting alternate motor control strategies for the movement response, for example, an alternate strategy for postural activation of the trunk muscles during limb movements or alternate back muscle activation during kinematically similar trunk movements.

Conceptualization of the relationship between chronic pain and motor control

According to the findings outlined above, a threat-based conceptualization of chronic pain and motor control is proposed. Three conceptual models have been drawn on that relate to the motoric dimension of chronic pain; from a perceptuo-motor perspective, the neuromatrix theory (Melzack 1989, 1990) and the reality–virtual reality theory (Wall & Melzack 1999), and from a behavioural perspective, the fear avoidance model (Vlaeyen & Linton 2000). Comprehensive discussion of these models is beyond the scope of this chapter.

A threat based model of chronic pain and motor control also has similarities with a model offered by Eccleston's group (Aldrich et al 2000), in which chronic pain is reconceptualized as chronic vigilance to threat. In their model, chronic vigilance to threat may lead to continued (unsuccessful) attempts to escape. That group and others have identified that chronic pain patients attend more readily to information related to pain or threat (Asmundson et al 1997, Eccleston et al 1997, Crombez et al 1999, Snider et al 2000).

The primary objective of the third model, the fear avoidance model (Vlaeyen & Linton 2000), was to provide a framework for understanding cognitive and behavioural aspects of chronicity, in particular chronic disability related to pain. It posits that in response to pain, patients either avoid movement due to fear of pain and/or (re)injury or perform the movement despite this fear. The former are reinforced in their choice because avoidance of the movement meant avoidance of pain, and thus they progress to chronicity. The latter learn that pain reduces over time and they progress to recovery.

Figure 16.6 Schematic representation of the physiological (A) and psychosocial (B) complexities associated with chronic pain as they may impact on motor control.

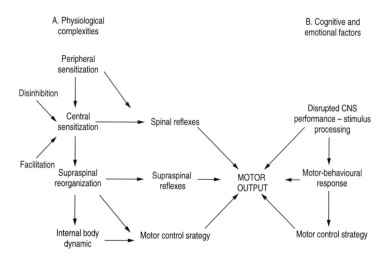

A new model of chronic pain and motor control: the threat response model

Figure 16.7 presents the threat response model. This model is a conceptual approach to chronic pain and motor control that incorporates the physiological and psychosocial complexities of chronic pain. In short, the threat response model proposes that pain, including its experiential and motor aspects, is produced by the CNS whenever the CNS considers it biologically prudent to do so, that is, the response occurs whenever the CNS concludes that a sufficient threat exists to warrant action. In this regard, physiological complexities associated with chronic pain have two main effects: first, the nociceptive system is highly sensitive, which means the kinematic margin for error is reduced, and second, proprioceptive acuity is reduced, which alters the internal body dynamic and disrupts motor control acuity. Psychosocial factors associated with chronic pain have a primary effect in maintenance of perceived threat. Assessment and management strategies can be organized according to the threat response model.

Assessment

According to the threat response model, the primary aim of motor control assessment is to identify factors that contribute to the perception of threat. Thus, assessment includes evaluation of the functional state of the nociceptive system, cognitive and emotional factors associated with chronic pain and the impact of psychosocial stressors on motor control.

Assessment of the state of the nociceptive system

Sensitization of the nociceptive system manifests clinically as allodynia and primary and secondary hyperalgesia. Evaluation of these clinical constructs uses pain pressure or pain thermal threshold tests, but there is debate about the accuracy of such tests to delineate between central or peripheral mechanisms (Doubell et al 1999). Regardless of the underlying mechanisms, assessment can be useful in order to identify movements or postures that should be avoided or approached with caution. The reader is referred to Chapter 15 for more information on assessment of allodynia and hyperalgesia.

Cognitive and emotional factors

There are three strategies that can be used to evaluate cognitive and emotional factors and the potential or actual impact of these factors on motor control: quantitative assessment, subjective interview and direct assessment.

Quantitative assessment

Pain cognitions, fear of pain and (re)injury, emotional characteristics of pain and somatic vigilance can all be assessed using self-report tools. Table 16.1 presents popular tools and the relevant construct they attempt to quantify. In general, these tools demonstrate strong psychometric properties. The primary application of quantitative analysis in the current context is identification of patients for whom cognitive and emotional factors may be directly disrupting motor control. Thus, these tools can provide direction for therapeutic strategies (e.g. fear reduction), and offer quantifiable reassessment options (see Table 16.1).

Interview

The interview permits specific questioning about the import of cognitive and emotional factors in both the production of pain and motor control changes, and the impact of pain on the patient's life. The interview provides an excellent opportunity to determine the patient's own explanatory model, which in turn is informative about pain and injury cognitions. 'Explanatory model' refers to the way in which the patient conceptualizes the cause of their pain. The importance of the explanatory model can readily be seen in patients who offer explanations such as 'I have a herniated disc that has slipped out the back of my spine and is pinching my spinal cord'. This is as devastating as it is inaccurate, because any movement is likely to be threatening for the individual who conceptualizes his LBP is this fashion.

'Illness information' offered by health and medical providers is potentially important in the development and establishment of an explanatory model. Certainly, inaccurate information based on outdated models of pain and injury can enhance an explanatory model that is inherently threatening. In this sense the provision of information that emphasizes tissue damage, 'positive' radiological results even though they are not clinically meaningful, or vulnerability of the body part, is regarded an important iatrogenic factor in chronicity (see, for example, Jones et al 1988, Nachemson 1992, Hirsch & Liebert 1998, Waddell 1998). However, accurate information emphasizing physiological, cognitive and behavioural responses to injury can have the opposite effect (see, for example, Symonds et al 1995, Burton et al 1999, Linton & Andersson 2000, Moseley 2002, 2003a, Moseley et al 2004c).

Unfortunately, there is a tendency for physiotherapists to underestimate the capacity of patients to understand an

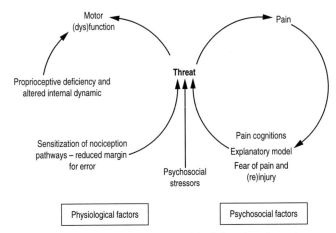

Figure 16.7 The threat response model of chronic pain and motor control.

Table 16.1 Assessment: examples of quantitative, subjective and physical assessment strategies

Construct	Quantitative analysis	Interview	Physical assessment
Fear of pain and (re)injury	Fear Avoidance Beliefs Questionnaire (FABQ)* (Waddell et al 1993) Tampa Scale of Kinesophobia (Kori et al 1990)	Are you afraid of performing any particular activities or movements?	Assessment during actual or virtual exposure to frightening movements.
Pain cognitions and thought processes	Survey of Pain Attitudes (SOPA) (Jensen et al 1987) Pain Catastrophizing Scale (PCS) (Sullivan et al 1995)	What does your pain mean?	
Emotional factors and somatic vigilance	Pain Anxiety Symptoms Scale (PASS) (McCracken et al 1992) Modified Somatic Perceptions Questionnaire (MSPQ) (Main 1983)	How does your pain make you feel?	Assessment during a recalled severe painful episode
Explanatory model		Tell me what is causing your pain	
Somatic vulnerability	Back Beliefs Questionnaire (Symonds et al 1996)	How vulnerable do you think your (neck) is?	
Psychosocial stressors	Psychosocial aspects of work (Symonds et al 1996)		Assessment during stress

*It is notable however that, because many of the items of the FABQ relate directly to vocational duties, the validity of this tool for unemployed patients is questionable.

accurate explanation for their pain (Moseley 2003b). Thus, 'simple' explanations and lay jargon (e.g. 'pinched nerve', 'locked joint', 'hypermobility') are often substituted. Arguably, this type of explanation is time and effort efficient in the short term. However, such statements may, at least in some patients, directly enhance the perceived threat associated with pain and effectively promote pain and motor dysfunction, notwithstanding disability and healthcare utilization (see Waddell 1998).

The interview can also provide important information about pain cognitions, the emotional impact of the pain, and the relationship between psychosocial stressors and pain. Careful and targeted questioning is required in order to obtain meaningful information in minimum time. Unfortunately, time resources are often insufficient for a comprehensive evaluation. In this regard, assessment tools which can be completed prior to initial assessment (e.g. in the waiting room) are helpful.

Physical assessment

The physical assessment should provide more specific information about the impact of cognitive and emotional factors on motor control. Specifics of motor control assessment are beyond the scope of this chapter but the subject is covered in depth elsewhere in this text. However, the general implication of the threat response model is that patient relevant threatening stimuli can be incorporated into the conventional assessment, for example: exposure to actual ('hold your contraction while you bend forwards') or virtual ('hold your contraction as you imagine bending forwards') frightening movements (motor planning mechanisms involved in actual and imagined movements are similar);

exposure to psychosocial stressors ('hold your contraction as you count backwards from 100 in lots of 7, out loud'); exposure to work-specific threatening stimuli ('hold your contraction as you imagine performing your normal work duty in front of your supervisor').

Obviously, these suggestions are not prescriptive and are highly specific to individual patients. Further, and importantly, the reliability and validity of these assessment approaches has not been verified and their utility is based on anecdotal evidence. This is not necessarily problematic because the assessment approach is intended to be exploratory rather than quantitative. Findings should be considered in light of the wider clinical assessment, quantitative tools and interview findings.

Progression of motor control training

In general, the implication of the threat response model is that threatening stimuli should be incorporated into the motor control training approach. This is done in much the same manner as motor control training is integrated into demanding postures and functional and vocational activities. The primary objective is to obtain proficiency in employing appropriate motor control strategies during threatening situations.

Schematic conceptualization of a typical approach is presented in Figure 16.8. Presuming that assessment strategies have been effective in identifying motor control function and threatening stimuli, initial strategies should target both of these factors. Specific and intensive education or specialist psychological intervention may be required to sufficiently resolve threatening psychosocial stimuli. Subsequently, and

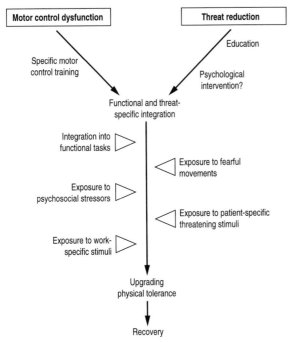

Figure 16.8   Schematic conceptualization of an approach to assessment and management based on the threat response model of chronic pain and motor control.

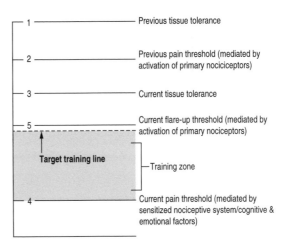

Figure 16.9   A working model suitable for patients that presents the impact of physiological changes on motor performance and highlights the need for a graded approach to management.

after basic motor control goals have been achieved, threatening stimuli can be gradually introduced with a focus on maintaining appropriate motor control strategies. This is critical because although exposure to movement is essential in reducing fear avoidance (see Vlaeyen & Linton 2000), threat is sufficient to both disrupt non-voluntary aspects of movement such as postural responses, and imperceptibly disrupt voluntary movement responses.

Implications of nociception sensitization for training progression

The physiological complexities associated with chronic pain have profound implications for the latter stages of exercise progression. In short, it is prudent to adhere to two primary principles:

- the nociceptive system is highly sensitive, which serves to protect the vulnerable body part
- the body is highly adaptable and will respond to demand.

Figure 16.9 presents a suitable framework with which to plan progression and consists of several components:

1. *Previous tissue tolerance*. Prior to the onset of pain the body was able to tolerate a certain amount of activity before it would hurt.
2. *Previous tissue mediated pain onset*. Pain is initiated by stimulation of primary nociceptive afferents, which served to protect from injury.
3. *Current tissue tolerance*. Because of alterations in activity and physical tasks since the onset of pain, the tolerance

to activity of the body part is reduced ('secondary disuse').

4. *Current protective pain onset*. Sensitization of the nociceptive system, and the import of cognitive and emotional factors that contribute to threat, means that the pain protective system is activated far earlier, potentially continuously during waking hours.
5. *Current tissue mediated pain onset*. The integrity of the primary afferent nociceptive system is maintained, or sensitized in the case of peripheral sensitization. This means that activation of primary nociceptors will still occur to protect the vulnerable part. Typically in a clinical situation this will manifest as a 'flare-up' and should be avoided by virtue of the flood of descending facilitation with which it is probably associated.

The objective of training progression is to; (a) find the line at which flare-up occurs (5); (b) structure the training plan to *conservatively* increase the exposure to activity, maintaining sufficient exposure to induce adaptation but avoiding flare-up ('the training zone'). Performing exercise and activity despite pain may require specific psychological training, for example learning coping strategies and distraction techniques. Should flare-up occur, the patient will need to be reminded of the sensitivity of the nociceptive system, and that flare-up does not indicate (re)injury.

Both physiological and cognitive-behavioural principles emphasize the importance of a structured approach to progression. Anecdotally, a detailed daily exercise diary is considered integral to progress, and frequency, duration and intensity of training should be planned at least a week in advance. Modification of the plan should not be based on resting pain levels. In the case of flare-up, the plan should be recommended at the previous level of exposure that did not elicit flare-up and then progressed in more conservative increments.

Finally, collaboration with other members of the rehabilitation team is critical. Ideally, for those patients who are reasonably disabled by pain, the team will include a psychologist and psychosocial goals will be fundamentally linked to motor control and physical goals. Thus, utilization of a consistent model is important and liaison and information management are critical. The role of the physiotherapist often includes educating other members of the team about the physiological complexities of chronic pain and using basic and clinical science evidence to guide therapeutic strategies.

CONCLUSION

Clinicians are well aware that management and rehabilitation of patients with chronic disabling pain is difficult and problematic. Fundamental changes in the function and properties of the nervous system, particularly the nociceptive system, and profound psychosocial impacts mean that conventional approaches to motor control training are often unsuccessful. The threat response model has been proposed, in which the particular challenges of chronic pain are incorporated to suggest an appropriate therapeutic approach. According to the model, the impact of threatening stimuli should be evaluated. Motor control then needs to be integrated into functionally and vocationally meaningful activities, and training should incorporate exposure to threatening stimuli. Finally, motor control is only one aspect of the clinical picture and motor control and physical intervention should be incorporated into a wider therapeutic plan according to the characteristics of individual patients.

Acknowledgements: GLM is supported by NHMRC fellowship ID 210348 and PWH is supported by NHMRC fellowship ID 157203.

KEYWORDS

sensitization	threat
trunk muscles	stress
postural adjustments	psychophysiology
fear	

References

Ahern D K, Follick M J, Council J R, Laser-Wolston N, Litchman H 1988 Comparison of lumbar paravertebral EMG patterns in chronic low back pain patients and non-patient controls. Pain 34(2): 153–160

Aldrich S, Eccleston C, Crombez G 2000 Worrying about chronic pain: vigilance to threat and misdirected problem solving. Behaviour Research and Therapy 38(5): 457–470

Allen D T, Kiernan J A 1994 Permeation of proteins from the blood into peripheral nerves and ganglia. Neuroscience 59(3): 755–764

Amir R, Devor M 1993 Ongoing activity in neuroma afferents bearing retrograde sprouts. Brain Research 630: 283–288

Andersen O K 1996 Physiological and pharmacological modulation of the human nociceptive withdrawal reflex. Centre for Sensory Motor Interaction, University of Aalborg, Aalborg, p 48

Arena J G, Blanchard E B 1996 Biofeedback and relaxation therapy for chronic pain disorders. In: Gatchel R, Turk D C (eds) Psychological approaches to pain management: a practitioner's handbook. Guilford Press, New York, pp 179–230

Arendt-Nielsen L, Graven-Nielsen T, Svarrer H, Svensson P 1996 The influence of low back pain on muscle activity and coordination during gait: a clinical and experimental study. Pain 64(2): 231–240

Asmundson G J, Kuperos J L, Norton G R 1997 Do patients with chronic pain selectively attend to pain-related information? Preliminary evidence for the mediating role of fear. Pain 72(1–2): 27–32

Behrends T, Schomburg E D, Steffens H 1983 Facilitatory interaction between cutaneous afferents from low threshold mechanoreceptors and nociceptors in segmental reflex pathways to alpha motoneurons. Brain Research 260: 131–134

Biedermann H J, Inglis J, Monga T N, Shanks G L 1989 Differential treatment responses on somatic pain indicators after EMG biofeedback training in back pain patients. International Journal of Pychosomatics 36(1–4): 53–57

Blanchard E B, Andrasik F, Arena J G, Teders S J 1982 Variation in meaning of pain descriptors for different headache types as revealed by psychophysical scaling. Headache 22(3): 137–139

Blenk K H, Michaelis M, Vogel C, Janig W 1996 Thermosensitivity of acutely axotomized sensory nerve fibers. Journal of Neurophysiology 76(2): 743–752

Bolles U, Fanselow M 1980 A perceptual-defensive recuperative model of fear and pain. Behavioral and Brain Sciences 3: 291–301

Brieg A 1978 Adverse mechanical tension in the central nervous system. Almqvist and Wiksell, Stockholm

Brown T L, Donnenwirth E E 1990 Interaction of attentional and motor control processes in handwriting. American Journal of Psychology 103(4): 471–486

Burton A K 1997 Spine update. Back injury and work loss: biomechanical and psychosocial influences. Spine 22(21): 2575–2580

Burton A K, Tillotson K M, Main C J, Hollis S 1995 Psychosocial predictors of outcome in acute and subchronic low back trouble. Spine 20(6): 722–728

Burton A K, Waddell G, Tillotson K M, Summerton N 1999 Information and advice to patients with back pain can have a positive effect: a randomized controlled trial of a novel educational booklet in primary care. Spine 24(23): 2484–2491

Bush C, Ditto B, Feuerstein M 1985 A controlled evaluation of paraspinal EMG biofeedback in the treatment of chronic low back pain. Health Psychology 4(4): 307–321

Bushnell M C 1995 Thalamic processing of sensory-discriminative and affective-motivational dimensions of pain. In: Besson J M, Guilbaud G, Ollat H (eds) Forebrain areas involved in pain processing Eurotext, Paris, pp 63–77

Bushnell M C, Duncan G H 1989 Sensory and affective aspects of pain perception: is medial thalamus restricted to emotional issues? Experimental Brain Research 67: 415–418

Butler D 2000 The sensitive nervous system. NOI Publications, Adelaide

Capra N F, Ro J Y 2000 Experimental muscle pain produces central modulation of proprioceptive signals arising from jaw muscle spindles. Pain 86(1–2): 151–162

Chen Y, Devor M 1998 Ectopic mechanosensitivity in injured sensory axons arises from the site of spontaneous electrogenesis. European Journal of Pain 2: 165–178

Coghill R C, Sang C N, Berman K F, Bennett G J, Iadarola M J 1998 Global cerebral blood flow decreases during pain. Journal of Cerebral Blood Flow and Metabolism 18(2): 141–147

Crombez G, Eccleston C, Baeyens F, Eelen P 1997 Habituation and the interference of pain with task performance. Pain 70(2–3): 149–154

Crombez G, Eccleston C, Baeyens F, Eelen P 1998a Attentional disruption is enhanced by the threat of pain. Behaviour Research and Therapy 36(2): 195–204

Crombez G, Eccleston C, Baeyens F, Eelen P 1998b When somatic information threatens, catastrophic thinking enhances attentional interference. Pain 75(2–3): 187–198

Crombez G, Eccleston C, Baeyens F, van Houdenhove B, van den Broek A 1999 Attention to chronic pain is dependent upon pain-related fear. Journal of Psychosomatic Research 47(5): 403–410

Derbyshire S W, Jones A K, Devani K et al 1994 Cerebral responses to pain in patients with atypical facial pain measured by positron emission tomography. Journal of Neurology, Neurosurgery, and Psychiatry 57(10): 1166–1172

Devor M, Seltzer Z 1999 Pathophysiology of damaged nerves in relation to chronic pain. In: Wall P, Melzack R (eds) The textbook of pain. Churchill Livingstone, Edinburgh, pp 129–164

Di Piero V, Ferracuti S, Sabatini U, Pantano P, Cruccu G, Lenzi G L 1994 A cerebral blood flow study on tonic pain activation in man. Pain 56(2): 167–173

Doubell T P, Mannion R J, Woolf C J 1999 The dorsal horn: state-dependent sensory processing, plasticity and the generation of pain. In: Wall P, Melzack R (eds) The textbook of pain. Churchill Livingstone, Edinburgh, pp 165–181

Dubner R, Ruda M A 1992 Activity-dependent neuronal plasticity following tissue injury and inflammation. Trends in Neurosciences 15(3): 96–103

Dufton B D 1989 Cognitive failure and chronic pain. International Journal of Psychiatry in Medicine 19(3): 291–297

Ebersbach G, Dimitrijevic M R, Poewe W 1995 Influence of concurrent tasks on gait: a dual-task approach. Perceptual and Motor Skills 81(1): 107–113

Eccleston C, Crombez G 1999 Pain demands attention: a cognitive-affective model of the interruptive function of pain. Psychological Bulletin 125(3): 356–366

Eccleston C, Crombez G, Aldrich S, Stannard C 1997 Attention and somatic awareness in chronic pain. Pain 72(1–2): 209–215

Ekberg K, Eklund J, Tuveson M 1995 Psychological stress and muscle activity during data entry at visual display units. Work Stress 9: 475–490

Fairbank J, Couper J, Davies J B, O'Brien J P 1980 The Oswestry Low Back Pain Disability Questionnaire. Physiotherapy 66: 271–273

Flor H, Birbaumer N 1993 Comparison of the efficacy of electromyographic biofeedback, cognitive-behavioral therapy, and conservative medical interventions in the treatment of chronic musculoskeletal pain. Journal of Consulting and Clinical Psychology 61(4): 653–658

Flor H, Turk D C 1989 Psychophysiology of chronic pain: do chronic pain patients exhibit symptom-specific psychophysiological responses? Psychological Bulletin 105(2): 215–259

Flor H, Haag G, Turk D C, Koehler H 1983 Efficacy of EMG biofeedback, pseudotherapy, and conventional medical treatment for chronic rheumatic back pain. Pain 17(1): 21–31

Flor H, Birbaumer N, Schugens M M, Lutzenberger W 1992 Symptom-specific psychophysiological responses in chronic pain patients. Psychophysiology 29(4): 452–460

Flor H, Braun C, Elbert T, Birbaumer N 1997 Extensive reorganization of primary somatosensory cortex in chronic back pain patients. Neuroscience Letters 224(1): 5–8

Grachev I D, Fredrickson B E, Apkarian A V 2000 Abnormal brain chemistry in chronic back pain: an in vivo proton magnetic resonance spectroscopy study. Pain 89(1): 7–18

Graven-Nielsen T, Svensson P, Arendt-Nielsen L 1997 Effects of experimental muscle pain on muscle activity and co-ordination during static and dynamic motor function. Electroencephalography and Clinical Neurophysiology 105(2): 156–164

Hasenbring M, Ulrich H W, Hartmann M, Soyka D 1999 The efficacy of a risk factor-based cognitive behavioral intervention and electromyographic biofeedback in patients with acute sciatic pain: an attempt to prevent chronicity. Spine 24(23): 2525–2535

Hides J A, Stokes M J, Saide M, Jull G A, Cooper D H 1994 Evidence of lumbar multifidus muscle wasting ipsilateral to symptoms in patients with acute/subacute low back pain. Spine 19(2): 165–172

Hides J A, Richardson C A, Jull J A 1996 Multifidus muscle recovery is not automatic after resolution of acute, first-episode low back pain. Spine 21(23): 2763–2769

Hirsch M S, Liebert R M 1998 The physical and psychological experience of pain: the effects of labeling and cold pressor temperature on three pain measures in college women. Pain 77(1): 41–48

Hodges P W 2001 Changes in motor planning of feed forward postural responses of the trunk muscles in low back pain. Experimental Brain Research 141(2): 261–266

Hodges P W, Richardson C A 1996 Inefficient muscular stabilization of the lumbar spine associated with low back pain: a motor control evaluation of transversus abdominis. Spine 21(22): 2640–2650

Hodges P W, Richardson C A 1998 Delayed postural contraction of transversus abdominis in low back pain associated with movement of the lower limb. Journal of Spinal Disorders 11(1): 46–56

Hodges P W, Richardson C A 1999 Transversus abdominis and the superficial abdominal muscles are controlled independently in a postural task. Neuroscience letters 265: 91–94

Hodges P W, Moseley G L, Gabrielsson A, Gandevia S C 2003 Experimental muscle pain changes feedforward postural responses of the trunk muscles. Experimental Brain Research 151: 262–271

Holroyd K A, Penzien D B, Hursey K G et al 1984 Change mechanisms in EMG biofeedback training: cognitive changes underlying improvements in tension headache. Journal of Consulting and Clinical Psychology 52(6): 1039–1053

Howe J F, Loeser J D, Calvin W H 1977 Mechanosensitivity of dorsal root ganglia and chronically injured axons: a physiological basis for the radicular pain of nerve root compression. Pain 3(1): 25–41

Hsieh J C, Belfrage M, Stone-Elander S, Hansson P, Ingvar M 1995 Central representation of chronic ongoing neuropathic pain studied by positron emission tomography. Pain 63(2): 225–236

Janig W, Levine J D, Michaelis M 1996 Interactions of sympathetic and primary afferent neurons following nerve injury and tissue trauma. Progress in Brain Research 113: 161–184

Jensen M P, Karoly P, Huger R 1987 The development and preliminary validation of an instrument to assess patients' attitudes toward pain. Journal of Psychosomatic Research 31(3): 393–400

Ji R R, Rupp F 1997 Phosphorylation of transcription factor CREB in rat spinal cord after formalin-induced hyperalgesia: relationship to c-fos induction. Journal of Neuroscience 17(5): 1776–1785

Jones G, Cale A 1997 Goal difficulty, anxiety and performance. Ergonomics 40(3): 319–333

Jones S L, Jones P K, Katz J 1988 Compliance for low-back pain patients in the emergency department: a randomized trial. Spine 13(5): 553–556

Keogh E, Ellery D, Hunt C, Hannent I 2001 Selective attentional bias for pain-related stimuli amongst pain fearful individuals. Pain 91(1–2): 91–100

Kimbrell T A, George M S, Parekh P I et al 1999 Regional brain activity during transient self-induced anxiety and anger in healthy adults. Biological Psychiatry 46(4): 454–465

Kippers V, Parker A W 1984 Posture related to myoelectric silence of erectores spinae during trunk flexion. Spine 9(7): 740–745

Kori S H, Miller R P, Todd D 1990 Kinesophobia: a new view of chronic pain behavior. Pain Management 3: 35–43

Lamoth C, Beek P, Meijer O G 2001a Pelvis-thorax coordination in the transverse plane during gait. Gait and Posture 16(2): 101–114

Lamoth C, Meijer O, Wuisman P I, van Dieen J H, Levin M F, Beek P J 2001b Pelvis-thorax coordination in the transverse plane during walking in non-specific low back pain. Spine 27(4): E92–99

Lamoth C, Daffertshofer A, Meijer O G, Lorimer Moseley G, Wuisman P I J M, Beek P J 2004 Effects of experimentally induced pain and fear of pain on trunk coordination and back muscle activity during walking. Clinical Biomechanics 19: 551–563

Linton S J, Andersson T 2000 Can chronic disability be prevented? A randomized trial of a cognitive-behavior intervention and two forms of information for patients with spinal pain. Spine 25(21): 2825–2831

Lund J P, Donga R, Widmer C G, Stohler C S 1991 The pain-adaptation model: a discussion of the relationship between chronic musculoskeletal pain and motor activity. Canadian Journal of Physiology and Pharmacology 69(5): 683–694

Luoto S, Taimela S, Hurri H, Alaranta H 1999 Mechanisms explaining the association between low back trouble and deficits in information processing: a controlled study with follow-up. Spine 24(3): 255–261

McCracken L M, Zayfert C, Gross R T 1992 The Pain Anxiety Symptoms Scale: development and validation of a scale to measure fear of pain. Pain 50: 67–73

Main C J 1983 The modified somatic perception questionnaire (MSPQ). Journal of Psychosomatic Research 27(6): 503–514

Main C J, Watson P J 1996 Guarded movements: development of chronicity. In: Allen M E (ed) Musculoskeletal pain emanating from the head and neck: current concepts in diagnosis, management and cost containment. Haworth Press, Chicago, pp 163–170

Mannion R J, Woolf C J 2000 Pain mechanisms and management: a central perspective. Clinical Journal of Pain 16(Suppl.): S144–156

Marras W S, Davis K G, Heaney C A, Maronitis A B, Allread W G 2000 The influence of psychosocial stress, gender, and personality on mechanical loading of the lumbar spine. Spine 25(23): 3045–3054

Marsh A P, Geel S E 2000 The effect of age on the attentional demands of postural control. Gait and Posture 12(2): 105–113

Matre D A, Sinkjaer T, Svensson P, Arendt-Nielsen L 1998 Experimental muscle pain increases the human stretch reflex. Pain 75(2–3): 331–339

Matre D A, Sinkjaer T, Knardahl S, Andersen J B, Arendt-Nielsen L 1999 The influence of experimental muscle pain on the human soleus stretch reflex during sitting and walking. Clinical Neurophysiology 110(12): 2033–2043

Matzner O, Devor M 1987 Contrasting thermal sensitivity of spontaneously active A and C fibres in experimental nerve end neuromas. Pain 30: 373–384

Mayer D J, Price D D 1976 Central nervous system mechanisms of analgesia. Pain 1: 51–58

Melzack R 1989 Phantom limbs, the self and the brain. Canadian Psychology 30: 1–16

Melzack R 1990 Phantom limbs and the concept of a neuromatrix. Trends in Neurosciences 13: 88–92

Melzack R 1996 Gate control theory: on the evolution of pain concepts. Pain Forum 5(1): 128–138

Melzack R 1999 Pain and stress: a new perspective. In: Gatchel R, Turk D C (eds) Psychosocial factors in pain: clinical perspectives. Guilford Press, New York, pp 89–106

Merskey H, Bogduk N 1994 Classification of chronic pain. IASP Press, Seattle

Michaelis M, Vogel C, Blenk K H, Janig W 1997 Algesics excite axotomised afferent nerve fibres within the first hours following nerve transection in rats. Pain 72(3): 347–354

Michaelis M, Vogel C, Blenk K H, Arnarson A, Janig W 1998 Inflammatory mediators sensitize acutely axotomized nerve fibers to mechanical stimulation in the rat. Journal of Neuroscience 18(18): 7581–7587

Middaugh S J, Kee W G 1987 Advances in electromyographic monitoring and biofeedback in the treatment of chronic cervical and low back pain. Advances in Clinical Rehabilitation 1: 137–172

Moseley G L 2001 Clinical and physiological investigation of the psychophysiology of pain and movement. In: Faculty of Medicine, University of Sydney, Sydney, p 446

Moseley G L 2002 Combined physiotherapy and education is effective for chronic low back pain: a randomised controlled trial. Australian Journal of Physiotherapy 48: 297–302

Moseley G L 2003a Joining Forces: combining cognition-targeted motor control training with group or individual pain physiology education: a successful treatment for chronic low back pain. Journal of Manual and Manipulative Therapy 11: 88–94

Moseley G L 2003b Unravelling the barriers to reconceptualisation of the problem in chronic pain: the actual and perceived ability of patients and health professionals to understand the neurophysiology. Journal of Pain 4(4): 184–189

Moseley G L 2004 Evidence for a direct relationship between cognitive and physical change during an education intervention in people with chronic low back pain. European Journal of Pain 8(1): 39–45

Moseley G L, Hodges P W, Gandevia S C 2002 Deep and superficial fibers of the lumbar multifidus muscle are differently active during voluntary arm movements. Spine 27(2): E29–36

Moseley G L, Hodges P W, Gandevia S C 2003 External perturbation of the trunk in standing humans results in differential activity of components of medial back muscles. Journal of Physiology 547: 581–587

Moseley G L, Hodges P W, Nicholas M K 2004a A randomized controlled trial of intensive neurophysiology education in chronic low back pain. Clinical Journal of Pain (in press)

Moseley G L, Nicholas M K, Hodges P W 2004b Pain differs from non-painful attention-demanding or stressful tasks in its effect on postural control patterns of trunk muscles. Experimental Brain Research 36: 64–71

Moseley G L, Nicholas M K, Hodges P W 2004c Does anticipation of back pain predispose to back trouble? Brain (in press)

Nachemson A L 1992 Newest knowledge of low back pain: a critical look. Clinical Orthopaedics and Related Research (279): 8–20

Newton-John T R, Spence S H, Schotte D 1995 Cognitive-behavioural therapy versus EMG biofeedback in the treatment of chronic low back pain. Behaviour Research and Therapy 33(6): 691–697

Nicholas M K, Wilson P H, Goyen J 1992 Comparison of cognitive-behavioral group treatment and an alternative non-psychological treatment for chronic low back pain. Pain 48(3): 339–347

Nordin M, Nystrom B, Wallin U, Hagbarth K E 1984 Ectopic sensory discharges and paresthesiae in patients with disorders of peripheral nerves, dorsal roots and dorsal columns. Pain 20(3): 231–245

Noteboom J T 2000 Acute stressor activate the arousal response and impair performance of simple motor tasks. Department of Kinesiology and Applied Physiology, University of Colorado, Denver, p 35

Nowicki B H, Haughton V M, Schmidt T A et al 1996 Occult lumbar lateral spinal stenosis in neural foramina subjected to physiologic loading. American Journal of Neuroradiology 17(9): 1605–1614

Osuch E A, Ketter T A, Kimbrell T A et al 2000 Regional cerebral metabolism associated with anxiety symptoms in affective disorder patients. Biological Psychiatry 48(10): 1020–1023

Panjabi M M 1992 The stabilizing system of the spine. I: Function, dysfunction, adaptation, and enhancement. Journal of Spinal Disorders 5(4): 383–389

Peyron R, Laurent B, Garcia-Larrea L 2000 Functional imaging of brain responses to pain: a review and meta-analysis (2000). Neurophysiologie Clinique 30(5): 263–288

Pinault D 1995 Backpropagation of action potentials generated at ectopic axonal loci: hypothesis that axon terminals integrate local environmental signals. Brain Research Reviews 21: 42–92

Price D D 2000 Psychological mechanisms of pain and analgesia. IASP Press, Seattle

Raja S N, Meyer R A, Ringkamp M, Campbell J N 1999 Peripheral neural mechanisms of nociception. In: Wall P, Melzack R (eds) The textbook of pain. Churchill Livingstone, Edinburgh, pp 11–57

Raminsky M 1978 Ectopic generation of impulses and cross-talk in spinal nerve roots of 'dystrophic' mice. Annals of Neurology 3: 351–357

Rokicki L A, Holroyd K A, France C R, Lipchick G L, France J L, Kvaal S A 1997 Change mechanisms associated with combined relaxation/EMG biofeedback training for chronic tension headache. Applied Psychophysiology and Biofeedback 22(1): 21–41

Sawamoto N, Honda M, Okada T, et al 2000 Expectation of pain enhances responses to nonpainful somatosensory stimulation in the anterior cingulate cortex and parietal operculum/posterior insula: an event-related functional magnetic resonance imaging study. Journal of Neuroscience 20(19): 7438–7445

Schade V, Semmer N, Main C J, Hora J, Boos N 1999 The impact of clinical, morphological, psychosocial and work-related factors on the outcome of lumbar discectomy. Pain 80(1–2): 239–249

Sherman R A, Arena J G 1992 Biofeedback in the assessment and treatment of low back pain. In: Basmajian J V, Nyberg R (eds) Spinal manipulative therapies. Williams and Wilkins, Baltimore, pp 177–197

Sihvonen T, Partanen J, Hanninen O, Soimakallio S 1991 Electric behavior of low back muscles during lumbar pelvic rhythm in low back pain patients and healthy controls. Archives of Physical Medicine and Rehabilitation 72(13): 1080–1087

Snider B S, Asmundson G J, Wiese K C 2000 Automatic and strategic processing of threat cues in patients with chronic pain: a modified stroop evaluation. Clinical Journal of Pain 16(2): 144–154

Stuckey S J, Jacobs A, Goldfarb J 1986 EMG biofeedback training, relaxation training, and placebo for the relief of chronic back pain. Perceptual and Motor Skills 63(3): 1023–1036

Sullivan M J L, Bishop S R, Pivik J 1995 The pain catastrophizing scale: development and validation. Psychological Assessment 7(4): 524–532

Svensson P, Graven-Nielsen T, Matre D, Arendt-Nielsen L 1998 Experimental muscle pain does not cause long-lasting increases in resting electromyographic activity. Muscle and Nerve 21(11): 1382–1389

Symonds T L, Burton A K, Tillotson K M, Main C J 1995 Absence resulting from low back trouble can be reduced by psychosocial intervention at the work place. Spine 20(24): 2738–2745

Symonds T L, Burton A K, Tillotson K M, Main C J 1996 Do attitudes and beliefs influence work loss due to low back trouble? Occupational Medicine (Oxford, England) 46(1): 25–32

Tracey D J, Walker J S 1995 Pain due to nerve damage: are inflammatory mediators involved? Inflammation Research 44(10): 407–411

Travell J, Rinzler S, Herman M 1942 Pain and disability of the shoulder and arm. Treatment by intramuscular infiltration with procaine hydrochloride. Journal of the American Medical Association 120: 417–422

van Dieen J H, Selen L P J, Cholewicki J 2003 Trunk muscle activation in low-back pain patients: an analysis of the literature. Journal of Electromyography and kinesiology 13(4): 333–351

van Galen G P, van Huygevoort M 2000 Error, stress and the role of neuromotor noise in space oriented behaviour. Biological Psychology 51(2–3): 151–171

Vlaeyen J W, Linton S J 2000 Fear-avoidance and its consequences in chronic musculoskeletal pain: a state of the art. Pain 85(3): 317–332

Vlaeyen J W, Seelen H A, Peters M et al 1999 Fear of movement/(re)injury and muscular reactivity in chronic low back pain patients: an experimental investigation. Pain 82(3): 297–304

Vogt B A, Sikes R W, Rogt L J 1993 Anterior cingulate cortex and the medial pain system. In: Vogt B A, Gabriel M (eds) Neurobiology of cingulate cortex and limbic thalamus: a comprehensive handbook. Birkhauser, Boston

Waddell G 1998 The back pain revolution. Churchill Livingstone, Edinburgh

Waddell G, Newton M, Henderson I, Somerville D, Main C J 1993 A fear-avoidance beliefs questionnaire (FABQ) and the role of fear-avoidance beliefs in chronic low back pain and disability. Pain 52(2): 157–168

Wadhwani K, Rapoport S 1987 Transport properties of vertebrate blood–nerve barrier: comparison with blood-nerve barrier. Progress in Neurobiology 43: 235–279

Wall P 1999 Pain: the science of suffering. Orion Publishing, London

Wall P, Gutnick M 1974 Ongoing activity in peripheral nerves: the physiology and pharmacology of impulses originating from a neuroma. Experimental Neurology 43: 580–593

Wall P D, Melzack R, (eds) 1999 Introduction. Textbook of pain. Churchill Livingstone, Edinburgh, pp xii, 1588

Watson P J, Booker C K, Main C J 1997 Evidence for the role of psychological factors in abnormal paraspinal activity in patients with chronic low back pain. Journal of Musculoskeletal Pain 5(4): 41–56

Weinberg R, Hunt V 1976 The interrelationships between anxiety, motor performance and electromyography. Journal of Motor Behavior 8: 219–224

Weisenfeld Z, Lindblom U 1980 Behavioural and electrophysiological effects of various types of peripheral nerve lesions in the rat: a comparison of possible models of chronic pain. Pain 8: 285–298

Willer J C, Boureau F, Albe-Fessard D 1979 Supraspinal influence on nociceptive flexion reflex and pain sensation in man. Brain Research 179: 61–68

Willer J C, Dehen H, Cambier J 1981 Stress-induced analgesia in humans: endogenous opioids and naloxone-reversible depression of pain reflexes. Science 212(4495): 689–691

Willis W D 1985 The pain system. Karger, New York

Woolf C J, Bennett G J, Doherty M et al 1998 Towards a mechanism-based classification of pain? Pain 77(3): 227–229

Xie Y, Xiao W, Li H Q 1993 The relationship between new ion channels and ectopic discharges from a region of nerve injury. Science in China B36: 68–74

Zedka M, Prochazka A, Knight B, Gillard D, Gauthier M 1999 Voluntary and reflex control of human back muscles during induced pain. Journal of Physiology 520(2): 591–604

Chapter **17**

Cervical vertigo

H. Heikkilä

DIZZINESS AND VERTIGO

Dizziness is a common complaint of patients presenting to the emergency department. In fact, dizziness is the third most common reason to seek medical advice in the USA (Kroenke & Mangelsdorff 1989). Dizziness increases in frequency with age and prevalence of dizziness ranges from 1.8% in young adults to more than 30% in the elderly (Sloane et al 2001). In Sweden a quarter of the middle-aged population have been shown to suffer from dizziness (Tibblin et al 1990). Vertigo and dizziness are also common complaints accompanying neck pain and are reported by up to 80–90% of patients suffering from chronic whiplash syndrome (Ommaya et al 1968, Oosterveld et al 1991). Life-threatening illnesses are rare in patients with dizziness, but many of these patients have serious functional impairment.

There are four main categories that patients describe: vertigo, near-syncope, disequilibrium, and lightheadedness. Of these four, vertigo is the most common (40–50%). Vertigo is a sensation of irregular or whirling motion, either of oneself or of external objects. When the symptom complex is of spinning or rotation, the cause is almost always the inner ear or peripheral vestibular system. Although it is true that some patients experience a definite sense of environmental spin or self-rotation, the majority do not present solely with true spinning vertigo. Vertigo is a subtype of dizziness which results from an imbalance within the vestibular system (Baloh 1998). The same author focuses on three common presentations of vertigo: prolonged spontaneous vertigo, recurrent attacks of vertigo and positional vertigo. Of these, the most common is benign positional vertigo, in which brief attacks are brought on by certain changes in head position (Sauron & Dobler 1994). Advances in recognizing different forms of canalolithiasis and cupulolithiasis, which are sometimes present with continuous positional nystagmus, have revealed a peripheral vestibular aetiology where central nervous system lesions were previously suspected. Treatments using repositioning manoeuvres are also successful in cases where there is no nystagmus (Magnusson & Karlberg 2002). In general, disorders of the vestibular nerve and end organs are the most common cause of vertigo. The importance of neck proprioceptors for maintaining balance is receiving increasing attention, since the function or malfunction of the otoliths may disturb equilibrium in certain head positions (Kogler et al 2000).

CERVICAL VERTIGO

The existence of cervical vertigo has continued to be controversial, debated and denied. Patients with cervical pain and with simultaneous complaints of dizziness or vertigo but normal findings at otoneurologic examination are not uncommon. While nearly all dizziness specialists agree that cervical vertigo does exist, there is controversy regarding the frequency with which it occurs (Brandt 1996). The incidence of cervical vertigo seems to be highest in the 30–50 year-old age group, and is reported to be more common in the female population (Kuilman 1959, Hülse 1983).

Vertigo due to neck disorders was termed 'cervical vertigo' by Ryan & Cope (1955). Most patients suggested to suffer from cervical vertigo do not experience vertigo (a sensation of movement) but a feeling of imbalance or unsteadiness (Brandt 1991, Brown 1992). The diagnosis of cervicogenic dizziness is dependent upon correlating symptoms of imbalance and dizziness with neck pain and excluding other vestibular disorders based on history, examination and vestibular function tests (Wrisley et al 2000). To complicate matters, patients with vertigo from vestibular disorders often suffer from cervical pain and tender muscles secondary to their vertigo. As movements of the head tend to increase vertigo in vestibular disorders, these patients adopt a rigid neck posture.

PATHOGENIC HYPOTHESES OF CERVICAL VERTIGO

Three hypotheses have been proposed to explain the mechanisms underlying cervical vertigo: the vascular hypothesis, the neurovascular hypothesis and the somatosensory input hypothesis. Also, a combination of these pathogenic factors has been suggested to give rise to dizziness.

The vascular hypothesis

The vascular hypothesis holds that the vertebral artery is affected by compression leading to episodic ischaemia of the brain stem or inner ear, and this is considered to be a common cause of vertigo (Brandt 1991). Pathophysiological explanations vary from vertebral artery injury resulting in vestibular dysfunction or vertebral nerve irritation producing a neural mediated spasm due to the close relation between the sympathetic trunk and the vertebral artery (Bogduk 1986). Tamura (1989) suggested that vertigo might be caused by ischaemia of the brain produced by sympathetic vasoconstriction of the internal carotid artery. Vertigo would probably not be the only sign of vertebrobasilar ischaemia, but would be accompanied by other symptoms

such as diplopia, dysarthria, ataxia and motor symptoms. These symptoms could be induced or triggered by the head position (e.g. head maximally rotated and/or extended) (Brandt 1991). Arteriosclerotic change is the main reason for vertebrobasilar insufficiency, the basilar artery being most commonly affected followed by the cervical portion of the vertebral artery (Myer et al 1960). Several reports have linked chiropractic manipulation of the neck to dissection or occlusion of the vertebral artery. Trauma to the atlanto-axial segment of the vertebral artery would be the most plausible mechanism. However, previous studies linking such strokes to neck manipulation consist primarily of uncontrolled case series. While some analysis is consistent with a positive association in young adults, potential sources of bias are also discussed (Rothwell et al 2001). The rarity of dissection or occlusion of the vertebral artery makes this association difficult to study despite high volumes of chiropractic treatment. Because of the popularity of spinal manipulation, high-quality research on both its risks and benefits is recommended.

The vertebral artery is susceptible to compression or angulation by laterally projecting osteophytes from the uncinate processes in the lower cervical spine (especially C4–6) causing verterobasilar insufficiency (Sheehan et al 1960, Bauer et al 1961). In a recent study using colour Doppler ultrasonograph (Strek et al 1998), a pathological decrease of vertebral artery flow/velocity was demonstrated to have a relationship with the presence of degenerative changes in the cervical spine. The correlation coefficient increased proportionally according to age, changing from 0 to 79%. Furthermore, subluxated osteoarthrotic superior articular prosesses can cause compression (Bogduk 1986, Rosenberg et al 1998). Occlusion of the atlanto-axial segment of the vertebral artery during head rotation has been observed in several cadaver studies (Tatlow & Bammer 1957, Brown & Tatlow 1963) but it is questionable how frequently they are the cause of verterobasilar symptoms (Brown & Tatlow 1963, Bogduk 1986, Cote et al 1996). Vertebral artery occlusion secondary to external compression during cervical rotation is also reported due to anomalies of the origin of the vertebral artery, bands of the deep cervical fascia crossing the artery and an anomalous course of the vertebral artery between fascicles of either longus colli or scalenus anterior (Bogduk 1986).

If clinical symptoms such as vertigo happen transiently and repeatedly with head movements, vascular insufficiency due to mechanical compression of the vertebral artery must be kept in mind as a cause. For unilateral mechanical compression of the vertebral artery to result in a significant decrease in the verterobasilar circulation, not only would communicating circulation in the circle of Willis need to be deficient, but there would also need to be a concomitant reduction of blood flow in the contralateral vertebral artery (Aschan & Hugosson 1966). The vascular mechanism must be considered particularly in elderly patients with known arteriosclerotic disease. However, the importance of ischaemia as a cause of vertigo in neck disorders may have been overestimated (Jongkees 1969).

The neurovascular hypothesis

Barré (1926) proposed that sympathetic plexus surrounding the vertebral arteries could be mechanically irritated by degenerative changes in the cervical and the sympathetic irritation could produce reflexive vasoconstriction in the verterobasilar system, thus accounting for the symptoms of disequilibrium. Tamura (1989) described 40 patients suffering from Barré–Lieou syndrome (headache, vertigo, tinnitus and ocular problems) after whiplash injury. The underlying theory was that lateral disc herniation at C3/4 causes irritation of the nerve root which in turn communicates with the superior cervical ganglion of the sympathetic chain, resulting in symptoms related to the sympathetic nervous system. Headache could then be seen as a result of a spasm of the internal and external carotid artery.

There are, however, contradictory results for the neurovascular hypothesis. Sympathetic stimulation has been suggested to decrease cochlear microphonics (Seymour & Tappin 1953) and to sensitize muscle spindles by increasing intrafusal muscle fibre contraction (Hubbart & Berkoff 1993). Increased muscle spindle sensitivity may be mediated by the sympathetic nervous system acting on the intrafusal fibres of the muscle spindles as a feedback loop (Hubbart & Berkoff 1993). The connection between interneurons and motoneurons in the spinal cord may also contribute to increased muscle tension (Carlsson & Pellettieri 1982). Assuming increased muscle tension and sensitized muscle spindles, the latter may give rise to erroneous proprioceptive signalling (Johansson & Sojka 1991), especially if spindles in different neck muscles or on different sides of the neck are unequally sensitized. Erroneous cervical proprioceptive information converges in the CNS with vestibular and visual signals, which could affect the mental perception of body orientation and the relation to the surroundings may be misinterpreted, resulting in a feeling of dizziness or unsteadiness. On the other hand, blocking of the cervical sympathetic chain by injections of local anaesthetic in patients with 'posterior sympathetic syndrome of Barré–Lieou' has induced vertigo, a tendency to fall, past-pointing, horizontal nystagmus and tinnitus, instead of diminishing the symptoms (Barré 1926, Lieou 1928). In several reports sympathetic stimulation has been shown to have little effect on the normal autoregulation of cerebral blood flow (Todd et al 1974, Alm 1975).

The somatosensory input hypothesis

The somatosensory input hypothesis (Fig. 17.1) suggests that symptoms in cervical vertigo are due to a disturbed sensory input from the proprioceptors of the neck (Ryan & Cope 1955, Brandt 1991, Brown 1992).

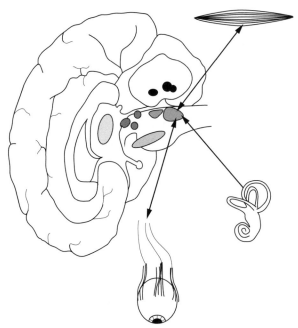

Figure 17.1 The somatosensory input hypothesis suggests that symptoms in cervical vertigo are due to a disturbed sensory input from the proprioceptors of the neck leading to a sensory mismatch. Dizziness results from a disturbance in the complex perceptive system containing interacting and integrating signals of the vestibular, visual and proprioceptive components.

The vestibular system constitutes one of the phylogenetically oldest CNS functions that in all species is especially developed to maintain posture and locomotion on land, sea or in the air. The vestibular part of the labyrinth consists of three semicircular canals and the otolith systems of the utricular and saccular maculae. The reflexes to the eye muscles and the trunk and limb muscles are developed to meet the needs of the system. The neck has been regarded as an important proprioceptive organ for postural processes since it was shown that tonic neck reflexes arise from receptors supplied by upper cervical segments (Magnus 1926). The purpose of the reflex from the labyrinth to the eye muscles, the vestibulo-ocular reflex (VOR), is to stabilize the visual field and for the vestibulocollic reflex (VCR), the purpose is to stabilize the head position (Norré 1990). The proprioceptive reflexes of the neck are the cervicocollic reflex (CCR) and the cervico-ocular reflex (COR). The CCR (Petersen et al 1985) and the COR (Hikosaka & Maeda 1973) have different functions. The CCR tends to stabilize the neck and protect over-rotation (Pyykkö et al 1989), and it counteracts the COR (Pompeiano 1988). The CCR is probably generated from the gamma muscle spindles of the deepest neck muscles (Hirai et al 1984) whereas the COR seems to be a 'helper reflex' if the labyrinth has been damaged (Botros 1979). Its function seems to be to provide information about the position of the neck and to cooperate with the VOR for clear vision during motion. The COR originates in proprioceptors in the neck muscles and in the cervical joints of the upper cervical spine (McLain 1994). Vestibulospinal reflexes (VSR) transmit correcting neural activity so as to establish an appropriate tone of the neck and body muscles for the purpose of balance – the feedback system.

Several studies in intact humans have shown that information from the cervical proprioceptors has significant effects on orientation and posture. Disturbances of gait have been provoked in experimental animals by interference with the upper cervical sensory supply by damaging (Longet 1845) or anaesthetizing neck muscles (Abrahams & Falchetto 1969, De Jong et al 1977) and by cutting the upper cervical dorsal roots (Cohen 1961, Richmond et al 1976).

The receptors for proprioception in the neck include the muscle spindles that are present in high density in the intervertebral muscles (Bakker & Richmond 1982) as well as the dorsal muscles (Richmond & Bakker 1982). Joint capsule receptors (pacinian corpuscles, Ruffini endings) and Golgi tendon organs at musculotendinous junctions may also contribute to proprioceptive sensation (Richmond & Bakker 1982).

The term proprioception was originally proposed by Sherrington (1906) to describe the sense of limb position and movements subserved by the deep receptors in the muscles, the tendons and the joints, and the receptors of the labyrinth. Since then, the term has been widely used to describe a number of different phenomena: to describe position sense only, or as a synonym of kinaesthesia, and movement and position sense. It has been used to describe the ability to detect, without visual input, the spatial position and/or movement of the limbs in relation to the rest of the body. Kinaesthesia generally refers to the perception of changes in the angles of joints, a function dependent upon mechanoreceptor input and a critical component in the proprioceptive system. Probably cervicocephalic kinaesthesia is linked to information coming from the extensive muscular and articular proprioceptive system (Wyke 1979, Taylor & McCloskey 1988, Norré 1990, Revel et al 1991, Lajoie et al 1993). Cervical kinaesthetic performance is not well described in healthy subjects. A method of evaluating cervicocephalic kinaesthesia was introduced by Revel et al (1991). The test evaluates the ability to appreciate both movement and the position of the head with respect to the trunk. It involves information from the cervical proprioceptive apparatus and from the vestibular system, but a number of experimental arguments point to a primarily cervical proprioceptive role (Revel et al 1991).

Loudon et al (1997) studied the ability to reproduce head position after whiplash injury and found inaccuracy in the assessment of neutral position of the head as well as in perception of rotational position. In a more recent study (Heikkilä et al 2000), impaired kinaesthetic performance was present in subjects with dizziness/vertigo of cervical origin, compared with healthy controls. It is likely that proprioception is primarily involved, either by lesioning or functional impairment of muscular and articular receptors, or by alteration in afferent integration and tuning (Wyke 1979, Taylor & McCloskey 1988, Lajoie et al 1993, Barnsley et al 1995). Altered kinaesthetic sensitivity has been implicated in functional instability of joints and their predisposition to re-injury, chronic pain and even degenerative joint disease (Revel et al 1991, Hall et al 1995). There is also evidence suggesting that removal of noxious or abnormal afferent input at the site of the articulation alone may result in improved proprioception and motor response (De Abdrade et al 1965, Slosberg 1988).

Postural control and vertigo

Postural equilibrium is ensured by a steady input to the brain of signals of vestibular, visual and proprioceptive origin. The postural control system of the upright standing human is in part a dynamic feedback control system (Johansson & Magnusson 1991). It is likely that proprioception is primarily involved in postural control and ocular motor control (Magnus 1924, de Jong & Bles 1986, Norré et al 1987, Karnath 1994). This sensory input is stored and integrated in a 'bank of memory pictures' (Roberts 1967), which may be located in the parapontine reticular formation of the brain stem. At every movement, 'sensory pictures' concerning the position and movement of the body are transmitted to the centre and efferent activity from this postural control centre is transmitted for adjustment to the muscles of the neck and the rest of the body. Vertigo and dizziness are the results of an abnormality of the sensory picture/sensory mismatch due to a disturbance in the complex perceptive system containing interacting and integrating signals of vestibular, visual and proprioceptive system origin (Brandt 1991, Karlberg et al 1995).

Patients with neck pain and concomitant dizziness have been reported to manifest impaired postural performance as compared to healthy subjects (de Jong & Bles 1986, Ålund et al 1993). Karlberg et al (1991) found that both postural control and voluntary eye movements were impaired in healthy subjects in whom cervical mobility was restricted by the application of a cervical collar.

Posturographic assessment of the dynamics of postural control function has been proposed to be a possible future tool for use in diagnosing cervical vertigo (Karlberg et al 1996b).

Disturbed eye movement and the neck

Oculomotor function tests have been used for detecting lesions affecting structures in the brain stem and cerebellum (Baloh & Honrubia 1979, Henriksson et al 1981, Wennmo et al 1983). The smooth pursuit and saccade are eye motility functions with important relay stations in the brain stem and cerebellum (Baloh & Honrubia 1979, Henriksson et al 1981, Wennmo et al 1983). Pathologic oculomotor dysfunction was reported in patients with whiplash trauma (Hildingsson et al 1989, Oosterveld et al

1991). In some patients with moderate oculomotor dysfunction (i.e. the smooth pursuit abnormalities) the disturbances may be explained by affection of the proprioceptive system in the cervical area (Hinoki 1984, Rosenhall et al 1987, Hildingsson et al 1989, Oosterveld et al 1991). The pronounced oculomotor dysfunction in some whiplash cases were possibly caused by medullar lesions (Hildingsson et al 1989). However, pathologic oculomotor dysfunction was also reported in patients with chronic primary fibromyalgia with dysaesthesia (Rosenhall et al 1987). In a recent study on whiplash subjects (Heikkilä & Wenngren 1998), 62% of the subjects showed pathological oculomotor test results in at least one of the smooth pursuit tests and one of the voluntary saccades tests at 2-year follow-up. There was a good association between the oculomotor functions and cervical kinaesthetic performance functions. Smooth pursuit tests were correlated with active range of cervical motion. These results suggest that restriction of cervical movements and changes in the quality of proprioceptive information from the cervical spine region affect voluntary eye movements. The same conclusion has been proposed by Karlberg et al (1991). Hikosaka & Maeda (1973) further showed that the vestibulo-ocular reflex could be modulated by sensory input from the region of neck vertebrae, but not from the large neck muscles.

VERTIGO IN DIFFERENT NECK DISORDERS

Oostveld et al (1991) reported presence of vertigo in 85% of whiplash subjects. None of them complained of real rotational sensations but merely of combinations of lightheadedness, spinning sensations and floating sensations. Floating sensations alone were present in 35% of subjects. In 18% of all patients vertiginous sensations appeared only during and after head and neck movements. Whiplash injuries usually result in neck pain due to myofascial trauma; this has been documented in both animal and human studies. Abnormalities in tests of vestibular and oculomotor functions are reported to be common (Hildingsson et al 1989, 1993, Oosterveld et al 1991). Visual disturbances mostly take the form of blurred vision and may be associated with retrobulbar pain. Other visual impairments may include photophobia and nystagmus. In some cases with pronounced oculomotor dysfunction, lesions of the brain stem might be a possible explanation, while in other patients with moderate oculomotor dysfunction it might be caused by an afferent proprioceptive dysfunction of the cervical spine (Hildingsson et al 1989, 1993). Gimse et al (1996) documented disturbed control of saccadic eye movements during reading as well as the smooth pursuit eye movements in a consecutive group of whiplash subjects. This last effect was augmented by neck torsion. This was interpreted as being caused by distorted neck proprioceptive activity which sends misleading information to the posture control system.

In another study, patients with chronic dysfunction following a whiplash trauma were significantly less accurate compared with a control group in their ability to relocate their head in space after an active displacement that turned the head away from the reference position (Heikkilä & Åström 1996). The whiplash subjects showed less accuracy in vertical plane repositioning movements, which might be explained by the hyperextension, hyperflexion trauma mechanism. However they showed significantly decreased relocation errors after undergoing a 6-week rehabilitation programme. A significant association between oculomotor dysfunction and head repositioning function occurred in whiplash subjects and significant correlations were observed between oculomotor dysfunction and active range of cervical range of motion 2 years after injury (Heikkilä & Wenngren 1998).

Vertigo and dizziness are common complaints accompanying neck pain. Patients with tension headache or tension neck syndromes often complain of dizziness (Blumenthal 1968, Carlsson & Rosenhall 1988), and patients with cervicogenic headache report dizziness in about 40% of cases (Jull 1986). Oculomotor disturbances have been reported in patients with tension headache (Carlsson & Rosenhall 1988). Complaints of vertigo and dizziness are also common in patients with cervical spondylosis who report symptoms in the neck and the extremities. In one study by Mangat & McDowall (1973), 50% of the patients had complained of vertigo and 20% also experienced positional nystagmus. Sandström (1962) found vertigo and positional nystagmus in about 20% of consecutive patients with cervicobrachial pain and cervical spondylosis. In patients with cervicobrachial pain, Karlberg et al (1995) reported a 50% incidence of vertigo and significantly poorer postural control than in the controls. A total of 83% of the patients showed signs of cervical root compression on MRI scans.

SYMPTOMS AND SIGNS IN CERVICAL VERTIGO

The diagnosis of cervicogenic dizziness is dependent upon correlating the symptoms of imbalance and dizziness with neck pain while excluding other vestibular disorders based on history, examination and vestibular function tests. It may be postulated that cervical vertigo is characterized not by rotatory vertigo but by a feeling of unsteadiness when standing and walking (Brandt 1991). Neck pain is an obligate symptom. The onset of neck pain commonly precedes the onset of dizziness. It is usually confined to the occipital region, but may radiate into the temporal or temporomandibular areas as well as to the forehead or the orbital region. Pain on palpation of the cervical muscles and findings of tender points and trigger points are also considered to be important. The short suboccipital muscles that run between the occiput and the atlas and axis can be particularly tense and painful. A feeling of dizziness and nausea might be provoked by palpation of the lateral mass of the atlas (Scherer 1985).

Headache is common. It is usually located in the back of the head, but patients also sometimes describe it as a band-like pressure around the head. Tinnitus is not uncommon and a low-frequency hearing loss has been reported (Hülse 1994). A direction-fixed or direction-changing positional nystagmus is reported to be common (Brown 1992). Visual disturbances mostly take the form of blurred vision and may be associated with retrobulbar pain. Other visual impairments may include photophobia and nystagmus. Attacks of more intense dizziness or even vertigo, with a duration of seconds to minutes, may be triggered by head movements such as rotation or extension of the neck. Imbalance may occur but patients with cervical vertigo may perform normally in the Romberg test, the Unterberger stepping test and other postural tests (Hülse 1983).

DIAGNOSTIC TESTS FOR CERVICAL VERTIGO

Every patient with vertigo or dizziness should be screened with a general physical examination during which particular attention should be paid to the vascular system by including the cranial and carotid pulses plus an evaluation for significant varicose veins. All patients with an undiagnosed disorder of equilibration should have a complete neurological examination. Baloh (1995) suggests that the examination of the dizzy patient should include a careful assessment of gait and balance and a search for spontaneous and positional nystagmus. The vestibulo-ocular reflex can be evaluated qualitatively at the bedside with Doll's eye, dynamic visual activity and ice water caloric tests, which provide different information about vestibular function.

Quantitative studies on the significance of disorders of the upper cervical spine as a cause of vertigo or impaired hearing are few. In one study (Galm et al 1998), the cervical spines of 67 patients who presented with symptoms of dizziness were examined. Of these, 31 were diagnosed with dysfunction of the upper cervical spine; 19 did not show signs of dysfunction. Dysfunction was found at level C1 in 14 cases, at level C2 in six cases and at level C3 in four cases. In seven cases more than one upper cervical spine motion segment was affected. A functional examination of motion segments of the upper cervical spine is important in diagnosing and treating cervical vertigo (Galm et al 1998).

The validity of the neck extension-rotation test as a clinical screening procedure to detect decreased vertebrobasilar blood flow associated with dizziness was studied by Cote et al (1996). Twelve subjects with dizziness reproduced by the extension-rotation test and 30 healthy control subjects had Doppler ultrasonography examination of their vertebral arteries with the neck extended and rotated. Vascular impedance to blood flow was measured and the presence of signs and symptoms of vertebrobasilar ischaemia was recorded. The positive predictive value of the test was found to be 0% and its negative predictive value ranged from 63 to 97%. Consequently, the value of this test for screening patients at risk of stroke after cervical manipulation is questionable (Brown & Tatlow 1963, Bogduk 1986, Cote et al 1996).

There are few clinical tests for postural instability and most patients perform normally in the Romberg test, the Unterberger stepping test and other postural test (Hülse 1983). Unfortunately, these tests have failed to distinguish patients with cervical vertigo from healthy subjects or from patients with other balance disorders (Norré et al 1987). The musculoskeletal physiotherapist also has to take into consideration the absence of any evaluation of otolith function in the classical examination techniques. Otoliths may have more influence on the results of the tests that include postural elements. Position of the head as well as erect standing rather than eye stabilization are more linked to otolith function than the semicircular canals (Norré 1990). In the Romberg test, a quiet stance is assessed by observing a subject's body sway when they are standing with eyes open or closed. The Unterberger stepping test puts further demands on the postural control systems by introducing a voluntary movement (stepping), to evaluate deviation or turning from the neutral position (Unterberger 1938). Increased postural sway with an extended neck in the standing position has been reported by some authors to have some correlation with cervical vertigo (de Jong & Bles 1986, Norré et al 1987, Kugler et al 2000) whereas others have not found differences in postural sway with extended head between healthy subjects and patients with suspected cervical vertigo (Ålund et al 1993). It has also been suggested that the head position with the neck extended puts the utricular otoliths in an unfavourable position with reduced sensitivity to movement relative to the gravitational field (Brandt et al 1981).

Hülse (1983) suggested the presence of cervical nystagmus or neck torsion nystagmus elicited by trunk movements relative to the fixated head to be diagnostic for cervical vertigo. Cervical nystagmus was found in about 50% of the patients with suspected cervical vertigo. Norré et al (1987) studied cervical nystagmus in healthy subjects and found a weak cervical nystagmus in 26% of those studied and a moderately strong nystagmus in another 26%. Cervically induced eye movements can be recorded by use of the neck torsion test, in which the trunk is rotated and the head is fixed. The cervical influence on oculomotor function has been studied in whiplash subjects with vertigo and dizziness (Tjell & Rosenhall 1998), in patients with whiplash associated disorders (Gimse et al 1996) and in patients with tension-type headache (Rosenhall et al 1996). The smooth pursuit neck torsion (SPNT) test was found to be useful for diagnosing cervical dizziness, at least in patients with whiplash associated disorders (Tjell & Rosenhall 1998). A method of evaluating cervicocephalic kinaesthesia was introduced by Revel et al (1991). The test concerns the ability to appreciate both movement and the position of the head with respect to the trunk. In a recent study (Heikkilä et al 2000), impaired kinaesthetic performance was present in subjects with dizziness/vertigo of cervical origin, compared with healthy controls. A good association between the oculomotor functions and cervical kinaesthetic performance functions has been reported by Heikkilä & Wenngren (1998).

Objective data on postural performance can be recorded by posturography, which measures the forces actuated by the subject's feet on the supporting surface (Aalto et al 1988). The movement of the centrepoint of forces does not represent the body motion but the forces applied to stabilize motion. In static conditions (static posturography) postural oscillations of the subject are recorded in the Romberg position, while in dynamic conditions motor responses are measured in response to destabilizing stimuli (dynamic posturography). Assessment of quiet stance does not seem to be very sensitive for distinguishing healthy subjects from patients with different balance disorders and various posture-perturbing stimuli have been introduced in order to put more demands on the postural systems. A vibratory stimulus applied to muscles or tendons (Enbom et al 1988), a galvanic stimulus applied to the vestibular nerves (Magnusson et al 1990), moving the support surface (Nashner 1977) or moving the visual surroundings (Voorhees 1989) have all been used. Ålund et al (1993) found that patients with suspected cervical vertigo showed significantly lower equilibrium scores for dynamic posturography than the controls when recorded in neutral position of the head, in rotation and in lateral flexion. The patients with vertigo also had significantly lower equilibrium scores in the position most likely to elicit their vertigo as compared with the patients with only neck pain. Using posturography in which stance was perturbed by a vibratory stimulus applied towards the calf muscles, Karlberg et al (1996a) studied 16 consecutive patients with recent onset of neck pain and concomitant complaints of vertigo or dizziness, 18 patients with recent vestibular neuritis and 17 healthy subjects. The results showed disturbed postural control in patients with cervical vertigo to differ from that in patients with recent vestibular neuritis, indicating posturographic assessment of human posture dynamics to be a possible future tool for use in diagnosing cervical vertigo.

TREATMENTS FOR CERVICAL VERTIGO

There are few published studies on the effects of treatment of the neck in patients with cervicogenic vertigo. Successful treatment of the neck disorder with pain reduction improves disturbed balance and reduces dizziness. Physiotherapy, traction of the neck, injection of local anaesthetics at tender points and immobilization of the neck with a collar have all been suggested as treatments for vertigo of cervical origin (de Jong & Bles 1986, Brown 1992). Temporomandibular disorder as a reason for tinnitus and dizziness has also been proposed and improvement following treatment with a dental orthotic and self-care instructions has been reported by Wright et al (2000).

In general, manual therapies have been demonstrated to be effective for mechanical neck pain and cervical vertigo in the short term. Safety is a prime consideration when applying these treatments even if the risk of increased symptoms resulting from manual therapy is low (in the range of 1–2%). In fact, the most common symptom aggravation reported is vertigo or dizziness (Gross et al 1996). Positive effects have been reported for manipulative treatments (Cronin 1997, Galm et al 1998, Hülse et al 2000) and acupuncture as a single therapy. There are no reported controlled studies where different physiotherapy methods have been compared. In a recent single-case study on 14 consecutive patients the effects of acupuncture, cervical manipulation and topical NSAID (non-steroidal anti-inflammatory drug) application were studied on dizziness/vertigo, neck pain and cervical kinaesthetic sensibility (Heikkilä et al 2000). Both acupuncture and manipulation reduced dizziness/vertigo and had positive effects on active head repositioning. Manipulation was the only treatment that shortened the duration of vertigo during the preceding 7 days. A manipulative thrust in the plane of normal movement of a joint would presumably be in such a plane as to affect the deep interarticular muscles. It is most likely that the observed effects are related more to changes in mechanoreceptor afferent input than to changes in the vestibular system. Although the risk of injury associated with manipulation of the cervical spine appears to be small, this type of therapy has the potential to expose patients to vertebral artery damage that can be avoided with the use of mobilization (non-thrust passive movements). Elderly people with arteriosclerosis and cervical spondylosis might be more vulnerable. It has been proposed that the benefits of cervical manipulation do not outweigh the risks (Di Fabio 1999).

Postural training has been advocated in patients with different vestibular disorders (Horak et al 1992, Shepard et al 1993). Vestibular rehabilitation is an increasingly popular treatment option for patients with persistent dizziness (Girardi & Konrad 1998). This treatment may contain head, eye, and body exercises designed to promote vestibular compensation. In a controlled study, improvement was reported for the treatment group compared to the control group with odds ratios for improvement 3.1:1 at 6 weeks and 3.8:1 at 6 months (Yardley et al 1998). Postural rehabilitation has been shown to have positive effects on postural stability but also on positional strategy in older people (Asai et al 1997). Recovery of postural stability has been reported following physiotherapy (de Jong & Bles 1986). In a randomized and controlled trial, Karlberg et al (1996a) studied the effects of physiotherapy in patients with dizziness of suspected cervical origin and found significantly reduced neck pain and reduced frequency of dizziness, as well as significantly improved postural performance. The majority of patients underwent several treatment modalities and treatment was given over a period of 5–20 weeks. Revel et al (1994) found that a rehabilitation programme based on eye–neck coordination exercises and aimed to improve neck proprioception significantly reduced neck pain in patients with chronic cervical pain syndromes and significantly improved cervicocephalic kinaesthesia and horizontal rotational active range of neck motion.

A combined approach for treatment of cervical vertigo including multiple modalities was proposed by Bracher et al (2000) to treat causal factors of vertigo including musculoskeletal complaints, mainly cervical pain, tension-type headache and shoulder girdle pain. When correctly diagnosed, cervical vertigo can be successfully treated using a combination of manual therapy and vestibular rehabilitation. Treatment should be directed at the underlying cause whenever possible. Further controlled studies are needed to assess the validity of earlier studies on the treatment of cervical vertigo.

SOME DIFFERENTIAL DIAGNOSES FOR CERVICAL VERTIGO

In addition to determining whether the symptom complex is episodic, the duration and length of symptoms and any associated complaints, the examiner should elicit an exact description of what the patient is experiencing. When the patient's complaints are actually of incoordination or clumsiness, the cause may be cerebellar dysfunction or peripheral neuropathology. If the symptom complex is of 'light-headedness', systemic factors such as postural hypotension, vasodepressor syncope or cardiac arrhythmia are possible. A history of episodic disequilibration accompanied by diplopia, slurred speech, periodic numbness, dimming of vision and occasional drop attacks would suggest transient vertebrobasilar ischaemia. If the patient has experienced severe episodes of imbalance in early life, followed by occipital or generalized headaches, the history would be suggestive of basilar artery migraine. Episodic positional vertigo with brief episodes of spinning while turning over in bed is suggestive of a common condition, benign paroxysmal vertigo. There are a significant number of patients whose balance disorder of disequilibration or dizziness is of long duration and could be aggravated or caused by anxiety. In some individuals there is decreased ability to compensate for peripheral vestibular abnormality. This inability could be congenital or an acquired central inability to compensate due to CNS lesions from conditions such as multiple sclerosis, a previous stroke, a fluctuating peripheral vestibular problem, as in Ménière's disease, relative inactivity without much afferent input and a peripheral vestibular apparatus providing inaccurate afferent information.

KEYWORDS	
balance	postural control
cervical pain	proprioception
dizziness	unsteadiness
kinesthesia	vertigo
neck disorders	

References

Aalto H, Pyykkö I, Starck J 1988 Computerized posturography, a development of the measuring system. Acta Otolaryngologica Supplementum 449: 71–76

Abrahams V C, Falchetto S 1969 Hind leg ataxia of cervical origin and cervico-lumbar interactions with a supratentorial pathway. Journal of Physiology 203: 435–447

Alm A 1975 The effect of stimulation of the cervical sympathetic chain on regional cerebral blood flow in monkeys: a study with radioactively labelled microspheres. Acta Physiologica Scandinavica 93: 483–489

Ålund M, Ledin T, Ödkvist L, Larsson S-E 1993 Dynamic postulography among patients with common neck disorders: a study of 15 cases with suspected cervical vertigo. Journal of Vestibular Research 3(4): 383–389

Asai M, Watanabe Y, Shimizu K 1997 Effects of vestibular rehabilitation on postural control. Acta Otolaryngologica Supplementum 528: 116–120

Aschan G, Hugosson R B 1966 Vestibular symptoms provoked by head and neck rotation after bilateral carotid ligation. Acta Otolaryngologica 61: 49–54

Bakker D A, Richmond R J R 1982 Muscle spindle complexes in muscles around upper cervical vertebrae in the cat. Journal of Neurophysiology 48: 62–74

Baloh R W 1995 Approach to the evaluation of the dizzy patient. Otolaryngology and Head and Neck Surgery 112(1): 3–7

Baloh R W 1998 Vertigo. Lancet 352 (9143): 1841–1846

Baloh R W, Honrubia V 1979 Clinical neurophysiologic of the vestibular system. F A Davis, Philadelphia.

Barnsley L, Lord S, Wallis B, Bogduk N 1995 The prevalence of chronic cervical zygapophysial joint pain after whiplash. Spine 20(1): 20–26

Barré M 1926 Sur un syndromes sympathique cervical postérieure et sa cause fréquente: l'arthrite cervicale. Revista de Neurologia 33: 1246–1248

Bauer R, Sheehand S, Meyer J S 1961 Arteriographic study of cerebrovascular disease. II: Cerebral symptoms due to kinking tortuousity, and compression of carotid and vertebral arteries of the neck. Archives of Neurology 4: 119–131

Blumenthal L S 1968 Tension headache. In: Vinken P J, Bruyn G W (eds) Handbook of clinical neurology. Headaches and cranial neuralgias. North-Holland Publ, Amsterdam, vol 5, pp 157–171

Bogduk N 1986 Cervical causes of headache and dizziness. In: Grieve G (eds) Modern Manual Therapy of the Vertebral Column. Churchill Livingstone, Edinburgh, pp 289–302

Botros G 1979 The tonic oculomotor function of the cervical joint and muscle receptors. Neuroscience 25: 214–220

Bracher E S, Almeida C I, Almeida R R, Duprat A C, Bracher C B 2000 A combined approach for the treatment of cervical vertigo. Journal of Manipulative and Physiological Therapeutics 23(2): 96–100

Brandt T 1991 Cervical vertigo. In: Brandt T Vertigo: its multisensory syndromes. Springer-Verlag, London, pp 277–281

Brandt T 1996 Cervical vertigo: reality or fiction? Audiology and Neuro-otology 1(4): 187–196

Brandt T, Krafczyk S, Malsbenden I 1981 Postural imbalance with head extension: improvement by training as a model for ataxia therapy. Annals of the New York Academy of Sciences 374: 636–649

Brown J J 1992 Cervical contribution to balance: cervical vertigo. In: Berthoz A, Vidal P P, Graf W (eds) The head-neck sensory motor system. Oxford University Press, New York, pp 644–647

Brown B S T J, Tatlow W F T 1963 Radiographic studies of the vertebral arteries in cadavers. Radiology 81: 80–88

Carlsson C, Pellettieri L 1982 A clinical view on pain physiology. Acta Chirurgica Scandinavica 148: 305–313

Carlsson J, Rosenhall U 1988 Oculomotor disturbances in patients with tension headache. Acta Otolaryngologica 106: 354–360

Cohen L A 1961 Role of eye and neck proprioceptive mechanisms in body orientation and motor coordination. Journal of Neurophysiology 24: 1–11

Cote P, Kreitz B G, Cassidy J D, Thiel H 1996 The validity of the extension-rotation test as a clinical screening procedure before neck manipulation: a secondary analysis. Journal of Manipulative and Physiological Therapeutics 19(3): 159–164

Cronin P C 1997 Cervicogenic vertigo. European Journal of Chiropractic 45: 65–69

De Abrade J R, Grant C, Dixon A 1965 Joint distension and reflex inhibition in the knee. Journal of Bone and Joint Surgery (American volume) 47: 313–322

de Jong J M B V, Bles W 1986 Cervical dizziness and ataxia. In: Bles W, Brandt T (eds) Disorders of posture and gait. Elsevier Science (Biomedical division), Amsterdam, pp 185–206

De Jong P T V M, de Jong J M B V, Cohen B, Jongkees L B W 1977 Ataxia and nystagmus induced by injection of local anaesthetic in the neck. Annals of Neurology 1: 240–246

Di Fabio R P 1999 Manipulation of the cervical spine: risks and benefits. Physical Therapy 79(1): 50–65

Enbom H, Magnusson M, Pyykkö I, Schalén L 1988 Presentation of a posturographic test with loading the proprioceptive system. Acta Otolaryngololologica Supplementum 455: 58–61

Galm R, Rittmeister M, Schmitt E 1998 Vertigo in patients with cervical spine dysfunction. European Spine Journal 7(1): 55–58

Gimse R, Tjell C, Bjorgen I A, Saunte C 1996 Disturbed eye movements after whiplash due to injuries to the posture control system. Journal of Clinical and Experimental Neuropsychology 18(2): 178–186

Girardi M, Konrad H R 1998 Vestibular rehabilitation therapy for the patient with dizziness and balance disorder. ORL Head and Neck Nursing 16(4): 13–22

Gross A R, Aker P D, Quartly C 1996 Manual therapy in the treatment of neck pain. Rheumatic Diseases Clinics of North America 22(3): 579–598

Hall M G, Ferell W R, Sturrock R D, Hamblen D L, Baxendale R H 1995 The effect of the hypermobility syndrome on knee joint proprioception. British Journal of Rheumatology 34: 121–125

Heikkilä H, Åström P-G 1996 Cervicocephalic kinesthetic sensibility in patients with whiplash injury. Scandinavian Journal of Rehabilitation Medicine 28: 133–138

Heikkilä H, Wenngren B-I 1998 Cervicocephalic kinesthetic sensibility, active range of cervical motion, and oculomotor function in patients with whiplash injury. Archives of Physical Medicine and Rehabilitation 79: 1089–1094

Heikkilä H, Johansson M, Wenngren B-I 2000 Effects of acupuncture, cervical manipulation and NSAID therapy on dizziness and impaired head repositioning of suspected cervical origin: a pilot study. Manual Therapy 5(3): 151–157

Henriksson N G, Hindfelt B, Pyykkö I, Schalén L 1981 Rapid eye movements reflecting neurological disorders. Clinical Otolaryngology and Allied Sciences 6 (2): 111–119

Hikosaka O, Maeda M 1973 Cervical effects on abducens motorneurons and their interaction with vestibulo-ocular reflex. Experimental Brain Research 18: 512–530

Hildingsson C, Wenngren B-I, Bring G, Toolanen G 1989 Oculomotor problems after cervical spine injury. Acta Orthopaedica Scandinavica 20: 513–516

Hildingsson C, Wenngren B-I, Toolanen G 1993 Eye motility dysfunction after soft-tissue injury of the cervical spine. Acta Orthopaedica Scandinavica 64: 129–132

Hinoki M 1984 Vertigo due to whiplash injury: a neurotological approach. Acta Otolaryngologica Supplementum 419: 9–29

Hirai N, Hongo T, Sasaki S, Yamashita M, Yoshida K 1984 Neck muscle afferent input to spinocerebellar tract cells of the central cervical nucleus in the cat. Experimental Brain Research 55: 286–300

Horak F B, Jones-Rycewicz C, Black F O, Shumway-Cook A 1992 Effects of vestibular rehabilitation on dizziness and imbalance. Otolaryngology and Head and Neck Surgery 106: 175–180

Hubbart D R, Berkoff G 1993 Myofascial trigger points show spontaneous needle EMG activity. Spine 18: 1803–1807

Hülse M 1983 Die zervikalen Gleichgewichtsstörungen. Springer-Verlag, Berlin

Hülse M 1994 Die zervikogene Hörstörung. HNO 42: 602–613

Hülse M, Holzel M 2000 Vestibulospinale reactionen bei der cervikogenen gleidigewichtstörnung. Die zervikogenen unsicherheit [Vestibulospinal reactions in cervicogenic dysequilibrium: cervicogenic imbalance.] HNO 48: 295–301

Johansson R, Magnusson M 1991 Human postural dynamics. Critical Reviews in Biomedical Engineering 18: 413–437

Johansson H, Sojka P 1991 Pathophysiological mechanisms involved in genesis and spread of muscular tension in occupational muscle pain and in chronic musculoskeletal pain syndromes: a hypothesis. Medical Hypotheses 35: 196–203

Jongkees L B W 1969 Cervical vertigo. Laryngoscope 79: 1473–1484

Jull G A 1986 Headaches associated with the cervical spine: a clinical review. In: Grieve G P (ed) Modern Manual Therapy of the Vertebral Column. Churchill Livingstone, New York, pp 322–329

Karlberg M, Magnusson M, Johansson R 1991 Effects of restrained cervical mobility on voluntary eye movements and postural control. Acta Otolaryngologica 111: 664–670

Karlberg M, Persson L, Magnusson M 1995 Impaired postural control in patients with cervico-brachial pain. Acta Otolaryngologica Supplementum 520(2): 440–442

Karlberg M, Magnusson M, Malmström E M, Melander A, Moritz U 1996a Postural and symptomatic improvement after physiotherapy in patients with dizziness of suspected cervical origin. Archives of Physical Medicine and Rehabilitation 77(9): 874–882

Karlberg M, Johansson R, Magnusson M 1996b Dizziness of suspected cervical origin distinguished by posturographic assessment of human postural dynamics. Journal of Vestibular Research 6(11): 37–47

Karnath H O 1994 Subjective body orientation in neglect and the interactive contribution of neck muscle proprioception and vestibular stimulation. Brain 117: 1001–1012

Kogler A, Lindfors J, Odkvist L M, Ledin T 2000 Postural stability using different neck positions in normal subjects and patients with neck trauma. Acta Otolaryngologica 120(2): 151–155

Kroenke K, Mangelsdorff A D 1989 Common symptoms in ambulatory care: incidence, evaluation, therapy, and outcome. American Journal of Medicine 86: 262–266

Kugler A, Lindfors J, Ödquist L M, Ledin T 2000 Postural stability using different neck positions in normal subjects and patients with neck trauma. Acta Otolaryngologica 120: 451–455

Kuilman J 1959 The importance of the cervical syndrome in otorhinolaryngology. Practica Otorhinolaryngologica 21: 174–185

Lajoie Y, Teasdale N, Bard C, Fleury M 1993 Attentional demands for static and dynamic equilibrium. Experimental Brain Research 97(1): 139–144

Lieou Y C 1928 Syndrome sympathique cervical posterieur et artrite cervicale chronique: étude clinique et radiologique. Schuler and Minh, Strasbourg

Longet F A 1845 Sur les troubles qui surviennet dans l'equilibration, la station et la locomotion des animaux après la section des parties molles de la nuque. Gazette Medicale de France 13: 565–567

Loudon J K, Ruhl M, Field E 1997 Ability to reproduce head position after whiplash injury. Spine 22(8): 865–868

McLain R F 1994 Mechanoreceptor endings in human cervical facet joints. Spine 19: 495–501

Magnus R 1924 Körperstellung. Julius Springer: Berlin

Magnus R 1926 Some results of studies in the physiology of posture. Cameron Prize lectures. Lancet 211: 531–536

Magnusson M, Karlberg M 2002 Peripheral vestibular disorders with acute onset of vertigo. Current Opinion in Neurology 15: 5–10

Magnusson M, Johansson R, Wiklund J 1990 Galvanically induced body sway in the anterior-posterior plane. Acta Otolaryngologica 110: 11–17

Mangat K S, McDowall G D 1973 Vertigo and nystagmus in cervical spondylosis and the role of 'anterior cervical decompression'. Journal of Laryngology and Otology 87: 555–563

Myer J S, Shehan S, Bauer R B 1960 An arteriographic study of cerebrovascular disease in man. Archives of Neurology 2: 27–44

Nashner L M 1977 Fixed pattern of rapid postural responses among leg muscles during stance. Experimental Brain Research 30: 13–24

Norré M E 1990 Posture in otoneurology. Acta Otorhinolaryngologica Belgica 44(I–III): 55–181

Norré M E, Forrez G, Stevans A, Beckers A 1987 Cervical vertigo diagnosed by postulography? Acta Otolaryngologica Belgica 41: 574–581

Ommaya A K, Faas F, Yarnell P 1968 Whiplash injury and brain damage. Journal of the American Medical Association 204: 285–289

Oosterveld W J, Kortschot H W, Kingma G G, de Jong H A A, Saacti M R 1991 Electronystagmographic findings following cervical whiplash injuries. Acta Otolaryngologica 111: 201–205

Petersen B W, Goldberg J, Biolotto G, Fuller J H 1985 Cervicocollic reflex: its dynamic properties and interactions with vestibular reflexes. Journal of Neurophysiology 54: 90–109

Pompeiano O 1988 The tonic neck reflex: supraspinal control. In: Peterson B W, Richmond F D (eds) Control of head movement. Oxford University Press, New York, pp 108–119

Pyykkö I, Aalto H, Seidel H, Starck J 1989 Hierachy of different muscles in postural control. Acta Otolaryngologica 468: 175–180

Revel M, Andre-Deshays C, Minguet M 1991 Cervicocephalic kinesthetic sensibility in patients with cervical pain. Archives of Physical Medicine and Rehabilitation 72: 288–291

Revel M, Minguet M, Gregoy P, Vaillant J, Manuel J L 1994 Changes in cervicocephalic kinesthesia after a proprioceptive rehabilitation program in patients with neck pain: a randomized controlled study. Archives of Physical Medicine and Rehabilitation 75: 895–899

Richmond F J R, Bakker D A 1982 Anatomical organisation and sensory receptor content of the soft tissue surrounding upper cervical vertebrae in the cat. Journal of Neurophysiology 48: 49–61

Richmond F J R, Anstee G C B, Sherwin E A, Abrahams V C 1976 Motor and sensory fibres of neck muscle nerves in the cat. Canadian Journal of Physiology and Pharmacology 54: 294–304

Roberts T D M 1967 Neurophysiology of postural mechanisms. Plenum Press, New York

Rosenberg W S, Salame K S, Sumrick K V Tew Jr 1998 Compression of the upper cervical cord causing symptoms of brainstem compromise: a case report. Spine 23: 1497–1500

Rosenhall U, Johansson G, Örndahl G 1987 Eye motility dysfunction in chronic primary fibromyalgia with dysesthesia. Scandinavian Journal of Rehabilitation Medicine 19(4): 139–145

Rosenhall U, Tjell C, Carlsson J 1996 The effect of neck torsion on smooth pursuit eye movements in tension type headache patients. Journal of Audiological Medicine 5: 130–140

Rothwell D M, Bondy S J, Williams J I 2001 Chiropractic manipulation and stroke: a population-based case-control study. Stroke 32(5): 1054–1060

Ryan G M S, Cope S 1955 Cervical vertigo. Lancet 31: 1355–1358

Sandström J 1962 Cervical syndrome with vestibular symptoms. Acta Otolaryngologica 54: 207–226

Sauron B, Dobler S 1994 Benign paroxysmal positional vertigo: diagnosis, course, physiopathology and treatment. Revue du Praticien 44: 313–318 [in French]

Scherer H 1985 Halsbedingter Schwindel. Archives of Otorhinolaryngology Supplement 2: 107–124

Seymour J C, Tappin J W 1953 Some aspects of the sympathetic nervous system in relation to the inner ear. Acta Otolaryngologica 43: 618–635

Sheehan S, Bauer R B, Meyer J S 1960 Vertebral artery compression in cervical spondylosis: arteriographic demonstration during life of vertebral artery insufficiency due to rotation and extension of the neck. Neurology 10: 968–986

Shepard N T, Telian S T, Smith-Wheelock M, Raj A 1993 Vestibular and balance rehabilitation therapy. Annals of Otology, Rhinology, and Laryngology 102: 198–205

Sherrington C S 1906 On the proprioceptive system, especially in its reflex aspect. Brain 29: 467–482

Sloane P D, Coeytaux R R, Beck R S, Dallara J 2001 Dizziness: state of the science. Annals of Internal Medicine 134: 823–832

Slosberg M 1988 Effects of altered afferent articular input on sensation, proprioception, muscle tone and sympathetic reflex responses. Journal of Manipulative and Physiological Therapeutics 11: 400–408

Strek P, Reron E, Maga P, Modrzejewski M, Szybist N 1998 A possible correlation between vertebral artery insufficiency and degenerative changes in the cervical spine. European Archives of Otorhinolaryngology 255(9): 437–440

Tamura T 1989 Cranial symptoms after cervical injury: aetiology and treatment of the Barré–Lieou syndrome. Journal of Bone and Joint Surgery (British volume) 72(2): 283–287

Tatlow W F T, Bammer H G 1957 Syndrome of vertebral artery compression Neurology 7: 331–340

Taylor J L, McCloskey D I 1988 Proprioception in the neck. Experimental Brain Research 70: 351–360

Tibblin G, Bengtsson C, Furunes B, Lapidus L 1990 Symptoms by age and sex: the population studies of men and women in Gothenburg, Sweden. Scandinavian Journal of Primary Health Care 8: 9–17

Tjell C, Rosenhall U 1998 Smooth pursuit neck torsion test: a specific test for cervical dizziness. American Journal of Otology 19: 76–81

Todd N W, Clairmont A A, Dennard J E, Jackson R T 1974 Sympathetic stimulation and otic blood flow. Annals of Otology, Rhinology, and Laryngology 83: 84–91

Unterberger S 1938 Neue objektive regisrierbare Vestibularis-Körber-Drehungen erhalten durch trenten auf der Stelle, Der 'Tretversuch'. Archiv Fur Ohren-, Nasen-, und Kehlkopfheilkunde 145: 4

Voorhees R L 1989 The role of dynamic posturography in neurootologic diagnosis. Laryngoscope 99: 995–1001

Wennmo C, Hindfelt B, Pyykkö I 1983 Eye movements in cerebellar and combined cerebello brainstem diseases. Annals of Otology, Rhinology, and Laryngology 92(2): 165–171

Wright E F, Syms C A, Bifano S L 2000 Tinnitus, dizziness, and nonotologic otalgia improvement through temporomandibular disorder therapy. Military Medicine 165(10): 733–736

Wrisley D M, Sparto P J, Whitney S L, Furman J M 2000 Cervicogenic dizziness: a review of diagnosis and treatment. Journal of Orthopaedic and Sports Physical Therapy 30(12): 755–766

Wyke B 1979 Cervical articular contribution to posture and gait: their relation to senile disequilibrium. Age and Ageing 8: 251–258

Yardley L, Beech S, Zander L, Evans T, Weinman J 1998 A randomized controlled trial of exercise therapy for dizziness and vertigo on primary care. British Journal of General Practice 48(429): 1136–1140

Chapter **18**

The cervical spine and proprioception

E. Kristjansson

INTRODUCTION

Clinical aspects of proprioceptive dysfunction in the cervical spine have not been researched extensively. Proprioception is a complex neurophysiological mechanism which plays a small but important role in motor control (Gandevia & Burke 1992). It is not possible or valid to separate proprioceptive function from other neural control mechanisms in the central nervous system (CNS). This complex matter is not covered here in depth. Rather this chapter will present the most important clinical theories of cervical proprioceptive function and dysfunction and their clinical utility. Theories about motor control and learning are increasing (Shumway-Cook & Woollacott 2001) and this growing field in movement science will be mentioned as it relates to clinical consideration of the cervical spine. Clinical measurement methods for the multifaceted consequences of altered proprioceptive function in the cervical spine will be explained and treatment alternatives outlined in order to introduce the clinician to existing tools and exercises as well as those being developed. The reader is referred to the basic science literature for an exploration of the more fundamental aspects of proprioception.

In contemporary practice, therapeutic exercises for common musculoskeletal disorders are being directed towards enhancing motor control of specific body parts and the body as a whole. This development is only beginning to occur in the cervical spine. This is somewhat surprising as the importance of the cervical spine as a reflex sensory organ has been known for a long time (Magnus & DeKleijn 1912, Magnus 1926, McCough et al 1951, Lindsay et al 1976). The cervical spine has great mobility at the expense of mechanical stability and a close neurophysiological connection to the vestibular and visual systems (Dutia 1991, Gimse et al 1996). As a consequence, the cervical spine is an extremely vulnerable structure and a source of a plethora of symptoms which do not arise from any other musculoskeletal region of the body. The important link is the powerful cervical proprioceptive system (Abrahams 1977, Richmond & Bakker 1982, Dutia 1991, McLain 1994) because it provides neuromuscular control to the cervical spine and allows efficient utilization of the vital organs in the head (Guitton et al 1986).

CLINICAL CONSIDERATIONS OF DIFFERENT THEORIES OF MOTOR CONTROL

Hierarchical models share a common theory to explain faults in the complex interaction and integration of the postural control system (PCS) (Roberts 1967, Lederman 1997, Schmidt & Lee 1999). A 'black box', where all possible motor strategies are pre-programmed and stored, is thought to be responsible for the initiation and selection of pre-existing motor strategies. These motor responses are controlled by continuous sensory inputs from various sources. This provides the CNS with ever changing 'sensory pictures' which are stored in the black box like a 'bank of memory pictures'. Under normal circumstances this ensemble of sensory information is recognized by the CNS and passes through at a subconscious level. This arrangement explains the feedforward mechanisms, which are essential for postural control prior to and during movement, especially rapid movement. Sensory conflict arises if the incoming information is unexpected, as in the case of altered mechanoreceptor input. If the incoming information is not recognized, then the results may be increased compensatory reflex activity, uncoordinated movement patterns and/or neural activity at the conscious level.

The strength of the hierarchical models is that different neural structures can be isolated in experimental research and their effect on motor control objectively observed (Loeb et al 1999, Pearson 2000). Hierarchical explanation models are also appropriate in a clinical context when examining and treating isolated dysfunction in neuromuscular control (Lederman 1997). One of the greatest objections to the hierarchical models is that it is just not possible to store all movement strategies and movement patterns as well as a combination of these so as to have them ready for play when needed (Bernstein 1967). Another objection is that these models cannot describe the great adaptability and flexibility of the neuromuscular system in unknown and ever changing circumstances. These models cannot therefore be used to explain the complexity of the coordinated movement patterns needed to perform diverse motor tasks. This has been called the 'degree of freedom' problem (Bernstein 1967). Treatments built on hierarchical ways of thinking (Knott & Voss 1968) have been accused of being too passive because the therapeutic interventions are more concerned with facilitation and inhibition than with functional training (Shumway-Cook & Woollacott 2001).

An alternative explanation of movement control is provided by the systems theories, which have evolved since the 1950s in many disciplines (Haken 1996). These models try to explain common natural phenomena in the real world including human movement. The premise common to all the systems models, which in other respects may be quite different, is that the functioning of a system as a whole, for example the neuro-musculo-skeletal system, is dependent on its interaction with other systems inside and outside the organism. This is accomplished by self-organization, a process by which the systems organize themselves without a superior control mechanism in the brain. This self-organization is generated by the same fundamental principles in physics which are responsible for the formation of effects such as ocean waves and tornados as well as other specific coordinated natural movement patterns. In humans, the movement patterns are influenced by certain constraints within the organism and in the environment as well as constraints related to the tasks performed. These constraints decide which movement patterns and movement strategies are the best for each individual as a whole (Shumway-Cook & Woollacott 2001). Many dysfunctions and compensatory mechanisms in the musculoskeletal system can be looked upon as a consequence of the choices the system as a whole has made. It is therefore important to understand all the other systems and their interaction with the musculoskeletal system.

The weakness of the system theories seems to be that movements are dependent upon so many conditions that it is very difficult to conduct research to verify their credibility. However, an important contribution of the system theories is that they can help us to deal with complex clinical problems such as balance disturbances caused by disordered proprioception function in the cervical spine. Of the many disciplines involved in the head–neck system, no one discipline provides a sufficient overview to understand the interaction between all different systems. The main clinical message to learn from system theories is that the physical treatment must be task dependent and functionally meaningful for the patient. Movement patterns and movement strategies processed and performed in this context will appeal to the patient's perception and cognition. These variables are essential in any treatment progression to enhance better motor control and motor learning.

UPPER VERSUS LOWER CERVICAL SPINE

The great mobility of the cervical spine allows us to fully utilize all the special senses contained in the head which connect us to our environment. The functional differences between the upper and the lower cervical spine, as well as the neurophysiological connections of the upper cervical spine to the vestibular and visual systems via complex neurological pathways, explain the special role of the cervical spine in musculoskeletal disorders.

Functional differences

The biogenetic evolution of the cervical spine is the key to understanding the biomechanical and neurophysiological functional peculiarities of the upper cervical spine (Wolff 1991, 1998). When the vertebrates evolved in the ocean from the chordates, the whole body, including the head, formed a spindle-like unity. This was necessary to utilize the hydrodynamic characteristics of the water, thereby enabling fast swimming. At this stage, spatial orientation was served by the peripheral vestibular system in cooperation with the visual system. The most fundamental development in the phylogeny of vertebrates took place when they climbed onto land about 350 million years ago. To survive on land, the head had to be able to move freely on the rest of the body. This was first accomplished through the development of a rudimentary relationship between the head and the rest of the body, allowing a nodding movement. This is what we know today as the atlanto-occipital joint. However, this simple movement was not satisfactory for survival on land. The need for rapid coordinated semi-cardinal head movement in all planes became urgent. This forced the most surprising evolution of the vertebral column at the segment below; the development of the dens axis enveloped by the ring of atlas (Wolff 1998) (Fig 18.1). The great range of movement in the transverse plane at this level facilitated an appreciation of the environment especially when in an upright position, with the axis for sight perpendicular to the axis of the body. The last major development took place at the C2/C3 segment, which facilitated coupled movements in the transverse and frontal planes to both the opposite and the same side. The upper cervical spine as a whole therefore behaves like a spherical joint enabling us to efficiently scan the environment by the sensory organs in the head.

These bony and articular adaptations were accompanied by a distinct development and special arrangement of the deep segmental musculature, which is unique for the upper cervical spine. However, it is the organization of the neurophysiological function of the upper cervical spine that allows us to understand the peculiarity of the upper cervical spine in the symptomatology of the musculoskeletal system. In terrestrial animals, the independent movements of the head, where the main sensory organs are placed, could only give information about the orientation of the head in space but not about the orientation of the head in respect to the rest of the body. A network of mechanoreceptors in the musculoskeletal tissue therefore evolved to provide this information. It is the mechanoreceptors in the upper cervical spine which are of special interest in this respect (Wolff 1991, 1998).

The cervical spine and the postural control system

In line with biogenetic evolution, the postural control system (PCS), the mechanism by which the body maintains balance and equilibrium, has been divided into several subsystems, namely the vestibular, visual and somatosensory subsystems (Johansson & Magnusson 1991). The information from these subsystems is processed and integrated at different levels within the central nervous system (CNS) to avoid mismatch in the efferent activity continuously created for optimal performance of movements (Karlberg 1995). The role of the upper cervical spine in motor control of the head, trunk, extremities and eyes is unique and has great clinical implications (Hülse 1998). Disorders in the vestibular system and lesions in the basal ganglia, brain stem and cerebellum have most often been considered responsible for deficit in postural control and are important differential diagnostic entities along with vertebrobasilar insufficiency (Hülse 1998).

The complex neurophysiological behaviour of different subsystems in the PCS and their complex interactions have been described well elsewhere (Berthoz et al 1992, Dietz 1992, Karlberg 1995, Tjell 1998). The impact that somatic dysfunctions in the cervical spine have on normal neurophysiological functioning of the PCS is still mostly speculative (Hülse 1998). However, advances in neuroanatomical research have increased our knowledge in this field. Experimental animal research shows that the upper cervical spine has certain neuroanatomical peculiarities in the processing of both proprioceptive and nociceptive inputs that may influence higher CNS centres (Hülse 1998, Sessle 2000). For a clinician it is important to have an overview of the most important neurological connections of the three subsystems as they relate to the cervical spine. This is imperative for understanding the rationale of different clinical measurement methods and treatment approaches for altered cervical proprioception function. This understanding will also enhance clinical reasoning for patients with upper cervical dysfunction as various symptoms from this area can be linked together in a more logical way.

The vestibular system

The vestibular system is specially developed to maintain posture and locomotion in higher ranked species. Trunk, limb and eye muscle reflexes are developed to meet these requirements. The specialized mechanoreceptors in the semicircular canals are sensitized during changes in rate of motion, that is, angular velocity and the specialized mechanoreceptors in the otolith systems of the utricular and saccular maculae provide information about the

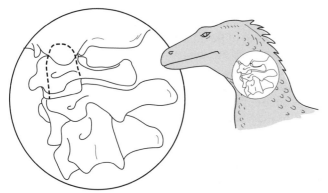

Figure 18.1 Moving onto land necessitated the special development of the cranial part of the vertebral column. (Drawing by Brian Pilkington.)

position of the head relative to the direction of the forces of gravity (i.e. linear velocity) and to head tilt (gravity) (Highstein 1996). Sensory information from these sources converges in all nuclei comprising the vestibular nuclear complex (VNC) via the vestibular nerve and in the cerebellum (Neuhuber & Bankoul 1992). A steady discharge of impulses from these sources maintains adequate postural tone in the trunk and extremities to maintain overall balance. The vestibulo- and reticular–spinal tracts are the final common pathways that serve this purpose through the vestibulospinal reflexes (VSR). Afferents from the trunk and extremities are mainly transmitted via the lateral vestibulospinal tract and via the reticulospinal tract originating in the lateral vestibular nucleus and the bulbar reticular formation respectively (Neuhuber 1998a). The mechanoreceptors in the upper cervical spine have indirect access to these tracts. The medial vestibulospinal tract, which originates from the medial part of the VNC, is the most important efferent pathway for the cervical spine and transmits impulses activated by stimulation of the semicircular canals, that is, the vestibulocollic reflexes (VCR) (Neuhuber 1998b). This tract receives direct input from the mechanoreceptors in the cervical spine.

The visual system and audition

Vision plays a dominant role in the guidance of movements and this is reflected by the fact that when somaesthetic inputs and vision disagree, it is usually the visual version of events that prevails. Over one-third of the brain in primates is devoted to visual processing (Stein & Glickstein 1992). The visual postural system consists of three different eye movement systems: the smooth pursuit system, the saccadic system and the optokinetic system (Tjell 1998). The smooth pursuit system stabilizes images of smooth moving targets on the fovea by slow eye movements such as when following a bird flying in the sky. The saccadic system on the other hand is responsible for rapid, small movements of both eyes simultaneously in changing a point of fixation. This enables us to visually target any movement in the visual periphery immediately, a function that is especially important, for example, when driving. The optokinetic system stabilizes images on the entire retina whenever the entire visual field is moving, for example when walking (Tjell 1998). In general, abnormalities in the optokinetic system mimic both the lesions affecting the smooth pursuit (slow phase) and saccadic (rapid phase) systems (Ruckenstein & Shepard 2000).

Sensory information from these eye movement systems converges at different places within the brain stem and cerebellum, notably also in the superior VNC (Neuhuber 1998a). The vestibular ocular reflexes (VOR) mediate the function of the three visual postural systems, that is to stabilize images on the retina under different conditions (Tjell 1998). The main route is from the labyrinth to the VNC via the vestibular nerve and from there via the ascending medial longitudinal fasciculus to the oculomotor muscle system (cranial nerves III, IV, VI) (Maeda & Hikosaka 1973). The main function of this arrangement is to integrate visual information and eye movements with information from the labyrinth to generate an estimate of head velocity in coordination with gaze (Cohen 1961, Lennerstrand et al 1996). The position and movement of the head in relation to the rest of the body and eye movements have also to be integrated to enhance clear vision during movement. This is accomplished by the interaction of the powerful VOR and the much weaker cervico-ocular reflex (COR), which originates in the mechanoreceptors of the upper cervical spine and acts on the extraocular muscles (Maeda & Hikosaka 1973, McLain 1994). However, in dysfunctional conditions, the COR becomes more active and this reflex can be used to diagnose altered upper cervical proprioceptive function (Neuhuber 1998a, Tjell 1998).

Like vision, audition requires spatial orientation of distant events through knowledge of the position of the head on the trunk The neuroanatomical interaction of the proprioceptive system of the cervical spine with the auditory system, via the ventral cochlear nucleus, carries out this function (Neuhuber 1998a). Research has found that cervical proprioception influences sound lateralization (Lewald et al 1999). This has also led to speculation that subjective hearing problems in some neck pain patients might be a reflex-mediated disturbance from the upper cervical mechanoreceptors (Neuhuber 1998a).

The somatosensory subsystem

The somatosensory subsystem of the upper cervical spine has an abundance of mechanoreceptors, like a receptor field, especially from the gamma muscle spindles in the deep segmental muscles (Abrahams 1977, Richmond & Bakker 1982, Dutia 1991). The mechanoreceptor impulses in the upper cervical spine are transmitted through nerve cells originating mainly in the C2 dorsal root ganglion but also in the C3 dorsal root ganglion (Neuhuber 1998b). These afferent nerve cells reach the brain stem cranially and the mid-thoracic segments caudally. Most importantly, the mechanoreceptor input from the C0–3 segments, at least from the muscles, has direct access to the vestibular nuclear complex (VNC), notably the medial and inferior part, through thick-calibre afferent fibres. This arrangement serves the need of the PCS to receive fast information about the position and movement of the head in relation to the body and to integrate this information with that from the labyrinth so that different information from these subsystems can be compared and equalled. In contrast, direct access to the VNC from the mechanoreceptors in the more caudal cervical segments gradually tapers off and is sparse or absent most caudally in the cervical spine (Neuhuber 1998a). The thoracic-lumbar mechanoreceptors have only indirect access to the VNC via second order afferent neurons. Afferents from the thoracolumbar spine can therefore be modulated at the spinal level. Mechanoreceptor input from the caudal cervical spine and the upper thoracic spine converges on the cuneatus nuclei, especially the external cuneatus nucleus, and travels from there to the cerebellum (Neuhuber 1998a).

The mechanoreceptor input from the upper cervical spine converges also in the important central cervical nucleus (CCN), which is situated at the C1–3 segments in the spinal cord (Neuhuber 1998a). The CCN serves as an origin for a crossed pathway to the flocculus of the cerebellum, which is a delicate integrator of vestibular, ocular and proprioceptive information (Tjell 1998). The CCN also has important connections to the VNC, especially the lateral vestibular nucleus, which receives information from the semicircular canals on the opposite side (Neuhuber 1998a). The lateral VNC is the origin for the powerful lateral vestibulospinal tract, which controls muscle tone in the trunk and extremities (Tjell 1998). The cervico-collic reflex (CCR) is mediated through these pathways and probably also through the medial vestibulospinal tract via the VNC (Peterson et al 1985). The CCR is stimulated by movements of the cervical spine and dampens the activity of the VOR and VCR that is stimulated via the semicircular canals. The CCR thereby protects the cervical spine against over-rotation (Peterson et al 1985). Patients who overshoot targets when position sense is measured may have disordered CCR inhibition. A simplified overview of the cervical PCS is presented in Figure 18.2.

The nociceptive system

The nociceptive system can potentially have a great influence on the neural processing of mechanoreceptor signals through various inflammatory substances. These substances stimulate the chemoreceptors in the muscles,

which in turn activate the gamma muscle system (Johansson et al 1993). Of special interest is the existence of a cervical-vestibulo-cervical loop found in experimental animals (Neuhuber & Bankoul 1992). The nociceptive system in the upper cervical spine projects on many cranial nerve afferents of which the trigeminal nucleus and the solitaritus nuclear complex (vagal nerve) may be the most important clinically. Neuroanatomical research indicates that nociceptive afferents from the upper cervical spinal cord are channelled via the parabrachial nuclei in the rostral pons to the limbic system (Feil & Herbert 1995). This opens the possibility that many symptoms that have been attributed to the post-concussion syndrome may in fact be caused by nociceptive input from the upper cervical spine. This has implications for clinical tests and the treatment of altered cervical proprioception function as poor concentration and memory loss may influence test results. These neuroanotomical peculiarities in nociceptive targeting have only been found in the upper cervical spinal cord (Neuhuber 1998b).

Coordination of movements is mainly the function of the cerebellum, where all spinal and brain stem reflexes directly or indirectly converge (Stein & Glickstein 1992). Ascending afferent signals are processed in the cerebral cortex to enhance conscious awareness of movements after they have been selectively gated at different levels in the CNS according to the relevance of the incoming information (Collins et al 1998). Disordered information from the somatosensory system of the upper cervical spine may cause balance and visual problems due to the close neurophysiological interaction with the vestibular and visual systems.

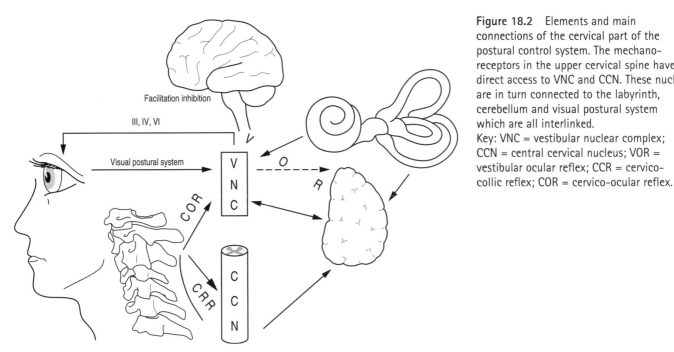

Figure 18.2 Elements and main connections of the cervical part of the postural control system. The mechanoreceptors in the upper cervical spine have direct access to VNC and CCN. These nuclei are in turn connected to the labyrinth, cerebellum and visual postural system which are all interlinked.
Key: VNC = vestibular nuclear complex; CCN = central cervical nucleus; VOR = vestibular ocular reflex; CCR = cervico-collic reflex; COR = cervico-ocular reflex.

BALANCE DISTURBANCES

Balance disturbances of cervical origin are accompanied by pain and dysfunction in the upper cervical spine. To complicate matters, patients with vertigo of vestibular origin often suffer from neck pain secondary to their vertigo (Karlberg 1995). Cervicogenic dizziness is characterized by the subjective feeling of unsteadiness, insecurity and light-headedness as a result of mismatch between the actual sensory information and the anticipatory sensory information (Karlberg 1995, Hülse 1998). Some patients also complain about a feeling of spinning but this is more like a feeling of 'spinning in the head' rather than spinning of the patient or the surroundings as in typical vertigo (Hülse 1998). These complaints are not described as strong attacks of dizziness but rather a tipsy-like state, which is a consequence of 'noise' in the PCS. Cervicogenic dizziness is often most pronounced in the morning and tapers gradually off in the course of the day. Common precipitating factors include variety of cervical movements but they also occur when watching a moving object or driving a car (Hülse & Hölzl 2000). These complaints tend to increase in intensity over time if the upper cervical dysfunctions are left untreated, because the mechanoreceptors are non-adaptive and their threshold for firing becomes lower with continuous irritation (Neuhuber 1998a). In less severe cases, the patients may not be aware that they have disordered balance. It seems that the vestibular and the somatosensory systems compensate by increasing the muscle stiffness in the body as a whole. This may explain the unrelenting hyperactivity in the musculature in some neck pain patients. This hypothesis has to be tested further. It may be one explanation for why so many patients develop fibromyalgia after whiplash-type distortion injuries to the neck (Buskila et al 1997). It is therefore important to screen neck pain patients with upper cervical dysfunctions for disordered balance despite a lack of subjective complaints about balance problems. In long-standing chronic cases, neurophysiological modulation in the CNS can occur due to its plasticity (Sessle 2000), which may explain why some chronic neck pain patients are therapy-resistant to common manual therapy approaches.

VISUAL DISTURBANCES

Visual disturbances as a consequence of altered mechanoreceptor input from the upper cervical spine are a controversial subject and not widely accepted by the medical profession. The main reason for this is that conventional ophthalmologic instruments cannot verify the patient's subjective complaints in most instances (Hülse 1998). These patients complain about diffuse visual problems. Of these, blurred vision, reduced visual field, grey spots appearing in the visual field, temporary blindness and disordered fusion are the most common (Hülse 1998). A common complaint when reading is that words or whole sentences 'jump'.

Diplopia, which is common in patients with vertebrobasilar insufficiency, is rare in somatic neck dysfunctions. If neck pain patients complain about double vision, it is most often not true diplopia but rather that the contours of objects are unclear (Hülse 1998). The visual disturbances in some neck pain patients may explain, for example, their reading problems (Gimse et al 1997). Dysfunction in the COR and CCR is thought to explain dizziness and visual disturbances of cervical origin in the tests described later in this chapter but unilateral vestibular lesions which influence the VOR might also be a cause (Tjell 1998).

CLINICAL MEASUREMENTS

Due to its complex neurophysiological processing, altered upper cervical proprioceptive function may have both regional and generalized influences on the functional capacity of the individual patient. Regional influences are thought to include reduced awareness of one's head–neck posture and altered conscious and unconscious control of cervical movements. This is thought to be an important factor in maintenance, recurrence or progression of local and referred symptoms (Glencross & Thornton 1981, Deusinger 1984, Bunton et al 1993, Parkhurst & Burnett 1994, Stone et al 1994, Hall et al 1995, Laskowski et al 1997, Lephart et al 1997), especially when the passive integrity of a joint is also compromised (O'Connor et al 1992). The generalized influences include balance and visual disturbances as well as unrelenting muscle hyperactivity. Correlating subjective complaints, physical examination findings and measurable functional impairment is important for deciding the diagnosis as well as the treatment progression in any musculoskeletal disorder. Many clinical measurement methods are available to ascertain the multifaceted consequences of altered proprioception function in the cervical spine.

Balance disturbances

The diagnosis of dizziness or balance disturbances of cervical origin is a diagnosis of exclusion as no test has been validated for cervicogenic dizziness. Questionnaires and many functional tests are available which help the clinician to screen patients with dizziness and vertigo. The Activities-Specific Balance Confidence Scale (Powell & Myers 1995) and the screening version of the Dizziness Handicap Inventory (Tesio et al 1999) are questionnaires that have been found to be clinically useful. The Dynamic Gait Index (Shumway-Cook & Woollacott 2001) and the Berg Balance Test (Berg et al 1992) are commonly used functional tests but they are not sensitive or specific for any particular lesion. One of the most popular screening tests is the Clinical Test for Sensory Interaction in Balance (CTSIB) which was introduced in 1986 as the 'foam and dome test' by Shumway-Cook & Horak. It tests how we integrate sensory information from the three subsystems in the PCS. Conventionally its foam portion is only used in a clinical setting (Weber & Cass 1993). The patient's ability to maintain quiet volitional stance under four different conditions is tested: on a flat firm surface with eyes open and then closed and on foam with eyes open and then closed (Weber & Cass 1993, Ruckenstein & Shepard 2000). Under the last condition the sensory input available is greatly reduced and the patient has to rely on their intact vestibular system (Ruckenstein & Shepard 2000, Shumway-Cook & Woollacott 2001). Research indicates that whiplash patients attempt to compensate for increased sway by greater reliance on visual rather than vestibular input, as their performance is much poorer with their eyes closed (Rubin et al 1995) (Fig. 18.3). This may reflect the fact that the somatosensory system of the upper cervical spine is the only part of the musculoskeletal system that has direct access to the VNC. The patient's postural sway and compensatory strategies while standing for 15 or 30 seconds are observed and quantified by various means (Shumway-Cook & Horak 1986, Weber & Cass 1993). These screening tools may provide important information concerning which patients will benefit from a laboratory study of postural control by means of posturography and other sophisticated medical tests.

Modern posturography is the high-technological version of the 'foam and dome' test. The six conditions tested on platform posturography are successively more difficult and represent the sensory organization test (SOT). Condition 5 in the SOT corresponds to the test in Figure 18.3. The functional consequences of suspected cervical balance disturbances have been measured by static posturography with simultaneous vibratory stimulus to the cervical extensors (Karlberg et al 1996, Koskimies et al 1997) or without such stimulation (Giacomini et al 1997). Vibratory stimuli signal that the muscles are lengthening and the patient gets an illusory feeling that the head and neck are moving forward when stimulation is applied to the cervical extensor muscles (Karlberg et al 1996). Posturography measures the force applied by the subject's feet to the supporting surface, thereby recording the compensatory strategies used by the patient (Karlberg et al 1996). In other posturography tests, different cervical spine positions have been used but the extended position has been found to be the most sensitive for detecting a cervicogenic balance disorder (Roth & Kohen-Raz 1998, Kogler et al 2000).

The question remains whether other stimuli are more appropriate for challenging cervical proprioceptive function. Vibration most likely stimulates the superficial muscles more than the deep segmental ones and cervical extension stimulates the utricular otoliths. To reach the deep segmental muscles, one option could be to perform the head-fixed, body-turned manoeuvre in advance of the static posturography measurements. In this test, the patient's head is held stationary while the body is rotated underneath. The COR and the CCR are both activated without activation of the mechanoreceptors in the semicircular canals. This test has been used in the clinic to provoke nystagmus and the patient's subjective feeling of dizziness (Hülse et al 1998). There is controversy, however, about the ability of this test to provoke cervical nystagmus (Hülse 1998). As the COR is a weak reflex, more pronounced responses could be provoked by activating the CCR by the head-fixed, body-turned manoeuvre and the patient's balance performance could be measured by static posturography immediately afterwards. Regardless of the perturbations used, supplementary electromyography (EMG) measurements and video recordings could be performed to register abnormal muscle activity and changes in joint angles related to the patient's compensatory strategies during the posturography measurements. The EMG measurements could provide information about the

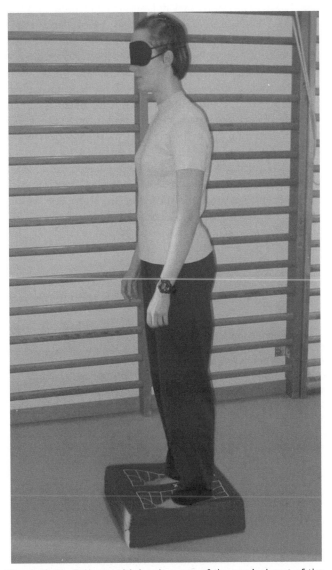

Figure 18.3 Patients with involvement of the cervical part of the postural control system have great difficulty on this test. They seem unable to utilize internal vestibular orienting information to resolve inaccurate information from the visual and somatosensory system. Reproduced with permission from the Whiplash Clinic, Reykjavik, Iceland.

unrelenting muscular hyperactivity observed in patients with balance disorders.

Visual disturbances

Many laboratory tests are available to test specific components of the visual and vestibular systems in order to gain knowledge of the extent and site of lesions that might be responsible for the patient's dizziness or vertigo. These are tests for the vestibular oculomotor loops (VOR) and they are important differential diagnosis entities for cervicogenic balance disorders. However, they do not test the functional consequences of a lesion. Commonly used laboratory and clinical tests are described in Table 18.1. The smooth pursuit neck torsion (SPNT) test is the most recent development in the diagnosis of cervical dizziness (Rosenhall et al 1996, Tjell & Rosenhall 1998). It tests the reflex interaction between the smooth pursuit system and the proprioceptive system of the cervical spine. Recordings are made on the subject's eye to register the velocity of the eye movements relative to the target stimulus and from this ratio, the mean gain parameter is calculated. Abnormal test results are found in the rotated neck positions and they are characterized by reduced gain in the same direction as the neck is rotated. Abnormal reflex activity in the upper cervical spine or in the VOR is thought to explain this response. When the trunk is rotated to the left beneath a stationary head, the neck is relatively rotated to the right. The COR helps the VOR to stimulate eye movements to the left in this position but for teleologic reasons, in order to look forward, the saccadic system moves the eyes to the mid-point. The VOR helped by an overactive COR moves the eyes again to the left and a right-directional nystagmus is induced (Tjell 1998, Tjell & Rosenhall 1998).

Cervicocephalic kinaesthetic sensibility

The term kinaesthesia (McCloskey 1978) or the terms joint position sense (JPS) and movement sense (MS) have all been used in measurement of regional proprioceptive activity to denote different qualities of proprioception (Clark et al 1986, Grigg 1994, Marks 1998). The rationale behind this dualism is the implication that JPS and MS may activate different neural structures (Clark et al 1986, Proske et al 1988, Eakin et al 1992, Clark & Deffenbacher 1996) and they are tested differently (Skinner et al 1984, Parkhurst & Burnett 1994, Swinkels & Dolan 1998). Clinically it is difficult to distinguish between position sense and movement sense in the strict meaning of these terms. For example, it is difficult to passively move the cervical, thoracic and lumbar spine sequentially and ask the person to detect when the movement starts, its direction and amplitude. Kinaesthesia, on the other hand, can be defined as a sensation which detects and discriminates between the relative weight of body parts, joint positions and movements, including direction, amplitude and speed (Newton 1982). This term indicates therefore all the qualities that are supposed to be a result of proprioception (McCloskey 1978, Rodier et al 1991,

Table 18.1 Commonly used tests for dizziness and vertigo

Test	Description
Electronystagmography (ENG)	The most established and widely used test for balance disorders. It consists of a battery of tests using electrodes placed around the eye to monitor eye movement. Recordings can also be made using infrared video cameras mounted on goggles which is superior to eye electrode ENG method. Various visual and vestibular stimuli are used to provoke nystagmus. These include oculomotor, gaze, positional and caloric stimuli. The vestibulo-ocular reflex (VOR) is assessed by this means
Caloric test	Each ear canal is stimulated with either water, equally above (warm) and below (cool) body temperature, or air pressure, positive and/or negative. The horizontal semicircular canals are stimulated and the resultant nystagmus is recorded by ENG
Rotational chair test	A physiological stimulus is induced for the semicircular canals by rotational chair movement at variant frequencies. This is performed in a dark room and the resultant nystagmus is recorded by ENG
Computerized dynamic posturography (CDP)	Designed to provide quantitative assessment of the relative contribution of visual, vestibular or somatosensory sensory system to postural stability. Recordings are made during or after a postural perturbation, as by moving the standing support or the visual surroundings. Eyes open and eyes closed conditions are also used
Motor coordination test (MCT)	A separate option of the CDP test. The floor plate is abruptly moved in different direction and the patient's motor responses measured
Dix–Hallpike test	A physical manoeuvre most commonly used to diagnose benign paroxysmal positional vertigo. The patient is in the long-sitting position on a treatment table and the therapist rotates the patient's head to 45° to the side to be tested. The patient is then moved quickly to a supine position with the patient's head about 30° over the end of the table. This brings the posterior semicircular canal in the plane of gravity during which the eyes are observed for a typical nystagmus

Gandevia et al 1992) and is tested actively in a clinical setting. This term is therefore the most appropriate in clinical measurements for altered cervical proprioceptive function.

The proprioceptive mechanisms controlling the head on the body have been tested clinically by simple target-matching tasks. The aim has been either to relocate the natural head posture (NHP) after an active movement (Revel et al 1991, Heikkilä & Åström 1996, Heikkilä & Wenngren 1998, Rix & Bagust 2001) or to actively relocate a set point in range (Loudon et al 1997, Kristjansson et al 2003). Studies have found reduced relocation accuracy in whiplash patients in comparison with asymptomatic people (Heikkilä & Åström 1996, Loudon et al 1997, Heikkilä & Wenngren 1998) but variable results exist regarding the presence of kinaesthetic deficits in people with insidious onset neck pain (Revel et al 1991, Rix & Bagust 2001, Kristjansson et al 2003). A recent reliability study found that relocating the NHP is the best test available for detecting disordered relocation accuracy, as tests that aim to relocate a set point in range seem to be too unreliable (Kristjansson et al 2001). The usefulness of a test is dependent on its ability to detect both the people with the impairment (sensitivity) and the people without the impairment (specificity). The test targeting the NHP after active movements in the transverse plane was plotted using the receiver operating characteristic (ROC) curve. The ROC curve shows the sensitivity and the false positive rate (1-specificity) for all possible cut-off points of a test. The relative frequency distribution for a chronic whiplash group ($n = 59$) versus an asymptomatic group ($n = 40$) and a cut-off value corresponding to 60% sensitivity and 80% specificity is shown in Figure 18.4 (E. Kristjansson, unpublished work, 2002).

Revel et al originally described the test for targeting the NHP in 1991. They used a laser light fixed on top of a helmet. The blindfolded patients were required to maximally move the head–neck in the transverse and sagittal planes, one direction at a time, and then to relocate the original start position (i.e. the NHP). The dependent variable was the mean deviation of the laser light from the starting NHP on a target. More sophisticated measuring equipment, for example the 3-Space Fastrak system, (Polhemus Navigation Science Division, Kaiser Aerospace, Vermont), is currently available. The Fastrak is a non-invasive electromagnetic measuring instrument, which tracks the positions of sensors relative to a source in three dimensions. A study has demonstrated that the 3-Space Isotrak system, which uses similar equipment, is accurate within ± 0.2 degrees (Pearcy & Hindle 1988). The Fastrak is connected to a PC and continually records the positions of the sensors relative to the source during the entire test sequence. The experimental set-up is shown in Figure 18.5. A software program formats and processes the data for three-dimensional analysis of movements in space. It converts the data directly into angle files and graphs to visualize the test process in real time on the screen from the starting position through to the excursion of movement. The primary movements in the movement plane and the simultaneous coupled rotations in the associated planes are recorded and represent the accuracy with which the subject can relocate the target (Kristjansson et al 2001).

Target-matching tasks have been those most widely used since their introduction by Slinger & Horsley in 1906. These tasks measure the awareness of, for example, head–neck posture (i.e. NHP) which is only one aspect of proprioceptive function (Barrack et al 1984, Grigg 1994, Clark et al 1996). When testing relocation accuracy, blindfolding subjects can eliminate visual input. The need for spatial orientation and overall balance can be reduced by a com-

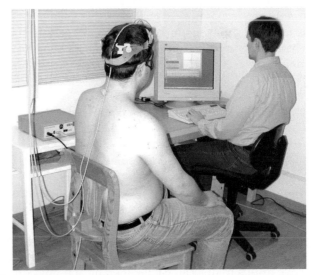

Figure 18.5 A research assistant operates the computer and applies a marker when the subject says, 'yes' to indicate that the natural head posture has been relocated. The subject is wearing a lightweight adjustable helmet which allows a Fastrak sensor to be attached to the forehead. Another sensor is placed over the C7 spinous process and fastened with double-sided sticky tape. The electromagnetic source is in the box of a wooden chair. Reproduced with permission from the Whiplash Clinic, Reykjavik, Iceland.

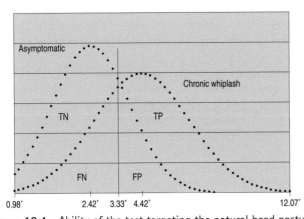

Figure 18.4 Ability of the test targeting the natural head posture to diagnose chronic whiplash patients by the Fastrak system. Key: TN = true negative; FN = false negative; FP = false positive; TP = true positive.

fortable and stable sitting position. All movements of the head in space stimulate the vestibular apparatus (Keshner & Peterson 1995). Movements in the transverse plane predominantly stimulate the semicircular canals, but movements in other planes stimulate also the utricular otoliths, which are sensitive to changes in gravitational orientation (Taylor & McCloskey 1990). Cervical proprioception is superior to the vestibular system for detecting slow movements of the head on the trunk due to the inertia of the cupula in the semicircular canals (Mergner et al 1983). Proprioceptive information from the cervical spine seems to overshadow the contribution of vestibular input under these conditions (Hassenstein 1988, Taylor & McCloskey 1988, 1990). For this reason, and because complex and rapid movements overstimulate the mechanoreceptors (Collins et al 1998, Prochazka & Gorassini 1998), it is essential to test cervical proprioceptive function by slow movements.

An important function of the proprioceptive system is to correct movements on a moment-to-moment basis, especially when learning new movements tasks (Gandevia & Burke 1992). A new test has been developed where subjects are required to follow a slowly moving object which appears on a computer screen by moving their head (Kristjansson et al 2004). The movement path is unpredictable and of short duration to avoid the programming and learning effects described by the hierarchical models (Shumway-Cook & Woollacott 2001). The sensors of the Fastrak system are attached to the patient's head so the patient can trace the movement patterns that appear on the screen (Fig. 18.6). A new software program called 'the Fly' was written for this purpose. As only the cursors from the new software program and the Fastrak system are visible on the screen it is not possible to predict the movement. This test seems to be more sensitive than Revel's test as it can better discriminate between asymptomatic subjects and chronic whiplash patients (Fig. 18.4), (Kristjansson et al 2003, 2004).

TREATMENT

No treatment has been optimized to enhance adequate neuromuscular control of the cervical spine. However, research has enabled the development of certain guidelines for the most important treatment strategies. Clinicians are encouraged to use and further develop these treatment modalities which are necessary for enhancing not only neuromuscular control of the cervical spine but also the body as a whole.

A few research studies have been conducted that show positive results from local manual therapy and physiotherapy approaches for improving dizziness or unsteadiness of suspected cervical origin (Wing & Hargrave-Wilson 1974, Karlberg et al 1996, Rogers 1997, Galm et al 1998, Hülse & Hölzl 2000). The positive responses are explained by the reduction in pain and the normalization of tissue compliance ensuring adequate stimulation of the mechanoreceptors in the tissue. However, in more difficult cases, as in

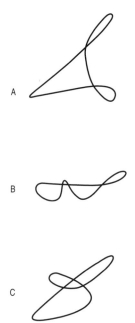

Figure 18.6 Movement patterns A, B and C traced by the 'Fly' which the participants were required to follow by moving their head. Reproduced with permission from Archives of Physical Medicine and Rehabilitation, Kristjansson et al 2004.

chronic whiplash associated disorders (WAD), the joint stability may be compromised, leading to more permanent changes in tissue compliance or direct damage to the receptors and their axons as they have lower tensile strength than the surrounding collagen fibres (Freeman et al 1965, Glencross & Thornton 1981, McLain 1994). Chemical changes brought about by ischaemic or inflammatory events may affect the sensitivity of the receptors (Barett et al 1991, Johannson et al 1993). The mechanical effects of effusion in a joint have also been found to influence the articular receptors such that they impose an inhibitory effect on the gamma motoneurons with potential muscle atrophy as a consequence (Spencer et al 1984, Stokes & Young 1984, Morrissey 1989, Hurley & Newham 1993). Patients who are affected by these conditions are unlikely to respond to conventional physiotherapy or manual therapy approaches alone.

Research on the lumbar spine (Hides et al 1996, Hodges & Richardson 1996) has demonstrated the importance of recruitment of the deep local spinal muscles. The same principles are thought to apply to the deep local cervical and shoulder girdle stabilizers. A pilot study found atrophy and fatty infiltration of the suboccipital muscles in chronic neck pain patients (Hallgren et al 1994). In the case of any cervical disorder, the first priority of any treatment progression for neuromuscular control is therefore to recruit the deep muscles with a neutral cervical and shoulder girdle alignment. This is carried out under low load to avoid activation of the powerful superficial torque producing muscles, which may have a lowered activation threshold

(Jull 2000). It has been suggested that altered cervical curvature may play an important role in the symptomatology of some neck pain patients (Harrison et al 2000). Correct segmental alignment of the spine is dependent on adequate functioning of the deep local muscles to provide a stable base for efficient limb and spinal movements (Wilke et al 1995, Cholewicki & McGill 1996). One study has found a decreased ratio between the lower versus the upper cervical spine lordosis in chronic whiplash patients (Kristjansson & Jónsson 2002). This may indicate dysfunction of the deep flexors in the upper cervical spine and of the deep extensors in the lower cervical spine. Enhancing appropriate recruitment patterns of the shoulder girdle and the upper extremity muscles is essential for proper functioning of the cervical spine as overactive shoulder girdle muscles will induce a constant strain on painful cervical segments.

The next stage of treatment is concerned with adequate movement control through range of motion. The treatment strategy used depends on whether the patient has decreased control of specific cervical segments and/or the cervical spine as a whole. In the former case it is important to determine whether the deficient control is in the upper, mid- or lower cervical spine. The patient is then first taught to keep the unstable area in neutral alignment while moving the cervical spine below and/or above. This is achieved by cognitive control over the deep segmental muscles. Having gained this, the next step is to recruit the local and global muscles that most efficiently bring the segmental motion under active control in a specific direction. The patient can be taught to move only the decontrolled area through controllable range or the whole cervical spine. The patient is specifically taught to gain control over the inner range and to move eccentrically from the inner range to the mid-range and in some cases to the outer range of the uncontrollable movement. This last option is necessary if the patient needs this movement for professional reasons (for example a house painter). The effectiveness of these treatment strategies has yet to be researched.

There has been little research into treatment strategies aimed at improving neuromuscular control of the cervical spine as a whole and improving awareness of carrying the head. Revel et al (1994) conducted a trial which was mainly concerned with eye–neck coordination exercises and awareness of movement. This found a significant improvement in neck pain patients after an 8-week period. A trial was recently conducted on chronic whiplash patients by using a modified 'awareness through movement' Feldenkrais approach (Ólafsdottir & Helgadottir 2001). In this approach the emphasis is on the patient's awareness of the quality of movement and all movements are performed slowly with integration of eye–neck movements (Feldenkrais 1991). Using the Fastrak instrument, a significant improvement in targeting the NHP was detected after a 4-week training period (mean 5.22 degrees ± 1.79 prior to treatment versus mean 3.32 degrees ± 1.27 after treatment). Moreover, some subjects gained a considerably lower pain score on a 100 mm visual analogue scale and a lower disability score on the Northwick Park Disability Index (Leak et al 1994) with use of the modified Feldenkrais approach alone. In order to improve overall dynamic neuromuscular control of the cervical spine it is recommended that treatment includes tasks in which the patient follows unpredictable movement paths, as proprioceptive function is challenged most when performing non-learned slow movements. Some other treatment suggestions for improving the functional status of patients with suspected cervical induced unsteadiness are shown in Table 18.2.

The consequences of altered proprioceptive processing from the upper cervical spine seem to have been greatly underestimated. To improve the functional status of chronic neck pain patients, it is urgent that new treatment modalities be developed and tested in appropriately designed research settings. Patients' unsteadiness and balance problems have to be managed. The question that has to be answered is whether treatment programmes that have been established in vestibular rehabilitation are also of value for patients with balance disturbances of cervical origin or

Table 18.2 Treatment suggestions for cervical induced unsteadiness

Exercise	Description
Eye–head coordination	A: Moving the eyeballs with the eyes open and closed. B: Visual tracking tasks with the head still. C: Keeping gaze fixed on a still object during progression of slow to fast head movements. D: Keeping gaze fixed on a target that is moving in phase with the patient's head in sitting, standing and walking. E: Moving the trunk or varying the surface conditions while maintaining the gaze on a fixed target
Balance exercises	A: Walking with sagittal and transverse plane movement of the head and neck. B: Walking a distance and turning rapidly and walking back. C: Standing on a balance board. D: Standing on a balance board making various head movements. E: Standing on a balance board while looking at a moving object. F: Walking on a treadmill detecting movements in the periphery without looking. G: Walking blindfolded
Task dependent exercises	Repeat the movement or task that provokes the feeling of unsteadiness, for example turning in bed, standing up from a chair, turning the head, etc.
General endurance exercise	Cardiovascular training

whether these treatment modalities have to be modified. New treatment strategies must also expose the patient to external perturbations in order to improve the reflex mediated neuromuscular responses of the cervical muscles (Gurfinkel et al 1988, Allum et al 1997). Similarly the shock absorbing properties of the cervical muscles have to be improved, for example by using a trampoline in the first instance. When developing new treatment approaches it is important to remember the close relationship between the masticatory system and the neck and the importance of visual feedback for performance of movements. In the near future, virtual reality programmes are likely to be developed which will ensure that the treatment regimes are more task dependent. This is perhaps the only way to fulfil the recommendations of the system theories.

CONCLUSION

The upper cervical spine is a very rich sensory organ with direct neurophysiological connections to the vestibular and visual systems. These connections explain the multifaceted consequences of altered proprioceptive processing from the upper cervical spine. In a clinical context it is important to be able objectively to verify all the different effects of altered cervical proprioceptive function and to be able to treat each of them successfully. More research activity is needed in this area as we are just beginning to understand this complex matter. This requires that therapists gain more knowledge of the head–neck system as a whole so as to understand the complex interaction between the different systems. This will facilitate the development of new treatment strategies where treatment of different aspects of altered proprioceptive function can be combined in various manners.

KEYWORDS

proprioception	motor control
cervical	diagnosis
kinaesthesia	treatment

References

Abrahams V C 1977 The physiology of neck muscles: their role in head movements and maintenance of posture. Canadian Journal of Physiology and Pharmacology 55: 332–339

Allum J H J, Gresty M, Keshner E, Scupert C 1997 The control of head movements during human balance corrections. Journal of Vestibular Research 7: 189–218

Barrack R L, Skinner H B, Cook S D 1984 Proprioception of the knee joint: paradoxal effect of training. American Journal of Physical Medicine 63: 175–181

Barrett D S, Cobb A G, Bentley G 1991 Joint proprioception in normal, osteoarthritic and replaced knees. Journal of Bone and Joint Surgery (British volume) 73: 53–56

Berg K O, Maki B E, Williams J I, Holliday P J, Wood-Dauphine S L 1992 Clinical and laboratory measure of postural balance in elderly population. Archives in Physical Medicine and Rehabilitation 73: 1073–1080

Bernstein N 1967 The coordination and regulation of movement. Pergamon Press, London

Berthoz A, Graf W, Vidal P P 1992 The head-neck sensory motor system. Oxford University Press, New York

Bunton E E, Pitney W A, Kane A.W, Cappaert T A 1993 The role of limb torque, muscle action and proprioception during closed kinetic chain rehabilitation of the lower extremity. Journal of Athletic Training 28: 10–20

Buskila D, Neumann L, Vaisberg G, Alkalay D, Wolfe F 1997 Increased rates of fibromyalgia following cervical spine injury. Journal of the American College of Rheumatology 40: 446–452

Cholewicki J, McGill S M 1996 Mechanical stability of the in vivo lumbar spine: implications for injury and low back pain. Clinical Biomechanics 11: 1–15

Clark F J, Burgess R C, Chapin J W 1986 Proprioception with the proximal interphalangeal joint of the index finger: evidence for a movement sense without a static-position sense. Brain 109: 1195–1208

Clark F J, Deffenbacher K A 1996 Models of behaviours when detecting displacements of joints. Experimental Brain Research 112: 485–495

Cohen L A 1961 Role of the eye and neck proprioceptive mechanisms in body orientation and motor coordination. Journal of Neurophysiology 24: 1–11

Collins D F, Cameron T, Gillard D M, Prochazka A 1998 Muscular sense is attenuated when humans move. Journal of Physiology 508: 635–643

Deusinger R H 1984 Biomechanics in clinical practice. Physical Therapy 64: 1860–1868

Dietz V 1992 Human neuronal control of automatic functional movements: interaction between central programs and afferent input. Physiological Reviews 72: 33–69

Dutia M B 1991 The muscles and joints of the neck: their specialisation and role in head movement. Progress in Neurobiology 37: 165–178

Eakin C L, Quesada P M, Skinner H 1992 Lower-limb proprioception in above-knee amputees. Clinical Orthopaedics and Related Research 284: 239–246

Feil K, Herbert H 1995 Topographical organization of spinal and trigeminal somatosensory pathways to the rat parabrachial and Kölliker–Fuse nuclei. Journal of Comparative Neurology 353: 506–528

Feldenkrais M 1991 Awareness through movement. Harper, San Francisco

Freeman M A R, Dean M R E, Hanham I W F 1965 The etiology and prevention of functional instability of the foot. Journal of Bone and Joint Surgery (British volume) 47: 678–685

Galm R, Rittmeister M, Schmidt E 1998 Vertigo in patients with cervical spinal dysfunction. European Spine Journal 7: 55–58

Gandevia S C, Burke D 1992 Does the nervous system depend on kinesthetic information to control natural limb movements Behavioural and Brain Sciences 15: 614–632

Gandevia S C, McCloskey D I, Burke D 1992 Kinaesthetic signals and muscle contraction. Trends in Neuroscience 15: 62–65

Giacomini P, Magrini A, Sorace F 1997 Changes in posture in whiplash evaluated by static posturography. Acta Otorhinolaryngologica Italica 17: 409–413

Gimse R, Tjell C, Bjørgen I A, Saunte C 1996 Disturbed eye movements after whiplash due to injuries to the postural control system. Journal of Clinical and Experimental Neurophysiology 18: 178–186

Gimse R, Bjørgen I A, Tjell C, Tyssedal J S, Bø K 1997 Reduced cognitive functions in a group of whiplash patients with demonstrated disturbances in the posture control system. Journal of Clinical and Experimental Neuropsychology 19: 838–849

Glencross D, Thornton E 1981 Position sense following joint injury. Journal of Sports Medicine 21: 23–27

Grigg P 1994 Peripheral neural mechanisms in proprioception. Journal of Sport Rehabilitation 3: 2–17

Guitton D, Kearney R E, Wereley N, Peterson B W 1986 Visual, vestibular and voluntary contribution to human head stabilization. Experimental Brain Research 64: 59–69

Gurfinkel V S, Lipshits M I, Lestienne F G 1988. Anticipatory neck muscle activity associated with rapid arm movements. Neuroscience Letters 94: 104–108

Haken H 1996 Principles of brain functioning: a synergetic approach to brain activity, behaviour and cognition. Springer, Berlin

Hall M G, Ferrell W R, Sturrock R D, Hamblen D L, Baxendale R H 1995 The effect of the hypermobility syndrome on knee joint proprioception. British Journal of Rheumatology 34: 121–125

Hallgren R C, Greenman P E, Rechtien J J 1994 Atrophy of suboccipital muscles in patients with chronic pain: a pilot study. Journal of the American Osteopathic Association 94: 1032–1038

Harrison D E, Harrison D D, Troyanovich S J, Harmon S 2000 A normal spinal position: it's time to accept the evidence. Journal of Manipulative and Physiological Therapeutics 23: 623–644

Hassenstein B 1988 Der Kopfgelenksbereich im Funktionsgefüge der Raumorientierung: systemtheoretische bzw. biokybernetische Gesichtspunkte. In: Wolff H D (ed) Die Sonderstellung des Kopfgelenksbereichs. Springer, Berlin

Heikkilä H, Åström P G 1996 Cervicocephalic kinesthetic sensibility in patients with whiplash injury. Scandinavian Journal of Rehabilitation Medicine 28: 133–138

Heikkilä H V, Wenngren B I 1998 Cervicocephalic kinesthetic sensibility, active range of cervical motion, and oculomotor function in patients with whiplash injury. Archives of Physical Medicine and Rehabilitation 79: 1089–1094

Hides J A, Richardson C A, Jull G 1996 Multifidus muscle recovery is not automatic after resolution of acute, first-episode low back pain. Spine 21: 2763–2769

Highstein S M 1996 How does the vestibular part of the inner ear work? In: Baloh R W, Halmagyi G M (eds) Disorders of the vestibular system. Oxford University Press, New York

Hodges P W, Richardson C A 1996 Inefficient muscular stabilization of the lumbar spine associated with low back pain: a motor control evaluation of transversus abdominis. Spine 21: 2640–2650

Hülse M, 1998 Klinik der Funktionsstörungen des Kopfgelengbereichs. In: Hülse M, Neuhuber W L, Wolff H D (eds) Der kranio-zervikale Übergang. Springer, Berlin, pp 43–98

Hülse M, Hölzl M 2000 Vestibulospinale Reaktionen bei der zervikogenen Gleichgewichtsstörung. Die zervikogene Unsicherheit. HNO 48: 295–301

Hurley M V, Newham D J 1993 The influence of arthrogenous muscle inhibition on quadriceps rehabilitation of patients with early, unilateral osteoarthritic knees. British Journal of Rheumatology 32: 127–131

Johansson R, Magnusson M 1991 Human postural dynamics. Critical Reviews in Biomedical Engineering 18: 413–436

Johanson H, Djupsjöbacka M, Sjölander P 1993 Influences on the gamma-muscle spindle system from muscle afferents stimulated by KCl and lactic acid. Neuroscience Research 16: 49–57

Jull G 2000 Deep cervical flexor muscle dysfunction in whiplash. Journal of Musculoskeletal Pain 8: 143–154

Karlberg M 1995 The neck and human balance. PhD Thesis, MERL 1039, Department of Otorhinolaryngology, Lund University Hospital, Sweden

Karlberg M, Magnusson M, Malmström E-M, Melander A, Moritz U 1996 Postural and symptomatic improvement after physiotherapy in patients with dizziness of suspected cervical origin. Archives of Physical Medicine and Rehabilitation 77: 874–882

Keshner E A, Peterson B W 1995 Mechanisms controlling human head stabilization. I: Head-neck dynamics during random rotations in the horizontal plane. Journal of Neurophysiology 73: 2293–2301

Knott M, Voss D 1968 Proprioceptive neuromuscular facilitation. Harper and Row, New York

Kogler A, Lindfors J, Odkvist L M, Ledin T 2000 Postural stability using different neck positions in normal subjects and patients with neck trauma. Acta Otolaryngologica 120: 151–155

Koskimies K, Sutinen P, Aalto H et al 1997 Postural stability, neck proprioception and tension neck. Acta Otolaryngologica Supplementum 529: 95–97

Kristjansson E, Jónsson H 2002 Is the sagittal configuration of the cervical spine changed in women with chronic whiplash syndrome? A comparative computer-assisted radiographic assessment. Journal of Manipulative and Physiological Therapeutics 25: 550–555

Kristjansson E, Dall'Alba P, Jull G 2001 Cervicocephalic kinesthesia: reliability of a new test approach. Physiotherapy Research International 6: 224–235

Kristjansson E, Dall'Alba P, Jull G 2003 A study of five cervicocephalic relocation tests in three different subject groups. Clinical Rehabilitation 17: 768–774

Kristjansson E, Hardardottir L, Asmundardottir M, Guðmundsson K 2004 A new clinical test for cervicocephalic kinesthetic sensibility: 'The Fly'. Archives of Physical Medicine and Rehabilitation 85: 490–495

Laskowski E R, Newcomer-Aney K, Smith J 1997 Refining rehabilitation with proprioception training. Physician and Sports Medicine 25: 89–102

Leak A M, Cooper J, Dyer S, Williams K A, Turner-Stokes L, Frank A O 1994 The Northwick Park Neck Pain Questionnaire, devised to measure neck pain and disability. British Journal of Rheumatology 33: 469–474

Lederman E 1997 Fundamentals of manual therapy: physiology, neurology and psychology. Churchill Livingstone, New York

Lennerstrand G, Han Y, Velay J-L 1996 Properties of eye movements induced by activation of neck muscle proprioceptors. Graefe's Archive for Clinical Experimental Ophthalmology 234: 703–709

Lephart S M, Pincivero D M, Giraldo J L, Fu F H 1997 The role of proprioception in the management and rehabilitation of athletic injuries. American Journal of Sports Medicine 25: 130–137

Lewald J, Karnath H-O, Ehrenstein W H 1999 Neck-proprioceptive influence on auditory lateralization. Experimental Brain Research 125: 389–396

Lindsay K W, Roberts T D, Rosenberg J R 1976 Asymmetric tonic labyrinth reflexes and their interaction with neck reflexes in the decerebrate cat. Journal of Physiology 261: 583–601

Loeb G E, Brown I E, Cheng E J 1999 A hierarchical foundation for models of sensorimotor control. Experimental Brain Research 126: 1–18

Loudon J K, Ruhl M, Field E 1997 Ability to reproduce head position after whiplash injury. Spine 22: 865–868

McCloskey D I 1978 Kinesthetic sensibility. Physiology Review 58: 763–820

McCough G P, Derring I D, Ling T H 1951 Location of receptors for tonic neck reflexes. Journal of Neurophysiology 14: 191–195

McLain R F 1994 Mechanoreceptor endings in human cervical facet joints. Spine 19: 495–501

Maeda M, Hikosaka O 1973 Cervical effects on abducens motoneurons and their interaction with vestibulo-ocular reflex. Experimental Brain Research 18: 512–530

Magnus R 1926 Some results of studies in the physiology of posture. Cameron prize lectures. Lancet 211: 531–536

Magnus R, DeKleijn A 1912 Die Abhängigkeit des Tonus der Extremitätenmuskleln von der Kopfstellung. Pflügers Archiv für die Gesamte Physiologie des Menschen und der Tiere 145: 455–548

Marks R 1998 The evaluation of joint position sense. New Zealand Journal of Physiotherapy 44: 20–28

Mergner T, Nardi G L, Becker W, Deecke L 1983 The role of canal-neck interaction for the perception of horizontal and head rotation. Experimental Brain Research 49: 198–208

Morrissey M C 1989 Reflex inhibition of thigh muscles in knee injury: causes and treatment. Sports Medicine 7: 263–276

Neuhuber W L 1998a Der kraniozervikale Übergang: Entwicklung, Gelenke, Muskulatur und Innervation. In: Hülse M, Neuhuber W L, Wolff H D (eds) Der kranio-zervikale Übergang. Springer, Berlin

Neuhuber W L 1998b Besonderheiten der Innervation des Kopf-Hals-Bereichs. Orthopäde 27: 794–801

Neuhuber W L, Bankoul S 1992 Der 'Halsteil' des Gleichgewichtsapparates-Verbindungen zervikaler Rezeptoren zu Vestibulariskernen. Manuelle Medizine 30: 53–57

Newton R A 1982 Joint receptor contribution to reflexive and kinaesthetic responses. Physical Therapy 62: 22–29

O'Conner B L, Densie V M, Brandt K D, Myres S L, Kalasinski L A 1992 Neurogenic acceleration of osteoarthrosis. Journal of Bone and Joint Surgery (American volume) 74: 367–376

Ólafsdottir E, Helgadottir S 2001 Effect of a modified Feldenkrais approach to improve position sense of the head and neck in women with chronic complaints after whiplash loading. BSc thesis, Unit of Physiotherapy, University of Iceland, Reykjavik

Parkurst T M, Burnett C N 1994 Injury and proprioception in the lower back. Journal of Orthopaedic Sports and Physical Therapy 19: 282–295

Pearcy M J, Hindle R J 1988 New method for non-invasive three-dimensional measurement of human back movement. Clinical Biomechanics 4: 73–79

Pearson K 2000 Motor systems. Current Opinion in Neurobiology 10: 649–654

Peterson B W, Goldberg J, Bilotto G, Fuller J H 1985 Cervicocollic reflex: its dynamic properties and interaction with vestibular reflexes. Journal of Neurophysiology 54: 90–109

Powell L E, Myers A M 1995 The activities-specific balance confidence (ABC) scale. Journal of Gerontology 50A: M23–M34

Prochazka A, Gorassini M 1998 Ensemble firing of muscle efferents recorded during normal locomotion in cats. Journal of Physiology 507: 293–304

Proske U, Schaible H-G, Schmidt R F 1998 Joint receptors and kinaesthesia. Experimental Brain Research 72: 219–224

Revel M, Andre-Deshays C, Minguet M 1991 Cervicocephalic kinesthetic sensibility in patients with cervical pain. Archives of Physical Medicine and Rehabilitation 72: 288–291

Revel M, Minguet M, Gergoy P, Vaillant J, Manuel J L 1994 Changes in cervicocephalic kinesthesia after a proprioceptive rehabilitation program in patients with neck pain: a randomized controlled study. Archives of Physical Medicine and Rehabilitation 75: 895–899

Richmond F J R, Bakker D A 1982 Anatomical organization and sensory receptor content of soft tissues surrounding upper cervical vertebrae in the cat. Journal of Neurophysiology 48: 49–61

Rix G D, Bagust J 2001 Cervicocephalic kinaesthetic sensibility in patients with chronic, nontraumatic cervical spine pain. Archives of Physical Medicine and Rehabilitation 82: 911–919

Roberts T D M 1967 Neurophysiology of postural mechanisms. Plenum Press, New York

Rodier S, Euzet J P, Gahery Y, Paillard J 1991 Crossmodal versus intramodal evaluation of the knee joint angle. Human Movement Science 10: 689–712

Rogers R G 1997 The effect of spinal manipulation on cervical kinesthesia in patients with chronic neck pain: a pilot study. Journal of Manipulative and Physiological Therapeutics 20: 80–85

Rosenhall U, Tjell C, Carlsson J 1996 The effect of neck torsion on smooth pursuit eye movements in tension-type headache patients. Journal of Audiological Medicine 5: 130–140

Roth V, Kohen-Raz R, 1998 Posturographic characteristics of whiplash patients. Proceedings of the XXth Regular Meeting of the Barany Society, Würzburg, Germany, 11-17 September

Rubin A M, Wolley S M, Dailey V M, Goebel J A 1995 Postural stability following mild head or whiplash injuries. American Journal of Otology 16: 216–221

Ruckenstein M J, Shepard N T 2000 Balance function testing: a rational approach. Otolaryngologic Clinics of North America 33: 507–518

Schmidt R A, Lee T D 1999 Central contribution to motor control. In: Schmidt R A, Lee T D (eds) Motor control and learning: a behavioural emphasis, 3rd edn. Human Kinetics, Champaign Illinois

Sessle B J 2000 Acute and chronic craniofacial pain: brainstem mechanisms of nociceptive transmission and neuroplasticity, and their clinical correlates. Critical Reviews in Oral Biology and Medicine 11: 57–91

Shumway Cook A, Horak F B 1986 Assessing the influence of sensory interaction on balance. Physical Therapy 66: 1548–1550

Shumway Cook A, Woollacott M H 2001 Motor control: theory and practical application. Lippincott, Williams and Wilkins, Philadelphia

Skinner H B, Barrack R L, Cook S D, Haddad R J 1984 Joint position sense in total knee arthroplasty. Journal of Orthopaedic Research 1: 276–283

Slinger R T, Horsley V 1906 Upon the orientation of points in space by the muscular, arthrodial, and tactile senses of the upper limbs in normal individuals and in blind persons. Brain 29: 1–27

Spencer J D, Hayes K C, Alexander I J 1984 Knee joint effusion and quadriceps reflex inhibition in man. Archives of Physical Medicine and Rehabilitation 65: 171–177

Stein J F, Glickstein M 1992 Role of the cerebellum in visual guidance of movement. Physiological Reviews 72: 967–1017

Stokes M, Young A 1984 The contribution of reflex inhibition to arthrogenous muscle weakness. Clinical Science 67: 7–14

Stone J A, Partin N B, Lueken J S, Timm K E, Ryan E J 1994 Upper extremity proprioceptive training. Journal of Athletic Training 29: 15–18

Swinkels A, Dolan P 1998 Regional assessment of joint position sense in the spine. Spine 23: 590–597

Taylor J L, McCloskey D I 1988 Proprioception in the neck. Experimental Brain Research 70: 351–360

Taylor J L, McCloskey D I 1990 Proprioceptive sensation in rotation of the trunk. Experimental Brain Research 81: 413–416

Tesio L Alpini D, Ceseranu A, Perucca L 1999 Short form of the Dizziness Handicap Inventory: construction and validation through Rasch analysis. American Journal of Physical Medicine and Rehabilitation 78: 233–241

Tjell C 1998 Diagnostic considerations on whiplash associated disorders. PhD Thesis, Karolinska Hospital, Stockholm, Sweden [ISBN 91-628-3139-9]

Tjell C, Rosenhall U 1998 Smooth pursuit neck torsion test: a specific test for cervical dizziness. American Journal of Otology 19: 76–81

Weber P C, Cass S P 1993 Clinical assessment of postural stability. American Journal of Otology 14: 566–569

Wilke H J, Wolf S, Claes L E, Arand M, Wiesend A 1995 Stability increase of the lumbar spine with different muscle groups: a biomechanical in vitro study. Spine 20: 192–198

Wing L W, Hargrave-Wilson W 1974 Cervical vertigo. Australian and New Zealand Journal of Surgery 44: 275–277

Wolff H D 1991 Kopfgelenke und Evolution. Manuelle Medizin 29: 41–46

Wolff H D 1998 Systemtheoretische Aspekte der Sonderstellung des kraniozervikalen Übergangs. In: Hülse M, Neuhuber W L, Wolff H D (eds) Der kranio-zervikale Übergang. Springer, Berlin

Chapter **19**

The vertebral artery and vertebrobasilar insufficiency

D. A. Rivett

INTRODUCTION

Neurovascular insult resulting from neck manipulation is almost always due to ischaemia of neural tissue supplied by the vertebrobasilar arterial system, following iatrogenic trauma to the vertebral artery (VA) (Assendelft et al 1996, Hurwitz et al 1996). The vertebrobasilar system provides 10–20% of the blood supply to the brain and branches to many vital neural structures, including the brain stem, cerebellum, spinal cord, cranial nerves III–XII and their nuclei and some of the cerebral cortex (Bannister et al 1995, Budgell & Sato 1997, Dommisse 1994, Refshauge 1995, Williams & Wilson 1962). Because of the risk associated with cervical spine manipulation (CSM), pre-manipulative screening tests designed to stress the VA and determine the patient's vulnerability to vertebrobasilar insufficiency (VBI) have been widely recommended (APA 1988). However, in order to understand the effects of cervical spine positional testing on the VA, it is first necessary to review the structural anatomy of the vessel and also consider the relevant neurological structures supplied by the vertebrobasilar system. It should be borne in mind that congenital anomalies of the vasculature and collateral routes of blood supply are important factors in determining whether pre-manipulative testing provokes symptoms or signs of VBI with a given patient (Mann 1995, Rivett 1997).

ANATOMY OF THE VERTEBROBASILAR ARTERIAL SYSTEM

Vertebral artery structure and anatomical relations

The VA is commonly described as comprising four parts. The first part usually arises from the superoposterior aspect of the first part of the subclavian artery and ascends back towards the ipsilateral transverse process of the sixth cervical vertebra (Argenson et al 1980, Hollinshead 1966) (Fig. 19.1). In 3–8% of cases the left VA may arise directly from the aortic arch between the subclavian and left common carotid arteries (Argenson et al 1980, Bannister et al 1995,

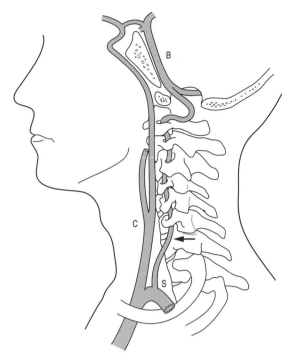

Figure 19.1 The course of the right vertebral artery (arrow) through the cervical transverse foramina, before joining with the opposite vessel to form the basilar artery (Freed et al 1998). Key: B = basilar artery; C = common carotid artery; S = subclavian artery.

Freed et al 1998, Heary et al 1996, Hollinshead 1966, Macchi et al 1995). The vessel normally travels superomedially between the longus colli and scalenus anterior and medius muscles, and sits posterior to the common carotid artery and the vertebral vein (Bannister et al 1995, Freed et al 1998, Hollinshead 1966, Macchi et al 1995). The inferior thyroid artery crosses this part of the VA anteriorly, while the stellate ganglion (or inferior cervical ganglion), the vertebral branch of the ganglion, and the seventh and eighth cervical ventral rami are situated posteriorly (Bannister et al 1995, Hollinshead 1966, Thiel 1991).

In the majority of cases the transverse process of the seventh cervical vertebra is also posterior to the artery (Freed et al 1998, Heary et al 1996). A small vertebral ganglion may be present anteromedial to the origin of the VA and its fibres join those of the stellate ganglion in enfolding the artery (Bannister et al 1995). In addition, the VA is usually enclosed in this region by the split posterior cord connecting the middle cervical ganglion to the stellate ganglion, and is invested by the deep cervical fascia (Argenson et al 1980, Bogduk 1994, Krueger & Okazaki 1980).

The second part of the VA normally commences with the vessel entering the transverse process of the sixth cervical vertebra. In about 90% of cases the VA enters at the C6 level, with the VA in the remainder of cases entering the transverse foramina at the C5 or C7 (or very occasionally higher) level (Argenson et al 1980, Bannister et al 1995, Bogduk

1994, Freed et al 1998, Hollinshead 1966, Macchi et al 1995, Mestan 1999). The vessel continues to ascend almost vertically through the transverse foramina of the vertebrae in a fibroperiosteal sheath, lateral to the neurocentral joints and anterolateral to the zygapophysial joints. It is accompanied by a plexus of veins, which later become the vertebral vein(s) (Argenson et al 1980, Bannister et al 1995, Carney 1981, Dan 1976, Hollinshead 1966, Hutchinson & Yates 1956, Krueger & Okazaki 1980, Terrett 1987b).

The artery also travels cranially with the vertebral sympathetic plexus, which is derived from the vertebral branch of the stellate ganglion posteriorly and branches of the vertebral ganglion or the cervical sympathetic trunk anteriorly (Carney 1981, Heary et al 1996, Hollinshead 1966, Thiel 1991). The artery fits tightly into the transverse foramen, with only 1–2 mm of the foraminal diameter remaining for the accompanying vertebral venous system and sympathetic elements (Argenson et al 1980). As the VA passes through the transverse process of the axis, its course deviates laterally to reach the more laterally projected atlantal transverse foramen (Pratt 1996, Roy 1994). The region of the VA between the transverse foramina of the axis and the atlas is described as a loop with a posterolateral convexity (Bannister et al 1995, Braakman & Penning 1971, Dumas et al 1996, Schmitt 1991, Thiel 1991).

The final extracranial segment or third part of the VA begins as the vessel emerges from the atlantal transverse foramen, deep to the semispinalis capitis, obliquus capitis inferior and rectus capitis posterior major muscles (Krueger & Okazaki 1980, Pratt 1996). The VA then abruptly turns posteriorly and medially behind the lateral mass, with the first cervical ventral spinal ramus situated medially (Terrett 1987b, Thiel 1991). The artery next traverses a wide groove in the upper surface of the posterior arch of the atlas directly posterior to the lateral mass, accompanied by the first cervical dorsal spinal ramus (suboccipital nerve) inferiorly and the venous plexus (Bannister et al 1995, Hollinshead 1966). The artery is held within the groove by a fibrous casing, reinforced by the transverse ligament and the retroglenoid ligament (Francke et al 1981). In about 33% of cases, there is a foramen (or retroarticular ring) instead of a groove, formed by bony spurs from the anterior and posterior margins of the groove (Lamberty & Zivanovic 1973). The atlanto-occipital joint capsule lies anteriorly and the posterior atlanto-occipital membrane is posterior to the vessel (Terrett 1987b). At this point the VA and the suboccipital nerve leave the atlas and enter the vertebral canal below the dense, fibrous (sometimes ossified) inferior border of the posterior atlanto-occipital membrane (Dvořák & Dvořák 1990, Hollinshead 1966, Thiel 1991). Notably, the VA is relatively fixed between the atlantal foramen and the membrane, as well as between the transverse foramina of the atlas and axis (Dumas et al 1996, Grant 1994b, Kunnasmaa & Thiel 1994).

The intracranial or fourth part of the VA penetrates the dura and arachnoid mater and enters the foramen magnum (Francke et al 1981). It then ascends sloping anterior to the medulla oblongata and unites medially with the contralateral VA at the lower pontine level to form the midline basilar artery (Bannister et al 1995, Barr 1979, Hollinshead 1966). The nerve supply for the VA is thought to arise from the postganglionic sympathetic fibres (originating from the superior, middle and inferior cervical ganglia) and myelinated fibres, which accompany it. A parasympathetic supply (from the facial nerve) has also been described (Barr 1979, Bogduk 1994, Nelson & Rennels 1970, Oostendorp et al 1992b, Thiel 1991).

Vertebral artery branches and structures supplied

The VA supplies a number of vital structures through its cervical and cranial branches. The cervical branches are further divided into spinal and muscular branches. The vessels, which supply the deep muscles of the upper cervical region, arise from the artery as it winds back and medially around the lateral mass of the atlas. The vessels also anastomose with the ascending and deep cervical arteries, as well as the occipital artery (Bannister et al 1995, Thiel 1991). The spinal branches (or segmental twigs) help to supply the spinal cord and related membranes and enter via the intervertebral foramina (Barr 1979, Braakman & Penning 1971). Furthermore, anastomoses are created with other spinal arteries to assist in the blood supply of the vertebral bodies, intervertebral joints and periosteum (Hollinshead 1966, Thiel 1991).

In addition to the basilar artery, the VA has several cranial branches:

1. posterior inferior cerebellar artery
2. posterior spinal artery
3. anterior spinal artery
4. medullary arteries
5. meningeal branches.

The medullary arteries and meningeal branches are minor vessels contributing to the supply of the medulla oblongata, cranial bone, dura, and the falx cerebelli (Thiel 1991). The posterior inferior cerebellar artery is the largest branch of the VA (Fig. 19.2), although sometimes it may arise from the basilar artery or is absent or even double (Bannister et al 1995, Hollinshead 1966, Terrett 1987b). It usually arises near the lower end of the olive of the medulla oblongata before following a tortuous route to arrive at the cerebellar vallecula, where it divides into medial and lateral branches. The medial branch supplies the cerebellar hemisphere and the inferior vermis, while the lateral branch supplies the inferior cerebellar surface. The trunk also provides blood to the lateral medulla oblongata, the choroid plexus of the fourth ventricle and the dentate nucleus of the cerebellum (Bannister et al 1995, Barr 1979, Hollinshead 1966, Thiel 1991). Disruption of the blood supply of the posterior inferior cerebellar artery may result in lateral medullary (or Wallenberg's) syndrome (Heary et al 1996). The posterior spinal artery usually arises from the posterior inferior cere-

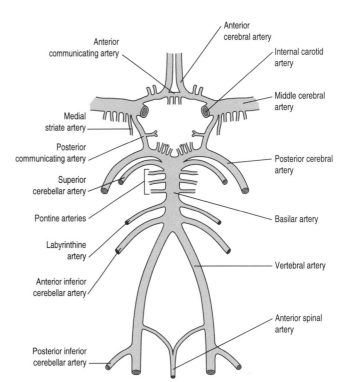

Figure 19.2 Depiction of the arteries at the base of the brain, demonstrating the circle of Willis (Bannister et al 1995).

bellar artery (or less frequently from the VA near the medulla oblongata). It forms two descending branches, which supply the dorsal roots of the spinal nerves and the posterolateral part of the spinal cord (Bannister et al 1995, Barr 1979, Dommisse 1994, Francke et al 1981, Hollinshead 1966, Thiel 1991).

The final branch of the VA is the anterior spinal artery, which arises near the end of the VA and descends anterior to the medulla oblongata to join with its counterpart at the mid-medulla level (Francke et al 1981). The united vessel then continues to descend on the anterior midline (median sulcus) of the spinal cord where it forms the anterior median artery with contributions from other vessels including small spinal rami from the VA (Barr 1979, Thiel 1991). The artery supplies about two-thirds of the cross-sectional area of the spinal cord via central branches (Barr 1979). The blood received by the spinal arteries from the VAs is sufficient for only the upper cervical portion of the spinal cord, although the segmental spinal arteries of the VAs also reinforce the supply (Barr 1979, Dommisse 1994). Branches from the anterior spinal arteries and their common vessel also contribute substantially to the blood supply of the medial medulla oblongata, disruption of which can produce medial medullary syndrome (Bannister et al 1995).

Basilar artery and branches

The basilar artery is formed by the joining of the two VAs and runs from the lower pontine border to the upper pontine border ventrally in the cisterna pontis in a shallow vertical median groove called the sulcus basilaris (Bannister et al 1995). It has five notable branches (see Fig. 19.2):

1. anterior inferior cerebellar artery
2. superior cerebellar artery
3. posterior cerebral artery
4. labyrinthine artery
5. pontine branches.

The anterior inferior cerebellar artery usually branches immediately after the two VAs join to form the basilar artery, but it may arise from the VA itself (Hollinshead 1966). It travels posterolaterally, commonly forming a variable loop into the internal acoustic meatus, from which it emerges to supply the anterolateral aspect of the inferior cerebellar surface. It also anastomoses with the posterior inferior cerebellar artery and supplies branches to the superior medulla oblongata and inferolateral region of the pons, including the vestibular nuclei (Bannister et al 1995, Barr 1979, Welsh et al 2000).

The superior cerebellar artery arises from near the end of the basilar artery, running laterally until it arrives at the superior cerebellar surface. Here it divides to anastomose with branches of the inferior cerebellar arteries to supply the superior aspect of the cerebellum. The pons, pineal body, colliculi of the mid-brain, superior medullary velum and tela choroidea of the third ventricle also receive supply from the superior cerebellar artery (Bannister et al 1995, Barr 1979).

The basilar artery divides into two relatively large posterior cerebral arteries. Each passes laterally and receives the ipsilateral posterior communicating artery. The posterior cerebral artery is frequently double and reaches the tentorial cerebral surface to supply cortical branches to the temporal and occipital lobes, including the visual area and other structures in the visual pathway (Carney 1981, Williams & Wilson 1962). It also supplies some of the medial and inferior cerebral surfaces (Bannister et al 1995, Barr 1979).

Several posteromedial central branches arise from the beginning of the vessel to supply the anterior thalamus, the globus pallidus and the lateral wall of the third ventricle. Small posterolateral central branches also supply the posterior thalamus, cerebral peduncle, colliculi of the mid-brain, and several other structures (Bannister et al 1995, Barr 1979).

The origin of the labyrinthine (or internal auditory) artery is variable. It sometimes branches from the lower part of the basilar artery, but more commonly branches from the anterior inferior cerebellar or superior cerebellar arteries (Bannister et al 1995, Bogduk 1994, Hollinshead 1966). It travels to the internal ear via the internal acoustic meatus.

Finally, the numerous pontine branches of the basilar artery assist in supplying the pons and nearby structures.

COLLATERAL CIRCULATION

An obstruction to blood flow in one VA may largely be compensated for by the contralateral artery, although this is somewhat contingent upon the calibre of the alternate vessel (Bogduk 1994, Terenzi & DeFabio 1996). Variation in the origin, calibre and course of the vessels of the vertebrobasilar system is very common (Bogduk 1994, Hollinshead 1966, Mestan 1999, Schmitt 1991). Notably, most individuals have a dominant VA, and therefore the consequences of an obstruction to flow may vary depending on whether the opposite vessel is the dominant one or not. Most frequently the left VA is dominant (Argenson et al 1980, Freed et al 1998, Heary et al 1996, Hollinshead 1966, Macchi et al 1996, Madawi et al 1997, Mitchell & McKay 1995). In an anatomic investigation, Argenson et al (1980) reported that the left VA diameter was larger than the right in 36% of cases, the right larger than the left in 26% of cases, with the remaining 38% of cases having VAs of equal diameter. About 10–20% of the general population have a hypoplastic (less than 2 mm in diameter) or congenitally absent VA, but can manage to function quite normally (Argenson et al 1980, Budgell & Sato 1997, Heary et al 1996, Keller et al 1976, Mestan 1999, Nicolau et al 2000). Termination of the VA in the posterior inferior cerebellar artery is another common anomaly (Heary et al 1996, Macchi et al 1995, Mestan 1999, Sturzenneger et al 1994).

In instances of VA flow obstruction, the internal carotid artery (ICA) may also provide compensatory blood supply by means of retrograde flow (Bogduk 1994). The posterior vertebrobasilar system is connected to the anterior carotid circulation via the circle of Willis anastomosis (see Fig. 19.2). Because the two VAs and the two ICAs provide the entire blood supply to the brain, the carotid circulation would therefore be required to perfuse the hindbrain to prevent neural tissue ischaemia in the event of deficient vertebrobasilar flow (Bannister et al 1995). This may occur through the connection of each posterior communicating artery with the ipsilateral posterior cerebral artery (branching directly from the basilar artery) and with the ipsilateral internal carotid artery (Hollinshead 1966, Terenzi & DeFabio 1996). Thus, the circle of Willis offers a potential shunt in abnormal circumstances, for example in the case of mechanical occlusion or vasospasm of the VA (Barr 1979, Carney 1981, Gillilan 1974, Hollinshead 1966, Sturzenneger et al 1994, Terenzi & DeFabio 1996).

Vessels in the arterial circle can vary considerably in calibre and can be partially developed, double or even absent, with only about 40% of circles fitting the textbook description (Bannister et al 1995, Barr 1979, Hollinshead 1966, Sturzenneger et al 1994, Williams & Wilson 1962). Most relevant to the present discussion is the finding of Fields et al (1965) that in about 90% of cases the circle is nevertheless complete, although in the majority one vessel in the circle is narrowed and not fully effective as a collateral route. In addition, the diameter of the pre-communicating portion of the posterior cerebral artery (in relation to the diameter of the posterior communicating artery) largely determines whether the carotid or the vertebrobasilar system is the primary blood supply to the occipital cortex (Van Overbeeke et al 1991). Furthermore, the carotid system is not uncommonly affected by atherosclerotic disease, limiting its collateral circulation capabilities (Freed et al 1998).

As well as giving rise to the internal carotid artery, the common carotid artery also divides into the external carotid artery, which in turn branches into the occipital artery. The deep ramus of the descending branch of the occipital artery anastomoses with the VA as it descends between the semispinales capitis and cervicis (Bannister et al 1995). This provides a potential channel for compensatory flow, depending on the location of the occlusion in the vertebrobasilar system (Bogduk 1994, Terenzi & DeFabio 1996). Similarly, the deep cervical artery (which usually arises from the costocervical trunk) anastomoses with branches of the VA, and the ascending cervical artery (which arises from the inferior thyroid artery) directly anastomoses with the VA (Bannister et al 1995, Bogduk 1994). The ascending cervical, occipital and deep cervical arteries may act individually or collectively to provide collateral circulation during an occlusion of the VA, although they require a certain amount of time to become haemodynamically effective (Dommisse 1994, Francke et al 1981, Sturzenneger et al 1994, Terenzi & DeFabio 1996).

It is feasible that minor compensatory flow to the cerebellum and brain stem is facilitated by the presence of superficial, and possibly deep, medullary anastomoses between branches of the three pairs of cerebellar arteries (Terenzi & DeFabio 1996, Williams & Wilson 1962). Terenzi & DeFabio (1996) also suggest that the leptomeningeal posterior collateral can act as an anastomotic pathway between the distal branches of the middle and posterior cerebral arteries. In addition, collateralization is recognized between the posterior cerebral and superior cerebellar arteries (Welsh et al 2000).

BIOMECHANICAL FACTORS

Serious vertebrobasilar complications following CSM are usually caused by trauma to the VA segment between the transverse foramina of the axis and the atlas during contralateral rotation (Aspinall 1989, Bogduk 1994, Fritz et al 1984, Frumkin & Baloh 1990, Grant 1994a, 1994b, 1996, Krueger & Okazaki 1980, Kunnasmaa & Thiel 1994, Mas et al 1989, Michaeli 1993, Raskind & North 1990, Rivett 1994, Roy 1994, Sherman et al 1981, Thiel et al 1994). Approximately 58% of cervical rotation occurs at the atlanto-axial joint, potentially stretching and compressing the adjacent region of the contralateral VA as the lateral mass of the atlas moves anteriorly, inferiorly and medially on the axis (Barton & Margolis 1975, Bogduk 1994, Bolton et al 1989, Corrigan & Maitland 1998, Di Fabio 1999, Dumas et al 1996, Grant 1987, 1994a, 1994b, Krueger & Okazaki 1980, Kunnasmaa & Thiel 1994, Licht et al 1999a, Petersen et al 1996, Rothrock et al 1991, Roy 1994, Schmitt 1991, Selecki 1969, Sherman et al 1981, Stevens 1991, Teasell & Marchuk 1994, Terrett 1987b, Weinstein & Cantu 1991, White & Panjabi 1990). The artery is also subjected to marked shearing forces during contralateral rotation because the atlantal transverse foramen is relatively removed from the axis of rotation and has a large excursion of movement (Assendelft et al 1996, Corrigan & Maitland 1998, Frumkin & Baloh 1990, Gutmann 1983, Lee et al 1995, Michaeli 1993, Pratt 1996, Stevens 1991).

The contralateral artery becomes increasingly angulated as rotation progresses, which is often associated with a corresponding decrease in luminal area and blood flow (Dvorák & Dvorák 1990, Petersen et al 1996, Pratt 1996, Weintraub & Khoury 1995) (Fig. 19.3). In fact, the VA may start to become 'kinked' at 30 degrees of rotation, with narrowing or occlusion of the vessel and possibly diminished blood flow to the hindbrain at 45 degrees (Bolton et al 1989, Brown & Tissington-Tatlow 1963, Corrigan & Maitland 1998, Dvorák & Dvorák 1990, Greenman 1991, Hedera et al 1993, Petersen et al 1996, Refshauge 1994, Selecki 1969, Stevens 1991, Toole & Tucker 1960). When stenosis happens it is mainly a result of compression at the level of the C2 transverse foramen, with the degree of reduction in blood flow dependent on intraluminal pressure, lumen diameter, angulation of the axial transverse foramen and the position of the axial foramen in relation to the atlantal foramen (Haynes et al 2002, Selecki 1969). The stresses applied to the VA during contralateral rotation are accentuated by attachment of the artery in the

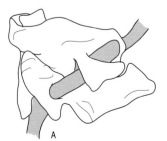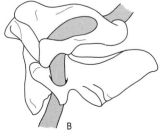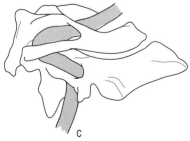

Figure 19.3 'Kinking' of the left vertebral artery as the atlas rotates contralaterally (c) on the axis from the neutral position (b). Kinking is less evident with ipsilateral rotation (a) Reproduced with permission from Dvorák & Dvorák 1990.

transverse foramina of the atlas and the axis, and also at the atlanto-occipital membrane (Bogduk 1994, Corrigan & Maitland 1998, Daneshmend et al 1984, Fast et al 1987, Grant 1987, 1994b, Kunnasmaa & Thiel 1994, Michaeli 1991, Robertson 1981, Terrett 1987b).

Stevens (1991) calculated that, upon full rotation, the VA may elongate by 45–75%, whereas Braakman & Penning (1971) estimated a 10% increase in length. However, the arterial wall in the extracranial region is somewhat adapted to the available range of movement, with a well-developed external elastic lamina and media (Grant 1994a, 1994b). In addition, the arterial loop between the atlas and the axis has a degree of redundancy that normally accommodates the large range of rotation at this segment, although loop deficiencies are present in some individuals (Braakman & Penning 1971, Haynes et al 2002, Johnson et al 1995, Roy 1994, Teasell & Marchuk 1994, Thiel 1991, Weinstein & Cantu 1991). Dumas et al (1996) used magnetic resonance angiography (MRA) to demonstrate that an underdeveloped atlanto-axial loop, combined with an atlanto-axial angle of opening exceeding 35 degrees, led to flow disturbances in the right VA at the C2 level in maximal left rotation. Recent work by Sheth et al (2001) using MRA with three-dimensional reconstructions suggests that the greatest anatomical distortion of the artery occurs where it turns most sharply as it exits the C1 transverse foramen.

The size of the lumen diameter may also be an important factor during stretching or compression of the artery, with smaller calibre vessels potentially at greater risk of stenosis and injury (Haynes 1995a, Macchi et al 1996, Mitchell & McKay 1995, Teasell & Marchuk 1994). Occlusion of the VA is thought to occur when a combination of tensile, shear and compressive forces exceeds the elastic properties of the vessel (Haynes & Milne 2000, Stevens 1991). Although the artery may occasionally be narrowed ipsilaterally, there is little evidence to suggest that the ipsilateral vessel is vulnerable with CSM (Faris et al 1963, Greenman 1991, Licht et al 1998, Selecki 1969, Symons et al 2002). In a recent, comprehensive investigation involving experiments with models and cadaveric specimens and in vivo Doppler ultrasound and magnetic resonance angiography, Haynes et al (2002) found no changes in the ipsilateral VA lumen during rotation.

Sagittal plane rotation is the primary movement at the atlanto-occipital joint (approximately 25–35 degrees). During the extension component, the VA may be compressed either as the occiput approximates the posterior arch of the atlas, or by folding of the atlanto-occipital membrane, or perhaps undergoes tensile strain as the occipital condyle glides anteriorly (Aspinall 1989, Grant 1996, Greenman 1991, Kunnasmaa & Thiel 1994, Michaud 2002, Okawara & Nibbelink 1974, Pratt-Thomas & Berger 1947, Schellhas et al 1980, Terrett 1987b, Thiel 1991, Tissington-Tatlow & Bammer 1957, Toole & Tucker 1960, White & Panjabi 1990, Worth 1988). It has also been suggested that the fibrous tissue ring surrounding the VA at the atlanto-

occipital junction can be distorted during extension with rotation, leading to arterial obstruction (Roy 1994, Thiel 1991). Nevertheless, clinical narrowing of the VA with extension has only occasionally been reported in the literature (Barton & Margolis 1975, Grant 1994a, 1994b, Hinse et al 1991, Nagler 1973, Okawara & Nibbelink 1974, Simeone & Goldberg 1968, Sturzenneger et al 1994).

SCREENING FOR VERTEBROBASILAR INSUFFICIENCY

The problem of vertebrobasilar complications resulting from manipulation of the cervical spine has been consistently reported for over half a century (Foster *v* Thornton 1934, Pratt-Thomas & Berger 1947, Rivett & Reid 1998, Terrett 1987a). Consequently, clinical testing procedures for VBI – which have remained essentially unchanged in that time – have been advocated for pre-manipulative screening purposes (Corrigan & Maitland 1998, De Kleyn & Nieuwenhuyse 1927, Terrett 1987b). The clinical value of pre-manipulative testing for VBI has, however, become a topic of increasing debate in the literature (Côté et al 1996, Refshauge 1994, Rivett et al 1998, Westaway et al 2003).

Interview

Prior to testing, questioning of the patient is recommended to ascertain the presence of symptoms suggestive of VBI, in particular dizziness and nausea (APA 1998, 2000, Grant 1994a, Grant & Trott 1991, Maitland 1986, Refshauge 1995). In this regard, the routine use of a self-administered or therapist-administered checklist for symptoms of VBI has been recommended by some authors (Grant 1996, Refshauge et al 2002, Rivett 1995b, 1997). If a symptom is elicited in the interview then further enquiry is conducted to determine its:

- nature, including degree, frequency and duration
- behaviour, especially its relationship to neck movements and sustained postures involving rotation and extension. Any reported provocative position or movement may be tested later in the physical examination
- status (improving, worsening or unchanged)
- history, particularly with respect to the presenting complaint (neck pain, headache, etc.). It is important to note that sudden, severe neck pain and occipital headache are often the first symptoms of VA dissection (Norris et al 2000). In addition, any effect on the symptom related to previous treatment is noted.

Pre-manipulative testing

The serious nature of neurovascular complications has led to the general recommendation that pre-manipulative testing for VBI be applied prior to the administration of any vigorous manual therapy procedure (in particular CSM and mobilization in end-range rotation) to detect patients at risk (Assendelft et al 1996, Côté et al 1996, Di Fabio 1999, Michaeli 1991, Refshauge 1995). These tests have also been recommended when a patient presents with a history suggestive of VBI (Corrigan & Maitland 1998, Gass & Refshauge 1995, Maitland 1986). The rationale of the tests is based on the assumption that neck positions involving rotation and/or extension may cause a reduction in blood flow through the VA, notably of the contralateral vessel (Kunnasmaa & Thiel 1994, Lewit 1992, Reif 1996). These flow changes are thought to be due to positionally induced mechanical stress causing vessel stenosis or occlusion (especially at the atlanto-axial region). These changes in blood flow may result in transient ischaemia manifesting as signs and symptoms of VBI (Grant 1994b, Haynes 1995b, Licht et al 1999a, Refshauge 1994, Weintraub & Khoury 1995). The clinical response elicited is presumed to be predictive of the likelihood of neurovascular complication associated with CSM.

Pre-manipulative clinical protocols or clinical guidelines which aim to identify vulnerable patients and prevent adverse outcomes have been endorsed by physiotherapy bodies in Australia, New Zealand, South Africa, Canada, the UK and the Netherlands (APA 1988, 2000, Barker et al 2000, Grant 1996, Oostendorp et al 1992a, SASP 1991). Pre-manipulative tests for VBI are also used and recommended by chiropractors, osteopaths and medical practitioners (Bolton et al 1989, Carey 1995, Combs & Triano 1997, Côté 1999, Haynes 1995b, 1996a, Ivancic et al 1993, Kleynhans & Terrett 1985, Licht et al 1999b). Nevertheless, there is a remote risk of neurological insult associated with pre-manipulative testing itself because of the stresses placed upon the VAs (Gass & Refshauge 1995, Grant 1994a, 1996, Grieve 1991, 1994, Meadows 1992). Indeed, instances of neurological complication due to testing have been documented (Bourdillon et al 1992, Edeling 1994, Grimmer 1998, Klougart et al 1996).

Responses to testing

The provocation on testing of symptoms or signs consistent with ischaemia in the vertebrobasilar distribution would normally constitute a positive response (APA 1988, Aspinall 1989, Barker et al 2000, Bourdillon et al 1992, Combs & Triano 1997, Grant 1994a, Kunnasmaa & Thiel 1994, Reif 1996) (Box 19.1).

Dizziness is probably the most frequent and earliest symptom of VBI and is generally regarded as being synonymous with vertigo, presenting as an illusion of self-rotation or environmental spin, or a sense of falling to one side (Aspinall 1989, Bogduk 1994, Corrigan & Maitland 1998, Côté et al 1996, Grant 1994a, 1994b, 1996, Michaeli 1991, Refshauge 1995, Williams & Wilson 1962). A positive response to testing for VBI is usually considered to indicate that end-range procedures and vigorous treatment should not be carried out, and that CSM is contraindicated (APA

Box 19.1 Potential positive responses to pre-manipulative testing

Anxiety
Ataxia
Blackouts
Changes in sweating
Clumsiness
Diplopia
Disorientation
Dizziness or vertigo
Drop attacks
Dysarthria
Dysphagia
Hearing disturbances
Hemianaesthesia
Hemiparesis
Incoordination
Light headedness
Loss of consciousness
Malaise
Nausea or vomiting
Nystagmus
Perioral dysaesthesia
Photophobia
Pupillary changes
Sensory changes extremities, face or head
Syncope
Tinnitus
Tremors
Unsteadiness
Visual disturbances
Weakness extremities, face or head

1988, Assendelft et al 1996, Bolton et al 1989, Carey 1995, Grant 1994a, Ivancic et al 1993, Licht et al 1999b, Petty & Moore 1998, Refshauge 1995). A negative response normally permits the clinician to manipulate. However, it is widely accepted that a negative response to testing does not guarantee an adverse outcome will not occur (Bolton et al 1989, Carey 1995, Corrigan & Maitland 1998, Di Fabio 1999, Grant 1994a, Grieve 1991, 1994, Ivancic et al 1993, Oostendorp et al 1992a, Refshauge 1995, Terrett 1987b).

There are a number of pre-manipulative tests recommended in the literature for eliciting signs and symptoms of VBI. The more commonly described tests include the following:

1. De Kleyn's test
In supine lying, the patient's head and neck are supported beyond the end of the treatment couch in sustained end-range cervical spine extension combined with end-range rotation (Fig. 19.4) (Bourdillon et al 1992, Carey 1995, Dvorák & Orelli 1985, Kunnasmaa & Thiel 1994, Maitland

1986). Lateral flexion may be added (Kleynhans & Terrett 1985). This test is frequently performed in sitting (Fig. 19.5) and is essentially the same as the Wallenberg test, Houle's test, Georges's test and the reclination test (Carey 1995, Combs & Triano 1997, Kleynhans & Terrett 1985, Thiel et al 1994). In addition, component movements of the test, that is sustained end-range rotation and end-range extension, may initially be tested individually (APA 1988, 2000).

2. Hautant's test

The seated patient stretches both arms forward to shoulder height, with the hands supinated and eyes closed. The cervical spine is then placed in combined extension and rotation by the examiner. In addition to provocation of possible signs or symptoms of brain stem ischaemia, if one hand sinks or pronates or deviates to one side then VBI is suspected (usually the arm affected is opposite to the rotation) (Carey 1995, Combs & Triano 1997, Kleynhans & Terrett 1985, Lewit 1992).

3. Underberger's walking test

The standing patient is asked to mark time by stepping on the spot (feet lifted high off the ground) with their eyes closed, arms stretched forward to shoulder height and their

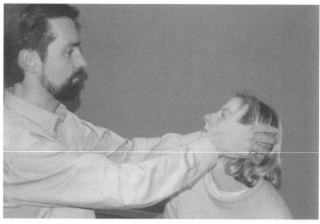

Figure 19.5 Combined end-range extension and rotation of the cervical spine applied in sitting.

hands supinated. The cervical spine is then moved into combined maximal rotation, extension and lateral flexion. Swaying or staggering of the body to one side is suggestive of VBI (Carey 1995, Kleynhans & Terrett 1985). Care is needed, as there is an obvious risk of the patient falling.

4. Simulated manipulation position test

The position for the proposed manipulation technique as adopted before thrusting is simulated and sustained (Fig. 19.6) (Carey 1995, Combs & Triano 1997, Kleynhans & Terrett 1985). This test is also known as Smith and Estridge's manoeuvre, as well as Maigne's manoeuvre or postural test (Combs & Triano 1997).

5. Passive accessory movement test

Unilateral anteroposterior or posteroanterior oscillatory movement is applied to the atlanto-axial articulation in a position of combined end-range rotation and extension to further stress rotation at this segment (Aspinall 1989, Grant 1988, Hutchison 1989).

The principal common element of all the pre-manipulative manoeuvres is the sustained position of combined end-range rotation and extension, with testing usually performed bilaterally, although the order of the component movements varies (Bolton et al 1989, Combs & Triano 1997, Côté et al 1996, Di Fabio 1999, Dvořák & Dvořák 1990, Grant 1996, Ivancic et al 1993, Kleynhans & Terrett 1985, Kunnasmaa & Thiel 1994, Lewit 1992, Licht et al 1999b, Terrett 1987b). Some authors also recommend that upper cervical spine extension be emphasized in tests involving extension (Aspinall 1989, Kunnasmaa & Thiel 1994, Rivett 1995b, 1997). During testing the patient is constantly questioned about any symptoms suggestive of VBI, especially dizziness, nausea and other volunteered symptoms, and observed for nystagmus (a sign of vestibular disorder) or any other relevant signs. Some authorities advocate performing pre-manipulative tests at each treatment session for which CSM is considered (APA 1988, 2000, Barker

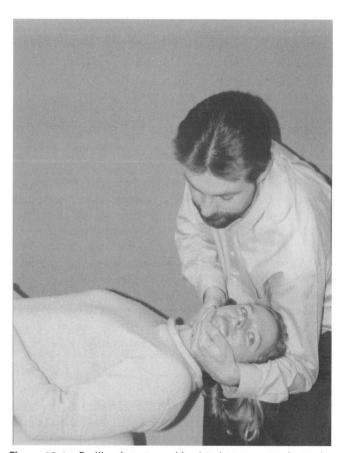

Figure 19.4 De Kleyn's test: combined end-range extension and rotation of the cervical spine applied in supine lying.

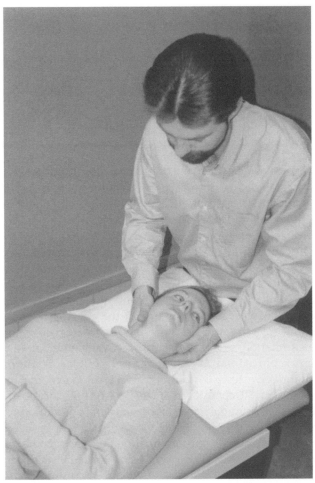

Figure 19.6 Simulated manipulation position test for left rotation manipulation of the right atlanto–axial joint using the cradle hold as described by Monaghan (2001).

et al 2000, Grant 1994a, 1996, Grant & Trott 1991, Oostendorp et al 1992a, Refshauge 1995, Terrett 1987b). This view gains some support from the studies of Hutchison (1989) and Powell (1990) which showed that a negative dizziness response to testing may change to a positive response between consecutive visits, possibly because of increased compromise of the VA with improved range of cervical spine motion.

The recommended time period for sustaining the test positions varies from 3 seconds to 55 seconds, but is usually for a minimum of 10 seconds. Testing is terminated immediately if a positive response is elicited (APA 1988, 2000, Aspinall 1989, Assendelft et al 1996, Bolton et al 1989, Bourdillon et al 1992, Brewerton 1986, Carey 1995, Corrigan & Maitland 1998, Di Fabio 1999, Dvorák & Dvorák 1990, Edeling 1994, Grant 1994a, 1996, Jaskoviak 1980, Kleynhans & Terrett 1985, Oostendorp 1988, Petty & Moore 1998, Reif 1996, Terrett 1987b, Thiel et al 1994). It is recommended that a short period separates each test to allow for the manifestation of latent responses (Grant &

Trott 1991, Reif 1996), with some authors suggesting at least 10 seconds (Aspinall 1989, Grant 1994a, Maitland 1986, Petty & Moore 1998). Recent sonographic research by Zaina et al (2003) lends some support for the use of a rest period between test positions. There also appears to be no consensus in the literature as to whether testing is preferably performed with the patient sitting or in supine lying or in both positions. The clinician should consider which position is most appropriate given the patient's presentation (APA 1988, Grant 1994a, Grant & Trott 1991, Refshauge 1995).

Differentiation of dizziness

If dizziness is provoked with rotation or rotation/extension, it is sometimes possible to implicate or exclude the vestibular apparatus of the inner ear as the source of the dizziness (APA 1988, Grant 1994a, Petty & Moore 1998). In the standing position, the therapist holds the patient's head steady as the patient turns the trunk while keeping the feet fixed, thus producing sustained end-range cervical spine rotation. Because the semicircular canal fluid is not disturbed by this test, a positive response then excludes the labyrinth (Edeling 1994) and suggests that the cause is either cervical (reflex) vertigo or compromise of the VA (Grant 1994a). However, pre-manipulative testing does not differentiate between VBI and cervical vertigo as the cause of elicited dizziness, unless it is accompanied by clear signs or symptoms of brain stem ischaemia, such as dysarthria (Dvorák & Orelli 1985, Grant 1988).

VALIDITY OF PRE-MANIPULATIVE TESTING

There is growing debate regarding the clinical value of premanipulatively testing for VBI, particularly with respect to its sensitivity and specificity in detecting the patient at increased risk of stroke following CSM (Assendelft et al 1996, Bolton et al 1989, Campbell 1994, Carey 1995, Combs & Triano 1997, Di Fabio 1999, Dvorák et al 1991, Edeling 1994, Gass & Refshauge 1995, Grieve 1993, Gross et al 1996, Haldeman et al 1999, Haynes 1996a, Ivancic et al 1993, Kunnasmaa & Thiel 1994, Mann 1995, Michaeli 1991, Oostendorp et al 1992a, Refshauge 1995, Rivett 1994, Robertson 1982, Terenzi & DeFabio 1996). It is considered by some that pre-manipulative procedures are valid tests of the adequacy of collateral flow to the hindbrain in the event of VA occlusion from manipulation but that they do not indicate the ability of the artery to withstand the force and speed of the manipulative thrust (Aspinall 1989, Assendelft et al 1996, Bogduk 1994, Mann 1995, Refshauge 1994, 1995, Rivett 1995a, Terenzi & DeFabio 1996, Terrett 1987b). Because the tests cannot simulate the stresses of the thrust (although they may reproduce some of the other stresses imposed on the VA during CSM), they cannot adequately predict an individual's susceptibility to vascular trauma (Rivett 1994, Terrett 1987b).

Cadaveric studies

The original rationale of the pre-manipulative tests for VBI was essentially derived from an understanding of the functional anatomy of the cervical spine and from the findings of dynamic cadaveric studies (Brown & Tissington-Tatlow 1963, Corrigan & Maitland 1998, Grant 1994b, Refshauge 1994). These investigations led to the conclusion that the VA was commonly narrowed or occluded during neck movement, principally with contralateral rotation or combined contralateral rotation and extension, and less frequently with extension or ipsilateral rotation (Brown & Tissington-Tatlow 1963, De Kleyn & Nieuwenhuyse 1927, Oppel et al 1989, Selecki 1969, Tissington-Tatlow & Bammer 1957, Toole & Tucker 1960). Stenosis usually occurred at, or above, the level of the axis, mostly adjacent to the atlanto-axial joint. A more recent instillation experiment using fresh spines has confirmed the findings of these earlier studies (Li et al 1999). However, it is not known how accurately these cadaveric studies represent the clinical situation, particularly considering post mortem tissue changes, flow pressure differences and absence of muscle tone (Bogduk 1994, Haynes 1996b, Licht et al 1998, Macchi et al 1996, Petersen et al 1996).

Ultrasonographic investigations

More recently, the effects of cervical spine movements on extracranial blood flow has been investigated in vivo using Doppler ultrasound. The findings of these studies have been somewhat conflicting, leading some researchers to question the validity of the pre-manipulative tests (Côté et al 1996, Grant 1996, Grant & Johnson 1997, Johnson et al 2000, Kunnasmaa & Thiel 1994, Li et al 1999, Refshauge 1994, Stevens 1991, Thiel et al 1994, Weingart & Bischoff 1992).

Early ultrasonographic studies employed continuous-wave Doppler ultrasound to demonstrate blood flow changes during rotation and extension of the neck. Arnetoli et al (1989) examined the VA flow velocity of 190 healthy volunteers and 60 patients diagnosed with VBI while in the position of combined rotation/extension. Continuous-wave ultrasonography revealed either loss of diastolic flow or absent Doppler signal of the contralateral VA in 6% of the control group, but in 33% of the patient group. Danêk (1989) also used continuous-wave ultrasound combined with rheoencephalographic tracings to demonstrate changes in both measures during sustained rotation/extension in 12 of 25 symptomatic patients. Furthermore, Stevens (1991) utilized continuous-wave Doppler to measure VA flow at the atlanto-axial level during positional testing. He reported that in 62% of 250 patients with an identified abnormal flow velocity pattern the VA flow velocity profile reduced in contralateral rotation, whereas in 20% of patients it increased. In addition, 18% exhibited decreased flow velocity in cervical extension.

More recent investigations have used duplex scanning, combining pulsed-wave Doppler ultrasound with real-time imaging of the VA. Refshauge (1994) used duplex scanning to measure extracranial blood flow velocity at the C2–3 level in 45 degrees contralateral rotation and in end-range contralateral rotation in 20 healthy volunteers. Flow changes (generally an increase) were observed at 45 degrees contralateral rotation, consistent with the in vitro findings of Toole & Tucker (1960). A significant trend for decreased VA blood velocity was demonstrated in full contralateral rotation. Two (10%) individuals exhibited no flow in 45 degrees contralateral rotation while remaining asymptomatic. Haynes (1996b) also found cessation of the Doppler signal during maximal contralateral rotation in 5% of 280 VAs.

In contrast, other studies have found no change in VA blood flow with positional testing of the cervical spine. Using continuous-wave ultrasound, Weingart & Bischoff (1992) failed to find any significant alteration in VA flow velocity at the level of the arch of the atlas in 30 normal volunteers with various positions of rotation and combined rotation/extension. Another investigation employed duplex ultrasound to ascertain the validity of some pre-manipulative tests by comparing the VA haemodynamic changes of 30 control volunteers with those of 12 individuals exhibiting signs and/or symptoms of VBI on testing (Thiel et al 1994). Blood flow velocity was measured during sustained extension, rotation and combined extension/rotation (Wallenberg test). No abnormal flow patterns were demonstrated during testing and no meaningful significant differences in mean velocity ratios were found between the two groups. The investigators concluded that the results failed to support the validity of the Wallenberg test in screening for VBI.

Côté et al (1996) performed a secondary analysis of the data of Thiel et al (1994). They evaluated the validity of the Wallenberg test to detect decreased vertebrobasilar arterial blood flow by measuring the impedance to blood flow of the VA during testing. Sensitivity for increased impedance to flow was reported as 0%, and specificity as 67–90% depending on the cut-off point and the artery (left or right). The positive predictive value was 0% and the negative predictive value ranged from 63% to 97%. It was similarly concluded that the test is of questionable value for pre-manipulative screening. Later research by Licht et al (2000) using colour duplex sonography (duplex scanning combined with simultaneous colour Doppler flow imaging) supports these findings. In this study, 15 patients with a positive pre-manipulative (extension/rotation) test response were scanned in 45 degrees rotation, maximal rotation and extension/rotation. There was no significant change in the peak flow velocity and the mean flow velocity of either VA in any test position.

A recent investigation described in two separate reports has produced further confusing results (Licht et al 1998, 1999a). Colour duplex ultrasound was used to determine the effect of both contralateral and ipsilateral rotation (45 degrees and maximal) on VA peak flow velocity in 20 healthy university students (Licht et al 1998). In both test positions, a significant but modest decrease was shown with contralateral rotation and a significant increase with ipsilateral rotation. However, volume blood flow data taken at the same time as the velocity data demonstrated no change with rotation, indicating that hindbrain perfusion was unaffected (Licht et al 1999a). This conclusion is supported by the recent work of Haynes & Milne (2000), who found that mean flow velocity and lumen diameter were not significantly changed during rotation in 20 patients using colour duplex sonography, and Zaina et al (2003) who reported no change in peak velocity or volume flow rate in 20 asymptomatic volunteers during rotation.

In contrast, Rivett et al (1999) used colour duplex ultrasound to demonstrate significant flow velocity changes in end-range positions involving rotation and extension. However, consistent with previous research (Côté et al 1996, Thiel et al 1994), there were no meaningful significant differences found between subjects testing either positive ($n = 10$) or negative ($n = 10$) to pre-manipulative testing. A subsequent larger study (100 patients) by the same investigators (Rivett et al 2000) using colour duplex ultrasound with power imaging capability to measure VA haemodynamics at the atlanto-axial level in neck positions involving rotation and extension produced similar findings. Notably, 20 patients exhibited total or partial occlusion during testing, but only two reported potential VBI symptoms at the time. The investigators concluded that pre-manipulative testing does not distinguish between patients with varying degrees of flow impedance and is unlikely to detect the patient at increased risk of stroke.

Differences in conclusions between these ultrasonographic studies may be attributable to a number of factors. Firstly, many investigations used continuous-wave Doppler which has the disadvantage that there is no visualization of the target vessel, potentially resulting in errors of vessel identification and sampling. There is also no capability for selective depth sampling of specific vessels (as with duplex ultrasound), resulting in superimposed Doppler shifts from all vessels insonated (Johnson et al 2000). Furthermore, the angle of insonation is unknown with continuous-wave Doppler and therefore any change in measured flow velocity may simply be attributable to a change in the Doppler angle (Haynes 1996b, Licht et al 1998). Secondly, despite the operator dependency of ultrasound examination (Grant & Johnson 1997), reliability studies were either limited in nature (Refshauge 1994, Stevens 1991) or not performed at all. Thirdly, different sites of the artery were sampled in the various studies, sometimes distant from the vulnerable atlanto-axial region (Johnson et al 2000). Fourthly, responses may vary depending on whether subjects were tested in supine lying or sitting (Zaina et al 2003). Finally, sample sizes were often small and few stud-

ies used a representative patient sample (Côté et al 1996, Johnson et al 2000).

Other haemodynamic investigations

The few angiographic studies of VA flow during neck rotation that have been undertaken have also produced contradictory results. Faris et al (1963) performed angiographic examination of 79 VAs in healthy males and reported an occlusion rate of 7.6% during contralateral rotation. Similarly, Dumas et al (1996) used MRA to show disturbance of flow in the right VA at the atlanto-axial level in four of 14 healthy individuals during left rotation, although blood flow downstream did not appear to be reduced. On the other hand, Takahashi et al (1994) failed to find evidence of VA occlusion or stenosis upon contralateral rotation at the atlanto-axial joint using angiography with 39 patients.

Reports using transcranial Doppler (TCD) sonography have focused more on the effects of neck rotation on intracranial circulation. Significant but inconsistent reductions in flow velocity of intracranial arteries during contralateral rotation have been related to posterior circulation anomalies, atherosclerosis or hypoplasia of the unilateral VA, and severe VA obstruction due to cervical joint pathology (Hedera et al 1993, Petersen et al 1996, Sturzenegger et al 1994). Nevertheless, a study of 50 healthy volunteers found intracranial flow velocity was decreased during combined rotation/extension and in extreme extension (Li et al 1999). However, no marked intracranial arterial flow velocity changes have been noted with TCD sonography in normal volunteers during rotation in other reports (Petersen et al 1996, Simon et al 1994). These studies suggest that VBI will manifest only if there is concomitant vascular anomaly or predisposing vascular or joint pathology involving the ipsilateral VA and the contralateral VA blood flow is embarrassed during rotation. Pre-manipulative testing may therefore provide an indication of the competence of the collateral pathways in the event of a unilateral reduction of VA flow (Grant 1996, Haynes 1995b, Mann 1995, Michaeli, 1991).

It is worth considering the predictive value of pre-manipulative testing in relation to arterial pathologies associated with manipulative complications. In cases of VA stenosis due to local vasospasm, intimal dissection or thrombus formation, neurological insult may be avoided because collateral flow is sufficient to maintain perfusion. Pre-manipulative testing in this situation may be of value in assessing the adequacy of the collateral pathways and therefore the probability of neurological ischaemia. However, testing cannot predict the likelihood or outcome of cranial projection of local traumatic pathology, in which the compensatory contribution of collateral vessels is markedly reduced. For example, VA intimal dissection may continue into the basilar artery, effectively negating the opposite VA as a collateral pathway. Alternatively, a thromboembolic event may ensue and cause obstruction in the distal circulation.

INTERPRETATION OF PRE-MANIPULATIVE TEST RESPONSES

The specificity of pre-manipulative testing is complicated by the fact that other structures stimulated by the tests can potentially produce responses that mimic VBI, notably the cervical spine and the vestibular/labyrinth system. It is likely that some patients experiencing somatic or vestibular disorders are needlessly alarmed and denied manipulative treatment because of false positive findings on testing (Combs & Triano 1997, Côté 1999, Côté et al 1996, Terenzi & DeFabio 1996, Terrett 1987b, Wing & Hargrave-Wilson 1974).

Clinical differential diagnosis of vestibular dysfunction may not always be possible for the manual therapist, particularly if dizziness is the only elicited symptom (Coman 1986, Grant 1987, Hutchison 1989, Refshauge 1995). Disturbances in the fluid in the affected semicircular canal can lead to nystagmus and vertigo with movement of the head, although flexion and lateral flexion are more commonly involved (Coman 1986). Symptoms and signs of vestibular dysfunction may be elicited by rapid inner range movements in the horizontal, coronal or sagittal plane, which are unlikely to cause vascular compromise and VBI (Laslett 1988). Differential diagnosis may also be facilitated by labyrinthine tests involving concurrent trunk and neck rotation without head movement (APA 1988, Grant 1994b, Meadows & Magee 1994), though the validity of this procedure has never been evaluated. Of course, the concomitant presence of clear neurological symptoms or signs, such as hemianopia or dysarthria, strongly suggests the presence of VBI (Coman 1986).

Cervical (or reflex) vertigo undoubtedly causes many false positive responses to pre-manipulative testing. The neck musculature and the capsules of the upper three cervical joints are thought to be the source of cervical vertigo, with joint hypomobility lesions and muscle spasm being the common clinical findings (Abrahams 1981, Aspinall 1989, Bogduk 1994, Bolton 1998, Bracher et al 2000, Corrigan & Maitland 1998, Grant 1994b, Refshauge 1995, Wing & Hargrave-Wilson 1974). Mechanoreceptors in these structures contribute to tonic neck reflexes for balance control, but can cause dizziness if proprioceptive afferent impulses to the vestibular nuclei in the brain stem become distorted (Bogduk 1994, Bolton 1998, Bracher et al 2000, de Jong et al 1977, Grant 1987). Cervical vertigo may also mimic other signs and symptoms associated with VBI, including light-headedness, nausea, nystagmus, blurring of vision, faintness, vomiting, hearing disturbances and ataxia (Bogduk 1994, Bolton 1998, Bracher et al 2000, Corrigan & Maitland 1998, Grant 1994b, Hutchison 1989). These symptoms are often provoked by neck movement (Bracher et al 2000, Corrigan & Maitland 1998, Hutchison 1989, Refshauge 1995).

Clinical differentiation between cervical and vascular vertigo is also very difficult (Aspinall 1989, Bogduk 1994, Coman 1986, Dvorák & Dvorák 1990, Dvorák & Orelli 1985, Grant 1994b, Grieve 1991, 1994, Hutchison 1989, Michaeli 1991, Refshauge 1995). Following gentle, non-provocative treatment to the upper cervical spine, repeated pre-manipulative testing might enable retrospective differential diagnosis (Grant 1994a, Hutchison 1989, Refshauge 1995). Changes from positive to negative may result from normalization of proprioceptive afferent input to the vestibular nuclei following treatment (Bogduk 1994, Hutchison 1989). It is also thought that cervical vertigo fatigues with sustained or repeated positional testing (unlike VBI). However, this entails increased risk to the patient (Aspinall 1989, Campbell 1994, Grant 1994b, Laslett 1988). In addition, it has been suggested sustained natural apophyseal glides (SNAGs) may assist in differential diagnosis (Rivett 1997). A sustained posteroanterior glide of the atlas or axis is applied while the patient is performing the provocative movement (Mulligan 1991, 1999). The glide is usually applied to the spinous process of the axis for symptomatic extension and to the lateral aspect of the arch of the atlas for symptomatic rotation (Fig. 19.7). If the symptoms are eliminated during the manoeuvre then cervical vertigo is probably responsible (Rivett 1997), although stresses imposed on the VA may be potentially reduced as well.

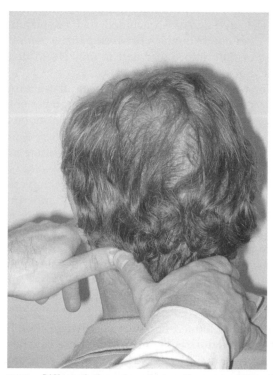

Figure 19.7 Differentiation of cervical vertigo versus VBI using a sustained natural apophyseal glide (SNAG). Sustained posteroanterior pressure is applied to the left aspect of the atlantal arch as the patient actively rotates to the right (Rivett 1997).

FUTURE DIRECTIONS

It is apparent that the validity of pre-manipulative testing is at best questionable, and its clinical value is limited (Corrigan & Maitland 1998, Di Fabio 1999, Dvorák & Orelli 1985, Grant 1994b, 1996, Grieve 1991, Maitland 1986, Refshauge 1995, Terrett 1987b). Certainly the capacity of the VA to withstand thrusting forces is not tested (Grant 1996, Middleditch 1991, Terrett 1987b), although it may test the adequacy of the collateral circulation to maintain hindbrain perfusion (Grant 1996, Mann 1995, Refshauge, 1994).

It has been argued by some that pre-manipulative testing should be abandoned because of its doubtful predictive validity and the risk it entails (Côté 1999, Côté et al 1996, Grieve 1991, 1993, 1994). Conversely, other authors contend that if testing occasionally prevents a stroke, then its use is warranted (Grant 1996, Kunnasmaa & Thiel 1994). Nevertheless, the development of alternative screening procedures is urgently needed. To this end, the clinical application of a hand-held Doppler velocimeter shows promise, but requires further study to determine its validity, reliability and clinical feasibility (Haynes 2000, Haynes et al 2000, Rivett 2001).

KEYWORDS	
vertebral artery	pre-manipulative testing
vertebrobasilar insufficiency	cervical spine

References

Abrahams V C 1981 Sensory and motor specialization in some muscles of the neck. Trends in Neurosciences 4: 24–27

Argenson C, Francke J P, Sylla S, Dintimille H, Papasian S, di Marino V 1980 The vertebral arteries (segments V1 and V2). Anatomia Clinica 2: 29–41

Arnetoli G, Amadori A, Stefani P, Nuzzaci G 1989 Sonography of vertebral arteries in De Kleyn's position in subjects and in patients with vertebrobasilar transient ischemic attacks. Angiology 40: 716–720

Aspinall W 1989 Clinical testing for cervical mechanical disorders which produce ischemic vertigo. Journal of Orthopaedic and Sports Physical Therapy 11: 176–182

Assendelft W J J, Bouter L M, Knipschild P G 1996 Complications of spinal manipulation: a comprehensive review of the literature. Journal of Family Practice 42: 475–480

Australian Physiotherapy Association (APA) 1988 Protocol for pre-manipulative testing of the cervical spine. Australian Journal of Physiotherapy 34: 97–100

Australian Physiotherapy Association (APA) 2000 Clinical guidelines for pre-manipulative procedures for the cervical spine. Australian Physiotherapy Association, Melbourne

Bannister L H, Berry M M, Collins P, Dyson M, Dussek J E, Ferguson M W J (eds) 1995 Gray's anatomy: the anatomical basis of medicine and surgery, 38th edn. Churchill Livingstone, New York

Barker S, Kesson M, Ashmore J, Turner G, Conway J, Stevens D 2000 Guidance for pre-manipulative testing of the cervical spine. Manual Therapy 5: 37–40

Barr M L 1979 The human nervous system: an anatomical viewpoint, 3rd edn. Harper and Row, Hagerstown

Barton J W, Margolis M T 1975 Rotational obstruction of the vertebral artery at the atlantoaxial joint. Neuroradiology 9: 117–120

Bogduk N 1994 Cervical causes of headache and dizziness. In: Boyling J D, Palastanga N (eds) Grieve's Modern Manual Therapy: the Vertebral Column, 2nd edn. Churchill Livingstone, Edinburgh

Bolton P S 1998 The somatosensory system of the neck and its effects on the central nervous system. Journal of Manipulative and Physiological Therapeutics 21: 553–563

Bolton P S, Stick P E, Lord R S A 1989 Failure of clinical tests to predict cerebral ischemia before neck manipulation. Journal of Manipulative and Physiological Therapeutics 12: 304–307

Bourdillon J F, Day E A, Bookhout M R 1992 Spinal manipulation, 5th edn. Butterworth Heinemann, Oxford

Braakman R, Penning L 1971 Injuries of the cervical spine. Excerpta Medica, New York

Bracher E S B, Almeida C I R, Almeida R R, Duprat A C, Bracher C B B 2000 A combined approach for the treatment of cervical vertigo. Journal of Manipulative and Physiological Therapeutics 23: 96–100

Brewerton D A 1986 The doctor's role in diagnosis and prescribing vertebral manipulation. In: Maitland G D Vertebral manipulation, 5th edn. Butterworths, London, pp 14–17

Brown B S J, Tissington-Tatlow W F 1963 Radiographic studies of the vertebral arteries in cadavers. Radiology 81: 80–88

Budgell B S, Sato A 1997 The cervical subluxation and regional cerebral blood flow. Journal of Manipulative and Physiological Therapeutics 20: 103–107

Campbell J 1994 The dangers of cervical spine manipulation. Journal of Orthopaedic Medicine 16: 1

Carey P F 1995 A suggested protocol for the examination and treatment of the cervical spine: managing the risk. Journal of the Canadian Chiropractic Association 39: 35–39

Carney A L 1981 Vertebral artery surgery: historical development, basic concepts of brain hemodynamics, and clinical experience of 102 cases. In: Carney A L, Anderson E M (eds) Advances in Neurology. Diagnosis and treatment of brain ischemia. Raven Press, New York, vol 30

Coman W B 1986 Dizziness related to ENT conditions. In: Grieve G P (ed) Modern Manual Therapy of the Vertebral Column. Churchill Livingstone, London

Combs S B, Triano J J 1997 Symptoms of neck artery compromise: case presentations of risk estimate for treatment. Journal of Manipulative and Physiological Therapeutics 20: 274–278

Corrigan B, Maitland G D 1998 Vertebral musculoskeletal disorders. Butterworth Heinemann, Oxford

Côté P 1999 Screening for stroke: let's show some maturity! Journal of the Canadian Chiropractic Association 43: 72–74

Côté P, Kreitz B G, Cassidy J D, Thiel H 1996 The validity of the extension-rotation test as a clinical screening procedure before neck manipulation: a secondary analysis. Journal of Manipulative and Physiological Therapeutics 19: 159–164

Dan N G 1976 The management of vertebral artery insufficiency in cervical spondylosis: a modified technique. Australian and New Zealand Journal of Surgery 46: 164–165

Danêk V 1989 Haemodynamic disorders within the vertebro-basilar arterial system following extreme positions of the head. Journal of Manual Medicine 4: 127–129

Daneshmend T K, Hewer R L, Bradshaw J R 1984 Acute brain stem stroke during neck manipulation. British Medical Journal 288: 189

de Jong P T V M, de Jong J M B V, Cohen B, Jongkees L B W 1977 Ataxia and nystagmus induced by injection of local anesthetics in the neck. Annals of Neurology 1: 240–246

De Kleyn A, Nieuwenhuyse P 1927 Schwindelanfaelle und nystagmus bei einer bestimmten stellung des kopfes. Acta Otolaryngolica 11: 155–157

Di Fabio R P 1999 Manipulation of the cervical spine: risks and benefits. Physical Therapy 79: 50–65

Dommisse G F 1994 The blood supply of the spinal cord and the consequences of failure. In: Boyling J D, Palastanga N (eds) Grieve's Modern Manual Therapy: the Vertebral Column, 2nd edn. Churchill Livingstone, Edinburgh

Dumas J-L, Salama J, Dreyfus P, Thoreux P, Goldlust D, Chevrel J-P 1996 Magnetic resonance angiographic analysis of atlanto-axial rotation: anatomic bases of compression of the vertebral arteries. Surgical and Radiologic Anatomy 18: 303–313

Dvorák J, Dvorák V 1990 Manual medicine diagnostics, 2nd edn. Thieme Medical, New York

Dvorák J, Orelli F V 1985 How dangerous is manipulation to the cervical spine? Case report and results of a survey. Journal of Manual Medicine 2: 1–4

Dvorák J, Baumgartner H, Burn L et al 1991 Consensus and recommendations as to the side-effects and complications of manual therapy of the cervical spine. Journal of Manual Medicine 6: 117–118

Edeling J 1994 Manual therapy for chronic headache, 2nd edn. Butterworth Heinemann, Oxford

Faris A A, Poser C M, Wilmore D W, Agnew C H 1963 Radiologic evaluation of neck vessels in healthy men. Neurology 13: 386–396

Fast A, Zinicola D F, Marin E L 1987 Vertebral artery damage complicating cervical manipulation. Spine 12: 840–842

Fields W S, Bruetman M E, Weibel J 1965 Collateral circulation of the brain. Williams Wilkins, Baltimore

Foster v Thornton 1934 Malpractice: death resulting from chiropractic treatment for headache. Journal of the American Medical Association 103: 1260

Francke J P, Marino V Di, Pannier M, Argenson C, Libersa C 1981 The vertebral arteries (arteria vertebralis): the V3 atlanto-axoidial and V4 intracranial segments-collaterals. Anatomia Clinica 2: 229–242

Freed K S, Brown L K, Carroll B A 1998 The extra-cranial cerebral vessels. In: Rumack C M, Wilson S R, Charbonneau J W (eds) Diagnostic ultrasound, 2nd edn. Mosby Year Book, St Louis, vol 1

Fritz V U, Maloon A, Tuch P 1984 Neck manipulation causing stroke: case reports. South African Medical Journal 66: 844–846

Frumkin L R, Baloh R W 1990 Wallenberg's syndrome following neck manipulation. Neurology 40: 611–615

Gass E M, Refshauge K M 1995 The use of information in clinical practice. In: Refshauge K M, Gass E M (eds) Musculoskeletal physiotherapy: clinical science and practice. Butterworth Heinemann, Oxford

Gillilan L A 1974 Potential collateral circulation to the human cerebral cortex. Neurology 24: 941–948

Grant E R 1987 Clinical testing before cervical manipulation: can we recognize the patient at risk? In: Proceedings of the Tenth International Congress of the World Confederation for Physical Therapy. World Confederation for Physical Therapy, Sydney

Grant R 1988 Dizziness testing and manipulation of the cervical spine. In: Grant R (ed) Clinics in Physical Therapy. Physical therapy of the cervical and thoracic spine. Churchill Livingstone, New York, vol 17

Grant R 1994a Vertebral artery concerns: premanipulative testing of the cervical spine. In: Grant R (ed) Clinics in Physical Therapy. Physical therapy of the cervical and thoracic spine, 2nd edn. Churchill Livingstone, New York, vol 17

Grant R 1994b Vertebral artery insufficiency: a clinical protocol for pre-manipulative testing of the cervical spine. In: Boyling J D, Palastanga N (eds) Grieve's Modern Manual Therapy: the Vertebral Column, 2nd edn. Churchill Livingstone, Edinburgh

Grant R 1996 Vertebral artery testing: the Australian Physiotherapy Association Protocol after 6 years. Manual Therapy 1: 149–153

Grant R, Johnson C L 1997 The variability of measurement of vertebral artery blood flow. In: Proceedings of the Tenth Biennial Conference of the Manipulative Physiotherapists Association of Australia. Manipulative Physiotherapists Association of Australia, Melbourne

Grant E R, Trott P H 1991 Pre-manipulative testing of the cervical spine: the A.P.A. protocol and its aftermath. In: Proceedings of the Eleventh International Congress of the World Confederation for Physical Therapy. World Confederation for Physical Therapy, London, book 1

Greenman P E 1991 Principles of manipulation of the cervical spine. Journal of Manual Medicine 6: 106–113

Grieve G P 1991 Mobilisation of the spine, 5th edn. Churchill Livingstone, Edinburgh

Grieve G P 1993 Scrutinizing tacit assumptions in manual therapy. Journal of Manual and Manipulative Therapy 1: 123–133

Grieve G P 1994 Incidents and accidents of manipulation and allied techniques. In: Boyling J D, Palastanga N (eds) Grieve's Modern Manual Therapy: the Vertebral Column, 2nd edn. Churchill Livingstone, Edinburgh

Grimmer K 1998 Cervical manipulation: compliance with, and attitudes to, the current Australian Physiotherapy Association protocol for pre-manipulative testing of the cervical spine: incidence of complications. University of South Australia, Centre for Physiotherapy Research, Adelaide

Gross A R, Aker P D, Quartly C 1996 Manual therapy in the treatment of neck pain. In: Lane N E, Wolfe F (eds) Rheumatic Disease Clinics of North America. Musculoskeletal medicine. W B Saunders, Philadelphia, vol 22

Gutmann G 1983 Injuries to the vertebral artery caused by manual therapy. Manuelle Medizin 21: 2–14

Haldeman S, Kohlbeck F J, McGregor M 1999 Risk factors and precipitating neck movements causing vertebrobasilar artery dissection after cervical trauma and spinal manipulation. Spine 24: 785–794

Haynes M J 1995a Are the effects of local joint movement on blood flow limited to the vertebral and internal carotid arteries? Doppler studies of the ulnar artery. Journal of Manipulative and Physiological Therapeutics 18: 569–571

Haynes M J 1995b Cervical rotational effects on vertebral artery flow: a case study. Chiropractic Journal of Australia 25: 73–76

Haynes M J 1996a Cervical spine adjustments by Perth chiropractors and post-manipulation stroke: has a change occurred? Chiropractic Journal of Australia 26: 43–46

Haynes M J 1996b Doppler studies comparing the effects of cervical rotation and lateral flexion on vertebral artery blood flow. Journal of Manipulative and Physiological Therapeutics 19: 378–384

Haynes M J 2000 Vertebral arteries and neck rotation: Doppler velocimeter and duplex results compared. Ultrasound in Medicine and Biology 26: 57–62

Haynes M J, Milne N 2000 Color duplex sonographic findings in human vertebral arteries during cervical rotation. Journal of Clinical Ultrasound 29(1): 14–24

Haynes M J, Hart R, McGeachie J 2000 Vertebral arteries and neck rotation: Doppler velocimeter interexaminer reliability. Ultrasound in Medicine and Biology 26: 1363–1367

Haynes M J, Cala L A, Melsom A, Mastaglia F L, Milne N, McGeachie J K 2002 Vertebral arteries and cervical rotation: modelling and magnetic resonance angiography studies. Journal of Manipulative and Physiological Therapeutics 25: 370–383

Heary R F, Albert T J, Ludwig S C et al 1996 Surgical anatomy of the vertebral arteries. Spine 21: 2074–2080

Hedera P, Bujdáková J, Traubner P 1993 Blood flow velocities in basilar artery during rotation of the head. Acta Neurologica Scandinavica 88: 229–233

Hinse P, Thie A, Lachenmayer L 1991 Dissection of the extra-cranial vertebral artery: report of four cases and review of the literature. Journal of Neurology, Neurosurgery, and Psychiatry 54: 863–869

Hollinshead W H 1966 Anatomy for surgeons: the head and neck. Hoeber-Harper International, New York, vol 1

Hurwitz E L, Aker P D, Adams A H, Meeker W C, Shekelle P G 1996 Manipulation and mobilization of the cervical spine: a systematic review of the literature. Spine 21: 1746–1760

Hutchinson E C, Yates P O 1956 The cervical portion of the vertebral artery: a clinico-pathological study. Brain 79: 319–331

Hutchison M S 1989 An investigation of premanipulative dizziness testing. In: Jones H M, Jones M A, Milde M R (eds) In: Proceedings of the Sixth Biennial Conference of the Manipulative Therapists Association of Australia. Manipulative Therapists Association of Australia, Adelaide

Ivancic J J, Bryce D, Bolton P S 1993 Use of provocational tests by clinicians to predict vulnerability of patients to vertebrobasilar insufficiency. Chiropractic Journal of Australia 23: 59–63

Jaskoviak P A 1980 Complications arising from manipulation of the cervical spine. Journal of Manipulative and Physiological Therapeutics 3: 213–219

Johnson C P, Scraggs M, How T, Burns J 1995 A necropsy and histomorphometric study of abnormalities in the course of the vertebral artery associated with ossified stylohyoid ligaments. Journal of Clinical Pathology 48: 637–640

Johnson C, Grant R, Dansie B, Taylor J, Spyropolous P 2000 Measurement of blood flow in the vertebral artery using colour duplex Doppler ultrasound: establishment of the reliability of selected parameters. Manual Therapy 5: 21–29

Keller H M, Meier W E, Kumpe D A 1976 Noninvasive angiography for the diagnosis of vertebral artery disease using Doppler ultrasound (vertebral artery Doppler). Stroke 7: 364–369

Kleynhans A M, Terrett A G J 1985 The prevention of complications from spinal manipulative therapy. In: Glasgow E F, Twomey L T, Scull E R, Kleynhans A M, Idczak R M (eds) Aspects of manipulative therapy. Churchill Livingstone, Melbourne

Klougart N, Leboeuf-Y de C, Rasmussen L R 1996 Safety in chiropractic practice. II: Treatment to the upper neck and the rate of cerebrovascular incidents. Journal of Manipulative and Physiological Therapeutics 19: 563–569

Krueger B R, Okazaki H 1980 Vertebral-basilar distribution infarction following chiropractic cervical manipulation. Mayo Clinic Proceedings 55: 322–332

Kunnasmaa K T T, Thiel H W 1994 Vertebral artery syndrome: a review of the literature. Journal of Orthopaedic Medicine 16: 17–20

Lamberty B G H, Zivanovic S 1973 The retro-articular vertebral artery ring of the atlas and its significance. Acta Anatomica 85: 113–122

Laslett M 1988 Vertigo and its relationship to the cervical syndrome. In: Proceedings of the Annual Conference of the New Zealand Manipulative Therapists Association. New Zealand Manipulative Therapists Association, Wellington

Lee K P, Carlini W G, McCormick G F, Albers G W 1995 Neurologic complications following chiropractic manipulation: a survey of California neurologists. Neurology 45: 1213–1215

Lewit K 1992 Clinical picture and diagnosis of vertebral artery insufficiency. Journal of Manual Medicine 6: 190–193

Li Y-K, Zhang Y-K, Lu C-M, Zhong S-Z 1999 Changes and implications of blood flow velocity of the vertebral artery during rotation and extension of the head. Journal of Manipulative and Physiological Therapeutics 22: 91–95

Licht P B, Christensen H W, Højgaard P, Høilund-Carlsen P F 1998 Triplex ultrasound of vertebral artery flow during cervical rotation. Journal of Manipulative and Physiological Therapeutics 21: 27–31

Licht P B, Christensen H W, Høilund-Carlsen P F 1999a Vertebral artery volume flow in human beings. Journal of Manipulative and Physiological Therapeutics 22: 363–367

Licht P B, Christensen H W, Svendsen P, Høilund-Carlsen P F 1999b Vertebral artery flow and cervical manipulation: an experimental study. Journal of Manipulative and Physiological Therapeutics 22: 431–435

Licht P B, Christensen H W, Hoilund-Carlsen P F 2000 Is there a role for premanipulative testing before cervical manipulation? Journal of Manipulative and Physiological Therapeutics 23: 175–179

Macchi C, Catini C, Gulisano M, Pacini P, Brizzi E, Bigazzi P 1995 The anatomical variations of the human extracranial vertebral arteries: a statistical investigation of 90 living subjects using MRI and color Doppler method. Italian Journal of Anatomy and Embryology 100: 53–59

Macchi C, Giannelli F, Cecchi F et al 1996 The inner diameter of human intracranial vertebral artery by color doppler method. Italian Journal of Anatomy and Embryology 101: 81–87

Madawi A A, Solanki G, Casey A T H, Crockard H A 1997 Variation of the groove in the axis vertebra for the vertebral artery: implications for instrumentation. Journal of Bone and Joint Surgery 79B: 820–823

Maitland G D 1986 Vertebral manipulation, 5th edn. Butterworths, London

Mann T W 1995 Mechanisms of non-traumatic vertebral artery injury from manipulation of the cervical spine: implications for the Australian Physiotherapy Association protocol for pre-manipulative testing. In: Proceedings of the Ninth Biennial Conference of the Manipulative Physiotherapists Association of Australia. Manipulative Physiotherapists Association of Australia, Gold Coast

Mas J-L, Henin D, Bousser M G, Chain F, Hauw J J 1989 Dissecting aneurysm of the vertebral artery and cervical manipulation: a case review with autopsy. Neurology 39: 512–515

Meadows J 1992 Safety considerations in vertebral artery testing. In: Proceedings of the Fifth International Conference of the International Federation of Orthopaedic Manipulative Therapists. International Federation of Orthopaedic Manipulative Therapists, Vail

Meadows J T S, Magee D J 1994 An overview of dizziness and vertigo for the orthopaedic manual therapist. In: Boyling J D, Palastanga N (eds) Grieve's Modern Manual Therapy: the Vertebral Column. Churchill Livingstone, Edinburgh

Mestan M A 1999 Posterior fossa ischemia and bilateral vertebral artery hypoplasia. Journal of Manipulative and Physiological Therapeutics 22: 245–249

Michaeli A 1991 Dizziness testing of the cervical spine: can complications of manipulations be prevented? Physiotherapy Theory and Practice 7: 243–250

Michaeli A 1993 Reported occurrence and nature of complications following manipulative physiotherapy in South Africa. Australian Journal of Physiotherapy 39: 309–315

Michaud T C 2002 Uneventful upper cervical manipulation in the presence of a damaged vertebral artery. Journal of Manipulative and Physiological Therapeutics 25: 472–483

Middleditch A 1991 The cervical spine: safe in our hands? In: Proceedings of the Eleventh International Congress of the World Confederation For Physical Therapy. World Confederation For Physical Therapy, London, book III

Mitchell J, McKay A 1995 Comparison of left and right vertebral artery intra-cranial diameters. Anatomical Record 242: 350–354

Monaghan M 2001 Spinal manipulation: a manual for physiotherapists. Aesculapius, Nelson

Mulligan B 1991 Vertigo: manual therapy may be needed. In: Proceedings of the Seventh Biennial Conference of the Manipulative Physiotherapists Association of Australia. Manipulative Physiotherapists Association of Australia, Blue Mountains

Mulligan B R 1999 Manual therapy 'NAGS', 'SNAGS', 'MWMS' etc., 4th edn. Plane View Services, Wellington

Nagler W 1973 Vertebral artery obstruction by hyperextension of the neck: report of three cases. Archives of Physical Medicine and Rehabilitation 54: 237–240

Nelson E, Rennels M 1970 Innervation of intra-cranial arteries. Brain 93: 475–490

Nicolau C, Gilabert R, Chamorro A, Vázquez F, Baragalló N, Concepció B 2000 Doppler sonography of the intertransverse segment of the vertebral artery. Journal of Ultrasound in Medicine 19: 47–53

Norris J W, Beletsky V, Nadareishvili Z G 2000 Sudden neck movement and cervical artery dissection. Canadian Medical Association Journal 163: 38–40

Okawara S, Nibbelink D 1974 Vertebral artery occlusion following hyperextension and rotation of the head. Stroke 5: 640–642

Oostendorp R A B 1988 Vertebrobasilar insufficiency. In: Proceedings of the Fourth International Conference of the International Federation of Orthopaedic Manipulative Therapists. International Federation of Orthopaedic Manipulative Therapists, Cambridge

Oostendorp R A B, Hagenaars L H A, Fischer A J E M, Keyser A, Oosterveld W J, Pool J J M 1992a Dutch standard for 'cervicogenic dizziness'. In: Proceedings of the Fifth International Conference of the International Federation of Orthopaedic Manipulative Therapists. International Federation of Orthopaedic Manipulative Therapists, Vail

Oostendorp R A B, van Eupen A A J M, Elvers J W H 1992b Aspects of sympathetic nervous system regulation in patients with cervicogenic vertigo: 20 years experience. In: Proceedings of the Fifth International Conference of the International Federation of Orthopaedic Manipulative Therapists. International Federation of Orthopaedic Manipulative Therapists, Vail

Oppel U, Fritz G, Struckhoff H J, Drüppel D 1989 Motion effects on blood flow of the vertebral artery and width of cervical intervertebral foramina. In: Louis R, Weidner A (eds) Cervical spine II. Springer-Verlag, New York

Petersen B, Maravic M von, Zeller J A, Walker M L, Kömpf D, Kessler C 1996 Basilar artery blood flow during head rotation in vertebrobasilar ischemia. Acta Neurologica Scandinavica 94: 294–301

Petty N J, Moore A P 1998 Neuromusculoskeletal examination and assessment: a handbook for therapists. Churchill Livingstone, Edinburgh

Powell V J 1990 An investigation of testing procedures for vertebrobasilar insufficiency. Australian Journal of Physiotherapy 36: 31

Pratt N 1996 Anatomy of the cervical spine. In: Beattie P (ed) Orthopaedic physical therapy home study course 96-1. Orthopaedic Section, American Physical Therapy Association, La Crosse

Pratt-Thomas H R, Berger K E 1947 Cerebellar and spinal injuries after chiropractic manipulation. Journal of the American Medical Association 133: 600–603

Raskind R, North C M 1990 Vertebral artery injuries following chiropractic cervical spine manipulation: case reports. Angiology 41: 445–452

Refshauge K M 1994 Rotation: a valid premanipulative dizziness test? Does it predict safe manipulation? Journal of Manipulative and Physiological Therapeutics 17: 15–19

Refshauge K M 1995 Testing adequacy of cerebral blood flow (vertebral artery testing). In: Refshauge K M, Gass E M (eds) Musculoskeletal physiotherapy: clinical science and practice. Butterworth Heinemann, Oxford

Refshauge K M, Parry S, Shirley D, Larsen D, Rivett D A, Boland R 2002 Professional responsibility in relation to cervical spine manipulation. Australian Journal of Physiotherapy 48: 171–179

Reif R A 1996 Evaluation and differential diagnosis of the cervical spine. In: Beattie P (ed) Orthopaedic physical therapy home study course 96-1. Orthopaedic Section, American Physical Therapy Association, La Crosse

Rivett D A 1995a Neurovascular compromise complicating cervical spine manipulation: what is the risk? Journal of Manual and Manipulative Therapy 3: 144–151

Rivett D A 1995b The premanipulative vertebral artery testing protocol: a brief review. New Zealand Journal of Physiotherapy 23(1): 9–12

Rivett D A 1997 Preventing neurovascular complications of cervical spine manipulation. Physical Therapy Reviews 2: 29–37

Rivett D A 2001 A valid pre-manipulative screening tool is needed. Australian Journal of Physiotherapy 47: 166

Rivett D A, Reid D 1998 Risk of stroke for cervical spine manipulation in New Zealand. New Zealand Journal of Physiotherapy 26(2): 14–17

Rivett D A, Milburn P D, Chapple C 1998 Negative pre-manipulative vertebral artery testing despite complete occlusion: a case of false negativity? Manual Therapy 3: 102–107

Rivett D A, Sharples K J, Milburn P D 1999 Effect of pre-manipulative tests on vertebral artery and internal carotid artery blood flow: a pilot study. Journal of Manipulative and Physiological Therapeutics 22: 368–375

Rivett D, Sharples K, Milburn P 2000 Vertebral artery blood flow during pre-manipulative testing of the cervical spine. In: Singer K P (ed) Proceedings of the International Federation of Orthopaedic and Manipulative Therapists Conference. International Federation of Orthopaedic and Manipulative Therapists, Perth

Rivett H M 1994 Cervical manipulation: confronting the spectre of the vertebral artery syndrome. Journal of Orthopaedic Medicine 16: 12–16

Robertson J T 1981 Neck manipulation as a cause of stroke. Stroke 12: 1

Robertson J T 1982 Neck manipulation as a cause of stroke [Letter]. Stroke 13: 260–261

Rothrock J F, Hesselink J R, Teacher T M 1991 Vertebral artery occlusion and stroke from cervical self-manipulation. Neurology 41: 1696–1697

Roy G 1994 The vertebral artery. Journal of Manual and Manipulative Therapy 2: 28–31

Schellhas K P, Latchaw R E, Wendling L R, Gold L H A 1980 Vertebrobasilar injuries following cervical manipulation. Journal of the American Medical Association 244: 1450–1453

Schmitt H P 1991 Anatomical structure of the cervical spine with reference to the pathology of manipulation complications. Journal of Manual Medicine 6: 93–101

Selecki B R 1969 The effects of rotation of the atlas on the axis: experimental work. Medical Journal of Australia 1: 1012–1015

Sherman D G, Hart R G, Easton J D 1981 Abrupt change in head position and cerebral infarction. Stroke 12: 2–6

Sheth T N, Winslow J L, Mikulis D J 2001 Rotational changes in the morphology of the vertebral artery at a common site of artery dissection. Canadian Association of Radiologists Journal 52: 236–241

Simeone F A, Goldberg H I 1968 Thrombosis of the vertebral artery from hyperextension injury to the neck: case report. Journal of Neurosurgery 29: 540–544

Simon H, Niederkorn K, Horner S, Duft M, Schröckenfuchs M 1994 The influence of head rotation on the vertebrobasilar system: a transcranial Doppler sonography study. HNO 42: 614–618

South African Society of Physiotherapy (SASP) 1991 Protocol for pre-manipulative testing of the cervical spine. South African Journal of Physiotherapy 41: 15–17

Stevens A 1991 Functional Doppler sonography of the vertebral artery and some considerations about manual techniques. Journal of Manual Medicine 6: 102–105

Sturzenneger M, Newell D W, Douville C, Byrd S, Schoonover K 1994 Dynamic transcranial Doppler assessment of positional vertebrobasilar ischemia. Stroke 25: 1776–1783

Symons B P, Leonard T, Herzog W 2002 Internal forces sustained by the vertebral artery during spinal manipulative therapy. Journal of Manipulative and Physiological Therapeutics 25: 504–510

Takahashi I, Kaneko S, Asaoka K, Harada T 1994 Angiographic examination of the vertebral artery at the atlantoaxial joint during head rotation. Neurological Surgery 22: 749–753

Teasell R W, Marchuk Y 1994 Vertebro-basilar artery stroke as a complication of cervical manipulation. Critical Reviews in Physical and Rehabilitation Medicine 6: 121–129

Terenzi T J, DeFabio D C 1996 The role of transcranial Doppler sonography in the identification of patients at risk of cerebral and brainstem ischemia. Journal of Manipulative and Physiological Therapeutics 19: 406–414

Terrett A G J 1987a Vascular accidents from cervical spine manipulation: report on 107 cases. Journal of the Australian Chiropractors' Association 17: 15–24

Terrett A G J 1987b Vascular accidents from cervical spine manipulation: the mechanisms. Journal of the Australian Chiropractors Association 17: 131–144

Thiel H W 1991 Gross morphology and pathoanatomy of the vertebral arteries. Journal of Manipulative and Physiological Therapeutics 14: 133–141

Thiel H W, Wallace K, Donat J, Yong-Hing K 1994 Effect of various head and neck positions on vertebral artery blood flow. Clinical Biomechanics 9: 105–110

Tissington-Tatlow W F, Bammer H G 1957 Syndrome of vertebral artery compression. Neurology 7: 331–340

Toole J F, Tucker S H 1960 Influence of head position upon cerebral circulation. Archives of Neurology 2: 616–623

Van Overbeeke J J, Hillen B, Tulleken C A F 1991 A comparative study of the circle of Willis in fetal and adult life: the configuration of the posterior bifurcation of the posterior communicating artery. Journal of Anatomy 176: 45–54

Weingart J R, Bischoff H-P 1992 Doppler sonography of the vertebral artery with regard to head positions appropriate to manual medicine. Journal of Manual Medicine 30: 62–65

Weinstein S M, Cantu R C 1991 Cerebral stroke in a semi-pro football player: a case report. Medicine and Science in Sports and Exercise 23: 1119–1121

Weintraub M I, Khoury A 1995 Critical neck position as an independent risk factor for posterior circulation stroke: a magnetic resonance angiographic analysis. Journal of Neuroimaging 5: 16–22

Welsh L W, Welsh J J, Lewin B 2000 Basilar artery and vertigo. Annals of Otology, Rhinology and Laryngology 109: 615–622

Westaway M D, Stratford P, Symons B 2003 False-negative extension/rotation pre-manipulative screening test on a patient with an atretic and hypoplastic vertebral artery. Manual Therapy 8: 120–127

White A A, Panjabi M M 1990 Clinical biomechanics of the spine, 2nd edn. J B Lippincott, Philadelphia

Williams D, Wilson T G 1962 The diagnosis of the major and minor syndromes of basilar insufficiency. Brain 85: 741–774

Wing L W, Hargrave-Wilson W 1974 Cervical vertigo. New Zealand Journal of Surgery 44: 275–277

Worth D R 1988 Biomechanics of the cervical spine. In: Grant R (ed) Clinics in Physical Therapy. Physical therapy of the cervical and thoracic spine. Churchill Livingstone, New York, vol 17

Zaina C, Grant R, Johnson C, Dansie B, Taylor J, Spyropolous P 2003 The effect of cervical rotation on blood flow in the contralateral vertebral artery. Manual Therapy 8: 103–109

Chapter 20

Mechanisms underlying pain and dysfunction in whiplash associated disorders: implications for physiotherapy management

M. Sterling, J. Treleaven, G. A. Jull

INTRODUCTION

The mechanisms underlying the persistence of pain and other symptoms following a whiplash injury are poorly understood and are controversial at present. Most people experiencing neck pain as a result of a motor vehicle crash recover quickly, but there are reports that indicate that between 4% and 42% of injured people will develop chronic pain and disability, often for many years (Eck et al 2001). The economic costs related to whiplash, and particularly to those who develop prolonged symptoms, are substantial. The costs to patients in terms of loss of quality of life likewise cannot be ignored.

Treatment strategies evaluated to date in both the acute and chronic stages of whiplash associated disorders (WAD) are yet to demonstrate efficacy in terms of decreasing the incidence of those who develop persistent symptoms (Borchgrevink et al 1998, Provinciali et al 1996, Rosenfeld et al 2000, Soderlund et al 2000). One reason for this may be the non-specific nature of the treatments that have been investigated which appear to view WAD as a homogenous condition with little consideration given to the potential mechanisms involved. It would appear that WAD is a more complex condition than previously assumed. Recently, investigations have begun to shed light on some of the mechanisms which may contribute to the persistence of symptoms in this condition.

This chapter will outline and discuss current evidence for mechanisms underlying persistent pain and disability in WAD, prognostic indicators of outcome, implications for management based on this evidence and directions for future research.

THE WHIPLASH INJURY

The cardinal feature of WAD is neck pain (Barnsley et al 1994, Sterling et al 2002a). It occurs typically in the posterior region of the neck but can also radiate to the head, shoulder and arm, thoracic, interscapular and lumbar regions. Symptoms such as headache, dizziness/loss of balance, visual disturbances, paraesthesia, anaesthesia, weakness and cognitive disturbances such as concentration and memory difficulties are common (Barnsley et al 1994, Radanov & Dvorak 1996, Treleaven et al 2003).

Diagnosis of the pathology involved is difficult due to the lack of findings with current radiological imaging techniques (Davis et al 1991, Pettersson et al 1994). However, evidence from cadaveric and animal studies indicates that lesions may occur to almost any cervical structure during a whiplash injury, including injury to the bony elements, discs and zygapophysial joints, ligaments, muscles and neural tissues (Table 20.1). The zygapophysial joint has been studied extensively, both in post mortem studies and at surgery (Barnsley et al 1998, Jonsson et al 1991, Taylor & Taylor 1996). Lord et al (1996) linked zygapophysial arthropathy with chronic WAD by achieving substantial pain relief in some patients with persistent pain following a whiplash injury using zygapophysial joint blocks. Fractures and dislocations of the atlanto-axial complex may cause death (Jonsson et al 1991), but injuries such as fractures of the odontoid peg, laminae and articular processes (Barnsley et al 1994, Schonstrom et al 1993) as well as injury to soft tissues such as synovial fold bruising (Schonstrom et al 1993), have been observed in survivors. Examination (manual) for alar ligament damage is commonly performed by physiotherapists (Swinkels & Oostendorp 1996) but the frequency

Table 20.1 Pathologies identified following whiplash injury

Pathology	References
Zygapophysial joints Haemarthroses Capsular tears Articular cartilage damage Joint fractures Joint capsule rupture	Jonsson et al 1991[1], Taylor & Taylor 1996[1], Yoganandan et al 2001[3], Lord & Bogduk 1996[4]
Intervertebral disc Rim lesions Bleeding – no disruption Disruption/avulsion Disc herniation	Jonsson et al 1991[1], Jonsson et al 1994[2], Taylor & Taylor 1996[1], Pettersson et al 1997[2]
Ligaments Anterior/posterior longitudinal ligament Ligamentum flavum	Taylor & Taylor 1996[1], Yoganandan et al 2001[3]
Muscles Prevertebral muscle injury Longus colli rupture	Jonsson et al 1991[1]
Atlanto-axial complex Synovial fold bruising Ligament ruptures Fractures	Jonsson et al 1991[1], Schonstrom et al 1993[1], Taylor & Taylor 1996[1]
Nerve tissue injury Bleeding around C2 nerve Nerve root injuries Dorsal root ganglia injuries Spinal cord/brain stem	Jonsson et al 1991[1], Seitz et al 1995[5], Taylor & Taylor 1996[1]
Fractures Vertebral bodies Transverse processes	Jonsson et al 1991[1], Taylor & Taylor 1996[1]
Other Vertebral artery damage	Taylor & Taylor 1996[1]

[1]Post mortem; [2]magnetic resonance imaging, [3]experimental (cadaver)/radiography, [4]controlled diagnostic blocks, [5]SPECT.

of alar ligament damage in WAD is controversial. Dvorak et al (1987), using cadaver material and computed tomography (CT), proposed that alar ligament lesions are present in 4.5% of whiplash patients. However, this was not confirmed by later studies using magnetic resonance imaging or CT (Patijn et al 2001, Willauschus et al 1995).

Pathology of nerve tissue has also been demonstrated in cadaver studies, including primary lesions to spinal nerves, nerve roots, dorsal root ganglia and even the spinal cord (Taylor & Taylor 1996). Irritation of nerve tissue may also occur as a consequence of inflammatory processes in damaged neighbouring structures including the zygapophysial joints and intervertebral discs (Eliav et al 1999, Taylor & Taylor 1996). In this case, nerve conduction often remains intact but the nerve tissue is highly mechanosensitive, most likely due to sensitization of C fibres from axons in continuity, producing ectopic discharge with little or no neuronal degeneration (Eliav et al 1999, 2001, Tal 1999). Due to intact nerve conduction, diagnosis is difficult and at this stage relies on clinical assessment. The presence of irritated or mechanosensitive nerve tissue has been demonstrated clinically in some subjects with persistent WAD using Tinel's test over various peripheral nerve trunk sites of the upper limb (Ide et al 2001) and the brachial plexus provocation test (Sterling et al 2002b).

Few cervical structures are immune from potential injury following whiplash. Despite the substantial evidence for the presence of pathology in WAD, the underlying mechanisms responsible for the persistence of symptoms in some people are not clear. As a consequence, recent research has begun to focus on and elucidate some features of chronic WAD that are suggestive of changes in physiological processes. From this research a model can be proposed which postulates that the initial injury leads to multifactorial inter-related changes in physiological systems which are apparent at 3 months post injury and contribute to persistent pain and disability (Fig. 20.1). The following sections will explore this model.

PAIN SYSTEM CHANGES

Peripheral nociception and central nervous system hypersensitivity

Whiplash injury is a trauma to peripheral tissues that may include articular structures, muscles and nerve tissue. It is now well known that tissue inflammation and/or peripheral nerve injury increases the sensitivity and lowers the threshold of peripheral nociceptors (Aδ and C fibres) resulting in the development of primary hyperalgesia (surrounding the site of injury) which is characterized by both mechanical and thermal hyperalgesia (Treede et al 1992). This leads to a cascade of events in the dorsal horn rendering second order neurons hyperexcitable. This sensitization of neurons in the dorsal horn of the spinal cord is believed to be the mechanism responsible for the phenomena of secondary hyperalgesia (outside the site of injury and characterized by mechanical hyperalgesia) and allodynia (pain with non-noxious stimuli such as light touch) (Ziegler et al 1999), both of which are familiar to the clinician treating patients with WAD.

Despite the explosion of knowledge regarding the plasticity of the nervous system in the presence of pain and tissue inflammation, it has only been fairly recently that these factors have been investigated in WAD. Sheather-Reid & Cohen (1998) demonstrated decreases in pain threshold

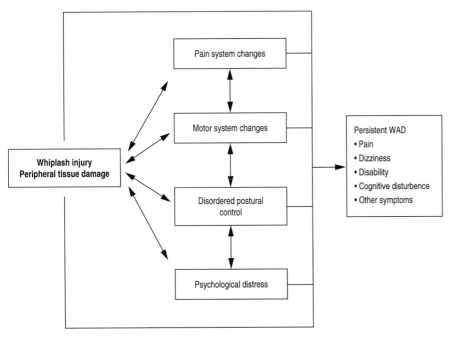

Figure 20.1 Proposed model of the development of chronic whiplash associated disorders.

and pain tolerance to electrocutaneous stimulation at sites within the cervical spine in chronic neck pain subjects (both WAD and non-traumatic neck pain). These authors hypothesized that because no overt peripheral pathology could be diagnosed, then these responses were evidence of secondary hyperalgesia as a result of sensitization of central pain processing pathways. Although this hypothesis may be valid, the possibility of ongoing local pathology being responsible for the findings could not be dismissed, as poor healing of some cervical structures and the persistence of local pathology have been demonstrated 18 months to 2 years post accident (Taylor & Taylor 1996). Further to the argument that the presence of an ongoing peripheral nociceptive source of pain may be a contributory factor to persistent symptoms in WAD are the findings that elimination of a peripheral nociceptive source of pain, using zygapophysial joint blocks, can alleviate pain in some cases (Lord et al 1996). Furthermore, hyperalgesic responses to heat stimuli have been demonstrated in the cervical spine of subjects with chronic WAD (Sterling & Jull 2001). Heat hyperalgesia is believed to be a feature of primary hyperalgesia or sensitization of peripheral nociceptors as it is not present in areas of secondary hyperalgesia (Koltzenburg 2000, Ziegler et al 1999). Although this evidence is preliminary, it nevertheless suggests that the presence of an ongoing peripheral source of pain in the cervical spine cannot and should not be overlooked as contributing to ongoing pain in these patients and has obvious implications for physiotherapy management.

Due to the evidence of plastic changes in the central nervous system following injury and inflammation, it is unlikely that a peripheral source of pain is the only contributor to persistence of pain following a whiplash injury. Spinal sensitization is likely also to play a role. Although Sheather-Reid & Cohen (1998) suggested this following their study using electrocutaneous stimuli within the cervical spine, later studies have taken this further by investigating responses to various stimuli at areas unrelated to the site of injury.

Koelbaek-Johansen et al (1999) demonstrated muscle hyperalgesia and larger referred pain areas following intramuscular saline injection into both local (infraspinatus) and remote (tibialis anterior) muscles to the site of pain. Similar results have been found using electrical stimuli, both transcutaneous and intramuscular (Curatolo et al 2001). These authors demonstrated that hypersensitivity was not decreased following local anaesthesia of tender neck muscles, which they interpreted as reinforcing the role of central nervous system mechanisms (Curatolo et al 2001). However, it should be noted that anaesthesia of deeper tissues such as articular structures was not performed so that ongoing nociceptive input from such tissues could not be ruled out as contributing to the hypersensitivity. In a larger study, Sterling et al (2002a) found widespread areas of lowered pain thresholds to mechanical stimuli using pressure algometry in 150 subjects with chronic WAD (Fig. 20.2).

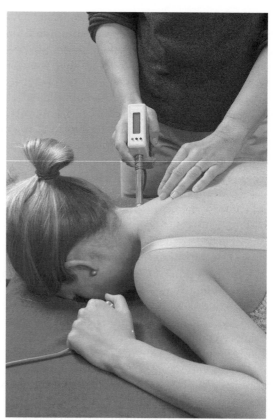

Figure 20.2 Measurement of mechanical hyperalgesia using pressure algometer.

Hypersensitivity was found over the posterior cervical region, over nerve tissue in the upper limbs and over a remote site in the lower limb (muscle belly of tibialis anterior). None of the subjects experienced pain in their lower limbs. While 50% of the subjects reported arm pain, there was no difference in pressure pain thresholds between those with and without arm symptoms. The lowered pressure pain thresholds within the cervical spine showed similar non-specificity with there being no difference in upper cervical spine sites (including the suboccipital nerve) between those who did and did not report headache. These widespread, generalized areas of mechanical hyperalgesia were suggested to be as a result of central nervous system hypersensitivity as a consequence of spinal cord sensitization (Sterling et al 2002a).

Allodynia is defined as pain to a stimulus that is normally not painful (such as light touch or brushing). It is believed to be mediated by activity in Aβ fibres with low threshold mechanoreceptors (Koltzenburg et al 1994). Although anecdotally this has been reported to be present in whiplash patients, it is yet to be extensively investigated. Preliminary evidence for the presence of allodynia comes from a study by Moog et al (1999) who demonstrated pain with vibration (a non-painful stimulus) in 28 of 43 chronic whiplash subjects. Interestingly, only one subject in this study reported pain with light touch, another feature of allodynia.

To date, only one longitudinal study has investigated hyperalgesic responses over time. Kasch et al (2001c) measured pressure pain thresholds over sites in the head and neck muscles and over a distant site in the hand and compared the results to a control group of subjects with acute ankle sprains. The whiplash subjects demonstrated decreased pressure pain thresholds in the head and neck at 1 and 3 months post injury but the groups were similar at 6 months. No difference between the groups existed at the distant site at any time frame (Kasch et al 2001c). At first examination of these results, it would appear that they are not supportive of the model of hypersensitivity in chronic WAD proposed by Koelbaek-Johansen et al (1999) and Sterling et al (2002b, 2002c). However in Kasch et al's (2001a) study, only 10% of the 141 whiplash subjects continued to report symptoms at 6-months post injury. These subjects were not analysed separately so the measures at the six month time frame were mainly of subjects who recovered and who would not be expected to demonstrate continuing hyperalgesia in the head and neck. Further investigation of the development of hyperalgesia and other evidence of altered pain processing is required in those who do not recover from their injury in the short term.

Hyperalgesia: motor manifestations

Alterations in the way pain is processed are not only represented by sensory responses. Hyperalgesic responses may also be manifested by changes in motor activity (Sterling et al 2001). One such motor response is the heightened flexor withdrawal response that occurs in the presence of nociceptive input from cutaneous, muscle and articular tissue. It has been observed in both animal and human studies (Andersen et al 2000, Wall & Woolf 1984). Although possibly a short lasting effect in the presence of transient pain (Andersen et al 2000), the flexor withdrawal response is believed to be more long lasting with ongoing pain (Andersen et al 2000, Gronroos & Pertovaara 1993). The loss of range of movement (usually elbow extension) seen clinically in the brachial plexus provocation test is likely to be due to a motor response to protect mechanosensitive nerve tissue (Elvey 1997, Hall & Elvey 1999). This response has been likened to a heightened flexor withdrawal response (Hall et al 1993, Wright et al 1994).

Hypersensitive responses (motor) to the brachial plexus provocation test (BPPT) have been demonstrated in 156 chronic whiplash subjects when compared to 95 healthy asymptomatic volunteers (Sterling et al 2002b). While whiplash subjects with clinical signs of mechanosensitive nerve tissue (25% of the cohort) demonstrated a greater loss of elbow extension at submaximal pain threshold, all whiplash subjects demonstrated significantly less elbow extension than the control group. In both groups these responses occurred bilaterally. These findings of generalized hypersensitive motor responses to the BPPT may represent motor correlates of central sensitization (Sterling et al 2002b).

A recent study has also demonstrated abnormalities in inhibitory, anti-nociceptive brain stem reflexes of the temporalis muscles of 82 subjects with acute post-traumatic headache following whiplash injury (Keidel et al 2001). The authors suggest this is further evidence of altered central pain control but it is as yet unknown whether it persists into the period of chronicity.

Sympathetic nervous system

Some patients with whiplash will report symptoms such as vasomotor changes, burning pain or cold hyperalgesia that may be suggestive of altered sympathetic nervous system activity. The sympathetic nervous system may become secondarily activated following whiplash injury. Peripheral nerve injury has been shown to be associated with sprouting of sympathetic nerve fibres into the dorsal root ganglia, thereby stimulating them when the sympathetic nervous system is activated (Munglani 2000). In addition, peripheral pain receptors can become sensitive to circulating noradrenaline (norepinephrine) that is released during stressful events (Devor 1991). Therefore activation of the sympathetic nervous system, as with weather changes or in times of stress and anxiety, may aggravate the pain and produce apparently bizarre symptoms (Munglani 2000). Evidence for sympathetic nervous system involvement in the maintenance of symptoms in WAD is at present mainly speculative. Ide et al (2001) in their study of whiplash showed that 58% of subjects who had evidence of nerve tissue irritation had high scores on the autonomic questions of the Cornell Medical Index Health Questionnaire. Adeboye et al (2000) reported on a single case history whereby the patient following a whiplash injury presented with circulatory disturbances of the hands believed to be due to cervical sympathetic chain dysfunction. In light of these findings further investigation of autonomic disturbances is required.

Summary

It would appear that the presence of hypersensitivity manifested by both sensory and motor responses, as a result of altered pain processing within the central nervous system, are likely to be a contributing factor to the persistence of pain in chronic WAD. The causes of the maintenance of this hypersensitive state are not completely understood; however, it is generally believed that ongoing peripheral nociceptive sources are a driving factor (Devor 1997, Gracely et al 1992). In the case of WAD, this could be the continued presence of pathology in injured cervical structures or perhaps secondary changes such as impaired neuromuscular and proprioceptive deficits perpetuating ongoing pain from cervical structures (Jull 2000). Why some people who have a whiplash injury go on to display these phenomena and others do not is not yet completely understood. Genetic differences may be one factor (Munglani 2000) while the temporal and spatial extent of the initial nociceptive barrage into the spinal cord may be another (Devor 1997).

MOTOR SYSTEM CHANGES

Motor system dysfunction has been reported in patients with persistent WAD (Dall'Alba et al 2001, Heikkilä & Astrom 1996, Jull 2000, Nederhand et al 2000). This dysfunction is reflected in changes in active range of cervical movement, increased electromyographic (EMG) activity in neck and shoulder girdle muscles, altered patterns of muscle recruitment and disturbances in postural control.

Active range of cervical movement

Arguably the most easily identified clinical finding in whiplash patients is that of restricted neck movement. Measures of range of cervical movement are often used to evaluate outcome following treatment and to quantify disability (American Medical Association 1993, Borchgrevink et al 1998). Reduced active range of movement in all the primary movement directions has been shown in subjects with persistent WAD when compared to healthy asymptomatic control subjects (Bono et al 2000, Dall'Alba et al 2001, Heikkilä & Wenngren 1998) and non-traumatic headache subjects (Dumas 2001). In our study, we also investigated conjunct (or associated) movements in WAD and found few differences when compared to an asymptomatic control group (Dall'Alba et al 2001). Where a difference existed, it was a reduction in the amount of movement as opposed to deviations from the coupling directions. However, the measurement of conjunct movement was in gross terms of active movement and not an indication of intersegmental movement. This study also demonstrated that when conjunct (or associated) range of movement, age and gender were taken into account, primary range of active movement could correctly classify 90% of subjects as either asymptomatic or those with WAD (Dall'Alba et al 2001). Decreased active range of movement has also been demonstrated in acute WAD (Kasch et al 2001b, Osterbauer et al 1996). Kasch et al (2001b) showed improvement in movement at 3 months post injury but no differentiation was made between those individuals who recovered and those with persistent symptoms. Research from our laboratories has demonstrated decreased cervical range of motion in subjects with acute WAD (less than 1 month post injury) with restoration of full movement by 3 months post injury in recovered subjects and those with persistent mild pain. However, those subjects with persistent moderate/severe symptoms at 3 months demonstrated continued loss of movement (Sterling et al 2003).

Although it can probably be expected that active range of movement will be decreased following whiplash injury, these studies do not provide information on the cause of the restricted active range of movement in WAD. Factors such as mechanical changes in the soft tissues themselves, pain inhibition, muscle spasm and guarding, altered movement patterns in response to pain, fear of movement or a combination of one or more of the above could be involved. Nevertheless, findings of our studies (Sterling et al 2003) have shown that loss of range of motion in patients with persistent moderate/severe symptoms of WAD is not totally explained by the subjects' fear of movement/reinjury, confirming suggestions that the relationship between fear avoidance beliefs and disability in cervical pain may be weaker than that for lumbar pain (George et al 2001).

Altered patterns of muscle recruitment

Many studies investigating motor activity in chronic WAD have sought to ascertain the presence of heightened or increased activity in muscles – a phenomenon purported to be seen in the clinical situation and to which treatment is often directed. Early evidence suggested a decreased ability to relax selected neck/shoulder muscles following high load endurance activities of the upper limbs or neck (Barton & Hayes 1996, Elert et al 2001, Fredin et al 1997). However, as most patients with chronic WAD tend to report pain and disability associated with more functional activities usually involving low load, a more relevant question may be to investigate muscle responses during tasks of low biomechanical load.

One such study by Nederhand et al (2000) investigated activity in upper trapezius following a functional low biomechanical load task of unilateral arm and hand movement between targets along a table in both chronic whiplash subjects and healthy asymptomatic control subjects. The whiplash subjects showed significantly higher electromyographic (EMG) activity in upper trapezius of the resting arm during the activity, and increased activity in both upper trapezius muscles after the subjects had ceased the activity. This decreased ability of the upper trapezius muscles of whiplash subjects to relax following a low load task was hypothesized by the authors as being due to a 'learned guarding response'. These findings could also support the recent proposal that increased activity in superficial muscles may be a measurable compensation for poor deep muscle or ligamentous control of the spinal segment during functional tasks (Cholewicki et al 1997).

In view of the knowledge of effects of joint injury and pain on muscle control in other musculoskeletal conditions (Cowan et al 2000, Hides et al 1996, Hodges et al 1996, Jull 1998, Pienimarki et al 1997), it is likely that patients with neck pain from a whiplash injury would display similar deficits. Jull (2000) demonstrated impaired motor control of the cervical flexors using the staged craniocervical flexion test in subjects with chronic WAD. The whiplash subjects demonstrated higher levels of EMG activity in the superficial neck flexor muscles (sternocleidomastoid) when compared to asymptomatic control subjects while performing the lower stages of the craniocervical flexion test. While acknowledging that the test is an indirect measure, it was suggested that these findings might be indicative of impaired function of the deep cervical flexors. Recently we have demonstrated that such altered patterns of muscle use during craniocervical flexion are apparent within 1 month of whiplash injury and persist to 3 months post injury. These changes occurred not only in those subjects continuing to report persistent pain but also in those who reported symptom resolution by 3 months post accident (Sterling et al 2003). Research of low back pain has shown that changes in the muscle system persist despite initial symptom resolution and may be one factor involved in the high rate of symptom recurrence in this condition (Hides et al 2001). To our knowledge, the frequency of recurrent episodes of neck pain following resolution of acute whiplash symptoms has not been investigated in a similar manner to that of acute first episode low back pain (Von Korff & Saunders 1996).

While changes in motor control result from pain and effusion, some evidence has been provided that suggests that those subjects with inherently less optimal muscle control may have a poorer outcome following a whiplash injury. Vibert et al (2001) investigated responses in asymptomatic participants submitted to brief abrupt changes of acceleration using a custom designed sled. They demonstrated that the subjects could be stereotyped into two groups: 'stiff' subjects and 'floppy' subjects. The stiff subjects were able to stabilize their head on their body using bilateral contractions of the axial muscles whereas the floppy subjects displayed passive behaviour of the head and neck or even inappropriate muscular synergies that might potentially increase the risk of injury. It seems that some people might be able to recruit effective, predefined motor strategies in order to compensate for the high frequency perturbations experienced during a motor vehicle crash. This was postulated as being a possible reason for the variability of neck injuries seen among different passengers and why low-amplitude accelerations can produce injury (Vibert et al 2001).

Disordered postural control mechanisms

Studies of subjects with persistent WAD have demonstrated deficits in cervical joint position error, standing balance and eye movement control which are likely to be a result of disturbed postural control. While there are many possible causes of disturbed postural control following a whiplash injury, disturbed cervical afferent input has been shown to be a likely common cause of these deficits.

Postural control relies on afferent information from the vestibular, visual and proprioceptive systems that converge in the central nervous system. Abnormal input from any of these systems can confuse the postural control system due to a mismatch between abnormal information from one source and normal information from the others. The symptom of dizziness is thought to be a consequence of this mismatch (Baloh & Halmagyi 1996). This has particular relevance to those with persistent WAD where after pain,

dizziness and unsteadiness are the next most frequent complaints. Data from our research on persons with persistent WAD (symptoms for more than 3 months post injury) indicated that 74% report these symptoms. The most common description of these symptoms was unsteadiness (90%). In addition, 48% of subjects reported at least one episode of loss of balance while 21% reported at least one associated fall, putting them at risk of incurring additional trauma (Treleaven et al 2003).

These symptoms are often attributed to medication and the anxiety caused by the ongoing problems (Ferrari & Russell 1999), or it is supposed that they reflect the high prevalence of dizziness in the normal population (Baloh & Halmagyi 1996). Recent evidence suggests that disturbances which may result from traumatic damage to any of the key elements of the postural control system might underlie these symptoms. The whiplash injury may damage vestibular receptors, neck receptors or the central nervous system directly via a mild head injury. The exact cause of the symptoms is often difficult to determine (Baloh & Halmagyi 1996, Chester 1991, Hildingsson et al 1993, Mallinson et al 1996, Rubin et al 1995, Schmand et al 1998, Sturzenegger et al 1994). When there is no traumatic brain injury, there are several lines of research which suggest that disturbed sensory properties of cervical joint and muscle mechanoreceptors and altered muscle spindle activity related to pain could be important in the development of symptoms after a whiplash injury. The disturbed afferentation may result from traumatic damage to the mechanoreceptors, functional impairment or from the effects of nociceptor sensitization, which may alter muscle spindle activity (Chester 1991, Gimse et al 1996, Heikkilä & Astrom 1996, Hildingsson et al 1989, 1993, Mallinson et al 1996, Rubin et al 1995, Thurnberg et al 2001, Tjell & Rosenhall 1998).

Proprioceptors located in the cervical joints and muscles are an important component of afferent information from the proprioceptive system to the postural control system. The deep neck muscles in particular have a vast density of muscle spindles of similar ratio to those in the hand (Peck et al 1984). Proprioceptive reflexes of the neck, the cervico-ocular reflex (COR) and the cervicocollic reflex (CCR) also originate from these cervical afferents and influence ocular control as well as vestibular and proprioceptive integration (Bolton 1998, Peterson et al 1985). The importance of cervical proprioceptive information in the control of posture, spatial orientation and coordination of the eyes and head has also been emphasized in experimental studies (Bolton 1998, Peterson et al 1985). Local anaesthetic injected into the deep tissues of the neck produces unsteadiness, ataxia and a tendency to fall in humans (Brandt 1996, DeJong & DeJong 1977). This demonstrates the potential potency of damage to cervical mechanoreceptors.

Nociceptive sensitization may also alter muscle spindle activity from neck structures and contribute to proprioceptive deficits. In animal studies, inflammatory mediators have been shown to activate chemosensitive nerve endings in both muscles and joints leading to altered muscle spindle activity and subsequent proprioceptive disturbances (Thurnberg et al 2001). There is also some evidence that experimental muscle pain produces central modulation of proprioceptive information from muscle spindles (Capra & Ro 2000). Therefore the influence of pain on muscle spindle afferents as well as its influence on central modulation of proprioceptive information may contribute to disturbed postural control.

Manifestations of disturbance to postural control are highlighted in studies of subjects with persistent WAD that have demonstrated deficits in cervical joint position error, standing balance and eye movement control. There is also suggestion that disturbed afferent input and the subsequent increased burden on the postural control system may also influence cognitive function (Gimse et al 1996, Tjell & Rosenhall 2002).

Cervical joint position error (JPE) is considered primarily to reflect afferent input from the neck joint and muscle receptors. This measure is based on the ability to relocate the natural head posture while vision is occluded (Revel 1991) (Fig. 20.3). Greater JPEs following both rotation and extension movements have been shown in subjects with persistent WAD compared to control subjects (Heikkilä & Astrom 1996, Heikkilä & Wenngren 1998, Kristjansson et al 2003, Treleaven et al 2003). Additionally, Treleaven et al (2003) demonstrated that WAD subjects who complained of dizziness had greater neck repositioning errors in rotation than WAD subjects with out this complaint.

Research investigating posturography and standing balance disturbance in subjects with persistent WAD has shown trends towards reduced standing balance but has been inconclusive (El-Kahky et al 2000, Mallinson et al 1996, Rubin et al 1995). Differences between studies in inclusion/exclusion criteria, methods of signal analysis and the tests investigated make it difficult to draw firm conclusions. Large inter-individual variations were also seen (El-Kahky et al 2000). In a recent study of WAD subjects who were reporting dizziness and unsteadiness we used the

method of sway trace analysis and observed differences in comfortable stance tests in subjects with persistent WAD as compared to control subjects. The total energy of the trace was significantly greater in the WAD group under all test conditions that included eyes open, eyes closed and visual conflict for both firm and soft surfaces (Treleaven et al 2004, unpublished data). These differences were seen in both the anterior–posterior direction and medial–lateral direction. In selected tandem stance tests, WAD subjects with dizziness/unsteadiness failed to complete the test significantly more often than did the control subjects. Deficits in standing balance have also been demonstrated in subjects with neck pain of insidious onset which adds evidence to the possible role of altered afferent input from the cervical afferents in altered balance responses (Alund et al 1993, Dieterich et al 1993, Karlberg et al 1996, Koskimies et al 1997, McPartland et al 1997).

Disturbances in eye movement control have been demonstrated in chronic WAD as well as other musculoskeletal conditions such as fibromyalgia (Hildingsson et al 1993, Mosimann et al 2000, Oosterveld et al 1991, Rosenhall et al 1987, 1996, Tjell & Rosenhall 1998). The underlying pathological basis for these disturbances is not clear but possible explanations include dysfunction within the central nervous system including frontal cortical structures and brain stem, vestibular dysfunction or from erroneous postural proprioceptive activity (Mosimann et al 2000, Tjell & Rosenhall 1998).

Tjell & Rosenhall (1998) compared smooth pursuit eye movement control in subjects with vestibular disorders, central nervous system dysfunction and chronic WAD. When the neck was in a torsioned position (45 degrees trunk rotation), the WAD subjects demonstrated altered smooth pursuit eye movement control compared to a neutral position with a greater loss in those WAD subjects complaining of dizziness. In contrast, although subjects with vestibular disorders and central nervous system dysfunction had greater overall deficits in eye movement control, they did not demonstrate any greater loss of eye movement control with the neck torsioned. This would suggest that altered afferent input from the cervical spine structures is more likely a cause of loss of eye movement control in WAD as opposed to vestibular or central nervous system dysfunction. In a follow-up study, these researchers reported on this test in subjects with non-traumatic neck pain, cervical spondylosis, cervicogenic dizziness and fibromyalgia (Tjell & Rosenhall 2002). Subjects with cervical dizziness and spondylosis demonstrated some differences from the control group. Although those with fibromyalgia had deficits in neutral, neck torsion did not influence this and thus the neck torsion differences were similar to the control group. Considering the two studies, WAD subjects displayed the greatest deficits, especially those subjects who reported dizziness. Tjell & Rosenhall (2002) proposed that the difference in eye movement control between atraumatic and traumatic origin neck pain subjects may be due

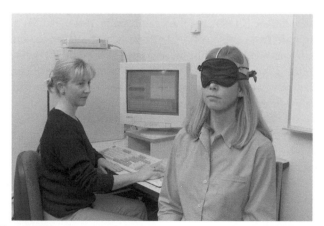

Figure 20.3   Measurement of joint position error using the Fastrak system

to the sudden acceleration and deceleration forces placed on the neck muscle attachments and their proprioceptors at injury, compounded by abnormal muscle activity as a response from the postural control system as well as pain.

Further to this, Gimse et al (1997) found a close correlation between technical reading ability, information uptake and abnormal results of the smooth pursuit neck torsion test. They suggested that disturbed postural control due to abnormal cervical afferent input might be a factor contributing to cognitive disturbances seen in WAD. It was hypothesized that like areas of the brain are overloaded by the abnormal proprioceptive activity, leading to decreased functional ability of areas controlling cognition (Gimse et al 1996, Tjell & Rosenhall 2002). However, it should be noted that cognitive disturbances are not uncommon complaints following whiplash injury and have been attributed to various other causes such as cerebral dysfunction, effects of medication and psychological factors including anxiety, post-traumatic stress or depression (Kessels et al 2000).

Thus there is evidence that disturbed cervical afferent input following a whiplash injury likely affects all three areas of JPE, balance and eye movement control, with some suggestion that this may be to a greater extent in those complaining of dizziness. Since this is a common complaint in WAD, the importance of adequate assessment and management of postural control disturbance in those with persistent WAD is emphasized.

PROGNOSIS FOLLOWING WHIPLASH INJURY

Despite growing evidence that changes in physiological mechanisms are present in chronic WAD, it remains unclear as to why some people develop persistent symptoms where others recover within a few weeks of injury. Many prospective studies investigating outcome following whiplash injury have suffered from poor methodology including inadequate description of source population, ill-defined outcome measures and non-report of loss to follow-up (Cote et al 2001). Nevertheless, some factors, mainly sociodemographic and symptomatic, consistently appear to be important predictors of recovery. Sociodemographic factors include a previous history of neck pain and headaches, older age and female gender (Cassidy et al 2000, Harder et al 1998, Radanov et al 1995, Satoh et al 1997, Suissa et al 2001). Symptomatic features associated with delayed recovery include the initial intensity of pain (neck pain and headache) post accident and neurological (radicular) signs and symptoms (Cassidy et al 2000, Radanov et al 1995, Sturzenegger et al 1995).

Investigation of the role accident related mechanisms plays in the outcome following whiplash injury provide inconsistent findings. A Swiss study of 117 acute whiplash subjects found that an inclined or rotated head position at the time of impact and the car being stationary when hit were associated with a poorer outcome (Radanov et al 1995, Suissa et al 2001). Other indicators which have been

reported to point to delayed recovery include: being a passenger, collision with a bus or truck, wearing or not of seatbelts, the presence of tow bars on the struck vehicle and being involved in a fatal collision (Cassidy et al 2000, Harder et al 1998, Kraft et al 2000). However, a longitudinal study by Cassidy et al (2000) failed to demonstrate any accident related mechanisms that were predictors of poor outcome. Further research is necessary before firm conclusions can be drawn with respect to the impact of accident related mechanisms and outcome (Cote et al 2001).

In comparison to other musculoskeletal conditions such as low back pain, the role that psychological factors play in the patient's outcome following whiplash injury are yet to be comprehensively investigated. Despite this lack of data, assertions have been made suggesting that psychological factors act to produce chronic symptoms in WAD with the inference that no underlying organic pathology exists or, if it did exist, has healed (Ferrari & Russell 1997). Psychological stress, affective disturbances and behavioural abnormalities have been found in patients with whiplash (Peebles et al 2001). These factors may be related to four different options: pre-existing psychological problems revealed by a stressful event; the consequence of prolonged pain and other symptoms; the direct effect of injury; and the expectation of compensation (Provinciali & Baroni 1999).

The available evidence to date demonstrates that the persistence of symptoms in WAD cannot be predicted from psychological traits (Borchgrevink et al 1997, Mayou & Bryant 1996, Radanov et al 1995). From a prospective Swiss study of 117 whiplash subjects, it was demonstrated that psychological problems most likely occur as a consequence of ongoing pain and disability (Radanov et al 1995, 1996). Gargan et al (1997) demonstrated that psychological disturbances were related to physical restriction of neck movement and did not become established until 3 months after injury. These results are supported by Wallis et al (1997) who demonstrated some resolution of psychological stress in patients with chronic WAD following pain relief using zygapophysial joint blocks.

The possible role that post-traumatic stress may play in persistent whiplash is at present unclear. Some patients may present with a post-traumatic stress disorder (Merskey 1993) but this has not been shown to predict the development of chronic symptoms (Provinciali & Baroni 1999). The effect that compensation and litigation factors have on outcome is controversial. A recent Canadian study showed that the retention of a lawyer soon after the accident and the type of insurance/compensation system were associated with a delayed recovery (Cassidy et al 2000). However, the outcome measure used in this study was 'time to claim closure' and although the authors assert an association between this measure and neck pain/physical function (recovery), other studies have noted no evidence that claim settlement is followed by significant changes in clinical status (Bryant et al 1997). Other studies have also demonstrated that compensation and litigation have no influence on outcome (Barnsley et al 1994, Kasch et al 2001a, Mayou & Bryant 1996). Until more studies provide evidence that litigation/compensation do influence recovery, it would appear that much of the scepticism directed toward individuals experiencing a whiplash injury is unfounded (Miller 1998).

Psychosocial factors, such as fear avoidance beliefs, attention, pain related beliefs and the use of coping strategies among others, are yet to be extensively investigated in WAD although they have been shown to be important in other musculoskeletal conditions such as low back pain (Linton 2000). However, it is suggested that a whiplash injury differs from low back pain in many respects, including physical and psychological trauma associated with the motor vehicle crash, the presence of many varied symptoms likely involving complex mechanisms, and therefore extrapolations between the two conditions cannot and should not be made at this stage.

Although sociodemographic and symptomatic factors as described may provide some indication of risk factors for poor outcome following a whiplash injury, they are of minimal benefit to the manual therapy clinician seeking the optimal treatment to reduce the risk of chronicity. Apart from active range of movement, there has been scant investigation of the predictive capacity of physical measures on outcome. Radanov et al (1994, 1995) found that restricted neck movement could predict outcome at 1 year but not 2 years post injury. More recently, Kasch et al (2001a) demonstrated that cervical active range of movement was the best predictor of handicap at 1 year post injury when evaluated against other factors such as pain intensity, non-painful neurological symptoms, strength of flexor and extensor muscles and psychometric tests. Further investigation of a wider range of physical measures is required.

Despite the number of studies investigating prognosis, there is still a dearth of conclusive predictors of outcome following whiplash injury. Little is known about the physiological mechanisms involved from the time of injury until recovery or the development of chronicity. The attainment of such knowledge is required such that factors contributing to the development of chronic symptoms are identified. At present the knowledge and understanding of involved mechanisms is mainly limited to those subjects who are already classified as having persistent or chronic symptoms, that is symptoms of more than 3 months' duration following the motor vehicle crash.

IMPLICATIONS FOR TREATMENT

Scientific evidence for the efficacy of physiotherapy treatment of whiplash is sparse. Evidence provided from systematic reviews would suggest that active interventions that stimulate the patient to return to daily activities as soon as possible are preferable to rest and wearing of a collar (Magee et al 2000, Peeters et al 2001, Scholten-Peeters et al 2002). However, trials of physical management such as range of movement exercises, advice to keep active and general exercise have generally failed to decrease the incidence of chronicity of this condition (Borchgrevink et al 1998, Rosenfeld et al 2000, Soderlund et al 2000).

As outlined in this chapter, evidence is now emerging which clearly demonstrates a complex array of mechanisms being involved in chronic WAD. In any condition it is likely that individualized treatment driven by mechanistic inferences will be more successful in delivering improved outcomes (Max 2000, Woolf et al 1998). The authors of these papers were referring to pharmaceutical treatment but the same approach must apply to the physiotherapy management directed to patients following a whiplash injury. In view of the many mechanisms involved in WAD, surely it is naive to believe that such non-specific treatments (as have so far been investigated) will be sufficient to reduce chronicity associated with this condition. It is suggested that the future management of WAD will need to be based on mechanisms, clinically identified in individual WAD patients. Such management is likely to be multidisciplinary as well as involving a multimodal physiotherapy approach.

A peripheral nociceptive source of pain may be accurately identified using manual examination skills – an underutilized tool in the diagnosis of whiplash but potentially useful considering the limited capacity of radiography to identify peripheral pathology. Alternatives such as diagnostic zygapophysial joint blocks are invasive and costly but, more importantly, skilled manual examination has been shown to be as accurate (Jull et al 1988) and reliable (Jull et al 1997). Manual therapy directed toward dysfunctional joints may help to relieve pain (Hurwitz et al 1996, Vicenzino et al 1998) but is unlikely to significantly improve the patient's overall outcome unless the presence of other physiological mechanisms is also addressed.

It is apparent that physiotherapy intervention aimed at addressing deficits in neuromuscular control and sensorimotor function will be necessary in the management of WAD. Non-specific exercise programmes are yet to demonstrate efficacy in reducing chronicity following a whiplash injury (Borchgrevink et al 1998, Rosenfeld et al 2000, Soderlund et al 2000), suggesting that future programmes may be more successful if specific motor impairments identified from individual assessment are identified and managed. Some success has been demonstrated for this approach using kinaesthetic retraining exercises in whiplash and non-traumatic neck pain (Provinciali et al 1996, Revel et al 1994) and specific re-education of deep neck flexor muscles in chronic neck pain and headache mainly of non-traumatic origin (Jull et al 2002). With evidence emerging that changes in muscle recruitment patterns and kinaesthetic deficits occur soon after injury, it would appear that specific physiotherapy intervention aimed at these deficits should be introduced early in the rehabilitation programme (Sterling et al 2003). Similarly, disordered balance and loss of eye movement control may need to be included in the rehabilitation programme if deficits in these areas are evident.

Evidence is emerging that a proportion of WAD patients demonstrate hypersensitivity consistent with alterations of central nervous system pain processing mechanisms. Other conditions with similar features, such as complex regional pain syndrome, are often recalcitrant to treatment interventions, including physical treatment approaches (Kingery 1997, Thimineur et al 1998). This suggests that whiplash patients displaying clinical signs of hypersensitivity might not respond successfully to physiotherapy interventions alone. These patients may be clinically identified as those with neuropathic-type pain features such as constant burning pain, cold hyperalgesia, allodynia and generalized lowered mechanical pain thresholds. Pharmaceutical interventions involving specific drugs to deal with the potential pain processes involved may be necessary. These may need to be commenced in the acute stage of injury with the goal being to prevent the development of chronic pain (Bonelli et al 2001). With respect to physiotherapy management of this group of patients, it would be important that any treatment is non-provocative in nature and pain-free such that this hypersensitivity is not further facilitated. As central sensitization is thought to be maintained by ongoing peripheral nociceptive input (Devor 1997, Gracely et al 1992), application of manual therapy or exercise techniques which are pain provocative may in fact result in maintenance of hypersensitivity and be detrimental to the patient's progress. However, evidence is accumulating that suggests gentle manual therapy techniques may act to influence supraspinal pathways involving descending inhibition of pain (Vicenzino et al 1998) and therefore demonstrate potential for use in the management of hypersensitivity.

Due to the complex, likely interactive, mechanisms involved in WAD the most successful management strategy is likely to be multidisciplinary. Psychological intervention will, of course, be necessary in patients with identified psychological disturbance. Behavioural treatment has shown efficacy in the treatment of chronic low back pain (Tulder et al 2000) but to our knowledge no specific evaluation has been made of its effect in WAD. Physiotherapists need to be aware of the psychological implications of whiplash injury and provide support and assurance as necessary. The patient's beliefs of fear of movement/reinjury may have particular relevance to physiotherapy interventions. Preliminary evidence suggests that the fear of movement/reinjury may have some influence on physical measures of motor function, this relationship occurring soon after injury (Sterling et al 2003). Physiotherapists may play an important role in allaying such fears and encouraging movement in modified and planned functional stages. However, as with all treatment interventions, psychological intervention alone, without taking into account other involved mechanisms, is also unlikely to succeed (Linton 2000).

CONCLUSION

The evidence to date points to the involvement of a complex set of mechanisms in the pathophysiology of chronic WAD. The development of these mechanisms and the timeframe for that development require investigation such that the incidence of chronicity from a whiplash injury may be reduced. Future treatment trials must take account of physiological mechanisms involved in both the acute and chronic stages of WAD in order to reduce chronicity associated with this condition.

KEYWORDS	
whiplash injury	psychological impairments
physical impairments	prediction

References

Adeboye K, Emerton D, Hughes T 2000 Cervical sympathetic chain dysfunction after whiplash injury. Journal of the Royal Society of Medicine 93: 378

Alund M, Ledin T, Odkvist L, Larsson S E 1993 Dynamic posturography among patients with common neck disorders: a study of 15 cases with suspected cervical vertigo. Journal of Vestibular Research, Equilibrium and Orientation 3: 383–389

American Medical Association 1993 Guides to the evaluation of permanent impairment. American Medical Association, Chicago

Andersen O, Graven-Nielsen T, Matre D, Arendt-Nielsen L, Schomburg E 2000 Interaction between cutaneous and muscular afferent activity in polysynaptic reflex pathways: a human experimental study. Pain 84: 29–36

Baloh R, Halmagyi G 1996 Disorders of the vestibular system. Oxford University Press, New York

Barnsley L, Lord S, Bogduk N 1994 Clinical review: Whiplash injury. Pain 58: 283–307

Barnsley L, Lord S, Bogduk N 1998 The pathophysiology of whiplash. Spine, State of the Art Reviews 12: 209–242

Barton P, Hayes K 1996 Neck flexor muscles strength, efficiency and relaxation times in normal subjects and subjects with unilateral pain and headache. Archives of Physical Medicine and Rehabilitation 77: 680–687

Bolton P 1998 The somatosensory system of the neck and its effects on the central nervous system. Journal of Manipulative and Physiological Therapeutics 21: 553–563

Bonelli R, Reisecker F, Koltringer P 2001 Prevention of chronic pain in whiplash injury. Journal of Pain and Symptom Management 21: 92–93

Bono G, Antonaci F, Ghirmai S, D'Angelo F, Berger M, Nappi G 2000 Whiplash injuries: clinical picture and diagnostic work-up. Clinical and Experimental Rheumatology 18: S23–S28

Borchgrevink G, Stiles T, Borchgrevink P, Lereim I 1997 Personality profile among symptomatic and recovered patients with neck sprain injury, measured by mcmi-i acutely and 6 months after car accidents. Journal of Psychosomatic Research 42: 357–367

Borchgrevink G, Kaasa A, McDonagh D, Stiles T, Haraldseth O, Lereim I 1998 Acute treatment of whiplash neck sprain injuries:

a randomized trial of treatment during the first 14 days after a car accident. Spine 23: 25–31

Brandt T 1996 Cervical vertigo: reality or fiction? Audiology and Neurootology 1: 187–196

Bryant B, Mayou R, Lloyd-Bostock S 1997 Compensation claims following road accidents: a six-year follow up study. Medicine, Science and the Law 37: 326–336

Capra N, Ro J 2000 Experimental muscle pain produces central modulation of proprioceptive signals arising from jaw muscle spindles. Pain 86: 151–162

Cassidy J D, Carroll L J, Cote P, Lemstra M, Berglund A, Nygren A 2000 Effect of eliminating compensation for pain and suffering on the outcome of insurance claims for whiplash injury. New England Journal of Medicine 20: 1179–1213

Chester J 1991 Whiplash, postural control, and the inner-ear. Spine 16: 716–720

Cholewicki J, Panjabi M, Khachatryan A 1997 Stabilizing function of trunk flexor-extensor muscles around a neutral spinal posture. Spine 22: 2207–2212

Cote P, Cassidy D, Carroll L, Frank J, Bombardier C 2001 A systematic review of the prognosis of acute whiplash and a new conceptual framework to synthesize the literature. Spine 26: E445–E458

Cowan S, Bennell K, Hodges P, Crossley K, McConnell J 2000 Delayed onset of electromyographic activity of vastus obliquus relative to vastus lateralis in subjects with patellofemoral pain syndrome. Archives of Physical Medicine and Rehabilitation 82: 183–189

Curatolo M, Petersen-Felix S, Arendt-Nielsen L, Giani C, Zbinden A, Radanov B 2001 Central hypersensitivity in chronic pain after whiplash injury. Clinical Journal of Pain 17: 306–315

Dall'Alba P, Sterling M, Trealeven J, Edwards S, Jull G 2001 Cervical range of motion discriminates between asymptomatic and whiplash subjects. Spine 26: 2090–2094

Davis S, Teresi L, Bradley W, Ziemba M, Bloze A 1991 Cervical spine hyperextension injuries: MR findings. Radiology 180: 245–251

DeJong P I V M, DeJong J M B V 1977 Ataxia and nystagmus induced by injection of local anaesthetics in the neck. Annals of Neurology 1: 240–246

Devor M 1991 Neuropathic pain and injured nerve: peripheral mechanisms. British Medical Bulletin 47: 619–630

Devor M 1997 Central versus peripheral substrates of persistent pain: which contributes more? Behavioral and Brain Sciences 20: 446–447

Dieterich M, Pollmann W, Pfaffenrath V 1993 Cervicogenic headache: electronystagmography, perception of verticality and posturography in patients before and after C2-blockade. Cephalalgia 13: 285–288

Dumas J 2001 Physical impairments in cervicogenic headache: traumatic versus non traumatic onset. Cephalalgia 21: 884–893

Dvorak J, Hayek J, Zehnder R 1987 CT-functional diagnostics of the rotatory instability of the upper cervical spine. 2: An evaluation of healthy adults and patients with suspected instability. Spine 12: 726–731

Eck J, Hodges S, Humphreys C 2001 Whiplash: a review of a commonly misunderstood injury. American Journal of Medicine 110: 651–656

Elert J, Kendall S, Larsson B, Mansson B, Gerdle B 2001 Chronic pain and difficulty in relaxing postural muscles in patients with fibromyalgia and chronic whiplash associated disorders. Journal of Rheumatology 28: 1361–1368

Eliav E, Herzberg U, Ruda M, Bennett G 1999 Neuropathic pain from an experimental neuritis of the rat sciatic nerve. Pain 83: 169–182

Eliav E, Benoliel R, Tal M 2001 Inflammation with no axonal damage of the rat saphenous nerve trunk induces ectopic discharge and mechanosensitivity in myelinated axons. Neuroscience Letters 311: 49–52

El-Kahky A, Kingma H, Dolmans M, De Jong I 2000 Balance control near the limit of stability in various sensory conditions in healthy subjects and patients suffering from vertigo or balance disorders:

impact of sensory input on balance control. Acta Oto-Laryngologica 120: 508–516

Elvey R 1997 Physical evaluation of the peripheral nervous system in disorders of pain and dysfunction. Journal of Hand Therapy 10: 122–129

Ferrari R, Russell A 1997 The whiplash syndrome: common sense revisited. Journal of Rheumatology 24: 618–623

Ferrari R, Russell AS 1999 Development of persistent neurologic symptoms in patients with simple neck sprain. Arthritis Care and Research 12: 70–76

Fredin Y, Elert J, Britschgi N, Nyberg V, Vaher A, Gerdle B 1997 A decreased ability to relax between repetitive muscle contractions in patients with chronic symptoms after whiplash trauma of the neck. Journal of Musculoskeletal Pain 5: 55–70

Gargan M, Bannister G, Main C, Hollis S 1997 The behavioural response to whiplash injury. Journal of Bone and Joint Surgery 79B: 523–526

George S, Fritz J, Erhard R 2001 A comparison of fear-avoidance beliefs in patients with lumbar spine pain and cervical spine pain. Spine 26: 2139–2145

Gimse R, Tjell C, Bjorgen I, Saunte C 1996 Disturbed eye movements after whiplash injury due to injuries to the posture control system. Journal of Clinical and Experimental Neurophysiology 18: 178–186

Gimse R, Bjorgen I, Tjell C, Tyssedal J, Bo K 1997 Reduced cognitive functions in a group of whiplash patients with demonstrated disturbances in the posture control system. Journal of Clinical and Experimental Neuropsychology 19: 838–849

Gracely R, Lynch S, Bennett G 1992 Painful neuropathy: altered central processing maintained dynamically by peripheral input. Pain 51: 175–194

Gronroos M, Pertovaara A 1993 Capsaicin-induced central facilitation of a nociceptive flexion reflex in humans. Neuroscience Letters 159: 215–218

Hall T, Elvey R 1999 Nerve trunk pain: physical diagnosis and treatment. Manual Therapy 4: 63–73

Hall T, Pyne E, Hamer P 1993 Limiting factors of the straight leg raise test. In: Singer K (ed) Eighth Biennial Conference of the Musculoskeletal Physiotherapists' Association of Australia. Manipulative Physiotherapists Association of Australia, Perth, pp 32–39

Harder S, Veilleux M, Sassa S 1998 The effect of socio-demographic and crash-related factors on the prognosis of whiplash. Journal of Clinical Epidemiology 51: 377–384

Heikkilä H, Astrom P 1996 Cervicocephalic kinesthetic sensibility in patients with whiplash injury. Scandinavian Journal of Rehabilitation 28: 133–138

Heikkilä H, Wenngren B 1998 Cervicocephalic kinesthetic sensibility, active range of cervical motion and oculomotor function in patients with whiplash injury. Archives of Physical Medicine and Rehabilitation 79: 1089–1094

Hides J, Richardson C, Jull G 1996 Multifidus muscle recovery is not automatic following resolution of acute first episode low back pain. Spine 21: 2763–2769

Hides J, Jull G, Richardson C 2001 Long term effects of specific stabilizing exercises for first episode low back pain. Spine 26: E243–248

Hildingsson C, Wenngren B, Bring G, Toolanen G 1989 Oculomotor problems after cervical spine injury. Acta Orthopaedica Scandinavica 60: 513–516

Hildingsson C, Wenngren B, Toolanen G 1993 Eye motility dysfunction after soft-tissue injury of the cervical spine. Acta Orthopaedica Scandinavica 64: 129–132

Hodges P, Richardson C, Jull G 1996 Evaluation of the relationship between the findings of a laboratory and clinical test of the function of transversus abdominis. Physiotherapy Research International 1: 30–40

Hurwitz E, Aker P, Adams A, Meeker W, Shekelle P 1996 Manipulation and mobilisation of the cervical spine: a systematic review of the literature. Spine 21: 1746–1760

Ide M, Ide J, Yamaga M, Takagi K 2001 Symptoms and signs of irritation of the brachial plexus in whiplash injuries. Journal of Bone and Joint Surgery (British volume) 83: 226–229

Jonsson H, Bring G, Rauschning W, Sahlstedt B 1991 Hidden cervical spine injuries in traffic accident victims with skull fractures. Journal of Spinal Disorders 4: 251–263

Jonsson H, Cesarini K, Sahlstedt B, Rauschning W 1994 Findings and outcome in whiplash-type neck distortions. Spine 19(24): 2733–2743

Jull G 1998 Characterization of cervicogenic headache. Physical Therapy Review 3: 95–105

Jull G 2000 Deep cervical flexor muscle dysfunction in whiplash. Journal of Musculoskeletal Pain 8: 143–154

Jull G A, Bogduk N, Marsland A 1988 The accuracy of manual diagnosis for cervical zygapophysial joint pain syndromes. Medical Journal of Australia 148: 233–236

Jull G, Zito G, Trott P, Potter H, Shirley D 1997 Inter-examiner reliability to detect painful upper cervical joint dysfunction. Australian Journal of Physiotherapy 43: 125–129

Jull G, Trott P, Potter H et al 2002 A randomized controlled trial of exercise and manipulative therapy for cervicogenic headache. Spine 27(17): 1835–1843

Karlberg M, Magnusson M, Malmstrom E M, Melander A, Moritz U 1996 Postural and symptomatic improvement after physiotherapy in patients with dizziness of suspected cervical origin. Archives of Physical Medicine and Rehabilitation 77: 874–882

Kasch H, Flemming W, Jensen T 2001a Handicap after acute whiplash injury. Neurology 56: 1637–1643

Kasch H, Stengaard-Pedersen K, Arendt-Nielsen L, Jensen T 2001b Headache, neck pain and neck mobility after acute whiplash injury. Spine 26: 1246–1251

Kasch H, Stengaard-Pedersen K, Arendt-Nielsen L, Staehelin Jensen T 2001c Pain thresholds and tenderness in neck and head following acute whiplash injury: a prospective study. Cephalalgia 21: 189–197

Keidel M, Rieschke P, Stude P, Eisentraut R, van Schayck R, Diener H 2001 Antinociceptive reflex alteration in acute posttraumatic headache following whiplash injury. Pain 92: 319–326

Kessels R, Aleman A, Verhagen W, Luijtelaar E 2000 Cognitive functioning after whiplash injury: a meta-analysis. Journal of the International Neuropsychological Society 6: 271–278

Kingery W 1997 A critical review of controlled clinical trials for peripheral neuropathic pain and complex regional pain syndromes. Pain 73: 123–139

Koelbaek-Johansen M, Graven-Nielsen T, Schou-Olesen A, Arendt-Nielsen L 1999 Muscular hyperalgesia and referred pain in chronic whiplash syndrome. Pain 83: 229–234

Koltzenburg M 2000 Primary afferent mechanisms of neuropathic pain. Journal of Back and Musculoskeletal Rehabilitation 14: 45–48

Koltzenburg M, Torebjork H, Wahren L 1994 Nociceptor modulated central sensitization causes mechanical hyperalgesia in acute chemogenic and chronic neuropathic pain. Brain 117: 579–591

Koskimies K, Sutinen P, Aalto H, et al 1997 Postural stability, neck proprioception and tension neck. Acta Oto-Laryngologica: Supplementum 529: 95–97

Kraft M, Kullgren A, Tingvall C 2000 How crash severity in rear impacts influences short and long term consequences to the neck. Accident Analysis and Prevention 32: 187–195

Kristjansson E, Dall'Alba P, Jull G 2003 A study of five cervicocephalic relocation tests in three different subject groups. Clinical Rehabilitation 17(7): 768–774

Linton S 2000 A review of psychological risk factors in back and neck pain. Spine 25: 1148–1156

Lord S, Bogduk N 1996 The cervical synovial joints as sources of post-traumatic headache. Journal of Musculoskeletal Pain 4: 81–94

Lord S, Barnsley L, Wallis B, Bogduk N 1996 Chronic cervical zygapophysial joint pain after whiplash: a placebo-controlled prevalence study. Spine 21: 1737–1745

McPartland J, Brodeur R, Hallgren R 1997 Chronic neck pain, standing balance, and suboccipital muscle atrophy: a pilot study. Journal of Manipulative and Physiological Therapeutics 20: 24–29

Magee D, Oborn-Barrett E, Turner S 2000 A systematic overview of the effectiveness of physical therapy intervention on soft tissue neck injury following trauma. Physiotherapy Canada (52): 111–130

Mallinson A, Longridge N, Peacock C 1996 Dizziness, imbalance, and whiplash. Journal of Musculoskeletal Pain 4: 105–112

Max M 2000 Is mechanism-based pain treatment attainable? Clinical trial issues. Journal of Pain 1: 2–9

Mayou R, Bryant B 1996 Outcome of whiplash neck injury. Injury 27: 617–623

Merskey H 1993 Psychological consequences of whiplash. Spine 7: 471–480

Miller L 1998 Motor vehicle accidents: clinical, neuropsychological and forensic considerations. Journal of Cognitive Rehabilitation (July/August): 10–23

Moog M, Zusman M, Quintner J, Hall T 1999 Allodynia and psychological profile in chronic whiplash patients. Ninth World Congress on Pain. IASP, Vienna

Mosimann U, Muri R, Felblinger J, Radanov B 2000 Saccadic eye movement disturbances in whiplash patients with persistent complaints. Brain 123: 828–835

Munglani R 2000 Neurobiological mechanisms underlying chronic whiplash associated pain. Journal of Musculoskeletal Pain 8: 169–178

Nederhand M, Ijzerman M, Hermens H 2000 Cervical muscle dysfunction in the chronic whiplash associated disorder grade II (WAD-II). Spine 25: 1938–1943

Oosterveld W, Kortschot H, Kingma G, de Jong H, Saatci M 1991 Electronystagmographic findings following cervical whiplash injury. Acta Oto-Laryngologica 111: 201–205

Osterbauer P, Long K, Ribaudo T, Petermann E, Fuhr A, Bigos S, Yamaguchi G 1996 Three-dimensional head kinematics and cervical range of motion in the diagnosis of patients with neck trauma. Journal of Manipulative and Physiological Therapeutics 19: 231–237

Patijn J, Wilmink J, ter Linden F, Kingma H 2001 CT study of craniovertebral rotation in whiplash injury. European Spine Journal 10: 38–43

Peck D, Buxton D, Nitz A 1984 A comparison of spindle contractions in large and small muscles acting in parallel concentrations. Journal of Morphology 180: 243–252

Peebles J, McWilliams L, MacLennan R 2001 A comparison of symptom checklist 90-revised profiles from patients with chronic pain from whiplash and patients with other musculoskeletal injuries. Spine 26: 766–770

Peeters G G, Verhagen A P, Bie R A, Oostendorp R A 2001 The efficacy of conservative treatment in patients with whiplash injury: a systematic review of clinical trials. Spine 26: E64–73

Peterson B, Goldberg J, Bilotto G, Fuller J 1985 Cervicocollic reflex: its dynamic properties and interaction with vestibular reflexes. Journal of Neurophysiology 54: 90–108

Pettersson K, Hildingsson C, Toolanen G, Fagerlund M, Bjornebrink J 1994 MRI and neurology in acute whiplash trauma. Acta Orthopaedica Scandinavica 65: 525–528

Pienimarki T, Kauranen K, Vanharanta H 1997 Bilaterally decreased motor performance of arms in patients with chronic tennis elbow. Archives of Physical Medicine and Rehabilitation 78: 1092–1095

Provinciali L, Baroni M 1999 Clinical approaches to whiplash injuries: a review. Critical Reviews in Physical and Rehabilitation Medicine 11: 339–368

Provinciali L, Baroni M, Illuminati L, Ceravolo M 1996 Multimodal treatment to prevent the late whiplash syndrome. Scandinavian Journal of Rehabilitation Medicine 28: 105–111

Radanov B, Dvorak J 1996 Spine update: impaired cognitive functioning after whiplash injury of the cervical spine. Spine 21: 392–397

Radanov B, Sturzenegger M, De Stefano G, Schnidrig A 1994 Relationship between early somatic, radiological, cognitive and psychosocial findings and outcome during a one-year follow-up in 117 patients suffering from common whiplash. British Journal of Rheumatology 33: 442–448

Radanov B, Sturzenegger M, Di Stefano G 1995 Long-term outcome after whiplash injury: a 2-year follow-up considering features of injury mechanism and somatic, radiologic, and psychological findings. Medicine 74: 281–297

Radanov B, Begre S, Sturzenegger M, Augustiny K 1996 Course of psychological variables in whiplash injury: a 2-year follow-up with age, gender and education pair-matched patients. Pain 64: 429–434

Revel M 1991 Cervicocephalic kinesthetic sensibility in patients with cervical pain. Archives of Physical Medicine and Rehabilitation 72: 288–291

Revel M, Minguet M, Gergory P, Vaillant J, Manuel J 1994 Changes in cervicocephalic kinesthesia after a proprioceptive rehabilitation program in patients with neck pain: a randomized controlled study. Archives of Physical Medicine and Rehabilitation 75: 895–899

Rosenfeld M, Gunnarsson R, Borenstein P 2000 Early intervention in whiplash-associated disorders: a comparison of two protocols. Spine 25: 1782–1787

Rosenhall U, Johansson G, Orndahl G 1987 Eye motility dysfunction in chronic primary fibromyalgia with dysesthesia. Scandinavian Journal of Rehabilitation Medicine 19: 139–145

Rosenhall U, Johansson G, Orndahl G 1996 Otoneurologic and audiologic findings in fibromyalgia. Scandinavian Journal of Rehabilitation Medicine 28: 225–232

Rubin A, Woolley S, Dailey V, Goebel J 1995 Postural stability following mild head or whiplash injuries. American Journal of Otology 16: 216–221

Satoh S, Naito S, Konishi T et al 1997 An examination of reasons for prolonged treatment in Japanese patients with whiplash injuries. Journal of Musculoskeletal Pain 5: 71–84

Schmand B, Lindeboom J, Schagen S, Heijt R, Koene T, Hamburger H 1998 Cognitive complaints in patients after whiplash injury: the impact of malingering. Journal of Neurology Neurosurgery and Psychiatry 64: 339–343

Scholten-Peeters G, Bekkering G, Verhagen A 2002 Clinical practice guideline for the physiotherapy of patients with whiplash associated disorders. Spine 27: 412–422

Schonstrom N, Twomey L, Taylor J 1993 The lateral atlanto-axial joints and their synovial folds: an in vitro study of soft tissue injuries and fractures. Journal of Trauma 35: 886–892

Seitz J, Unguez C, Corbus H, Wooten W 1995 SPECT of the cervical spine in the evaluation of neck pain after trauma. Clinical Nuclear Medicine 20(8): 667–673

Sheather-Reid R, Cohen M 1998 Psychophysical evidence for a neuropathic component of chronic neck pain. Pain 75: 341–347

Soderlund A, Olerud C, Lindberg P 2000 Acute whiplash-associated disorders (WAD): the effects of early mobilisation and prognostic factors in long term symptomatology. Clinical Rehabilitation 14: 457–467

Sterling M, Jull G 2001 Altered pain processing in WAD. Manipulative Physiotherapists' Association of Australia Biennial Conference. Manipulative Physiotherapists Association of Australia, Adelaide

Sterling M, Jull G, Wright A 2001 The effect of musculoskeletal muscle pain on motor activity and control. Journal of Pain 2(3): 135–145

Sterling M, Jull G, Vicenzino B, Kenardy J, Darnell R 2003 Development of motor system dysfunction following whiplash injury. Pain 103: 65–73

Sterling M, Treleaven J, Edwards S, Jull G 2002a Pressure pain thresholds in chronic whiplash associated disorder: further evidence of altered central pain processing. Journal of Musculoskeletal Pain 10(3): 69–79

Sterling M, Treleaven J, Jull G 2002b Responses to nerve a tissue provocation test in whiplash associated disorders. Manual Therapy 7(2): 89–94

Sturzenegger M, DiStefano G, Radanov B, Schnidrig A 1994 Presenting symptoms and signs after whiplash injury: the influence of accident mechanisms. Neurology 44: 688–693

Sturzenegger M, Radanov B, Stefano G D 1995 The effect of accident mechanisms and initial findings on the long-term course of whiplash injury. Journal of Neurology 242: 443–449

Suissa S, Harder S, Veilleux M 2001 The relation between initial symptoms and signs and the prognosis of whiplash. European Spine Journal 10: 44–49

Swinkels R, Oostendorp R 1996 Upper cervical instability: fact or fiction. Journal of Manipulative and Physiological Therapeutics 19: 185–194

Tal M 1999 A role for inflammation in chronic pain. Current Reviews of Pain 3: 440–446

Taylor J, Taylor M 1996 Cervical spinal injuries: an autopsy study of 109 blunt injuries. Journal of Musculoskeletal Pain 4: 61–79

Thimineur M, Sood P, Kravitz E, Gudin J, Kitaj M 1998 Central nervous system abnormalities in complex regional pain syndrome (CRPS): clinical and quantitative evidence of medullary dysfunction. Clinical Journal of Pain 14: 256–267

Thurnberg J, Hellstrom F, Sjolander P, Bergenheim M, Wenngren B-I, Johansson H 2001 Influences on the fusimotor-muscle spindle system from chemosensitive nerve endings in cervical facet joints in the cat: possible implications for whiplash induced disorders. Pain 91: 15–22

Tjell C, Rosenhall U 1998 Smooth pursuit neck torsion test: a specific test for cervical dizziness. Americian Journal of Otology 19: 76–81

Tjell C, Rosenhall U 2002 Smooth pursuit neck torsion test: a specific test for WAD. Journal of Whiplash and Related Disorders 1(2): 9–24

Treede R, Meyer R, Raja S, Campbell J 1992 Peripheral and central mechanisms of cutaneous hyperalgesia. Progressive Neurobiology 38: 397–421

Treleaven J, Jull G, Sterling M 2003 Dizziness and unsteadiness following whiplash injury: characteristic features and relationship with cervical joint position error. Journal of Rehabilitation 35(1): 36–43

Treleaven J, Murison R, Jull G, Low Choy N 2004 Is signal analysis important for measuring standing balance in chronic whiplash? Gait and Posture (in press)

Tulder M, Ostelo R, Vlaeyen J, Linton S, Morley S, Assendelft W 2000 Behavioural treatment for chronic low back pain: a systematic review within the framework of the Cochrane Back Review Group. Spine 26: 270–281

Vibert N, MacDougall H, de Waele C et al 2001 Variability in the control of head movements in seated humans: a link with whiplash injuries. Journal of Physiology 532: 851–868

Vicenzino B, Collins D, Benson H, Wright A 1998 An investigation of the interrelationship between manipulative therapy induced hypoalgesia and sympathoexcitation. Journal of Manipulative and Physiological Therapeutics 21: 448–453

Von Korff M, Saunders K 1996 The course of back pain in primary care. Spine 21: 2833–2839

Wall P, Woolf C 1984 Muscle but not cutaneous C-afferent input produces prolonged increases in the excitability of the flexion reflex in the rat. Journal of Physiology 356: 443–458

Wallis B, Lord S, Bogduk N 1997 Resolution of psychological distress of whiplash patients following treatment by radiofrequency neurotomy: a randomised, double-blind, placebo controlled trial. Pain 73: 15–22

Willauschus W, Kladny B, Beyer W, Gluckert K, Arnold H, Scheithauer R 1995 Lesions of the alar ligaments: in vivo and in vitro studies with magnetic resonance imaging. Spine 20: 2493–2498

Woolf C, Bennett G, Doherty M et al 1998 Towards a mechanism-based classification of pain. Pain 77: 227–229

Wright A, Thurnwald P, O'Callaghan J, Smith J, Vincenzino B 1994 Hyperalgesia in tennis elbow patients. Journal of Muscoluskeletal Pain 2: 83–97

Yoganandan N, Cusick J, Pintar F, Rao R 2001 Whiplash injury determination with conventional spine imaging and cryomicrotomy. Spine 26(22): 2443–2448

Ziegler E, Magerl W, Meyer R, Treede R 1999 Secondary hyperalgesia to punctate mechanical stimuli. Brain 122: 2245–2257

Chapter 21

The cervical spine and headache

G. A. Jull, K. R. Niere

INTRODUCTION

Headache is a common and often incapacitating condition. It is estimated that a headache in some form is experienced by at least 90% of the population at some stage of their lives, often leading to a visit to a general practitioner or time lost from work (Leonardi et al 1998, Philips 1977, Rasmussen et al 1991a). Headaches may arise when nociceptive input is received from the head or structures that can refer pain to the head. Headache may also arise when there is dysfunction in the areas of the central nervous system involved in the processing and perception of head pain. Consequently, the number of structures and disorders capable of causing headache is considerable.

Healthcare practitioners involved in the management of patients with cervical spine disorders have an interest in the relationship between headaches and disorders of the neck. Many practitioners of manual therapy worldwide act as first-contact practitioners. As a result, patients with headache from a variety of causes may present for management. Niere (1998) has exemplified this in a clinical study of 112 headache patients presenting for manipulative physiotherapy treatment. He found that 17% fulfilled the subjective criteria for cervicogenic headache as described at that time by Sjaastad et al (1990). In a further study, 36% of 111 headache patients presenting to physiotherapy fulfilled Sjaastad et al's (1998) criteria, 30% were diagnosed with tension-type headache, 14% as having migraine without aura and 7% as suffering from migraine with aura (Quin & Niere 2001). Rather than treat headache patients indiscriminately, the challenge for manual therapy practitioners is to identify those headache patients for whom their management methods are appropriate. In the main, these are patients with cervicogenic headache. However, rather than being black and white, this area is greyed by the symptomatic overlap of common benign headache forms such as migraine, tension-type headache and cervicogenic headache, the presence of mixed headache forms, as well as some common aggravating features.

The evidence base is growing for the effectiveness of manual therapy and therapeutic exercise for the management of headache which is associated with cervical musculoskeletal dysfunction (Boline et al 1995, Jull et al 2002, Nilsson et al 1997). There is no evidence to suggest that headaches which have no association with cervical musculoskeletal pathology can be effectively managed by these modalities. This chapter will explore the topic of headache with a focus on cervicogenic headache. It will consider the classification of the three more common benign headache types, namely migraine, tension-type and cervicogenic headache, epidemiological aspects and headache mechanisms which might underlie the overlap of symptoms and common aggravating factors. An emphasis is placed on differential diagnosis towards appropriate, safe and effective management of the headache patient by the primary contact manual therapy practitioner.

CLASSIFICATION OF HEADACHE

In 1988, the Headache Classification Committee of the International Headache Society (IHS) published *Classification and Diagnostic Criteria for Headache Disorders, Cranial Neuralgias and Facial Pain* (IHS 1988). The broad categories of this classification system are listed in Table 21.1 and these categories highlight the number of structures and disorders capable of causing headache.

Diagnostic criteria

The differential diagnosis of headache is guided largely, in the first instance, by the history, temporal pattern and behaviour of the headache, especially in the cases of migraine, tension-type headache and cervicogenic headache. Manual therapy practitioners need to be able to differentiate between these headache forms. The diagnostic criteria for migraine without aura and tension-type headache are presented in Tables 21.2 and 21.3 respectively. Migraine with aura is distinguished from migraine without aura by the reversible neurological symptoms that usually precede the headache.

In 1983, Sjaastad and colleagues first characterized features of a headache type that they felt was very likely to originate in the cervical spine and applied the term 'cervicogenic headache' (Sjaastad et al 1983). The diagnostic criteria were documented by Sjaastad and colleagues in 1990 (Sjaastad et al 1990), and revised in 1998 (Sjaastad et al 1998) (Table 21.4). They were recognized by the International Association for the Study of Pain (IASP) in 1994 (Merskey & Bogduk 1994). In a later revision of the criteria, Sjaastad et al (1998) noted that, while the criteria describe a unilateral headache, cervicogenic headache might spread across the midline, although the pain remains greater on the usually affected side. Criteria I and III are considered obligatory for diagnosis, with criterion II (positive response to anaesthetic blockades) obligatory only for scientific work.

In accord with Sjaastad's et al (1998) criterion II, diagnostic blocks are proposed by many as a gold standard to identify cervicogenic headache (Bogduk 1997, Bovim et al 1992a). Bovim & Sand (1992) found that cervicogenic headache patients were more likely to respond to greater occipital nerve blocks than were patients with either migraine without aura or tension-type headache. Seventeen of 22 subjects with cervicogenic headache achieved at least 40% pain relief, as opposed to only one of the 14 subjects

Table 21.1 Headache types categorized by the IHS classification committee (IHS 1988)

	Headache classification categories
1	Migraine
2	Tension-type headache
3	Cluster headache and chronic paroxysmal hemicrania
4	Miscellaneous headaches unassociated with structural lesion
5	Headache associated with head trauma
6	Headache associated with vascular disorders
7	Headache associated with non-vascular intracranial disorder
8	Headache associated with substances or their withdrawal
9	Headache associated with non-cephalic infection
10	Headache associated with metabolic disorder
11	Headache or facial pain associated with disorder of cranium, neck, eyes, ears, nose, sinuses, teeth, mouth or other facial or cranial structures
12	Cranial neuralgias, nerve trunk pain and deafferentation pain
13	Headache not classifiable

Table 21.2 IHS classification of migraine without aura (IHS 1988, pp 19–20)

A At least five attacks fulfilling B–D
B Headache attacks lasting 4–72 hours
C Headache has at least two of the following characteristics:
   1. Unilateral location
   2. Pulsating quality
   3. Moderate or severe intensity (inhibits or prohibits daily activities)
   4. Aggravation by walking stairs or similar routine activity
D During headache at least one of the following:
   1. Nausea and/or vomiting
   2. Photophobia and phonophobia
E At least one of the following:
   1. History, physical and neurological examinations do not suggest one of the disorders listed in groups 5–11*
   2. History and/or physical and/or neurological examinations do suggest such disorder, but it is ruled out by appropriate investigations
   3. Such disorder is present, but migraine attacks do not occur for the first time in close temporal relation to the disorder

*Groups 5–11 referred to in criterion E.1 refer to the headache categories given in Table 21.1.

Table 21.3 IHS classification of tension-type headache (IHS 1988, pp 29–30)

Section A in the criteria for tension-type headache relates to the frequency of the headaches for the purposes of classification into episodic or chronic tension-type headache.

B Headaches lasting from 30 minutes to 7 days

C At least 2 of the following pain characteristics:
1. Pressing/tightening (non-pulsating) quality
2. Mild or moderate intensity (may inhibit, but does not prohibit activities)
3. Bilateral location
4. No aggravation by walking stairs or similar routine physical activity

D Both of the following:
1. No nausea or vomiting (anorexia may occur)
2. Photophobia and phonophobia are absent, or one but not the other is present

E At least one of the following:
1. History, physical and neurological examinations do not suggest one of the disorders listed in groups 5–11*
2. History and/or physical and/or neurological examinations do suggest such disorder, but it is ruled out by appropriate investigations
3. Such disorder is present, but tension-type headache does not occur for the first time in close temporal relation to the disorder

*Groups 5–11 referred to in criterion E.1 refer to the headache categories given in Table 21.1.

Table 21.4 Diagnostic criteria for cervicogenic headache (Sjaastad et al 1998, pp 42–43)

Major criteria of cervicogenic headache	

1. Symptoms and signs of neck involvement
  i. Precipitation of comparable head pain by:
    – neck movement or sustained awkward head postures, and/or
    – external pressure over the upper cervical or occipital region on the symptomatic side
  ii. Restriction of range of motion in the neck
  iii. Ipsilateral neck, shoulder or arm pain
	One or more of the points 1 (i–iii) should be present

2. Confirmatory evidence by diagnostic blocks 3. Unilaterality of head pain, without sideshift	

4. Head pain characteristics
  i. Moderate-severe, non-throbbing and non-lancinating pain, usually starting in the neck
  ii. Episodes of varying duration
  iii. Fluctuating continuous pain
	None of the single points in 4 are obligatory

Other characteristics of some importance	

5. i. Only marginal effects or lack of effect of idomethician
  ii. Only marginal effect or lack of effect of ergotamine and sumatriptan
  iii. Female sex
  iv. Not infrequent history of head or indirect neck trauma, usually of more than medium severity
	None of the single points in 5 are obligatory

Other features of lesser importance	

6. Various attack-related phenomena, only occasionally present, and/or moderately expressed when present
  i. Nausea
  ii. Phonophobia and photophobia
  iii. Dizziness
  iv. Ipsilateral blurred vision
  v. Difficulties on swallowing
  vi. Ipsilateral oedema, mostly in the periocular area	

with migraine and none of the subjects with tension-type headache. However, there are limitations to diagnostic blocks. These include: the sensitivity and specificity of single blocks, validity of interpretation of results, the time taken for the procedure as well as associated cost when performed under X-ray control or placebo conditions, operator skill in the diagnostic method and widespread community applicability (Anthony 2000, Barnsley et al 1993, Edmeads 1996, Lord et al 1995a, Pearce 1995a, Pollmann et al 1997). Additionally, blocks aimed at the greater occipital nerve (C2) or the C1–2 or C2–3 joints will not necessarily implicate headaches arising from structures supplied by the C1 nerve. Nerve blocks can also be positive when there is abnormal central nervous system (CNS) processing of non-nociceptive afferent information carried by that nerve (Sheather-Reid & Cohen 1998). Positive responses to nerve blocks might confirm that the cervical spine is implicated in a headache but they cannot identify the origin or mechanism (peripheral or central) of pain.

Validity of cervicogenic headache criteria

Several studies have investigated the reliability of the IHS criteria for the common headache types (Granella et al 1994, Leone et al 1994), but understandably, it is only in more recent times that the diagnostic criteria for cervicogenic headache have been tested. Vincent & Luna (1999) investi-

gated the sensitivity and specificity of Sjaastad et al's 1990 criteria in relation to tension-type headache and migraine without aura. They tested 33 subjects fulfilling the criteria for cervicogenic headache with the IHS criteria for migraine and tension-type headache and also tested 29 episodic tension-type headache patients and 65 migraine patients with the criteria for cervicogenic headache. None of the patients with migraine fulfilled the criteria for cervicogenic headache although 30% of the subjects with cervicogenic headache fulfilled the criteria for migraine. Criterion I of cervicogenic headache, addressing signs and symptoms of neck involvement, was found to be a key differentiating factor between cervicogenic headache and migraine. None of the subjects with tension-type headache met criterion III for cervicogenic headache (unilaterality without sideshift) while 3% of the subjects with cervicogenic headache fulfilled the criteria for tension-type headache. Criterion III (unilateral pain without sideshift) and the finding of pain starting in the neck and spreading to the fronto-ocular area were the key differentiating factors between tension-type headache and cervicogenic headache.

The sensitivity and specificity of criterion III has been challenged. Blau & Macgregor (1994) reported that 62% of 50 subjects with migraine suffered associated neck pain or stiffness during the headache attack although the symptoms were unilateral in only 11 of these subjects (22% of total sample). However, Sjaastad et al (1992) found that 75% of 32 subjects diagnosed with migraine had unilateral headache with sideshift, while only 16% of the subjects had side-locked unilateral headaches. Side-locked unilaterality could be expected in between 6% (Vincent & Luna 1999) and 21% (D'Amico et al 1994) of patients with migraine although some of the subjects in the latter study may have had misdiagnosed cervicogenic headache. Sjaastad et al (1989) proposed that the localization of the initial pain of the headache attack might differentiate the unilateral pain of migraine from that of cervicogenic headache. They found that of 22 patients diagnosed as having migraine with aura, 91% felt the initial pain in the forehead and temporal regions while 73% of the 11 patients diagnosed with cervicogenic headache felt the initial pain in the neck.

The inter-observer reliability for applying the diagnostic criteria for cervicogenic headache was studied by van Suijlekom et al (1999). Six physicians examined 24 patients with migraine, tension-type headache or cervicogenic headache. Kappa values for agreement between pairs of physicians ranged from 0.83 for expert headache neurologists and 0.43 for 'other physicians'. Reliability for diagnosing cervicogenic headache (76% agreement) was similar to migraine (77% agreement) and better than that for tension-type headache (48% agreement).

Thus clinicians can use the headache classification criteria with some confidence, being cognisant of the potential difficulty particularly with differential diagnosis of cervicogenic headache and tension headache.

Prevalence of cervicogenic headache

Any study of headache prevalence will depend on the population studied and the validity of the classification system used. Epidemiological studies have indicated that most benign, idiopathic headaches can be diagnosed as either migraine or tension-type headache although headache arising from the cervical spine is rarely considered as a diagnostic category in these studies (Marcus 1992, Rasmussen et al 1991a, 1991b, Scher et al 1999). Nilsson (1995) found the prevalence of cervicogenic headache to be 2.5% in a random population sample of 20–59-year-olds in Denmark, although 17.8% of 45 subjects with frequent headache fulfilled the IHS criteria for cervical headache. Pfaffenrath & Kaube (1990) determined that the prevalence

of cervicogenic headache was 13.8% in a population of 5520 primary headache sufferers. They also found that 56.4% of the 430 cervicogenic headache sufferers also suffered from other types of headache such as tension headache and migraine.

HEADACHE MECHANISMS

The most likely explanation for pain referral from the neck to the head is convergence of afferent impulses from the upper three cervical nerves and the trigeminal nerve in the dorsal horn grey matter of the upper cervical segments. The pars caudalis of the trigeminal nucleus is continuous with the dorsal horn grey matter of the upper cervical spine and extends at least functionally to the second cervical level (Falconer 1949, Kerr 1961, Taren & Khan 1962). The area of overlap forms a single functional nucleus, which is termed the 'trigemino-cervical nucleus' (Bogduk 1995a) (Fig. 21.1). Electrophysiological studies performed on cats (Goadsby et al 1997, Kerr & Olafson 1961) have demonstrated the convergence of trigeminal and upper cervical afferents. Although this convergence has not been replicated in humans, it is the most likely explanation of the experimental and clinical observations of the association between the cervical spine and headaches. Stimulation studies (Aprill et al 2002, Feinstein et al 1954, Hunter & Mayfield 1949, Kerr 1961, Piovesan et al 2001) and clinical observations of headache associated with cervical dysfunction (Niere 1998, Watson & Trott 1993) suggest that predominantly, the oph-

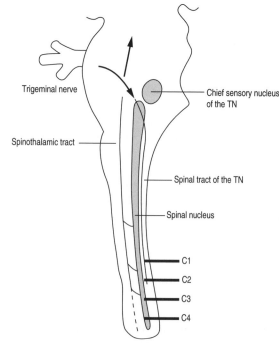

Figure 21.1 A schematic illustration of the trigeminocervical nucleus. The pars caudalis of the trigeminal nucleus is continuous with the grey matter of the upper cervical spinal cord, extending at least to the second cervical level.
Key: TN = trigeminal nerve.

thalmic division of the trigeminal nerve is involved in the mechanism of cervicogenic headache.

Rather than fitting neatly into discrete diagnostic categories, many headaches in the clinical setting can satisfy the criteria for, or have components of, more than one headache type (Nelson 1994, Niere 2002, Rasmussen et al 1992). The concept that migraine without aura and tension-type headache reflects different points on a headache continuum is not new (Marcus 1992) although the issue has been the cause of many debates (Leston 1996, Rasmussen 1996). Nelson (1994) proposed that cervicogenic headache, migraine and tension-type headache share many features and have considerable overlap because of the unique anatomy and physiology of the trigeminocervical nucleus. Cognitive and attentional processes notwithstanding, the perception of any headache will depend on the degree of excitation of the trigeminocervical nucleus. It has been proposed that nociceptive activity in the trigeminocervical nucleus is normally inhibited by descending neural pathways arising from the ventrolateral peri-aqueductal grey matter (vPAG) in the brain stem via the rostro ventromedial medulla. These pathways primarily use serotonin as their neurotransmitter (Fields 1997, Lance et al 1983). This inhibitory action is balanced by noradrenergic pathways arising in the hypothalamus, locus coeruleus and dorsomedial peri-aqueductal grey matter (dPAG) (Joseph et al 1989, Lance et al 1983).

From a psychosocial perspective, pain processing and perception can be influenced by past experiences, culture, attitudes and beliefs about pain (Gifford 1998, Melzack 1999a, Petrovic & Ingvar 2002). It would seem that despite the headache type, factors that may affect sensitivity of the trigeminocervical nucleus in susceptible individuals include allergies, dietary intolerances, sleep disturbances, stress, anxiety and hormonal changes. Visual, olfactory and somatosensory stimulation may also be significant for some patients. With altered pain processing through any of these factors, there may be responses to the headache experience either from a behavioural or physiological point of view.

Figure 21.2 depicts the some of the likely influences on, and outputs of, the trigeminocervical nucleus. For convenience, nociceptive input has been divided into musculoskeletal and visceral sources. Where normal supraspinal pain processing exists, nociceptive input from upper cervical spine musculoskeletal dysfunction could be perceived as a headache. If nociceptive input is inhibited, then mild or moderate levels of dysfunction may be asymptomatic. Where nociceptive activity is enhanced, input from minimal cervical dysfunction or non-painful afferents may be sufficient to trigger and maintain a headache. Increased CNS sensitivity has been shown in chronic neck pain populations (Sheather-Reid & Cohen 1998) and whiplash populations (Curatolo et al 2001, Johansen et al 1999, Sterling et al 2002a, 2002b). It is also possible that abnormal central processing can be maintained by ongoing peripheral input. Gracely et al (1992) demonstrated, on four patients with

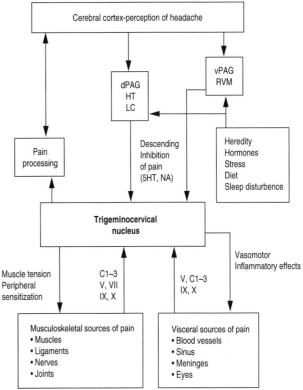

Figure 21.2 Transmission of nociceptive impulses from the trigeminocervical nucleus will be dependent on the level of afferent input from either musculoskeletal or visceral sources as well as the level of descending inhibition. Sensitization of the trigeminocervical nucleus could also lead to peripheral changes in both musculoskeletal and visceral sources of headache.
Key: dPAG= dorsal peri-aqueductal grey matter; HT = hypothalamus; LC = locus coeruleus; vPAG = ventral peri-aqueductal grey matter; RVM = rostro ventromedial medulla; 5-HT = 5-hydroxytryptamine (serotonin); NA = noradrenaline (norepinephrine).

reflex sympathetic dystrophy, that blocking peripheral nociceptive input could normalize central processing. It is likely that many patients become caught in a 'vicious circle' of peripheral nociception that contributes to central sensitivity, which then causes secondary peripheral sensitization and dysfunction, leading to further peripheral nociception. This scenario supports the argument of Schoenen & Maertens de Noordhout (1994) that cervicogenic headache could be triggered initially by peripheral dysfunction but caused in its chronic form by central mechanisms. This argument could apply to the 28% of 150 chronic cervicogenic headache patients who, in a recent clinical trial, failed to achieve a 50% reduction in headache frequency with manipulative therapy and/or specific therapeutic exercise (Jull et al 2002).

The neurogenic model of migraine proposes that certain extrinsic or intrinsic triggers act in combination or alone to desensitize the trigeminocervical nucleus (Burstein 2001, Buzzi et al 1995, Hargreaves 2000). A consequence of this desensitization is the secondary sterile inflammatory reaction and vasodilatation affecting primarily the dural blood vessels, which then contribute strong nociceptive input to an already over-sensitive trigeminocervical nucleus and CNS. The common accompaniments of migraine such as nausea, vomiting, photophobia and phonophobia are produced upon activation of associated central pathways. Although the exact pathogenesis of migraine is unknown, a strong genetic factor is likely that predisposes the trigeminocervical nucleus to this increased reactivity (Russell 2001, Sandor et al 2000).

While tension-type headache may have myofascial factors and sensitization of peripheral nociceptors in its episodic form, central sensitization has been demonstrated consistently in its chronic form (Bendtsen 2000, Jensen 2001). There is also evidence of a hereditary component in chronic tension-type headache (Ostergaard et al 1997), possibly contributing to sensitization of the trigeminocervical nucleus. Thus, chronic tension-type headache and migraine are both likely to have their aetiology within the central nervous system, although peripheral nociception may occur in conjunction with the central sensitization.

Possible output mechanisms due to painful stimuli need to be considered in any headache presentation. These may include altered muscle activity, autonomic, neuro-endocrine and neuro-immune and behavioural changes (Gifford 1998, Melzack 1999a, 1999b). It is possible that cervical musculoskeletal dysfunction could also arise as a consequence of other headache types where central sensitization occurs. Cervical dysfunction may be a secondary effect of the headache, whatever the primary cause. If the cervical dysfunction then becomes a source of nociceptive input, there may be a cervical contribution to the headache. Therefore, there may be a secondary cervical component to other headache types that may in turn lead to ongoing sensitization of the trigeminocervical nucleus.

It is recommended that physiotherapists approach the assessment of a patient presenting with headache from a biopsychosocial perspective. This involves consideration of descending central nervous system influences on headache processing and perception, peripheral inputs to the trigeminocervical nucleus, possible outputs of the trigeminocervical nucleus and psychosocial factors that could affect both peripheral and central mechanisms of headache and its perception.

EXAMINATION OF THE HEADACHE PATIENT

Consistent with the assessment and treatment of any patient presenting for physiotherapy, examining a patient presenting with headache involves gathering and interpreting information in the following clinical reasoning categories (Jones et al 2000):

- pathobiological mechanisms
- functional limitation and disability
- physical and psychosocial impairments and their sources

- contributing factors
- precautions and contraindications
- management and treatment
- prognosis.

The aims of a physiotherapy examination of a headache patient are:

- to determine if the patient's condition is suitable for physiotherapy management
- to elicit a pattern of headache consistent with the criteria for cervicogenic headache, or components of headache consistent with a cervical component
- to elicit a pattern of cervical neuromusculoskeletal impairment which is comparable to the patient's presenting headache complaint
- to determine the most appropriate management approach for that patient
- to identify future treatment and management strategies for that patient
- to gain an idea of the likely prognosis.

Initial examination

During the initial interview, information is sought regarding the history of the headache, its temporal pattern, and the area, nature and behaviour of the headache and related symptoms. Of particular importance is information relating to diagnosis, activity restriction and impact on quality of life, and outcome measures. The physical examination must reveal a relevant and comparable pattern of cervical pain and musculoskeletal dysfunction to either make a diagnosis of cervicogenic headache, or to decide provisionally that cervical dysfunction plays a role in the patient's headache syndrome and the condition is suitable for physiotherapy management. The physiotherapist should also be formulating hypotheses regarding the pain mechanisms and non-mechanical factors that could be contributing to the symptoms. The initial examination should detect the presence of serious pathology necessitating medical referral.

Red flags

As primary contact practitioners in many countries, manual therapy practitioners must be alert for danger signs or 'red flags' that may be indicators of serious or life-threatening pathology that may underlie the patient's headache. Failure to recognize these danger signs could lead to a delay in the correct diagnosis and management of the condition, which in some cases (e.g. subarachnoid haemorrhage) may prove fatal.

Severe headache of sudden onset

Acute subarachnoid haemorrhage is typically associated with sudden onset of severe headache that may be associated with neck stiffness, photophobia, nausea and vomiting (Silberstein 1992). The headache may also be precipitated by exertion or other physical activity. In some cases, an aneurysm may 'leak' hours, days or even weeks prior to major rupture. In these cases, nausea and vomiting are common accompanying complaints (Silberstein 1992). Although relatively uncommon (an annual incidence of 4–5 per 100 000), vertebral artery and internal carotid artery dissections may cause headaches before the onset of neurological signs and symptoms. Such headaches often have accompanying neck pain (Mokri 1997). In a series of 161 patients with spontaneous dissections of the internal carotid or vertebral arteries, Silbert et al (1995) reported that ipsilateral headache was the initial symptom in 47% of the carotid artery and 33% of the vertebral artery groups. The median interval from headache onset to development of neurological symptoms was 4 days (internal carotid) and 14.5 hours (vertebral artery). Posterior neck pain was experienced by 46% of the vertebral artery group while the neck pain experienced by the internal carotid group (26%) tended to be anterolateral.

Subacute headache progressively worsening

Although many patients presenting with undiagnosed headaches are fearful that the cause of their pain is a brain tumour, Pfund et al (1999), in a series of 279 patients with brain tumours, found that half of the patients did not have headache as the initial complaint. Of the 164 patients who did experience headaches at some stage of the disease, the intensity of pain was described as severe by 55%, the quality as throbbing by 63% and shooting by 38% and the headaches were constant in only 12%. The signs that raise the probability of an intracranial tumour include a change in the headache, new symptoms, progression of the headache and abnormal neurological signs. A common finding in studies reviewed by Edmeads (1997) was that posterior fossa tumours are more likely to cause headaches and cause them earlier in the course of the disease.

Severe headache associated with nausea and vomiting

Nausea and vomiting are common accompaniments of migraine although past history of migraine should clarify the diagnosis. If it is the first time the patient has experienced nausea and vomiting with a headache, acute subarachnoid haemorrhage should be excluded by medical examination. Silbertsein (1992) describes 'the first or worst headache of the patients life' as a potential danger sign requiring investigation. If associated with a fever, the headache may be due to an infective condition such as meningitis or encephalitis.

Headache associated with neurological signs or changes in consciousness

Such headaches could be indicative of an intracranial lesion, stroke or acute subarachnoid haemorrhage and emergency medical evaluation is essential.

Temporal headache with onset after the age of 50

This may indicate the presence of giant cell arteritis, particularly if the headache is throbbing in nature and accompanied by tenderness on palpation of the temple. Identification of this condition is important, as blindness is a common complication if left untreated (Caselli & Hunder 1997).

Headache not associated with identifiable aetiology

Cervical musculoskeletal dysfunction may coexist with serious pathology, possibly as a secondary phenomenon. If there is any doubt about the headache aetiology, or the patient is not responding as expected to physiotherapy treatment, they should be referred for appropriate medical investigation and management.

The headache features and history

The length of history of cervicogenic headache is often prolonged (Fredriksen et al 1987, Jull 1986a, Pfaffenrath et al 1987, Sjaastad et al 1998). In the early stages, the headache is characterized by episodes of varying duration but over time, headaches become more continuous with exacerbations and remissions (Merskey & Bogduk 1994). Onset can occur at any age (Fredriksen et al 1987), and while onset in the young adult and middle aged is well recognized (Merskey & Bogduk 1994), Pearce (1995b) contends cervicogenic headache is the most common form of headache in people over 50 years of age. Onset may be related to neck trauma often related to a motor vehicle accident, but it is commonly insidious, possibly reflecting an accumulation of mechanical strain or symptomatic degenerative joint disease.

The studies of Vincent & Luna (1999) and Bono et al (1998) established that the criteria for cervicogenic headache (see Table 21.4) have high sensitivity and good specificity in differential diagnosis from migraine and tension-type headache, provided that at least seven features were present. The features that most distinguished cervicogenic headache were unilateral, side-locked headache with neck pain and headache association with neck postures or movements, in agreement with Sjaastad et al's (1998) major criteria.

In the examination, the practitioner is therefore seeking a pattern of headache suggestive of a cervical cause and not every criterion will be present in every patient. For example, although neck movements or sustained postures would be expected as aggravating or precipitating factors when a headache is arising from the neck, previous studies of patients diagnosed on IHS (1988) or Sjaastad's et al criteria (1990) as cervicogenic headache have shown that this is not always the case. Watson & Trott (1993) found that 69.8% of 30 subjects related the onset of their headaches to neck movements or sustained postures. Jull et al (2002) determined that 60% of 200 cervicogenic headache subjects reported mechanical precipitants for headache onset, although in the physical examination, all subjects reported pain on one or more active cervical movements.

In the differential diagnosis of the headache patient, cervical dysfunction has been reported in other headache types such as migraine or tension-type headache (Kidd & Nelson 1993, Tuchin & Pollard 1998, Vernon et al 1992a). Although some of the reported cases in these studies could have been unrecognized cervicogenic headache, it is possible that the dysfunction was secondary or even incidental to the migraine or tension-type headache. While the cervical dysfunction may not be the source of the headache, cervical nociceptive input into the trigeminocervical nucleus could contribute to the symptoms. When the trigeminocervical nucleus is in a sensitized state, any input (nociceptive or non-nociceptive) from activities or postures usually thought to indicate a mechanical component could be painful. For example, in migraine, physical activity is often painful and is one of the diagnostic criteria, yet the mechanism is not aggravation of a cervical musculoskeletal disorder. Thus, physiotherapists must use information gained from the subjective and physical examination (and treatment outcome) to determine the likely degree of musculoskeletal contribution to the headache as well as the state of excitability of the trigeminocervical nucleus and the other pathways and systems involved in pain processing and perception.

Non-mechanical considerations

During the subjective examination, the physiotherapist should ascertain whether there are any non-musculoskeletal factors affecting the patient's headache. The effect of medication may assist in the diagnostic process (Criterion 5 i, ii, Table 21.4) and give an indication of the possible pain mechanisms involved in the production and maintenance of the headaches. Non-musculoskeletal factors which precipitate or aggravate particular headache types may also aggravate cervicogenic headache when the entity of pain and a sensitized trigeminocervical system are considered. Practitioners should be aware of the possible effects that such factors as stress, hormonal changes in women and diet may have on management of the headache patient.

Stress

The relationship between pain and stress has been reviewed by Melzack (1999b). Of particular interest is the activation of the hypothalamic–pituitary–adrenal and locus coeruleus–noradrenaline (norepinephrine) systems by pain and stress leading to characteristic central and peripheral changes. Reynolds & Hovanitz (2000) found a significant positive relationship between negative life event stress and headache frequency in 1289 undergraduate psychology students. The link between stress and cervicogenic headache was explored by Bansevicius & Sjaastad (1996) who measured EMG of shoulder–neck and facial muscles as well as pain levels in cervicogenic headache patients and group-matched controls before, during and after a stressful reaction time test. They found that in the headache patients, pain values for the shoulder increased markedly during the test, while pain values for the temple and neck increased in the post-test period. There were no significant changes in pain levels for the controls. Similarly, trapezius EMG increased significantly in the headache patients during the test while there was no significant increase in trapezius EMG in control subjects. These results suggest that in susceptible individuals,

stress can affect the periphery (increased trapezius EMG), possibly at the same time as sensitizing the trigeminocervical nucleus, thus causing ongoing headache (increased post-test temple and neck pain).

Practitioners of manual therapy must be aware of the effect that altered stress levels may have on their patients' headaches. For example, decreased stress and headaches following a holiday or altered work situation may lead the treating physiotherapist to mistakenly believe that the treatment given has caused the improvement in the patient's condition. Alternatively, increased stress and headaches could mask the effect of a successful treatment or management approach. Of 91 subjects studied by Niere & Robinson (1997) 2 months after their initial physiotherapy consultation for headache, 20 felt that altered stress levels had affected their headaches during the treatment period. Of these, 10 indicated that decreased stress levels had improved their headaches, six felt that increased stress had aggravated their headaches, while four did not specify an effect. Once the patient recognizes that stress is a significant component to their headaches, they can often begin to control or manage stressful situations. In some cases, referral to another health professional (e.g. clinical psychologist) specializing in stress management and relaxation techniques may be appropriate.

Hormonal changes

The main times when hormonal changes are more likely to influence a woman's headaches are during the menstrual cycle, during pregnancy and at menopause. There have been a number of proposed mechanisms by which hormonal changes during the menstrual cycle can affect headaches. These include reduced magnesium, progesterone withdrawal, prostaglandin release and oestrogen withdrawal (MacGregor 1996). Pregnancy is usually associated with a sustained increase in oestrogen levels, and migraine sufferers appear to be more likely than sufferers of tension-type headache to experience a reduction in their levels of headache (Rasmussen 1993). In some women, headache may increase or begin during pregnancy, particularly in the first trimester when oestrogen levels are less stable. Similar variability exists with oral contraceptive use and during menopause where existing headaches (including possibly cervicogenic headache) may be exacerbated or ameliorated, or new headaches generated (Silberstein & Merriam 1991).

Diet

Not unexpectedly, relatively low percentages of patients presenting for physiotherapy management of headache implicate diet as a precipitating factor (Jull 1986a, Niere 1998), a factor not uncommon in other headache types. The classic food triggers of migraine are chocolate, oranges, red wine and cheese although glutamates (e.g. MSG), aspartame (artificial sweetener) and coffee have also been associated with the triggering of migraines and other headache types (Scharff et al 1995). The identification of a dietary component to a patient's headaches may be difficult. Scharff et al (1995) commented that specific dietary substances alone might not necessarily trigger a headache but predispose the sufferer to an attack when other factors are present. Some signs that may indicate a dietary component to the headaches include the presence of other symptoms of food allergy such as bowel irritability, eczema or persistent skin itchiness, intermittent fluid retention or lethargy. If a dietary component to the headache is likely, referral to a dietitian specializing in food allergies or to a specialist allergist may be appropriate.

The physical examination of the headache patient

In the face of the possible symptomatic overlap between cervicogenic headache, migraine and tension-type headache as well as the occurrence of combined or mixed headache forms, the physical examination assumes considerable importance to confirm or refute the diagnosis of cervicogenic headache or determining a cervical contribution to headache. The descriptions and criteria for musculoskeletal dysfunction in cervicogenic headache nominated by Sjaastad et al (1998), the IHS (1988) and IASP (Merskey & Bogduk 1994) are limited and, to a large extent, many are non-specific (Table 21.5). However, recent and continuing research is beginning to build a clearer picture of impairments in the neuro-musculo-articular systems that are associated with cervicogenic headache. In the clinical reasoning process, there can be an expectation that there will be interrelated impairment in the systems as is found in extremity musculoskeletal disorders.

The articular system

Restriction of cervical motion has been listed as a characteristic of cervicogenic headache. Painful cervical joint dysfunction is considered as one of the primary features of cervicogenic headache (Bogduk & Marsland 1985, Bogduk et al 1985, Bovim et al 1992a, Dreyfuss et al 1994, Ehni & Benner 1984, Lord et al 1994, Trevor-Jones 1964), even though the precise pathology may not be clearly evident (Bogduk 1992). Relevant dysfunction should be evident within the upper three segments (C0–1, C1–2, C2–3) for a

diagnosis of cervicogenic headache, in accordance with their neural access to the trigeminocervical system. Upper cervical dysfunction may be accompanied by joint dysfunction in other regions of the cervical or thoracic spines (Bovim et al 1992a, Jensen et al 1990a). In some cases, headache has been related to pathology in the lower cervical region (Michler et al 1991, Perez-Limonte et al 1999, Persson & Carlsson 1999).

Zwart (1997) conducted a pivotal study and quantified cervical range of movement in cervicogenic, tension-type and migraine headache sufferers against a control population. Strict inclusion criteria, according to IHS and IASP guidelines for each headache, were used in the formation of study groups. Zwart (1997) confirmed that motion was restricted in the cervicogenic headache group in flexion/extension and rotation and was a characteristic of this group only. Notable was the lack of difference in range of movement between the control, tension headache and migraine groups despite the mean age and length of history of headache of subjects in these groups. Gijsberts et al (1999a) also determined that cervicogenic headache could be distinguished from other headache forms by movement restriction. Caution may be required in viewing results of past studies in which strict inclusion criteria have not been used for headache groups, yet causative relationships have been inferred between musculoskeletal dysfunction and headache. The presence of movement restriction in studies of tension-type headache (Kidd & Nelson 1993, Tuchin & Pollard 1998, Vernon et al 1992a) may reflect the fact that such groups were inclusive of some unrecognized cervicogenic headache sufferers.

Diagnostic nerve or joint blocks are advocated for the medical diagnosis of cervicogenic headache (Criterion 2, Table 21.4). The limitations of these blocks have been discussed, but notably, they cannot be used for large population groups as encountered in general practice. Practitioners of manual therapy use the conservative method of manual examination to detect the presence or absence of symptomatic upper cervical joint dysfunction to identify cervicogenic headache patients or a possible cervical component to headache. Various studies have demonstrated good to high levels of accuracy of manual

Table 21.5 Current criteria for physical dysfunction in headache classifications

International Headache Society (1988)	International Association for the Study of Pain (Merskey & Bogduk 1994)	Sjaadstad et al (1998)
Resistance to or limitation of passive neck movements	Reduced range of motion in the neck	Restriction of range of movement in the neck
Changes in neck muscle contour, texture or tone or response to active stretching or contraction	–	–
Abnormal tenderness in neck muscles	–	Pressure over the ipsilateral upper cervical or occipital region reproduces headache

examination conducted by skilled manipulative physiotherapists to detect the presence or absence of painful upper cervical joint in headache populations (Gijsberts et al 1999b, Jull et al 1994, 1988, 1997). Furthermore, Gijsberts et al (1999b) and Zito et al (unpublished data) have shown that the presence of upper cervical joint pain and dysfunction as detected by manual examination could successfully differentiate subjects with cervicogenic headache from migraine and tension-type headache groups and asymptomatic control subjects. The results provide evidence that the conservative non-invasive method of manual examination could be used as an equivalent to diagnostic blocks in identifying the cervicogenic headache patient.

There is a note of caution. Upper cervical joint mobility as assessed by manual examination decreases with increasing age (Jull 1986b). Tenderness in neck muscles overlying the joints has been observed in patients with cervicogenic headache, migraine and tension headache as well as in asymptomatic populations (Bovim et al 1992b, Graff-Radford et al 1987, Jaeger 1989, Jensen & Rasmussen 1996, Jensen et al 1992, Langermark et al 1989, Marcus et al 1999, Vernon et al 1992b). The muscle tenderness may represent a specific primary hyperalgesia (Davidoff 1998) or a secondary hyperalgesia of a centrally sensitized state in the trigeminocervical system (Sheather-Reid & Cohen 1998) in a variety of headache types. True joint dysfunction must present as a combination of abnormal motion, abnormal tissue resistance to motion in association with local or referred pain. In addition, as elsewhere in the body, this joint dysfunction should be associated with muscle dysfunction to ensure that there is a musculoskeletal cause of headache.

The muscle system

Sjaastad et al (1998) did not nominate muscle dysfunction as a diagnostic criterion of cervicogenic headache (see Table 21.4). The IHS (1988) did so, but the criteria listed for muscle dysfunction in cervicogenic headache were expressed in general terms (see Table 21.5). The criteria reflect expected changes in the muscle system in reaction to pain and joint pathology and research is growing to better define the problems. Research has been directed towards several aspects of cervical muscle function, including aspects of neuromuscular control, muscle strength and endurance and flexibility.

Neuromotor control

Cervical neuromuscular control is a comparatively new field of clinical measurement with investigations into the control of the craniocervical flexion movement, measurement of muscle activity in defined tasks and cervical kinaesthesia.

Investigations of the interactions between the deep and superficial neck flexor synergy in the craniocervical flexion movement were stimulated by several factors. These included knowledge of the importance of the deep seg-

mental muscles for control of the cervical curve and segments (Mayoux-Benhamou et al 1994, 1997, Winters & Peles 1990), clinical theories of weakness in the deep cervical flexors in neck pain patients (Janda 1994) and discoveries in low back pain patients of motor control disturbances affecting the deep trunk and back muscles (Hodges & Richardson 1996). Disturbances in the neck flexor synergy have been documented in patients with cervicogenic headache and whiplash associated disorders using the craniocervical flexion clinical test (Jull 2000, Jull et al 1999, 2002). These studies found that the neck pain patients, as compared to asymptomatic control subjects, were less able to perform and hold progressively increasing ranges of craniocervical flexion (the action of longus capitus in synergy with longus colli). This deficit in the deep neck flexors was accompanied by increased activity in the superficial neck flexors (Jull 2000), which may be a compensatory strategy (Cholewicki et al 1997). The results suggest altered strategies of neuromuscular control in the cervical region seemingly as a reaction to pain and pathology, which may compromise the active support of the cervical spinal segments. Changes have also been documented in the deep suboccipital extensors. Andrey et al (1998), Hallgren et al (1994) and McPartland et al (1997) identified atrophy and fatty infiltration in the deep suboccipital muscles with magnetic resonance imaging in subjects with chronic upper cervical dysfunction which may further compound problems of control of the upper cervical segments.

Altered patterns of muscle activity and neuromuscular control have been documented in patients with chronic neck pain. Nederhand et al (2000) studied subjects with neck pain following a whiplash injury and found higher levels of trapezius activity (EMG) during and following low load upper limb tasks as compared to control subjects. The inability to relax the trapezius muscle following the activity was particularly notable. Barton & Hayes (1996) also noted that some subjects with cervicogenic headache had prolonged EMG relaxation times in the sternocleidomastoid muscles following cervical flexor strength tests. As mentioned previously, the study of cervicogenic headache subjects by Bansevicius & Sjaastad (1996) also demonstrated increased EMG activity in the upper trapezius while subjects performed a computer based task requiring concentration. These muscle reactions to physical or psychological stress have the potential to impact on both movement patterns and pain perception.

Deficits in cervical kinaesthetic sense (joint position error) have been documented in several studies of patients with neck pain of both traumatic and insidious onset (Heikkilä & Astrom 1996, Heikkilä & Wenngren 1998, Kristjansson et al 2003, Loudon et al 1997, Revel et al 1991, Treleaven et al 2003). The abnormal afferent activity from the neck joint and muscle receptors confuses the postural control system. A relationship has been found between the magnitude joint position error and the symptom of dizziness (Heikkilä & Wenngren 1998, Treleaven et al 2003), which may accompany cervicogenic headache (see Table 21.4).

Muscle strength, endurance and extensibility

Deficits in cervical flexor and extensor muscle strength and particularly endurance have been documented in patients with cervicogenic headache (Barton & Hayes 1996, Placzek et al 1999, Silverman et al 1991, Treleaven et al 1994, Watson & Trott 1993). Most studies have focused on the cervical flexors in line with the long-standing clinical interest in these muscles. Vernon et al (1992b) measured flexion/extension strength ratios, and found a progressive reduction in strength of the flexors relative to the extensors in the neck pain patients compared to the symptomatic group, vindicating this clinical interest.

Research into the prevalence of muscle tightness in cervicogenic headache subjects is limited which probably reflects the difficulty in developing quantitative measures to represent the length of selected muscles in the cervicothoracic region. Three studies (Jull et al 1999, Treleaven et al 1994, Zito et al unpublished data) have used conventional clinical tests of muscle length (Evjenth & Hamberg 1984, Janda 1994) to assess the upper trapezius, levator scapulae, scalene and upper cervical extensor muscle groups. The results of these studies revealed that muscle tightness could be present in cervicogenic headache subjects but it was not universal and normal responses to stretch were commonly found. Incidences of tightness were found in all muscle groups but more frequently in the upper trapezius. This might relate clinically to the findings of increased EMG activity in the upper trapezius muscle in cervicogenic headache sufferers found by Bansevicius & Sjaastad (1996) and Nederhand et al (2000).

Postural form

A forward head posture is the postural anomaly that has commonly been associated with neck pain and cervicogenic headache (Janda 1994). However, the evidence suggests that the relationship may be tenuous. Watson & Trott (1993) found that the cervicogenic headache subjects had a significantly more forward head posture than asymptomatic control subjects, as did Griegel-Morris et al (1992). However, the latter researchers also found that the severity of postural abnormality did not correlate with severity and frequency of pain. Treleaven et al (1994) failed to find a significant association between posture and headache and Haughie et al (1995) found no difference in postural shape in erect sitting. However, when posture was measured in subjects' natural sitting posture to work at a computer, the group with most symptoms had a significantly more forward head position.

The neural structures

Direct physical compromise of neural structures can contribute to the pathogenesis of some cervicogenic headaches and nerves may become physically painful.

Greater occipital nerve and C2 root allodynia may be present in cervicogenic headache (Pollmann et al 1997), and Sjaastad et al (1998) rate this sign as important in diagnosis (see Table 21.4). Nevertheless the sensitivity of the sign, and indeed the accuracy with which allodynic nerves can be differentiated from other painful myofascial and articular structures in the occipital, suboccipital region, has been questioned (Bogduk 1995a, Leone et al 1998, Pearce 1995a).

Cervicogenic headache is principally recognized as a referred pain (Bogduk 1995a) but a neurogenic origin from physical compromise of the upper cervical nerve roots or the dorsal root ganglion and the greater occipital nerve has been recorded in a few cases. Various causes have been identified surgically. These include: fibrosis of the greater occipital nerve, spondylitic changes or scar tissues around the nerve root and compression of the C2 root by vascular structures (Hildebrandt & Jansen 1984, Jansen 2000, Jansen et al 1989a, 1989b, Pikus & Philips 1995, 1996, Sjaastad et al 1986).

The dura mater of the upper cervical cord and the posterior cranial fossa receives innervation from branches of the upper three cervical nerves (Bogduk 1995a) and is capable of being a source of cervicogenic headache if they or related neural structures become mechanosensitive. Anatomical studies have demonstrated fibrous connections between the rectus capitus posterior minor and the cervical dura mater (Hack et al 1995) and continuity has been observed between the ligamentum nuchae and the posterior spinal dura at the first and second cervical levels (Mitchell et al 1998), indicating the mechanical interdependence of neural, ligamentous and muscular structures. The incidence of mechanosensitivity of neural tissues in cervicogenic headache has not been studied widely but two studies have documented incidences of 10% and 8% respectively (Jull 2001, Zito et al unpublished data). In these studies, the neural tissue provocation test was passive upper cervical flexion, subsequently sensitized by presetting the subject in the positions of the brachial plexus provocation test and straight leg raise.

The diagnosis of cervicogenic headache

Research is increasing to characterize the physical impairment in the cervical musculoskeletal system towards the diagnosis of cervicogenic headache or a cervical component of headache. Table 21.6 summarizes knowledge to date. As with symptoms, not all patients will have every impairment, but a pattern of physical dysfunction in the articular and muscle systems is mandatory. The practitioner must not be swayed by the mere presence of neck pain or tenderness to make a diagnosis of cervicogenic headache, as these may be present in several headache types. Rather, a pattern of relevant dysfunction in the cervical musculoskeletal system must be added to the pattern of symptoms (see Table 21.4) to make this diagnosis.

Table 21.6 Physical criteria for cervicogenic headache

System	Impairment	
Articular	Decreased cervical range of motion	✓
	Upper cervical segmental joint dysfunction	✓
Muscle	Altered neuromuscular control	✓
	Reduced strength and endurance	✓
	Muscle tightness	±
Postural form	Forward head posture	±
Neural	Neural tissue mechanosensitivity	±

MANAGEMENT OF CERVICOGENIC HEADACHE

When the literature is reviewed, it becomes evident that many treatments have been trialed for cervicogenic headache. Conservative treatments have included pharmaceutical agents (simple analgesics and non-steroidal anti-inflammatory drugs) (Bogduk 1995b, Pollmann et al 1997, Sjaastad et al 1997, van Suijlekom et al 1998) and a variety of physical therapies. Those tested include manipulative therapy, traction, trigger point therapy, muscle stretching, cold packs, heat packs and transcutaneous electrical stimulation (Beeton & Jull 1994, Farina et al 1986, Jaeger 1989, Jensen et al 1990b, Martelletti et al 1995, Nilsson et al 1997, Schoensee et al 1995, Vernon 1991, Whittingham et al 1994). Cognitive behavioural programmes have also been tested (Graff-Radford et al 1987). In addition, a variety of medical and surgical procedures have been used. These include: anaesthetic blocks to muscle trigger points, joints and nerves; percutaneous radiofrequency neurotomies; radiofrequency therapy to the external surface of the occipital bone; C2 ganglionectomy; and surgical decompression or fusion (Bogduk & Marsland 1985, Bovim et al 1992b, Graff-Radford et al 1987, Jansen et al 1998, Lord et al 1995b, Pikus & Philips 1996, Sjaastad et al 1995, van Suijlekom et al 1998, Vincent 1998). Such an extensive list either attests to the fact that the optimal treatment has not been discovered or it may reflect the spectrum of pathologies and physical reactions that are present in the cervicogenic headache syndrome.

Sjaastad et al (1997) recently reviewed the therapies for cervicogenic headache and presented them in a hierarchical order. Treatments begin with the most uncomplicated measures inclusive of physiotherapy, non-steroidal anti-inflammatory drugs (NSAIDs) or mild analgesics, the use of repeated (e.g. weekly) injections of local anaesthetics, with or without corticosteroids, into the greater or lesser occipital nerves, and progress toward invasive procedures for the more severe and recalcitrant headaches. Towards the development of an evidence base for the conservative management of cervicogenic headache, manipulative therapy has been the physical therapy that has received most attention in studies of the conservative management of cervicogenic headache or a cervical component of headache (Boline et al 1995, Jensen et al 1990b, Martelletti et al 1995,

Nilsson et al 1997, Schoensee et al 1995, Vernon 1991, Whittingham et al 1994). In systematic reviews, Hurwitz et al (1996) and Vernon et al (1999) found that there was preliminary evidence to suggest that manipulative therapy had some benefit at the short-term follow-up times tested in the trials, but the scarcity and quality of evidence precluded definitive recommendations about its effectiveness.

Evidence is increasing for a better effect of combined treatments in the management of cervical musculoskeletal dysfunction (Aker et al 1996, Bronfort et al 2001). As previously discussed, research into the physical characteristics of cervicogenic headache is establishing that cervicogenic headache is associated with impairment in both the muscle and articular systems. In response, Jull et al (2002) tested a multimodal management programme consisting of manipulative therapy and specific therapeutic exercise against each modality used alone and a control non-treatment group, in a cohort of 200 cervicogenic headache sufferers. The therapeutic exercise programme, in contrast to strength training, used specific low load endurance exercises to train muscle control of the cervicoscapular region. It aimed to address impairments in neuromotor control found in cervicogenic headache subjects (Jull et al 1999). The exercise programme is detailed in Chapter 33. The results of the trial indicated that the multimodal and single modality therapies all significantly reduced the neck pain and headache compared to the control group. The relief was sustained in the long term, over the 12-month follow-up period. A beneficial outcome was not related to the age or gender of the patient nor to the length of history of headache (population mean, 6.1 years). Although the results did not reach statistical significance, subjects receiving the multimodal programme achieved a 10% greater reduction in the frequency of their headaches compared to those who received single modality treatment, which is clinically relevant. While there was overlap in the effects of the three treatments, particular treatments had a better effect on one outcome than another. For example, manipulative therapy used alone did not improve performance in the craniocervical muscle test. This trial has added to the evidence base for the effectiveness of physiotherapy management for cervicogenic headache and reinforces the contemporary argument and clinical logic for the need to address all systems in a multimodal management approach.

While positive results of treatment effectiveness are reassuring to the practitioner in the evidence based treatment climate, it is possibly the unexpected and negative outcomes of clinical trials such as the cervicogenic headache trial that stimulate most thought. Manipulative therapy and therapeutic exercise at first glance appear quite different treatment methods, but both achieved similar outcomes, suggesting that both produce similar responses in the pain system. Both are specific treatment methods and both could induce quite local afferent input to modulate pain perception. Research suggests that the afferent input induced by manipulative therapy procedures may stimulate neural inhibitory systems at various levels in the spinal cord (Allen et al 1984, Christian et al 1988) as well as activating descending inhibitory pathways from, for example, the lateral peri-aqueductal grey area of the midbrain (Vicenzino et al 1994, 1998, Wright 1995, Wright et al 1994). Furthermore, Thabe (1986) measured a reduction in electrical activity in the small suboccipital extensors which overlie C1–2 in response to joint mobilization and high velocity manipulation, a response that could also be achieved through reciprocal relaxation with exercise of the deep neck flexors. Such factors point to the need to research and consider in clinical practice multi-mechanisms to explain the pain relief gained by these physical treatments. A negative finding of the clinical trial was that 28% of patients at the 12-month follow-up failed to achieve the benchmark of at least a 50% reduction in headache frequency. No baseline characteristics clearly identified this group. It is possible that these patients had other factors maintaining the sensitization of the trigeminocervical nucleus which were not addressed by the physical treatments (see Fig. 21.2), that central mechanisms were more dominant in the pain state, or that the neck pathogenesis of the headache was not amenable to conservative care (Jansen et al 1989b, Lord et al 1995b, Pikus & Philips 1996, van Suijlekom et al 1998). This patient group exemplifies the need for the clinician to critically evaluate patient outcomes and refer the patient for specific medical management if desired results are not being achieved.

There are case reports and clinical trials of manipulative therapy which have specifically addressed other headache forms such as migraine or tension headache with the underlying assumption that there is a purported cervical cause or component to the headache form (Boline et al 1995, Bove & Nilsson 1998, Hammill et al 1995, Hoyt et al 1979, Parker et al 1978, Tuchin & Pollard 1998). Neither the pathogenesis of migraine nor tension-type headache resides primarily in cervical musculoskeletal dysfunction. However, as previously discussed, concurrent cervical dysfunction may further sensitize the trigeminocervical nucleus or cervical musculoskeletal dysfunction may arise as a consequence of other headache types where central sensitization occurs. Partial or temporary relief may be achieved with physical therapies. Accurate diagnosis is the key. The clinician must recognize the place of physical treatments in the overall management of these headache types and discuss prognosis with the patient. It is inappropriate to provide prolonged ongoing treatment and this situation emphasizes the essential need for use of valid outcome assessments in the management of the headache patient.

OUTCOME ASSESSMENT

It is essential to be able to determine whether or not the management approach to the headache patient is of benefit. In clinical practice patient and/or therapist estimates are often sought as an indicator of treatment efficacy. However, the reactivity or potential for bias of patient and therapist estimates should be considered (Turk et al 1993).

Headache symptoms

Most benign headache types are characterized by intermittent bouts of head pain of finite duration. Intervening periods are usually pain-free or have a lower level of baseline pain. The headache characteristics of intensity, frequency and duration are therefore often used as outcome measures. These parameters are usually measured in the clinical setting by retrospective patient reports, either through interview or by questionnaire (Andrasik 1992, Niere & Robinson 1997), although headache diaries are the preferred method of data collection for research projects (IHS 1995). Regardless of the method, measurement of headache is dependent on patient report with its potential for bias or inaccuracy. Niere & Jerak (2002) studied 40 headache sufferers and found that when compared to the use of a headache diary, patient estimations of headache frequency (rho = 0.80), and duration (rho = 0.72) were reasonably accurate. There was a tendency for subjects to underestimate headache frequency, but overestimate duration. Memory for headache intensity was relatively poor (rho = 0.51), with 75% of subjects overestimating headache intensity. A reason for this inaccuracy could be the multidimensional nature of pain (as opposed to the temporal nature of frequency and duration). However, other studies have found that retrospective reporting of chronic headache may be dependent on current pain intensity (Eich et al 1985) or that bias might exist towards remembering more severe or recent headache episodes (Rasmussen et al 1991c).

Given the possible inaccuracy of memory for headache intensity, if headache intensity were used to determine the efficacy of treatment, larger changes would be necessary to be certain of a treatment effect. Headache frequency seems to be more intuitively important to headache sufferers as a measure of treatment success. A study by Niere (1997) found that of 154 patients presenting to physiotherapy clinics for physiotherapy treatment of their headaches, 66% indicated that reduced headache frequency was the most important indicator of treatment success, as opposed to 21% for intensity and 5% for duration.

If a patient's headaches are infrequent or inconsistent the physiotherapist should establish the longest period of time the patient can be headache free and the length of time since their last headache. There will then be less likelihood of wrongly attributing a headache attack or headache-free period to the physiotherapy treatment administered. Where the headaches are constant or semi-continuous the number of headache days in a typical week or over the previous month should be ascertained. Other outcome measures that may be of use include the amount and type of medication taken, time missed from work, school or home duties and pain measurement scales such as the McGill

Pain Questionnaire (MPQ) or the Short Form MPQ (Melzack 1983, 1987).

Headache related activity restriction

Cavallini et al (1995) demonstrated that headache sufferers experienced a reduction in their functional capabilities during headache attacks. The study also demonstrated that subjects suffered from diminished motor performance, disturbed interpersonal relationships and feelings of inadequacy. The headaches also had a negative impact on well-being during headache-free periods. Subjects reported distress from imminence of attacks and also disturbed relationships with family, friends and colleagues, often influencing the planning of their social lives.

A number of measures have been designed to measure headache related disability. However, these have related either to specific headache types such as migraine or were developed within secondary referral headache clinics (Jacobsen et al 1994). In order to measure the activity restriction experienced by headache patients attending physiotherapy clinics, Quin & Niere (2001) reduced a 16-item migraine-specific questionnaire (Stewart et al 1998) into a nine-item questionnaire based on responses made by a population of 111 subjects receiving physiotherapy treatment for their headaches. The suggested items, detailed in Box 21.1, are measured using an 11-point Likert scale with

---

Box 21.1 Items derived by Quin & Niere (2001) for inclusion in a headache specific disability questionnaire

1. How would you rate the average pain from your headache on a scale from 0 to 10?
2. When you have headaches, how often is the pain severe?
3. On how many days in the last month did you actually lie down for an hour or more because of your headaches?
4. When you have a headache, how often do you miss work or school for all or part of the day?
5. When you have a headache while you work (work or school), how much is your ability to work reduced?
6. How many days in the last month have you been kept from doing housework or chores for at least half of the day because of your headaches?
7. How much is your ability to do housework or chores reduced?
8. How many days in the last month have you been kept from non-work activities (family, social or recreational) because of your headaches?
9. When you have a headache, how much is your ability to engage in non-work activities (family, social or recreational) reduced?

---

scores ranging from 0 to 10 for each item. The questionnaire was found to have good construct validity and internal consistency and is currently undergoing investigation of test–retest reliability and sensitivity to change.

Physical outcomes

Quality of life outcomes are most important outcomes to the patient and indeed can be regarded as the major factor in assessing the effectiveness of a therapy. Also of importance for physiotherapists is the link between pain, physical impairment and disability (Fitzgerald et al 1994, Jette 1995). Physiotherapists are used to reassessing the patient's physical signs in order to evaluate current and guide continuing treatment. What is needed is more ordered and better quantification of these physical impairments in routine clinical practice. There are simple and relatively inexpensive devices on the market to measure, for example, range of movement with an accompanying pain rating and to make a clinical evaluation of the neck flexor synergy in the craniocervical flexion test. Pain provocation on manual examination of the upper cervical joints can be documented as an outcome measure. Preliminary evidence of their sensitivity to change was demonstrated in a recent trial of management of cervicogenic headache (Jull et al 2002).

Physical outcome measures are necessary to evaluate the effectiveness of a particular treatment technique on neuromuscular–articular pain and impairment. They are also valuable in guiding decisions about the primary or secondary role of cervical musculoskeletal dysfunction in headache. The pattern and magnitude of the painful cervical dysfunction should fit the pattern of headache frequency, intensity and duration. There should be some relationship between improvement in physical signs and improvement in headache in a progressive way in a cervicogenic headache patient. If improvement occurs in physical signs without improvement in headache, it is possible that the musculoskeletal dysfunction is incidental to the headache. If initial improvement occurs in physical signs but cannot be sustained and headaches continue, it is probable that the musculoskeletal dysfunction is a secondary phenomenon to a primary headache of non-musculoskeletal origin. Lasting change must occur in symptoms and signs to justify continuing physical therapy treatment.

CONCLUSION

Headache is a common and often debilitating condition. Cervicogenic headache probably accounts for between 10 and 20% of the common benign headache types. The efficacy of physical therapy management is being evaluated within the framework of evidence based health care. The evidence for effectiveness of multimodal physical therapy programmes for cervicogenic headache is growing. The first criterion for successful outcomes is to treat the patient for whom the intervention is appropriate. Fundamental to successful management is the differential diagnosis of headache. The diagnostic criteria for cervicogenic headache present a pattern of headache symptoms suggestive of a cervical cause. These, together with emerging evidence of the physical impairments in the cervical musculoskeletal system, provide the practitioner of manual therapy with a 'package' of symptoms and signs to guide their diagnosis.

References

Aker P D, Gross A R, Goldsmith C H, Peloso P 1996 Conservative management of mechanical neck pain: systematic overview and meta-analysis. British Medical Journal 313: 1291–1296

Allen C J, Terrett D, Vernon H 1984 Manipulation and pain tolerance. American Journal of Physical Medicine 63: 217–225

Andrasik F 1992 Assessment of patients with headache. In: Turk D C, Melzack R (eds) Handbook of pain assessment. Guilford Press, New York, pp 344–361

Andrey M T, Hallgren R C, Greenman P E, Rechtien J J 1998 Neurogenic atrophy of suboccipital muscles after a cervical injury. American Journal of Physical Medicine and Rehabilitation 77: 545–549

Anthony M 2000 Cervicogenic headache: prevalence and response to local steroid therapy. Clinical and Experimental Neurology 18: S59–S64

Aprill C, Axinn M J, Bogduk N 2002 Occipital headaches stemming from the lateral atlanto-axial (C1–2) joint. Cephalalgia 22: 15–22

Bansevicius D, Sjaastad O 1996 Cervicogenic headache: the influence of mental load on pain level and EMG of shoulder-neck and facial muscles. Headache 36: 372–378

Barnsley L, Lord S, Wallis B, Bogduk N 1993 False-positive rates of cervical zygapophysial joint blocks. Clinical Journal of Pain 9: 124–130

Barton P M, Hayes K C 1996 Neck flexor muscle strength, efficiency, and relaxation times in normal subjects and subjects with unilateral neck pain and headache. Archives of Physical Medicine and Rehabilitation 77: 680–687

Beeton K, Jull G A 1994 The effectiveness of manipulative physiotherapy in the management of cervicogenic headache: a single case study. Physiotherapy 80: 417–423

Bendtsen L 2000 Central sensitization in tension-type headache-possible pathophysiological mechanisms. Cephalalgia 20: 486–508

Blau J N, MacGregor E A 1994 Migraine and the neck. Headache 34: 88–90

Bogduk N 1992 The anatomical basis for cervicogenic headache. Journal of Manipulative and Physiological Therapeutics 15: 67–70

Bogduk N 1995a Anatomy and physiology of headache. Biomedicine and Pharmacotherapy 49: 435–445

Bogduk N 1995b Neck pain: assessment and management in general practice. Modern Medicine of Australia (September): 102–108

Bogduk N 1997 Headache and the neck. In: Goadsby P J, Silberstein S D (eds) Headache. Butterworth Heinemann, Boston, pp 369–381

Bogduk N, Marsland A 1985 Third occipital headache. Cephalalgia 5(Suppl. 3): 310–311

Bogduk N, Corrigan B, Kelly P, Schneider G, Farr R 1985 Cervical headache. Medical Journal of Australia 143: 202–207

Boline P D, Kassak K, Bronfort G, Nelson C, Anderson A V 1995 Spinal manipulation vs amitriptyline for the treatment of chronic tension-type headaches: a randomized clinical trial. Journal of Manipulative and Physiological Therapeutics 18: 148–154

Bono G, Antonaci F, Ghirmai S, Sandrini G, Nappi G 1998 The clinical profile of cervicogenic headache as it emerges from a study based on the early diagnostic criteria (Sjaastad et al 1990). Functional Neurology 13: 75–77

Bove G, Nilsson N 1998 Spinal manipulation in the treatment of episodic tension-type headache. Journal of the American Medical Association 280: 1576–1579

Bovim G, Sand T 1992 Cervicogenic headache, migraine without aura and tension-type headache: diagnostic blockade of greater occipital and supra-orbital nerves. Pain 51: 43–48

Bovim G, Berg R, Dale L G 1992a Cervicogenic headache: anesthetic blockades of cervical nerves (C2–C5) and facet joint (C2/C3). Pain 49: 315–320

Bovim G, Fredriksen T A, Nielsen A S, Sjaastad O 1992b Neurolysis of the greater occipital nerve in cervicogenic headache: a follow up study. Headache 32: 175–179

Bronfort G, Evans R, Nelson B, Aker P D, Goldsmith C H, Vernon H 2001 A randomized clinical trial for patients with chronic neck pain. Spine 26: 788–799

Burstein R 2001 Deconstructing migraine into peripheral and central sensitisation Pain 89: 107–110

Buzzi M G, Bonamini M, Moskowitz M A 1995 Neurogenic model of migraine. Cephalalgia 15: 277–280

Caselli R J, Hunder G G 1997 Giant cell (temporal) arteritis as a cause of headache in the elderly. In: Goadsby P J, Silberstein S D (eds) Headache. Butterworth Heinemann, Boston, pp 299–311

Cavallini A, Micieli G, Bussone G, Rossi F, Nappi G 1995 Headache and quality of life. Headache 35: 29–35

Cholewicki J, Panjabi M M, Khachatryan A 1997 Stabilizing function of the trunk flexor-extensor muscles around a neutral spine. Spine 22: 2207–2212

Christian G F, Stanton G J, Sissons D et al 1988 Immunoreactive ACTH, beta-endorphins and cortisol levels in plasma following spinal manipulative therapy. Spine 13: 1411–1417

Curatolo M, Petersen-Felix S, Arendt-Nielsen L, Giani C, Zbinden A M, Radanov B P 2001 Central sensitivity in chronic pain after whiplash injury. Clinical Journal of Pain 17: 306–315

D'Amico D, Leone M, Bussone G 1994 Side-locked unilaterality and pain localisation in long-lasting headaches: migraine, tension-type headache and cervicogenic headache. Headache 34: 526–530

Davidoff R A 1998 Trigger points and myofascial pain: toward understanding how they affect headaches. Cephalalgia 18: 436–448

Dreyfuss P, Rogers J, Dreyer S, Fletcher D 1994 Atlanto-occipital joint pain: a report of three cases and description of an intra-articular joint block technique. Regional Anesthesia 19: 344–351

Edmeads J 1996 Plenary session on headache cervicogenic headache. Pain Research and Management 1: 119–122

Edmeads J 1997 Brain tumours and other space-occupying lesions In: Goadsby P J, Silberstein S D (eds) Headache. Butterworth Heinemann, Boston, pp 313–326

Ehni G, Benner B 1984 Occipital neuralgia and C1–C2 arthrosis. New England Journal of Medicine 310: 127

Eich E, Reeves J L, Jaeger B, Graff-Radford S B 1985 Memory for pain: relation between past and present intensities. Pain 23: 375–379

Evjenth O, Hamberg J 1984 Muscle stretching in manual therapy. Alfta Rehab Forlag, Alfta, vols 1–2

Falconer M A 1949 Intramedullary trigeminal tractotomy and its place in the treatment of facial pain. Journal of Neurology, Neurosurgery and Psychiatry 12: 297

Farina S, Granella F, Malferrari G, Manzoni G C 1986 Headache and cervical spine disorders: classification and treatment with transcutaneous electrical nerve stimulation. Headache 26: 431–433

Feinstein B, Langton J B K, Jameson R M, Schiller F 1954 Experiments on referred pain from deep somatic tissues. Journal of Bone and Joint Surgery 36A: 981–997

Fields H L 1997 Pain modulation and headache In: Goadsby P J, Silberstein S D (eds) Headache. Butterworth Heinemann, Boston, pp 39–57

Fitzgerald G K, McClure P W, Beattie P, Riddle D L 1994 Issues in determining the effectiveness of manual therapies. Physical Therapy 74: 227–233

Fredriksen T A, Hovdal H, Sjaastad O 1987 Cervicogenic headache: clinical manifestations. Cephalalgia 7: 147–160

Gifford L 1998 Pain, the tissues and the nervous system: a conceptual model. Physiotherapy 84: 27–36

Gijsberts T J, Duquet W, Stoekart R, Oostendorp R 1999a Impaired mobility of cervical spine as tool in diagnosis of cervicogenic headache [Abstract]. Cephalalgia 19: 436

Gijsberts T J, Duquet W, Stoekart R, Oostendorp R 1999b Pain-provocation tests for C0–4 as a tool in the diagnosis of cervicogenic headache [Abstract]. Cephalalgia 19: 436

Goadsby P J, Knight Y E, Hoskin K L 1997 Stimulation of the greater occipital nerve increases metabolic activity in the trigeminal nucleus and cervical dorsal horn of the cat. Pain 73: 23–28

Gracely R H, Lynch S A, Bennett G J 1992 Painful neuropathy: altered central processing maintained dynamically by peripheral input. Pain 51: 175–194

Graff-Radford S B, Reeves J L, Jaeger B 1987 Management of chronic head and neck pain: effectiveness of altering factors perpetuating myofascial pain. Headache 27: 186–190

Granella F, D'Alessandro R, Manozi G 1994 International Headache Society classification: interobserver reliability in diagnosis of primary headache. Cephalalgia 14: 16–20

Griegel-Morris P, Larson K, Mueller-Klaus K, Oatis C A 1992 Incidence of common postural abnormalities in the cervical, shoulder, and thoracic regions and their association with pain in two age groups of healthy subjects. Physical Therapy 72: 425–431

Hack G D, Koritzer R T, Robinson W L, Hallgren R C, Greenman P E 1995 Anatomic relation between the rectus capitis posterior minor muscle and the dura mater. Spine 20: 2484–2486

Hallgren R C, Greenman P E, Rechtien J J 1994 Atrophy of suboccipital muscles in patients with chronic pain: a pilot study. Journal of American Osteopathic Association 94: 1032–1038

Hammill J M, Cook T M, Rosecrance J C 1995 Effectiveness of a physical therapy regimen in the treatment of tension-type headache. Headache 36: 149–153

Hargreaves R J 2000 Pharmacology and potential mechanisms of action of rizatriptan. Cephalalgia 20(Suppl. 1): 2–9

Haughie L J, Fiebert I M, Roach K E 1995 Relationship of forward head posture and cervical backward bending to neck pain. Journal of Manual and Manipulative Therapy 3: 91–97

Heikkilä H V, Astrom P G 1996 Cervicocephalic kinesthestic sensibility in patients with whiplash injury. Scandinavian Journal of Rehabilitation Medicine 28: 133–138

Heikkilä H, Wenngren B 1998 Cervicocephalic kinesthetic sensibility, active range of cervical motion and oculomotor function in patients with whiplash injury. Archives of Physical Medicine and Rehabilitation 79: 1089–1094

Hildebrandt J, Jansen J 1984 Vascular compression of the C2 and C3 roots: yet another cause of chronic intermittent hemicrania. Cephalalgia 4: 167–170

Hodges P W, Richardson C A 1996 Inefficient stabilisation of the lumbar spine associated with low back pain: a motor control evaluation of transversus abdominis. Spine 21: 2640–2650

Hoyt W H, Shaffer F, Bard D A et al 1979 Osteopathic manipulation in the treatment of muscle-contraction headache. Journal of American Osteopathic Association 78: 322–325

Hunter C R, Mayfield F H 1949 Role of the upper cervical roots in the production of pain in the head. American Journal of Surgery 78: 743–749

Hurwitz E L, Aker P D, Adams A H, Meeker W C, Shekelle P G 1996 Manipulation and mobilization of the cervical spine: a systematic review of the literature. Spine 21: 1746–1760

International Headache Society Committee on Clinical Trials 1995 Guidelines for trials of drug treatments in tension-type headache. Cephalalgia 15: 165–179

International Headache Society Headache Classification Committee 1988 Classification and diagnostic criteria for headache disorders, cranial neuralgias and facial pain. Cephalalgia 8(7S): 1–96

Jacobsen G P, Ramadan N M, Aggarwal S K, Newman C W 1994 The Henry Ford Hospital headache disability inventory (HDI). Neurology 44: 837–842

Jaeger B 1989 Are cervicogenic headaches due to myofascial pain and cervical spine dysfunction? Cephalalgia 9: 157–164

Janda V 1994 Muscles and motor control in cervicogenic disorders: assessment and management. In: Grant R (ed) Physical therapy of the cervical and thoracic spine. Churchill Livingstone, New York, pp 195–216

Jansen J 2000 Surgical treatment of non responsive cervicogenic headache. Clinical and Experimental Neurology 18: S67–S70

Jansen J, Bardosi A, Hilderbrandt J, Lucke A 1989a Cervicogenic, hemicranial attacks associated with vascular irritation or compression of the cervical nerve root C2: clinical manifestations and morphological findings. Pain 39: 203–212

Jansen J, Markakis E, Rama B, Hildebrandt J 1989b Hemicranial attacks or permanent hemicrania: a sequel of upper cervical root compression. Cephalalgia 9: 123–130

Jansen J, Vadokas V, Vogelsang J P 1998 Cervical peridural anaesthesia: an essential aid for the indication of surgical treatment of cervicogenic headache triggered by degenerative diseases of the cervical spine. Functional Neurology 13: 79–81

Jensen R 2001 Mechanisms of tension-type headache. Cephalalgia 21: 786–789

Jensen R, Rasmussen B K 1996 Muscular disorders in tension-type headache Cephalalgia 16: 97–103

Jensen O K, Justesen T, Nielsen F F, Brixen K 1990a Functional radiographic examination of the cervical spine in patients with post-traumatic headache. Cephalalgia 10: 295–303

Jensen O, Nielsen F F, Vosmar L 1990b An open study comparing manual therapy with the use of cold packs in the treatment of post-traumatic headache. Cephalalgia 10: 241–250

Jensen R, Rasmussen B K, Pedersen B, Lous I, Olesen J 1992 Cephalic muscle tenderness and pressure pain threshold in a general population. Pain 48: 197–203

Jette A M 1995 Outcomes research: shifting the dominant research paradigm in physical therapy. Physical Therapy 75: 965–970

Johansen M K, Graven-Nielsen T G, Olesen A S, Arendt-Nielsen L 1999 Generalised muscular hyperalgesion in chronic whiplash syndrome. Pain 83: 229–234

Jones M A, Jensen G, Edwards I 2000 Clinical reasoning in physiotherapy. In: Higgs J, Jones M A (eds) Clinical reasoning in the health professions, 2nd edn. Butterworth Heinemann, Oxford, pp 118–127

Joseph R, Welch K M A, D'Andrea G 1989 Serotonergic hypofunction in migraine: a synthesis of evidence based on platelet dense body dysfunction. Cephalalgia 9: 293–299

Jull G A 1986a Headaches associated with the cervical spine: a clinical review. In: Grieve G P (ed) Modern Manual Therapy of the Vertebral Column. Churchill Livingstone, Edinburgh, pp 322–329

Jull G A 1986b Clinical observation of upper cervical mobility. In: Grieve G P (ed) Modern Manual Therapy of the Vertebral Column. Churchill Livingstone, Edinburgh, pp 315–321

Jull G A 2000 Deep cervical neck flexor dysfunction in whiplash. Journal of Musculoskeletal Pain 8: 143–154

Jull G A 2001 The physiotherapy management of cervicogenic headache: a randomised clinical trial. PhD Thesis, University of Queensland, Australia

Jull G, Bogduk N, Marsland A 1988 The accuracy of manual diagnosis for cervical zygapophysial joint pain syndromes. Medical Journal of Australia 148: 233–236

Jull G A, Treleaven J, Versace G 1994 Manual examination of spinal joints: is pain provocation a major diagnostic cue for dysfunction? Australian Journal of Physiotherapy 40: 159–165

Jull G, Zito G, Trott P, Potter H, Shirley D, Richardson C 1997 Inter-examiner reliability to detect painful upper cervical joint dysfunction. Australian Journal of Physiotherapy 43: 125–129

Jull G, Barrett C, Magee R, Ho P 1999 Further characterisation of muscle dysfunction in cervical headache. Cephalalgia 19: 179–185

Jull G, Trott P, Potter H, et al 2002 A randomized controlled trial of exercise and manipulative therapy for cervicogenic headache. Spine 27: 1835–1843

Kerr F W L 1961 Mechanisms, diagnosis and treatment of some cranial and facial pain syndromes. Surgical Clinics of North America 43: 951–961

Kerr F W L, Olafson R A 1961 Trigeminal and cervical volleys. Archives of Neurology 5: 171–178

Kidd R F, Nelson R 1993 Musculoskeletal dysfunction of the neck in migraine and tension headache. Headache 33: 566–569

Kristjansson E, Dall'Alba P, Jull G 2003 A study of five cervicocephalic relocation tests in three different subject groups. Clinical Rehabilitation 17: 768–774

Lance J W, Lambert G A, Goadsby P J, Duckworth J W 1983 Brainstem influences on the cephalic circulation: experimental data from cat and monkey of relevance to the mechanism of migraine. Headache 23: 258–265

Langermark M, Jensen K, Jensen T S, Olesen J 1989 Pressure-pain thresholds and thermal nociceptive thresholds in chronic tension-type headache. Pain 38: 203–210

Leonardi M, Musicco M, Nappi G 1998 Headaches as a major public health problem: current status. Cephalalgia 18(Suppl. 21): 66–69

Leone M, Filippini G, D'Amico D, Farinotti M, Bussone G 1994 Assessment of International Headache Society diagnostic criteria: a reliability study. Cephalalgia 14: 280–284

Leone M, D'Amico D, Grazzi L, Attanasio A, Bussone G 1998 Cervicogenic headache: a critical review of current diagnostic criteria. Pain 78: 1–5

Leston J A 1996 Migraine and tension-type headache are not separate disorders. Cephalalgia 16: 220–222

Lord S M, Barnsley L, Wallis B J, Bogduk N 1994 Third occipital nerve headache: a prevalence study. Journal of Neurology, Neurosurgery and Psychiatry 57: 1187–1190

Lord S M, Barnsley L, Bogduk N 1995a The utility of comparative local anesthetic blocks versus placebo-controlled blocks for the diagnosis of cervical zygapophyseal joint pain. Clinical Journal of Pain 11: 208–213

Lord S M, Barnsley L, Bogduk N 1995b Percutaneous radiofrequency neurotomy in the treatment of cervical zygapophysial joint pain: a caution. Neurosurgery 36: 732–329

Loudon J K, Ruhl M, Field E 1997 Ability to reproduce head position after whiplash injury. Spine 22: 865–868

MacGregor E A 1996 'Menstrual' migraine: towards a definition. Cephalalgia 16: 11–21

McPartland J M, Brodeur R R, Hallgren R C 1997 Chronic neck pain, standing balance, and suboccipital muscle atrophy: a pilot study. Journal of Manipulative and Physiological Therapeutics 20: 24–29

Marcus D A 1992 Migraine and tension-type headaches: the questionable validity of current classification systems. Clinical Journal of Pain 8: 28–36

Marcus D A, Scharff L, Mercer S, Turk D C 1999 Musculoskeletal abnormalities in chronic headache: a controlled comparison of headache diagnostic groups. Headache 39: 21–27

Martelletti P, LaTour D, Giacovazzo M 1995 Spectrum of pathophysiological disorders in cervicogenic headache and its therapeutic indications. Journal of the Neuromusculoskeletal System 3: 182–187

Mayoux-Benhamou M A, Revel M, Vallee C, Roudier R, Barbet J P, Bargy F 1994 Longus colli has a postural function on cervical curvature. Surgical Radiologic Anatomy 16: 367–371

Mayoux-Benhamou M A, Revel M, Vallee C 1997 Selective electromyography of dorsal neck muscles in humans. Experimental Brain Research 113: 353–360

Melzack R 1983 The McGill Pain Questionnaire. In: Melzack R (ed) Pain measurement and assessment. Raven Press, New York, pp 41–47

Melzack R 1987 The short-form McGill Pain Questionnaire. Pain 30: 191–197

Melzack R 1999a From the gate to the neuromatrix. Pain 6(Suppl.): S121–S126

Melzack R 1999b Pain and stress: a new perspective In: Gatchel R J, Turk D C (eds) Psychosocial factors in pain. Guildford Press, New York, pp 89–106

Merskey H, Bogduk N 1994 Classification of chronic pain. IASP Press, Seattle, pp 94–95

Michler R P, Bovim G, Sjaastad O 1991 Disorders in the lower cervical spine: a cause of unilateral headache? A case report. Headache 31: 550–551

Mitchell B S, Humphries B K, O'Sullivan E 1998 Attachments of ligamentum nuchae to cervical posterior dura and the lateral part of the occipital bone. Journal of Manipulative and Physiological Therapeutics 21: 145–148

Mokri B 1997 Headache in spontaneous carotid and vertebral artery dissections In: Goadsby P J and Silberstein S D (eds) Headache. Butterworth Heinemann, Boston, pp 327–353

Nederhand M J, Ijerman M J, Hermens H J, Baten C T, Zilvold G 2000 Cervical muscle dysfunction in chronic whiplash associated disorder Grade 11 (WAD-11). Spine 25: 1939–1943

Nelson C F 1994 The tension headache, migraine headache continuum: a hypothesis. Journal of Manipulative and Physiological Therapeutics 17: 156–167

Niere K R 1997 Expectations of physiotherapy treatment in headache patients. In: Focusing Ahead: Proceedings of the 10th biennial conference of the Manipulative Physiotherapists' Association of Australia. MPAA Publishers, Melbourne, pp 136–137

Niere K R 1998 Can characteristics of benign headache predict manipulative physiotherapy treatment outcome? Australian Journal of Physiotherapy 44: 87–93

Niere K R 2002 Pain descriptors used by headache patients presenting for physiotherapy. Physiotherapy 88(7): 409–416

Niere K R, Jerak A 2001 Memory for headache frequency and duration is more accurate than for headache intensity. In Singer K P (ed) Proceedings of the 7th Scientific Conference of the International Federation of Orthopaedic Manipulative Therapists. University of Western Australia, Perth, pp 353–356

Niere K R, Robinson P M 1997 Determination of manipulative physiotherapy treatment outcome in headache patients. Manual Therapy 2: 199–205

Nilsson N 1995 The prevalence of cervicogenic headache in a random population sample of 20–59 year olds. Spine 20: 1884–1888

Nilsson N, Christensen H W, Hartvigsen J 1997 The effect of spinal manipulation in the treatment of cervicogenic headache. Journal of Manipulative and Physiological Therapeutics 20: 326–330

Ostergaard S, Russell M B, Bendtsen L, Olesen J 1997 Comparison of first degree relatives and spouses of people with chronic tension headache. British Medical Journal 314: 1092–1093

Parker G B, Tupling H, Pryor D S 1978 A controlled trial of cervical manipulation for migraine. Australian and New Zealand Journal of Medicine 8: 589–593

Pearce J M S 1995a Cervicogenic headache: a personal view. Cephalalgia 15: 463–469

Pearce J M S 1995b The importance of cervicogenic headache in the over-fifties. Headache Quarterly, Current Treatment and Research 6: 293–296

Perez-Limonte L, Bonati A, Perry M et al 1999 Lower cervical pathology as a recognizable cause of cervicogenic headaches [Abstract]. Cephalalgia 19: 435

Persson G C L, Carlsson J Y 1999 Headache in patients with neck-shoulder-arm pain of cervical radicular origin. Headache 39: 218–224

Petrovic P, Ingvar M 2002 Imaging cognitive modulation of pain processing. Pain 95: 1–5

Pfaffenrath V, Kaube H 1990 Diagnostics of cervicogenic headache. Functional Neurology 5: 159–164

Pfaffenrath V, Dandekar R, Pollmann W 1987 Cervicogenic headache: the clinical picture, radiological findings and hypotheses on its pathophysiology. Headache 27: 495–499

Pfund Z, Szapary L, Jaszberenyi O, Nagy F, Czopf J 1999 Headache in intracranial tumors. Cephalalgia 19: 787–790

Philips C 1977 Headache in general practice. Headache 16: 322–329

Pikus H J, Phillips J M 1995 Characteristics of patients successfully treated for cervicogenic headache by surgical decompression of the second cervical root. Headache 35: 621–629

Pikus H J, Philips J M 1996 Outcome of surgical decompression of the second cervical root for cervicogenic headache. Neurosurgery 39: 63–71

Piovesan E J, Kowacs P A, Tatsui C E, Lange M C, Ribas L C, Werneck L C 2001 Referred pain after painful stimulation of the greater occipital nerve in humans: evidence of convergence of cervical afferences on trigeminal nuclei. Cephalalgia 21: 107–109

Placzek J D, Pagett B T, Roubal P J et al 1999 The influence of the cervical spine on chronic headache in women: a pilot study. Journal of Manual and Manipulative Therapy 7: 33–39

Pollmann W, Keidel M, Pfaffenrath V 1997 Headache and the cervical spine: a critical review. Cephalalgia 17: 801–816

Quin A, Niere K R 2001 Development of a headache-specific disability questionnaire for physiotherapy patients. In: Magarey M E (ed) Proceedings of the Twelfth Biennial Conference Musculoskeletal Physiotherapy Australia MPA, Adelaide, South Australia, pp 34–37

Rasmussen B K 1993 Migraine and tension-type headache in a general population: precipitating factors, female hormones, sleep pattern and relation to lifestyle. Pain 53: 65–72

Rasmussen B K 1996 Migraine and tension-type headache are separate disorders. Cephalalgia 16: 217–220

Rasmussen B K, Jensen R, Olesen J 1991a A population-based analysis of the diagnostic criteria of the International Headache Society. Cephalalgia 11: 129–134

Rasmussen B K, Jensen R, Schroll M, Olesen J 1991b Epidemiology of headache in a general population: a prevalence study. Journal of Clinical Epidemiology 11: 1147–1157

Rasmussen B K, Jensen R, Olesen J 1991c Questionnaire versus clinical interview in the diagnosis of headache. Headache 31: 290–295

Rasmussen B K, Jensen R, Schroll M, Olesen J 1992 Interrelations between migraine and tension-type headache in the general population. Archives of Neurology 49: 914–918

Revel M, Andre-Deshays C, Minguet M 1991 Cervicocephalic kinesthetic sensibility in patients with cervical pain. Archives of Physical Medicine and Rehabilitation 72: 288–291

Reynolds D J, Hovanitz C A 2000 Life event stress and headache frequency revisited. Headache 40: 111–118

Russell M B 2001 Genetics of migraine without aura, migraine with aura, migrainous disorder, head trauma migraine without aura and tension-type headache. Cephalalgia 21: 778–780

Sandor P S, Afra J, Proietti Cecchini A P, Albert A, Schoenen J 2000 From neurophysiology to genetics: cortical information processing in migraine underlies familial influences – a novel approach. Functional Neurology 15(Suppl. 3): 68–72

Scharff L, Turk D C, Marcus D A 1995 Triggers of headache episodes and coping responses of headache diagnostic groups. Headache 35: 397–403

Scher A I, Stewart W F, Lipton R B 1999 Migraine and headache: a meta-analytic approach. In: Crombie I K, Croft P R, Linton S J, LeResche L, Von Korff M (eds) Epidemiology of pain. IASP Press, Seattle, pp 159–170

Schoenen, J, Maertens de Noordhout A 1994 Headache. In: Wall P D, Melzack R (eds), Textbook of pain. Churchill Livingstone, Edinburgh, pp 495–521

Schoensee S K, Jensen G, Nicholson G, Gossman M, Katholi C 1995 The effect of mobilization on cervical headaches. Journal of Orthopaedic and Sports Physical Therapy 21: 184–196

Sheather-Reid R B, Cohen M L 1998 Psychophysical evidence for a neuropathic component of chronic neck pain. Pain 75: 341–347

Silberstein S D 1992 Evaluation and emergency treatment of headache. Headache 32: 396–407

Silberstein S D, Merriam G R 1991 Estrogens, progestins and headache. Neurology 41: 786–793

Silbert P L, Mokri B, Schievink W I 1995 Headache and neck pain in spontaneous internal carotid and vertebral artery dissections. Neurology 45: 1517–1522

Silverman J, Rodriquez A, Agre J 1991 Quantitative cervical flexor straining in healthy subjects and in subjects with mechanical neck pain. Archives of Physical Medicine and Rehabilitation 72: 679

Sjaastad O, Saunte C, Hovdahl H, Breivik H, Gronbaek E 1983 'Cervicogenic headache': an hypothesis. Cephalalgia 3: 249–256

Sjaastad O, Fredriksen T A, Stolt-Nielsen A 1986 Cervicogenic headache, C2 rhizopathy and occipital neuralgia: a connection? Cephalalgia 6: 189–195

Sjaastad O, Fredriksen T A, Sand T 1989 The localisation of the initial attack: a comparison between classic migraine and cervicogenic headache. Functional Neurology 4: 73–78

Sjaastad O, Fredriksen T A, Pfaffenrath V 1990 Cervicogenic headache: diagnostic criteria. Headache 30: 725–726

Sjaastad O, Bovim G, Stovner L J 1992 Laterality of pain and other migraine criteria in common migraine: a comparison with cervicogenic headache. Functional Neurology 7: 289–294

Sjaastad O, Stolt-Nielsen A, Blume H, Zwart J, Fredriksen T A 1995 Cervicogenic headache: long-term results of radiofrequency treatment of the planum nuchale. Functional Neurology 10: 265–271

Sjaastad O, Fredriksen T A, Stolt-Nielsen A et al 1997 Cervicogenic headache: a clinical review with a special emphasis on therapy. Functional Neurology 12: 305–317

Sjaastad O, Fredriksen T A, Pfaffenrath V 1998 Cervicogenic headache: diagnostic criteria. Headache 38: 442–445

Sterling M, Treleaven J, Edwards S, Jull G 2002a Responses to a clinical test of nerve tissue provocation in whiplash associated disorders. Manual Therapy 7: 89–94

Sterling M, Treleaven J, Edwards S, Jull G 2002b Pressure pain thresholds in chronic whiplash associated disorder: further evidence of altered central pain processing. Journal of Musculoskeletal Pain 10: 69–81

Stewart W F, Lipton R B, Simon D, Von Korff M, Liberman J 1998 Reliability of an illness severity measure for headache in a population of migraine sufferers. Cephalalgia 18: 44–51

Taren J A, Khan E A 1962 Anatomic pathways related to pain in the face and neck. Journal of Neurosurgery 19: 116–121

Thabe H 1986 Electromyography as a tool to document diagnostic findings and therapeutic results associated with somatic dysfunctions in the upper cervical spinal joints and sacro-iliac joints. Manual Medicine 2: 53–58

Treleaven J, Jull G, Atkinson L 1994 Cervical musculoskeletal dysfunction in post-concussional headache. Cephalalgia 14: 273–279

Treleaven J M, Jull G A, Sterling M 2003 Dizziness and unsteadiness following whiplash injury: characteristic features and relationship to cervical joint position error. Journal of Rehabilitation Medicine 35: 36–43

Trevor-Jones R 1964 Osteoarthritis of the paravertebral joints of the second and third cervical vertebrae as a cause of occipital headache. South African Medical Journal 38: 392–394

Tuchin P J, Pollard H 1998 Does classic migraine respond to manual therapy? A case series. Physical Therapy Reviews 3: 149–162

Turk D C, Rudy T E, Sorkin B A 1993 Neglected topics on chronic pain treatment outcome studies: determination of success. Pain 53: 3–16

van Suijlekom J A, van Kleef M, Barendse G A, Sluijter M E, Sjaastad O, Weber W E 1998 Radiofrequency cervical zygapophyseal joint neurotomy for cervicogenic headache: a prospective study of 15 patients. Functional Neurology 13: 297–303

van Suijlekom J A, de Vet H C W, van den Berg S G M, Weber W E J 1999 Interobserver reliability of diagnostic criteria for cervicogenic headache. Cephalalgia 19: 817–823

Vernon H 1991 Spinal manipulation and headaches of cervical origin: a review of literature and presentation of cases. Journal of Manual Medicine 6: 73–79

Vernon H, Steiman I, Hagino C 1992a Cervicogenic dysfunction in muscle contraction headache and migraine: a descriptive study. Journal of Manipulative and Physiological Therapeutics 15: 418–429

Vernon H T, Aker P, Aramenko M, Battershill D, Alepin A, Penner T 1992b Evaluation of neck muscle strength with a modified sphygmomanometer dynamometer: Reliability and validity. Journal of Manipulative and Physiological Therapeutics 15: 343–349

Vernon H, McDermaid C, Hagino C 1999 Systematic review of randomized clinical trials of complementary/alternative therapies in the treatment of tension-type and cervicogenic headache. Complementary Therapies and Medicines 7: 142–155

Vicenzino B, Collins D, Wright A 1994 Sudomotor changes induced by neural mobilisation techniques in asymptomatic subjects. Journal of Manual and Manipulative Therapy 2: 66–74

Vicenzino B, Collins D, Benson H, Wright A 1998 An investigation of the interrelationship between manipulative therapy-induced hypoalgesia and sympathoexcitation. Journal of Manipulative and Physiological Therapeutics 21: 448–453

Vincent M 1998 Greater occipital nerve blockades in cervicogenic headache. Functional Neurology 13: 78–79

Vincent M B, Luna R A 1999 Cervicogenic headache: a comparison with migraine and tension-type headache. Cephalalgia 19(Suppl. 25): 11–16

Watson D H, Trott P H 1993 Cervical headache: an investigation of natural head posture and upper cervical flexor muscle performance. Cephalalgia 13: 272–284

Whittingham W, Ellis W B, Molyneux T P 1994 The effect of manipulation (toggle recoil technique) for headaches with upper cervical joint dysfunction: a pilot study. Journal of Manipulative and Physiological Therapeutics 17: 369–375

Winters J M, Peles J D 1990 Neck muscle activity and 3-D head kinematics during quasi-static and dynamic tracking movements. In: Winters J M, Woo S L Y (eds) Multiple muscle systems: biomechanics and movement organization. Springer-Verlag, New York, pp 461–480

Wright A 1995 Hypoalgesia post-manipulative therapy: a review of the potential neurophysiological mechanisms. Manual Therapy 1: 11–16

Wright A, Thurnwald P, O'Callaghan J, Smith J, Vicenzino B 1994 Hyperalgesia in tennis elbow patients. Journal of Musculoskeletal Pain 2: 83–97

Zwart J A 1997 Neck mobility in different headache disorders. Headache 37: 6–11

Chapter **22**

'Clinical instability' of the lumbar spine: its pathological basis, diagnosis and conservative management

P. B. O'Sullivan

INTRODUCTION

Back related injury is a growing problem in the Western industrialized world, placing an increasing burden on the health budget (Indahl et al 1995). Estimates of lifetime incidence of low back pain range from 60 to 80% (Long et al 1996) and although most low back pain episodes (80–90%) subside within 2–3 months, recurrence is common (Croft et al 1998). Of major concern are the 5–10% of people who become disabled with a chronic back pain condition and who account for up to 75–90% of the cost (Indahl et al 1995). In spite of the large number of pathological conditions that can give rise to back pain, in most cases (85%) a definitive diagnosis is difficult to achieve (Waddell 1995). Patients within this group are frequently classified as having 'non-specific low back pain' (Dillingham 1995). More recently there has been increased focus on the identification and classification of different subgroups within this population (Bogduk 1995, Coste et al 1992). One of the proposed subgroups is that of 'clinical instability' of the lumbar spine (Nachemson 1985).

STABILIZATION OF THE LUMBAR SPINE

The ligamentous lumbar spine, without the influence of muscles, becomes unstable under very low levels of compressive load (Cholewicki & McGill 1996). The intervertebral disc acts as the main loadbearing structure of the lumbar spine and is well designed to withstand vertical loading forces, but it is vulnerable to shear and rotational forces (Bogduk 1997). The intervertebral disc is protected from these forces by the lumbar facet joints which limit rotation and anterior shear forces, and also by the muscles that control the spine (Bogduk 1997).

There is a close relationship between the passive anatomical restraints of the lumbar spine and the muscles that control it. At the end of spinal range of motion, the restraints to bending, rotation and shear forces are provided largely by tension and compression on the spine's passive structures (Bogduk 1997), with an associated reflex reduction in spinal muscle activity (O'Sullivan et al 2002b, Valencia & Munro 1985). Within its neutral zone of motion (region of high flexibility around the mid-zone of motion), the restraints and control for bending, rotation and shear force are largely provided by the muscles that surround and act on the spinal segment (Panjabi 1992).

In this light, Panjabi proposed that the concept of the neutral zone was central to the understanding of spinal stability. This neutral zone increases with intersegmental injury and intervertebral disc degeneration, and decreases with simulated muscle forces across a motion segment (Panjabi et al 1989, Wilke et al 1995). Thus Panjabi proposed that the size and control of the neutral zone be considered to be an important measure of spinal stability. It is influenced by the interaction between what was described as the passive, active and neural control systems:

- the passive system comprising the vertebrae, intervertebral discs, zygapophysial joints and ligaments
- the active system comprising the muscles and tendons surrounding and acting on the spinal column
- the neural system comprising the peripheral nerves and central nervous system which direct and control the active system in providing dynamic stability (Panjabi 1992).

Bergmark (1989) hypothesized the presence of two muscle systems that act in the maintenance of spinal stability:

1. The 'global' muscle system consisting of large torque producing muscles that act on the trunk and spine without directly attaching to it. These muscles include rectus abdominis, external oblique and the thoracic part of lumbar iliocostalis and provide general trunk stabilization, but are not capable of having a direct segmental influence on the spine.
2. The 'local' muscle system consisting of muscles that directly attach to the lumbar vertebrae and are responsible for providing segmental stability and directly controlling the lumbar segments. By definition lumbar multifidus, psoas major, quadratus lumborum, the lumbar parts of the lumbar iliocostalis and longissimus, transversus abdominis, the diaphragm and the posterior fibres of internal oblique all form part of this local muscle system as well as smaller muscles such as interspinalis and intertransversarii.

Growing evidence is emerging to support the hypothesis forwarded by Bergmark (1989) that the local system muscles function differently to global system muscles (O'Sullivan et al 1997b). Furthermore the relationship between the two muscle systems alters depending on the loading conditions placed on the spine (Daneels et al 2001, Essendrop et al 2002, O'Sullivan et al 1997b).

Coordinated patterns of muscle recruitment are essential between the global and local system muscles of the trunk in order to compensate for the changing demands of daily life to ensure that the dynamic stability of the spine is pre-

served (Cholewicki & McGill 1996, Gardener-Morse et al 1995). To accomplish this the neuromuscular system must provide the necessary compressive forces along the spine to ensure stability, while controlling its curvature at a segmental level (Aspden 1992). In this way the muscle forces act to maintain and stabilize the arch-like structure of the lumbar spine. The activation of the erector spinae and psoas major, known to significantly increase the compressive loading to the lumbar spine when active (Bogduk 1992, Bogduk et al 1992), enhances the segmental stiffness and hence stability of the spine. The segmental stabilizing role of muscles such as lumbar multifidus, with separate segmental innervation, acts to maintain the lumbar lordosis and ensure control of individual vertebral segments particularly within the neutral zone (Paajanen & Tertti 1991, Panjabi et al 1989, Wilke et al 1995). Lumbar multifidus is also provides spinal proprioception, critical for safe functioning of the lumbar spine (Brumagne et al 2000). The transverse abdominal wall muscles (transversus abdominis and the transverse fibres of internal oblique), while applying some compressive forces to the spine (McGill & Norman 1987) and pelvis (Richardson et al 2002), are primarily active in providing rotational and lateral stability to the spine via the thoracolumbar fascia while maintaining levels of intra-abdominal pressure (IAP) (Cresswell et al 1992, McGill 1991). The intra-abdominal pressure mechanism, primarily controlled by the diaphragm, transversus abdominis and pelvic diaphragm, also provides an important stabilizing role in the lumbar spine (Aspden 1992, McGill & Norman 1987).

During low levels of spinal loading, such as static postures and dynamic movements, the spine's local system muscles, such as the transverse abdominal wall and lumbar multifidus, display tonic muscle activation (Cresswell et al 1992, Daneels et al 2001, O'Sullivan et al 2002b, Valencia & Munro 1985). This occurs throughout all ranges of motion irrespective of direction of movement, suggesting a stabilizing function of these muscles (Cresswell 1993, Hodges & Richardson 1997). On the other hand, global system muscles such as external oblique, rectus abdominis and the erector spinae display activity consistent with torque production and movement initiation, and therefore their function is more direction-specific (Hodges & Richardson 1996, Valencia & Munro 1985).

Under high-level spinal loading significant co-activation of both the local and global system muscles occurs, with an increase in intra-abdominal pressure, to stiffen the thorax on the pelvis thereby meeting the increased demands for spinal stability (Essendrop et al 2002, McGill 1992). During rapid movement initiation or sudden loading of the spine the neuromuscular system utilizes strategies of pre-activation of muscles such as transversus abdominis, lumbar multifidus and the diaphragm, in conjunction with increases in intra-abdominal pressure. This provides a stable base upon which other torque-producing trunk muscles can safely act (Cresswell et al 1994, Essendrop et al

2002, Hodges & Richardson 1996). Inappropriate timing or altered control of these complex patterns of muscle co-contraction could result in tissue damage rather than the provision of stability to the motion segment (Gardener-Morse et al 1995, McGill & Sharratt 1990).

INJURY RISK TO THE LUMBAR SPINE

Cholewicki & McGill (1996) reported that the lumbar spine is more vulnerable to instability (non-physiological buckling) in its neutral positions, at low load and when the muscle forces are low. They confirmed that under these conditions lumbar stability is maintained in vivo by increasing the activity (stiffness) of the lumbar segmental muscles (local muscle system). Furthermore they highlighted the importance of motor control to coordinate muscle recruitment between large trunk muscles (the global muscle system) and small intrinsic muscles (the local muscle system) during functional activities to ensure that mechanical stability is maintained. Under such conditions they suggest that intersegmental muscle forces as low as 1–3 % maximal voluntary contraction may be sufficient to ensure dynamic stability. While the global muscle system provides the bulk of stiffness to the spinal column, the activity of the local muscle system is considered necessary to maintain the mechanical stability of the whole spine. In situations where the passive stiffness of a motion segment is reduced, the vulnerability of the spine towards instability is increased (Cholewicki & McGill 1996). This mechanism of injury explains how someone can injure or exacerbate their spine carrying out trivial through range movements such as bending to pick up a light object.

Under higher levels of spinal compression and muscle forces the spine is more stable (Gardener-Morse et al 1995). However, under these conditions the spine is vulnerable to tissue strain if the spine is loaded at the end of range (McGill & Cholewicki 2001). This has been shown in the case of power lifters who are capable of lifting loads far greater than body weight as long as the motor control system prevents end-range spinal loading (Cholewicki and McGill 1992). Under these loading conditions the neuromuscular control over the neutral zone of spinal motion is critical to ensure end-range loading of the spinal motion segment does not occur (McGill & Cholewicki 2001). This is brought about with the coordinated function of the local and global muscle systems acting in co-contraction with the generation of high levels of IAP (Essendrop et al 2002).

DYSFUNCTION OF THE NEUROMUSCULAR SYSTEM IN THE PRESENCE OF LOW BACK PAIN

The scientific literature reports varying disruptions in the patterns of recruitment and co-contraction within and between different muscle synergies (O'Sullivan et al 1997a). There is growing evidence that the transverse abdominal wall muscles and lumbar multifidus are prefer-

entially adversely affected in the presence of low back pain (Hides et al 1996), chronic low back pain (Daneels et al 2000) and lumbar instability (Lindgren et al 1993, Sihvonen & Partanen 1990), although it appears that the manner of the dysfunction within lumbar multifidus may vary with different lumbar pathology (Daneels et al 2000, Stokes et al 1992). There have also been reports that in the presence of local muscle system dysfunction, there is a compensatory substitution to adopt of global system muscle strategies of stabilization with generation of high levels of IAP (O'Sullivan 2002a). In this sense, motor control strategies normally observed under high level spinal loading conditions are observed under low levels of spinal loading (O'Sullivan 2002a). This appears to be the neural control system's attempt to maintain the stability demands of the lumbopelvic region when there is a deficit in the passive or local muscle systems (Edgerton et al 1996, O'Sullivan 2002a). There is also evidence to suggest that the presence of chronic low back pain often results in changes to the neural control system, affecting timing of patterns of co-contraction, balance, reflex and righting responses (O'Sullivan et al 1997c).

Generalized changes to the trunk musculature such as a loss of strength, endurance and muscle atrophy are believed to result from disuse and inactivity in this population. The more specific and segmental changes are considered to result from either motor or sensory nerve damage, or altered habitual movement patterns of activity, and reflex excitation or inhibition of the muscles proximal to the site of pathology (Grabiner et al 1992, Stokes et al 1992). The altered mechanoceptive and proprioceptive afferent input into the neural system is likely to result in further disruption to patterns of muscle activation, leaving the subject biomechanically vulnerable to further injury or increased chronicity.

MOVEMENT BASED PAIN DISORDERS OF THE LUMBAR SPINAL SEGMENT

Movement based pain disorders of the lumbar spinal segments have been reported by manual therapists for many years (Maitland 1986). However, there is a great deal of controversy regarding the discriminative validity of classifying movement based pain disorders. Both hypo- and hypermobile spinal segments have been reported in both pain and pain-free populations (Friberg 1987, Pearcy & Shepherd 1985). It is clear from this evidence that the mobility of a spinal segment in isolation is not predictive or diagnostic in classifying a pain disorder. Rather it is the association between the mobility and control of the spinal segment, and its relationship to the pain disorder, which appears to be critical. It is proposed that movement based pain disorders of the lumbar spinal segment can be classified into different subgroups (see Ch. 34).

At one end of the spectrum, movement based pain disorders may be associated with a painful loss of spinal segment mobility or 'hypomobility'. This could occur secondary to connective tissue changes and/or muscle guarding around the spinal segment. However, a spinal segment with normal movement parameters may become sensitized and symptomatic from repetitive end-range of spinal loading. This may develop from a loss of motor control of the spinal segment within the neutral zone, resulting in an 'overstrain' pain disorder. If the repetitive strain of the spinal segment at the end of range were to continue, it could result in connective tissue adaptation with resultant segmental symptomatic 'hypermobility' presenting as a 'hypermobility overstrain' pain disorder.

Clinical instability of a spinal segment represents a loss of functional competence of a spinal segment within its neutral zone of motion with a resultant loading and movement based pain disorder associated with this loss of control. Clinical instability is more likely to occur in association with a pathological increase in spinal segment flexibility or hypermobility (Gardener-Morse et al 1995), resulting in an increase in the spinal segment neutral zone, with an associated loss of motor control of the segment within this zone.

A loss of dynamic control of the spinal segment within the neutral zone of motion could leave the spinal segment vulnerable to tissue strain, from repetitive end-range loading of the spinal segment (overstrain), as well as to non-physiological loading and movement within its neutral zone of motion (clinical instability). It appears that clinical instability of the spinal segment is frequently the end-stage of a chronic mechanical low back pain disorder. This may result from repeated or traumatic end-range strain of a spinal segment with associated tissue damage, pain and associated loss of motor control of the segment within its neutral zone of motion.

Pain associated with a functional loss of neutral zone control may manifest in:

1. through range movement pain due to non-physiological motion of the spinal segment
2. loading based pain due to non-physiological loading of the spinal segment
3. end of range pain or overstrain due to repetitive strain of the spinal motion segment at the end of range.

Evidence of a functional loss of neutral zone control of the lumbar spine in subjects with CLBP and clinical signs of LSI has recently been reported (O'Sullivan et al 2003).

PATHO-ANATOMICAL BASIS OF CLINICAL INSTABILITY

Historically, instability of a spinal segment was defined by the finding of excessive movement of the spinal segment beyond physiological limits (Frymoyer & Selby 1985). Because of this, the diagnosis was historically based on the finding of increased translation or angulation of a spinal segment during flexion-extension or lateral bending radi-

ographs. However, problems with this definition of instability arose with the findings of increased intersegmental motion in subjects without a back pain condition (Boden & Wiesel 1990). This led to an increased focus on the significance of the neuromuscular control of the spinal motion segment (Panjabi 1992).

The radiological diagnosis of spondylolisthesis in subjects with chronic low back pain attributable to these findings has been considered to be one of the most obvious manifestations of lumbar instability (Nachemson 1991). This has been supported by a number of studies reporting increased translational and rotational motion occurring segmentally in the presence of this condition and also with spondylolysis (Friberg 1989, Mimura et al 1994, Montgomery & Fischgrund 1994, Wood et al 1994), as well as altered centres of rotation of the spinal segment (Schneider 2001). However, spondylolisthesis is also present in pain-free populations indicating that the presence of this finding in isolation is not diagnostic of clinical instability (Saraste 1987).

Other patho-anatomical findings of the lumbar spine have also been reported to potentially implicate an underlying instability disorder of the spinal segment. These include degenerative spondylolisthesis, retrolisthesis, the presence of traction spurs, annular tears and degenerative change of the intervertebral disc (Taylor 2000). However, the predictive value of these findings in isolation, to identify pain disorders or diagnose clinical instability, is limited as all these pathologies have also been reported in pain-free populations (Nachemson 1999).

Clinical instability of the lumbar spine is also reported to occur following decompression spinal surgery such as laminectomy. The compromised function of the facet joints combined with well documented damage to the lumbar multifidus following this form of surgery has been suggested to render the motion segment vulnerable to instability (Taylor 2000).

Furthermore clinical instability in the absence of patho-anatomical changes to structure of the lumbar spine has also been cited as a significant cause of chronic low back pain (Long et al 1996). A number of studies have reported the presence of increased and abnormal intersegmental motion in subjects with chronic low back pain, often in the absence of other radiological findings (Gertzbein 1991, Lindgren et al 1993, Sihvonen & Partanen 1990).

One of the limitations in the diagnosis of clinical instability still lies in the difficulty in measuring accurately the functional control of the spinal segment within its neutral zone. Conventional radiological testing is static and assesses the spinal segment mobility at its end of range (outside the neutral zone of motion), and is often reported to be insensitive and unreliable in the diagnosis of these disorders (Dvorak et al 1991, Pope et al 1992). In light of this, the finding of increased and abnormal intersegmental motion of a single motion segment on radiological examination is considered to be significant only if it confirms the finding of clinical instability at the corresponding level (Kirkaldy-Willis 1983).

Clinical instability of the lumbar spine most often affects the lower two spinal segments and may or may not be associated with patho-anatomical findings. A patho-anatomical weakness of the motion segment such as isthmic or degenerative spondylolisthesis, retrolisthesis, annular tear or degenerative disc disease may render the motion segment vulnerable to repetitive strain or trauma, particularly if the motor control of the spinal segment is compromised. Similarly a mobile spinal segment without gross pathological changes may become clinically unstable with a loss of motor control within neutral zone control (Gertzbein et al 1985).

DIAGNOSIS OF CLINICAL INSTABILITY OF THE LUMBAR SPINE

Because of the lack of sensitivity and specificity of any one test to accurately identify these conditions, the diagnosis of clinical instability requires the presence of a concurrent number of diagnostic criteria based on findings from the subjective and physical examination.

Subjective characteristics

Questionnaire data completed by subjects diagnosed with clinical instability involved in recent clinical trials revealed that half of the subjects developed their back pain condition secondary to a single event injury and the other half developed their back pain gradually in relation to multiple minor traumatic incidents (O'Sullivan 1997). The subjects' main complaint was of chronic and recurrent low back pain with increasing levels of functional disability over time. Their means of controlling the symptoms was to reduce their level of activity. Subjects also reported a poor conservative treatment response with either aggravation from spinal manipulation and mobilization or only short-term relief from this form of therapy, which did not alter the natural history of the condition.

The back pain was most commonly described as recurrent (70%), constant (55%), 'catching' (45%), 'locking' (20%), 'giving way' (20%) or accompanied by a feeling of 'instability' (35%). The most frequently reported aggravating postures were sustained sitting (85%), prolonged standing (70%) and semi-flexed postures (70%). The most common aggravating movements were forward bending (75%), sudden unexpected movements (75%), returning to an upright position from forward bending (65%), lifting (65%) and sneezing (60%) (O'Sullivan 1997). These symptoms and signs are commonly reported as consistent with the presence of clinical instability (Kirkaldy-Willis 1983, Nachemson 1985), and are consistent with the presence of a loading and movement based pain disorder – particularly within the neutral zone of motion.

Physical examination

Active spinal movement commonly reveals good ranges of spinal mobility but with aberrant quality of motion (O'Sullivan et al 1997a). This is often associated with the presence of through range pain or a painful arc with or without a painful end of range pain. The aberrant movement is commonly associated with a sudden acceleration, hesitation, or lateral movement within the mid-range of spinal motion. This may be associated with the need to assist the movement with the use of the hands. Segmental hinging of the symptomatic segment is commonly observed to be associated with the painful movement. Another common feature is the reported abolition or significant reduction of pain with transverse abdominal wall muscle contraction (or attempts to normalize the movement pattern) during the pain provocative movement. Also noted in the physical examination is the absence of abnormal neurological examination findings in all the subjects. Similarly neural tissue provocation tests such as straight leg raise, slump and prone knee bend are generally normal (O'Sullivan 1997).

Signs of abnormal increased movement between one vertebra and the next are detected by inspection and confirmed by palpation. Confirmation that the abnormally mobile segment detected is in fact symptomatic and reproductive of the patients symptoms is essential. Passive physiological motion segment testing is used to detect increased segmental motion. Flexion/extension and rotation were reported to be the most sensitive movement tests to detect excessive intersegmental motion. For spondylolisthesis and spondylolysis the excessive segmental motion was detected at the level above the pars defects (O'Sullivan 1997). All these physical examination findings have also been reported by other authors as indicative of clinical instability (Kirkaldy-Willis 1983, Nachemson 1985). However, the sensitivity, specificity and predictive value of these signs are largely unproven (Nachemson 1991).

Neuromuscular examination

The neuromuscular examination determines the relationship between the motor control of the spinal segment and the pain disorder. The model of examination described outlines three different components of the examination, which assess different aspects of the motor control of the spinal segment:

Posture and movement analysis

The first component of the examination employs the careful analysis of aggravating and easing postures and functional movements of the lumbopelvic region. This is a qualitative form of examination and demands a high level of therapist observational skill for accurate detection and interpretation. There is growing evidence that skilled therapists are capable of detecting subtle changes in the functional movement of the spine (Newman et al 1996). The critical aspect of this part of the examination is to analyse the strategy of postural dynamic stabilization that the patient has adopted and its relationship to the pain disorder. The second is to identify whether there is a directional basis to the pain disorder (Fig. 22.1).

Specific postural and movement control tests

The second component of the examination involves a number of specific movement and postural loading tests. These tests aim to determine the motor control strategies that the patient presents with, the neutral zone control of the spinal segment and the relationship between the motor control of the lumbopelvic region and the patient's symptoms. These tests are directed by the findings of the first aspect of the neuromuscular examination. They involve tests of spinal proprioception and thoraco-lumbo-pelvic control (Fig. 22.2). If the patient is capable of altering their spinal posture and movement patterns based on these tests, then the therapist seeks to determine the relationship between altering specific postures and movements that are pain provocative, to determine the relationship between the control of the lumbopelvic region and the subject's symptoms. For example, if pain is reproduced in a specific posture or functional

	Flexion	Lateral shift/ flexion	Extension (passive)	Extension (active)	Multidirectional
Standing posture	Flattened lumbar lordosis at 'unstable' segment	Flattened lumbar lordosis at 'unstable' segment Lateral shift	Thorax posterior to pelvis Increased segmental lordosis at 'unstable' segment	Thorax anterior to pelvis Increased segmental lordosis at 'unstable' segment	Variable
Stabilizing strategy	Thoracic ES Upper abdominal wall (RA, EO, upper TO)	Asymmetrical thoracic ES, quadratus lumborum, upper, abdominal ipsilateral to shift	Upper abdominal wall (RA, EO, upper IO)	Lumbar ES, psoas +/- LM	Co-contraction / guarding of global trunk muscles
Spinal segment loading	Anterior	Anterior / lateral	Posterior	Posterior	Variable / alternating
Forward bending in standing	Increased flexion at 'unstable' segment Extension thoraco-lumbar spine Increased posterior pelvic rotation (+/- arc of pain)	Increased flexion and lateral deviation of trunk above 'unstable' segment	-	Delayed or loss of reverse lordosis (delayed or absence of flexion relaxation) Hyperextension of 'unstable' segment Excessive anterior pelvic rotation	Increased flexion at 'unstable' segment
Return to neutral from forward bending	Extension thoraco-lumbar spine 'Unstable' segment remains flexed (+/- arc of pain)	Extension thoracolumbar spine 'Unstable' segment remains flexed and deviated (+/- arc of pain)	Tendency to overextend at 'unstable' segment, and sway pelvis anteriorly on assuming upright position	Tendency to hyperextend 'unstable' segment early on return to upright position (+/- arc of pain)	Variable / alternating
Lumbar:hip ratio	3:1	3:1	-	1:3	3:1
Centre of rotation of spinal segment	Anterior	Anterolateral	-	Posterior	Anterior
Backward bending in standing	Increased extension above 'unstable' segment Reduced extension at 'unstable' segment	Increased extension above 'unstable' segment with lateral deviation Reduced extension at unstable segment	Increased extension at 'unstable' segment Reduced extension above 'unstable' segment Excessive pelvic sway	Increased extension at 'unstable' segment Anterior pelvic rotation	Increased extension at 'unstable' segment
Lumbar:hip ratio	1:3	1:3	3:1	3:0	3:1
Centre of rotation of spinal segment	Anterior	Anterolateral	Posterior	Posterior	Posterior
Single leg stand / gait	-	Lateral shift of thorax, relative to pelvis +/- Trendelenberg	Anterior sway of pelvis relative to thorax +/- Trendelenberg Internal hip rotation	Posterior sway of pelvis relative to thorax Internal hip rotation	Variable / alternating
Squat	Increased flexion at 'unstable' segment Posterior pelvic rotation	As with flexion pattern + Lateral deviation	-	Increased extension of 'unstable' segment Anterior pelvic rotation	Variable / alternating
Lumbar:hip ratio	3:1	3:1	1:3	-	Variable
Sitting	Flexed lower lumbar spine Posterior pelvic rotation Extended thoraco-lumbar spine	As with flexion + deviation	Slumped posture	Hyperlordotic lumbar posture Anterior rotation of pelvis	Variable / alternating
Sit-Stand	Increased flexion at 'unstable' segment Extension thoraco-lumbar spine Increased posterior pelvic rotation (+/- arc of pain)	Increased flexion and lateral deviation of 'unstable' segment (+/- arc of pain)	Hyperextension of 'unstable' segment and excessive anterior pelvic, sway on assuming erect, position	'Unstable' segment maintained in hyper-lordosis throughout the movement (+/- arc of pain)	Either flexed or extended
Lumbar:hip ratio	3:1	3:1	-	1:3	Variable / alternating

Figure 22.1 Posture and movement analysis.

	Flexion	Lateral shift/flexion	Extension (passive)	Extension (active)	Multidirectional
Standing posture correction (for loading pain)	Anterior rotation of pelvis Increase lower lumbar lordosis	As with flexion + correct deviation	Correct sway posture	Reduce lordosis / posterior pelvic rotation / relax thorax	As indicated
Forward bending correction (for movement pain)	Anterior rotation of pelvis Increase lower lumbar lordosis Flex thoracolumbar spine	As with flexion + Correct deviation	-	Enhance posterior pelvic rotation and lumbar flexion Enhance return to neutral with gluteal activation	As with flexion
Backward bending correction (for movement pain)	-	Correct deviation	Reduces sway Enhance extension of upper lumbar spine with control of sway and posterior pelvic rotation to minimize hinging	Enhance posterior pelvic rotation via hips	As with 'passive' extension
Single leg stand correction (for loading pain)	Enhance anterior rotation of pelvis Increase lower lumbar lordosis	Correct deviation with focus on keeping head central with weight transference via hip	Correct postural sway aligning thorax over pelvis	Reduce lordosis / posterior pelvic rotation / relax thorax	As indicated
Squat correction (for loading +/- movement pain)	Enhance anterior rotation of pelvis Increase lower lumbar lordosis	Correct deviation with focus on keeping head central with weight transference via hip	-	Reduce lordosis/ posterior pelvic rotation / relax thorax	As indicated
Sitting correction (for loading pain)	Anterior rotation of pelvis Increase lower lumbar lordosis Relax thorax	As with flexion + correct deviation	-	Reduce lordosis / posterior pelvic rotation / relax thorax	As indicated
Erect and slump sitting	Erect sitting associated with thoracolumbar extension. Unstable segment remains in flexion	As with flexion + deviation	Hyperextension unstable segment	Erect sit associated with hyperlordosis Inability to slump sit	Hyperextension lower lumbar spine
Neutral zone re-positioning test Place into neutral lordosis- (a) fully slump and ask to return to neutral position	Tendency to reposition into flexion at unstable segment	Tendency to reposition into deviation	Tendency to reposition into extension	Tendency to reposition into extension	Variable
(b) maintain neutral lordosis and bend forward through the hips	Tendency to flex at 'unstable' region	Tendency to flex and laterally deviate at 'unstable' region	Tendency to extend at 'unstable' region	Tendency to hyperextend lumbar spine	Variable
Sit-stand Place spine in neutral lordosis–assess ability to hold neutral spinal position during task (for loading and movement pain)	Tendency to flex at 'unstable' region	Tendency to flex and laterally deviate at 'unstable' region	Tendency to extend at 'unstable' region	Tendency to hyperextend lumbar spine	Variable
Sit-stand – single leg loading	-	Excessive lateral shift of thorax over the pelvis when loading the affected side	-	-	-
Anterior posterior pelvic rotation (supine)	Inability to anterior rotate pelvis and extend low lumbar spine independent of thorax	As with flexion + asymmetrical pelvic rotation	Inability to extend thoracolumbar spine independent of pelvis	Inability to posterior rotate pelvis and flex lumbar spine independent of hip flexion	
Lumbopelvic lateral rotation independent from hip and thorax (supine)	-	Inability to rotate lumbopelvic region independent of thorax and hip–on side of shift	-	-	As with lateral shift
Prone hip extension	-	-	Excessive segmental extension Absence of gluteal activation	Excessive lumbar lordosis and trunk rotation Minimal hip extension	Excessive segmental extension
Four-point kneeling anterior / posterior pelvic rotation	Inability to anterior rotate pelvis and extend lumbar spine independent of thorax	As with flexion with associated lateral deviation	Inability to extend thoracolumbar spine independent of pelvis and 'unstable' segment	Inability to posterior rotate pelvis and flex lumbar spine	Variable
Lateral leg lower (supine)	-	Inability to maintain lumbopelvic position on side of shift Asymmetrical rotation	Tendency to hyper-extend and rotate lower lumbar spine and flex thoracolumbar spine	Tendency to hyper-extend and rotate lumbar spine	Excessive rotation and extension of lumbar–pelvic region

Figure 22.2   Specific postural and movement control tests.

movement test, then correction of the posture, movement pattern or activation of stabilizing muscles allows assessment of the relationship between the manner in which the spine loads or moves and the pain disorder. If correction of the posture or movement pattern results in a reduction of symptoms, then this supports the notion that motor control has a direct relationship to the pain disorder. If, on the other hand, the symptoms are exacerbated with the correction of the loading or movement pattern, this may indicate that the motor control deficit is being driven by some other process.

Specific muscle tests

Specific muscle testing forms the third part of the neuromuscular examination (Fig. 22.3). It should be noted that these are relatively non-functional cognitive tests and therefore lack diagnostic specificity. This aspect of the examination seeks to specifically assess the patient's ability to consciously isolate the activation of the local muscle system without dominant activation of the global muscle system, under low load conditions. More specifically, it tests the ability of the patient to co-contract the transverse abdominal wall and pelvic floor muscles with segmental multifidus in a neutral lordotic posture while controlling relaxed respiration. This aspect of the examination seeks to identify the presence of local muscle system dysfunction and faulty patterns of global muscle substitution. Muscle length tests may also be included in this aspect of the examination. This

form of examination has been described in detail previously (Richardson & Jull 1995).

DIRECTIONAL PATTERNS OF CLINICAL INSTABILITY

The directional nature of instability based upon the mechanism of injury and resultant site of tissue damage is well understood in the knee and shoulder, but poorly understood in the lumbar spine. As the motion within the spine is three-dimensional and involves coupled movements, tissue injury in a specific movement plane may result in pain sensitization, motor dysfunction and resultant movement dysfunction specific to that movement direction. Dupuis and co-workers (Dupuis et al 1985) stated, on the basis of experimental and radiological data, that the location of the dominant lesion in the motion segment determines the pattern of instability manifested. Hence, if the dominant lesion is anterior primary restraint failure, posterior horizontal translation in extension films and increased lateral shearing in side bending films are detected. If the dominant lesion is primary posterior restraint failure, anterior horizontal displacement in the flexion film and radiologically detectable patterns of coupling in the posterior elements are detected. Frymoyer & Selby classified lumbar instability as axial rotational, translational, retrolisthetic, or post-surgical (Frymoyer & Selby 1985).

Clinical experience has revealed five common but distinctly different patterns of presentation observed in

	Flexion	Flexion / lateral shift	Extension (passive)	Extension (active)	Multidirectional
Pelvic floor and transverse abdominal wall (supine, side-lying, sitting)	Global abdominal wall contraction with tendency to flex lower lumbar spine and posteriorly rotate pelvis (loss of LM co-contraction)	As with flexion + lateral deviation Asymmetrical weakness	Tendency to flex thorax and upper lumbar spine dominant upper abdominal wall activation Associated breath holding or apical breathing	Tendency to hyperextend lower lumbar spine Anterior pelvic rotation Global bracing of the abdominal wall Breath holding or apical breathing	Variable
Lumbar multifidus with co-contraction with transverse abdominal wall muscles in neutral lordosis (prone, side-lying, four-point kneel, sitting)	Inability to activate LM Tendency to flex lower lumbar spine and posteriorly rotate pelvis	Asymmetrical activation of LM Deficit on contralateral side to shift	Inability to activate LM at and above unstable segment	Inability to co-contract LM with TrA in neutral spine position Tendency to hyperextend lower lumbar spine with dominant ES +/– LM activity	Inability to co-contract in neutral lordosis
Gluteus maximus (prone)	Bilateral weakness	Unilateral weakness	Bilateral weakness	Inner range weakness	Bilateral weakness
Iliopsoas (hip flexion sitting) (anterior pelvic rotation –supine and sitting)	Inner range weakness Tendency to posterior rotate pelvis and flex lower lumbar spine	Unilateral inner range weakness Excessive lateral deviation and rotation on side of shift	Inability to maintain upper lumbar lordosis	Overactive psoas Tendency to hyper-extend lumbar spine and anterior rotate pelvis	Variable
Hip flexor length test (Thomas position)	Long 'short hip flexors'	Long 'short hip flexors'	Long 'short hip flexors'	Short hip flexors	Long 'short hip flexors'

Figure 22.3 Specific muscle testing.

patients with clinical instability. These patterns are also observed in 'hypermobility overstrain' pain disorders, without the presence of loading and movement pain within the neutral zone of motion. It is important to note that these patterns are observations of the author and the validity of the patterns is currently under scientific investigation. Furthermore, they do not represent the only clinical patterns to be seen with patients with clinical instability, as some patients may present with different combinations of these patterns. Rather the following descriptions serve to illustrate common clinical patterns observed by the author and help the reader to identify these patients in the clinical situation. The clinical patterns are reported on a directional basis of flexion, lateral shift, passive extension, active extension and multidirectional. This is not to say that the problem is only manifested in a unidirectional manner, but rather altered motion segment coupling and loading can be observed in a movement zone such as flexion/rotation/side bending.

1. Flexion pattern

This appears to be the most common pattern. These patients primarily complain of central back pain. They commonly relate their injury to either a single flexion/rotation injury or to repetitive strains relating to flexion/rotational activities. They predominantly report the aggravation of their symptoms and exhibit their control problems in flexed spinal postures and movements, with a reported difficulty to perform or sustain flexion and in particular semiflexed postures. Conversely they report relief of their symptoms in lordotic or upright postures.

Posture and movement analysis reveals a loss of segmental lumbar lordosis at the level of the unstable motion segment. This is sometimes noticeable in standing and is accentuated in sitting postures with an associated tendency to hold the pelvis in a degree of posterior pelvic tilt. This loss of segmental lordosis is accentuated in flexed postures and is usually associated with increased tone in the upper lumbar and lower thoracic erector spinae muscles with an associated increase in lordosis present in the thoracic region (Figs 22.4, 22.5). Movements into forward bending are commonly associated with the initiation of movement and a tendency to flex more at the symptomatic level than at the adjacent levels and hold the upper lumbar spine in lordosis, with an associated lack of hip flexion. This movement is often associated with an arc of pain into flexion and an inability to return from flexion to neutral without use of the hands to assist the movement. During backward bending one frequently observes a tendency to preferentially extend above the symptomatic segment with an associated loss of extension at the affected segment.

Specific movement testing reveals an inability to differentiate anterior pelvic tilt and low lumbar spine extension independent of upper lumbar and thoracic spine extension (sitting, supine and four-point kneeling). Also commonly

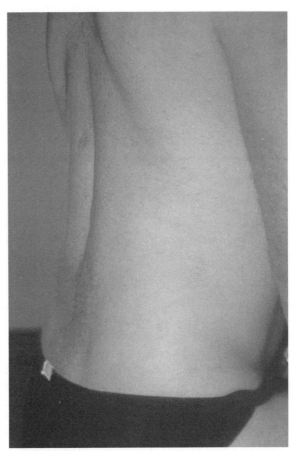

Figure 22.4 Flexion pattern: patient who sustained a L5/S1 flexion injury complains of flexion related pain. Note in sitting the posterior tilt of the pelvis and a segmental loss of lower lumbar lordosis with upper lumbar and lower thoracic compensatory lordosis. Reproduced from Taylor & O'Sullivan 2000.

noted is the inability to control the lumbar lordosis in forward-loaded postures. The quality of the movement during attempts to initiate segmental lordosis and independent anterior pelvic tilt motion from the upper lumbar and thoracic spine is usually associated with jerky and staccato

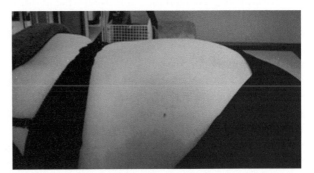

Figure 22.5 Flexion pattern: patient in four-point kneeling in 'their' neutral resting position. Note the regional loss of lumbar lordosis accentuated at the L3/4 symptomatic level associated with posterior tilt of the pelvis and thoracic compensatory lordosis.

movements rather than smooth controlled movement. This is most accentuated on the eccentric phase of these movement tests. Movement tests such as squatting, sitting with knee extension and hip flexion, and 'sit- to -stand' test usually reveal an inability to control segmental lordosis and an anterior pelvic tilt position, with a tendency to segmentally flex at the unstable motion segment and posteriorly tilt the pelvis. Tests of position sense in sitting reveal an inability to reposition within the neutral zone of motion, with a tendency to 'overshoot' into flexion at the unstable segment.

Specific muscle tests reveal an inability to activate lumbar multifidus and psoas in co-contraction with the transverse abdominal wall muscles at the unstable motion segment. Many of the patients are unable to assume a start position of a neutral lordotic lumbar spine, particularly in four-point kneeling and sitting, due to an inability to initiate anterior pelvic tilt and lordose the lower lumbar spine (see Fig. 22.5). These patients' attempts to activate these muscles are commonly associated with a Valsalva manoeuvre and bracing of the abdominal muscles with a loss of breathing control and excessive co-activation of the thoracolumbar erector spinae muscles. Attempts to specifically activate the transverse abdominal wall muscles usually result in excessive recruitment of external oblique, rectus abdominis, the vertically orientated fibres of internal oblique and the diaphragm with a loss of breathing control and a further flattening of the segmental lordosis, often resulting in pain. Indeed a common observation is an inability to diaphragm breathe with an apical respiration pattern being assumed. It appears that the diaphragm preferentially functions as a stabilizing muscle, thereby compromising its respiratory function.

Passive physiological motion testing reveals a segmental increase in flexion and rotation mobility at the symptomatic motion segment. Extension may appear to be 'stiff'. Palpatory examination in prone may reveal a decrease in posteroanterior accessory motion at the unstable motion segment.

Dynamic stabilizing strategy

These patients present with segmental dysfunction of the lumbar multifidus, psoas major, the transverse abdominal muscles. Their strategy for dynamically stabilizing the lumbar spine appears to be the excessive activation of the thoracolumbar erector spinae and upper abdominal wall muscles with associated bracing with the diaphragm. In this case the dominant activation of the thoracolumbar erector spinae and superficial abdominal muscles appears to stabilize the motion segment by 'locking' it into an end of range flexion position rather than providing stabilization to the motion segment within the neutral zone. Sacroiliac joint dysfunction is also noted to be common in this patient group and this appears to be closely related to dysfunction of the lumbar multifidus, transverse abdominal wall and pelvic floor muscles and associated loss of pelvic control and force closure mechanisms (Fig. 22.6)

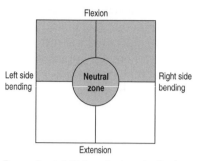

Figure 22.6 Dynamic stabilizing strategy in flexion pattern. Reproduced from O'Sullivan 2000.

2. Lateral shift pattern

A second presentation is the lateral shift. This is usually associated with a flexion/lateral shift movement disorder, but in rare situations where there has been a rotation/extension injury it may present as an extension/lateral shift pattern. In the flexion/lateral shift patterns, patients commonly report a history of a traumatic injury or repetitive strain into flexion/rotation. This is usually associated with unilateral low back pain. These patients commonly relate a vulnerability to reaching or rotating in one direction in association with flexion postures and/or movements. They usually report relief in extended or lordotic postures. These patients report that with minimal precipitation their spine may deviate into a lateral shift position in flexion.

Posture and movement analysis in standing reveals a loss of lumbar segmental lordosis at the affected level (similar to the flexion pattern) but with an associated lateral shift in the lower lumbar spine. Palpation of the lumbar multifidus muscles in standing commonly reveals atrophy and the absence of resting tone on the contralateral side to the shift. The lateral shift is accentuated when standing on the foot ipsilateral to the shift and during gait (Fig. 22.7). This may also be associated with a Trendelenberg hip pattern. Sagittal spinal movements reveal a tendency to laterally deviate at mid-range flexion and this is commonly associated with an arc of pain (Fig. 22.8). Side bending in the direction of the shift commonly reveals a lateral translatory motion rather than a side bending motion at the unstable level.

Specific movement tests reveal dominant activation of the thoracolumbar erector spinae and lumbar multifidus on the ipsilateral side of the shift and a loss of rotary and lateral trunk control in the direction of the shift. This can be observed in supine postures with a lateral leg lowering and in four-point kneeling when flexing one arm. Single leg standing reveals an inability to load the thoracolumbar spine vertically over the pelvis. Sitting to standing and squatting usually reveal a tendency towards lateral trunk shift during the movement with increased weight bearing on the lower limb on the side of the shift. Tests of position sense in sitting reveal an inability to reposition the lumbar

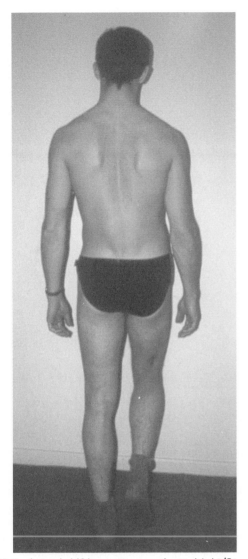

Figure 22.7 Lateral shifting pattern: patient with L5/S1 grade 1 spondylolisthesis complaining of flexion/rotation related pain and presenting with a left lateral shifting pattern accentuated when single leg standing on the left foot. Reproduced from Taylor & O'Sullivan 2000.

spine within the neutral zone of motion, with a tendency to overshoot into flexion and laterally deviate in the direction of the shift.

Specific muscle testing reveals an inability to bilaterally activate segmental lumbar multifidus in co-contraction with the transverse abdominal wall muscles, with an inability to activate the muscles on the contralateral side to the shift.

Palpatory examination reveals a unidirectional increase in intersegmental motion at the symptomatic level into flexion and rotation and side bending in the direction of the shift.

Dynamic stabilizing strategy

These patients usually present with a loss of co-contraction of the lumbar multifidus and deep abdominal muscles on the side contralateral to the segmental lateral shift.

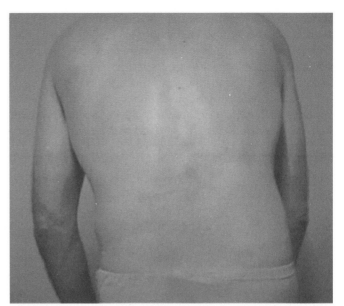

Figure 22.8 Lateral shifting pattern: patient with L4/5 pain associated with flexion/rotation activities reports mid-range arc of pain with observed lateral deviation of the spine to the left during mid-range of forward bending.

Attempts at dynamically stabilizing the lumbar spine appear to be carried out by dominant activation of the lumbar erector spinae, quadratus lumborum and in some cases the lumbar multifidus on the ipsilateral side to the shift and associated bracing with the diaphragm and abdominal muscles. This appears to represent the tendency in these patients to stabilize the motion segment by 'holding' it into a flexed and lateral shift position rather than providing stabilization to the motion segment within the neutral zone (Fig. 22.9)

3.   Active extension pattern

A third group of patients report central low back pain aggravated by extension movements and activities. There are two distinct extension clinical patterns that can be observed. The first of these is described as an 'active' pattern, as the lumbar spine is actively held into extension

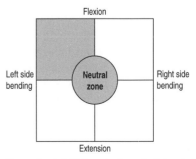

Figure 22.9 Dynamic stabilizing strategy in lateral shift pattern. Reproduced from O'Sullivan 2000.

with high levels of concentric muscle activity from the segmental back extensors and iliopsoas. These patients commonly recount their injury as resulting from an extension/rotation incident or repetitive trauma frequently associated with sporting activities involving extension activities. However, in some situations these patients may report that they injured their back during forward bending activities (where they actively fixed their spines into extension). Frequently reported provocative activities include standing, erect sitting, forward bending postures (where the tendency is to hold the lumbar spine in segmental hyperextension), carrying out overhead activities and an inability to walk fast, run and swim. These patients relate that their symptoms are relieved with flexion postures of the lumbar spine such as crook lying.

Posture and movement analysis reveals the tendency is for the lumbar spine to be held into segmental hyperlordosis at the unstable level during all upright postures and functional tasks. In the standing position these patients commonly exhibit an increase in segmental lordosis at the unstable motion segment, with an increased level of segmental muscle activity at this level. The pelvis is often positioned in anterior pelvic tilt with the thorax positioned relatively anterior to the pelvis (Fig. 22.10). Forward bending movements commonly reveal increased hip flexion and a tendency to hold the lumbar spine in hyperlordosis (particularly at the level of the unstable motion segment) with or without a sudden loss of lordosis at mid-range flexion commonly associated with an arc of pain (Fig. 22.11). Return to neutral again reveals a tendency to hyperlordose the spine at the unstable segment before the upright posture is achieved, with pain on returning to the erect posture and the necessity to assist the movement with the use of the hands. In sitting the spine is held in segmental hyperlordosis and the patient displays difficulty in relaxing the lumbar spine and posteriorly tilting the pelvis. Segmental hyperlordosis of the lumbar spine is again accentuated in functional tests such as sit–stand, squat and gait.

Specific movement tests reveal an inability to initiate posterior pelvic tilt independent of hip flexion and activation of the hip flexors, rectus abdominis and external obliques in standing and supine. Similarly, hip extension and knee flexion movement tests in prone reveal a loss of co-contraction of the deep abdominal muscles and dominant patterns of inner range activation of the lumbar erector spinae, iliopsoas (and in some cases the superficial lumbar multifidus). This results in excessive segmental lumbar spine extension at the unstable level. Tests of position sense in sitting and four-point kneeling reveal an inability to reposition the unstable spinal segment within the neutral zone of motion, with a tendency to overshoot into extension.

Specific muscle tests reveal an inability to co-contract segmental lumbar multifidus with the transverse abdominal muscles in a neutral lumbar posture – with a tendency to posture the lumbar spine into extension. Attempts to iso-

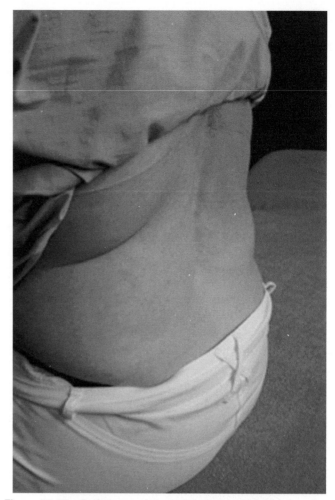

Figure 22.10 Active extension pattern: patient complaining of extension related pain at L5/S1. The patient's usual sitting posture with an anterior pelvic tilt and increased lower lumbar lordosis with associated hyperactivity of the superficial lumbar multifidus and erector spinae muscles.

late transverse abdominal muscle activation are commonly associated with excessive activation of the segmental spinal extensors, the upper abdominal wall and an inability to control diaphragmatic breathing.

Passive physiological intervertebral motion testing reveals a segmental increase in extension and rotation mobility at the symptomatic motion segment. Flexion may feel 'stiff'. Palpatory examination in prone reveals a painful increase in posteroanterior motion at the unstable motion segment.

Dynamic stabilizing strategy

These patients' dynamic stabilizing strategy for the lumbar spine appears to be associated with dominant activation of the lumbar erector spinae, iliopsoas and in some cases the superficial fibres of lumbar multifidus, with associated bracing with the diaphragm and global activation of the abdominal muscles. In this case it appears that segmental bending activities and postures as they do reverse their lordosis.

Posture and movement analysis reveals that in standing these patients tend to sway their thorax posterior to the pelvis (Fig. 22.12), with resultant hinging of the 'unstable' spinal segment into extension (Fig. 22.13). This 'passive' posture is associated with a reduction in tone in the transverse abdominal wall, lumbar multifidus, erector spinae and gluteal muscles, with tonic activation of the rectus abdominis and external oblique muscles (O'Sullivan 2002b). These patients tend to complain of extension loading pain in standing. In standing, compression through the shoulders enhances the segmental hinging at the unstable segment and increases the symptoms. Extension activities and movements of the lumbar spine usually reveal hinging at

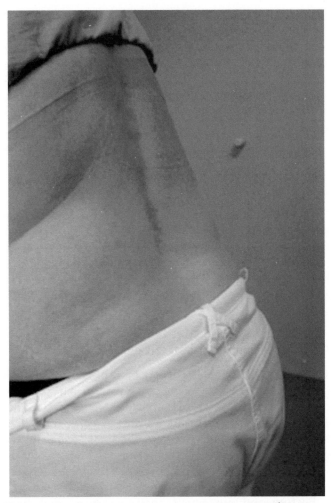

Figure 22.11   Active extension pattern: patient with L5/S1 extension related pain reports arc of pain in forward bending and on return to upright. Note the lack of reverse lordosis in forward bending and the tendency to fix the spine in extension and flex at the hips.

and global extensors of the spine (with the absence of co-contraction with the transverse abdominal muscles) stabilize the motion segment by 'locking' it into end of range extension rather than providing stabilization to the motion segment within the neutral zone.

4.   Passive extension pattern

The other extension pattern is described as 'passive' as opposed to the 'active' extension group. These patients present with very low tone of the lumbar multifidus, iliopsoas and erector spinae muscles of the lumbar spine. Similar to the active extension group they report a traumatic or repetitive injury to the spine in extension. They report that they are aggravated by extension activities and postures, and relieved with flexion activities and postures. Unlike the active extension group, these patients do not usually report aggravation of symptoms with forward

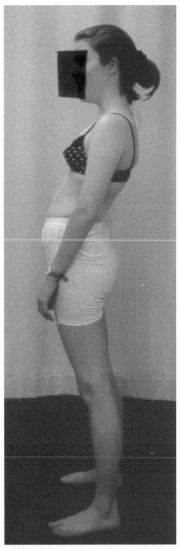

Figure 22.12   Passive extension pattern: patient with L5/S1 extension pain pattern in usual standing posture. Note the postural sway of thorax posterior to pelvis, with associated lower lumbar lordosis, thoracic kyphosis and upper abdominal wall tone.

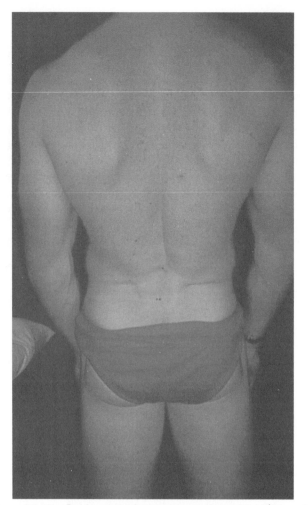

Figure 22.13 Passive extension pattern: patient with L5/S1 grade 1 spondylolisthesis complaining of extension related pain and presenting with a segmental hinging pattern with backward bending. Reproduced from Taylor & O'Sullivan 2000.

the affected segment with a loss of lordosis above this level and associated 'sway' posture. This may be associated with an arc of pain as well as end-range symptoms. In sitting, unlike the 'active' group, these patients sit with a slump posture. Forward bending is usually pain free, but on return to neutral they tend to overshoot and hinge into extension. This is also the case with sit–stand test.

Specific movement tests (sitting, four-point kneeling) reveal an inability to extend the thoracolumbar spine above the unstable segment with a tendency to hinge into extension at this segment. Attempts to posteriorly rotate the pelvis show an inability to do so without dominant activation of the upper abdominal wall muscles and flexion of the thorax. Tests of position sense in sitting and four-point kneeling reveal an inability to reposition the lumbar spine within the neutral zone of motion, with a tendency to overshoot into extension at the unstable segment and flex the upper lumbar and thoracic spine.

Specific muscle testing reveals an inability to co-contract the pelvic floor and transverse abdominal wall muscles, with a tendency to dominate with activation of the upper abdominal wall and associated flexion of the thoracolumbar spine. These patients also present with an inability to co-contract lumbar multifidus, at and above the level of the unstable motion segment, with the transverse abdominal wall muscles.

Passive physiological intervertebral motion testing reveals a segmental increase in extension as with the active extension group.

Dynamic stabilization strategy

Dynamic stabilization of the lumbopelvic region in patients with this pain disorder is associated with dominant activation of the upper abdominal wall (rectus abdominis, external oblique, upper internal oblique), with inhibition of the lumbar multifidus, the transverse abdominal wall muscles and psoas. This results in extension hinging of the unstable segment. (Fig. 22.14)

4.   Multidirectional pattern

This is the most debilitating of the clinical presentations and is usually associated with a significant traumatic injury. Patients complain of high levels of pain and functional disability. They describe their provocative movements as being multidirectional in nature. All weight bearing postures are painful and difficulty is reported in obtaining relieving positions during weight bearing. 'Locking' of the spine is commonly reported following sustained flexion and extension postures.

Posture and movement analysis reveals that these patients may assume a flexed, extended or laterally shifted spinal posture, and may frequently alternate them. Excessive segmental shifting and hinging patterns may be observed in all movement directions, with associated jerky movement patterns and reports of stabbing pain on movement in all directions with observable lumbar erector spinae muscle spasm.

These patients have great difficulty assuming neutral lordotic spinal positions. Neutral zone repositioning tests reveal overshooting into flexion, extension or lateral shift postures.

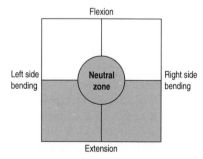

Figure 22.14 Dynamic stabilizing strategy in passive extension. Reproduced from O'Sullivan 2000.

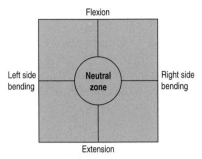

Figure 22.15 Dynamic stabilizing strategy in multidirection pattern. Reproduced from O'Sullivan 2000.

Attempts to facilitate lumbar multifidus and transverse abdominal wall muscle co-contraction (especially during weight bearing positions) are usually associated with a tendency to flex, extend or laterally shift the spine segmentally, with associated global muscle substitution, bracing of the diaphragm and pain. These patients, if they have high levels of irritability, present with an inability to tolerate compressive loading in any position and have the poorest prognosis for conservative exercise management.

Dynamic stabilizing strategy

The dynamic stabilizing strategy of patients in this group may be variable and associated with muscle spasm and splinting of the thoracolumbar spine. These patients present with difficulty stabilizing the spine in neutral positions and may revert to end-range flexion, extension or laterally shifted postures in an attempt to achieve stability (Fig. 22.15).

A common observation noted with all patients with clinical instability is the tendency to hold the lumbar spine out of the neutral zone (as in flexion, extension or a lateral shifted position), although the patient may describe these resting positions as their 'normal neutral' spinal posture. This loss of position sense and segmental control appears greatest within the neutral zone. It appears that the neuromuscular system strategy in these patients is to stabilize the motion segment out of the neutral position (in flexion, extension or in a lateral shifted posture) in an attempt to maintain stability.

MANAGEMENT OF CLINICAL INSTABILITY OF THE LUMBAR SPINE

Motor learning model

On the basis of the growing body of knowledge, a recent focus in the physiotherapy management of chronic mechanical low back pain patients is the identification of a subgroup of subjects whose pain disorder appears to relate to an underlying motor control disorder of the spinal segment. In these cases the specific motor control deficits that maintain the pain disorder are identified. The primary focus of management is to correct postures and movement patterns that are linked to maintaining the pain disorder.

This approach is based on a motor control model whereby the faulty movement pattern or patterns are identified, the components of the movement are isolated and retrained into functional tasks specific to the patients' individual needs (O'Sullivan et al 1997a). This approach to management is different to conditioning approaches to exercise, where the prime focus is on the recruitment of motor units. The motor learning approach to exercise training focuses more on the quality and control of segmental spinal posture and movement. This frequently involves inhibiting dominant muscle activity. This model also encompasses specific training of muscles whose primary role is considered to be the provision of dynamic stability and segmental control to the spine, that is, transverse abdominal wall muscles and lumbar multifidus (Richardson & Jull 1995). This is based on the identification of specific motor control deficits in the movements and postures that these muscles control (O'Sullivan 2000). This specific exercise intervention represents, in its simplest form, the process of motor learning described by Fitts and Posner (Shumway-Cook & Woollacott 1995) who reported three stages in learning a new motor skill: cognitive, associative and autonomous. There is growing evidence to suggest that this model of management is effective with long-term reductions in pain and functional disability in subjects with chronic low back pain with a diagnosis of clinical instability of the low back (O'Sullivan et al 1997b, 1997c) and sacroiliac joints (O'Sullivan et al 2001).

First stage of training

The first stage of training is the cognitive stage. Initially it is critical to ensure the patient is educated so that they develop an understanding and awareness of the relationship between their pain disorder and the way in which they habitually control their spine during postural loading and movement tasks. The use of palpatory and visual feedback with the use of mirrors and video is often critical to augment this process.

The first aim in the motor learning process is to achieve a neutral lordosis by developing control of the lumbopelvic region independent from the thorax and hips. Many subjects with profound motor control dysfunction of the lumbopelvic region will initially be unable to assume a neutral lordotic posture of the lumbopelvic region in any loading position. The initial training to assume a neutral lordosis is different for each clinical pattern.

For patients with flexion or lateral shift patterns of instability, training is usually needed to facilitate anterior pelvic tilt and low lumbar spine lordosis independent from the hips and upper lumbar and thoracic spine extension. This is due to motor control strategies where these patients hold the pelvis in posterior tilt with an associated loss of low lumbar lordosis, due to dysfunction of the iliopsoas and lumbar multifidus muscles, and dominant activation of the erector spinae muscles and hamstrings (see Figs 22.1 and 22.2). This is best taught in supine crook lying, four-point kneeling and sitting. For the lateral shift pattern, establishing central loading of the thoracolumbar spine over the pelvis (correction of the shift) is critical when training is carried out in sitting.

For the 'active' extension pattern, initial training is needed to facilitate posterior pelvic tilt and flex the spine towards a more neutral lordosis. To achieve this, inhibition of the dominant activation of superficial lumbar multifidus and iliopsoas is best achieved in supine crook lying with a focus on disassociating posterior pelvic tilt from the hips and inhibiting the hip flexors (iliopsoas).

For the 'passive' extension pattern the focus is to facilitate a neutral lordosis above the unstable segment while maintaining the pelvis and the unstable segment within a neutral position. To achieve this, inhibition of the dominant upper abdominal wall muscles must occur. This can be best achieved in sitting while ensuring the thorax is positioned anterior to the pelvis, to minimize facilitation of the upper abdominal wall from the influence of gravity (O'Sullivan et al 2002b).

Once the neutral lordosis is achieved in sitting, it is often observed that reflex activation of the lumbar multifidus and transverse abdominal wall muscles occurs automatically (O'Sullivan et al 2002b). If this is the case the therapist can progress directly to the functional training programme without specific muscle training. If reflex activation of these muscles does not occur, these positions become the start position for specific training of the lumbar multifidus in co-contraction with the transverse abdominal wall muscles within the neutral lordosis. This must be achieved in a neutral lordosis, at low levels of maximal voluntary contraction and with controlled relaxed respiration, and without dominant activation of the vertically orientated abdominal wall muscles (rectus abdominis, external oblique, vertical fibres of internal oblique).

For each clinical pattern the focus for the specific exercise training is different. For the flexion pattern the focus is more on the lumbar multifidus and psoas (to facilitate lower lumbar lordosis), with co-activation of the pelvic floor and transverse abdominal wall muscles without dominant activation of the erector spinae. For the lateral shift pattern the emphasis is on achieving activation of the unilaterally inhibited lumbar multifidus and psoas in co-activation of the transverse abdominal wall muscles while maintaining optimal spinal alignment. For the active extension pattern, the focus is on the pelvic floor and transverse abdominal wall (to reduce the lumbar lordosis), without dominant activation of the segmental spinal extensors. In the passive extension pattern the focus is on the lumbar multifidus and psoas in co-activation with the transverse abdominal wall muscles, while inhibiting the dominant upper abdominal wall muscles. The start position selected by the therapist to facilitate the activation of the local system muscles is based on that which best isolates the activation of these muscles in a neutral lordotic posture, identified in the physical examination.

Where reflex muscle activation is not automatic, attempts to isolate the activation of the pelvic floor, transverse abdominal wall and lumbar multifidus are commonly associated with bracing of the abdominal wall, breath holding and bearing down of the pelvic floor. This appears to reflect a dysfunction in the dual respiratory and stabilizing roles of the diaphragm, where the motor control system adopts splinting of the diaphragm, global abdominal wall activation with associated intra-abdominal pressure generation during attempts to contract the pelvic floor muscles. This represents a high load stabilizing strategy, but observed under low spinal loading conditions (O'Sullivan et al 2002a). To break this pattern, training diaphragm breathing with independent activation of the pelvic floor and transverse abdominal wall muscles is necessary.

It is important to note that the activation of the transverse abdominal wall muscles is a focused contraction of the muscles of the lower and middle abdomen (below the level of the lateral ribcage). No dominant abdominal muscle activation is encouraged above a level of about midway between the umbilicus and the xiphisternum. If abdominal muscle activation occurs above this level it will result in activation of the vertically orientated abdominal wall muscles (rectus abdominis, external oblique and upper internal oblique) with resultant spinal compression, fixation of the ribcage, restriction of respiration and the generation of intra-abdominal pressure. The pattern of muscle activation focuses on a 'drawing up' of the pelvic floor, and lower and mid-belly in towards the spine while controlling lateral costal breathing and maintaining a neutral lordotic posture. In weight bearing positions such as sitting and standing there is a greater vertical loading of the abdominal contents on the pelvic floor and lower abdomen, so the focus is more of a 'lifting' contraction with a drawing in contraction of the lower abdominal wall. If it is noted that the neutral lumbar lordosis is lost, controlled lateral costal diaphragm breathing ceases, activation of the upper abdominal wall or flexion of the thorax occurs, then the patient is instructed to stop the contraction.

Specific facilitation of the lumbar multifidus (for flexion and lateral shift patterns) is often best achieved in sitting, once pelvic control and a neutral lordosis has been achieved. Palpating the spinous process of the unstable segment provides a feedback for the patient to draw the lumbar spine into lordosis. The patient will have a sense of the lower abdomen and the lumbar spine being drawn together without dominant activation of the thoracic erector spinae or upper abdominal wall. The focus for the lumbar multifidus training is on accurate control of the segmental lumbar lordosis during upright postures and low level loading activities.

These co-contractions involve a high level of specificity, patient compliance and low levels of voluntary contraction. It is important to educate the patient that the exercises are more 'brain' exercises than 'muscle' exercises in the early stages of training, and the focus is on control. Some chronic subjects take up to 4 or 5 weeks of specific training before an accurate pattern of co-contraction can be achieved in weight bearing postures. The greater the effort or higher the level of voluntary contraction to the motor task, the more likely subjects are to substitute with other synergistic muscles.

In the early stages the patient is not given set holding times. Rather the instruction is to hold the contraction only until global muscle substitution occurs, breathing control is lost or muscle fatigue occurs. This training must be performed in a quiet environment without interruption over a 10–15 minute period as a high level of concentration is required. Training should be carried out a minimum of once a day. Once this pattern of muscle activation has been isolated then the contractions must be performed in sitting and standing and the holding contraction increased until the patient experiences fatigue. Holding contractions of up to 5 minutes are ideal prior to integrating this muscle control into functional tasks and aerobic activities such as walking. It should be noted that throughout this training period there should be no increase or aggravation of back pain at any time.

Once low level co-contraction of the transverse abdominal wall muscles with lumbar multifidus has been achieved in a neutral lordosis in sitting and standing, with good breathing control and without global muscle substitution, the patient will usually describe pain relief in these postures. This provides a powerful biofeedback for the patient and helps to reduce activity-based fear.

This early form of training is consistent with assertions that motor learning and control are not a process of strength training, but depend on patterning and inhibition of inappropriately active motoneurons. The acquisition of skills occurs through selective inhibition of unnecessary muscular activity, as well as the activation and synchronization of additional motor units (Edgerton et al 1996).

Second stage of training

The second phase of motor learning is the associative stage, where the focus is on refining a particular movement pattern. Once the ability to assume a neutral lordosis in weight bearing with co-contraction of the local system muscles is achieved, it is immediately incorporated into dynamic tasks or static holding postures. This is based on the patient's individual presentation, movement disorder and primary movement and postural faults detected in the clinical examination. The pain provocative faulty loading or movement pattern is identified and broken down into simple steps. The patient is taken through these steps while maintaining neutral zone control and isolating the co-contraction of the local muscle system. First this is carried out while maintaining the spine in a neutral lordotic posture and finally with normal spinal movement while ensuring pain.

For example, if the patient complains of pain when transferring from sitting to standing then the components

of the movement are isolated and trained. Initially the patient is taught to hold the co-contraction within a neutral spine position in sitting and then to move the weight forward maintaining the same spinal position while flexing at the hips, and then during weight transference from sitting to standing. At all times the co-contraction pattern is maintained as neutral zone control is imperative. If the patient loses segmental control – either with a loss or increase of segmental lordosis or a lateral shifting pattern – then the movement is ceased and retraining to this point is repeated until it can be performed with normal segmental pain-free movement. Once this has been achieved this becomes the training exercise. When it can be carried out with relative ease, the patient is trained to flex the spine beginning with the cervical spine, then the thoracic spine, then the hips and finally the lumbar spine, while maintaining the pattern of co-contraction in a pain-free manner. In this manner neutral zone control is established with normal movement patterns rather than a rigid movement pattern of 'fixing' the spine in a neutral position. For patients with a flexion pattern the tendency is to lose low lumbar lordosis and anterior pelvic tilt control with an accentuated increased lordosis in the upper lumbar spine. Patients with a lateral shifting pattern usually have a similar tendency and during weight transference will shift their trunk laterally over the pelvis. For patients with extension patterns, the tendency will be to increase the segmental lordosis during load transfer and lose the transverse abdominal wall muscle contraction. This must be carefully monitored and corrected by the therapist.

The aim of the therapist is to identify two or three primary faulty and pain provocative movement patterns, and break them down into component movements with high repetitions (40–50). This breakdown of movement components for retraining motor control strategies can be performed for walking, lifting, forward bending, backward bending, twisting, etc. The patients carry out the movement components at home on a daily basis with pain control and gradually increase the speed and complexity of the movement pattern until they can move in a smooth, free and controlled manner without pain. Patients are also encouraged to carry out regular aerobic exercise such as walking while maintaining optimal postural alignment with low-level co-contraction of the local muscle system. Therefore if the patient goes for a 30-minute walk, they have performed a 30-minute low-level contraction of the muscles. This helps to increase the tone within the muscles and aids in developing an automatic pattern of control.

Subjects are also encouraged to be aware of optimal postural alignment throughout the day and to be aware of their movement patterns in situations where they experience or anticipate pain or feel 'unstable'. This is essential, so that the postures and movement patterns eventually occur automatically without need for conscious control during activities and habitual postures of daily living, with resultant automatic activation of the local muscle system. Once the loading and movement patterns are isolated with appropriate muscle co-contraction, patients report a reduction in symptoms when integrating this control into static postures (such as sitting, standing and sustained flexion), functional activities (such as bending, twisting and lifting), and aerobic activities (such as walking, swimming or running). This ability to control pain, reported by many subjects when performing the corrected motor control patterns, appears to act as a powerful biofeedback to reinforce the integration of this muscle control into functional tasks. This stage can last from weeks to months depending on the performer, the complexity of the task, the degree and nature of the pathology and the intensity of practice before the motor pattern is learned and becomes automatic. At this point patients commonly report an ability to carry out (with minimal discomfort) the regular aerobic, general exercise or loaded physical or recreational activities that previously aggravated their condition. It is at this stage that patients are able to cease the formal specific exercise programme but are instructed to maintain control functionally with postural awareness, while maintaining regular levels of general exercise.

Third stage of training

The third stage is the autonomous stage where a low degree of attention is required for the correct performance of the motor task (Shumway-Cook & Woollacott 1995). The third stage is the aim of the specific exercise intervention, whereby subjects can dynamically stabilize their spines in an automatic manner during the functional demands of daily living. It is at this stage that higher load conditioning and cardiovascular programmes can be introduced. Evidence that this automatic change was achieved in the trial groups lies in the results of the surface EMG data and

in the long-term outcome in subjects who had undergone this treatment intervention (O'Sullivan et al 1997d) (Fig. 22.16).

The design of examination based specific exercise programmes address the specific motor dysfunction of each subject in a functional manner, while taking into account the level at which they experience pain or sense instability. However, this management approach requires a high degree of skill and expertise on the part of the treating physiotherapist, to initially train the motor control patterns and then to integrate this new motor skill into the previously painful postures and activities which were a part of the patient's normal lifestyle. This approach is also dependent on a high level of patient motivation, awareness and compliance. A possible reason for the high levels of compliance and motivation observed in subjects with this exercise approach may relate to the knowledge that this approach allows the exercises to be performed during normal daily activities and that it focuses on the subject's ability to control their own symptoms.

CONCLUSION

The successful management of chronic low back pain conditions greatly depends on the accurate identification and classification of subgroups within the population who respond to specific interventions. An individual motor learning exercise approach, designed to enhance segmental spinal control for patients with clinical instability, is a logical management strategy for this condition. The success of this approach depends on the skill and ability of the physiotherapist to accurately identify the clinical pattern and specific motor control dysfunction present and to facilitate the correction of the faulty movement strategies. It will also be greatly influenced by the severity of the patient's condi-

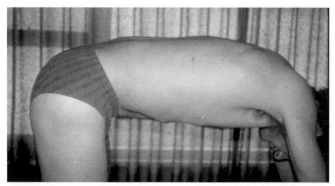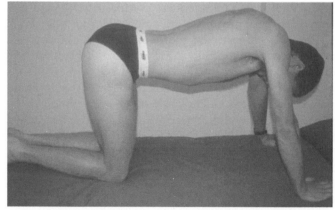

Figure 22.16 A and B: Multidirectional pattern: patient with L5/S1 grade 1 spondylolisthesis in 'natural' four-point kneeling posture with flexed lower lumbar spine (A). Note in post treatment picture (B) the change in 'natural' spinal posture in four-point kneeling with 'neutral lordosis' of the lumbar spine.

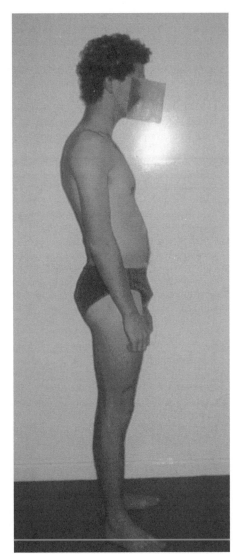 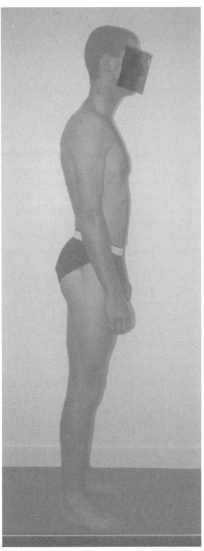

Figure 22.16 C and D: Multidirectional pattern: patient with L5/S1 grade 1 spondylolisthesis in 'usual' standing posture. Note the sway posture and laxity of the lower abdominal wall prior to intervention (C), and the change in 'usual' standing posture with no postural sway, improved lower abdominal wall and gluteal tone at 18-month follow-up (D). Reproduced from Taylor & O'Sullivan 2000.

tion and their level of compliance. Research is currently ongoing to determine the validity of the different movement disorders proposed. Evidence for the efficacy of this approach is growing although clinical trials, comparing this to other exercise approaches, are required.

KEYWORDS

low back pain
instability
motor control

exercise
trunk muscles

References

Aspden R 1992 Review of the functional anatomy of the spinal ligaments and the lumbar erector spinae muscles. Clinical Anatomy (New York) 5: 372–387

Bergmark A 1989 Stability of the lumbar spine: a study in mechanical engineering. Acta Orthopaedica Scandinavica Supplementum 230(60): 20–24

Boden S, Wiesel S 1990 Lumbosacral segmental motion in normal individuals: have we been measuring instability properly? Spine 15: 571–576

Bogduk N 1992 Anatomy and biomechanics of psoas major. Clinical Biomechanics 7: 109–119

Bogduk N 1997 Clinical anatomy of the lumbar spine and sacrum, 3rd edn. Churchill Livingstone, New York

Bogduk N, Macintosh J, Pearcy M 1992 A universal model of the lumbar back muscles in the upright position. Spine 17(8): 897–913

Brumagne S, Cordo P, Lysens R, Verschueren S, Swinnen S 2000 The role of paraspinal muscle spindles in lumbosacral position sense in individuals with and without low back pain. Spine 25: 989–994

Cholewicki J, McGill S 1992 Lumbar posterior ligament involvement during extremely heavy lifts estimated from fluoroscopic measurements. Journal of Biomechanics 25(1): 17–28

Cholewicki J, McGill S 1996 Mechanical stability of the in vivo lumbar spine: implications for injury and chronic low back pain. Clinical Biomechanics 11(1): 1–15

Coste J, Paolaggi J, Spira A 1992 Classification of non-specific low back pain. II: Clinical diversity of organic forms. Spine 17(9): 1038–1042

Cresswell A 1993 Responses of intra-abdominal pressure and abdominal muscle activity during dynamic loading in man. European Journal of Applied Physiology 66: 315–320

Cresswell A, Grundstrom H, Thorstensson A 1992 Observations on intra-abdominal pressure and patterns of abdominal intra-muscular activity in man. Acta Physiologica Scandinavica 144: 409–418

Cresswell A G, Blake P L, Thorstensson A 1994 The effect of an abdominal muscle training program on intra-abdominal pressure. Scandinavian Journal of Rehabilitation Medicine 26: 79–86

Croft P R, McFarlane G J, Papageorgiow A C, et al 1998 Outcome of low back pain in the general population. British Medical Journal 316: 1356–1359

Daneels L, Vanderstraeten G, Cambier D, Witvrouw E, Cuyper H D 2000 CT imaging of trunk muscles in chronic low back patients and healthy control subjects. European Spine Journal 9: 266–272

Daneels L, Cuyper H D, Vanderstraeten G, Cambier D, Witvrouw E, Stevens V 2001 A functional subdivision of hip, abdominal and back muscles during asymmetrical lifting. Spine 26: E114–121

Dillingham T 1995 Evaluation and management of low back pain: and overview. State of the Art Reviews 9(3): 559–574

Dupuis P, Yong-Hing K, Cassidy D, Kirkaldy-Willis W 1985 Radiological diagnosis of degenerative spinal instability. Spine 10(3): 262–276

Dvorak J, Panjabi M, Novotny J, Chang D, Grob D 1991 Clinical validation of functional flexion-extension roentgenograms of the lumbar spine. Spine 16(8): 943–950

Edgerton V, Wolf S, Levendowski D, Roy R 1996 Theoretical basis for patterning EMG amplitudes to assess muscle dysfunction. Medicine and Science in Sports and Exercise 28(6 June): 744–751

Essendrop M, Anderson T, Schibye B 2002 Increase in spinal stability obtained at levels of intra-abdominal pressure and back muscle activity realistic to work situations. Applied Ergonomics 33: 471–476

Friberg O 1987 Lumbar instability: a dynamic approach by traction-compression radiography. Spine 12(2): 119–129

Friberg O 1989 Functional radiography of the lumbar spine. Annals of Medicine 21(5): 341–346

Frymoyer J, Selby D 1985 Segmental instability. Spine 10(3): 280

Gardener-Morse M, Stokes I, Laible J 1995 Role of muscles in lumbar spine stability in maximum extension efforts. Journal of Orthopaedic Research 13(5): 802–808

Gertzbein S 1991 Segmental instability of the lumbar spine. Seminars in Spinal Surgery 3(2): 130–135

Gertzbein S, Sligman J, Holtby R et al 1985 Centrode patterns and segmental instability in degenerative disc disease. Spine 10(3): 257–261

Grabiner M, Koh T, Ghazawi A E 1992 Decoupling of bilateral paraspinal excitation in subjects with low back pain. Spine 17(10): 1219–1223

Hides J, Richardson C, Jull G 1996 Multifidus recovery is not automatic following resolution of acute first episode of low back pain. Spine 21(23): 2763–2769

Hodges P, Richardson C 1996 Inefficient muscular stabilisation of the lumbar spine associated with low back pain: a motor control evaluation of transversus abdominis. Spine 21(22): 2640–2650

Hodges P, Richardson C 1997 Contraction of the abdominal muscles associated with movement of the lower limb. Physical Therapy 77(2): 132–143

Indahl A, Velund L, Reikeraas O 1995 Good prognosis for low back pain when left untampered. Spine 20(4): 473–477

Kirkaldy-Willis W 1983 Managing low back pain. Churchill Livingstone, New York

Lindgren K, Sihvonen T, Leino E, Pitkanen M 1993 Exercise therapy effects on functional radiographic findings and segmental electromyographic activity in lumbar spine instability. Archives of Physical Medicine and Rehabilitation 74: 933–939

Long D, BenDebba M, Torgenson W 1996 Persistent back pain and sciatica in the United States: patient characteristics. Journal of Spinal Disorders 9(1): 40–58

McGill S 1991 Electromyographic activity of the abdominal and low back musculature during the generation of isometric and dynamic axial trunk torque: implications for lumbar mechanics. Journal of Orthopaedic Research 9: 91–103

McGill S 1992 A myoelectrically based dynamic three-dimensional model to predict loads on lumbar spine tissues during lateral bending. Journal of Biomechanics 25(4): 395–414

McGill S, Cholewicki J 2001 Biomechanical basis for stability: an explanation to enhance clinical utility. Journal of Orthopaedic and Sports Physical Therapy 31(2): 96–100

McGill S, Norman R 1987 Reassessment of the role of intra-abdominal pressure in spinal compression. Ergonomics 30(11): 1565–1688

McGill S, Sharratt M 1990 Relationship between intra-abdominal pressure and trunk EMG. Clinical Biomechanics 5: 59–67

Maitland J 1986 Vertebral manipulation, 5th edn. Butterworths, London

Mimura M, Panjabi M, Oxland T, Crisco J, Yamamoto I, Vasavada A 1994 Disc degeneration affects the multidirectional flexibility of the lumbar spine. Spine 19(12): 1371–1380

Montgomery D, Fischgrund J 1994 Passive reduction of spondylolisthesis on the operating room table: a prospective study. Journal of Spinal Disorders 7(2): 167–172

Nachemson A 1985 Lumbar spine instability. Spine 10(3): 290–291

Nachemson A 1991 Instability of the lumbar spine. Neurosurgery Clinics of North America 2(4): 785–790

Nachemson A 1999 Back pain: delimiting the problem in the next millenium. International Journal of Law and Psychiatry 22(5–6): 473–480

Newman N, Gracovetsky S, Itoi M et al 1996 Can the computerized physical examination differentiate normal subjects from abnormal subjects with benign mechanical low back pain? Clinical Biomechanics 11(8): 466–473

O'Sullivan P 1997 The efficacy of specific stabilising exercises in the management of chronic low back pain with radiological diagnosis of lumbar segmental instability. PhD Thesis, Curtin University of Technology, Perth

O'Sullivan P 2000 Lumbar segmental instability: clinical presentation and specific exercise management. Manual Therapy 5(1): 2–12

O'Sullivan P, Twomey L, Allison G, Taylor J 1997a Specific stabilising exercise in the treatment of chronic low back pain with a clinical and radiological diagnosis of lumbar segmental 'instability'. In: Manipulative Physiotherapists Association of Australia Tenth Biennial Conference, Melbourne, Australia

O'Sullivan P, Twomey L, Allison G 1997b Dynamic stabilisation of the lumbar spine. Critical Reviews in Physical and Rehabilitation Medicine 9: 315–330

O'Sullivan P, Twomey L, Allison G 1997c Dysfunction of the neuro-muscular system in the presence of low back pain: implications for physical therapy management. Journal of Manual and Manipulative Therapy 5(1): 20–26

O'Sullivan P, Twomey L, Allison G 1997d Evaluation of specific stabilising exercise in the treatment of chronic low back pain with radiological diagnosis of spondylolysis and spondylolisthesis. Spine 22(24): 2959–2967

O'Sullivan P, Beales D, Avery A 2001 Normalisation of aberrant motor patterns in subjects with sacroiliac joint pain following a motor learning intervention. In: Proceedings of the 4th Interdisciplinary World Congress of Low Back and Pelvic Pain. Montreal, Canada

O'Sullivan P, Beales D, Beetham J et al 2002a Altered motor control in subjects with sacro-iliac joint pain during the active straight leg raise test. Spine 27(1): E1–E8

O'Sullivan P, Grahamslaw K, Kendell M, Lapenskie S, Möller N, Richards K 2002b The effect of different standing and sitting postures on trunk muscle activity in a pain free population. Spine 27: 1238–1244

O'Sullivan P, Burnett A, Floyd A et al 2003 Lumbar repositioning deficit in a specific low back pain population. Spine 28(10): 1074–1079

Paajanen H, Tertti M 1991 Association of incipient disc degeneration and instability in spondylolisthesis. Archives of Orthopaedic and Trauma Surgery 111: 16–19

Panjabi M 1992 The stabilizing system of the spine. 2: Neutral zone and instability hypothesis. Journal of Spinal Disorders 5(4): 390–397

Panjabi M, Abumi K, Duranceau J, Oxland T 1989 Spinal stability and intersegmental muscle forces: a biomechanical model. Spine 14(2): 194–199

Pearcy M, Shepherd J 1985 Is there instability in spondylolisthesis? Spine 10(2): 175–177

Pope M, Frymoyer J, Krag M 1992 Diagnosing instability. Clinical Orthopaedics and Related Research 296: 60–67

Richardson C A, Jull G A 1995 Muscle control–pain control. What exercises would you prescribe? Manual Therapy 1(1): 2–10

Richardson C, Snijders C, Hides J et al 2002 The relation between the transversus abdominis muscles, sacroiliac joint mechanics, and low back pain. Spine 27: 399–405

Saraste H 1987 Long-term clinical and radiological followup of spondylolysis and spondylolisthesis. Journal of Paediatric Orthopaedics 7: 631

Schneider G 2001 The biomechanical basis of instability in spondylolytic spondylolisthesis is not excessive translation, but rather, segments operating around an abnormal point of axial compression. In: Maagerey M (ed) Musculoskeletal Physiotherapy Association, Twelfth Biennial Conference, Adelaide, South Australia, pp 42–49

Shumway-Cook A, Woollacott M 1995 Motor control: theory and practical applications. Williams and Wilkins, Baltimore

Sihvonen T, Partanen J 1990 Segmental hypermobility in lumbar spine and entrapment of dorsal rami. Electromyography and Clinical Neurophysiology 30: 175–180

Stokes M, Cooper R, Jayson M 1992 Selective changes in multifidus dimensions in patients with chronic low back pain. European Spine Journal 1: 38–42

Taylor J, O'Sullivan P B 2000 Pathological basis, clinical presentation and specific exercise management of lumbar segmental instability. In: Twomey L T, Taylor J R (eds) Clinics in Physical Therapy: Physical therapy of the low back, 3rd edn. Churchill Livingstone, Edinburgh, pp 201–248

Valencia F, Munro R 1985 An electromyographical study of the lumbar multifidus in man. Electromyography and Clinical Neurophysiology 25: 205–221

Waddell G 1995 Modern management of spinal disorders. Journal of Manipulative and Physiological Therapeutics 18(9): 590–596

Wilke H, Wolf S, Claes L, Arand M, Wiesend A 1995 Stability increase of the lumbar spine with different muscle groups. Spine 20(2): 192–198

Wood K, Popp C, Transfeldt E, Geissele A 1994 Radiographic evaluation of instability in spondylolisthesis. Spine 19(15): 1697–1703

Chapter **23**

Abdominal pain of musculoskeletal origin

V. Sparkes

INTRODUCTION

Abdominal pain is a common clinical problem, which may have many causes. Fifty percent of patients attending gastroenterological clinics have abdominal pain of unknown origin (Manning et al 1978, Thompson & Heaton 1980). In all cases where patients present with abdominal pain it is essential that serious visceral pathology be excluded.

The importance of the musculoskeletal system as a cause of abdominal pain is recognized in the literature. Studies of referred pain demonstrate that the structures around the spine are capable of producing symptoms, including cutaneous tenderness, in the abdomen (Feinstein et al 1954, Kellgren 1938, 1939, Lewis & Kellgren 1939, McCall et al 1979). More recent work has emphasized the need to examine the spine as a source of abdominal pain. In some of these cases the pain can be relieved by therapeutic blocks (Ashby 1977, Jorgensen & Fossgreen 1990, Mollica et al 1986, Perry 2000, Stolker & Groen 2000). Carnett (1926) recognized that a lesion in the abdominal wall itself could cause abdominal pain. Other recent studies have stressed the importance of examining the abdomen for musculoskeletal lesions and have proposed treatment methods (Bourne 1980, Gallegos & Hobsley 1989, 1992, Gray et al 1988, Greenbaum & Joseph 1991, Heinz & Zavala 1977, Thomson et al 1991). When abdominal symptoms persist and a serious visceral cause has been excluded the musculoskeletal system should be assessed.

DIFFICULTIES OF IDENTIFICATION: IS IT VISCERAL OR SOMATIC PAIN?

When assessing patients with abdominal pain the key question to answer is, 'Is the pain of musculoskeletal or visceral origin?' The differentiation between visceral and somatic pain is far from clear. Thoracic spinal pain in particular presents a diagnostic puzzle. The thoracic spine has been described as having the 'capacity for much mischief' (Grieve 1994b) and as 'an enigma within the vertebral column' (Singer & Edmondston 2000). Vigilance and care are required when assessing the thoracic spine so as to avoid misinterpretation of the signs and symptoms (Singer & Edmondston 2000). Musculoskeletal disorders of the thoracic spine can mimic gastrointestinal, pulmonary and cardiac conditions (Mennell 1966) but, conversely, the viscera, which have been described as the 'masqueraders', can produce symptoms that appear to be musculoskeletal (Errico et al 1997, Grieve 1986b, 1994b, Mennell 1966). The clinical presentation of many visceral disorders can mislead even the most experienced clinician. Grieve (1994b) summarizes: 'Things are not always what they seem initially – be informed and keep awake.'

Does the description of pain help?

Does a patient's description of their pain help differentiate its origin? There are some discernible differences between the appreciation of visceral and somatic pain. Cutaneous pain is usually a distinct pain, focal, sharp, stabbing, burning and within well-defined boundaries (Mense 1993). Muscular pain has been described as cramping and aching (Mense 1993). Deep pain may arise from muscle, viscera, fascia, bone and vascular tissue (Baker 1993, Ness & Gebhart 1990).

Pain that comes from visceral tissue is described as dull, aching, cramping, burning, gnawing, wave-like, ill defined, often initially poorly localized and diffuse (Cervero 1991, 1999, Gebhart & Ness 1991, Goodman & Snyder 1995, McMahon 1997, Proccaci et al 1986). Pain from muscle tissue is also generally poorly localized and ill defined and of an aching quality similar to visceral pain (Baker 1993, Mense 1993). Both visceral and musculoskeletal pains can develop into stabbing and cramping pain as the intensity of noxious stimuli increases (Baker 1993). These pains can also be accompanied by autonomic sensations, including nausea and general unwellness, and can produce strong emotional, autonomic and motor reflexes, which can be long-lasting (Feinstein et al 1954), whereas cutaneous pain does not show these associations. Both somatic and visceral pain can be intermittent or constant (Goodman & Snyder 1995).

Referred pain and hyperalgesia

When assessing patients with pain it is imperative to appreciate the 'behaviour and vagaries of referred pain . . . and problems of referred tenderness' (Grieve 1986a). Both the viscera and somatic tissue can produce referred pain (Cervero 1988, 1999, Cervero & Tattersall 1986, Lewis & Kellgren 1939, Mense 1993, Ruch 1946). Willis (1986) notes that 'a hallmark of visceral pain is its tendency to be confused with somatic sensation'. Referred muscle pain is felt at a remote site from the lesion and it may be referred to other tissues and into other dermatomes, similar to visceral pain (Mense 1993, Schaible & Grubb 1993). Referral patterns from both muscle and viscera do not follow rigid

maps and may be spread over wider areas with much overlap (Brodal 1981, Groen 2000, McCall et al 1979). Although often felt in the midline of the abdomen, one of the characteristics of visceral pain is its frequent reference to somatic areas that are innervated from the same spinal segments as the diseased organ. Its referral is superficial to the skin or muscle and always to proximal regions and not to distal body parts (Hobbs et al 1992, Procacci et al 1986). The area of referred pain may mask the original site of visceral pain (McMahon 1997) and may become the dominant area of complaint (Mollica et al 1986).

Stimulation of the visceral and somatic tissues will cause an increase in the somatic receptive field of spinal cord neurons. The area of referral is amplified due to convergence of visceral and somatic fibres onto the same neurons (McMahon 1997). These changes appear to be a central phenomenon in both somatic and visceral tissues (Cervero & Laird 1999, Dubner 1992, Meyer et al 1985, Ness & Gebhart 1990, Woolf 1989).

Referred pain may or may not be accompanied by hyperalgesia (Giamberardino & Vecchiet 1995, McMahon 1997, Procacci et al 1986). Visceral hyperalgesia typically arises in the absence of tissue injury and inflammation, unlike somatic hyperalgesia. It is, however, like somatic hyperalgesia in that it can be maintained by peripheral and central mechanisms (Gebhart 2000). Repeated episodes of visceral pain produce a greater area of hyperalgesia (Vecchiet et al 1989) and the hyperalgesia often remains when the visceral pathology has been resolved (Cervero & Laird 1999, Giamberardino & Vecchiet 1995, Vecchiet et al 1989).

Areas of hyperalgesia may demonstrate (Slocumb 1990):

- trigger points, which may also refer pain to other dermatomes
- hyperaesthesia of the skin
- tender points within the skin, muscle and fascia.

In subjects who exhibited hyperalgesia, even when the visceral disorder had resolved, changes in the subcutaneous tissues and muscle were demonstrated. In all cases muscle was involved, whereas the skin and other subcutaneous tissue was not. A reduction in thickness of muscle wall and thickening of subcutaneous tissue was noted (Vecchiet et al 1992). These trophic changes may have implications for the development of musculoskeletal disorders in the future or the persistence of joint and muscle sensitivity. Referred hyperalgesia arises in part from a sensitization of primary sensory nociceptors (McMahon 1997). The maintenance of this hyperalgesic state does not necessitate a persistent drive from the periphery but the brain stem nuclei and viscerosomatic neuron in the spinal cord play a more important role in maintenance of central excitability (Cervero & Laird 1999, Giamberardino & Vecchiet 1995, Woolf 1991).

Neurophysiological connections

There is considerable experimental evidence that there is viscerosomatic convergence of impulses onto spinal cord neurons in the thoracic spine (Cervero 1987, Cervero & Connell 1984, Cervero & Tattersall 1985, 1986, Milne et al 1981, Tattersall & Cervero 1987). The thoracic spine appears to be a 'junction box' where the spinal cord neurons can receive a convergent input from the visceral and somatic afferent fibres. The thoracic spine has both somatic neurons driven only by somatic afferents and viscerosomatic neurons driven both by somatic and visceral afferents (Cervero & Tattersall 1985). This convergence of impulses onto the same neurons makes it difficult to differentiate between visceral and somatic pain (Choi & Chou 1995, Holzi et al 1999, Kumar 1996, McMahon 1994, Ness & Gebhart 1990, Perry 2000). Equally difficult is the differentiation between pains from two different visceral organs (Garrison et al 1992, Ness & Gebhart 1990). Visceral pathology can produce changes in the somatic nerves and present as local tenderness in the thoracic spine. Conversely, soft tissue pathology can present as visceral disorders (Perry 2000).

There are still many unanswered questions about the differences in neurophysiological processes between somatic and visceral pain. Studies utilizing functional magnetic resonance imaging (fMRI) and positron emission tomography (PET) have identified specific areas of the brain involved in the processing and modulation of deep somatic and visceral pain. Most studies have identified multiple components to this process (Aziz et al 2000, Baciu et al 1999, Cervero & Laird 1999, Clement et al 2000, McMahon 1997). This new knowledge will further the understanding of these complex issues.

PATHOLOGY OF THE THORACIC SPINE

The following sections outline musculoskeletal pathologies in the thoracic region that clinicians should consider as a potential source of abdominal pain when serious visceral pathology has been excluded.

Zygapophysial, costovertebral and costotransverse osteoarthrosis

The zygapophysial, costovertebral and costotransverse joints and immediate local soft tissues can be responsible for both local and referred pain (Bogduk & Valencia 1994, Dreyfuss et al 1994a, 1994b, Feinstein et al 1954, Nathan et al 1964, Shealy 1975, Skubic & Kostuik 1991, Wilson 1987). Pain patterns originating from the zygapophysial joints in the thoracic spine have been demonstrated as being unilateral or bilateral and can radiate to and from the spine and anteriorly (Dreyfuss et al 1994a, 1994b, Feinstein et al 1954, Kellgren 1939, Lewis & Kellgren 1939, Valencia 1988). Thoracic zygapophysial arthropathy has highest frequency at C7–T1, T3–5 and T11–L1 (Boyle et al 1998, Nathan 1962, Nathan et al 1964, Shore 1985).

Nathan identified a predominance of anterior osteophytes as well as fusion in the thoracic spine, particularly at levels 9 and 10 and on the right side (Nathan 1962). Figure

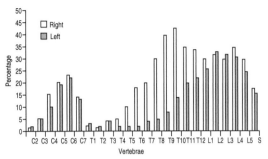

Figure 23.1 The distribution of right-sided and left-sided osteophytes of the vertebral column in 346 skeletons of white and black people of both sexes. This shows a preponderance of osteophytes along the right side of the fifth to twelfth thoracic vertebrae and that the highest frequency is to be found in the thoracic region. Reproduced with permission of the British Editorial Society of Bone and Joint Surgery, London, from Nathan 1962.

23.1 shows the distribution of right-sided and left-sided osteophytes throughout the spine. Other studies have identified that the costovertebral joints presenting with full facets, particularly at T1, T11 and T12, appear to be most affected by arthritic changes (Malmivaara et al 1987, Nathan et al 1964, Schmorl & Junghanns 1971). Degeneration of the disc, vertebral body osteophytes and Schmorl's nodes in the lower thoracic region have been identified which could refer symptoms to the abdomen (Malmivaara et al 1987). The anterior disc height reduces with age, which will accentuate the thoracic kyphosis, and may be compounded with the presence of osteoporosis (Schmorl & Junghanns 1971). Disc calcification and peripheral margin osteophyte formation often accompany disc degeneration, particularly in the thoracolumbar region (Melnick & Silverman 1963, Vernon-Roberts 1992). Thoracic canal stenosis, although uncommon, can have serious consequences due to the combination of a narrow canal and critical vascular supply, particularly at levels T3–9 (Errico et al 1997, Mitra et al 1996, Panjabi et al 1991). The site of the cord compression may be central within the canal, lateral recess or the neural foramen or a combination of these. Rheumatoid arthritis can also affect the costotransverse, costovertebral and zygapophysial joints and the disc (Bywaters 1974, Simpson & Booth 1992).

The close relationship of the intercostal nerves and the sympathetic plexus to these arthritic changes could account for radiating symptoms along the line of the peripheral nerve to the abdominal wall, with accompanying altered sensations and autonomic disturbances (Lipschitz et al 1988, Mollica et al 1986, Nathan et al 1964). Patients with joint dysfunction in the thoracic region caused by any of the above pathologies may present with simple backache but can also complain of abdominal and chest wall pain (Mollica et al 1986, Slocumb 1984). Their back pain may not be mentioned due to the dominance of the abdominal pain, as symptoms at the source may be inconsequential for the patient. The pain may be described as 'deep', 'dull ache', 'boring', 'cramp-like', 'nauseating' and 'similar to delayed muscle soreness' (Dreyfuss et al 1994a, 1994b). Autonomic symptoms, including nausea and sweating, may accompany thoracic pain (Grieve 1986b, Maigne 1996). Other symptoms may include radiculopathy, myelopathy and pseudo-claudication, which can develop gradually. Acute myelopathy may present after minor trauma to the area (Mitra et al 1996).

The onset of pain may be sudden, for instance after lifting or twisting, or of gradual onset. It may be accentuated by movements of the thorax, including deep breathing and coughing (Maitland 1988, Mennell 1966, Mollica et al 1986). Examination can often detect faulty postural mechanics with an accentuated thoracic kyphosis and restricted range of movement (Grieve 1988, Maitland 1988, Mollica et al 1986). The pain may manifest itself when the patient returns from a flexion manoeuvre and, in the case of zygapophysial degeneration, is often accentuated by hyperextension or rotation of the spine. In examining the thoracic spine, tenderness is often located over the zygapophysial and costotransverse articulation and this tenderness may follow the line of the intercostal nerve. Clinically, there may be sensory changes on the surface of the abdomen (Cyriax & Cyriax 1993).

Muscular guarding reactions are a common phenomenon when musculoskeletal or visceral tissue is stressed or damaged (Van Buskirk 1990). A model of dysfunction is proposed by Van Buskirk (1990) where prolonged muscular guarding causes musculoskeletal dysfunction, with accompanying alterations in the surrounding tissues. This proposes that stretching these tissues into normal range of motion will re-stimulate the nociceptor, reflexly reinforcing the somatic dysfunction.

Prolapsed intervertebral disc and discitis

Disc prolapses in the thoracic spine are rare but may account for a higher proportion of thoracic pain than is often realized (Currier et al 1992, Cyriax & Cyriax 1993) and can account for abdominal pain (Bland 2000, Cedoz et al 1996, Whitcomb et al 1995, Xiong et al 2001). In one-third of cases the disc herniation was associated with trauma (Stillerman et al 1998), with T11–12 being the most common site for disc herniation (Singer 1997). Patients may present with pain which can be midline, unilateral or bilateral, sensory disturbances, cold feet, weakness, tightness around the chest or abdomen, bladder and bowel dysfunction, hyper-reflexia, spasticity and gait disturbance (Benson & Byrnes 1975, Stillerman et al 1998, Whitcomb et al 1995). Compression of T11 and T12 roots may cause symptoms in the iliac fossa or the testicles and can simulate ureteral calculi, pelvic disorders or renal disease (Bland 2000, Currier et al 1992, Errico et al 1997, Taylor 1964, Whitcomb et al 1995).

Discitis is an inflammatory lesion affecting the intervertebral disc and can affect both children and adults (Stambough & Saenger 1992). The disc space becomes narrowed and there is associated fever and elevated erythrocyte sedimentation rate. The disc narrowing occurs mainly in the lumbar spine but can occur in the thoracic spine (Menelaus 1964, Stambough & Saenger 1992). Its aetiology is unclear, but may be caused by a traumatic separation of the vertebral end-plate (Alexander 1970, Stambough & Saenger 1992). Others believe it is of bacterial aetiology, with *Staphylococcus aureus* being identified (Boston et al 1975, Doyle 1960, Wenger et al 1978). Patients often describe severe unremitting thoracic pain which can radiate to the abdomen with associated symptoms of nausea and fever. They may have difficulty walking and sitting. The pain may be present at night, with the patient not being able to sit up or get out of bed. The pain will become constant regardless of position or movement, but active movements may aggravate the pain. Patients are often misdiagnosed, initially with appendicitis or pyelonephritis (Goodman & Snyder 1995, Kurz et al 1992).

On examination, patients have limited spinal movements, paravertebral muscle spasm and localized spinal tenderness and restricted straight leg raise. Abdominal examination in most cases is unremarkable. Most symptoms respond to antibiotics and rest. After initial X-rays, which are often negative, X-rays at a later date show narrowing of disc space and, in some cases, spinal fusion (Leahy et al 1984, Stambough & Saenger 1992).

Other spinal disorders

In cases of Scheuermann's disease, osteoporosis, ankylosing spondylitis, diffuse idiopathic skeletal hyperostosis and Paget's disease an accentuated thoracic kyphosis is often characteristic. This, together with bony and soft tissue changes, may lead to referred pain presenting in the abdomen. In Scheuermann's disease, which is normally painless, X-rays may demonstrate wedging of the thoracic spine, end-plate irregularity, disc lesions, Schmorl's nodes and osteophytic overgrowth (Balague et al 1989, Bohlman & Zdeblick 1988, Errico et al 1997, Yablon et al 1988). If the intercostal nerve is affected this pain can be sharp and incapacitating, with effects on respiration. As well as pain, patients may present with limited extension and rotation of the thoracic spine (Cassidy & Petty 1995, Cyriax & Cyriax 1993).

With ankylosing spondylitis the posterior, interspinous and supraspinous ligaments together with all the spinal joints are affected as the disease progresses (Bessette et al 1997, Bywaters 1974, Le T et al 2001, Singer 2000). As well as the lumbar spine becoming more flattened and rigid, the thoracic spine becomes more kyphotic with potential for irritation of the intercostal nerve (Cyriax & Cyriax 1993, Simpson & Booth 1992, Wollheim 1993). Osteoporosis affects the trabecular bone resulting in wedging of the vertebrae and is most common in the thoracic spine, particularly the mid-thoracic segments (Singer 2000, Singer et al

1995). Wedging of the vertebrae results in increased abdominal creases. The distance between the tenth rib and the iliac crest is reduced to the point of impact, which can be painful (Hall & Einhorn 1997, Woolf & St John-Dixon 1988).

In both Paget's disease and diffuse idiopathic skeletal hyperostosis (DISH) skeletal changes can result in accentuated thoracic kyphosis. Patients with Paget's disease may demonstrate signs and symptoms of spinal stenosis (Hall & Einhorn 1997). Vertebral changes noted in patients with DISH demonstrate osteophytes in the anterior longitudinal ligament as well as osteoporosis, disc disease, Schmorl's nodes and thickened syndesmophytes which bridge the disc space (Vernon-Roberts 1974). These changes may result in thoracic spinal and abdominal pain and reduction in spinal movement (Resnick & Niwayama 1976).

Slipping rib syndrome

Slipping rib syndrome occurs when the medial fibrous attachments of the eighth, ninth and tenth ribs are inadequate or ruptured allowing the cartilage tip to slip superiorly and anteriorly. This may lead to impingement on the adjacent rib or the nearby intercostal nerve (Cyriax 1919, McBeath & Keene 1975, Mooney & Shorter 1997). This condition may cause a variety of somatic and visceral complaints, is often confused with a gall bladder disorder and there may be a perception of a slipping movement of the ribs or an audible click (Lum-Hee & Abdulla 1997). Clinically, patients have pain in the inferior costal regions and will complain of 'pain under my ribs' or 'clicking under the ribs'. The area of pain anteriorly can be located easily and there may be accompanying pain in the back or around the axilla. The pain can vary in quality and severity but is often sharp and aggravated by deep breathing and physical activity. Hyperaesthesia can often be found along the line of the intercostal nerve (Vincent 1978).

Although generally regarded as affecting middle-aged people it can also affect children (Lum-Hee & Abdulla 1997, Mooney & Shorter 1997, Porter 1985). Diagnosis is made by reproducing the pain on palpation of the appropriate rib or cartilage. The hooking manoeuvre is often used to aid diagnosis (Heinz & Zavala 1977, Vincent 1978). As this syndrome is always unilateral, the hooking manoeuvre will be pain-free on the asymptomatic side. The examiner curves their fingers, hooking them under the inferior rib margins and pulls them anteriorly. If the costal cartilages are causing the condition, the patient will recognize their characteristic pain and a clicking sound may be heard as the cartilages rub against one another. Exhaustive investigations and X-rays are of little value except in ruling out other disorders (Lum-Hee & Abdulla 1997, Mooney & Shorter 1997, Wright 1980). Injection with local anaesthetic is first line treatment and nerve blocks are sometimes useful (Vincent 1978). In some cases surgical excision of the affected rib and costal cartilage can be successful treatment for those with persistent pain (Copeland et al 1984).

The abdominal wall

The entire nerve supply of the anterior abdominal wall comes from the sixth to twelfth intercostal nerves and the first lumbar nerve (Williams et al 1989). About eighty years ago Carnett (1926) described simulation of visceral pain by 'intercostal neuralgia'. His key signs were tenderness persisting when the abdominal muscles were tensed, combined with palpation. This procedure is only applicable where the pain is able to be located clearly with the tip of the finger.

The patient is examined supine, the clinician palpates the maximum area of tenderness. Patients fold their arms across their chest and sit halfway up. If continued palpation at the same point elicits similar or increased pain then the test is said to be positive. Carnett hypothesized that if the cause of the pain was intra-abdominal then the tensed muscle would now protect the viscera and the tenderness should diminish. If the abdominal wall is to blame, the pain will be at least as severe or increase (Carnett 1926). Infiltration of local anaesthetic is the treatment of choice for focal tender points (Slocumb 1984).

Amended versions of the test have been devised to put less muscular stress on the patient so less fit people are able to complete the test. The patient is examined as before but they only need to lift their head and shoulders from the pillow, just enough to tense the abdominal muscles without flexing the trunk, while the clinician continues to palpate (Ashby 1977, Gallegos & Hobsley 1992, Sharpstone & Colin-Jones 1994). This revised test has been found to be sensitive and specific (Gray et al 1988, Greenbaum & Joseph 1991, Greenbaum et al 1994, Thomson et al 1991). However, the possibility exists that this test could implicate the thoracic vertebrae and other structures in that region which may produce abdominal symptoms. Therefore, a positive Carnett sign is not infallible and should be interpreted alongside a full history taking and physical examination, including examination of the dorsal spine and any peripheral areas that are relevant (Hall et al 1991, Thomson et al 1991).

Muscular lesions

Tears of the external oblique aponeurosis and superficial inguinal ring have been shown to cause lower abdominal pain in hockey players. The pain can have a gradual onset and be aggravated by ipsilateral hip extension and contralateral trunk rotation. The pain can be worse in the morning, especially hip extension from a sitting position. Surgical exploration revealed tears of the external oblique aponeurosis and the superficial inguinal ring (Simonet et al 1995). The ilioinguinal nerve may be trapped in scar tissue formed at the area of the torn aponeurosis and it is felt that this plays a major part in the symptom presentation (Lacroix et al 1998).

Sandford & Barry (1987) report a case of latissimus dorsi strain presenting as right upper quadrant abdominal wall pain which radiated to the back, in which gastrointestinal screening was negative. Musculoskeletal assessment revealed tender areas over the right mid-thoracic back inferior to the scapula and reproduction of the symptoms by shoulder internal rotation, extension and adduction. The onset was precipitated by playing on slot machines for up to 6 hours the previous week. Symptoms were resolved following physical therapy intervention.

Intercostal neuralgia and abdominal cutaneous nerve entrapment syndrome

Intercostal neuralgia and abdominal cutaneous nerve entrapment syndrome are terms used to describe pain and symptoms caused by compromise of the abdominal cutaneous nerves (Applegate 1972, Applegate & Buckwalter 1997, Carnett 1926). Symptom presentation can lead clinicians to a mistaken diagnosis of gall bladder disease or appendicitis. The sixth to tenth right intercostal nerves supply the right upper quadrant of the anterior abdominal wall and irritation of these nerves is often mistaken for biliary lesions (Williams et al 1989).

Entrapment of the abdominal cutaneous nerve can occur at any place along its length but most commonly occurs where the nerve is anchored at the following five locations (Applegate 1972, Applegate & Buckwalter 1997):

- the spinal cord
- the origination point of the posterior cutaneous branch
- the origination point of the lateral branch
- where the nerve makes an almost 90 degree turn to enter the rectus channel
- the skin.

Figure 23.2 shows in detail the site of anterior abdominal cutaneous nerve entrapment and the area for infiltration of local anaesthetic.

The pathology appears to be ischaemia of the affected nerve (Applegate & Buckwalter 1997). It is suggested that the peripheral nerve gets compressed in a narrow space by a fibrous band or becomes kinked when turning sharply before suddenly changing course. This can arise when the anterior cutaneous branch of the thoraco-abdominal nerve becomes entrapped in the fascial sheath of the rectus abdominis (Applegate 1972, Applegate & Buckwalter 1997, Doouss & Boas 1975, Mehta & Ranger 1971).

Bony conditions that can cause compression and abnormal stretch on the nerve include degenerative disc and joint disease resulting in angulation of the vertebrae and osteo-

Figure 23.2 Site of anterior abdominal cutaneous nerve entrapment. Reproduced with permission from Johansen et al 2001, Bonica's management of pain, 3rd edn. Lippincott, Williams & Wilkins, Philadelphia, p. 1326. Key: ARS = anterior rectus sheath; PRS = posterior rectus sheath.

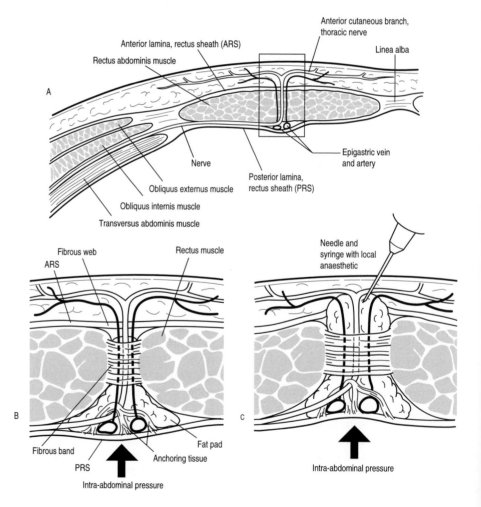

porosis leading to collapse of the vertebrae and scoliosis, where the apex of the concave section may compromise the nerve. Scar tissue from surgery or trauma can compress the nerve and the T8 or T9 nerves can be entrapped in a cholecystectomy scar. Cases of biliary pain have been mimicked by neurofibroma of the seventh and eighth spinal nerve roots on the right side. Thoracic lateral cutaneous nerve entrapment has been cited as causing disabling abdominal wall pain in pregnant women (Peleg et al 1997).

Damage to the ilioinguinal and iliohypogastric nerves (T12–L1) may be a source of pelvic pain. These are nerves that are likely to be damaged during surgery, such as in appendectomy, hernia repair and Pfannensteil incision, as can any cutaneous nerves in abdominal and thoracic surgery (Lacroix et al 1998). Other nerves that can be involved include the genitofemoral (L1–2) and obturator (L2–4). In cases of genitofemoral disorders the pain may appear to radiate from the back to the abdomen and may radiate to the labial or scrotal region.

Symptoms of nerve entrapment include localized tender spots at the site of entrapment, which can be experienced as stabbing, cramping, severe, burning, intermittent pain but can also be dull. It may or may not be affected by rest or exercise, although twisting and flexion movements often aggravate the pain (Applegate & Buckwalter 1997). Symptoms may be relieved by inactivity (Bonica & Graney 2001). Flexion of the hip may give relief in the cases of ilioinguinal and iliohypogastric nerve entrapment. Generally, there is no systemic upset. Paraesthesia and hyperaesthesia may be present and a patient may be unable to tolerate tight-fitting clothes such as belts and waistbands (Doouss & Boas 1975). The abdomen needs to be examined specifically for tenderness localized to the anterior abdominal wall, the lower ribs or superior pubis, particularly in or adjacent to incision sites (Roberts 1962). The onset is generally insidious but direct trauma, intense abdominal muscle training or inflammatory conditions could also lead to entrapment of the nerve as it passes through or close to the abdominal muscle layers (Lacroix et al 1998). Nerve entrapments are often treated with nerve blocks and with local anaesthetic (Applegate & Buckwalter 1997, Hall & Lee 1988, Mehta & Ranger 1971, Peleg et al 1997, Perry 2000).

Diabetic radiculopathy

Thoracic diabetic radiculopathy causing abdominal bulging and abdominal and trunk pain is a rare complication of diabetes (Chaudhuri et al 1997). There may be associated cutaneous hypersensitivity. There is electromyographic evidence of nerve root denervation in some patients (Longstreth 1997). The condition predominantly affects the right side of the abdominal wall, although it may be bilateral, involving three or four adjacent nerve roots in the region of T6–12 (Chaudhuri et al 1997, Longstreth 1997). The pain can be of various types, and may be aggravated at night, increased by light touch and accompanied by local-

ized abdominal wall paresis with protrusion of the abdominals. Weight loss may be a feature; this normally resolves as the pain is eased. Spontaneous recovery is the norm, but some patients have recurrent polyradiculopathy. Early recognition is essential to avoid expensive and extensive investigations of the viscera (Chaudhuri et al 1997, Longstreth 1997).

Trigger points

Myofascial trigger points are defined as a locus of hyperirritability or point of hypertonicity associated with a taut band located within a muscle. An active trigger point is always tender and found as a palpable band of muscle fibres, which seem to prevent full lengthening of the fibres caused by associated spasm (Maigne 1996, Travell & Simon 1983). Palpation of the points is painful and can produce referred pain, tenderness and autonomic changes (Slocumb 1990, Travell & Simon 1983). Within the abdomen, myofascial trigger points are often found in rectus abdominis, transversus abdominis and the external obliques. Figures 23.3 and 23.4 show patterns of referred pain from trigger points in the abdominal muscles. Symptoms referred from these trigger points can sometimes mimic visceral disease (Johansen et al 2001). Patterns of pain from trigger points in the abdominal muscles are less consistent from patient to patient than patterns in other muscles.

Trigger points may be the result of a primary musculoskeletal dysfunction and, for complete relief of the symptoms, the musculoskeletal system should be thoroughly assessed and treated accordingly (Slocumb 1984).

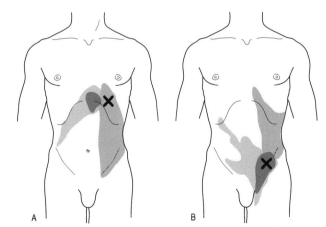

Figure 23.3 Pain patterns produced by trigger points (X) in the abdomen. A: Trigger point in the external oblique muscle overlying the lower part of the abdominal wall. B: Pain in the groin and testicle, with radiation to the upper lateral abdominal caused by a trigger point in the lower lateral abdominal wall musculature. The solid black depicts the essential zone and stippled pattern depicts the spillover zone. Reproduced with permission from Johansen et al 2001, Bonica's management of pain, 3rd edn. Lippincott Williams & Wilkins, Philadelphia, p. 1345.

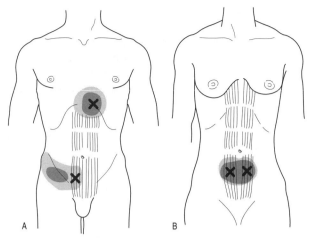

Figure 23.4 Pain patterns produced by trigger point (X) in the rectus abdominis muscle. A: Right lower quadrant pain in the region of McBurney's point caused by a trigger point in the lateral border in the ipsilateral rectus abdominis muscle and by a trigger point at the upper attachment of the rectus abdominis muscle that occasionally causes lower oesophageal spasm. The solid black line represents the essential zone and the stippled pattern represents the spillover zone. Reproduced with permission from Johansen et al 2001, Bonica's management of pain, 3rd edn. Lippincott, Williams & Wilkins, Philadelphia, p. 1326.

Viscerofascial and myofascial system

The viscerofascial and myofascial systems, although often regarded as a separate entity, should be seen as an integral part of the whole human organism (Robertson 1999). The fascial system provides support and framework to the visceral, nervous, lymphatic and muscular systems (Barral & Mercier 1988). Several studies have focused on the role of the thoracolumbar fascia as a stabiliser of the spine and its ability to transfer loads between the spine, pelvis, upper and lower limbs (Gracovetsky et al 1977, Tesh et al 1987, Vleeming et al 1995). Deficits in innervation of the thoracolumbar fascia have been noted in patients with back pain (Bednar et al 1995). With links between the visceral and musculoskeletal fascia an assessment of the fascial system is recommended when assessing patients with abdominal or musculoskeletal pain (Robertson 1999).

Rectus sheath haematoma

Rectus sheath haematoma is a rare cause of abdominal pain, but is a recognized complication of abdominal trauma or surgery (Choi & Chou 1995, Finnance et al 1995). Its location and presentation may lead the clinician to investigate the viscera (Hill et al 1995). Common causes include acute coughing attacks, anticoagulant therapy, muscular exertion, trauma, over-training of the abdominal muscles and hypertension (Hill et al 1995, Maffuli et al 1992). More uncommon instances can arise as a complication following marrow transplantation. This group of patients may be at

risk due to prolonged inactivity, thrombocytopenia and administration of high doses of corticosteroids (Zainea & Jordan 1988). It has been noted in pregnancy (Humphrey et al 2001) and suspected abruptio placentae can be misdiagnosed by clinical and ultrasound examination with rectus sheath haematoma only detected at surgery. This type of haematoma is produced by disruption of a deep epigastric vessel (Rimkus et al 1996).

Patients may present with localized abdominal tenderness, guarding and a palpable mass (Berna et al 1996, Fukuda et al 1996, Hill et al 1995). Dysuria may present at a later stage as a secondary symptom from bladder compression (Finnance et al 1995). Abdominal rigidity may develop due to irritation of the parietal peritoneum. Carnett's test may be used to distinguish between the abdominal wall and viscera (Carnett 1926, Gallegos & Hobsley 1992, Greenbaum & Joseph 1991, Thomson et al 1991). Diagnostic studies to confirm the diagnosis include ultrasonography and magnetic resonance imaging (Berna et al 1996, Finnance et al 1995, Fukuda et al 1996, Hill et al 1995, Maffuli et al 1992). Haematomas normally resolve spontaneously or may require aspiration (Siddiqui et al 1992).

Pelvic pain

It is often difficult to differentiate between pelvic pain due a musculoskeletal disorder and pelvic pain due to a gynaecological disorder as the clinical presentation can be similar for both (Baker 1993). Structures that should be considered because they can refer to the pelvic region include the lower thoracic and lumbar spine, pelvis and the hip. The local soft tissues, including pelvic fascia, muscles and ligaments, must be considered. Any structures receiving innervation from T12–L4 spinal nerves can elicit pain in the lower abdomen. Muscles that should be considered include the abdominals, iliopsoas, piriformis, quadratus lumborum, obturators and pubococcygeus. Pelvic control, leg length and spinal posture, including hypermobility, must be assessed (Kendal et al 1993, King et al 1991, Richardson et al 1999, Sinaki et al 1977). Pelvic pain has been associated with poor posture, unilateral standing, prolonged sitting and deconditioned abdominals (King et al 1991, Paradis & Marganoff 1969, Sinaki et al 1977). Symptoms associated with this disorder include heaviness in the legs and thighs, and pain in the perineum (King et al 1991). It is important to remember that the reproductive organs are innervated from T10–S4, and can refer pain to the low back, thighs and posterior pelvis (Baker 1993). Muscular pathologies to consider are trigger points and nerve entrapment, particularly when the patient has undergone surgery in the painful area.

Other disorders to consider include osteitis pubis, particularly in athletes presenting with pubic and adductor pain. This is often associated with pelvic malalignment and sacroiliac dysfunction (McDonald & Rapkin 2001). Inflammation of the adductor tendons which attach to the pubic ramus should be considered when patients present with pubic pain. The pain will often feel of bony origin and can mislead the clinician with its radiation laterally. Exquisite pain on palpation of the tendon at its insertion will confirm the diagnosis. Injection of local anaesthetic is the recommended treatment (McDonald & Rapkin 2001).

IDENTIFYING PATIENTS WITH ABDOMINAL PAIN OF MUSCULOSKELETAL ORIGIN

The question to try and answer is, 'Are the symptoms of musculoskeletal or visceral origin?' It is important not to make the clinical features fit a diagnosis when they do not. As Groen (2000) maintains, it is important to remember that the description of the quality, 'location and distribution of the pain are not absolute criteria for reliable identification of the primary source of pain'. Generally, patients presenting with visceral disorders will have accompanying symptoms, although this is not always the case. Accompanying symptoms of visceral disorders include:

- abdominal bloating
- abdominal cramps
- belching
- change in bowel/bladder habit
- dark urine
- decreased appetite
- dysuria
- faecal incontinence
- fatigue/malaise
- feeling unwell
- fever and sweating
- flatulence
- generalized weakness
- jaundice
- loss of weight
- melaena or light coloured stools
- migratory arthralgias
- nausea and vomiting
- night sweats
- pain relieved by passing stool
- symptoms affected by food
- uveitis.

Generally, benign musculoskeletal disorders have no accompanying signs. However, dysfunction of the thoracic spine may have accompanying autonomic signs and symptoms that may confuse the clinician (Choi & Chou 1995, Grieve 1986). Occasionally stimulation of trigger points may cause sweating and nausea (Kirkaldy-Willis 1983).

Musculoskeletal physiotherapists must be alert to the fact that visceral disorders can present symptoms typical of musculoskeletal pain. Gastrointestinal disorders can refer pain to a wide range of areas including shoulder, scapular, hip, groin, thoracic and lumbar spine. For example, epigastric pain radiating to the back can be related to a gastrointestinal ulcer and Crohn's disease can radiate

pain to the thigh causing limping (Bonica & Graney 2001, Meyers 1995). The stomach, duodenum and pancreas can all refer pain to the back; in some cases of pancreatic cancer back pain is the only pain presentation. Kidney disease should be considered where flank pain is aggravated by spinal extension (Bonica & Graney 2001).

Patients presenting with abdominal pain due to a musculoskeletal cause may fail to mention their vague backache as their abdominal pain is the more dominant (Mollica et al 1986). Conversely, the referred pain or hyperalgesia from the viscera is so dominant it may mask the true visceral pain (Holzi et al 1999). A musculoskeletal dysfunction, for instance, in the thoracic spine can present as a local area of abdominal pain and a visceral disorder can present as spinal pain with local spinal tenderness. The interpretation of symptoms and identification of the causes is problematic. This is further compounded when both a thoracic spinal disorder and visceral disorder exist at the same time. When determining aggravating and easing factors of pain clinicians need to remember that visceral disorders can mimic musculoskeletal disorders. They can often be relieved by certain movements (Grieve 1994a, 1994b), for example, gall bladder pain may decrease when leaning forwards and pancreatic pain can decrease when sitting upright (Goodman & Snyder 1995).

Once visceral disease has been excluded it is important for a positive diagnosis to be made to ensure appropriate and timely treatment. King (1998) designed a study to determine whether certain questions in the history taking could be useful as indicators of abdominal pain of musculoskeletal origin. In this study self-administered questionnaires were designed. These included questions concerned with musculoskeletal factors that were determined by Maitland (1988) and also included additional questions on bowel habit and dietary information. These questionnaires were tested for validity and repeatability and were subsequently applied to subjects attending a gastroenterology clinic with abdominal pain of unexplained origin, after screening for serious visceral disease. All subjects underwent a complete physical examination including spinal, sacroiliac and hip examination. In those patients where there was agreement of diagnoses by the physician and physiotherapist the history-taking information was analysed.

The following questions and responses were found to be a useful indicator of a musculoskeletal cause of abdominal symptoms (King 1998):

'Yes' response by patient:

- 'Does coughing, sneezing or taking a deep breath make your pain feel worse?'
- 'Do activities such as bending, sitting, lifting, twisting or turning over in bed make your pain feel worse?'
- 'Was the start of your symptoms connected with a fall, an accident or lifting something?'

'No' response by patient:

- 'Does eating certain foods make your pain feel worse?'
- 'Has there been any change in your bowel habit since the start of your symptoms?'
- 'Has there been any change in your weight since your symptoms began?'

These questions help decide the basis for further investigation and examination to determine the nature of the problem. These questions could be included in the routine history taking in gastroenterology clinics to alert clinicians to the possibility of a musculoskeletal cause of abdominal symptoms.

CONCLUSION

There is substantial evidence in the literature that the musculoskeletal system is capable of producing abdominal symptoms. Most authors agree that the vast majority of cases of abdominal pain have a visceral origin and, in the first instance, visceral pathology must be excluded. However, when routine visceral screening investigations are negative, clinicians should consider the musculoskeletal system as a potential cause of symptoms (Ashby 1977, Mollica et al 1986, Stoddard 1983).

Abdominal pain of musculoskeletal origin should be suspected where:

- pain is aggravated by bending or lifting
- pain is aggravated by coughing or sneezing
- pain is not aggravated by eating
- the patient's weight is steady
- there is no change in bowel habit since onset of symptoms

- there are areas of abdominal hyperaesthesia
- physical examination of the musculoskeletal system reproduces/aggravates the pain (King 1998, Mollica et al 1986).

Patients with musculoskeletal causes of abdominal pain may complain of localized abdominal pain alone or abdominal pain with accompanying back pain. It is important to remember that clinical diagnosis based on patients' symptoms is rarely straightforward. The viscera are known for their capacity to present misleading symptoms and have been described as the 'great deceivers' in terms of the patterns of pain presentation (Grieve 1986b). Due to the convergence of afferents from somatic and visceral structures on the same dorsal horn cells in the thoracic spinal ganglia (Cervero & Connell 1984), visceral pathology may be misinterpreted as musculoskeletal. Of course, both a musculoskeletal and a visceral cause of pain may coexist. Correct interpretation of the symptoms through a careful history and physical examination is important for an accurate diagnosis and treatment (Perry 2000, Procacci 1996).

Given the incidence of patients with abdominal pain that remains unexplained following gastroenterological investigations, it is vital to investigate the musculoskeletal system and, where appropriate, treat accordingly (King 1998).

KEYWORDS	
abdominal pain	visceral pain
musculoskeletal	somatic pain
thoracic spine	

References

Alexander C J 1970 The aetiology of juvenile spondyloarthritis (discitis). Clinical Radiology 21: 178–187

Applegate W V 1972 Abdominal cutaneous nerve entrapment syndrome. Surgery 71: 118–124

Applegate W V, Buckwalter N R 1997 Microanatomy of the structures contributing to abdominal cutaneous nerve entrapment syndrome. Journal of the American Board of Family Practitioners 10(5): 329–332

Ashby E C 1977 Abdominal pain of spinal origin. Annals of the Royal College of Surgeons of England 59: 242–246

Aziz Q, Schnitzler A, Enck P 2000 Functional neuroimaging of visceral sensation. Journal of Clinical Neurophysiology 17(6): 604–612

Baciu M V, Bonaz B L, Papillon E et al 1999 Central processing of rectal pain: a functional MR imaging study. American Journal of Neuroradiology 20(10): 1920–1924

Baker P K 1993 Musculoskeletal origins of chronic pelvic pain. Obstetrics and Gynecology Clinics of North America 20(4): 719–742

Balague F, Fankhauser H, Rosazza A, Waldburger M 1989 Unusual presentation of thoracic disk herniation. Clinical Rheumatology 8(2): 269–273

Barral J P, Mercier P 1988 Visceral manipulation. Eastland Press, Washington

Bednar D A, Orr F W, Simon G T 1995 Observations on the pathomorphology of the thoracolumbar fascia in chronic mechanical back pain. A microscopic study. Spine 20(10): 1161–1164

Benson M K, Byrnes D P 1975 The clinical syndromes and surgical treatment of thoracic intervertebral disc prolapse. Journal of Bone and Joint Surgery 57B: 471–477

Berna J D, Garcia-Medina V, Guirao J, Garcia-Medina J 1996 Rectus sheath haematoma: diagnostic classification by CT. Abdominal Imaging 21(1): 62–64

Bessette L, Katz J N, Liang M H 1997 Differential diagnosis and conservative treatment of rheumatic disease. In: Frymoyer J W (ed) The spine: principles and practice, 2nd edn. Lippincott Raven, Philadelphia, pp 803–826

Bland J H 2000 Diagnosis of thoracic pain syndromes. In: Giles L G F, Singer K P (eds) Clinical anatomy and management of thoracic spine pain. Butterworth Heineman, Oxford, pp 145–156

Bogduk N, Valencia F 1994 Innervation and pain patterns of the thoracic spine. In: Grant R (ed) Physical therapy of the cervical and thoracic spine, 2nd edn. Churchill Livingstone, London, pp 77–87

Bohlman H H, Zdeblick T A 1988 Anterior excision of herniated thoracic discs. Journal of Bone and Joint Surgery 70A: 1038–1047

Bonica J J, Graney D O 2001 General considerations of abdominal pain. In: Loeser J D (ed) Bonica's management of pain, 3rd edn. Lippincott, Williams and Wilkins, Philadelphia, pp 1235–1268

Boston H C, Bianco Jr A J, Rhodes K J 1975 Disc space infections in children. Orthopedic Clinics of North America 6: 953–964

Bourne I H J 1980 Treatment of painful conditions of the abdominal wall with local injections. Practitioner 224: 921–925

Boyle J W W, Milne N, Singer K P 1998 Clinical anatomy of the cervico thoracic junction. In: Giles L G F, Singer K P (eds) Clinical anatomy and management of cervical spine pain. Butterworth Heinemann, Oxford, pp 40–52

Brodal A 1981 Neurological anatomy in relation to clinical medicine, 3rd edn. Oxford University Press, Oxford, p 375

Bywaters E G L 1974 Rheumatoid discitis in the thoracic region due to spread from costovertebral joints. Annals of the Rheumatological Diseases 33: 408–409

Carnett J B 1926 Intercostal neuralgia as a cause of abdominal pain and tenderness. Surgery, Gynecology and Obstetrics 42: 625–632

Cassidy J T, Petty R E 1995 Textbook of paediatric rheumatology, 3rd edn. W B Saunders, Philadelphia, p 120

Cedoz M E, Larbre J P, Lequin C, Fischer G, Llorca G 1996 Upper lumbar disk herniations. Revue du Rhematisme (English edition) 63(6): 421–426

Cervero F 1987 Fine afferent fibres from viscera and visceral pain: anatomy and physiology of viscero somatic convergence. In: Schmidt R F, Schaible H-G, Vahle-Hinz C (eds) Fine afferent nerve fibers and pain. V C H Verlagsgesellschaft, Weinheim, pp 322–331

Cervero F 1988 Neurophysiology of gastrointestinal pain. Baillieres Clinical Gastroenterology 2(1): 183–199

Cervero F 1991 Mechanism of acute visceral pain. British Medical Bulletin 47(3): 549–560

Cervero F, Connell L A 1984 Distribution of somatic and visceral primary afferent fibres within the thoracic spinal cord of the cat. Journal of Comparative Neurology 230: 88–98

Cervero F, Laird J M 1990 Visceral pain. The Lancet 353: 2145–2148

Cervero F, Tattersall J E H 1985 Cutaneous receptive fields of somatic and viscero-somatic neurones in the thoracic spinal cord of the cat. Journal of Comparative Neurology 237: 325–332

Cervero F, Tattersall J E H 1986 Somatic and visceral sensory integration in the thoracic spinal cord. In: Cervero F, Morrison J F B (eds) Progress in brain research Vol. 67. Elsevier, London

Cervero F, Laird J M A, Pozo M A 1992 Selective changes of receptive field properties of spinal nociceptive neurones induced by noxious visceral stimulation in the cat. Pain 51: 335–342

Chaudhuri K R, Wren D R, Werring D, Watkins P J 1997 Unilateral muscle herniation with pain: a distinctive variant of diabetic radiculopathy. Diabetic Medicine 14(9): 803–807

Choi Y K, Chou S 1995 Rectus syndrome: another cause of upper abdominal pain. Regional Anesthesia 20(4): 347–351

Clement C I, Keay K A, Podzebenko K, Gordon B D, Bandler R 2000 Spinal sources of noxious visceral and noxious deep somatic afferent drive onto the ventrolateral periaqueductal gray of the rat. Journal of Comparative Neurology 425(3): 323–344

Copeland G P, Machin D G, Shennan J M 1984 Surgical treatment of the 'slipping rib syndrome'. British Journal of Surgery 71(7): 522–523

Currier B L, Eismont F J, Green B A 1992 Thoracic disk disease. In: Rothman R H, Simeone F A (eds) The spine, 3rd edn. W B Saunders, Philadelphia, vol 1, pp 655–670

Cyriax E M 1919 On various conditions that may simulate the referred pains of visceral disease and a consideration of these from the point of view of cause and effect. Practitioner 102: 314–322

Cyriax J H, Cyriax P J 1993 Cyriax Illustrated manual of orthopaedic medicine. Butterworth Heinemann, Oxford, pp 181–196

Doouss J D, Boas R A 1975 The abdominal cutaneous nerve entrapment syndrome. New Zealand Medical Journal 81: 473–475

Doyle J R 1960 Narrowing of the intervertebral disc space in children: presumably an infectious lesion of the disc. Journal of Bone and Joint Surgery 42A: 1191–1200

Dreyfuss P, Tibiletti C, Dreyer S J 1994a Thoracic zygapophyseal joint pain patterns: a study in normal volunteers. Spine 19(7): 807–811

Dreyfuss P, Tibiletti C, Dreyer S J, Sobel J 1994b Thoracic zygapophyseal pain: a review and description of an intra-articular block technique. Pain Digest 4: 44–52

Dubner R 1992 Hyperalgesia and expanded receptive fields. Pain 48: 3–4

Errico T J, Stecker S, Kostuik J P 1997 Thoracic pain syndromes. In: Frymoyer J W (ed) The spine: principles and practice, 2nd edn. Lippincott-Raven, Philadelphia, vol 2, pp 1623–1637

Feinstein B, Langton J B K, Jameson R M, Schiller F 1954 Experiments on referred pain from deep somatic tissues. Journal of Bone and Joint Surgery 36A (2): 981–997

Finnance N, Sullivan K M, Tobin R, Rice K W, McDonald G B 1995 A female bone marrow recipient with abdominal pain. Physician Assistant 19(5): 106–109

Fukuda T, Sakamoto I, Kohzaki S et al 1996 Spontaneous rectus sheath haematomas: clinical and radiological features. Abdominal Imaging 21(1): 58–61

Gallegos N, Hobsley M 1989 Recognition and treatment of abdominal wall pain. Journal of the Royal Society of Medicine 82: 343–344

Gallegos N, Hobsley M 1992 Abdominal pain: parietal or visceral? Journal of the Royal Society of Medicine 85: 379

Garrison D W, Chandler M J, Foreman R D 1992 Viscerosomatic convergence onto feline spinal neurones from esophagus, heart and somatic fields: effects of inflammation. Pain 49: 373–382

Gebhart G F 2000 Pathobiology of visceral pain: molecular mechanisms and therapeutic implications. IV: Visceral afferent contributions to the pathobiology of visceral pain. American Journal of Gastrointestinal and Liver Physiology 278(6): G834–838

Gebhart G F, Ness T J 1991 Central mechanisms of visceral pain. Canadian Journal of Physiology and Pharmacology 69(5): 627–634

Giamberardino M A, Vecchiet L 1995 Visceral pain, referred hyperalgesia and outcome: new concepts. European Journal of Anaesthesiology Supplement 10: 61–66

Goodman C C, Snyder T E K 1995 Differential diagnosis in physical therapy, 2nd edn. W B Saunders, Philadelphia, pp 215–283, 522–585

Gracovetsky S, Farfan H F, Lamy C 1977 A mathematical model of the lumbar spine using an optimised system to control muscle and ligaments. Orthopedics Clinics of North America 8: 135–153

Gray D W R, Seabrook G, Dixon J M, Colin J 1988 Is abdominal wall tenderness a useful sign in the diagnosis of non-specific abdominal pain? Annals of the Royal College of Surgeons 70: 233–234

Greenbaum D S, Joseph J G 1991 Abdominal wall tenderness test [Letter]. Lancet 337: 1607

Greenbaum D S, Greenbaum R B, Joseph J G, Natale J E 1994 Chronic abdominal wall pain: diagnostic validity and costs. Digestive Diseases and Sciences 39(9): 1935–1941

Grieve G P 1986a Referred pain and other clinical features. In: Grieve G P (ed) Modern Manual Therapy of the Vertebral Column. Churchill Livingstone, Edinburgh, pp 233–249

Grieve G P 1986b Thoracic joint problems and simulated visceral disease. In: Grieve G P (ed) Modern Manual Therapy of the Vertebral Column. Churchill Livingstone, Edinburgh, pp 377–396

Grieve G P 1988 Common vertebral joint problems, 2nd edn. Churchill Livingstone, Edinburgh, pp 243–248, 487–489

Grieve G P 1994a Counterfeit clinical manifestations. MACP Journal 26(2): 17–19

Grieve G P 1994b The masqueraders. In: Boyling J D, Palastanga N (eds) Grieve's Modern Manual Therapy: the Vertebral Column, 2nd edn. Churchill Livingstone, Edinburgh, pp 841–856

Groen G J 2000: Neural maps of the spine: confronting accepted knowledge. In: Singer K P (ed) Proceedings of the Seventh Scientific

Conference of the International Federation of Orthopaedic Manipulative Therapists in Conjunction with the IFOMT, Albany, Auckland, New Zealand, pp 179–181

Hall J C, Einhorn T A 1997 Metabolic bone disease of the adult spine. In: Frymoyer J W (ed) The spine: principles and practice, 2nd edn. Lippincott Raven, Philadelphia, pp 783–803

Hall P N, Lee A P B 1988 Rectus nerve entrapment causing abdominal pain. British Journal of Surgery 75: 917

Hall M W, Sowden D S, Gravestock N 1991 Abdominal wall tenderness test [Letter]. Lancet 337: 1606

Heinz III G J, Zavala D C 1977 Slipping rib syndrome. Journal of the American Medical Association 237: 794–795

Hill S A, Jackson M A, Fitzgerald R 1995 Abdominal wall haematoma mimicking visceral injury: the role of CT scanning. Injury 26(9): 605–607

Hobbs S F, Chandler M J, Bolser D C, Foreman R D 1992 Segmental organisation of visceral and somatic input onto C3-T6 spinothalamic tract cells of the monkey. Journal of Neurophysiology 68(5): 1575–1588

Holzi R, Moltner A, Neidig C W 1999 Somatovisceral interactions in visceral perception: abdominal masking of colonic stimuli. Integrative Physiological and Behavioural Science 34(4): 269–284

Humphrey R, Carlan S J, Greenbaum L 2001 Rectus sheath haematoma in pregnancy. Journal of Clinical Ultrasound 29(5): 306–311

Johansen et al 1990 Bonica's Management of pain, 2nd edn. Lipincott, Philadelphia,

Johansen K H, Dellinger E P, Loeser J D 2001 Abdominal pain caused by other diseases. In: Loeser J D (ed) Bonica's Management of pain, 3rd edn. Lippincott, Williams and Wilkins, Philadelphia, pp 1326–1348

Jorgensen L S, Fossgreen J 1990 Back pain and spinal pathology in patients with functional upper abdominal pain. Scandinavian Journal of Gastroenterology 25: 1235–1241

Kellgren J H 1938 Observations on referred pain arising from muscle. Clinical Science 3: 175–190

Kellgren J H 1939 On the distribution of pain arising from deep somatic structures with charts of segmental pain areas. Clinical Science 4: 35–46

Kendall F D, McCreary E K, Provance P G 1993 Muscles testing and function, 4th edn. Williams and Wilkins, Baltimore

King V 1998 Irritable bowel syndrome: a case for musculoskeletal assessment. PhD Thesis, Loughborough University, Loughborough

King P M, Myers C A, Ling FW 1991 Musculoskeletal factors in chronic pelvic pain. Journal of Psychosomatic Obstetrics and Gynecology 12: 87–98

Kirkaldy-Willis W H 1983 Managing low back pain. Churchill Livingstone, New York

Kumar S 1996 Right sided low inguinal pain in young women. Journal of the Royal College of Surgeons 41(2): 93–94

Kurz L T, Simeone F A, Dillin W H et al 1992 Cervical disc disease. In: Rothman R H, Simeone F A (eds) The spine, 3rd edn. W B Saunders, Philadelphia, vol 1, pp 547–591

Lacroix V J, Kinnear D G, Mulder D S, Brown R A 1998 Lower abdominal pain syndrome in national hockey league players: a report of 11 cases. Clinical Journal of Sports Medicine 8: 5–9

Le T, Biundo J, Aprill C, Deiparine E 2001 Costovertebral joint erosion in ankylosing spondylitis. American Journal of Physical Medical Rehabilitation 80(1): 62–64

Leahy A L, Fitzgerald R J, Regan B F 1984 Discitis as a cause of abdominal pain in children. Surgery 95: 412–414

Lewis T, Kellgren J H 1939 Observations relating to referred pain, viscero-motor reflexes and other associated phenomena. Clinical Science 4: 47–71

Lipschitz M, Bernstein-Lipschitz L, Nathan H 1988 Thoracic sympathetic trunk compression by osteophytes associated with arthritis of the costovertebral joint. Acta Anatomica 132: 48–54

Longstreth G F 1997 Diabetic thoracic polyradiculopathy: ten patients with abdominal pain. American Journal of Gastroenterology 92(3): 502–505

Lum-Hee N, Abdulla A J 1997 Slipping rib syndrome: an overlooked cause of chest and abdominal pain. International Journal of Clinical Practice 51(4): 252–253

McBeath A A, Keene J S 1975 The rib-tip syndrome. Journal of Bone and Joint Surgery 57A: 795–797

McCall I W I, Park W M, O'Brien J P 1979 Induced pain referral from posterior lumbar elements in normal subjects. Spine 4(5): 441–446

McDonald J S, Rapkin A J 2001 Pelvic pain: general considerations. In: Loeser J D (ed) Bonica's Management of pain, 3rd edn. Lippincott, Williams and Wilkins, Philadelphia, pp 1351–1387

McMahon S B 1994 Mechanisms of cutaneous, deep and visceral pain. In: Wall P D, Melzack R (eds) Textbook of pain, 3rd edn. Churchill Livingstone, London, pp 129–151

McMahon S B 1997 Are there fundamental differences in the peripheral mechanisms of visceral and somatic pain? Behavioural Brain Science 20(3): 381–391

Maffuli N, Petri G J, Pintore E 1992 Rectus sheath haematoma in a canoeist. British Journal of Sports Medicine 26(4): 221–222

Maigne R 1996 Diagnosis and treatment of pain of vertebral origin: a manual medicine approach. Williams and Wilkins, Baltimore, pp 81–87

Maitland G D 1988 Vertebral manipulation, 5th edn. Butterworths, London

Malmivaara A, Videman T, Kuosma E, Troup J D 1987 Facet joint orientation, facet and costovertebral joint osteoarthrosis, disc degeneration, vertebral body osteophytosis and Schmorl's nodes in the thoracolumbar junctional region of cadaveric spines. Spine 12: 458–463

Manning A P, Thompson WG, Heaton K W, Morris A F 1978 Towards a positive diagnosis of the irritable bowel. British Medical Journal 2: 653–654

Mehta M, Ranger I 1971 Persistent abdominal pain: treatment by nerve block. Anaesthesia 263: 330–333

Melnick J C, Silverman F 1963 Intervertebral disc calcification in childhood. Radiology 80: 399–402

Menelaus M B 1964 Discitis: an inflammation affecting the intervertebral discs in children. Journal of Bone and Joint Surgery 46B: 16–23

Mennell J M 1966 Differential diagnosis of visceral from somatic back pain. Journal of Occupational Medicine 8(9): 477–480

Mense S 1993 Nociception from skeletal muscle in relation to clinical muscle pain. Pain 54: 241–289

Meyer R A, Campbell J N, Raja S N 1985 Peripheral neural mechanisms of cutaneous hyperalgesia. Advances in Pain Research 9: 53–71

Meyers S 1995 Crohn's disease: clinical features and diagnosis. In: Haubrich W S, Schaffner F, Berk J E (eds) Bockus Gastroenterology, 5th edn. W B Saunders, Philadelphia, vol 2, pp 1410–1428

Milne R J, Foreman R D, Giesler Jr G T, Willis W D 1981 Convergence of cutaneous pelvic, visceral nociceptive inputs onto primate spinothalamic neurons. Pain 11: 163–183

Mitra S R, Gurjar S G, Mitra K R 1996 Degenerative disease of the thoracic spine in central India. Spinal Cord 34(6): 333–337

Mollica Q, Ardito S, Russo T C 1986 Pseudovisceral pain due to posterior joint pathology in the dorso lumbar spine. Italian Journal of Orthopedics and Trauma 12(4): 467–471

Mooney D P, Shorter N A 1997 Slipping rib syndrome in children. Journal of Paediatric Surgery 32(7): 1081–1082

Nathan H 1962 Osteophytes of the vertebral column. Journal of Bone and Joint Surgery 44(2): 243–264

Nathan H, Weinberg H, Robin G C, Aviad I 1964 The costovertebral joints: anatomical-clinical observations in arthritis. Arthritis and Rheumatism 7(3): 228–240

Ness T J, Gebhart G F 1990 Visceral pain: a review of experimental studies. Pain 41: 167–234

Ness T J, Metcalf A M, Gebhart G F 1990 A psychophysiological study in humans using phasic colonic distension as a noxious visceral stimulus. Pain 43: 377–386

Panjabi M M, Takata K, Goel V, Federico D, Oxland T, Duranceau J, Krag M 1991 Thoracic human vertebrae. Qualitative 3 dimensional anatomy. Spine 16: 888–900

Paradis H, Marganoff H 1969 Rectal pain of extrarectal origin. Diseases of the Colon and Rectum 12: 306–312

Peleg R, Gohar J, Koretz M, Peleg A 1997 Abdominal wall pain in pregnant women caused by lateral thoracic cutaneous nerve entrapment. European Journal of Obstetrics, Gynaecology and Reproductive Biology 74(2): 169–171

Perry C P 2000 Peripheral neuropathies causing chronic pelvic pain. Journal of the American Association of Gynecologic Laparoscopists 7(2): 281–287

Porter G E 1985 Slipping rib syndrome: an infrequently recognised entity in children: A report of three cases and review of the literature. Paediatrics 76(5): 810–813

Procacci P, Zoppi M M, Maresca M 1986 Clinical approach to visceral sensation. In: Cervero F, Morrison J F B (eds) Progress in brain research. Elsevier, Amsterdam.

Procacci P, Zoppi M, Maresca M 1986 Clinical approach to visceral sensation. In: Cervero F, Morrison J F B (eds) Progress in brain research. Elsevier, Amsterdam, pp 21–28

Resnick D, Niwayama G 1976 Radiographic and pathological features of spinal involvement in diffuse idiopathic skeletal hyperostosis (DISH). Radiology 119: 559–563

Richardson C, Jull G, Hodges P, Hides J 1999 Therapeutic exercises for spinal segmental stabilisation in low back pain. Churchill Livingstone, Edinburgh

Rimkus D S, Ashok G, Jamali M H 1996 Bone scan in strenuous abdominal musculature exercise. Clinical Nuclear Medicine 21(8): 648

Roberts H J 1962 Atypical abdominal syndromes due to systemic disease I and II. American Journal of Gastroenterology 37: 139–276

Robertson S 1999 Neuroanatomical review of visceral pain. Journal of Manual and Manipulative Therapy 7(3): 131–140

Ruch T C, 1946 Visceral sensation and referred pain. In: Fulton J F (ed) Howell's textbook of physiology 15th edn. Saunders, Philadelphia, pp 385–401

Sandford P R, Barry D T 1987 Acute somatic pain can refer to sites of chronic abdominal pain. Archives of Physical Medicine and Rehabilitation 68: 532–533

Schaible H G, Grubb B D 1993 Afferent and spinal mechanisms in joint pain. Pain 55: 5–54

Schmorl G, Junghanns H 1971 The human spine in health and disease, 2nd edn. Grunne and Stratton, New York, p 10

Sharpstone D, Colin-Jones D G 1994 Chronic, non-visceral abdominal pain. Gut 35: 833–836

Shealy C N 1975 Percutaneous radiofrequency denervation of spinal facets: treatment for chronic low back pain and sciatica. Journal of Neurosurgery 43: 448

Shore L R 1985 On osteo-arthritis in the dorsal intervertebral joints. British Journal of Surgery 22: 833–839

Siddiqui M N, Qasseem T, Ahmed M, Abid Q, Hameed S 1992 'Spontaneous' rectus sheath haematoma: a rare cause of abdominal pain. Journal of Royal Society of Medicine 85: 420–421

Simonet W T, Saylor III H L, Sim L 1995 Abdominal wall muscle tears in hockey players. International Journal of Sports Medicine 16(2): 126–128

Simpson J M, Booth R E 1992 Arthritis of the spine. In: Rothman R H, Simeone F A (eds) The spine, 3rd edn. W B Saunders, Philadelphia, vol 1, pp 515–545

Sinaki M, Merritt J L, Stillwell G W 1977 Tension myalgia of the pelvic. Mayo Clinic Proceedings 52: 717–720

Singer K P 1997 Pathomechanics of the ageing thoracic spine. In: Lawrence D (ed) Advances in chiropractic. Mosby, St Louis, pp 129–153

Singer K P 2000 Pathology of the thoracic spine. In: Giles L G F, Singer K P (eds) Clinical anatomy and management of the thoracic spine. Butterworth Heinemann, Oxford, pp 62–83

Singer K P, Edmondston S J 2000 Introduction: the enigma of the thoracic spine. In: Giles L G F, Singer K P (eds) Clinical anatomy and management of the thoracic spine. Butterworth Heinemann, Oxford, pp 3–15

Singer K P, Edmondston S J, Day R, Breidhal P, Price R 1995 Prediction of thoracic and lumbar vertebral body compressive strength; correlation with bone mineral density and vertebral region. Bone 17: 167–174

Skubic J W, Kostuik J P 1991 Thoracic pain syndromes and thoracic disc herniation. In: Frymoyer J W (ed) The adult spine. Raven Press, New York, vol 2, pp 1443–1461

Slocumb J C 1984 Neurological factors in chronic pelvic pain: trigger points and the abdominal pelvic pain syndrome. American Journal of Obstetrics and Gynecology 149: 536–543

Slocumb J C 1990 Chronic somatic, myofascial and neurogenic abdominal pelvic pain. Clinical Obstetrics and Gynecology 33(1): 145–153

Stambough J L, Saenger E L 1992 Discitis. In: Rothman R H, Simeone R H (eds) The spine, 3rd edn. W B Saunders, Philadelphia, vol 1, pp 365–371

Stillerman C B, Chen T C, Couldwell W T, Zhang W, Weiss M H 1998 Experience in the surgical management of 82 symptomatic herniated thoracic discs and review of literature. Journal of Neurosurgery 88: 623–633

Stoddard A 1983 Manual of osteopathic practice, 2nd edn. Hutchinson, London, p 16

Stolker R J, Groen G J 2000 Medical and invasive management. In: Giles L G F, Singer K P (eds) Clinical anatomy and management of the thoracic spine pain. Butterworth Heineman, Oxford, pp 205–222

Tattersall J E H, Cervero F 1987 Somatic and visceral inputs to the superficial dorsal horn (laminae I–III) of the lower thoracic spinal cord of the cat. In: Schmidt R F, Schaible H-G, Vahle-Hinz C (eds) Fine afferent nerve fibers and pain. V C H Verlagsgesellschaft, Weinheim, pp 315–320

Taylor T K F 1964 Thoracic disc lesions. Journal of Bone and Joint Surgery 68B: 788

Tesh K M, Dunn J S, Evans J H 1987 The abdominal muscles and vertebral stability. Spine 12(5): 501–508

Thompson W G, Heaton K W 1980 Functional bowel disorders in apparently healthy people. Gastroenterology 79: 283–288

Thomson W H F, Dawes R F H, Carter S St C 1991 Abdominal wall tenderness: a useful sign in chronic abdominal pain. British Journal of Surgery 78: 223–225

Travell J G, Simon D G 1983 Myofascial pain and dysfunction: the trigger point manual. Williams and Wilkins, Baltimore

Valencia F 1988 Biomechanics of the thoracic spine. In: Grant R (ed) Physical therapy of the cervical and thoracic spine. Churchill Livingstone, London, p 44

Van Buskirk R L 1990 Nociceptive reflexes and the somatic dysfunction: a model. Journal of the American Osteopathic Association 90(9): 792–809

Vecchiet L, Giamberardino M A, Dragani L, Albe-Fessard D 1989 Pain from renal/ureteral calculosis: evaluation of sensory thresholds in the lumbar area. Pain 36: 289–295

Vecchiet L, Giamberardino M A, Dragani L, Galletti R, Albe-Fessard D 1990 Referred muscular hyperalgesia from viscera: clinical approach. In: Lipton S (ed) Advances in pain research and therapy. Raven Press, New York, vol 13, pp 175–182

Vecchiet L, Giamberardino M A, de Bigonitina P 1992 When symptoms persist despite the extinction of the visceral focus. In: Sicuteri F (ed) Advances in pain research and therapy. Raven Press, New York, vol 20, pp 101–119

Vernon-Roberts B, Pirie C J, Trenwith V 1974 Pathology of the dorsal spine in ankylosing hyperostosis. Annals of the Rheumatic Diseases 33: 281–288

Vernon-Roberts B 1992 Age related and degenerative pathology of the intervertebral discs and apophyseal joints. In: Jayson M I V (ed) The lumbar spine and back pain, 4th edn. Churchill Livingstone, Edinburgh, pp 17–42

Vincent F M 1978 Abdominal pain and slipping rib syndrome. Annals of Internal Medicine 88(1): 129–130

Vleeming A, Pool-Goudzwaard A L, Stoeckart R, van Wingerden J P, Snijders CJ 1995 The posterior layer of the thoracolumbar fascia. Its function in load transfer from spine to legs. Spine 20(7): 753–758

Wenger D R, Bobechki W P, Gilday D L 1978 The spectrum of intervertebral disc-space infections in children. Journal of Bone and Joint Surgery 64A: 100–108

Whitcomb D C, Martin S P, Schoen R E, Jho H 1995 Chronic abdominal pain caused by thoracic disc herniation. American Journal of Gastroenterology 90: 835–837

Williams P L, Warwick R, Dyson M, Bannister L H (eds) 1989 Gray's Anatomy, 37th edn. Churchill Livingstone, London

Willis W D Jr 1986 Visceral inputs to sensory pathways in the spinal cord. In: Cervero F, Morrison J F B (eds) Progress in brain research. Elsevier, Amsterdam, vol 67, pp 207–223

Wilson P R 1987 Thoracic facet joint syndrome: a clinical entity? Pain 4(Suppl.): S87

Wollheim F A 1993 Ankylosing spondylitis. In: Kelly W N, Harris E D, Ruddy S, Sledge C B (eds) Textbook of rheumatology, 4th edn. W B Saunders, Philadelphia, vol 1, pp 943–960

Woolf C J 1989 Afferent induced alterations of receptive field properties. In: Cervero F, Bennett G J, Harding P M (eds) Processing of sensory information in the superficial dorsal horn of the spinal cord. Plenum Press, New York, pp 443–462

Woolf C J 1991 Central mechanisms of acute pain. In: Bond M, Charlton J, Woolf C (eds) Pain research and clinical management. Proceedings of the Sixth World Congress on Pain. Elsevier, Amsterdam, vol 4, pp 25–34

Woolf A D, St John-Dixon A 1988 Osteoporosis: a clinical guide. Martin Dunitz, London, pp 73–109

Wright J T 1980 Slipping rib syndrome. Lancet 2(8195/1): 632–634

Xiong Y, Lachman E, Marini S, Nagler W 2001 Thoracic disk herniation presenting as abdominal and pelvic pain: a case report. Archives of Physical Medicine and Rehabilitation 82(8): 1142–1144

Yablon J S, Kasdon D L, Levine H 1988 Thoracic cord compression in Scheurmann's disease. Spine 13(8): 896–898

Zainea G G, Jordan F 1988 Rectus sheath haematomas: their pathogenesis, diagnosis and management. American Surgeon 54: 630–633

Chapter 24

Osteoporosis

K. Bennell, J. Larsen

INTRODUCTION

Osteoporosis is a metabolic bone disorder characterized by low bone mass and micro-architectural deterioration leading to skeletal fragility and increased fracture risk (Consensus Development Conference 1993). Although osteoporosis affects the entire skeleton, the most common sites for osteoporotic fractures are the proximal femur, distal radius and vertebral bodies. Fractures at these sites result in pain, loss of function, loss of quality of life and increased mortality (Cooper & Melton 1992). Osteoporosis is a major public health problem and one that is expected to increase with the significant ageing of the population (Kannus et al 1999). It is more common in women than men. Osteoporosis consumes a large portion of the health care budget, the majority of the cost being attributable to hip fractures (Randell et al 1995).

The epidemiology of spine fractures is less well documented than that of hip fractures because these fractures may not receive clinical attention. Fracture rates differ depending on factors such as geography, gender, ethnicity and race. In the USA and UK, the lifetime risk of clinical vertebral fracture calculated at age 50 is 16% and 11% for women respectively and 5% and 2% for men (Cooper 1997). Vertebral fracture incidence is virtually zero before age 50 but increases exponentially with age. Approximately half of those who suffer vertebral fracture will develop multiple fractures.

Health practitioners have a role to play in osteoporosis through exercise prescription and strategies to maximize function, reduce the risk of falls and manage pain. This chapter will provide an overview of the role of physiotherapy in the prevention and management of osteoporosis with an emphasis on vertebral fractures.

BONE ANATOMY AND PHYSIOLOGY

Bone is a specialized connective tissue consisting of cells, fibres and ground substance. Unlike other connective tissues, its extracellular components are mineralized giving it the property of marked strength. This makes bone ideally suited to its principal responsibility of supporting loads that are imposed on it. Bone is a dynamic tissue that adapts its structure throughout life by the actions of osteoblasts (bone forming cells) and osteoclasts (bone resorbing cells) in the processes of modelling and remodelling. Bone modelling is predominant during growth and refers to the change in bone size or shape in response to external factors, such as mechanical strains. This occurs due to the addition and removal of bone by strategically placed, non-adjacent activity of osteoblasts and osteoclasts. Modelling improves bone strength not only by adding mass but also by expanding the periosteal (outer) and endocortical (inner) diameters of bone (Cordey et al 1992). In contrast, in adult bone, remodelling is the main process by which bone tissue is turned over (Eriksen et al 1994). Remodelling is a cyclic process of bone resorption followed by bone formation at roughly the same location. When the amount of bone resorbed equals that formed, they are said to be coupled, resulting in maintenance of bone mass. However, a net deficit or increase in bone results if there is an imbalance between the amount of resorption and the amount of formation (Parfitt 1988).

During physical activity, contact with the ground and muscle activity generate forces within the body. Ground reaction forces can vary from 2–3 times body weight with running (Cavanagh & LaFortune 1980) up to 12–22 times body weight with jumping activities (Heinonen et al 2001). This leads to bone strain, which affects bone's adaptive response. The 'mechanostat theory' as proposed by Frost is the most widely accepted paradigm of bone biology that explains how the bone adapts to load (Frost 1988). This theory claims that in order to elicit an osteogenic response, strain must exceed a minimal effective strain (MES) before there is an increase in bone modelling and/or bone remodelling. The MES varies at different bone sites and is lower for bone remodelling than bone modelling. During old age or in times of oestrogen deficiency, the MES becomes less sensitive and thus greater strains are required to elicit an osteogenic response.

FACTORS INFLUENCING THE RISK OF FRACTURE

Bone strength and falls are two major determinants of the risk of fracture (Lespessailles et al 1998, Petersen et al 1996). As with most structures, the strength of bone is influenced by the inherent material properties of its constituents and the way in which these constituents are arranged and interact, referred to as structural properties (Einhorn 1996). Overall, 75–80% of the variance in ultimate strength of bone can be accounted for by its mineral mass and density (Bouxsein et al 1999, Lespessailles et al 1998). Smaller contributions to bone strength come from variations in structural geometry. Geometric characteristics of bone include size, shape, cortical thickness, cross-sectional area and trabecular architecture. Appendicular bone adapts to mechan-

ical loads by endosteal resorption and periosteal apposition of bone tissue. This increases bone diameter, cortical thickness, or both, and thus provides greater resistance to loading (Nordin & Frankel 1989).

There are three stages of life in women, and two in men, that are most relevant to the risk of osteoporotic fractures in later life. These are the stages in life when bone mass or density is most subject to change. Approximately 40% of total body bone mineral accumulates over several years in late childhood and early adolescence (Bailey 1997) with an individual's peak bone mass reached around the late teens and early twenties (Bailey 1997, Young et al 1995). Approximately 60–80% of peak bone mass is determined by genes (Zmuda et al 1999) but other determinants include hormones, mechanical loading, nutrition, body composition and lifestyle factors such as smoking and alcohol intake. It is now thought that one's peak bone mass is a better predictor of the risk of osteoporosis in later life than the amount of bone lost with age. Therefore, in addition to steps for minimizing bone loss, prevention strategies for osteoporosis are focusing on maximizing peak bone mass.

In women, the menopause is the next life-stage when major changes in bone mass occur due to the cessation of oestrogen production. Here rates of loss may be as great as 5–6% per year and are highest in the years immediately post menopause (Riggs & Melton 1986). Menopausal bone loss is a major reason for the higher incidence of fractures in older women than men, though a greater propensity of older women to fall also contributes to their fracture risk.

In the elderly a further phase of accelerated bone loss has been demonstrated, particularly at the proximal femur. The pathogenesis of this phase of bone loss is multifactorial and involves poor vitamin D and calcium nutrition, probably also reduced levels of physical activity and changes in body composition, specific disease states and medication use (Pfeifer et al 2001). A greater propensity to fall in the elderly (Campbell et al 1989, Hill et al 1999, Tinetti et al 1988) will increase the risk of fracture (Parkkari et al 1999), especially non-spinal fractures. Many risk factors for fall initiation have been identified. These can be classified into intrinsic factors, for example poor eyesight, reduced balance and reduced lower limb strength, and extrinsic factors such as home hazards, multiple drug use and inappropriate footwear (Lord et al 1991, 1994). Thus attention to preventing falls is necessary for preventing osteoporotic fracture in the elderly.

In addition to osteoporosis risk factors found broadly in populations, there are specific risk factors that put specific subgroups at risk. Examples include pharmacotherapy with glucocorticoids, various causes of premature loss of ovarian function, male hypogonadism and other endocrinopathies. Therapists need to be aware of risk factors for osteoporosis as well as medical conditions and pharmacological agents that predispose to secondary osteoporosis (Table 24.1).

Table 24.1 Risk factors for osteoporosis and medical conditions predisposing to secondary osteoporosis (reproduced with permission from Bennell et al 2000)

Risk factors for osteoporosis

- A family history of osteoporosis/hip fracture
- Postmenopausal without hormone replacement therapy
- Late onset of menstrual periods
- A sedentary lifestyle
- Inadequate calcium and vitamin D intake
- Cigarette smoking
- Excessive alcohol
- High caffeine intake
- Amenorrhoea – loss of menstrual periods
- Thin body type
- Caucasian or Asian race

Medical conditions predisposing to secondary osteoporosis

- Anorexia nervosa
- Rheumatological conditions, e.g. rheumatoid arthritis, ankylosing spondylitis
- Endocrine disorders, e.g. Cushing's syndrome, primary hyperparathyroidism, thyrotoxicosis
- Malignancy
- Gastrointestinal disorders (malabsorption, liver disease, partial gastrectomy)
- Certain drugs (corticosteroids, heparin)
- Immobilization (paralysis, prolonged bed rest, functional impairment)
- Congenital disorders (Turner's syndrome, Kleinfelter's syndrome)

MEASUREMENT OF BONE MINERAL DENSITY

Although fracture incidence is the clinically important endpoint in osteoporosis, for research purposes it is a difficult outcome to measure. For this reason, bone mineral density (BMD) is used as a surrogate measure to diagnose and grade osteoporosis and to predict an individual's short-term fracture risk.

Dual energy X-ray absorptiometry (DXA) is the technique of choice to measure bone density (Blake & Fogelman 1998). It is relatively inexpensive, has excellent measurement precision and accuracy and is widely available. DXA uses a small amount of radiation (Lewis et al 1994) but the effective dose delivered is less than 1–3% of the annual natural background radiation one receives from living in a major city (Huda & Morin 1996). This makes it ideal for both clinical and research purposes.

DXA converts a three-dimensional body into a two-dimensional image and provides an integrated measure of both cortical and trabecular bone. The measurement of bone mineral density (BMD) is calculated by dividing the total bone mineral content (BMC) in grams by the projected area of the specified region. It is therefore an area density expressed in g/cm^2 and not a true volumetric density. This has limitations particularly for paediatric populations where bone size rapidly changes during growth.

DXA scans are generally indicated if the individual is at risk for osteoporosis, if information is needed to help make a decision about pharmacological treatments, or to monitor the success of treatment (Wark 1998). Repeat scans should be performed not less than 12 months apart as changes in bone density occur slowly. Furthermore, the same machine should be used each time as machines are calibrated differently. Bone density changes for an individual need to be more than 2–3% in order to represent true change and not simply measurement error.

Another method used in some centres is ultrasound measurements of the heel. These ultrasound machines do not measure bone density per se but measure the speed of sound across the bone. This gives an indication of the elasticity of the bone, which is related in part to bone density, but also to other factors such as bone micro-architecture (Hans et al 1999). At this stage, the technology is not regarded as a substitute for DXA. Those diagnosed with low bone density by ultrasound would need to have a DXA scan to confirm the results.

Interpretation of DXA scans

The results of DXA scans are used to diagnose osteoporosis and can be used to help guide patient management. There are three common methods of reporting a person's BMD from DXA. The most direct method provides the unadjusted score in g/cm^2 but this is less useful as it is influenced by the age of the subject. The two most useful BMD scores are the Z- and T-scores. The Z-score compares the person's BMD with that of an age-matched group (calculated as the deviation from the mean result for the age- and sex-matched group divided by the standard deviation of the group). This score indicates whether one is losing bone more rapidly than one's peers. The T-score is similarly defined but uses the deviation from the mean peak bone density of a young, healthy sex-matched group. The World Health Organization had defined bone mass clinically based on T-scores (World Health Organization 1994) and has categorized it into normal, osteopenia, osteoporosis and established osteoporosis (Table 24.2) although, given that there is a continuous relationship between bone density and fracture risk, these cut-off values are arbitrary. DXA-derived BMD scores have been shown clinically to predict fracture risk. There is a 1.9-fold increase in risk of vertebral fracture with each standard deviation decrease in lumbar spine BMD, while there is a 2.6-fold increase in risk of hip fracture with each SD decrease in femoral neck BMD (Cummings et al 1993).

However, one very important patient related factor not captured completely by bone density testing is a history of previous low trauma fracture. Previous fracture increases the risk of further fractures about 3-fold, independently of bone density, and is therefore important in grading a patient's future risk of fracture.

Table 24.2 Diagnostic criteria for osteoporosis (reproduced with permission from Bennell et al 2000)

Classification	DXA result
Normal	BMD greater than 1 standard deviation (SD) below the mean of young adults (T-score > −1)
Osteopenia	BMD between 1 and 2.5 SD below the mean of young adults (T-score −1 to −2.5)
Osteoporosis	BMD more than 2.5 SD below the mean of young adults (T-score ≤ −2.5)
Severe or established osteoporosis	BMD more than 2.5 SD below the mean of young adults plus one or more fragility fractures

Key: BMD = bone mineral density; DXA = dual X-ray absorptiometry.

SIGNS, SYMPTOMS AND CONSEQUENCES OF OSTEOPOROSIS

Low bone density per se is asymptomatic and many individuals are unaware that they have osteopenia or osteoporosis until a fracture occurs. The common fracture sites are the hip, vertebrae and wrist and less commonly the ribs, pelvis and upper arm (Sanders et al 1999).

The most frequently fractured vertebrae are the lower six thoracic vertebrae and all of the lumbar vertebrae. There are three main types of osteoporotic vertebral fractures:

1. Compression, where the entire vertebral body collapses. This can be a slow process that occurs over time.
2. Anterior wedge – reduction of anterior height results when the anterior cortex collapses. The posterior height remains unchanged.
3. Biconcave – a concave deformity results after collapse of the superior or inferior end-plate. Posterior and inferior heights may remain unchanged. The majority of fractures are considered stable.

Vertebral fractures are associated with a range of non-specific symptoms. Approximately 33% lead to medical visits, 8% to hospitalization and 2% to nursing care (Ross 1997). The risk of mortality is also increased even after adjusting for other known predictors (Ensrud et al 2000). Although not all vertebral fractures are symptomatic, acute pain associated with vertebral fracture leads to an increased risk of days of bed rest and days of limited activity. Chronic pain may persist for years (Ross 1997). The risk of pain generally increases progressively with the number and severity of vertebral fractures. A large prospective study showed that a single vertebral fracture increased the odds of back pain by 2.8 times while two and three fractures increased the odds by 7.8 and 21.7 times respectively (Huang et al 1996).

Vertebral compression fractures can cause loss of height and this may occur suddenly or gradually over time.

Height loss of more than 4 cm over 10 years has been found to be a clinical marker of reductions in bone density in postmenopausal women (Sanila et al 1994). A common clinical sign of advanced spinal osteoporosis is thoracic kyphosis or the 'dowager's hump'. This is due to anterior wedge fractures of the vertebral bodies (Ensrud et al 1997) but muscle weakness and pain may contribute (Cutler et al 1993). Postural changes may cause patients to complain of a 'pot belly' with a bulging stomach and concertina-like skin folds. These postural changes also result in less space within the thorax and abdominal region and increased intra-abdominal pressure. This can cause shortness of breath and reduced exercise tolerance, hiatus hernia, indigestion, heartburn and stress incontinence (Larsen 1998).

Patients with vertebral fractures have significantly weaker back extensors, less thoracic and lumbar range of motion, poorer balance and reduced mobility compared with age-matched individuals (Lyles et al 1993). Another common complaint in people with a history of vertebral fracture is a feeling of chronic back tiredness or fatigue (Shipp et al 2000). The odds of physical impairment are increased 2–3 times for fractures identified on radiographic population surveys and 3–4 times for clinically diagnosed fractures. Depression and low self-esteem accompany the loss of functional capabilities and independence. Of major concern to individuals with vertebral fracture is a fear of falling and of additional fractures (Cook et al 1993). Overall this leads to a reduction in quality of life (Cooper 1997).

PHYSIOTHERAPY ASSESSMENT

The choice of questions and procedures in the subjective and objective examination depends on several factors including inpatient or outpatient status, the age of the patient, severity of the condition, coexisting pathologies, functional status, cognitive status and reasons for consultation. Specific questions that could be included in the subjective assessment for osteoporosis are shown in Table 24.3.

It is important to use reliable and standardized measurement tools to gain a more accurate assessment of the patient's needs (Table 24.4). The following section describes the key assessment procedures including those outlined in the excellent guidelines from the UK Chartered Society of Physiotherapy (1999). However, in patients with an acute vertebral fracture some of these may not necessarily be relevant at this stage.

Pain and function

The risk of physical and functional limitation is doubled in those with a history of osteoporotic fracture at any site (Greendale et al 1995b). Simple functional tests that can be administered in a clinical setting to establish the extent of disability and handicap include the timed up-and-go (Podsiadlo & Richardson 1991) and the timed 6 m walk test (Hageman & Blanke 1986). Assessing ability to transfer and

Table 24.3 Relevant questions for subjective assessment in the area of bone health (reproduced with permission from Bennell et al 2000)

Category	Specific questions
DXA results	Date performed?
	T- and Z-scores?
	Amount of change with serial scans?
Family history of osteoporosis	Which family member?
	Which sites?
Fracture status	Site?
	When?
	Related to minimal trauma?
Falls history	Number of falls in past year?
	Mechanism of falls?
	Associated injuries?
	Risk factors, e.g. eyesight, home hazards?
Medical history	Particularly with relation to risk factors including ovariectomy, eating disorder, endocrine disorder
Medication	Current or past, especially long-term steroids, hormone replacement therapy, bisphosphonates
Menstrual history	Age of onset of periods?
	Ever ≤ 8 periods per year and number of years?
	Menopausal status including age at menopause and number of years since menopause?
Smoking habits	Number of cigarettes per day and number of years smoked currently or in past?
Diet	Dietary restrictions such as vegetarianism, low fat?
	Sources of daily calcium – yoghurt, cheese, milk?
	Calcium supplementation – type and daily dose?
	Amount of caffeine?
	Number of glasses of alcohol per week?
Exercise status	Amount and type of activity during youth?
	Current exercise – type, intensity, duration, frequency?
	Interests and motivational factors?
	Exercise tolerance and shortness of breath?
Posture	Noticed any loss of height?
	Difficulty lying flat in bed?
	Number of pillows needed?
	Any activities encouraging bad posture?
Musculoskeletal problems and functional status	Pain, weakness, poor balance, incontinence functional limitations?
Social history	Occupation – full time/part time?
	Hobbies?
	Family?

to undertake activities of daily living such as climbing stairs, reaching, lifting and dressing will provide further indication of functional status.

There are several disease-specific, self-administered questionnaires that have been developed for use with patients with osteoporosis (Marquis et al 2001, Silverman 2000). The Osteoporosis Functional Disability Questionnaire and the QUALEFFO are two valid and reliable questionnaires developed for patients with back pain due to vertebral compression fractures (Helmes et al 1995, Lips et al 1999). Use of other generic validated self-reported questionnaires that assess health related qualify of life, such as the SF-36, allow comparison of the impact of disease and intervention across multiple studies and conditions.

Pain can also be assessed using visual analogue scales, the McGill pain questionnaire (Melzack 1975) and the monitoring of daily analgesic intake (Chartered Society of Physiotherapy 1999).

Posture and range of motion

In elderly patients, serial height measures should be recorded to gauge significant loss of height (Gordon et al 1991). The severity of cervical and thoracic deformity can be assessed by measuring the distance of the tragus or the occiput to wall in standing (Laurent et al 1991) (Fig. 24.1) as well as by measuring range of shoulder elevation (Crawford & Jull 1993). A kyphometer or a flexicurve ruler are simple, reliable and cost-effective alternatives to X-rays for measuring spinal kyphosis (Lundon et al 1998). A digital camera may also provide a pictorial record of serial postural changes. Other relevant movements to assess include cervical rotation and lateral flexion, and hand behind back and head. Limitation of ankle dorsiflexion may increase the risk of falling and is best assessed in weight bearing (Bennell et al 1998).

Muscle strength and endurance

Function of the quadriceps, ankle dorsiflexors, scapula retractors, trunk extensors, hip extensors and abdominals (especially transversus abdominis) are of most relevance for osteoporosis. Various isometric, isotonic or isokinetic methods can be used to assess strength. Trunk extensors may be assessed using the trunk extension endurance measurement (Toshikazu et al 1996) although this is contraindicated in those with a severe thoracic kyphosis. The function of transversus abdominis can be assessed visually while the patient performs abdominal bracing in a variety of positions (Richardson & Jull 1995). Grip strength using a hand-held dynamometer provides a useful indicator of overall muscle strength while other functional tests such as bridging, sit-to-stand and ability to stair climb give an indication of lower limb strength.

To assess combined trunk and arm endurance in people with vertebral osteoporosis, Shipp et al (2000) developed a reliable and valid test called the timed loaded standing (TLS). This test measures the time a person can stand while

Table 24.4   Summary of outcome measurements that can be used to design and evaluate physiotherapy programmes for the prevention and treatment of osteoporosis

Variable	Measurement
Pain	• 10 cm visual analogue scale
	• McGill Pain Questionnaire (Melzack 1975)
	• Daily analgesic use
Function and aerobic capacity	• Timed up-and-go (Podsiadlo & Richardson 1991)
	• Timed 6 m walk test (Hageman & Blanke 1986)
	• Adapted shuttle walk (Singh et al 1994)
Self-reported function and health related quality of life	• SF-36 Questionnaire
	• Osteoporosis Functional Disability Questionnaire (Helmes et al 1995)
	• Quality of Life Questionnaire of the European Foundation for Osteoporosis (QUALEFFO) (Lips et al 1999)
Balance	• Balancing on one leg or in stride standing – eyes open/closed, on hard surface/foam (Shumway-Cook & Horak 1986)
	• Step test (Hill et al 1996)
	• Functional reach (Duncan et al 1990)
Muscle strength	• Main muscles of interest include the quadriceps, ankle dorsiflexors, scapula retractors, trunk extensors, hip extensors and abdominals
	• Isometric, isotonic or isokinetic methods
	• Grip strength using a hand-held dynamometer
	• Timed loaded standing test (Shipp et al 2000)
Posture and range of motion	• Distance from the tragus of the ear to the wall with the patient standing back against the wall to determine thoracic and cervical posture
	• Range of shoulder elevation, cervical spine movement, ankle dorsiflexion

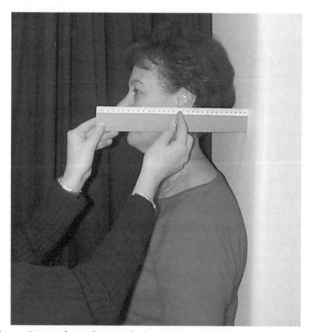

Figure 24.1   Assessing cervical and thoracic posture by measuring the distance of the tragus to the wall in standing. A more severe kyphosis will be reflected by a greater distance from the wall.

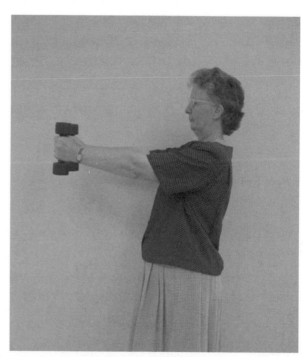

Figure 24.2   Timed loaded standing test: a measure of combined trunk and arm endurance.

holding a 1 kg dumbbell in each hand with the arms at 90 degrees of shoulder flexion and the elbows extended (Fig. 24.2).

Aerobic capacity

Simple tests which require minimal equipment such as the 6 minute walk (Steele 1996), the adapted shuttle walk test

(Singh et al 1994), the timed 6 m walk and the 'timed up-and-go' test (Podsiadlo et al 1991) are more suitable for older patients. If one is concerned about exercise tolerance, more sophisticated lung function tests such as forced vital capacity and forced expiratory volume in 1 second may be requested. A sub-maximal progressive exercise test using a treadmill or bike can provide an estimate of aerobic capacity in relatively fit individuals.

Balance

Reliable and valid measures of balance, depending on the person's functional level, include:

- aspects of the clinical test of sensory interaction of balance (Cohen et al 1993, Shumway-Cook & Horak 1986) where the longest duration that the person can balance under different test conditions (eyes open/closed, standing on floor/foam) is timed
- step test (Hill et al 1996) where the number of times the person can place the foot onto and off a step (7.5 or 15 cm high) in a 15-second period is counted
- functional reach (Duncan et al 1990) which measures the maximal anterior–posterior distance that the person can reach in standing with the arm outstretched (Fig. 24.3). This can also be measured in the lateral direction.

MANAGEMENT OF VERTEBRAL FRACTURES AND SPINAL OSTEOPOROSIS

Medical management

Following an acute vertebral fracture, many patients will initially require bed rest or at least limitation to their activity. This is usually guided by pain. Extended periods of bed

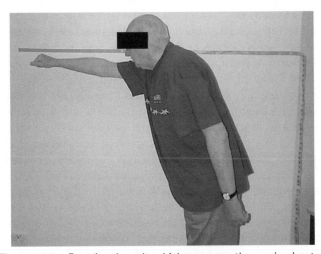

Figure 24.3 Functional reach, which measures the maximal anterior–posterior distance that the person can reach in standing with the arm outstretched, is a simple clinical measure of balance. Reproduced with permission from Bennell et al 2000.

rest has the disadvantage of having further detrimental effects on bone density, overall fitness and psychological well-being. Some patients may require hospitalization in the acute stage depending on the severity of pain, their functional capacity and the availability of home support services. Standard pharmacotherapy is used to assist with pain relief. Some patients find that nasal calcitonin is effective in relieving pain at this time.

There are several surgical augmentation procedures that are currently being used to treat pain associated with vertebral compression fractures (Watts et al 2001). Vertebroplasty and kyphoplasty involve percutaneous injection of bone cement into a collapsed vertebrae to stabilize the fractured end-plates. Unlike vertebroplasty where the technique makes no attempt to restore the height of the collapsed vertebral body, kyphoplasty involves the introduction of inflatable bone tamps into the vertebral body. Once inflated, the bone tamps restore the vertebral body back towards its original height while creating a cavity that can be filled with bone cement. Case studies suggest that these procedures are associated with early clinical improvement of pain and function but controlled trials are needed to determine short- and long-term safety and efficacy.

Drug therapies are available to assist in improving bone density and preventing fracture. Calcium supplementation, usually to a total intake of 1250–1500 mg daily, has been shown to lessen bone loss, particularly in late post-menopausal women with a low dietary calcium intake at baseline. The major alternative to hormone-replacement therapy (HRT) in treating osteoporosis is the bisphosphonates, which act primarily by suppressing bone resorption resulting in a net increase in bone density (average approximately 5% at the lumbar spine) in the first several years of therapy. Furthermore, the new bisphosphonates have been shown to reduce the risk of new fractures by approximately 50% and the risk of multiple vertebral fractures by 80%. The frail elderly (including many patients in aged care institutions) can often be managed using calcium and vitamin D supplementation (Bolognese 2002).

Physiotherapy management

There are few clinical trials to provide evidence for best physiotherapy practice in patients with spinal osteoporosis with or without vertebral fracture. In these patients the management focus shifts from specifically loading bone to reducing pain (if necessary), preventing falls, encouraging mobility and function, and improving posture and flexibility. Figure 24.4 shows how a patient's bone density and fracture status may influence management (Forwood & Larsen 2000). However, it must be remembered that the divisions are relatively arbitrary and should only be used as a guide. Other factors that will influence the choice of treatment programme include the patient's age, previous fractures, co-morbid musculoskeletal or medical conditions, lifestyle, interests and current fitness level. Activities to

Figure 24.4   Devising an exercise programme based on DXA determined fracture risk. Reproduced with permission from Bennell et al 2000.

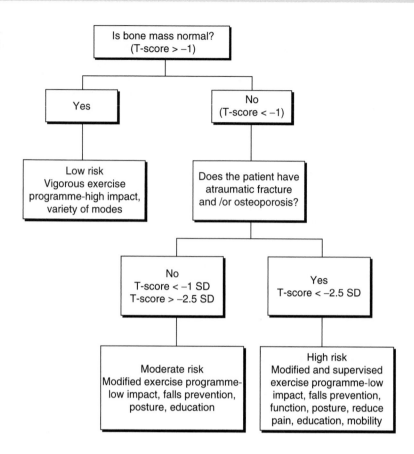

avoid in osteoporotic patients include high-impact loading, abrupt or explosive movements, trunk flexion, twisting movements and dynamic abdominal exercises.

Pain management

Acute pain accompanying a vertebral fracture may be debilitating. The physiotherapist will need to bring many skills to the patient–therapist relationship that deals with acute pain. An understanding of the relationship between pain and motivation and of the need to push gently yet not to lose the patient's confidence is essential. Responding appropriately and giving correct verbal and tactile cues to promote early rehabilitation is important. Patients should be encouraged to set some short-term realistic goals that are achievable (Larsen 1998). To deal more positively with chronic pain, cognitive and behavioural strategies or relaxation techniques may be employed by the physiotherapist.

Pain relieving modalities can be used including ice packs or ice massage, superficial heat in the form of heat packs, and pulsed shortwave. Some patients will find that transcutaneous electrical nerve stimulation (TENS) offers significant pain relief although it may be more effective in relieving chronic pain found in the older patient. Skin care with TENS electrodes is necessary, particularly in those patients who may have been on long-term steroids and whose skin is, as a consequence, very papery or transparent.

Various forms of massage including effleurage and gentle muscle rolling may be useful in decreasing protective muscle spasm in the paraspinal muscles or reducing patient anxiety prior to exercise and mobilization. The massage can be incorporated into gentle passive and then active assisted movements of the trunk and limbs.

As a result of pain and protective spasm other segments of the spine will become stiff and immobile. This can increase pain and lack of function. Gentle spinal mobilization techniques have been used to decrease these signs in the segments above and below the fracture. However, forceful joint manipulation is obviously contraindicated.

The value of spinal braces in relieving pain is unclear. Braces generally help to stabilize and immobilize the spine to allow earlier mobility with less pain. The design of these devices is such that they restrict flexion and encourage extension of the spine. Braces may be considered if the patient is slow to progress and pain is a problem or persists. There is a range of suitable braces and corsets for these fractures but the type of brace will depend on the level of the fracture. All braces should be individually made and fitted as poor compliance is often related to ill-fitting devices. Patients need to be educated that these appliances are an interim measure and that the body needs to re-activate its natural 'bracing' mechanisms, including the back, neck and hip extensors and the abdominals so that they in time will take over from the artificial brace and better support the spine. The patient must be well educated to activate the extensors and the flexors either when the brace is removed or while it is on by pulling the abdomen and back away from the support and bracing naturally (Larsen 1998).

Postural taping (Fig. 24.5) may also be required to assist with maintenance of correct posture and for pain relief. Tape can be applied diagonally across the upper back starting from the anterior aspect of the shoulder.

Exercise has been shown to reduce back pain and improve psychological well-being in postmenopausal women with osteopenia (Bravo et al 1996, Preisinger et al 1996) and with established osteoporosis (Malmros et al 1998). In a randomized placebo-controlled trial of 53 women with a history of spinal crush fracture and back pain, a 10-week physiotherapy programme consisting of balance training, muscle strengthening and lumbar stabilization exercises was effective in decreasing analgesic use and back pain and increasing quality of life and level of daily function (Malmros et al 1998).

Mobility and transfers

In the acute phase following a vertebral fracture, positions of comfort individual to each patient will need to be discussed. Often flexed positions will be more comfortable.

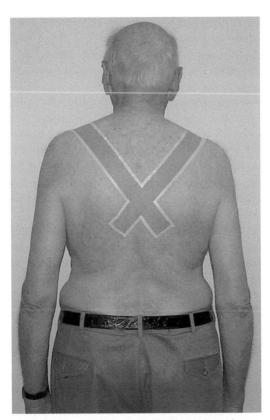

Figure 24.5 Taping may be used to facilitate thoracic extension and improve posture. Reproduced with permission from Bennell et al 2000.

Side lying with pillow support for trunk and pillow between the knees or crook lying with a pillow under the knees may be preferable. Purpose-designed mattress covers to decrease pressure and promote circulation may be useful. As soon as pain allows, the patient must be encouraged to extend out of these positions into ones that encourage less flexion. The patient should be taught how to change positions in bed as well as to transfer to chair and toilet with minimal stress and pain. Log rolling and sitting from side lying with hips in a flexed position and no trunk movement are important skills to minimize pain. Some will prefer moving off the bed backwards from prone (Larsen 1998).

The patient should stand out of bed for at least 10 minutes every hour. This should be progressed daily if possible. Any amount of mobilization should be encouraged and if necessary, a gait aid can be used as this may have the effect of reducing pain in some patients, possibly due to an unloading effect. The use of activity charts to record daily activity and exercise can be encouraging and motivational. The patient will be able to see progression over a period of time even if they are unaware of daily progression. Pain on a scale of 0–10 and pain management techniques can also be mapped on this chart.

Exercise

Initial exercises during the acute phase following a vertebral fracture will be directed at reducing pain and maintaining good circulation including preventing pressure areas and promoting good lung expansion. Pain will inhibit movement in all areas including the ribcage and chest expansion. The physiotherapist must be guided by the patient's pain tolerance, particularly to avoid further damage and also to maintain the patient's confidence in the physiotherapist. However, the reality is that the patient must move to prevent further bone loss, deterioration of other systems and an increased likelihood of falling.

Spinal extension exercises should be commenced as early as possible. Initially, these may comprise isometric contractions in the position of comfort such as side lying. These should then be progressed to active exercises. For some patients it may be more comfortable to begin extension in a chair. Bridging will be difficult at first but should be encouraged as pain allows. In the bridging starting position gentle rocking of the knees from side to side within pain limits will allow the beginning of functional rotation as an exercise (Larsen 1998). The patient can then progress to standing and may be able to extend their leg, initially in a pain-free range. If possible, they may be able to lie in the prone position although in some patients kyphotic changes will prevent prone lying. Initially resting in this position for short periods may be all that can be tolerated but some patients will be able to progress to hip extension in this position and possibly extension of the head and shoulders. As the patient improves, postural re-education and dynamic stabilization for the trunk and limb girdles are particularly important to normalize mechanical forces. Furthermore, stronger back extensors have been shown to be related to smaller thoracic kyphosis (Sinaki et al 1996).

In most patients there will be weakness in other muscles, particularly the scapular stabilizers and shoulder extensors, and exercises to strengthen these should be included (Bravo et al 1997, Chartered Society of Physiotherapy 1996). Patients are often concerned about their abdominal bulge or pot belly. Therefore they need to be educated as to the risk of dynamically exercising the abdominal flexors and predisposing themselves to increased risk for future wedge fractures (Sinaki & Mikkelsen 1984). Static abdominal exercises should be taught to the patient, particularly to train the transversus abdominis in its role as a stabilizer. These exercises can be made more difficult by adding movement once an isolated contraction has been learned.

Aquatic physiotherapy should be considered particularly as an early treatment option following a vertebral fracture. Warmth and the effects of gravity reduction on pain will often allow early movement that the patient is unable to achieve on land. The hydrotherapy pool is often a less clinical environment and allows the patient to relax a little and yet still achieve both exercise and pain reduction. Aquatic physiotherapy should be considered as soon as the patient can be transferred to the pool in a wheelchair.

Falls reduction

Where falls risk factors have been identified treatment should be directed towards reducing falls and their consequences. Patients who report multiple falls may benefit from referral to a falls clinic or to medical specialists for further evaluation and multifaceted interventions. Such interventions may be effective in reducing fall frequency (Tinetti et al 1994), depending upon the programme and setting (McMurdo et al 2000). Home hazard modification may be required, often in consultation with an occupational therapist. Consideration should be given to prescription of gait aids and external hip protectors in appropriate patients. Hip protectors have been shown to attenuate fall impact (Parkkari et al 1995, 1997) and to halve the incidence of hip fractures in institutionalized older persons (Lauritzen et al 1993) although compliance in wearing the protectors may be an issue. Specific deficits, such as restrictions in range of ankle dorsiflexion, may be improved through therapist techniques or self-stretches.

Various forms of land and water based exercise have positive effects on balance and strength deficits in elderly individuals (Bravo et al 1997, Kronhed & Moller 1998, Lord 1996, McMurdo & Rennie 1993, Morganti et al 1995, Nelson et al 1994, Simmons & Hansen 1996). However, of the ran-domized controlled trials of exercise in older persons using falls as an outcome measure (Buchner et al 1997, Campbell et al 1997, 1999, Lord et al 1995, McMurdo et al 1997, McRae et al 1994, Mulrow et al 1994, Reinsch et al 1992, Wolf et al 1996), only a few report significant reductions in falls with exercise. The effective exercise programmes included Tai Chi (Wolf et al 1996) and physiotherapy prescribed combined lower limb strengthening and balance training (Buchner et al 1997, Campbell et al 1997, 1999). The fact that other studies have failed to show significant results may be partly due to differences in exercise dimensions (type, duration, frequency and intensity), populations studied and falls definition.

At this stage, no definitive exercise prescription guidelines to prevent falls can be made on the basis of published studies. However, there is sufficient evidence to recommend a broad-based exercise programme comprising balance training, resistive exercise, walking and weight transfer as part of a multifaceted intervention to address all falls risk factors (American College of Sports Medicine 1998).

Education

A large part of the physiotherapist's role is to provide osteoporosis education and to empower the individual to take control of the condition. In many cases, patients may be anxious and require reassurance and advice about safe activities. Advice can be given about correct ways to lift as well as correct posture during standing, lying, sitting and bending. Information about lifestyle behaviours such as diet and smoking should be provided and there is an abundance of printed literature and websites available for this purpose. Physiotherapists should continually update their knowledge about self-help groups, community programmes and reputable gymnasiums and exercise classes in the local area. Osteoporosis organizations are found in many countries and states and provide a range of useful services and resources. The physiotherapist may need to liase with other medical and health professionals for overall patient care.

However, despite the amount of material available, the ability of various educational/self-help strategies to change diet, exercise and other lifestyle behaviours is not clear (Jamal et al 1999, Kessinich et al 2000). One study showed that provision of educational material changed behaviours in premenopausal women (Jamal et al 1999) while another found that an 8-week support group intervention with regular telephone calls had little impact on health related quality of life in women with a history of vertebral fracture (Kessinich et al 2000). Both tailored and non-tailored educational interventions changed calcium intake in older women whereas neither intervention had an effect on exercise habits (Blalock et al 2002). Further research is needed to investigate strategies that will enhance motivation and compliance.

THE ROLE OF EXERCISE IN THE PREVENTION OF OSTEOPOROSIS

In many instances physiotherapists can advise about the role of exercise in normal healthy individuals to help prevent osteoporosis in the future. However, while exercise influences bone material and structural properties, it is not known whether exercise reduces fracture rates, the ultimate goal. There are no randomized controlled trials to answer this question probably because of methodological difficulties. Some, but not all, large-scale epidemiological studies suggest that physical activity is associated with a lower risk of fracture in both men and women (Greendale et al 1995a, Joakimsen et al 1999, Kujala et al 2000, Paganini-Hill et al 1991). Numerous studies highlight the positive effects of exercise on bone mineral density (Bennell et al 1997, Karlsson et al 1993). Thus it seems prudent to advise individuals about the need for regular physical activity throughout life.

The skeletal effects of exercise at different ages

The prevailing view is that exercise in childhood and adolescence produces much higher gains in bone mass than does exercise in adulthood. There are an increasing number of studies evaluating the effects of mechanical loading during growth. Cross-sectional and longitudinal cohort studies show greater bone mass in physically active children than in less active controls (Bailey et al 1999, Cassell et al 1993, Grimston et al 1993, Lehtonen-Veromaa et al 2000, McCulloch et al 1992, Slemenda et al 1991). In intensely training élite athletes such as gymnasts and weight-lifters, the increases in bone mass can be as high as 30–80% (Bass et al 1998, Conroy et al 1993). Intervention studies in pre- and peri-pubertal girls (Heinonen et al 2000, McKay et al 2000, Morris et al 1997) and boys (Bradney et al 1998) show that even moderate levels of exercise have skeletal benefits. In addition, it appears that childhood exercise stimulates the bone modelling process expanding the bone size to produce a larger, possibly stronger bone (Bradney et al 1998, Haapasalo et al 1996, Petit et al 2002). This phenomenon is generally not possible once growth has ceased. Skeletal exercise effects are not confined to healthy children. Exercise programmes in paediatric populations with disability, such as cerebral palsy, have led to improvements in bone density (Chad et al 1999).

There seems to be increasing evidence in favour of a fairly narrow critical period in childhood, probably determined by sexual maturation, where activity has a maximal positive effect on rapidly growing bone. This critical period appears to be in the peri-pubertal years (Tanner stages II and III) rather than the pre-pubertal years (Tanner stage I) but further research is required as current data conflict somewhat (Bass et al 1998, Haapasalo et al 1998, Petit et al 2002) (Fig. 24.6). Certainly the skeleton is less responsive after menarche (Heinonen et al 2000, Witzke & Snow 2000).

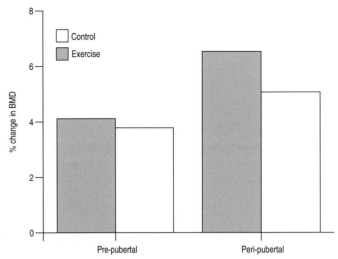

Figure 24.6   Percentage change in femoral neck bone mineral density comparing pre- and peri-pubertal girls in the exercise and control groups. Reproduced from MacKelvie et al (in press).

It is unknown whether skeletal gains can be maintained into the elderly years when fractures occur as there has been no long-term exercise intervention study following children over this time. Evidence to suggest that this is possible comes from the site-specific higher bone density related to unique loading patterns reported in retired athletes (Bass et al 1998, Kirchner et al 1996) and from exercise detraining studies (Kontulainen et al 1999, 2001). However, this issue is still unresolved as recent authors have suggested a gradual diminution of exercise effects over time (Karlsson et al 2000).

Exercise in adulthood mainly results in conservation of bone but this is important considering that the adult skeleton is much more responsive to the adverse effects of unloading than to the beneficial effects of overloading. Attention to lifestyle factors such as diet is also important during this time as the skeletal effects appear to be modulated by calcium intake (Specker 1996).

There are a large number of exercise trials in pre- and postmenopausal women. A recent meta-analysis concluded that exercise prevented or reversed about 1% of bone loss per year at both the lumbar spine and femoral neck (Wolff et al 1999). This was supported by other meta-analyses in postmenopausal women (Berard et al 1997, Kelley 1998) although Berard et al (1997) claimed that the exercise effect was confined to the lumbar spine. Postmenopausal women do not seem to be as responsive to the same loading stimulus as premenopausal women (Bassey et al 1998). Based on the mechanostat theory, it has been proposed that oestrogen deficiency increases the set points for bone adaptation meaning that a greater loading stimulus is needed than in an oestrogen-replete state (Dalsky 1990).

Much less attention has been paid to the effects of exercise in men. Results of the small number of trials showed that targeted exercise can cause bone mass gains in the order of 2.6% at both the spine and hip in men over the age of 31 years (Kelley et al 2000).

A small number of studies have evaluated the effect of exercise in individuals with diagnosed osteopenia (Bravo et al 1996, Chien et al 2000, Hartard et al 1996) or osteoporosis (Malmros et al 1998, Preisinger et al 1996). While the emphasis in these groups is on preventing falls, improving function and reducing pain, exercise has been shown to conserve bone density.

In adulthood, exercise must be continued in order to maintain exercise induced BMD levels (Dalsky et al 1988). Attrition rates from exercise are high even in supervised clinical trials (Bassey & Ramsdale 1994, Kerschan et al 1998). This reinforces the importance of developing strategies to improve compliance and encourage lifelong participation in physical activity.

What types of exercise are best for improving bone strength?

Different activities will provide bone tissue with different strain environments and hence influence the overall adaptive response. Animal studies show that maximal skeletal effects are achieved with dynamic loads that are high in magnitude and rate, and unusual in distribution (Judex and Zernicke 2000, Lanyon et al 1982, O'Connor et al 1982, Rubin & Lanyon 1984, 1985). Relatively few loading cycles are necessary (Umemura et al 1997). It is also known that bone changes are localized to the areas directly loaded (Bennell et al 1997).

In humans, high impact exercises, which generate ground reaction forces greater than two times body weight, are more osteogenic than low impact exercises (Bassey & Ramsdale 1994, Heinonen et al 1996, 1998). Exercise programmes reported in the literature have included various combinations of stair climbing, aerobics, skipping, jumping, sprinting, dancing and jogging. These can be safely prescribed for healthy younger individuals.

Weight training has been advocated for skeletal health at all ages. Loss of muscle mass and strength with age is well documented especially after the sixth decade (Harries & Bassey 1990, Rutherford & Jones 1992) and progressive weight training, even in the frail elderly, can lead to large strength gains (Fiatarone et al 1990). Furthermore, lean mass (Flicker et al 1995, Young et al 1995) and muscle strength (Madsen et al 1993) are positively correlated with bone density. In premenopausal women, weight training has generally been shown to be of benefit at the lumbar spine (Gleeson et al 1990, Lohmann et al 1995, Snow-Harter et al 1992), with an effect size similar in magnitude to that gained with running (Snow-Harter et al 1992). The benefits of weight training for the hip region are unclear (Lohmann et al 1995, Snow-Harter et al 1992) although a significant improvement in bone density at the trochanter was seen following an 18-month programme (Lohmann et al 1995).

Skeletal benefits of weight training in healthy postmenopausal women have been reported by some authors (Kerr et al 1996, 2001, Nelson et al 1994) but not others (Nichols et al 1995, Pruitt et al 1992), which may relate partly to the type of exercise regimen. Effects have been noted with programmes using high loads and low repetitions and with progressive increases in load (Kerr et al 1996, 2001). Weight training has also been shown to increase bone density in men (Ryan et al 1994) and to conserve bone in women with osteoporosis and osteopenia (Hartard et al 1996).

Walking is frequently recommended in clinical practice to maintain skeletal integrity but controversy exists in the literature regarding its efficacy. Some larger epidemiological studies have found lifetime walking to be of some skeletal benefit (Cummings et al 1995) but overall the results of clinical trials have not demonstrated significant effects of walking on spine or hip bone density (Ebrahim et al 1997, Hatori et al 1993, Humphries et al 2000, Martin & Notelovitz 1993). This may relate to the fact that walking imparts relatively low magnitude, repetitive and customary strain to the skeleton. Although walking is an excellent exercise for its numerous health benefits, it may be a more effective exercise for bone in those with restricted mobility than in healthy ambulant individuals. For example, Jorgensen et al found that relearning to walk within the first 2 months after stroke, even with the support of another person, reduced the bone loss after immobilization (Jorgensen et al 2000).

Non-weight-bearing activities such as cycling and swimming do not seem to stimulate bone adaptation despite increases in muscle strength (Orwoll et al 1989, Rico et al 1993, Taaffe et al 1995, Warner et al 2002). This suggests that these activities do not generate sufficient strain to reach the threshold for bone adaptation.

Exercise dosage

The exact exercise dose required for maximal skeletal effects is not yet known. For an elderly or previously sedentary population, exercise should be gradually introduced to minimize fatigue and prevent soreness or injury (Forwood & Larsen 2000). Animal studies suggest that exercise performed 2–3 times per week is as effective for bone as daily loading (Raab-Cullen et al 1994). Recently it has been shown that daily exercise may be more beneficial if broken down into smaller sessions separated by recovery periods (Robling et al 2002).

For aerobic exercise, sessions should last between 15 and 60 minutes. The average conditioning intensity recommended for adults without fragility fractures is 70–80% of their functional capacity. Individuals with a low functional capacity may initiate a programme at 40–60% (Forwood & Larsen 2000).

Adults commencing a weight-training programme may perform a few weeks of familiarization (Kerr et al 1996) followed by a single set of 8–10 repetitions at an intensity of 40–60% of one repetition maximum (1 RM). This can be progressed to 80%, even in the very elderly (American College of Sports Medicine 1998, Fiatorone et al 1994). In a study of postmenopausal women with diagnosed osteopenia, strength training at 70% 1 RM was safe and effective for maintaining hip and spine bone mass (Hartard et al 1996). Programmes should include 8–10 exercises involving the major muscle groups. Supervision, particularly in the beginning, and attention to safe lifting technique is paramount.

Bone adaptation will cease if the exercise dosage is not periodically progressed (Kerr et al 2001). Increasing the intensity or weight bearing is probably more effective than increasing the duration of the exercise. A periodic increase in a step-like fashion may be better than progression in a linear fashion (Forwood & Larsen 2000). Nevertheless, there comes a point where gains in bone mass will slow and eventually plateau. This is because each person has an individual biological ceiling that determines the extent of a possible training effect (American College of Sports Medicine 1995).

In women, the intensity and volume of exercise should not compromise menstrual function. The incidence of menstrual disturbances in athletes is greater than that in the general female population (Malina et al 1978, Skierska 1998). Amenorrhoea (loss of menstrual cycles) and oligomenorrhoea (3–8 cycles per year) are associated with bone loss, particularly at the lumbar spine, which has a high proportion of trabecular bone (Drinkwater et al 1984, Pettersson et al 1999, Rutherford 1993). Endurance athletes are more susceptible to bone loss than athletes involved in high-impact sports (Robinson et al 1995). Of concern is evidence that even long-term resumption of regular menses may not restore the bone deficits (Keen & Drinkwater 1997, Micklesfield et al 1998). Patients with menstrual disturbances should be referred to an appropriate medical practitioner for further investigation.

CONCLUSION

Physiotherapists have a role to play in both the prevention and management of osteoporosis. Appropriate treatment goals can be established following a thorough assessment. Since the aim is to maximize peak bone mass in children and adolescents, participation in a variety of high-impact activities should be encouraged. In the middle adult years, small increases in bone mass may be achieved by structured weight training and weight-bearing exercise. In the older adult years, particularly if osteopenia or osteoporosis is present, the aim is to conserve bone mass, reduce the risk of falls, promote extended posture, reduce pain and improve mobility and function. Management consists of various physiotherapy techniques and specific exercise prescription. Education is an essential part of the physiotherapist's role in promoting skeletal health throughout the lifespan.

KEYWORDS	
osteoporosis	exercise
minimal trauma fracture	bone density
physical therapy	falls

References

American College of Sports Medicine (ACSM) 1995 Position stand on osteoporosis and exercise. Medicine and Science in Sports and Exercise 27: i–vii

American College of Sports Medicine (ACSM) 1998 Position stand on exercise and physical activity for older adults. Medicine and Science for Sports and Exercise 30: 992–1008

Bailey D A 1997 The Saskatchewan pediatric bone mineral accrual study: bone mineral acquisition during the growing years. International Journal of Sports Medicine 18: S191–194

Bailey D A, McKay H A, Mirwald R L, Crocker P R E, Faulkner R A 1999 A six-year longitudinal study of the relationship of physical activity to bone mineral accrual in growing children: the University of Saskatchewan bone mineral accrual study. Journal of Bone and Mineral Research 14: 1672–1679

Bass S, Pearce G, Bradney M et al 1998 Exercise before puberty may confer residual benefits in bone density in adulthood: studies in active prepubertal and retired female gymnasts. Journal of Bone and Mineral Research 13: 500–507

Bassey E J, Ramsdale S J 1994 Increase in femoral bone density in young women following high impact exercise. Osteoporosis International 4: 72–75

Bassey E J, Rothwell M C, Littlewood J J, Pye D W 1998 Pre- and postmenopausal women have different bone mineral density responses to the same high-impact exercise. Journal of Bone and Mineral Research 13: 1805–1813

Bennell K L, Malcolm S A, Khan K M et al 1997 Bone mass and bone turnover in power athletes, endurance athletes and controls: a 12-month longitudinal study. Bone 20: 477–484

Bennell K, Talbot R, Wajswelner H, Techovanich W, Kelly D 1998 Intra-rater and inter-rater reliability of a weight-bearing lunge measure of ankle dorsiflexion. Australian Journal of Physiotherapy 44: 175–180

Bennel K, Khan K, McKay 2000 The role of physiotherapy in the prevention and management of osteoporosis. Manual Therapy 5: 198–213

Berard A, Bravo G, Gauthier P 1997 Meta-analysis of the effectiveness of physical activity for the prevention of bone loss in postmenopausal women. Osteoporosis International 7: 331–337

Blake G M, Fogelman I 1998 Applications of bone densitometry for osteoporosis. Endocrinology and Metabolism Clinics of North America 27: 267–288

Blalock S J, DeVellis B M, Patterson C C, Campbell M K, Orenstein D R, Dooley M A 2002 Effects of an osteoporosis prevention program incorporating tailored educational materials. American Journal of Health Promotion 16: 146–156

Bolognese M 2002 Effective pharmacotherapeutic interventions for the prevention of hip fractures. Endocrinologist 12: 29–37

Bouxsein M L, Coan B S, Lee S C 1999 Prediction of the strength of the elderly proximal femur by bone mineral density and quantitative ultrasound measurements of the heel and tibia. Bone 25: 49–54

Bradney M, Pearce G, Naughton G et al 1998 Moderate exercise during growth in prepubertal boys: changes in bone mass, size, volumetric density, and bone strength – a controlled prospective study. Journal of Bone and Mineral Research 13: 1814–1821

Bravo G, Gauthier P, Roy P M et al 1996 Impact of a 12-month exercise program on the physical and psychological health of osteopenic women. Journal of the American Geriatrics Society 44(7): 756–762

Bravo G, Gauthier P, Roy P, Payetter H, Gaulin P 1997 A weight-bearing, water-based exercise program for osteopenic women: its impact on bone, functional fitness, and well-being. Archives of Physical Medicine and Rehabilitation 78: 1375–1380

Buchner D M, Cress M E, de Lateur B J et al 1997 The effect of strength and endurance training on gait, balance, fall risk, and health services use in community-living older adults. Journals of Gerontology 52(4): M218–M224

Campbell A J, Borrie M J, Spears G F 1989 Risk factors for falls in a community-based prospective study of people 70 years and older. Journal of Gerontology 44: M112–117

Campbell A J, Robertson M C, Gardner M M, Norton R N, Tilyard M W, Buchner D M 1997 Randomised controlled trial of a general practice programme of home based exercise to prevent falls in elderly women. BMJ 315(7115): 1065–1069

Campbell A J, Robertson M C, Gardner M M, Norton R N, Buchner D M 1999 Falls prevention over 2 years: a randomized controlled trial in women 80 years and older. Age and Ageing 28(6): 513–518

Cassell C, Benedict M, Uetrect G, Ranz J, Ho M, Specker B 1993 Bone mineral density in young gymnasts and swimmers. Medicine and Science in Sports and Exercise 25: 49

Cavanagh P R, LaFortune M A 1980 Ground reaction forces in distance running. Journal of Biomechanics 13: 397–406

Chad K E, Bailey D A, McKay H A, Zello G A, Snyder R E 1999 The effect of a weight-bearing physical activity program on bone mineral content and estimated volumetric density in children with spastic cerebral palsy. Journal of Pediatrics 135: 115–117

Chartered Society of Physiotherapy 1999 Physiotherapy guidelines for the management of osteoporosis. UK Chartered Society of Physiotherapy, London

Chien M Y, Wu Y T, Hsu A T, Yang R S, Lai J S 2000 Efficacy of a 24-week aerobic exercise program for osteopenic postmenopausal women. Calcified Tissue International 67: 443–448

Cohen H, Blatchly C, Gombash L 1993 A study of the clinical test of sensory interaction and balance. Physical Therapy 73: 346–351

Conroy B P, Kraemer W J, Maresh C M et al 1993 Bone mineral density in elite junior Olympic weight lifters. Medicine and Science in Sports and Exercise 25: 1103–1109

Consensus Develoment Conference (CDC) 1993 Diagnosis, prophylaxis and treatment of osteoporosis. American Journal of Medicine 94: 646–650

Cook D J, Guyatt G H, Adachi J D et al 1993 Quality of life issues in women with vertebral fractures due to osteoporosis. Arthritis and Rheumatism 36: 750–756

Cooper C 1997 The crippling consequences of fractures and their impact on quality of life. American Journal of Medicine 103: 12S–17S

Cooper C, Melton L 1992 Epidemiology of osteoporosis. Trends in Endocrinology and Metabolism 3: 224–229

Cordey J, Schneider M, Belendez C et al 1992 Effect of bone size, not density, on the stiffness of the proximal part of the normal and osteoporotic human femora. Journal of Bone and Mineral Research 2: S437–S444

Crawford H J, Jull G A 1993 The influence of thoracic posture and movement on range of arm elevation. Physiotherapy Theory and Practice 9: 143–148

Cummings S R, Black D M, Nevitt M C et al 1993 Bone density at various sites for prediction of hip fractures. Lancet 341: 72–75

Cummings S R, Nevitt M C, Browner W S et al 1995 Risk factors for hip fractures in white women. New England Journal of Medicine 332: 767–773

Cutler W B, Friedmann E, Genovese-Stone E 1993 Prevalence of kyphosis in a healthy sample of pre- and postmenopausal women. American Journal of Physical Medicine and Rehabilitation 72: 219– 225

Dalsky G P 1990 Effect of exercise on bone: permissive influence of estrogen and calcium. Medicine and Science in Sports and Exercise 22: 281–285

Dalsky G P, Stocke K S, Ehansi A A, Slatopolsky E, Lee W C, Birge S J 1988 Weight-bearing exercise training and lumbar bone mineral content in postmenopausal women. Annals of Internal Medicine 108: 824–828

Drinkwater B L, Nilson K, Chesnut III C H, Bremner W J, Shainholtz S, Southworth M B 1984 Bone mineral content of amenorrheic and eumenorrheic athletes. New England Journal of Medicine 311(5): 277–281

Duncan P, Weiner K, Chandler J, Studenski S 1990 Functional reach: a new clinical measure of balance. Journal of Gerontology 45: M192–197

Ebrahim S, Thompson P, Baskaran V, Evans K 1997 Randomized placebo-controlled trial of brisk walking in the prevention of postmenopausal osteoporosis. Age and Ageing 26: 253–260

Einhorn T A 1996 Biomechanics of bone. In: Bilezikian J P, Raisz L G, Rodan G A (eds) Principles of bone biology. Academic Press, San Diego

Ensrud K E, Black D M, Harris F, Ettinger B, Cummings S R 1997 Correlates of kyphosis in older women. Journal of the American Geriatrics Society 45: 682–687

Ensrud K E, Thompson D E, Cauley J A et al 2000 Prevalent vertebral deformities predict mortality and hospitalization in older women with low bone mass. Journal of the American Geriatrics Society 48: 241–249

Eriksen E F, Axelrod D W, Melsen F 1994 Bone histomorphometry. Raven Press, New York

Fiatarone M, Marks E, Ryan N, Meredith C, Lipsitz L, Evans W 1990 High-intensity training in nonagenarians. JAMA 263: 3029–3034

Fiatarone M A, O'Neill E F, Ryan N D et al 1994 Exercise training and nutritional supplementation for physical frailty in very elderly people. New England Journal of Medicine 330: 1769–1775

Flicker L, Hopper J L, Rodgers L, Kaymakci B, Green R M, Wark J D 1995 Bone density determinants in elderly women: a twin study. Journal of Bone and Mineral Research 10: 1607–1613

Forwood M, Larsen J 2000 Exercise recommendations for osteoporosis: a position statement for the Australian and New Zealand Bone and Mineral Society. Australian Family Physician 29: 761–764

Frost H M 1988 Vital biomechanics: proposed general concepts for skeletal adaptations to mechanical usage. Calcified Tissue International 42: 145–156

Gleeson P, Protas E, LeBlanc A, Schneider V, Evans H 1990 Effects of weight lifting on bone mineral density in premenopausal women. Journal of Bone and Mineral Research 5: 153–158

Gordon C C, Cameron Chumlea W C, Roche A F 1991 Stature, recumbent length, and weight. In: Lohman T G, Roche A F, Martorell R (eds). Anthropometric standardization reference manual, abridged edn. Human Kinetics, Champaign, Illinois, pp 3–8

Greendale G A, Barrettconnor E, Edelstein S, Ingles S, Haile R 1995a Lifetime leisure exercise and osteoporosis: the Rancho Bernado study. American Journal of Epidemiology 141: 951–959

Greendale G A, Barrettconnor E, Ingles S, Haile R 1995b Late physical and functional effects of osteoporotic fracture in women: the Rancho Bernado study. Journal of the American Geriatrics Society 43: 955–961

Grimston S K, Willows N D, Hanley D A 1993 Mechanical loading regime and its relationship to bone mineral density in children. Medicine and Science in Sports and Exercise 25: 1203–1210

Haapasalo H, Sievanen H, Kannus P, Heinonen A, Oja P, Vuori I 1996 Dimensions and estimated mechanical characteristics of the humerus after long-term tennis loading. Journal of Bone and Mineral Research 11: 864–872

Haapasalo H, Kannus P, Sievanen H et al 1998 Effect of long-term unilateral activity on bone mineral density of female junior tennis players. Journal of Bone and Mineral Research 13: 310–319

Hageman P, Blanke D J 1986 Comparison of gait of young women and elderly women. Physical Therapy 66: 1382–1387

Hans D, Wu C, Njeh C F et al 1999 Ultrasound velocity of trabecular cubes reflects mainly bone density and elasticity. Calcified Tissue International 64: 18–23

Harries U J, Bassey E J 1990 Torque-velocity relationships for the knee extensors in women in their 3rd and 7th decades. European Journal of Applied Physiology 60: 187–190

Hartard M, Haber P, Ilieva D, Preisinger E, Seidl G, Huber J 1996 Systematic strength training as a model of therapeutic intervention. American Journal of Physical Medicine and Rehabilitation 75: 21–28

Hatori M, Hasegawa A, Adachi H et al 1993 The effects of walking at the anaerobic threshold level on vertebral bone loss in postmenopausal women. Calcified Tissue International 52: 411–414

Heinonen A, Kannus P, Sievänen H et al 1996 Randomised, controlled trial of effect of high-impact exercise on selected risk factors for osteoporotic fractures. Lancet 348: 1343–1347

Heinonen A, Oja P, Sievänen H, Pasanen M, Vuori I 1998 Effect of two training regimens on bone mineral density in healthy perimenopausal women: a randomised, controlled trial. Journal of Bone and Mineral Research 13: 483–490

Heinonen A, Sievänen H, Kannus P, Oja P, Pasanen M, Vuori I 2000 High-impact exercise and bones of growing girls: a 9-month controlled trial. Osteoporosis International 11: 1010–1017

Heinonen A, Sievänen H, Kyröläinen H, Perttunen J, Kannus P 2001 Mineral mass, size and estimated mechanical strength of the lower limb bones of triple jumpers. Bone 29(3): 279–285

Helmes E, Hodsman A, Lazowski D et al 1995 A questionnaire to evaluate disability in osteoporotic patients with vertebral compression fractures. Journals of Gerontology Series A, Biological Sciences and Medical Sciences 50: M91–M98

Hill K, Bernhardt J, McGann A, Maltese D, Berkovits D 1996 A new test of dynamic standing balance for stroke patients: reliability, validity, and comparison with healthy elderly. Physiotherapy Canada 48: 257–262

Hill K, Schwarz J, Flicker L, Carroll S 1999 Falls among healthy, community-dwelling, older women: a prospective study of frequency, circumstances, consequences and prediction accuracy. Australian and New Zealand Journal of Public Health 23: 41–48

Huang C, Ross P D, Wasnich R D 1996 Vertebral fractures and other predictors of back pain among women. Journal of Bone and Mineral Research 11: 1026–1032

Huda W, Morin R L 1996 Patient doses in bone mineral dosimetry. British Journal of Radiology 69: 422–425

Humphries B, Newton R U, Bronks R et al 2000 Effect of exercise intensity on bone density, strength, and calcium turnover in older women. Medicine and Science in Sports and Exercise 32: 1043–1050

Jamal S A, Ridout R, Chase C, Fielding L, Rubin L A, Hawker G A 1999 Bone mineral density testing and osteoporosis education improve lifestyle behaviors in premenopausal women: a prospective study. Journal of Bone and Mineral Research 14: 2143–2149

Joakimsen R M, Fonnebo V, Magnus J H, Stormer J, Tollan A, Sogaard A J 1999 The Truomso study: physical activity and the incidence of fractures in a middle-aged population. Journal of Bone and Mineral Research 13: 1149–1157

Jorgensen L, Jacobsen B K, Wilsgaard T, Magnus J H 2000 Walking after stroke: does it matter? Changes in bone mineral density within the first 12 months after stroke: a longitudinal study. Osteoporosis International 11: 381–387

Judex S, Zernicke R F 2000 High-impact exercise and growing bone: relation between high strain rates and enhanced bone formation. Journal of Applied Physiology 88: 2183–2191

Kannus P, Niemi S, Parkkari J, Palvanen M, Vuori I, Jarvinen M 1999 Hip fractures in Finland between 1970 and 1997 and predictions for the future. Lancet 353: 802–805

Karlsson M K, Johnell O, Obrant K J 1993 Bone mineral density in weight lifters. Calcified Tissue International 52: 212–215

Karlsson M K, Linden C, Karlsson C, Johnell O, Obrant K, Seeman E 2000 Exercise during growth and bone mineral density and fractures in old age. Lancet 355: 469–470

Keen A D, Drinkwater B L 1997 Irreversible bone loss in former amenorrheic athletes. Osteoporosis International 7: 311–315

Kelley G A 1998 Exercise and regional bone mineral density in postmenopausal women: a meta-analytic review of randomized trials. American Journal of Physical Medicine and Rehabilitation 77: 76–87

Kelley G A, Kelley K S, Tran Z V 2000 Exercise and bone mineral density in men: a meta-analysis. Journal of Applied Physiology 88: 1730–1736

Kerr D, Morton A, Dick I, Prince R 1996 Exercise effects on bone mass in postmenopausal women are site-specific and load-dependent. Journal of Bone and Mineral Research 11(2): 218–225

Kerr D, Ackland T, Maslen B, Morton A, Prince R 2001 Resistance training over 2 years increases bone mass in calcium-replete post-menopausal women. Journal of Bone and Mineral Research 16: 175–181

Kerschan K, Alacamlioglu Y, Kollmitzer J et al 1998 Functional impact of unvarying exercise program in women after menopause. American Journal of Physical Medicine and Rehabilitation 77: 326–332

Kessinich C R, Guyatt G H, Patton C L, Griffith L E, Hamlin A, Rosen C I 2000 Support group intervention for women with osteoporosis. Rehabilitation Nursing 25: 88–92

Kirchner E M, Lewis R D, O'Connor P J 1996 Effect of past gymnastics participation on adult bone mass. Journal of Applied Physiology 80: 226–232

Kontulainen S, Kannus P, Haapasalo H et al 1999 Changes in bone mineral content with decreased training in competitive young adult tennis players and controls: a prospective 4-yr follow-up. Medicine and Science in Sports and Exercise 31: 646–652

Kontulainen S, Kannus P, Haapasalo H et al 2001 Good maintenance of exercise-induced bone gain with decreased training of female tennis and squash players: a prospective 5-year follow-up study of young and old starters and controls. Journal of Bone and Mineral Research 16: 195–201

Kronhed A, Moller M 1998 Effects of physical exercise on bone mass, balance skill and aerobic capacity in women and men with low bone mineral density, after one year of training - a prospective study. Scandinavian Journal of Medicine and Science in Sports 8: 290–298

Kujala U M, Kaprio J, Kannus P, Sarna S, Koskenvuo M 2000 Physical activity and osteoporotic hip fracture risk in men. Archives of Internal Medicine 160: 705–708

Lanyon L E, Goodship A E, Pye C J, MacFie J H 1982 Mechanically adaptive bone remodelling. Journal of Biomechanics 15: 141–154

Larsen J 1998 Osteoporosis. In: Sapsford R, Bullock-Saxton J, Markwell S (eds) Women's health: a textbook for physiotherapists. WB Saunders, London, pp 412–453

Laurent M R, Buchanon W W, Bellamy N 1991 Methods of assessment used in ankylosing spondylitis clinical trials: a review. British Journal of Rheumatology 30: 326–329

Lauritzen J B, Petersen M M, Lund B 1993 Effect of external hip protectors on hip fractures. Lancet 341: 11–13

Lehtonen-Veromaa M, Mottonen T, Nuotio I, Heinonen O J, Viikari J 2000 Influence of physical activity on ultrasound and dual-energy X-ray absorptiometry bone measurements in peripubertal girls: a cross-sectional study. Calcified Tissue International 66: 248–254

Lespessailles E, Jullien A, Eynard E et al 1998 Biomechanical properties of human os calcanei: relationships with bone density and fractal evaluation of bone microarchitecture. Journal of Biomechanics 31: 817–824

Lewis M K, Blake G M, Fogelman I 1994 Patient dose in dual X-ray absorptiometry. Osteoporosis International 4: 11–15

Lips P, Cooper C, Agnusdei D et al 1999 Quality of life in patients with vertebral fractures: validation for the quality of life questionnaire of the European Foundation for Osteoporosis (QUALEFFO). Osteoporosis International 10: 150–160

Lohmann T, Going S, Pamenter R et al 1995 Effects of resistance training on regional and total bone mineral density in premenopausal women: a randomized prospective study. Journal of Bone and Mineral Research 10(7): 1015–1024

Lord S 1996 The effects of a community exercise program on fracture risk factors in older women. Osteoporos International 6: 361–367

Lord S R, Clark R D, Webster I W 1991 Physiological factors associated with falls in an elderly population. Journal of the Geriatrics Society 39: 1194–1200

Lord S R, Sambrook P N, Gilbert C et al 1994 Postural stability, falls and fractures in the elderly: results from the Dubbo osteoporosis epidemiology study. Medical Journal of Australia 160: 684–691

Lord S R, Ward J A, Williams P, Strudwick M 1995 The effect of a 12-month exercise trial on balance, strength, and falls in older women: a randomized controlled trial. Journal of the American Geriatrics Society 43(11): 1198–1206

Lundon K M A, Li A M W, Bibershtein S 1998 Interrater and intrarater reliability in the measurement of kyphosis in postmenopausal women with osteoporosis. Spine 23: 1978–1985

Lyles K W, Gold D T, Shipp K M et al 1993 Association of osteoporotic vertebral compression fractures with impaired functional status. American Journal of Medicine 94: 595–601

McCulloch R G, Bailey D A, Whalen R L, Houston C S, Faulkner R A, Craven B R 1992 Bone density and bone mineral content of adolescent soccer athletes and competitive swimmers. Pediatric Exercise Science 4: 319–330

McKay H A, Petit M A, Schutz R W, Prior J C, Barr S I, Khan K M 2000 Augmented trochanteric bone mineral density after modified physical education classes: a randomized school-based exercise intervention study in prepubescent and early pubescent children. Journal of Pediatrics 136: 156–162

MacKelvie K J, McKay H A, Khan K M, Crocker P R E 2001 A school-based loading intervention augments bone mineral accrual in early pubertal girls. Journal of Pediatrics 139:501–508

McMurdo M, Rennie L 1993 A controlled trial of exercise by residents of old people's homes. Age and Ageing 22: 11–15

McMurdo M E, Mole P A, Paterson C R 1997 Controlled trial of weight bearing exercise in older women in relation to bone density and falls. BMJ 314(7080): 22

McMurdo M E T, Millar A M, Daly F 2000 A randomized controlled trial of fall prevention strategies in old people's homes. Gerontology 46: 83–87

MacRae P G, Feltner M E, Reinsch S 1994 A 1-year exercise program for older women: effects on falls, injuries and physical performance. Journal of Ageing and Physical Activity 2: 127–142

Madsen O R, Schaadt O, Bliddal H, Egsmose C, Sylvest J 1993 Relationship between quadriceps strength and bone mineral density of the proximal tibia and distal forearm in women. Journal of Bone and Mineral Research 8: 1439–1444

Malina R M, Spriduso W W, Tate C, Baylor A M 1978 Age at menarche and selected menstrual characteristics in athletes at different competitive levels and in different sports. Medicine and Science in Sports and Exercise 10: 218–222

Malmros B, Mortenson L, Jensen M B, Charles P 1998 Positive effects of physiotherapy on chronic pain and performance in osteoporosis. Osteoporosis International 8: 215–221

Marquis P, Cialdella P, De la Loge C 2001 Development and validation of a specific quality of life module in post-menopausal women with osteoporosis: the QUALIOST (TM). Quality of Life Research 10: 555–566

Martin D, Notelovitz M 1993 Effects of aerobic training on bone mineral density of postmenopausal women. Journal of Bone and Mineral Research 8: 931–936

Melzack R 1975 The McGill Pain Questionnaire: major properties and scoring methods. Pain 1: 277–299

Micklesfield L K, Reyneke L, Fataar A, Myburgh K H 1998 Long-term restoration of deficits in bone mineral density is inadequate in premenopausal women with prior menstrual irregularity. Clinical Journal of Sport Medicine 8: 155–163

Morganti C M, Nelson M E, Fiatorone M A et al 1995 Strength improvements with 1 yr of progressive resistance training in older women. Medicine and Science in Sports and Exercise 27: 906–912

Morris F L, Naughton G A, Gibbs J L, Carlson J S, Wark J D 1997 Prospective ten-month exercise intervention in premenarcheal girls: positive effects on bone and lean mass. Journal of Bone and Mineral Research 12: 1453–1462

Mulrow C D, Gerety M B, Kanten D et al 1994 A randomized trial of physical rehabilitation for very frail nursing home residents [see comments]. JAMA 271(7): 519–524

Nelson M, Fiatarone M, Morganti C, Trice I, Greenberg R, Evans W 1994 Effects of high-intensity strength training on multiple risk factors for osteoporotic fractures: a randomized controlled trial. JAMA 272: 1909–1914

Nichols J F, Nelson K P, Sartoris D J 1995 Bone mineral responses to high-intensity strength training in active older women. Journal of Ageing and Physical Activity 3: 26–38

Nordin M, Frankel V H 1989 Basic biomechanics of the musculoskeletal system, 2nd edn. Lea and Febiger, Philadelphia

O'Connor J A, Lanyon L E, MacFie H 1982 The influence of strain rate on adaptive bone remodelling. Journal of Biomechanics 15: 767–781

Orwoll E S, Ferar J, Oviatt S K, McClung M, Huntington K 1989 The relationship of swimming exercise to bone mass in men and women. Archives of Internal Medicine 149: 2197–2200

Paganini-Hill A, Chao A, Ross R K, Henerson B 1991 Exercise and other factors in the prevention of hip fracture: the Leisure World study. Epidemiology 2: 16–25

Parfitt A M 1988 Bone remodeling: relationship to the amount and structure of bone, and the pathogenesis and prevention of fractures. In: Riggs B L, Melton III L J (eds) Osteoporosis: etiology, diagnosis, and management. Raven Press, New York

Parkkari J, Kannus P, Heikkilä J, Poutala J, Sievanen H, Vuori I 1995 Energy-shunting external hip protector attenuates the peak femoral impact force below the theoretical fracture threshold: an in vitro biomechanical study under falling conditions of the elderly. Journal of Bone and Mineral Research 10: 1437–1442

Parkkari J, Kannus P, Heikkilä J et al 1997 Impact experiments of an external hip protector in young volunteers. Calcified Tissue International 60: 354–357

Parkkari J, Kannus P, Palvanen M et al 1999 Majority of hip fractures occur as a result of a fall and impact on the greater trochanter of the femur: a prospective controlled hip fracture study with 206 consecutive patients. Calcified Tissue International 65: 183–187

Petersen M M, Jensen N C, Gehrchen P M, Nielsen P K, Nielsen P T 1996 The relation between trabecular bone strength and bone mineral density assessed by dual photon and dual energy X-ray absorptiometry in the proximal tibia. Calcified Tissue International 59: 311–314

Petit M A, McKay H A, MacKelvie K J, Heinonen A, Khan K M, Beck T J 2002 A randomized school-based jumping intervention confers site and maturity-specific benefits on bone structural properties in girls: a hip structural analysis study. Journal of Bone and Mineral Research 17: 363–372

Pettersson U, Stalnacke B M, Ahlenius G M, Henriksson-Larsen K, Lorentzon R 1999 Low bone mass density at multiple skeletal sites, including the appendicular skeleton in amenorrheic runners. Calcified Tissue International 64: 117–125

Pfeifer M, Begerow B, Minne H W et al 2001 Vitamin D status, trunk muscle strength, body sway, falls, and fractures among 237 postmenopausal women with osteoporosis. Experimental and Clinical Endocrinology and Diabetes 109: 87–92

Podsiadlo D, Richardson S 1991 The timed 'up and go': a test of basic functional mobility for frail elderly persons. Journal of the American Geriatric Society 39: 142–148

Preisinger E, Alacamlioglu Y, Pils K et al 1996 Exercise therapy for osteoporosis: results of a randomised, controlled trial. British Journal of Sports Medicine 30: 209–212

Pruitt L A, Jackson R D, Bartels R L, Lehnhard H J 1992 Weight-training effects on bone mineral density in early post-menopausal women. Journal of Bone and Mineral Research 7: 179–185

Raab-Cullen D M, Akhter M P, Kimmel D B, Recker R R 1994 Bone response to alternate-day mechanical loading of the rat tibia. Journal of Bone and Mineral Research 9: 203–211

Randell A, Sambrook P N, Nguyen T V et al 1995 Direct clinical and welfare costs of osteoporotic fracture in elderly men and women. Osteoporosis International 5: 427–432

Reinsch S, Macrae P, Lachenbruch P A, Tobis J S 1992 Attempts to prevent falls and injury: a prospective community study. Gerontologist 32: 450–456

Richardson C A, Jull G A 1995 Muscle control – pain control. What exercises would you prescribe? Manual Therapy 1: 2–10

Rico H, Revilla M, Hernandez E R, Gomez-Castresana F, Villa L F 1993 Bone mineral content and body composition in postpubertal cyclist boys. Bone 14: 93–95

Riggs B L, Melton L J I 1986 Involutional osteoporosis. New England Journal of Medicine 314: 1676–1686

Robinson T L, Snow-Harter C, Taaffe D R, Gillis D, Shaw J, Marcus R 1995 Gymnasts exhibit higher bone mass than runners despite similar prevalence of amenorrhea and oligomenorrhea. Journal of Bone and Mineral Research 10: 26–35

Robling A G, Hinant F M, Burr D B, Turner C H 2002 Shorter, more frequent mechanical loading sessions enhance bone mass. Medicine and Science in Sports and Exercise 34: 196–202

Ross P D 1997 Clinical consequences of vertebral fractures. American Journal of Medicine 103: 30S–43S

Rubin C T, Lanyon L E 1984 Regulation of bone formation by applied dynamic loads. Journal of Bone and Joint Surgery 66A: 397–402

Rubin C T, Lanyon L E 1985 Regulation of bone mass by mechanical strain magnitude. Calcified Tissue International 37: 411–417

Rutherford O M 1993 Spine and total body bone mineral density in amenorrheic endurance athletes. Journal of Applied Physiology 74: 2904–2908

Rutherford O M, Jones D A 1992 The relationship of muscle and bone loss and activity levels with age in women. Age and Ageing 21: 286–293

Ryan A S, Trueth M S, Rubin M A et al 1994 Effects of strength training on bone mineral density: hormonal and bone turnover relationships. Journal of Applied Physiology 77: 1678–1684

Sanders K M, Nicholson G C, Ugoni A M, Pasco J A, Seeman E, Kotowicz M A 1999 Health burden of hip and other fractures in Australia beyond 2000: projections based on the Geelong osteoporosis study. Medical Journal of Australia 170: 467–470

Sanila M, Kotaniemi A, Viikare J, Isomake H 1994 Height loss rate as a marker of osteoporosis in post-menopausal women with rheumatoid arthritis. Clinical Rheumatology 13: 256–260

Shipp K M, Purser J L, Gold D T et al 2000 Time loaded standing: a measure of combined trunk and arm endurance suitable for people with vertebral osteoporosis. Osteoporosis International 11: 914–922

Shumway-Cook A, Horak F 1986 Assessing the influence of sensory interaction on balance: suggestions from the field. Physical Therapy 66: 1548–1550

Silverman S L 2000 The Osteoporosis Assessment Questionnaire (OPAQ): a reliable and valid disease-targeted measure of health-related quality of life (HRQOL) in osteoporosis. Quality of Life Research 9: 767–774

Simmons V, Hansen P D 1996 Effectiveness of water exercise on postural mobility in the well elderly: an experimental study on balance enhancement. Journal of Gerontology 51A: M233–M238

Sinaki M, Mikkelsen B A 1984 Postmenopausal spinal osteoporosis: flexion versus extension exercises. Archives of Physical Medicine and Rehabilitation 65: 593–596

Sinaki M, Ito E, Rogers J W, Bergstralh E J, Wahner H W 1996 Correlation of back extensor strength with thoracic hyphosis and lumbar lordosis in estrogen-deficient women. American Journal of Physical Medicine and Rehabilitation 75: 370–374

Singh S J, Morgan S J, Hardman A E, Rowe A E, Bardsley P A 1994 Comparison of oxygen uptake during a conventional treadmill test and the shuttle walking test in chronic airflow limitation. European Respiratory Journal 11: 2016–2020

Skierska E 1998 Age at menarche and prevalance of oligo/amenorrhea in top Polish athletes. American Journal of Human Biology 10: 511–517

Slemenda C W, Miller J Z, Hui S L, Reister T K, Johnston Jr C C 1991 Role of physical activity in the development of skeletal mass in children. Journal of Bone and Mineral Research 6: 1227–1233

Snow-Harter C, Bouxsein M L, Lewis B T, Carter D R, Marcus R 1992 Effects of resistance and endurance exercise on bone mineral status of young women: a randomized exercise intervention trial. Journal of Bone and Mineral Research 7: 761–769

Specker B L 1996 Evidence for an interaction between calcium intake and physical activity on changes in bone mineral density. Journal of Bone and Mineral Research 11(10): 1539–1544

Steele B 1996 Timed walking tests of exercise capacity in chronic cardiopulmonary illness. Journal of Cardiopulmonary Rehabilitation 16: 25–33

Taaffe D R, Snow-Harter C, Connolly D A, Robinson T L, Brown M D, Marcus R 1995 Differential effects of swimming versus weight-bearing activity on bone mineral status of eumenorrheic athletes. Journal of Bone and Mineral Research 10: 586–593

Tinetti M E, Speechley M, Ginter S F 1988 Risk factors for falls among elderly persons living in the community. New England Journal of Medicine 319: 1701–1707

Tinetti M, Baker D, McAvay G et al 1994 A multifactorial intervention to reduce the risk of falling among elderly people living in the community. New England Journal of Medicine 331: 822–827

Toshikazu I, Shirado O, Suzuki H, Takahashi M, Kanedo K, Strax T E 1996 Lumbar trunk muscle endurance testing: an inexpensive alternative to a machine for evaluation. Archives of Physical Medicine and Rehabilitation 77: 75–79

Umemura Y, Ishiko T, Yamauchi T, Kurono M, Mashiko S 1997 Five jumps per day increase bone mass and breaking force in rats. Journal of Bone and Mineral Research 12: 1480–1485

Wark J D 1998 How to prevent and treat osteoporosis. Australian Doctor (July): I–VII

Warner S E, Shaw J M, Dalsky G P 2002 Bone mineral density of competitive male mountain and road cyclists. Bone 30: 281–286

Watts N B, Harris S T, Genant H K 2001 Treatment of painful osteoporotic vertebral fractures with percutaneous vertebroplasty or kyphoplasty. Osteoporosis International 12: 429–437

Witzke K A, Snow C M 2000 Effects of plyometric jump training on bone mass in adolescent girls. Medicine and Science in Sports and Exercise 32: 1051–1057

Wolf S L, Barnhart H X, Kutner N G, McNeely E, Coogler C, Xu T 1996 Reducing frailty and falls in older persons: an investigation of Tai Chi and computerized balance training. Journal of the American Geriatrics Society 44(5): 489–497

Wolff I, van Croonenborg J J, Kemper H C G, Kostense P J, Twisk J W R 1999 The effect of exercise training programs on bone mass: a meta-analysis of published controlled trials in pre- and postmenopausal women. Osteoporosis International 9: 1–12

World Health Organization 1994 Assessment of fracture risk and its application to screening for ostoeporosis. Report of WHO Study Group. World Health Organization, Geneva

Young D, Hopper J L, Nowson C A et al 1995 Determinants of bone mass in 10- to 26-year-old females: a twin study. Journal of Bone and Mineral Research 10: 558–567

Zmuda J M, Cauley J A, Ferrell R E 1999 Recent progress in understanding the genetic susceptibility to osteoporosis. Genetic Epidemiology 16: 356–367

SECTION 4

Clinical science and practices of manual therapy

Chapter **25**

Neurophysiological effects of spinal manual therapy

T. Souvlis, B. Vicenzino, A. Wright

INTRODUCTION

Healthcare practitioners frequently use spinal manual therapy (SMT) techniques to treat conditions of musculoskeletal pain and dysfunction (Jull 2002). Recent meta-analyses and randomized controlled trials have confirmed that spinal manual therapy is efficacious in the treatment of spinal pain (Aker et al 1996, Gross et al 1996, Koes et al 1992, Shekelle 1996). However, there is only a developing understanding of the mechanisms by which these treatments exert their effects. The outcomes of spinal manual therapy have most commonly been described in terms of the biomechanical response to application of the treatment technique; that is, numerous studies that investigate parameters of forces applied to the spine, such as load, deformation, vibration, as well as the movement responses to those forces, have been performed (Allison et al 1998, Herzog 2000, Keller et al 2000, Latimer et al 1998, Lee & Liversidge 1994, Lee et al 1993, 1995, Vicenzino et al 1999b). Studies such as these are important to gain a perspective of the nature of the stimulus applied during SMT interventions but in themselves do not provide insight into possible neurophysiological mechanisms of action.

It is implicit in the practice of SMT that the direct manual contact and movement of the underlying and surrounding structures produced during the application of techniques activates cutaneous, articular, muscular and neurovascular afferents. While it is tempting to explain the mechanisms of SMT in biomechanical terms, to underestimate the powerful input to the central nervous system via these afferent neurons would be to fail to appreciate the potential neurophysiological influence of SMT. Although Maitland (1986) alluded to the potential for manual therapy to modulate pain via gating mechanisms, a more comprehensive model to describe the potential neurophysiological response to SMT has gradually evolved (Wright 1995, Wyke 1985, Zusman et al 1989). Activation of the descending pain inhibitory systems (DPIS) and local segmental pain inhibitory mechanisms as well as psychological effects were suggested as some of the possible mechanisms for the production of SMT related effects (Wright 1995, Wright & Vicenzino 1995).

A number of studies have been performed to characterize the pain modulation response to SMT (Christian et al 1988, McGuiness et al 1995, Petersen et al 1993, Sanders et al 1990, Souvlis et al 1999, 2000a, 2000b, Sterling et al 2000, Vernon et al 1986, Vicenzino et al 1994, 1995, 1996, 1998a, 1998b, 1999a, 2000, 2001).

The emphasis of this chapter will be on reviewing the evidence pertaining to the neurophysiological effects produced by SMT. Firstly, somatosensory innervation of the spine will be presented so that the responses to SMT such as changes in pain perception, motor function and sympathetic nervous system response can be discussed in the context that SMT can be viewed as a physiological stimulus. The effects of both high velocity thrust low amplitude manipulation type techniques (HVT) and low velocity oscillatory techniques (MOB) will be reviewed and possible mechanisms of action involved in these responses will be highlighted.

SOMATOSENSORY INPUT FROM THE SPINE

The tissues of the spine, including skin, joint, muscle, tendon, discs and ligaments, are all extensively innervated and provide afferent input to the central nervous system (Groen et al 1990). It is thought that these fibres are mostly afferent with some efferent sympathetic fibres responsible for vasomotor control (Bolton 1998).

As well as normal afferent input, structures capable of signalling nociceptive information have been located in spinal tissue. In a study of unmyelinated afferents associated with the deep paraspinal tissues of the sacrum and tail in rats, Bove & Light (1995) noted the receptive fields for these afferents were located in a number of structures including the nerve sheaths and associated connective tissue, as well as that of muscles, tendons and tissue under the skin. Therefore it was proposed that these afferents signal nociceptive information from these tissues. The following sections will highlight the specific characteristics of somatosensory input from the spine.

Cervical spine

Structures of the cervical spine such as capsules, ligaments, intervertebral discs and paraspinal musculature are innervated with afferents that project both directly and indirectly to many levels of the neuraxis. The afferent input from the cervical spine is complex due to the interrelationship with other systems such as the vestibular, sympathetic and optic systems. A multifaceted neurophysiological response may be expected from afferent input occurring during SMT induced movement and perturbations to the head and neck.

Both cutaneous receptors and receptors from deeper tissues play a role in reflex response to touch and movement which are both key features of SMT. It is assumed that the receptors of the skin overlying the axial skeleton are similar in nature to receptors found in non-glabrous skin in other parts of the body, detecting mechanical deformation, hot, cold and nociception (free nerve endings) (Bolton 1998). However, in the neck, both animal and human studies have described the muscle spindle as the most common encapsulated nerve ending (Amonoo-Kuofi 1982, Richmond & Bakker 1982).

Paciniform capsules were also located in muscles in cats but were much more common in the connective tissue surrounding joints, particularly in the joint capsules on the external surface of the vertebrae, and Golgi tendon organs were located at musculotendinous junctions (Richmond & Bakker 1982).

In a study of the mechanoreceptive endings in human cervical zygapophysial joints, McLain (1994) demonstrated the presence of both encapsulated receptors (predominantly types I and II according to the 1967 classification by Freeman & Wyke) along with free nerve endings in the capsules indicating that afferent input from these zygapophysial capsules may subserve a role in proprioceptive and nociceptive input to the central nervous system. However, an interesting study by Bolton & Holland (1996) showed that vertebral displacement of C2 in the cat was accompanied by activation of primary and secondary afferents to the muscle spindles indicating both a dynamic and static response to vertebral displacement. Interestingly, activation of zygapophysial joint afferents did not occur frequently, suggesting that these afferents provide relatively little information regarding passive movement in the neck. Hence these data suggest that vertebral movement is signalled mainly by afferent innervation from deep intervertebral muscle where most of the spindles are located (Bolton 2000).

Afferents from the receptors terminate as expected in the spinal cord with cutaneous afferents synapsing in laminae I–IV, low threshold afferents from muscles terminating in laminae IV–VI as well as the ventral horn, and those from zygapophysial joint afferents synapsing in laminae I and II (Bolton 1998). In addition, primary afferents from the cervical spine also project higher to nuclei within the medulla including the ipsilateral cuneate nucleus and vestibular nuclei providing a relay for afferent information to the contralateral thalamus, cerebellum and sensorimotor cortex (Bolton & Tracey 1992), signalling both proprioceptive and nociceptive information (Bolton 1998).

There is a strong relationship between head and neck movement, the optical and the vestibular system. This is due to activation of neck afferents being part of a very complex collection of sensory afferent input to the central nervous system as movement of the neck, eyes and activation of the vestibular system usually accompanies movement of the head.

The response to this multifaceted afferent input is also diverse and complex. Both noxious stimulation to the skin of the neck in cats (Kaufman et al 1977) and non-noxious neck movements are associated with a number of postural reflexes such as the cervicocollic, vestibulocollic and opti-cokinetic reflexes (Bolton 1998). These reflexes are generally integrated in the intact nervous system but are apparent in the newborn and in brain-injured adults. They are responsible for the integrated movements of head and eye and head on body and the appropriate physiological responses to these movements.

Thoracic and lumbar spines

In the thoracic and lumbar spines, similar types of receptors were located in the zygapophysial joints as for the cervical spine in humans (McLain & Pickar 1998). Type I and II fibres were found as well as free nerve endings. However, the number of receptors was found to be lower than in the cervical spine and their distribution inconsistent (McLain & Pickar 1998). The low number and large receptive fields of the receptors compared with the cervical spine suggests that the proprioceptive function in this part of the spine requires less precision (McLain & Pickar 1998). Pickar & McLain (1995) have demonstrated that receptors lying outside the facet capsule in peri-articular and paraspinal tissues may be sensitive to facet movement. This is similar to the cervical spine where the muscles were sensitive to movement of the joint. It is of considerable interest that Pickar & McLain (1995) were also able to demonstrate that some fibres showed direction sensitivity to movement. Mechanosensitive receptors were also located in the facet joints and peri-articular tissue of rabbits by Cavanaugh et al (1996). These receptors responded to compressive loading, which induced a dorsolateral movement that stretched the facet joint capsules with low load (300–500 g) producing activation of the low threshold receptors and higher loads (3–5.5 kg) producing activity in the high threshold receptors (presumably nociceptors).

There are differences in connections within the spinal cord for afferents from the lumbar spine as opposed to those from the cervical spine, particularly afferents from muscle spindles. Keirstead & Rose (1988) identified that the connections in the lumbar spine were monosynaptic with motoneurons as opposed to some cervical spine endings that projected supraspinally. Neurophysiological responses to activation of lumbar spine afferents might therefore be expected to be different to that of the cervical spine.

In a single case study, Colloca et al (2000) were able to demonstrate that mechanical manipulation (less than 0.1 ms duration and 150 N of peak force application) applied to lower lumbar and sacral spines produced action potentials in a mixed nerve unilaterally at S1 the magnitude of which was direction-specific. Although it is impossible to generalize results from single case study, it is of interest to note that there was a specific mixed nerve response to SMT techniques that varied with changes in the stimulus parameters (Colloca et al 2000).

In summary, data presented in this section indicate that SMT which produces movement of the vertebral column

and its associated structures can potentially influence multiple receptors and generate afferent input to the spinal cord and supraspinal projection neurons. In the cervical spine particularly, there are also complex interactions with other systems such as the vestibular and optic systems that may also be activated in the presence of head and neck movements with some SMT techniques. As such, there is a neuroanatomical basis through which a multifaceted neurophysiologic response may occur with SMT.

ANALGESIC EFFECTS OF SPINAL MANUAL THERAPY

One of the main indications for the use of SMT is in the treatment of painful conditions of the musculoskeletal system. Both HVT and MOB can be used in the treatment of spinal pain. There are studies investigating the analgesic effect of both types of SMT. The essential differences between the two techniques are the velocity of the technique and amount and type of force used. A manipulation in the context of this review will relate to a high velocity thrust technique usually administered at the end of the available range of movement. This type of technique is usually accompanied by a 'pop' or 'crack' sound (i.e. audible release). Mobilization therapy is described as a low velocity oscillatory movement administered with a frequency range of approximately 0–2 Hz. These techniques can be mainly passive in nature (Maitland 1986) or may be accompanied by active movement such as the mobilization with movement techniques devised by Mulligan (1999).

A qualitative review of the effect of manipulation on pain mechanisms was undertaken by Vernon (2000) who suggested that less than 1% of indexed literature on manipulation studied the effect of this modality on pain by using physiological measures. This research has typically used pain measures before and after a treatment or combination of treatments and some have examined putative mechanisms of action, for example measuring the presence of neuropeptides such as β-endorphins which are known to contribute to various forms of endogenous analgesia. In many cases, however, analgesic outcomes of SMT have been described in terms of the biomechanical effect, that is, a reduction in pain can be ascribed to improvement in joint range of movement (Zusman 1994) or altered joint alignment (Gal et al 1997).

An early study of manipulation-induced analgesia was conducted by Glover et al (1974) using pinprick over the skin of paraspinal muscle adjacent to the participants' painful spinal segment. They noted a decrease in the size of the painful receptive field for pinprick in participants receiving a single rotary manipulation of the lumbar spine compared to controls receiving detuned short-wave diathermy. Based on the findings of this study, Terret & Vernon (1984) investigated the effect of a spinal manipulation to the thoracic spine in 50 normal subjects on electrically induced cutaneous pain thresholds. They located at least one painful spinal segment from T3–10 and half the subjects were given a manipulation with the other half being given pre-manipulation oscillatory palpation without the thrust. The researchers noted an increase in pain tolerance at 10 minutes (up to 130%) after the manipulative procedure that was significantly different ($P<0.05$) to that following the oscillatory movement without thrust.

Using algometry as an outcome measure, Vernon et al (1990) investigated pain relief following spinal manipulation in nine sufferers of chronic neck pain. Pre-manipulation oscillatory mobilization was used as a control condition and a rotational manipulation was performed as the treatment technique. A blinded investigator performed the measurements over standardized tender points in the paraspinal areas adjacent to the treated level. There was a statistically significant increase in pressure pain thresholds (PPT) in the manipulation group compared to control. The mean increase in PPT was 45% compared to no change in the control group. In another study by Cote et al (1994), PPT was used to examine the effect of manipulation over specified points in the lumbar area in 30 subjects with chronic low back pain. As in the above study, the control condition was mobilization and PPT was measured prior to, immediately after, and 15 and 30 minutes after the intervention. There was no difference demonstrated between groups or across time.

A multifactorial model to explain the rapid hypoalgesic effect produced by SMT was developed by Wright (1995). A number of potential mechanisms for analgesia were described including: stimulation of healing, modification of the chemical milieu of peripheral nociceptors, activation of segmental pain inhibitory mechanisms and activation of descending inhibitory pain control systems in addition to positive psychological influences. It has been suggested that the descending pain inhibitory system (DPIS) in particular could be responsible for mediating this immediate analgesic response. Both animal and human studies have demonstrated that a key locus of control for mediation of endogenous analgesia is the peri-aqueductal grey area of the midbrain (PAG) (Cannon et al 1982, Hosobuchi et al 1977, Reynolds 1969). The PAG plays an important integrative role for behavioural responses to pain, stress and other stimuli by coordinating responses of a number of systems including the nociceptive system, autonomic nervous system and motor system (Fanselow 1991, Lovick 1991, Morgan 1991). The PAG has a columnar structure (dorsomedial, dorsolateral, lateral and ventrolateral columns). The lateral (lPAG) and ventrolateral (vlPAG) subdivisions of the caudal PAG have been extensively investigated (Bandler & Shipley 1994, Bandler et al 1991, Carrive 1991, Farkas et al 1998, Jansen et al 1998, Lovick 1991), and Lovick (1991) described a set of complex responses following stimulation of these PAG subdivisions. This research highlighted that stimulation of vlPAG in rodents produces a tripartite effect including inhibition of the sympathetic nervous system, freezing of movement and analgesia

which is opioid in nature. Stimulation of lPAG appears to result in a non-opioid form of analgesia accompanied by sympatho-excitation and movement facilitation. Hence she suggested that lPAG coordinates a 'flight or fight' response to threatening or nociceptive stimuli whereas vlPAG activates more recuperative behaviour involving the opioid system. The 'flight' response usually occurs first and its activity inhibits the vlPAG neurons (Behbehani 1995). A study by Jansen et al (1998) has also confirmed the presence of local interconnections between the columns of the PAG. As such, it appears that PAG is responsible for co-coordinating responses that ensure survival rather than solely modulating pain perception (Fanselow 1991). Low threshold mechanoreceptors from joint and muscles project to the PAG and therefore non-noxious afferent input might also elicit components of this reaction (Yezierski 1991). Consequently, SMT may be an adequate stimulus to activate key regions of the PAG. It has been predicted that the response to SMT may not only involve analgesia but also incorporate changes in other aspects of nervous system function that are modulated by the PAG, that is, motor system and sympathetic nervous system responses (Wright 1995, Wright & Vicenzino 1995).

In order to investigate the characteristics of hypoalgesia following SMT, several studies have used quantitative sensory testing to investigate the effect of mobilization therapy in the cervical spine in both symptomatic and asymptomatic participants (Slater & Wright 1995, Souvlis et al 1999, 2000a, 2000b, Sterling et al 2000, Vicenzino et al 1995, 1996, 1998b, 1999a). Within subject placebo controlled studies were performed in participants suffering from unilateral lateral epicondylalgia (LE) (Souvlis et al 2000b, Vicenzino et al 1996) and non-traumatic cervical spine pain (Sterling et al 2000). Two treatment techniques were tested, posteroanterior mobilization at C5 and the lateral glide technique performed at C5–6. The measures included pressure pain threshold (PPT), pain-free grip threshold, thermal pain thresholds, neural tissue provocation test and a visual analogue scale (VAS) for pain. To control for the non-specific effects related to manual contact and pre-manipulation joint set-up position, all studies in this series incorporated a manual contact control condition with no joint movement as well as a no contact control condition.

This series of studies has shown that a rapid onset hypoalgesic response follows treatment in both asymptomatic and symptomatic participants. In a study of 24 asymptomatic participants Vicenzino et al (1995) evaluated pressure pain and thermal pain thresholds following the lateral glide technique described by Elvey (1986) at C5–6. A 22% improvement in PPT was noted with no concomitant change in thermal pain thresholds. This finding demonstrated the specificity of effect of SMT in that changes in mechanical pain but not thermal pain thresholds were produced. A study by Sterling et al (2000) also showed a specific effect of SMT in producing mechanical but not thermal hypoalgesia in treatment of neck pain. Using the lateral glide technique in 15 patients with unilateral LE, Vicenzino et al (1996) demonstrated improvements in PPT (approximately 25%), pain-free grip threshold (30%) and neural tissue provocation test (approximately 40%) and VAS for pain (1.9 cm). These findings were replicated in a study investigating the interrelationship between analgesic and sympathetic nervous system effects following SMT in patients with LE (Vicenzino et al 1998b). Importantly, with these studies it was shown that the participants were not able to distinguish treatment interventions from the control conditions. Both asymptomatic and symptomatic groups were naive to the effects of SMT. From these studies of HVT thrust and MOB techniques, it appears manual therapy produces a robust hypoalgesic effect that is reproducible across a number of studies using different techniques and patient populations.

Dhondt et al (1999) studied the effect of manual oscillations on pain in sufferers of rheumatoid arthritis (RA). These oscillations consisted of left and right rotations and ventral–dorsal translation that were performed at a variety of frequencies (1.5–0.5 Hz) and amplitudes (small amplitude at the beginning of range and large amplitude in midrange) at T12 and L4. A relative rise in the PPT was evident after the use of manual oscillations. A significant effect was seen in the paraspinal areas of T6, L1 and L3 with a trend towards a significant difference at T3, T10 and L5. The authors suggest a global inhibition mechanism as well as potential spinal gating due to the widespread nature of the effect (Dhondt et al 1999).

One of the possible mechanisms of manipulation-induced analgesia (MIA) is the release of endogenous opioids. Opioids include peptides such as endorphins, enkephalins and dynorphins. A method used to investigate SMT has been to characterize the response by measuring levels of endorphins as well as evaluating the effects of opioid antagonism by naloxone and tolerance development with SMT.

In an early study by Vernon et al (1986), the effect of spinal manipulation at the cervical spine was compared with a sham manipulation and a no contact control condition. Blood samples were taken by venepuncture at various intervals from 20 minutes prior to treatment up to 30 minutes post intervention to detect levels of β-endorphins in normal males. They showed a small but statistically significant increase in the level of serum β-endorphin level in the manipulation group at 5 minutes post treatment.

A study by Sanders et al (1990) compared manipulation in the lumbar spine with sham (light touch) and no contact control conditions and showed pain relief with manipulation compared to placebo and control conditions. The outcome measure used was a VAS. However, they also measured β-endorphin levels but were unable to detect a difference between the three conditions. Manipulation of the cervical and thoracic spines was conducted in both symptomatic and asymptomatic populations by Christian et al (1988) and they were not able to demonstrate a signif-

icant difference in β-endorphin levels between manipulation and a sham manipulation control. Methodological issues in using assays to test the plasma levels of circulating β-endorphin rather than the levels in the cerebrospinal fluid may have influenced the outcome of these studies (Vernon 2000).

Using a rather different approach to investigate the premise that endogenous opioids were involved in analgesia post SMT, Zusman et al (1989) compared the administration of naloxone to a saline control on the response to SMT. Naloxone is an opioid antagonist and reverses the effect of opioids, thereby reducing or eliminating the analgesic response. SMT was administered to 21 patients with spinal pain, following which the intervention was administered (10 naloxone, 11 saline). The authors used a VAS to detect differences in a pain provoking movement pre and post SMT; however, the treatment techniques were not described. There was a statistically significant improvement in pain VAS that was not different between conditions. That is, there was no antagonism of the hypoalgesic effect by naloxone. Administration of the intervention after SMT and the small dose of naloxone may have contributed to the lack of response (Wright 1995).

In a more recent study by Vicenzino et al (2000), the influence of naloxone on pain relief following administration of the lateral glide technique to C5–6 in patients with LE was compared with saline and no drug control conditions. No influence of naloxone on the hypoalgesic response was shown in this study. To further assess the possible contribution of opioid mechanisms to the analgesic response, the effect of repeated administration of lateral glide to C5–6 in LE subjects was undertaken to determine whether tolerance developed to the initial hypoalgesic effect of SMT (Souvlis & Wright 1997, Souvlis et al 1999). Development of tolerance is considered to be a key characteristic of opioid analgesia. Results demonstrated that no tolerance developed to the initial effect when the technique was applied over six sessions.

Thus, the only study performed to date that was able to show potential evidence of opioid mediated analgesia following SMT as indicated by significantly elevated plasma levels of β-endorphin levels was the initial one by Vernon et al (1986). No studies have shown naloxone reversibility of the immediate analgesic effect that follows SMT. Considered together, the studies provide very little evidence to support the potential involvement of opioid systems in manipulation-induced analgesia. However, inherent limitations in the non-invasive study of the role of opioids in SMT mean that the involvement of endogenous opioids cannot be entirely ruled out. Table 25.1 provides a summary of the potential analgesic effects produced by SMT.

MOTOR EFFECTS OF SPINAL MANUAL THERAPY

There are a number of studies investigating the effect of SMT on aspects of motor function. The majority of these

Table 25.1 Summary of the potential effects of spinal manual therapy on the nociceptive, motor and sympathetic nervous systems

Analgesia	Motor system	Sympathetic nervous system
Decreased area of pain perception	Transient increase EMG	Increase in heart rate
Increased mechanical pain thresholds	Decrease in size of H-reflex	Increase in blood pressure
No effect on thermal pain threshold	Decrease in muscle inhibition	Increase in respiratory rate
Non-opioid characteristics	Increased motor evoked potential	Increased peripheral blood flow
– no change in β-endorphin levels		Increase in skin conductance
– not reversible by naloxone		Decrease in skin temperature
– no tolerance to repeated applications		

have involved the use of HVT techniques. It is often assumed by clinicians that pain of spinal origin is accompanied by what is often termed hyperactivity, hypertonicity or spasm of the surrounding muscles. Thus there exists a biased position taken by the investigators towards evaluating the motor effects of SMT. One of the consequences of this assumption is that SMT is researched in terms of its ability to inhibit muscle hyperactivity (Herzog et al 1999, Knutson 2000).

The effect of SMT on the motor system

It has been proposed that one of the mechanisms by which pain relief is obtained is by breaking the pain/spasm/pain cycle as a result of SMT induced reflex inhibition of muscle (Dishman et al 2002a, Zusman 1992). Wright (1995) suggested that the initial neurophysiological response to SMT might incorporate a motor effect that can occur concurrently but not result from pain relief produced by SMT. A number of studies have been conducted to investigate the effects of SMT on the motor system, some of which have reported inhibitory effects while others have reported excitatory effects.

Inhibition of motor activity

An early study by Thabe (1986) showed that EMG activity in the paraspinal musculature of patients with restricted sacroiliac motion could be decreased following a local anaesthetic injection as well as following manipulation of the joint. Murphy et al (1995) tested the theory that altered afferent input from structures in and around the joint being manipulated leads to a reduction in excitability of motoneurons, consequently breaking the pain/spasm/pain cycle. In their study, the H-reflex amplitude was measured pre and post interventions in asymptomatic participants. The treatments consisted of a manipulation to the ipsilateral and contralateral sacroiliac joints (SIJ) as well as a sham procedure involving manual contact. There was a significant decrease in the magnitude of the H-reflex in the ipsilateral soleus muscle compared to contralateral and sham

conditions. In a further study in 14 asymptomatic subjects, EMLA anaesthetic cream was applied to the skin over the SIJ prior to manipulation, to eliminate the contribution from the cutaneous afferents to the response. The results once again showed a significant decrease in reflex response for the manipulation on the ipsilateral side compared with contralateral and sham conditions, demonstrating that the effect was mediated not only by cutaneous afferents but also by deeper mechanoreceptors.

Zhu et al (2000) investigated the relationship between evoked potentials by magnetic stimulation and palpable muscle spasm, low back pain and activity. They noted that cerebral evoked potentials (CEPs) were lower in patients who had palpable muscle spasm on clinical evaluation. These potentials were re-evaluated after 2 weeks of treatment (3–5 visits per week) incorporating HVT spinal manipulation in the side lying position, ischaemic compression/massage, intermittent traction, general advice and home exercises. Results showed that the cerebral evoked potentials returned to published normal values following treatment. The authors gave the rationale for reduced cerebral evoked potentials with muscle spasm as being related to a decrease in the number of afferents available for stimulation by the magnetic device (Zhu et al 2000). As spasm decreases, the number of Ia afferents available for stimulation would increase, thereby increasing the amplitude of the CEP (Zhu et al 2000). As there was no control group used in the study, it is difficult to ascertain whether these effects are related to time, learning and/or treatment effects.

The effects of performing SMT on the cervical and lumbar spines may be substantially different. As indicated above, the neck has a larger population of muscle spindles and mechanoreceptors than the lumbar spine. There is also convergence of cervical somatic afferents on vestibular nuclei that could facilitate or inhibit motor activity. Dishman et al (2002b) compared the effect of SMT at the cervical and lumbar spines on the tibial nerve H-reflex to investigate the relationship between potential cortical and segmentally controlled responses to SMT. Using both a between groups and within groups design, an experienced clinician performed a unilateral right-sided manipulation at either L5–S1, C5–6 (between group), or at both levels (within group). They demonstrated a small but significant decrease in the size of the reflex following lumbar manipulation. Conversely, there was no effect of SMT performed at the cervical spine on the H-reflex. The authors suggest a segmental rather than global effect produced by SMT on the motoneuron pool. This effect was transient, lasting only 60 seconds after manipulation (Dishman et al 2002b).

The effects of SMT and massage on motoneuron excitability have been compared. Dishman & Bulbulian (2001) noted that the amplitude of the H-reflex was significantly decreased following spinal manipulation compared with massage and control. The interventions (lumbar manipulation and paraspinal and limb massage) were performed in asymptomatic participants.

Facilitation of motor activity

Keller & Colloca (2000) were able to demonstrate a positive increase in the maximum voluntary contraction of erector spinae muscles using EMG following a mechanical SMT technique compared to a sham technique or control interventions in 20 patients with low back pain. In this study a clinical assessment and treatment protocol was used and this was followed by 'stiffness assessment' involving high velocity PA thrusts at a number of sites: 20 thrusts were delivered at sites from sacrum to T8 on both spinous and bilateral transverse processes. Algometry measures were taken but these were not reported in the results. No other pain related measures were taken. It is therefore difficult to determine whether the short-term effect produced by SMT resulted from pain relief or was a primary change in motor function. Similar results were reported by Colloca & Keller (2001) with HVT thrusts in a number of areas showing a positive effect on the paraspinal muscles. They suggest that as the time from manipulation to EMG response was 2–4 ms, this response was in line with conduction speed for an intraspinal reflex loop (Colloca & Keller 2001).

Using a different approach to their previous studies, mentioned above, Dishman et al (2002a) studied the effect of manipulation on motor evoked potentials (MEPs). They used transcranial magnetic stimulation to produce MEPs at the gastrocnemius muscle and compared the effects of an L5–S1 spinal manipulation (high velocity, low amplitude) and a sham condition (side positioning, no manipulation) on the size of the MEPs. They considered that the MEPs were indicative of postsynaptic central motor changes rather than the presynaptic peripheral changes that are reportedly associated with changes in the H-reflex. They concluded that the manipulation condition significantly increased the amplitude of the MEP compared with the sham condition. This facilitation was short lived with the effects being significant only for a period of up to 120 seconds post manipulation. There were no significant differences between sham and manipulation after 5 or 10 minutes.

The authors concluded that the manipulative thrust facilitated the central motor system due to a postsynaptic facilitation of both alpha and cortical motoneurons. These results appear in conflict with the results of the earlier studies using H-reflex measurement. However, the authors suggest that the outcome measurement (H-reflex vs MEPs) and the difference in methodology may produce different effects. They also proposed that central facilitation may require a decreased activation of motoneurons peripherally and therefore are different measures of the same outcome.

A number of studies have used EMG output of paraspinal muscles following SMT to measure the effect of SMT on motor function. Herzog et al (1999) used SMT at various areas in the spine and evaluated the EMG response post treatment in 10 asymptomatic participants. HVT thrusts were used and an initial local transient increase of EMG in both spinal and limb musculature was noted. It was suggested that the reflex response might be related to a decrease in pain and decrease in hypertonicity, presumably through post-activation inhibition of muscle. No sham or control procedures were used during this study and the use of asymptomatic subjects makes it difficult to substantiate these proposals.

In contrast to the relatively large number of studies reporting motor effects following SMT, there has only been one study to date that has investigated the effect of mobilization therapy on motor responses. Sterling et al (2000) used mobilization of the cervical spine in patients with neck pain to look at the concurrent effects on motor responses, sympathetic nervous system function and analgesia. The effect of a PA technique on the craniocervical flexion test was assessed. A decreased activation of superficial musculature of the cervical spine that was interpreted as facilitation of the deeper neck flexors gives some confirmation that motor responses are altered following SMT. The patients in this study showed pain relief as measured by algometry thus indicating concurrent hypoalgesic and motor effects.

In summary, the effect of SMT on the motor system is inconclusive. There are various theories on how pain is related to changes in motor function and studies of SMT-induced motor effects report both facilitatory and inhibitory effects (see Table 25.1 for summary). The measures of neural system function (e.g. H-reflex versus motor evoked potential) may partially explain contradictory findings. Alternatively, rather than being inconsistent these findings may point to a number of possible responses of the motor system following SMT, possibly depending on the origin, location and nature of the pain, the muscles tested and the treatment technique.

EFFECTS OF SPINAL MANUAL THERAPY ON THE SYMPATHETIC NERVOUS SYSTEM

As well as analgesic and motor effects following SMT, the effects on the sympathetic nervous system (SNS) have been investigated. The effect of non-noxious stimulation of both cutaneous and deep somatic afferents on SNS function has been studied using mainly animal models and, along with SMT studies, will be reported in the following sections.

To understand the SMT literature on SNS effects, it is important to acknowledge that there are two perspectives on SMT-induced SNS changes. The long held tenet of osteopathy/chiropractic is that SMT will alter ANS outflow to the organs and viscera and that this will rectify any dysfunction of the end-organs (appendicitis, angina, etc.). This view is still widely held despite a lack of scientific validation (Jamison et al 1992). A more recent approach has taken SNS changes produced by SMT to be indicators of a multifaceted CNS response to the manual therapy stimulus. Consequently this approach has used SNS changes to develop an understanding of potential mechanisms of action of SMT (Souvlis et al 2001, Vicenzino et al 1994, 1995, 1998a, 1998b).

Cardiorespiratory effects

Some investigators have used animal models to study the response of the SNS to innocuous stimulation of spinal structures in order to investigate the relationship between somatic and sympathetic nervous systems. (Bolton et al 1998, Budgell et al 1997). Previous evidence suggested that only activation of high threshold receptors with noxious mechanical cutaneous stimulation produced changes in heart rate and blood pressure in rats (Kimura et al 1995) and heart rate in cats (Kaufman et al 1977). However, Bolton et al (1998) showed that non-noxious stimulation of neck afferents could produce changes in sympathetic nerve activity. Movements of the head–neck complex have been shown to induce changes in heart rate, arterial pressure, vascular resistance and limb blood flow (Fujimoto et al 1999, Hume & Ray 1999, Shortt & Ray 1997). The human study by Fujimoto et al (1999) involved innocuous movement of the neck that would be similar to those performed during clinical physical examination of the spine and found both increases and decreases in heart rate and arterial pressure in participants, depending on whether the subject was alert or drowsy. So evidence from both animal and human studies demonstrates a cardiovascular response to non-noxious neck movement.

A study by Knutson (2001) using both between and within groups study design investigated the changes in systolic blood pressure following upper cervical adjustment to determine the influence on the cervicosympathetic and pressor reflexes. Participants in the treatment group (vectored upper cervical adjustment in side lying) demonstrated a significant lowering of systolic blood pressure compared with the control group. A similar finding was demonstrated in the within groups study. In these studies there was no blinding of the subjects and control interventions were performed in the same sessions.

Heart rate and blood pressure have been used to detect changes in SNS activity following somatic stimulation in animals and humans. Innocuous cutaneous stimulation does not appear to produce a change in the blood pressure of anaesthetized rats (Adachi et al 1990). However, noxious stimulation of the skin produced an increase in the heart rate and blood pressure (Adachi et al 1990, Kimura et al 1995).

Mechanical stimulation such as stretch of muscle by passive or active movement produced a small decrease in heart rate and blood pressure whereas a noxious stimulus to the muscle produced a pressor response (Tallarida et al 1981). In a study investigating the effects of mechanical stimulation of the spine, Sato & Swenson (1984) demonstrated that stimulation of isolated thoracic and lumbar vertebrae in anaesthetized rats produced decreases in blood pressure and heart rate. The changes in blood pressure were larger than those in heart rate. Spinalization of the animals at C1–2 reversed the changes and produced an increase in blood pressure therefore providing support for this effect being mediated supraspinally (Sato & Swenson 1984).

In contrast, innocuous rhythmic passive movement of the knee joint within normal physiological range of movement did not significantly affect blood pressure or heart rate in anaesthetized cats (Sato et al 1984). However, increases in blood pressure and heart rate were demonstrated in both non-anaesthetized (Barron & Coote 1973) and anaesthetized cats (Sato et al 1984) following noxious stimulation to the knee joint and also to end of range joint movement (Sato et al 1984). Sensitization of the knee joint afferents by induced inflammation also produced an increase in the pressor response following previously innocuous movements within the limits of joint range (Sato et al 1984).

The effect of adjustment of the lower cervical spine was investigated by Nansel et al (1991) in 24 asymptomatic males demonstrating lateral flexion passive end-range asymmetry. Outcome measures were taken for blood pressure, heart rate and plasma catecholamine (noradrenaline (norepinephrine), adrenaline (epinephrine) and dopamine) levels. There was a significant change in the lateral flexion movement in the treatment group compared to the control group. However, no significant changes were noted in any of the other measures. This result may be as a consequence of a number of factors in this study. All participants were asymptomatic and there were a relatively small number of subjects per group. This may have reduced the power of the study to detect differences. The sampling of plasma may not be a suitable technique to detect changes in catecholamine levels following SMT.

Vicenzino et al (1998a) measured indices of SNS function, namely cardiovascular and respiratory function, during application of the lateral glide (LG) technique to C5–6 in 24 asymptomatic subjects. A significant increase ($P<0.05$) in heart rate and both diastolic and systolic blood pressure of the order of approximately 14% was observed in the treatment condition in comparison with 1–2% in the placebo and control conditions. The respiratory rate also showed an increase of about 36% that was significantly larger than the control conditions. McGuiness et al (1997) measured central SNS markers following posteroanterior (PA) technique at C5 and also demonstrated an increase in heart rate, blood pressure (diastolic > systolic) and respiratory rate.

Sudomotor/vasomotor systems

Activation of the sudomotor system occurs following an increase in body temperature such as during exercise. Kuno (1956) described this phenomenon as 'thermal sweating' as opposed to 'mental sweating' which was described as the activation of the sweat glands particularly in the palms of the hands and soles of the feet following mental exertion or stress. Regulation of body temperature in response to an increase in temperature involves the inactivation of the cutaneous sympathetic vasoconstrictors and activation of cutaneous sudomotor fibres (Sato et al 1997). Activation of the sweat glands can be measured by a change of impedance of the skin (e.g. skin conductance or galvanic skin response).

An early study by Harris & Wagnon (1987) investigated skin temperature of the fingertips before and immediately after spinal adjustment in 196 patients. When the lumbar and cervical spines were manipulated, a significant increase in skin temperature from baseline of about 0.42°F was noted. In contrast, a significant decrease in temperature from baseline of about 0.25°F was seen following manipulation of the thoracic spine. The treatments at a range of spinal levels were administered to patients on the basis of their condition and no specific technique was investigated for its effect. Also the effects were not compared to placebo or control interventions with the authors concluding that the differential result was related to the area of spine manipulated such that lumbar and cervical spine areas were considered anatomically 'non-sympathetic' whereas the sympathetic nerves exit the thoracic spine and manipulation could directly stimulate these fibres.

Clinton & McCarthy (1993) evaluated the effects of spinal manipulation on the sudomotor system by measuring electric skin response (ESR). In a study involving 20 male chiropractic students with asymptomatic fixation of the first rib, ESR was measured at ipsilateral and contralateral forearms following manipulation of the first rib. The effect was compared with the response following set-up, sham manipulation and auditory shock. There was no significant difference between the responses for any intervention.

Based on the hypothesis that multisystem responses are evoked by SMT (Wright 1995, Wright & Vicenzino 1995), several studies have specifically investigated the effect of MOB on the sympathetic nervous system. Studies have investigated the effect of posteroanterior and lateral glide mobilization of the cervical spine and of neural tissue.

Outcome measures for SNS function in these studies were sudomotor, cutaneous vasomotor and cardiorespiratory functions (McGuiness et al 1995, 1997, Petersen et al 1993, Souvlis et al 2001, Vicenzino et al 1994, 1995, 1998a, 1998b, 1999a).

Grade III posteroanterior mobilization of C5 produced a change in SNS function which was significantly different to that produced by placebo and control conditions in a suite of studies using a within subjects controlled design.

Petersen et al (1993) investigated sudomotor and cutaneous vasomotor responses to SMT. They found an increase in skin conductance of the order of 60% and a small but significant decrease in skin temperature measured at the hand, in comparison with placebo and control techniques representing an excitatory response of the SNS following the SMT stimulus. Vicenzino et al (1994, 1996, 1998b, 1999a) investigated the effect of SMT on SNS function in groups of both symptomatic and asymptomatic subjects. In a study of 24 asymptomatic patients, a LG technique was applied to C5–6. A comparison was made between LG incorporating either upper limb tension test positions 1 or 2b, in comparison with control conditions. LG2b produced the greatest increase in skin conductance. This effect was not significantly larger than that produced by the LG1 technique but was significantly larger than control effects (Vicenzino et al 1994). The effects of lateral glide mobilization on cutaneous vasomotor responses were also studied. Skin temperature was measured at both the pileous skin of the elbow and the glabrous skin of the hand. Differential responses of these measures were noted, with the skin temperature of the hand showing a significant decrease in comparison with control interventions whereas skin temperature at the elbow did not change. A significant increase in elbow blood flux was noted; however, the decrease in flux measurement at the hand was non-significant. The changes in effects produced in these studies are indicative of an excitatory response of the peripheral indicators of SNS function (Vicenzino et al 1998b).

Souvlis et al (2001) evaluated the effect of dose of treatment on the initial sympatho-excitatory response to SMT. They investigated the SNS response to three different applications of LG2b at C5–6 and showed that there was no difference in response to 3 × 30 second, 3 × 60 second or 6 × 30 second applications of the technique in asymptomatic subjects. However, there were significant differences between treatment and manual contact and no contact control conditions (Souvlis et al 2001). In this study the SNS indicators were measured for up to 1 hour post treatment and it was evident that there was a return to baseline measures within 20 minutes of the treatment. There was no evidence of post-treatment sympatho-inhibition that has been cited in some chiropractic studies (Harris & Wagnon 1987, Knutson 1997).

Activation of the SNS in response to stress is a well-known phenomenon (flight/fight response) and it is necessary to determine whether the sympatho-excitatory effects noted following SMT are related to stress. To this end, a study was conducted by Vicenzino et al (1999a) to establish whether the study participants perceived that the manual therapy treatment technique produced stress and pain in comparison with placebo and control interventions. Twenty-four asymptomatic participants were asked to complete a stress rating scale and a stress VAS. Pain during application of the technique was measured using a pain VAS and the McGill Pain Questionnaire. The results suggest that application of the technique was not linked with stress and pain. However, stress levels, although very small, were noted to decrease over the time course of the study. This was not related to the treatment but more to familiarization with the environment as the conditions were randomized to prevent such an order effect (Vicenzino et al 1999a).

Data from both basic animal studies and human studies support the premise that non-noxious afferent stimulation can induce SNS responses which are specific in nature and related to the type of stimulus and have both a supraspinal and spinal component. Studies from our laboratories have demonstrated that SMT is a sufficient stimulus to induce an SNS response. These predominantly excitatory responses appear to be reproducible independent of technique or subject population. There is little conclusive evidence to date as to the effect of HVT thrust techniques on SNS function.

The premise that the PAG may be the locus of control of the initial analgesic effect of SMT (Wright 1995, Wright & Vicenzino 1995) is strengthened by the findings from the above studies investigating SNS response to MOB. Animal studies have demonstrated that activation of lPAG produces a response incorporating non-opioid analgesia and excitation of motor and sympathetic nervous systems (Lovick 1991). Using confirmatory factor analysis, Vicenzino et al (1998b) were able to demonstrate a significant relationship ($P<0.05$), between the hypoalgesic and SNS responses to SMT. The analgesia following MOB did not display opioid characteristics as it was not reversed by naloxone (Vicenzino et al 2000) and did not become tolerant to repeated application (Souvlis et al 1999). Limited evidence is available on the motor effects of MOB. However, Sterling et al (2000) were able to demonstrate concurrent effects of MOB on analgesia, motor and SNS function. Nevertheless, to fully establish the role of supraspinal structures in the neurophysiological effects of SMT, further research is required which directly investigates these mechanisms.

KEYWORDS	
spinal manual therapy	hypoalgesia
manipulation	motor system
mobilization	sympathetic nervous system

References

Adachi T, Meguro K, Sato A, Sato Y 1990 Cutaneous stimulation regulates blood flow in cerebral cortex in anesthetized rats. Neuroreport 1: 41–44

Aker P D, Gross A R, Goldsmith C H, Peloso P 1996 Conservative management of mechanical neck pain: systematic overview and meta-analysis. British Medical Journal 313: 1291–1296

Allison G, Edmondston S, Roe C, Reid S, Toy D, Lundgren H 1998 Influence of load orientation on the posteroanterior stiffness of the lumbar spine. Journal of Manipulative and Physiological Therapeutics 21: 534–538

Amonoo-Kuofi H S 1982 The number and distribution of muscle spindles in human intrinsic postvertebral muscles. Journal of Anatomy 135: 585–599

Bandler R, Shipley M T 1994 Columnar organization in the midbrain periaqueductal gray: modules for emotional expression. Trends in Neurosciences 17: 379–389

Bandler R, Carrive P, Depaulis A 1991 Emerging principles of organisation of the midbrain periaqueductal gray matter. In: Depaulis A, Bandler R (eds) The midbrain periaqueductal gray matter. Plenum Press, New York, pp 1–8

Barron W, Coote J H 1973 The contribution of articular receptors to cardiovascular reflexes elicited by passive limb movement. Journal of Physiology (London) 235: 423–436

Behbehani M M 1995 Functional characteristics of the midbrain periaqueductal gray. Progress in Neurobiology 46: 575–605

Bolton P S 1998 The somatosensory system of the neck and its effect on the central nervous system. Journal of Manipulative and Physiological Therapeutics 21: 553–563

Bolton P S 2000 Reflex effects of vertebral subluxations: the peripheral nervous system. An update. Journal of Manipulative and Physiological Therapeutics 23: 101–103

Bolton P S, Holland C T 1996 Afferent signaling of vertebral displacement in the neck of the cat. Neuroscience Abstracts 22: 1802

Bolton P S, Tracey D J 1992 Neurons in the dorsal column nuclei of the rat respond to stimulation of neck mechanoreceptors and project to the thalamus. Brain Research 595: 175–179

Bolton P S, Kerman I A, Woodring S F, Yates B J 1998 Influences of neck afferents on sympathetic and respiratory nerve activity. Brain Research Bulletin 47: 413–419

Bove G M, Light A R 1995 Unmyelinated nociceptors of rat paraspinal tissues. Journal of Neurophysiology 73: 1752–1762

Budgell B, Sato A, Suzuki A, Uchida S 1997 Responses of adrenal function to stimulation of lumbar and thoracic interspinous tissues in the rat. Neuroscience Research 28: 33–40

Cannon J T, Prieto G J, Lee A, Liebeskind J C 1982 Evidence for opioid and non-opioid forms of stimulation produced analgesia in the rat. Brain Research 243: 315–321

Carrive P 1991 Functional organisation of PAG neurons controlling regional vascular beds. In: Depaulis A, Bandler R (eds) The midbrain periaqueductal gray matter. Plenum Press, London, pp 67–100

Cavanaugh J M, Ozaktay A C, Yamashita H T, King A I 1996 Lumbar facet pain: biomechanics, neurophysiology and neuroanatomy. Journal of Biomechanics 29: 1117–1129

Christian G H, Stanton G J, Sissons D et al Immunoreactive ACTH, β-endorphin and cortisol levels in plasma following spinal manipulative therapy. Spine 13: 141–147

Clinton E M F, McCarthy P W 1993 The effect of a chiropractic adjustment of the first rib on the electric skin response in ipsilateral and contralateral human forelimbs. Complementary Therapies in Medicine 1: 61–67

Colloca C J, Keller T S 2001 Electromyographic reflex responses to mechanical force, manually assisted spinal manipulative therapy. Spine 26: 1117–1124

Colloca C J, Keller T S, Gunzburg R, Vandeputte K, Fuhr A W 2000 Neurophysiologic response to intraoperative lumbosacral spinal manipulation. Journal of Manipulative and Physiological Therapeutics 23: 447–457

Cote P, Mior S A, Vernon H T 1994 The short term effect of a spinal manipulation on pain/pressure threshold in patients with chronic mechanical low back pain. Journal of Manipulative and Physiological Therapeutics 17: 364–368

Dhondt W, Willaeys T, Verbruggen L A, Oostendorp R A, Duquet W 1999 Pain threshold in patients with rheumatoid arthritis and effect of manual oscillations. Scandinavian Journal of Rheumatology 28: 88–93

Dishman J D, Bulbulian R 2001 Comparison of effects of spinal manipulation and massage on motoneuron excitability. Electromyography and Clinical Neurophysiology 41: 97–106

Dishman J D, Ball K A, Burke J 2002a Central motor excitability changes after spinal manipulation: a transcranial magnetic stimulation study. Journal of Manipulative and Physiological Therapeutics, 25: 1–9

Dishman J D, Cunningham B M, Burke J 2002b Comparison of tibial nerve H-Reflex excitability after cervical and lumbar spine manipulation. Journal of Manipulative and Physiological Therapeutics 25: 318–325

Elvey R 1986 Treatment of arm pain associated with abnormal brachial plexus tension. Australian Journal of Physiotherapy 32: 225–230

Fanselow M S 1991 The midbrain periaqueductal gray as a coordinator of action in response to fear and anxiety. In: Depaulis A, Bandler R (eds) The midbrain periaqueductal gray matter. Plenum Press, New York, pp 151–173

Farkas E, Jansen A S P, Loewy A D 1998 Periaqueductal gray matter input to cardiac-related sympathetic premotor neurons. Brain Research 792: 179–192

Freeman M A R, Wyke B D 1967 The innervation of the knee joint: an anatomical and histological study in the cat. Journal of Anatomy 101: 505

Fujimoto T, Budgell B, Uchida S, Suzuki A, Meguro K 1999 Arterial tonometry in the measurement of the effects of innocuous mechanical stimulation of the neck on heart rate and blood pressure. Journal of the Autonomic Nervous System 75: 109–115

Gal J, Herzog W, Kawchuk G N, Conway P, Zhang J M 1997 Movements of vertebrae during manipulative thrusts to unembalmed human cadavers. Journal of Manipulative and Physiological Therapeutics 20: 30–40

Glover J R, Morris J G, Khosla T 1974 Back pain: a randomised clinical trial of rotational manipulation of the trunk. British Journal of Industrial Medicine 31: 59–64

Groen G J, Baljet B, Drukker J 1990 Nerve and nerve plexuses of the human vertebral column. American Journal of Anatomy 188: 282–296

Gross A R, Aker P D, Quartly C 1996 Manual therapy in the treatment of neck pain. Rheumatic Disease Clinics of North America 22: 579–598

Harris W, Wagnon R J 1987 The effects of chiropractic adjustments on distal skin temperature. Journal of Manipulative and Physiological Therapeutics 10: 57–60

Herzog W 2000 Clinical biomechanics of spinal manipulation. Churchill Livingstone, Edinburgh

Herzog W, Scheele D, Conway P 1999 Electromyographic responses of back and limb muscles associated with spinal manipulative therapy. Spine 24: 146–153

Hosobuchi Y, Adams J E, Linchitz R 1977 Pain relief by electrical stimulation of the central gray matter in human and its reversal by naloxone. Science 197: 183–186

Hume K M, Ray C A 1999 Sympathetic responses to head-down rotations in humans. Journal of Applied Physiology 86: 1971–1976

Jamison J R, McEwen A P, Thomas S J 1992 Chiropractic adjustment in the management of visceral conditions: a critical appraisal. Journal of Manipulative and Physiological Therapeutics 15: 171–180

Jansen A S P, Farkas E, Sams J M, Loewy A D 1998 Local connections between the columns of the periaqueductal gray matter: a case for intrinsic neuromodulation. Brain Research 784: 329–336

Jull G 2002 Use of high and low velocity cervical manipulative therapy procedures by Australian manipulative physiotherapists. Australian Journal of Physiotherapy 48: 189–193

Kaufman A, Sato A, Sato Y, Sugimoto H 1977 Reflex changes in heart rate after mechanical and thermal stimulation of the skin at various segmental levels in the cat. Neuroscience 2: 103–109

Keirstead S A, Rose P K 1988 Structure of the interspinal projections of single identified muscle spindle afferents from the neck of the cat. Journal of Neuroscience 8: 3413–3426

Keller T S, Colloca C J 2000 Mechanical force spinal manipulation increases trunk muscle strength assessed by electromyography: a comparative clinical trial. Journal of Manipulative and Physiological Therapeutics 23: 585–595

Keller T S, Colloca C J, Fuhr A W 2000 In vivo transient vibration assessment of the normal human thoracolumbar spine. Journal of Manipulative and Physiological Therapeutics 23: 521–530

Kimura A, Ohsawa H, Sato A, Sato Y 1995 Somatocardiovascular reflexes in anesthetized rats with the central nervous system intact or acutely at the cervical level. Neuroscience Research 22: 297–305

Knutson G A 1997 Thermal asymmetry of the upper extremity in scalenus anticus syndrome, leg length inequality and response to chiropractic adjustment. Journal of Manipulative and Physiological Therapeutics 20: 476–481

Knutson G A 2000 The role of the γ-motor system in increasing muscle tone and muscle pain syndromes: a review of the Johannson/Sojka hypothesis. Journal of Manipulative and Physiological Therapeutics 23: 564–572

Knutson G A 2001 Significant changes in systolic blood pressure post vectored upper cervical adjustments vs resting control groups: a possible effect of the cervicosympathetic and/or pressor reflex. Journal of Manipulative and Physiological Therapeutics 24: 101–109

Koes B W, Bouter L M, Vanmameren H et al 1992 Randomized clinical-trial of manipulative therapy and physiotherapy for persistent back and neck complaints: results of one year follow-up. British Medical Journal 304: 601–605

Kuno Y 1956 Human perspiration. Thomas, Springfield

Latimer J, Lee M, Adams R D 1998 The effects of high and low loading forces on measured values of lumbar stiffness. Journal of Manipulative and Physiological Therapeutics 21: 157–163

Lee M, Liversidge K 1994 Posteroanterior stiffness at three locations in the lumbar spine. Journal of Manipulative and Physiological Therapeutics 17: 511–516

Lee M, Latimer J, Maher C 1993 Manipulation: investigation of a proposed mechanism. Clinical Biomechanics 8: 302–306

Lee M, Maher C, Simmonds M J, Kumar S, Lechelt E 1995 Spinal models: use of a spinal model to quantify the forces and motion that occur during therapists' test of spinal motion. Physical Therapy 75: 638–641

Lovick T A 1991 Interactions between descending pathways from the dorsal and ventrolateral periaqueductal gray matter in rats. In: Depaulis A, Bandler R (eds) The midbrain periaqueductal gray matter. Plenum Press, New York, pp 101–120

McGuiness J, Vicenzino B, Wright A 1995 The effects of a postero-anterior cervical mobilisation technique on central nervous system function. Physiotherapy Theory and Practice

McGuiness J, Vicenzino B, Wright A 1997 The influence of a cervical mobilisation technique on respiratory and cardiovascular function. Manual Therapy 2: 216–220

McLain R F 1994 Mechanoreceptor endings in human cervical facet joints. Spine 19: 495–501

McLain R F, Pickar J G 1998 Mechanoreceptor endings in human thoracic and lumbar facet joints. Spine 23: 168–173

Maitland G D 1986 Vertebral manipulation. Butterworths, London

Morgan M M 1991 Differences in antinociception evoked from dorsal and ventral regions of the caudal periaqueductal gray matter. In: Depaulis A, Bandler R (eds) The midbrain periaqueductal gray matter. Plenum Press, New York, pp 139–150

Mulligan B R 1999 Manual therapy: NAGS, SNAGS, MWM, etc. Plane View Services, Wellington, New Zealand

Murphy B A, Dawson N J, Slack J 1995 Sacroiliac joint manipulation decreases the H-reflex. Electromyography and Clinical Neurophysiology 35: 87–94

Nansel D, Jansen R, Cremata E, Dhami M S I, Holley D 1991 Effects of cervical adjustments on lateral-flexion passive end-range asymmetry and on blood pressure, heart rate and plasma catecholamine levels. Journal of Manipulative and Physiological Therapeutics 14: 450–456

Petersen N P, Vicenzino G T, Wright A 1993 The effects of a cervical mobilisation technique on sympathetic outflow to the upper limb in normal subjects. Physiotherapy Theory and Practice 9: 149–146

Pickar J G, McLain R F 1995 Responses of mechano-sensitive afferents to manipulation of the lumbar facet in the cat. Spine 20: 2379–2385

Reynolds D V 1969 Surgery in the rat during electrical analgesia induced by focal brain stimulation. Science 164: 444–445

Richmond F J R, Bakker D A 1982 Anatomical organisation and sensory receptor content of soft tissues surrounding upper cervical vertebrae in the cat. Journal of Neurophysiology 48: 49–61

Sanders G E, Reinnert O, Tepe R, Maloney P 1990 Chiropractic adjustive manipulation on subjects with acute low back pain: visual analog scores and plasma β-endorphin levels. Journal of Manipulative and Physiological Therapeutics 13: 391–395

Sato A, Swenson R S 1984 Sympathetic nervous system response to mechanical stress of the spinal column in rats. Journal of Manipulative and Physiological Therapeutics 7: 141–147

Sato A, Sato Y, Schmidt R F, Torigata Y 1984 Changes in blood pressure and heart rate induced by movements of normal and inflamed knee joints. Neuroscience Letters 52: 55–60

Sato A, Sato Y, Schmidt R F 1997 The impact of somatosensory input on autonomic functions. Reviews of Physiology, Biochemistry and Pharmacology 130: 1–328

Shekelle P 1996 Point of view: Spinal manipulation for low back pain: an updated systematic review of randomised clinical trials. Spine 21: 2872

Shortt T L, Ray C A 1997 Sympathetic and vascular responses to head-down neck rotation in humans. American Journal of Physiology 272: H1780–H1784

Slater H, Wright A 1995 An investigation of the physiological effects of the sympathetic slump on peripheral sympathetic nervous system function in patients with frozen shoulder. Moving in on Pain, Adelaide

Souvlis T, Wright A 1997 The tolerance effect: Its relevance to analgesia produced by physiotherapy interventions. Physical Therapy Reviews 2: 227–237

Souvlis T, Kermode F, Williams E, Collins D, Wright A 1999 Does the initial analgesic effect of spinal manual therapy exhibit tolerance? Ninth World Congress on Pain, Book of Abstracts, Vienna

Souvlis T, Pearce L, Jull G, Wright A 2000a Later analgesic effects of spinal manual therapy on chronic 'tennis elbow' Pre-Olympic Conference. International Congress on Sport Science, Sports Medicine and Physical Education, Brisbane

Souvlis T, Pearce L, Vicenzino B, Jull G A, Wright A 2000b Spinal manual therapy induced hypoalgesia is not naloxone reversible. International Federation of Orthopaedic Manipulative Therapists (IFOMT), Perth

Souvlis T, Vicenzino B, Wright A 2001 Dose of spinal manual therapy influences change in SNS function. Musculoskeletal Physiotherapy Australia (MPA) Biennial Conference, Adelaide

Sterling M, Jull G, Wright A 2000 Cervical mobilisation: concurrent effects on pain, sympathetic nervous system activity and motor activity. Manual Therapy 6: 72–81

Tallarida G, Baldoni F, Peruzzi G, Raimondi G, Massaro M, Sangiorgi M 1981 Cardiovascular and respiratory reflexes from muscles during dynamic and static exercise. Journal of Applied Physiology 50: 784–791

Terrett A J C, Vernon H T 1984 Manipulation and pain tolerance: a controlled study of the effect of spinal manipulation on paraspinal cutaneous pain tolerance levels. American Journal of Physical Medicine 63: 217–225

Thabe H 1986 Electromyography as tool to document diagnostic findings and therapeutic results associated with somatic dysfunctions in the upper cervical spinal joints and sacroiliac joints. Manual Medicine 2: 53–58

Vernon H T 2000 Qualitative review of studies of manipulation-induced hypoalgesia. Journal of Manipulative and Physiological Therapeutics 23: 134–138

Vernon H T, Dhami M S, Howley T P, Annett R 1986 Spinal manipulation and beta-endorphin: a controlled study of the effect of a spinal manipulation on plasma beta-endorphin levels in normal males. Journal of Manipulative and Physiological Therapeutics 9: 115–123

Vernon H T, Aker P D, Burns S, Viljakaanen S, Short L 1990 Pressure pain threshold evaluation of the effect of spinal manipulation in the treatment of chronic neck pain: a pilot study. Journal of Manipulative and Physiological Therapeutics 13: 13–16

Vicenzino B, Collins D, Wright A 1994 Sudomotor changes induced by neural mobilization techniques in asymptomatic subjects. Journal of Manual and Manipulative Therapy 2: 66–74

Vicenzino B, Gutschlag F, Collins D, Wright A 1995 An investigation of the effects of spinal manual therapy on forequarter pressure and thermal pain thresholds and sympathetic nervous system activity in asymptomatic subjects. Moving In On Pain, Adelaide

Vicenzino B, Collins D, Wright A 1996 The initial effects of a cervical spine manipulative physiotherapy treatment on the pain and dysfunction of lateral epicondylalgia. Pain 68: 69–74

Vicenzino B, Collins D, Cartwright T, Wright A 1998a Cardiovascular and respiratory changes produced by lateral glide mobilisation of the cervical spine. Manual Therapy 3: 67–71

Vicenzino B, Collins D, Benson H, Wright A 1998b An investigation of the interrelationship between manipulative therapy-induced hypoalgesia and sympathoexcitation. Journal of Manipulative and Physiological Therapeutics 21: 448–453

Vicenzino B, Cartwright T, Collins D, Wright A 1999a An investigation of stress and pain perception during manual therapy in asymptomatic subjects. European Journal of Pain 3: 13–18

Vicenzino B, Neal R, Collins D, Wright A 1999b The displacement, velocity and frequency profile of the frontal plane motion produced by the cervical lateral glide treatment technique. Clinical Biomechanics 14: 515–521

Vicenzino B, O'Callaghan J, Felicity K, Wright A 2000 No influence of naloxone on the initial hypoalgesic effect of spinal manual therapy. Ninth World Congress on Pain, Vienna

Vicenzino B, Paungmali A, Buratowski S, Wright A 2001 Specific manipulative therapy treatment for chronic lateral epicondylalgia produces uniquely characteristic hypoalgesia. Manual Therapy 6: 205–212

Wright A 1995 Hypoalgesia post manipulative therapy. Manual Therapy 1: 11–16

Wright A, Vicenzino B 1995 Central mobilisation techniques, sympathetic nervous system effects and their relationship to analgesia. Moving in on Pain, Adelaide

Wyke B D 1985 Articular neurology and manipulative therapy. In: Glasgow E F (ed) Aspects of manipulative therapy. Churchill Livingstone, Edinburgh, pp 72–77

Yezierski R P 1991 Somatosensory input to the periaqueductal gray: a spinal relay to a descending control center. In: Depaulis A, Bandler

R (eds) The midbrain periaqueductal gray matter. Plenum Press, New York, pp 365–386

Zhu Y H, Haldeman S, Hsieh C J, Pingjia W, Starr A 2000 Do cerebral potentials to magnetic stimulation of paraspinal muscles reflect changes in palpable muscle spasm, low back pain, and activity scores. Journal of Manipulative and Physiological Therapeutics 23: 458–464

Zusman M 1992 Central nervous contribution to mechanically produced motor and sensory responses. Australian Journal of Physiotherapy 38: 245–255

Zusman M 1994 What does manipulation do? The need for basic research. In: Boyling J D, Palastanga N (eds) Grieve's Modern Manual Therapy: the Vertebral Column. Churchill Livingstone, Edinburgh, pp 651–659

Zusman M, Edwards B, Donaghy A 1989 Investigation of a proposed mechanism for the relief of spinal pain with passive joint movement. Journal of Manual Medicine 4: 58–61

Chapter **26**

Manual therapy and tissue stiffness

D. Shirley

MANUAL THERAPY

Manual therapy involves manual application of forces and is commonly used in the assessment and treatment of low back pain (LBP) (Grieve 1984, Maitland et al 2001). These forces are often applied in a posteroanterior (PA) direction. The use of manually applied forces in treatment relies on judgements made by the clinician during the application of PA forces in assessment. While forces have been used in this way since the time of Hippocrates (Schiotz & Cyriax 1975), until recently there had not been any substantial changes to the method of application or in the understanding of their mechanism of effect. Nevertheless, manual therapy is an effective treatment for LBP. Recent evidence based guidelines recommend that manual therapy is most effective in the management of acute LBP although its use in chronic LBP remains controversial (Bigos et al 1994, Clinical Standards Advisory Group 1994, Waddell et al 1996). In response to the need for evidence to explain the underlying mechanisms of manual therapy, there has been a marked increase in research in this area. This recent research has made a significant contribution to our understanding of the spine's responses to manually applied forces. It is anticipated that this growing body of knowledge will lead to suggestions of how to optimize the use of manual therapy techniques and allow the identification of subgroups of people with LBP for whom manual therapy may be most effective.

Manual therapy includes both passive mobilization and manipulation techniques. Passive mobilization is the application of passive movements to the spine in a rhythmical oscillating fashion. These movements are under the voluntary control of the patient and can be prevented by the patient (Maitland et al 2001). Manipulation is a high velocity, low amplitude thrust performed with a minimum of force applied at or near the end of available range of movement. Manipulation is not under the voluntary control of the patient (Maitland et al 2001). Mobilizations are described by grades of movement (i.e. grade I–IV) depending on where they are performed in range. A manipulation could be described as a higher grade of mobilization (e.g.

grade V) (Maitland et al 2001). Both mobilization and manipulation are often applied over the posterior structures of the spine and the techniques involve applying forces in a PA direction.

The mechanisms by which manual therapy techniques are effective are not fully understood. Proposed mechanisms include mechanical effects and neurophysiological effects (Zusman 1986). Mechanical effects could involve a permanent or temporary change in length of connective tissue structures, such as the joint capsule of the zygapophysial joints, ligaments and muscle. It seems unlikely that any observed changes in mobility associated with mobilization are due to permanent changes in the length of connective tissue. To achieve permanent changes in a single treatment session the force used would have to be great enough to cause micro-failure of the tissue (Threlkeld 1992). Threlkeld (1992) suggests that the forces used in manual therapy techniques are not great enough to result in microfailure of tissue and are more likely to cause temporary length changes due to creep which is reversible over time. Therefore, mechanical effects on the passive tissues do not adequately explain the dramatic changes in mobility that are observed in the clinic and maintained between treatments.

Neurophysiological mechanisms have also been postulated to account for changes in PA mobility observed in response to the application of PA forces. One of these neurophysiological mechanisms may be modulation of the afferent input such that the perception of pain is diminished (Zusman 1986). While the mechanisms are still not fully understood, there is growing evidence to support the notion that the reduction of pain following manual therapy is due at least in part to activation of the descending inhibition system (Wright 1995). In addition, muscle activity is thought to occur in response to pain (Mennell 1960, Travell & Simons 1983) and increased muscle excitability in response to joint pathology or pain provocation has been demonstrated in animal models (Ferrell et al 1988, Qing-Ping & Woolff 1995). If increased muscle activity occurs in response to pain, then it would be expected that muscle activity might reduce if the level of pain reduces (Katavich 1998). As it is a common belief that muscle activity contributes to stiffness detected by applied PA forces, reducing pain and subsequently associated muscle activity may lead to a decrease in PA stiffness.

POSTEROANTERIOR (PA) STIFFNESS

Posteroanterior (PA) stiffness is the term used by physiotherapists and other practitioners of manual therapy to describe the resistance to movement felt when a force is applied in the PA direction to the spinous process of a vertebra in the lumbar spine (Maitland et al 2001). When a PA force is applied the therapist obtains information about the reproduction of the patient's symptoms, any increase in PA stiffness and whether any muscle spasm is present

(Maitland et al 2001). This information is then used to determine the most appropriate technique to use for treatment. A common method of choosing treatment is to use the passive accessory technique that most closely reproduces the patient's symptoms during assessment (Maitland et al 2001). It is believed that applying the technique, as a treatment, will result in a decrease in pain, PA stiffness and muscle activity. Although this belief has not been fully investigated, understanding of the relationship between pain, stiffness and muscle activity is continually improving.

Stiffness is the relationship between force and displacement – i.e. the force required to move a tissue through a given displacement. In manual therapy terms PA stiffness is the resistance to movement perceived by a therapist when applying a PA force manually to the spine (Maitland et al 2001). Stiffness as assessed manually in the clinic is a complex phenomenon. For many years it was believed that stiffness represented the resistance to movement at the particular intervertebral level at which the force was being applied and has often been referred to as intersegmental stiffness. However, when a force is applied to the spine a complex movement occurs which includes anterior rotation of the pelvis, extension of the spine, compression of the ribcage, compression of the abdominal contents, increase in intra-abdominal pressure and a small amount of intervertebral movement (Lee et al 1996). Therefore, it is important to be aware that manual examination of PA stiffness provides information about the response of the spine and associated structures to PA force applied at a particular level.

MEASUREMENT OF STIFFNESS

Manual assessment

The assessment of the response of the spine to applied PA forces is generally carried out manually in the clinic. However, mechanical devices have also been devised to produce an objective measure of the spine's response. Clinicians assess the spine manually with PA forces to obtain an impression of the status of the soft tissues and stiffness (compliance) of the spine. The information about stiffness of the spine is based on a subjective judgement of the spine's response when PA forces are applied.

Manual assessment has been shown to be unreliable in determining whether there is increased stiffness (Maher & Adams 1994, Matyas & Bach 1985). An early study determined that students are unreliable in judging stiffness but that they are reliable in determining the pain response (Matyas & Bach 1985). This work has been criticized because those making stiffness judgements were physiotherapy students who were inexperienced in the use of these techniques. However, further studies using experienced manipulative physiotherapists have found similar results, indicating that experience does not improve reliability of stiffness judgements. Experienced manipulative physiotherapists demonstrated good reliability for making pain judgements but were unreliable with stiffness judgements on patients with LBP being tested with the range of forces used by physiotherapists in clinical practice (Binkley et al 1995, Maher & Adams 1994). The value of identifying painful segments is highlighted by the ability of some therapists to accurately detect symptomatic levels of the cervical or lumbar spine compared to spinal level diagnosis with segmental nerve blocks when manual examination is accompanied by the patient's verbal response (Jull et al 1988, Phillips & Twomey 1996). In contrast, a manipulative physiotherapist demonstrated excellent agreement when identifying symptomatic segments of the cervical spine without feedback of the pain response from the patient suggesting that pain may not be the only important factor (Jull et al 1994). Furthermore, the identification of some asymptomatic individuals as symptomatic (Jull et al 1977) suggests that the clinical picture is also important to give manual findings clinical relevance.

The ability to make judgements about spinal PA stiffness is a complex task that is influenced by many variables. Standardizing some of the variables that affect the judgement may result in better reliability of this process. These variables can be described in the following categories: the perception of stiffness; variations in technique; and patient variations (Lee et al 1996).

Judgements about PA stiffness of the spine are made from a subjective interpretation of the information perceived when applying PA forces to the lumbar spine. However, it is not known exactly which information the therapist focuses on when making judgements of PA stiffness. Stiffness judgements may involve the therapist focusing on either abnormal tissue stiffness, which could be due to muscle reactivity, qualities of the response through range (Jull et al 1994) or other patient or therapist related factors.

Perception of stiffness could relate to the responses of the spine early in range or the stiffness characteristics later in range. Patients with LBP have decreased displacement of the spine early in range as well as increased stiffness later in range during an episode of LBP (Latimer et al 1996), suggesting that the responses of the spine throughout the entire range of force application are worthy of further consideration. Although the importance of the non-linear phase early in range is still not fully understood, the addition of a non-linear toe region to non-biological elastic stimuli did not alter the ability to discriminate stiffness (Nicholson et al 1998) compared to elastic stimuli alone (Nicholson et al 1997). It is possible that different therapists focus on different aspects of the response when they apply a PA force to make their stiffness judgement. Variations in the focus of attention of the spine's response to PA loading could lead to different judgements of stiffness and therefore contribute to the poor inter-rater reliability.

Variation in therapist technique during manual application of a PA force can also influence perception and reliability of spinal PA stiffness. Variations in therapist technique include the direction of force application (Allison et al 1998, Caling & Lee 2001, Viner & Lee 1995), the vertebral level tested (Lee & Liversidge 1994, Viner et al 1997), the contact grip used (Maher & Adams 1996a, Squires et al 2001), the frequency of force application (Lee & Svensson 1993, Squires et al 2001), the magnitude of the applied force (Latimer et al 1998) and vision (Maher & Adams 1996b). The evidence that variations in therapist technique can influence PA stiffness highlights the importance of standardizing the methods of application which in turn may lead to increased inter-therapist reliability.

Patient variations that influence PA stiffness include body mass index (BMI) and vertebral level. People with a low BMI tend to increased PA stiffness compared to those with a higher BMI (Viner et al 1997). In addition, PA stiffness varies between vertebral levels (Viner et al 1997) and between individuals (Shirley et al 2002). Therefore, interpreting PA stiffness judgements by comparison to levels above and below the level being tested as well as to the therapists understanding of stiffness in the population (Maitland et al 2001) is probably of limited value.

Muscle activity is another factor that influences PA stiffness. Activation of various trunk muscles (Lee et al 1993, Shirley et al 1999) and muscles of respiration (Shirley et al 2003a) increases lumbar PA stiffness. Therefore, if the patient is not relaxed and there is activation of their trunk muscles during stiffness assessment it is possible that this activation could increase stiffness.

Many factors influence the PA stiffness of people measured with a mechanical device and also affect the perception of stiffness in manual assessment. Understanding the factors that influence judgements of PA stiffness highlights the aspects of manual stiffness testing that it is important to standardize to improve reliability. Improving reliability will also increase therapists' confidence that changes in PA stiffness observed clinically reflect true changes in stiffness.

Mechanical assessment

Mechanical devices were developed in the various professions utilizing manual therapy as assessment and treatment techniques to overcome the problems with reliability of manual assessment and to more accurately quantify the effects of applying forces to the spine. Some of the earlier devices include the tissue compliance meter (Fischer 1987) and the spinal physiotherapy simulator (SPS) (Lee & Svensson 1990). Similar devices were also developed by a number of researchers in the area of manual therapy (Edmondston et al 1998, Keller & Colloca 2000, Lee 1995). More recently, portable and more sophisticated versions of these devices have been developed. A portable version of the SPS was described by Latimer et al (1996a) and was the first of its kind to be easily transported to the clinic to study subjects with LBP (Fig. 26.1). In addition, Colloca et al (2001) report the development of a hand-held stiffness measurement device also suitable for testing people with LBP in the clinical setting.

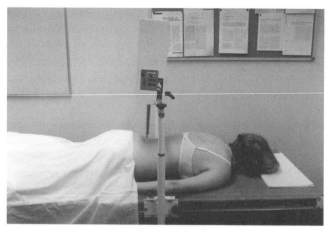

Figure 26.1 Portable mechanical stiffness testing device. The device consists of a mechanical component housing a servo-controlled motor, a strain gauge to measure force and a linear potentiometer to measure displacement. The device is supported on a frame that can be moved in a caudad and cephalad direction along the rigid plinth so that it can be positioned over the target level. The device can also be set at the required angle for application of force. An indentor moves downward from the mechanical device to make contact with the skin over a spinous process. When the device is activated the indentor moves up and down in a rhythmical manner. Adapted from Shirley et al 2002.

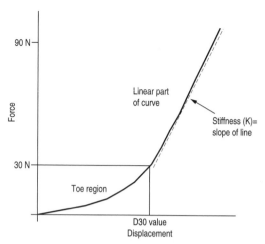

Figure 26.2 Schematic diagram of part of a force displacement curve (loading to 90 N) showing stiffness coefficient K and D30. Stiffness coefficient K is the slope of a regression line fitted to the curve between 30 and 90 N. Displacement D30 is the displacement between 2 and 30 N of force. Reproduced from Shirley et al 2002.

Mechanical devices provide reliable (Latimer et al 1996a, Lee & Svensson 1990) and accurate measures of stiffness (Keller et al 1999, Latimer et al 1996a) thus making them suitable for evaluating the stiffness responses of the spine. It is not clear, however, how closely the application of force to the spine replicates that used in the manual assessment of stiffness, suggesting comparison between manual and mechanically assessed stiffness may not be appropriate. Nevertheless, the investigations with mechanical devices have enabled a greater understanding of the mechanical responses of the spine to PA loading and have allowed investigation of factors that contribute to stiffness, such as muscle activity.

The key elements of these devices are that they apply forces to the spine and measure the resulting displacement. These variables can then be used to make force displacement curves from which stiffness can be calculated (Fig. 26.2). A common method of calculating PA stiffness involves fitting a regression line to the force displacement curve between 30 and 90 N of force (Latimer et al 1996a, Shirley et al 2002). This range of force has been used because the force displacement curve is usually linear in this range. Variation in experimental methodology has led to variations in the calculated stiffness values according to the maximum force applied, the number of loading cycles and the range of forced used in the calculation of stiffness (Shirley et al 2002). The variation in methodology between researchers means that comparison of absolute stiffness values between studies is not valid. However, the individual results provide some very useful information about the responses of the spine to PA loading.

Mechanical assessment is especially useful for research purposes and provides information that helps to explain the responses to manual therapy observed clinically. These devices have not been developed for routine use clinically and most are too cumbersome and time-consuming for everyday use. Therefore, practitioners of manual therapy still primarily rely on their manual skills for assessment and treatment of patients. Information provided by studies using mechanical devices has led to refinement of manual techniques and has provided explanations for some clinical observations.

LUMBAR RESPONSES TO PA FORCES

In addition to understanding factors that influence judgements of PA stiffness, there is a growing interest in the area of manually applied forces, with an increasing body of work discussing the responses of the lumbar spine to applied PA forces in both asymptomatic and symptomatic subjects. The responses examined include PA stiffness, displacement and muscle activity, with measurements made while the subjects were at rest or performing tasks involving activation of trunk and respiratory muscles. It is interesting to consider the findings of recent studies and speculate on their implications for the understanding of mechanisms related to manual therapy and clinical practice.

Normal lumbar PA response

When PA forces are applied to the lumbar spine there is a time-dependent behaviour similar to the cyclic response previously described in cadaveric and living tissues (Lee &

Evans 1992, Yahia et al 1991). This response was also demonstrated uniformly in a group of asymptomatic individuals (Shirley et al 2002), and therefore could be termed the normal response to PA loading. The normal response of PA loading to the lumbar spine is stable over short periods of time (e.g. 5 minutes), and also over a longer period (up to 8 days) (Shirley et al 2002). Furthermore, the PA response of asymptomatic subjects did not change over much longer periods of up to 7 months (Shirley et al 2003b). Therefore, the lumbar PA responses generally do not vary over time in asymptomatic individuals if the testing conditions are constant.

The response during the first loading cycle is different from that of subsequent cycles, that is, stiffness was less and displacement was greater (Shirley et al 2002). This response was consistent each time PA stiffness was measured, even after a short interval of 5 minutes. Therefore, this finding indicates that it may be important to omit the first cycle from analysis of research data. In addition, if comparisons of data from different studies are undertaken, it is important to make sure equivalent testing procedures and analyses are compared. Comparison of stiffness data between studies that have included the first cycle and those that have excluded the first cycle is not recommended as those that have reported results using the first cycle will report a lower stiffness. It is suggested that the variation between the first and subsequent cycles during application of PA forces should be considered as a normal response of the tissues of the lumbar spine to cyclic loading in asymptomatic subjects.

The normal responses of the lumbar spine to loading with PA forces have implications for the use of these forces in clinical examination of patients with LBP as well as for research purposes. As the lumbar spine exhibits time-dependent behaviour to mechanical loading within a series of loading cycles, the clinical application of PA forces to assess PA stiffness may result in the short-term decreases in PA stiffness perceived during assessment with PA forces. These effects due to testing the lumbar spine with PA forces are no longer apparent after 5 minutes. An important implication is that mechanisms other than the time-dependent behaviour of tissues may be responsible for changes in PA stiffness lasting for longer periods of time (e.g. between treatments).

Muscle activity and lumbar PA stiffness

Much of the research on the effects of manual therapy has involved investigating the muscle responses that occur during high velocity manipulative (thrust) techniques. These techniques provoke a reflex response in the muscles adjacent to the spine and in some cases also distant from the spine (Herzog et al 1999). Alternate approaches have reported an increase in mean amplitude of EMG in response to a slow sustained load (8 seconds) and a reduction in the mean amplitude after a manipulative thrust in asymptomatic subjects (Kawchuk & Fauvel 2001). In addi-

tion, recent studies provide the first evidence of a relationship between muscle responses (measured by reflex activity and mean amplitude) and PA stiffness in the lumbar spine in both a population with acute LBP and asymptomatic individuals (Colloca & Keller 2001, Shirley et al 2003b).

Muscle activation and PA forces have been investigated in two ways: first, the response of PA stiffness to PA forces applied during voluntary activation of various trunk and respiratory muscles in asymptomatic subjects; and second, the response to applied PA forces in passive symptomatic and asymptomatic subjects. The effects of various voluntary activities, including activation of the erector spinae muscles, abdominal muscles, respiratory muscles and associated intra-abdominal pressure on lumbar PA stiffness, have been determined in addition to the responses of the erector spinae in the resting subject with LBP.

Voluntary activation of muscles that act on the lumbar spine increases lumbar PA stiffness (Shirley et al 1999, 2003a). Voluntary activation of the lumbar extensor muscles significantly increased lumbar PA stiffness by 12% even when the activation was as low as 10% MVC (Shirley et al 1999). The increase in stiffness was in the range of elastic stiffness able to be detected manually by some manipulative physiotherapists (Maher & Adams 1995, Nicholson et al 1997), that is, about 8–11%. Therefore, stiffness increases of 12% due to small amounts of voluntary activity are in the range that could be detected during examination with PA forces by some physiotherapists.

Respiratory muscle activation during voluntary respiratory manoeuvres influenced lumbar PA stiffness (Beaumont et al 1991, Shirley et al 2003a). There was no increase in PA stiffness with breath holding at different inspiratory lung volumes when subjects were instructed to hold their breath with the glottis closed (Shirley et al 2003a). It is a natural response to close the glottis to maintain lung volume during breath holding, as less respiratory effort is required (inspiratory muscles are able to relax). Confirming this, a further study demonstrated that breath holding at the same lung volumes with the glottis held closed significantly decreased PA stiffness compared to breath holding with the glottis open (Shirley et al 2003a). The difference between these manoeuvres was greater activation of the respiratory, abdominal and erector spinae muscles with the glottis open (Fig. 26.3). In addition, there was an increase in trans-diaphragmatic pressure with the glottis open.

Increases in PA stiffness occur during dynamic tasks such as tidal breathing (Shirley 2002) and other tasks that involve activation of the respiratory muscles (Shirley et al 2003a), lending support to the theory that it is muscle activity rather than lung volume that increases lumbar PA stiffness during these voluntary tasks. While there was no difference in PA stiffness with breath held at different lung volumes with the glottis closed, there were changes in stiffness between inspiratory and expiratory cycles during dynamic breathing with corresponding changes in respiratory muscle activity (Shirley 2002). In addition, the finding that

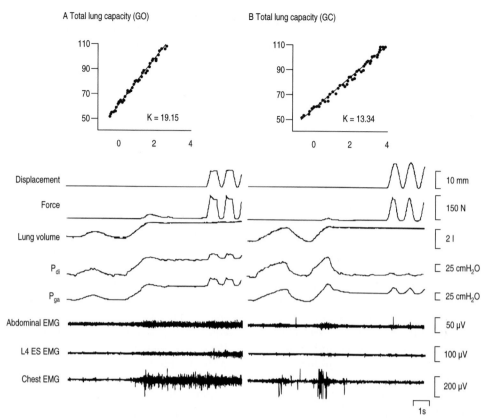

Figure 26.3 Representative data for the total lung capacity (TLC) condition with (A) the glottis open (GO) and (B) closed (GC). At TLC with the glottis open there is a marked increase in stiffness. The data show an increased lung volume along with increases in EMG and pressures during the period of loading. By comparison when testing was carried out at TLC with the glottis closed the stiffness decreased. The lung volume remains high; however, there is less activity in the EMG and P_{di} is decreased. P_{ga} does not decrease significantly. These data suggest increased lung volume does not lead to increased stiffness but that EMG and pressure play a major role. Reproduced from Shirley et al 2003a.

there is greater stiffness when loading is applied at the L2 level, where there is a direct attachment of the diaphragm, than at L4 provides further evidence that the diaphragm may contribute to lumbar PA stiffness (Fig. 26.4). Furthermore, the evidence that factors including trunk and respiratory muscle activity and intra-abdominal and trans-diaphragmatic pressures contribute to lumbar PA stiffness is added support for the multifactorial nature of stiffness (Shirley et al 2003a).

Voluntary activation of trunk and respiratory muscles increases PA stiffness and the mechanism is likely to be due to a combination of many factors and involve contributions from various muscles that contribute to lumbar stability, either by their direct actions on the lumbar spine or indirectly via the thoracolumbar fascia or by increasing intra-abdominal pressure. In summary, the evidence indicates that muscle activity increases PA stiffness, even when activation is small (Shirley et al 1999), and particularly when there is maximal activity of the muscles (Shirley et al 1999, 2003a).

The implication of these findings for clinical practice is that it is important to standardize the respiratory effort of

patients during testing of PA stiffness. If the patient is holding their breath with a closed glottis the lung volume does not appear to be important. However, it may be easier for subjects to breath-hold at volumes greater than functional residual capacity (FRC) as they will not be as oxygen depleted. In addition, specific instructions about glottis closure should be given as there is more muscle activity and greater stiffness with the glottis held open. It is also important for the patient to be relaxed during assessment of PA stiffness because activation of the lumbar extensors or other trunk muscles will potentially affect stiffness of the lumbar spine.

Stiffness is greatest when the breath is held at maximal expiration with an open glottis (Shirley et al 2003a). People often breath-hold or breathe out during tasks involving considerable exertion such as lifting, weight-lifting, etc. While there is no demonstrated relationship between PA stiffness in prone to stability during tasks in other positions it is interesting to speculate on the purpose of breathing out during exertion. This practice may have come about because it increases stiffness of the spine and it may be a natural mechanism to attempt to stabilize the spine. Shirley

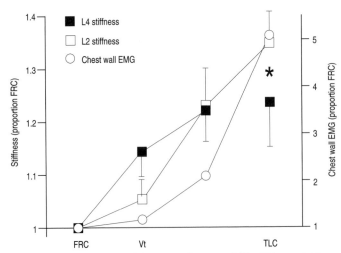

Figure 26.4 Proportional increases in mean (SE) stiffness at L2 and L4. There was a different pattern of increase in stiffness when the spine was loaded at L2 to when loaded at L4 (mean ± SD). The increase when loaded at L4 is most marked between functional residual capacity (FRC) and end tidal inspiration (Vt) and then plateaus with increasing effort (50% inspiration (50% insp) and total lung capacity (TLC)). In contrast the increase at L2 is more gradual over the range of respiratory tasks chosen. The pattern of increase in stiffness at L2 is similar to the pattern of increase in chest wall EMG. *Significant difference in stiffness between L2 and L4 at TLC. Reproduced from Shirley et al 2003a.

et al (2003a) provide the first evidence that activity of erector spinae, abdominal muscles and the diaphragm, which contribute to the stabilization of the spine during active tasks (Hodges & Richardson 1997, Hodges et al 1997), also contribute to PA stiffness.

The diaphragm is active during tasks that require stabilization of the lumbar spine (Hodges et al 1997). The diaphragm produces phasic activity related to the breathing pattern as well as tonic activity while the task is performed (Hodges & Gandevia 2000). In asymptomatic subjects without respiratory compromise, the diaphragm is able to perform both of these functions simultaneously (Hodges & Gandevia 2000). The implications of respiratory disease on the function of the diaphragm and its role in stability of the spine have not yet been investigated. However, people with respiratory disease are more susceptible to LBP (Synnot & Williams 2001) or may be more likely to develop chronic LBP. Therefore, the link between respiratory compromise and the role of the diaphragm in relation to its stabilizing function in the presence of LBP is an interesting direction for future research.

PA STIFFNESS, MUSCLE ACTIVITY AND LOW BACK PAIN

A further important aspect of understanding the relationship between manual therapy and tissue stiffness is to examine whether there is a relationship between PA stiffness, lumbar muscle activity and LBP. Investigation of individuals with LBP indicates that those with LBP have increased lumbar PA stiffness (Latimer et al 1996b). However, the effect is only small. An important finding of recent work is the evidence that a combination of stiffness and variables of muscle activity are associated with low back pain during an acute episode of LBP (Shirley et al 2003b). In addition, the presence of pain many months later is also associated with a combination of stiffness and muscle activity factors during the episode of pain (Shirley 2002). The association is interesting because, during the acute episode of LBP, higher pain intensity is associated with higher stiffness. However, over the longer term, low stiffness in the acute phase appears to be associated with longer lasting pain. There was also a trend for lower muscle activity during the initial episode to be associated with ongoing symptoms.

Increased stiffness during an episode of LBP may be the body's mechanism to protect the spine against further damage. It is interesting to note that low stiffness and lower muscle activity during the initial episode seem to be associated with longer lasting pain. While only erector spinae activity has been measured during applied PA forces, it is possible there was also decreased activity of other spinal stabilizing muscles that were not measured (e.g. multifidus and transversus abdominis). These muscles may be recruited to stabilize the spine in response to externally applied PA forces. It is possible that there is inhibition of muscle activity due to pain. Transversus abdominis and multifidus do not activate as early during voluntary activity in people with LBP (Hides et al 1994, Hodges & Richardson 1998, 1999) and decreased cross-sectional area of multifidus is associated with acute LBP (Hides et al 1994). Consideration of the importance of decreased muscle activity and low stiffness allows speculation of the implications for treatment of acute LBP. When stiffness is low, exercises aimed at improving the function of stabilizing muscles may be more appropriate than manual therapy as exercises should help to stabilize and stiffen the spine.

Reflex muscle responses to the application of manipulation to the spine have been described both for people with and for people without LBP (Colloca & Keller 2001, Herzog et al 1999). These studies have applied fast manipulative thrust techniques to the spine using mechanical devices. In contrast, when slower forces are applied to the lumbar spine (0.5–1 Hz), a stretch reflex response is not triggered in all subjects (Shirley et al 2003b). A stretch reflex response was elicited in some individuals, although these responses were observed in both symptomatic and asymptomatic subjects. However, there was a trend for increased stretch reflex responses in people with pain during an episode of LBP (Shirley et al 2003b). These results suggest that while reflex responses of the erector spinae may occur in response to a manipulative thrust or mobilization procedure, they may be a normal response to forces applied to the spine in some people irrespective of their pain status. Therefore, at least in the resting patient, reflex activity of the erector spinae may not be a major contributing factor to PA stiffness.

The relationship between reflex responses and stiffness in people with pain should be interpreted with caution at this time. In the study by Colloca & Keller (2001) approximately two-thirds of the subjects were classified as having reflex responses to manipulative forces applied in a PA direction. However, the majority of subjects (63.7%) were in the lower quarter for magnitude of reflex response. This information is supported by the findings of Shirley et al (2003b) that some people are responders and some are not. In addition there appeared to be no difference in the stiffness between those with reflex response and those without for PA forces delivered to the spinous processes (Colloca 2001). This also is consistent with the results of other work that demonstrated no difference in PA stiffness between subjects with pain and those without pain (Shirley et al 2003b).

Voluntary activity of the erector spinae as low as 10% of MVC increased PA stiffness by approximately 11% (Shirley et al 1999). However, the increase in stiffness related to voluntary activation of the erector spinae does not necessarily indicate that spontaneous activity occurring in people with LBP will also increase stiffness. An increase in the mean amplitude of activity of the erector spinae in response to applied PA forces has been described in subjects with LBP (Shirley et al 2003b). It is possible that the increases in erector spinae activity detected in pain subjects in response to applied PA forces are not of great enough magnitude to result in clinically relevant increases in stiffness. While a contraction of 10% MVC of erector spinae results in a significant increase in PA stiffness, it is interesting to note that the level of activity in response to applied PA forces in people with pain was only approximately 4.4% of an MVC (Shirley et al 2003b), which may not be big enough to influence PA stiffness. Clearly, there is scope for further research in this area to more comprehensively investigate the relationship between PA stiffness, muscle activity and LBP.

CHARACTERIZATION OF PA STIFFNESS

In many studies reporting PA stiffness derived from data provided by mechanical stiffness testing devices, the stiffness has been calculated from the loading part of the force displacement curve. Typically force values between 30 and 90 N have been used and it is likely that this range of force only depicts elastic stiffness in the early part of the loading

cycle. Therefore, this method of calculating PA stiffness does not take into account the full range of the loading curve or involve the unloading curve. The stiffness responses are usually termed stiffness coefficient K and displacement D30. Other researchers have used different methods to calculate PA stiffness which involve force and acceleration properties (Colloca & Keller 2001).

In an attempt to more accurately describe the loading curve a method of calculation of the stiffness responses including viscous and elastic properties has been developed (Nicholson et al 2001). Examining the muscle responses in relation to the viscous and elastic properties of the complete loading/unloading curve may provide a more complete picture of the relationship between PA stiffness, muscle activity and LBP. In addition, a greater understanding of the properties of the loading cycle may highlight the components that are most critical in clinical manual assessment, thus indicating a direction for further research.

CONCLUSION

Interpretation of the responses of the spine to applied PA forces is a complex process. However, a marked increase in research in this area of manual therapy in recent years has made significant contributions to understanding responses and mechanisms. With greater understanding of stiffness responses and methods of application it is possible that reliability and accuracy of stiffness assessment may be improved. The focus of recent research has been investigation of the relationship between spinal stiffness and muscle activity. Voluntary muscle activation plays a key role in influencing stiffness of the spine. Furthermore, reflex muscle responses to applied PA forces have been described in symptomatic and asymptomatic people but are variable and do not consistently relate to pain, although increased mean amplitude of erector spinae activity is associated with LBP. Finally, further investigation of the relationship between factors relating to increased stiffness and muscle activity in individuals with LBP may lead to more appropriate treatment selection involving combinations of manual therapy techniques and muscle activation/stabilizing techniques.

KEYWORDS	
manual therapy	spinal stiffness
tissue stiffness	PA stiffness
muscle activity	reflex response

References

Allison G T, Edmondston S J, Roe C P, Reid S E, Toy D A, Lundgren H E 1998 Influence of load orientation on the posteroanterior stiffness of the lumbar spine. Journal of Manipulative and Physiological Therapeutics 21: 534–538

Beaumont A, McCrum C, Lee M 1991 The effects of tidal breathing and breath-holding on the postero-anterior stiffness of the lumbar spine.

In: Seventh Biennial Conference of the Manipulative Physiotherapists Association of Australia, Blue Mountains, New South Wales, pp 244–251

Bigos S, Bowyer O, Brean G 1994 Acute low back problems in adults. Clinical Practice Guideline no. 14. ACHPR publication no. 95-0642. Agency for Health Care Policy and Research, Public Health

Service, US Department of Health and Human Services, Rockville, Maryland

Binkley J, Stratford P W, Gill C 1995 Interrater reliability of lumbar accessory motion mobility testing . . . including commentary by Maher C with author response. Physical Therapy 75: 786–795

Caling B, Lee M 2001 Effect of direction of applied mobilization force on the posteroanterior response in the lumbar spine. Journal of Manipulative and Physiological Therapeutics 24: 71–78

Colloca C J, Keller T S 2001 Stiffness and neuromuscular reflex response of the human spine to posteroanterior manipulative thrusts in patients with low back pain. Journal of Manipulative and Physiological Therapeutics 24: 489–500

Clinical Standards Advisory Group (CSAG) 1994. Back pain: report of a CSAG committee on back pain. Clinical Standards Advisory Group, HMSO, London

Edmondston S J, Allison G T, Gregg C D, Purden S M, Svansson G R, Watson A E 1998 Effect of position on the posteroanterior stiffness of the lumbar spine. Manual Therapy 3: 21–26

Ferrell W R, Wood L, Baxendale R H 1988 The effect of acute joint inflammation on flexion reflex excitability in the decerebrate, low spinal cat. Quarterly Journal of Experimental Physiology 73: 103–111

Fischer A 1987 Clinical use of tissue compliance meter for documentation of soft tissue pathology. Clinical Journal of Pain 3: 23–30

Grieve G 1984 Mobilisation of the spine: notes on examination, assessment and clinical method. Churchill Livingstone, Edinburgh

Herzog W, Scheele D, Conway P J 1999 Electromyographic responses of back and limb muscles associated with spinal manipulative therapy. Spine 24: 146–152; discussion, 153

Hides J A, Stokes M J, Saide M, Jull G, Cooper D H 1994 Evidence of lumbar multifidus muscle wasting ipsilateral to symptoms in patients with acute/subacute low back pain. Spine 19: 165–172

Hodges P W, Gandevia S C 2000 Activation of the human diaphragm during a repetitive postural task. Journal of Physiology 522: 165–175

Hodges P W, Richardson C A 1997 Contraction of the abdominal muscles associated with movement of the lower limb. Physical Therapy 77: 132–142; Discussion 142–144

Hodges P W, Richardson C A 1998 Delayed postural contraction of transversus abdominis in low back pain associated with movement of the lower limb. Journal of Spinal Disorders 11: 46–56

Hodges P W, Richardson C A 1999 Altered trunk muscle recruitment in people with low back pain with upper limb movement at different speeds. Archives of Physical Medicine and Rehabilitation 80: 1005–1012

Hodges P W, Butler J E, McKenzie D K, Gandevia S C 1997 Contraction of the human diaphragm during rapid postural adjustments. Journal of Physiology 505: 539–548

Jull G, Zito G, Trott P, Potter H, Shirley D, Richardson C 1977 Inter-examiner reliability to detect painful upper cervical joint dysfunction. Australian Journal of Physiotherapy 43(2): 125–129

Jull G, Bogduk N, Marsland A 1988 The accuracy of manual diagnosis for cervical zygapophyseal joint pain syndromes. Medical Journal of Australia 148: 233–236

Jull G, Treleaven J, Versace G 1994 Manual examination: is pain provocation a major cue for spinal dysfunction? Australian Journal of Physiotherapy 40: 159–165

Katavich L 1998 Differential effects of spinal manipulative therapy on acute and chronic muscle spasm: a proposal for mechanics and efficacy. Manual Therapy 3: 132–139

Kawchuk G N, Fauvel O R 2001 Sources of variation in spinal indentation testing: indentation site relocation, intra-abdominal pressure, subject movement, muscular response, and stiffness estimation. Journal of Manipulative and Physiological Therapeutics 24: 84–91

Keller T S, Colloca C J 2000 Mechanical force spinal manipulation increases trunk muscle strength assessed by electromyography: a comparative clinical trial. Journal of Manipulative and Physiological Therapeutics 23: 585–595

Keller T S, Colloca C J, Fuhr A W 1999 Validation of the force and frequency characteristics of the activator adjusting instrument: effectiveness as a mechanical impedance measurement tool [Comment]. [Erratum appears in Journal of Manipulative and Physiological Therapeutics 22(6): 367.] Journal of Manipulative and Physiological Therapeutics 22: 75–86

Latimer J, Lee M, Goodsell M, Maher C, Wilkinson B, Adams R 1996a Instrumented measurement of spinal stiffness. Manual Therapy 1: 204–209

Latimer J, Lee M, Moran C 1996b An investigation of the relationship between low back pain and lumbar posteroanterior stiffness. Journal of Manipulative and Physiological Therapeutics 19: 587–591

Latimer J, Lee M, Adams R D 1998 The effects of high and low loading forces on measured values of lumbar stiffness. Journal of Manipulative and Physiological Therapeutics 21: 157–163

Lee R Y 1995 The biomechanical basis of spinal manual therapy. Thesis, University of Strathclyde, Glasgow

Lee R, Evans J 1992 Load-displacement-time characteristics of the spine under posteroanterior mobilisation. Australian Journal of Physiotherapy 38: 115–123

Lee M, Liversidge K 1994 Posteroanterior stiffness at three locations in the lumbar spine. Journal of Manipulative and Physiological Therapeutics 17: 511–516

Lee M, Svensson N 1990 Measurement of stiffness during simulated spinal physiotherapy. Clinical Physics and Physiological Measurement 11: 201–207

Lee M, Svensson N L 1993 Effect of loading frequency on response of the spine to lumbar posteroanterior forces. Journal of Manipulative and Physiological Therapeutics 16: 439–446

Lee M, Esler M A, Mildren J, Herbert R 1993 Effect of extensor muscle activation on the response to lumbar posteroanterior forces. Clinical Biomechanics 8: 115–119

Lee M, Steven G, Crosbie J, Higgs J 1996 Towards a theory of lumbar mobilisation: the relationship between applied force and movements of the spine. Manual Therapy 1: 67–75

Maher C, Adams R 1994 Reliability of pain and stiffness assessments in clinical manual lumbar spine examination. Physical Therapy 74: 801–811

Maher C, Adams R 1995 A psychophysical evaluation of manual stiffness discrimination. Australian Journal of Physiotherapy 41: 161–167

Maher C, Adams R 1996a A comparison of pisiform and thumb grips in stiffness assessment. Physical Therapy 76: 41–48

Maher C G, Adams R D 1996b Stiffness judgments are affected by visual occlusion. Journal of Manipulative and Physiological Therapeutics 19: 250–256

Maitland G, Banks K, English K, Hengeveld E (eds) 2001 Maitland's Vertebral manipulation. Butterworth Heinemann, Oxford

Matyas T, Bach T 1985 The reliability of selected techniques in clinical arthrometrics. Australian Journal of Physiotherapy 31: 175–199

Mennell J M 1960 Back pain: diagnosis and treatment using manipulative techniques. Little, Brown, Boston

Nicholson L, Adams R, Maher C 1997 Reliability of a discrimination measure for judgements of non-biological stiffness. Manual Therapy 2: 150–156

Nicholson L, Maher C, Adams R 1998 Hand contact area, force applied and early non-linear stiffness (toe) in a manual stiffness discrimination task. Manual Therapy 3: 212–219

Nicholson L, Maher C, Adams R, Phan-Thien N 2001 Stiffness properties of the human lumbar spine: a lumped parameter model. Clinical Biomechanics 16: 285–292

Phillips D R, Twomey L T 1996 A comparison of manual diagnosis with a diagnosis established by a uni-level lumbar spinal block procedure. Manual Therapy 1: 82–87

Qing-Ping M, Woolff C J 1995 Noxious stimuli induce an N-methyl-D-aspartate receptor-dependent hypersensitivity of the flexion withdrawal reflex to touch: implications for treatment of mechanical allodynia. Pain 61: 383–390

Schiotz E, Cyriax J 1975 Manipulation past and present. Heinemann, London

Shirley D 2002 Muscle activity and lumbar PA stiffness. PhD thesis, University of Sydney, Sydney

Shirley D, Lee M, Ellis E 1999 The relationship between submaximal activity of the lumbar extensor muscles and lumbar posteroanterior stiffness. Physical Therapy 79: 278–285

Shirley D, Lee M, Ellis E 2002 The response of postero-anterior lumbar stiffness to repeated loading. Manual Therapy 7: 19–25

Shirley D, Hodges P W, Eriksson A E, Gandevia S C 2003a Spinal stiffness changes throughout the respiratory cycle. Journal of Applied Physiology 95: 1467–1475

Shirley D, Lee M, Ellis E, O'Dwyer N J 2003b The relationship between lumbar postero-anterior stiffness, muscle activity and low back pain. Fourteenth International World Confederation of Physical Therapy Congress, Barcelona, Spain, p 104

Squires M C, Latimer J, Adams R D, Maher C G 2001 Indenter head area and testing frequency effects on posteroanterior lumbar stiffness and subjects' rated comfort. Manual Therapy 6: 40–47

Synnot A, Williams M 2001 Prevalence of low back pain in subjects with chronic airflow limitation: a preliminary study. Australian Journal of Physiotherapy 47: 281

Threlkeld A J 1992 The effects of manual therapy on connective tissue. Physical Therapy 72: 893–902

Travell J G, Simons D G 1983 Myofascial pain and dysfunction: the trigger point manual. Williams and Wilkins, Baltimore

Viner A, Lee M 1995 Direction of manual force applied during assessment of stiffness in the lumbosacral spine. Journal of Manipulative and Physiological Therapeutics 18: 441–447

Viner A, Lee M, Adams R 1997 Posteroanterior stiffness in the lumbosacral spine: the correlation between adjacent vertebral levels. Spine 22: 2724–2730

Waddell G, Feder G, McIntosh A, Lewis M, Hutchinson A 1996 Low back pain evidence review. Royal College of General Practitioners, London

Wright A 1995 Hypoalgesia post-manipulative therapy: a review of a potential neurophysiological mechanism. Manual Therapy 1: 11–16

Yahia L, Audet J, Drouin G 1991 Rheological properties of the human lumbar spine ligaments. Journal of Biomedical Engineering 13: 399–406

Zusman M 1986 Spinal manipulative therapy: review of some proposed mechanisms, and a new hypothesis. Australian Journal of Physiotherapy 32: 89–99

Chapter **27**

Clinical reasoning in the diagnosis and management of spinal pain

N. Christensen, M. Jones, I. Edwards

INTRODUCTION

The past decade has been one of evolution within the physiotherapy profession, and one of the catalysts in the changing nature of physiotherapy has been the quest for professional autonomy. Achievement of true professional autonomy requires, in part, that physiotherapists are accountable for their own actions and capable of independent, accurate, appropriate and responsible clinical decisions (Higgs & Hunt 1999). Thus, the promotion of professional autonomy within physiotherapy has provided a strong impetus for continued interest in the understanding and development of superior clinical reasoning skills among practising clinicians and those responsible for educating future clinicians.

To illustrate the clinical reasoning involved in the diagnosis and management of patients, consider the following patient case scenario involving spinal pain:

CASE STUDY

Sandra, a 29-year-old secretary at a university, is suffering from lower back and left leg pain. An avid cyclist and tennis player, Sandra has not participated in either of these activities since the pain began. Her symptoms started 6 weeks ago when, after a long bike ride, she lifted her bicycle onto the rack on the roof of her car. Although Sandra has had episodes of lower back pain in the past, which she relates to long periods working at her computer, this is the first time she has experienced pain radiating into her leg. After consulting with her physician, Sandra was sent home with anti-inflammatory and muscle relaxant medications as well as orders to rest from all strenuous physical activities. After a month of persistent back and leg pain, the physician ordered X-rays and subsequently referred Sandra to physiotherapy with a diagnosis of left L5/S1 grade I spondylolisthesis.

What types of knowledge, thinking, and associated clinical actions are involved when a physiotherapist enters into a collaborative working relationship with a patient? We will consider Sandra's case later in this chapter, after examining in some detail the concept of clinical reasoning and factors which have come to shape our current understanding of this complex process.

Clinical reasoning has been consistently defined as the thinking and decision making processes which occur throughout the evaluation, diagnosis and management of patient problems. Although the definition of clinical reasoning has not changed within the past decade, the description of the factors involved in the clinical reasoning process has changed significantly. For example, in the last edition of this book, Jones (1994, p. 473) described the clinical reasoning process as 'the actions and evolving thoughts used by a clinician to arrive at a diagnostic and management decision and subsequently administer and advance the patient's treatment'. In recent literature, Higgs & Jones (2000, p. 11) have expanded this definition, describing the clinical reasoning process as 'the process in which the clinician, interacting with significant others (client, caregivers, health care team members), structures meaning, goals and health management strategies based on clinical data, client choices, and professional judgement and knowledge'.

This chapter will describe the implications for clinical reasoning that have resulted from changes in the physiotherapy profession over the past 10 years. These changes have been brought about by the evidence based health care (EBHC) movement and by the pain science movement. In addition, the contribution of research will be discussed, specifically in regard to the growth in the conceptualization of clinical reasoning as an interactive, collaborative process that reflects a more holistic appreciation of the role of patients/clients and their personal perspectives or beliefs. This chapter will review a method of organizing clinical knowledge into hypothesis categories, within a clinical reasoning framework. Finally, various orientations or strategies of reasoning will be presented, and their interaction across the broad range of clinical activities related to diagnosis, management and ethical problem solving will be discussed. Our patient with spinal pain, Sandra, introduced above, will serve to provide examples of how hypothesis categories and clinical reasoning strategies are employed by the physiotherapist to guide diagnosis and management decision making.

EVOLUTION IN THE PHYSIOTHERAPY PROFESSION

Two of the most powerful catalysts for change at work within the physiotherapy profession during the past decade have been, and continue to be, the evidence based health care movement and the emergence of biopsychosocial theory from within the pain science literature. As a result of this ongoing change, the following brief examination of the literature will be neither complete nor current by the time this chapter reaches publication. The intention is to provide a framework for the ensuing discussion of how

these changes have contributed to current models of clinical reasoning.

Evidence based health care

The concepts and approach to clinical practice – consolidated and termed evidence based medicine (EBM) or evidence based health care (EBHC) by Guyatt and colleagues (Evidence-Based Medicine Working Group 1992)—originated from a group of clinical epidemiologists originally led by Sackett (Sackett et al 2000). Sackett et al (2000, p. 1) have defined evidence based medicine as 'the integration of best research evidence with clinical expertise and patient values' which results in optimal clinical outcomes and quality of life. Included within the phrase 'clinical expertise' are clinical knowledge, skills and memories of past experiences (Sackett et al 2000). This definition of EBHC in itself does not conflict with the components included in our definition of the clinical reasoning process and therefore should provide no fuel for contention within the academic or clinical practice communities on that basis. However, controversy has arisen over EBHC, in part due to the medical paradigm shift it advocates. This paradigm stresses the importance of examination of evidence from clinical research as the basis of clinical decision making. Traditional clinical decision making in physiotherapy, for most of our professional history, has been based on experiential knowledge. We have not limited our clinical decisions solely to empirically generated evidence. The hierarchy, or rating system, for strength of evidence presented in EBM, however, places a lower value on expert opinion and intuition than does the traditional medical paradigm (Guyatt et al 2002).

Interpretations of what is meant by the term EBHC have varied, as has the reaction to suggestions for practical application of EBHC principles to the clinical research and practice of physiotherapy (Cibulka & Aslin 2001, DiFabio 1999, Fritz 2001, Koes & Hoving 1998). Much of this variability and the resultant controversy can be explained by a common misinterpretation of EBHC as being a call to reject the clinical use of all knowledge other than that generated within a positivist, empirico-analytical, quantitative research paradigm (e.g. via randomized controlled trials). EBHC includes the adoption of a hierarchy of evidence system, which rates the evidence from randomized controlled trials as the strongest and therefore most desirable, evidence upon which to base clinical decisions. A cause for concern and a subject for discussion within the current literature has been the over-emphasis by some on the characterization of the whole of EBHC as clinical decision making based only on quantitative, research based evidence (Binkley 2000, DiFabio 1999, 2000, Fritz 2001, Jones & Higgs 2000, Moore & Petty 2001). Much of the response within the clinical reasoning and education literature has been focused on a call for a broader definition of what is considered 'strong' evidence within an EBHC framework in the allied health professions (Higgs & Titchen 1995, Higgs et al 2001, Jones & Higgs 2000,

Parry 2001). These authors stress the value of evidence including different types of knowledge (such as propositional, professional craft and personal knowledge) emerging from the full spectrum of empirico-analytical and interpretive and critical research paradigms. The knowledge generated from the interpretive and critical research paradigms is often more suitable for answering many of the clinically relevant questions pertaining to patients' pain experiences (i.e. their personal perspectives/beliefs regarding their pain, disability and effects on their lives) as required in the broader biopsychosocial approach (Higgs & Titchen 1998, Higgs et al 2001, Ritchie 1999).

There is great incentive for health researchers to generate and demonstrate the value of clinically relevant qualitative research, since many of our clinical practice tasks require understanding the person as well as the physical problem (Edwards 2000, Jones et al 2000, 2002).

Biopsychosocial theory

The biopsychosocial model of disability is a way of conceptualizing the multifactorial and complex system that shapes a person's experience of pain and disability. This system comprises the pain itself, the person's attitudes and beliefs about the pain, elements of psychological distress experienced and illness behaviours exhibited, and parameters of the social environment in which the person functions (Waddell & Main 1998, Watson 2000). Biopsychosocial theory states that the degree of disability a person develops will be based upon the reaction of that person to the pain experienced far more than on the physical experience of pain itself (Watson 2000). The biopsychosocial model places a complaint of pain into a more holistic context, and views the pain as important not in isolation, but in relation to any disability the person with pain is experiencing as a result of that pain (Gifford 2001, Watson 2000). This is consistent with contemporary learning theory in which peoples' perceptions, and the basis of those perceptions, are recognized as being critical to shaping their beliefs, emotions and behaviours (Mezirow 1991). As Mezirow (1991, p. xiii) has stated, 'it is not so much what happens to people but how they interpret and explain what happens to them that determines their actions, their hopes, their contentment and emotional well-being, and their performance'.

Manual therapists recognize complaints of pain as the most common reason patients give for seeking treatment. Physiotherapy training and practice have been traditionally based in the biomedical model, which views a patient's pain and associated disability as symptoms of underlying tissue pathology. Operating within this model, the main focus of the patient interview and physical examination is to identify physical impairments within the tissues of the neuro-musculoskeletal system, and to determine the appropriate treatment of this tissue (Butler 2000, Gifford 1998c, 1998d, Jones et al 2002, Main & Watson 1999). While attention to psychosocial factors is not new, physiotherapists

have generally learned the skills of psychosocial assessment and management (for example, listening, communicating, negotiating, counselling and motivating) to effect positive changes in their patients' health understanding, beliefs and behaviours through personal experience. As such, physiotherapists have lacked a structured framework of reasoning in which to evaluate their findings and actions in these areas. Consequently the knowledge and interpersonal skills required are often tacit and less developed in some therapists.

This is not a call to abandon assessment and management of physical disability and impairment. Rather, the biopsychosocial approach should be viewed as recognizing the potential relevance of the interaction between biomedical and psychosocial factors in the development of patients' functional limitations and/or disabilities and the associated impairments (Gifford 2001).

Integration of emerging evidence, in this case from the pain sciences and biopsychosocial theory literature, into the clinical reasoning process is one example of movement within the physiotherapy profession towards a more evidence based approach to clinical practice. However, practical application of the biopsychosocial model to physiotherapy practice has been challenging, in that it forces clinicians to expand the scope of factors explicitly assessed and overtly addressed as part of comprehensive patient management. Several authors have suggested models and methods with which to incorporate knowledge of the biopsychosocial model into clinical practice (Butler 2000, Christensen et al 2002, Gifford 1998c, Gifford & Butler 1997, Jones 1995, Jones et al 2002, Main & Watson 1999, Watson 2000, Watson & Kendall 2000). Some of these suggestions, relative to the evolution in the conceptualization of clinical reasoning and the development of models of a more holistic nature, will be discussed in further detail in the next section of this chapter.

EVOLUTION IN MODELS OF CLINICAL REASONING

How have clinical reasoning models in physiotherapy developed in the light of the biopsychosocial theory outlined above? An examination of models of the clinical reasoning process that appear in the physiotherapy clinical reasoning literature reveals a progressive shift in focus and evolution in the research paradigms from which they are derived.

Early models

Early descriptions of clinical reasoning in physiotherapy literature were diagnostically based and drew conclusions suggesting that the clinical reasoning process used by physiotherapists was similar to that described in the medical clinical reasoning research of that time (Payton 1985, Thomas-Edding 1987). At that time, much of the medical education literature was based on a cognitive science paradigm and clinical reasoning was characterized as either pattern recognition or hypothetico-deductive reasoning (see, for example, Elstein et al 1978, Patel & Groen 1986). Whether a medical clinician uses pattern recognition or generates and tests multiple hypotheses depends upon that clinician's level of familiarity with a particular clinical presentation. The emphasis on clinical reasoning within an empirico-analytical reasoning paradigm was shared in the physiotherapy literature, as illustrated by the hypothesis-oriented algorithm proposed by Rothstein & Echternach (1986).

Jones (1992) adapted a model from the medical literature (Barrows & Tamblyn 1980) to depict the clinical reasoning process of physiotherapists. Models or descriptions of the clinical reasoning process in medicine were primarily focused on the diagnostic nature of the initial patient encounter. Jones's model (1994) illustrated the cycle of hypothesis generation, testing, and subsequent modification of hypotheses that occurs throughout the initial evaluation as well as throughout ongoing management of all components of a patient problem.

This representation of the clinical reasoning process also highlights the interaction of all components of the process with the clinician's knowledge base, cognition and metacognition. The knowledge base includes basic science and biomedical knowledge (typically based on research evidence) acquired through formal education. In addition, the knowledge base includes clinical (craft) knowledge (for example clinical patterns, assessment, reasoning and management related knowledge) acquired from previous clinical experiences, personal knowledge acquired from life and social experiences, and tacit knowledge. Tacit knowledge is professional knowledge acquired through experience, but 'not processed in a focused cognitive manner', which 'lies at a not quite conscious level', and is acted upon but not easily verbalized (Fleming & Mattingly 2000, p. 55). The clinician's knowledge base affects and is affected by every phase of the clinical reasoning process.

Cognition refers to the perception, analysis, synthesis and evaluation of the data collected. The clinician processes clinical data against the knowledge base in memory. Metacognition refers to the self-monitoring processes clinicians employ to think about their thinking. Metacognitive skills enable clinicians to detect when incoming clinical information matches or is inconsistent with existing clinical patterns or expectations, based on prior learning (Higgs & Jones 2000). In addition, metacognition allows clinicians to critique aspects of their own clinical reasoning process relating to accuracy, reliability, validity, logic, scope, client relevance, efficiency and creativity (Higgs & Jones 2000). Importantly, it is clinicians' metacognitive abilities that enable them to recognize any limitations in their own skills and knowledge. It is this reflective capacity, combined with open-mindedness and healthy scepticism, that leads expert clinicians, skilled in clinical reasoning, to learn from their own experiences and shift their personal perspectives when the evidence (both research and experience based) indicates a shift is needed. While experts do not know everything,

they are metacognitive; in other words, they are aware of what they do not know and are therefore always learning.

Implicit in this portrayal of clinical reasoning is the interplay that takes place between pure hypothesis testing, or deductive reasoning (more characteristic of reasoning through unfamiliar patient presentations), and pattern recognition, or inductive reasoning (characteristic of more expert reasoning). Both hypothesis testing and pattern recognition can occur during different stages in the overall hypothetico-deductive process employed in the management of a patient (Jones 1995).

Hypothesis categories system

Jones (1992) also introduced a system of categorization of clinical hypotheses and organization of clinical knowledge. The hypothesis categories system demonstrates the many interrelated components of a patient's problem that physiotherapists must consider and manage in addition to the initial diagnosis of the physical problem. This system has been expanded upon in recent years (Butler 2000, Gifford & Butler 1997, Jones 1995, Jones et al 2002). The expansion reflects the trend towards defining the physiotherapy profession in the context of various models of disablement (see, for example, Guide to Physical Therapist Practice 2001, Main et al 1999), and growing awareness of pain science and the biopsychosocial factors that must be considered in the clinical reasoning process. The hypothesis categories system currently comprises seven categories:

1. Functional limitation and/or disability (physical or psychological limitations in functional activities and the associated social, occupational and economic consequences).
2. Pathobiological mechanisms (includes consideration of tissue healing mechanisms and pain mechanisms).
3. Physical and psychosocial impairments and their associated sources.
4. Contributing factors.
5. Precautions and contraindications to physical examination and treatment.
6. Management and treatment.
7. Prognosis.

For a more detailed description of each of the above hypothesis categories, see Jones & Rivett (2004).

Collaborative models

The most recent clinical reasoning research in physiotherapy has focused on the study of expert practice (Beeston & Simons 1996, Edwards 2000, Embrey et al 1996, Jensen et al 1990, 1992, 1999, Rivett & Higgs 1997). This research, by providing deeper understanding of what characterizes the practice of experts, facilitates ongoing attempts to define the physiotherapy profession. In response to growing interest in the investigation of clinical practice activities other than initial diagnosis, as they occur in realistic clinical settings, research in other allied health professions also considered the development of expertise and the nature of clinical reasoning. This research includes that done in nursing (Agan 1987, Benner & Tanner 1987, Benner et al 1992, Rew & Barrow 1987) and in occupational therapy (Crepeau 1991, Fleming 1991, Hagedorn 1996, Mattingly 1991). Designing research intended to describe clinical reasoning as it occurs in various clinical practice activities necessitated a paradigm shift in both focus and methodology. Researchers recognized that much of clinical practice is, by nature, non-diagnostic. As such, the study of expertise and the clinical reasoning of experts requires interpretive, qualitative methods of inquiry. In physiotherapy, the work of Jensen and colleagues (1990, 1992, 1999) illustrates this newer interpretive methodology, with conclusions which describe the qualities of expert physiotherapists and expert clinical practice. One of the many findings of Jensen et al (1992, 1999) is that all expert physiotherapists, in various fields of specialty practice, demonstrate a more interactive, collaborative approach to patient management than do novice practitioners.

Collaborative clinical reasoning model

Edwards (1995) and Jones et al (2000) expanded upon Jones's early model and made explicit the role of the patient, highlighting the importance of collaboration in the clinical reasoning process (Fig. 27.1).

This model helps to shift the conceptualization of the clinical reasoning process from one occurring solely inside the clinician's head to one that includes the interaction between the clinician's thoughts and those of the patient (Jones 1995). This shift in the conceptualization of the clinical reasoning process also reflects the growing awareness within the pain science literature (discussed previously) of the impact of biopsychosocial factors on the process. Through this collaborative process, physiotherapists are able to enrich their clinical knowledge base by learning how multiple factors, in addition to the physical structures involved in a patient's problem, interact and produce variations upon classic clinical patterns (Jones et al 2000). This type of learning by the clinician thus contributes to the formation of a more holistic concept of clinical practice.

The collaboration of the physiotherapist with the patient throughout the clinical reasoning process not only increases the growth in knowledge or learning of the physiotherapist, but also contributes to significant patient learning (for example altered understanding, beliefs, attitudes and health behaviours) (Christensen et al 2002, Jones et al 2000). The collaborative clinical reasoning model makes explicit that a main goal of the process is an increased understanding of the problem, and that participation in the management of the problem by the patient results in increased self-efficacy. This collaboration, and the learning that results in transformation of a patient's perspective of the problem, is thought to have a significant positive impact on treatment outcomes (Gifford 1998c, Jones et al 2002, Main & Watson 1999, Watson 2000).

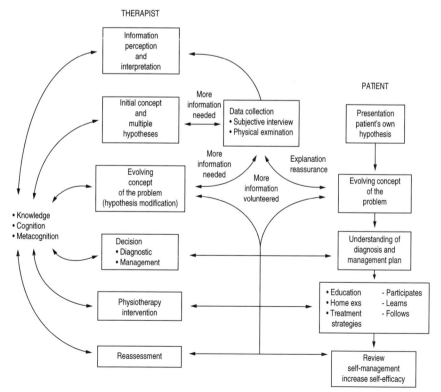

Figure 27.1 Collaborative clinical reasoning process. Reproduced with permission from Jones et al 2000, p. 119.

Client centred model

The view of clinical reasoning as collaborative and interactive has also been illustrated by Higgs & Jones (2000), in their model of client centred clinical reasoning (Fig. 27.2 and 27.3).

The upward and outward spiral (Fig. 27.2) represents the cyclical nature of clinical reasoning as the process develops over time. The cross-sectional view of the model (Fig. 27.3) represents the interaction between the components of clinical reasoning occurring 'within the clinician's mind' – including cognition or reflective inquiry, discipline-specific knowledge base and metacognition – and components active in the reasoning process that are characteristic of each individual client and the client's problem. This model shows clearly the importance of the context within which each individual client's problem places the clinical reasoning process. This context is provided, in part, by the role each individual client plays in the decision making process, which in turn reflects and impacts upon that client's personal circumstances (physical home/work environment, culture, family, finances). The impact of the nature of the clinical problem itself (simple, multifactorial, degree of certainty or changeability inherent in the nature of the problem) will influence the clinical reasoning process. In addition, the situation or clinical environment within which the decision making is occurring affects the clinical reasoning process (Higgs & Jones 2000).

Clinical reasoning strategies

A recent interpretive study by Edwards (2000) has added another dimension to the understanding of expert physiotherapy practice. He described the clinical reasoning of experts in three different practice specialties: manual therapy, neurophysiotherapy and domiciliary care physiotherapy. The findings of this study are that, regardless of practice setting, physiotherapists demonstrate foci of thinking and acting across a range of diagnostic, management and ethical problem-solving activities in clinical practice. These different foci or orientations of reasoning are termed clinical reasoning strategies (see Jones et al 2002 for more

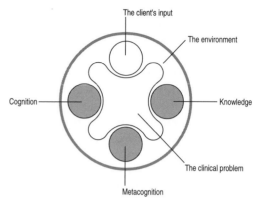

Figure 27.3 Client centred clinical reasoning. Reproduced with permission from Higgs & Jones 2000, p. 11.

detail), and include the following, under the headings of diagnosis, management and ethical problem solving:

Diagnosis

- *Diagnostic reasoning:* formation of a diagnosis related to physical disability/functional limitation and associated impairment(s), with consideration of associated pain mechanisms, tissue pathology and the broad scope of potential contributing factors.
- *Narrative reasoning:* understanding a patient's illness experience, 'story', context, beliefs and culture.

Management

- *Procedural reasoning:* determination and carrying out of treatment procedures.
- *Interactive reasoning:* establishing therapist–patient rapport.
- *Collaborative reasoning:* nurturing a consensual approach towards the interpretation of examination findings, the setting of goals and priorities and the implementation and progression of treatment.
- *Reasoning about teaching:* planning, carrying out and evaluating individualized and context-sensitive teaching.
- *Predictive reasoning:* envisioning future scenarios with patients and exploring their choices and the implications of those choices.

Ethical problem-solving

- *Ethical reasoning:* apprehension and resolution of ethical and pragmatic dilemmas.

In addition, the study found that each of the strategies was seldom applied in isolation, or applied separately for particular tasks in clinical practice. Instead, as will be evident in the following patient case, the study found that the strategies were often applied in combination, overlapping in various ways, according to the particular clinical situation at hand.

Dialectical reasoning

Furthermore, the manner in which the clinical reasoning strategies are approached by physiotherapists can be described as representative of different reasoning para-

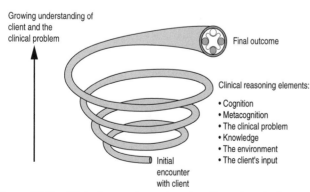

Figure 27.2 Clinical reasoning – overview. Reproduced with permission from Higgs & Jones 2000, p. 11.

digms (Edwards 2000, Jones et al 2002), that is, at times the reasoning and/or clinical action of clinicians is employed in a manner where its 'outcome' is tested and measured in an empirical manner. As discussed previously, this is the manner in which much of the earlier medical and physiotherapy clinical reasoning literature has traditionally characterized the nature of clinical reasoning.

At other times, the reasoning and/or clinical action is more communicatively oriented and its outcome is evaluated quite differently. In such instances reasoning is characterized by a more interpretive, qualitative paradigm. In these situations, physiotherapists seek to understand the patient's experience within that patient's individual life context, and establish the validity of this understanding by consensus with the patient.

Such differences in reasoning are analogous to the differences in quantitative and qualitative research methods. The interplay in clinical practice between these two distinct paradigms of reasoning is termed dialectical reasoning (Edwards 2000).

This complex interplay of different reasoning processes (empirico-analytical vs. interpretive paradigms) occurs in every task of clinical practice (Edwards 2000, Jones et al 2002). One way to characterize this interplay of reasoning in clinical practice is the thinking and actions oriented toward understanding the patient's physical problem versus the thinking and actions directed toward understanding the person. Although there is overlap (and while understanding the problem requires understanding the person and vice versa), such a general distinction is useful to highlight the different reasoning strategies, management strategies and knowledge sources required when attempting to holistically understand and collaboratively manage patients' problems.

APPLICATION TO DIAGNOSIS AND MANAGEMENT OF SPINAL PAIN

The following section will highlight several examples of how a physiotherapist might reason through aspects of the case of Sandra, the patient with spinal pain introduced earlier. Although one chapter cannot adequately address every aspect of the reasoning a therapist would use in comprehensively managing this patient case, by presenting several of the clinical reasoning strategies a physiotherapist might employ while working with Sandra we will illustrate how principles of EBHC, pain science and biopsychosocial theory and organization of knowledge via hypothesis categories all come into play at various times in the collaborative clinical reasoning process.

Diagnosis

Diagnosis in the context of clinical reasoning and biopsychosocial theory has multiple dimensions incorporating the therapist's understanding of the patient and their prob-

lem(s). Some of this understanding will be reached using reasoning in an empirico-analytical (diagnostic reasoning) paradigm and some will be reached through reasoning in an interpretive (narrative reasoning) paradigm. If we refer to the collaborative clinical reasoning model (Fig. 27.1), the therapist and Sandra will develop their understanding concurrently as they progress through the various elements of the collaborative clinical reasoning cycle. These elements include: formation of an initial concept and generation of hypotheses; data collection through the interview and physical examination; exploration, consideration and incorporation of Sandra's own interpretation of her problem; and the resultant evolution and expansion of the initial concept of the problem.

Diagnostic reasoning

In forming the basis of a 'diagnosis', the therapist will employ a diagnostic reasoning strategy based on an empirical reasoning process as he endeavours to identify Sandra's functional limitations and/or disabilities and any physical impairments. A narrative reasoning process is required, even at this early stage of diagnostic reasoning, when the therapist is beginning to determine the dominant pain mechanisms in the presentation and whether there are potential psychological impairments. Listed below are examples of several of the hypothesis categories that the therapist may consider in the early stages of the interview. These categories can assist the therapist in organizing clinical knowledge, recognizing clinical patterns and generating hypotheses at this stage in the reasoning process. When indicated, additional information the therapist has attained through the interview and physical examination is provided before a discussion of the therapist's hypotheses for each category.

CASE STUDY (Contd)

Functional limitation and/or disability

During the subjective interview, Sandra tells the therapist she has not participated in bicycling or tennis since the onset of her symptoms 6 weeks ago. When the therapist asks why not, Sandra reveals that she initially stopped these activities because she was in too much pain. Although her symptoms have lessened in frequency and intensity since the time of onset, she has not resumed the activity because her physician instructed her to rest in order to get better. Sandra 'doesn't want to do anything to make it worse again'. Sandra also mentions that she is a bit worried about resuming tennis ever again. She explains that there are times when she must bend backwards in order to reach for an overhead shot and to serve properly, and just recently her physician told her she should avoid bending backwards. He said this was so that 'the fractured bone in my spine won't slide any further forward'. Sandra cannot sit at her computer for more than 30 minutes without experiencing pain into her left leg. Although she attempts to pace herself, she is not able to get all of her work done. This is now causing her some stress at work. Providing she is careful to avoid prolonged flexion and any activities that require arching her back, Sandra reports she is not limited from performing any of her other normal daily activities.

From the data the therapist has gathered by interview, he can be confident that Sandra's main functional limitations/disabilities are a limited sitting tolerance at work and that she is unable to participate in bicycling or tennis. In other words, Sandra is no longer able to carry out her work duties in her usual manner or fully participate in her normal fitness recreational activity. At this stage, the therapist cannot say if these limitations in activity are due more to psychological/behavioural factors (such as maladaptive beliefs about pain and further damage and fear-avoidance behaviour), physical factors (such as inability to physically perform these activities due to pain and/or impaired mobility, etc.), or a combination of both. He will continue to investigate these hypotheses through the physical examination (to identify any physical barriers to these functional activities) and, as discussed below, can further explore (through narrative reasoning) the maladaptive beliefs/fear-avoidance behaviour hypothesis.

CASE STUDY (Contd)

Pathobiological mechanisms

Sandra's symptoms began 6 weeks ago, and were related to a specific incident when, after a 2-hour ride, she lifted her bicycle up onto the rack on the top of her car. Sandra felt a strong pull in the centre of her low back as she lifted the bike from the ground up to shoulder height, and before she raised it above her head to place it in the rack. During the 30-minute drive home, Sandra reports she began to feel a bit stiff and sore in the same central lower back area, and by the next morning she had significant constant deep aching pain that now radiated from her lower back down into her lateral left thigh. Initially, all movements were painful, and bending forwards and sitting were, and still are, the most aggravating activities. Lying supine with hips and knees bent is her most comfortable position. Sandra consulted with her physician and for the first week rested at home, mostly supine with legs supported, while taking anti-inflammatory and muscle-relaxant medications. Within the first 5 days following the injury, her symptoms became intermittent, less intense and less frequent. They have continued to improve so that now she has intermittent symptoms in the low back and left lateral thigh, which she rates as 3/10 at the worst, after sitting for 30 minutes, and which settle completely after standing and moving around for 5 minutes. Sandra reports no problems with sleeping at night, and on days when she does

not sit for more than 10–15 minutes at a time she has no build-up of symptoms through the day. Her symptoms have been at their current level for about 10 days.

When generating hypotheses in the category of pathobiological mechanisms, the therapist considers the mechanisms by which Sandra's symptoms are being initiated and maintained by her nervous system. In considering the tissue mechanisms component of this hypothesis category, the therapist's goal is twofold. First, the therapist attempts to determine whether or not Sandra's presentation matches the pattern he expects for the degree of tissue 'injury' or inflammation that may be present. In addition, the therapist must determine whether or not the presentation matches the associated normal progression of healing for her injury (Gogia 1992, Hardy 1989). The therapist recognizes that Sandra has a 6-week old lifting injury, which has become progressively better. At first her symptoms were inflammatory and irritable in nature and they progressed to stable mechanical symptoms of low irritability. The area and characteristics of her central low back pain with radiation to the lateral left thigh are typical of an injury to local spinal structures at the L4 segment. In other words, the information the therapist has gathered thus far supports that Sandra has progressed through normal phases of tissue healing, and that her presentation fits with what he would expect for someone with an injury in the remodelling/maturation phase (Gogia 1992, Hardy 1989).

The tissue mechanisms hypothesis is integral to hypothesis generation about pain mechanisms. Pain mechanisms relate to particular physiologic/pathophysiologic processes that give rise to pain in sensory, cognitive, emotional and behavioural dimensions (Butler 2000, Gifford 1998a, 1998b, 1998d, Gifford & Butler 1997). These mechanisms have been broadly categorized as being adaptive or maladaptive in nature (Gifford 1998c). When an adaptive pain mechanism is dominant, the pain the patient is experiencing is attributed to the physiological processes that govern the typical, appropriate, protective response of the nervous system to an acute injury. When pain is adaptive, the source of the pain is related to impairments in the involved tissues and fits with the hypothesized tissue mechanism hypothesis. One adaptive pain mechanism is nociceptive pain, where the pain originates from target tissues of nerves, such as muscle, ligament, disc, bone and tendon. Another is peripheral neurogenic pain, where the pain originates in the neural tissue 'outside' the dorsal horn.

Maladaptive pain mechanisms become dominant when the central nervous system becomes sensitized due to altered processing of afferent input, and the pain itself becomes the source of the problem – pathology local to the tissues that were initially injured is no longer driving the person's pain experience. Examples of pain mechanisms that may be maladaptive include central pain, and mechanisms that involve abnormal output from the motor, autonomic, neuroendocrine, and neuroimmune systems. The concept of pain mechanisms is closely linked to biopsychosocial theory. It is beyond the scope of this chapter to provide an adequate description and explanation of maladaptive pain mechanisms and central sensitization; for more information, the reader is referred to the literature by Gifford and Butler (Butler 2000, Gifford 1998a, 1998b, 1998d, Gifford & Butler 1997).

At this stage of the inquiry there are several clues that suggest Sandra's understanding, her health behaviours and the stress she now finds herself under while at work may be contributing to her problem, or at least may represent obstacles to her recovery. As is often the case, the full story does not emerge in the first appointment and the therapist will need to further investigate his hypothesis regarding the potential contribution of maladaptive beliefs, fear-avoidance behaviour and work-related stress to her disability and pain presentation (i.e. possible central sensitization and inappropriate self-management). The presence of any distortion in her beliefs and behaviours would then need to be addressed in the management.

CASE STUDY (Contd)

Physical and psychosocial impairments and their associated sources

Sandra's physical examination findings include abnormal static posture and movement patterns, with a tendency to maintain a flattened lumbar spine. She also demonstrates decreased segmental mobility throughout the lumbar spine for transitional movements such as sit-to-stand and bending and reaching motions. Sandra is able to assume a better postural alignment with cueing. Lumbar extension is limited by stiffness, and Sandra expresses mild apprehension about bending backwards. Flexion is mildly painful in the central low back at end-range. Repeated flexion in standing results in a worsening of the intensity of the low back symptoms and a mild ache into the left buttock. Passive segmental mobility testing results indicate hypomobility at L4/5 both centrally and unilaterally, with left greater than right-sided involvement. Her neurological screening examination was clear. Sandra demonstrates poor awareness of spinal posture, movement and motor control as evaluated through her ability to control her spine through both static postures and movement (e.g. sitting, standing, sit-to-stand, etc.). She is also unable to recruit her transversus abdominis muscle in isolation, and demonstrates external oblique abdominal muscle co-contraction with the attempt. Her left lower lumbar multifidi muscles are less active when compared to her right side.

The therapist, when comparing Sandra's physical presentation with all of the interview data (area and behaviour of symptoms, mechanism of injury, progression), might begin to recognize a clinical pattern. In this case, the clinical pattern is typical of an L4/L5 motion segment impairment, which is characterized by increased mechanical sensitivity and reduced segmental movement combined with reduced general motor awareness/control and local stabilization.

Her movement patterns and impaired motor control also fit with someone who is afraid to move for fear of worsening the pathology present in her spine. At this stage, the best the therapist can rightly deduce is that there is evidence of both physical impairment and psychosocial influences, and that both may be contributing to Sandra's pain perception and pain experience.

This therapist could consult recent evidence in the literature in order to assist him in the diagnosis of this component of Sandra's problem. Moller et al (2000) investigated the presence of specific symptoms, signs or functional disabilities that can be associated with adult spondylolisthesis. These authors found that the clinical pattern for adult spondylolisthesis is similar to that seen with other patients with low back pain of non-specific origin. Thus, it is likely that patients with spondylolisthesis experience symptoms due to many of the same sources and causes as do patients without a radiological diagnosis of spondylolisthesis. The therapist can use this information to strengthen his hypothesis that the source(s) of Sandra's physical impairments may not be directly attributable to the radiological diagnosis of grade I spondylolisthesis, and may be more related to injured or sensitized (peripheral or central) motion segment tissues. The hypothesis category of contributing factors is important here, as physical and psychological factors may be contributing to any peripheral or central sensitization that may be present. Physical factors may include things like restricted mobility and poor motor control, while psychological factors can include unhelpful beliefs and behaviours.

CASE STUDY (Contd)

The therapist, by specifically inquiring throughout the interview, learned that Sandra had taken time away from her work during the first week following the injury, but since then has been back to work. She has never before taken time off of work as a result of back pain. As described previously, the therapist discussed with Sandra her understanding of the cause of her back pain ('spondylolisthesis') and discovered that, based on what her physician had told her, she expects to be given exercises to 'stabilize' her spine. She expects to be pain-free soon, but feels she will need to avoid bending backwards or 'over-arching' her back from now on, and 'might never be able to return to playing tennis or other vigorous exercise if I want the pain to stay away'.

This information attained by the therapist is the result of screening for what has been referred to in the biopsychosocial literature as 'yellow flags', or typical psychosocial factors shown to be predictive of poorer outcomes when demonstrated by patients with low back pain (Main &

Watson 1999, Watson & Kendall 2000). Similarly, the ongoing narrative reasoning required to further understand Sandra's pain experience will need to delve deeper into the potential work related issues. Main and colleagues have categorized work factors that may impact on recovery as 'black' and 'blue' flags (Main & Burton 2000).

This is another example of integrating evidence, in this case from the pain sciences and biopsychosocial theory literature, into clinical practice. This therapist can now identify issues he needs to overtly address (i.e. Sandra's misperception of the nature of her problem and its implications for her future) as part of the overall management of Sandra's problem. By identifying and subsequently addressing all components of the problem, from both a biomedical and a psychosocial perspective, the likelihood that Sandra will go on to develop a maladaptive or centralized chronic pain state is minimized.

Contributing factors

The therapist, when considering potential causes for Sandra's problem and any factors that might be maintaining her symptoms, could generate a number of hypotheses. Examples include the following:

- The radiological findings of grade I spondylolisthesis could contribute to the development of a physical impairment/sensitization in an adjacent spinal segment. This could possibly be the result of the mild structural segmental instability due to the bony defect or abnormal forces/extra stresses placed on the affected segment due to the dysfunction at an adjacent segment.
- If the poor spinal segmental motor control was present prior to this injury (possibly due to a pre-existing structural defect or previous episodes of minor low back), this impairment could also be a factor that could have contributed to injury with the lifting activity. The motor control impairment is also likely to be contributing to the maintenance of Sandra's current symptoms.
- Hypotheses related to poor habitual posture while working on the computer, poor lifting technique or poor cycling technique would need to be investigated further.
- Avoidance of movement due to fear may also be contributing to the current impairments in mobility and motor control/movement patterns.

Narrative reasoning

In order to form an accurate and comprehensive diagnosis the therapist will attempt to develop a concept of Sandra's own hypotheses and interpretations of the problem itself, the reason for its development and the related consequences.

This understanding can generate new hypotheses or provide additional data to strengthen or weaken existing hypotheses generated within the diagnostic reasoning strategy. For example, when Sandra explained why she had not resumed her bicycling or tennis, the therapist was able to get an idea of the way in which Sandra has interpreted

the information she has received from her physician and the results of her X-rays. One hypothesis at this stage is that while initially avoiding these activities due to pain, Sandra is now avoiding these activities more from the fear that she could worsen what she believes to be the source of her symptoms, namely the 'fracture' (spondylolisthesis) in her spine. In order to further explore Sandra's 'story' or perspective, the therapist could engage her in a more in-depth, interactive discussion about her understanding of the nature of grade I spondylolisthesis and what she believes to be the implications of this problem now and for the future. This discussion is more than simply listening to Sandra telling her story. To truly represent narrative reasoning, this discussion must involve interactive communication between the therapist and Sandra, and the resultant interpretation by the therapist of Sandra's experience must be validated by consensus between the therapist and Sandra.

This example is but one illustration of how clinical reasoning strategies often overlap and are applied in combination during particular clinical activities. In this case, not only does narrative reasoning provide the therapist with an understanding of Sandra as a person, it also informs the reasoning about her physical problem in that it supports the notion that the limitation in her function at this stage is in part influenced by her beliefs about her pathology and fear of worsening it through continued extension movements.

Management

Considering again the collaborative clinical reasoning model (Fig. 27.1), at this stage the therapist is able to use his 'diagnosis', or the understanding of Sandra's physical problem and of Sandra as a person, to direct his decisions and actions within reasoning strategies directed toward management.

Collaborative reasoning

When examining the therapist's reasoning through Sandra's 'diagnosis', it becomes apparent that she and the therapist have already entered into a collaborative relationship. By soliciting the information she has given him and demonstrating that he values and understands her 'story' the therapist has already established the foundation for a collaborative approach towards deciding and implementing goals of Sandra's physiotherapy treatment. The collaboration that will continue throughout the rest of the therapeutic interaction is an integral factor in the skilful employment of all other reasoning strategies, and ultimately guarantees that Sandra and the therapist move together through the management of her problem, as partners in decision making, action and learning.

Procedural reasoning

The therapist will use procedural reasoning to choose and prioritize appropriate treatment techniques and approaches.

This reasoning includes the reassessment of each intervention's effect on Sandra's impairments (both physical and psychosocial) and functional limitations/disability in order to determine whether the chosen treatment approaches are yielding the optimal desired outcomes. In Sandra's case, in addition to addressing the physical impairments identified, intervention will include graded exposure to functional activities involving lumbar spinal extension so as to address her fear, and gradually increase her confidence that by doing these activities in an appropriate manner she will not worsen her condition.

Another example of applying principles of EBHC to clinical practice could come into play here if Sandra's physiotherapist had little or no experience with management of patients with low back pain and a demonstrated impairment in motor control. The therapist could consult the evidence to assist him in making his treatment decision. The therapist would consult the evidence to answer a clinical question such as: 'In patients with subacute low back pain (with or without a diagnosed spondylolisthesis) and impairment in motor control, is exercise an effective intervention?' In this case, the therapist would find the available evidence helpful, in that it supports a therapeutic exercise approach. This is a growing area of research in physiotherapy. While the effectiveness of one approach over another is still unclear, both clinical and research-based evidence is growing in support of motor control management when such impairment is present (see, for example, Maher et al 1999, O'Sullivan et al 1997, Richardson et al 1999, Tulder et al 2002).

Reasoning about teaching

The use of teaching in the management of Sandra's problem may in fact be the most important of all interventions in terms of potential long-term outcome. Teaching will naturally occur in conjunction with treatment interventions such as motor control re-education, body mechanics instruction for lifting, postural education and home exercise instruction. Most importantly, however, is the teaching that the therapist will do in order to educate Sandra about the nature of grade I spondylolisthesis (her initial understanding and a basis of her fear of movement), and how this structural problem may or may not be related to her current symptoms. As Sandra begins to understand more about the nature of her problem she is able to reflect on her situation in a more realistic way. The end result is a revised perspective on her problem with a reduction in fear and avoidance of movement. What Sandra learns will enable her to make appropriate decisions about how to manage her own situation, and the outcome is not likely to include any residual disability.

While not brought out in this particular patient case, it is also important to acknowledge the role of predictive and ethical reasoning, particularly in situations where a patient's disability may either be long term and/or uncertain (Edwards 2000).

CONCLUSION

Successfully managing patients' problems requires a breadth of understanding, reasoning and skills. The application of biopsychosocial theory in contemporary manual therapy is facilitated through further development of reasoning skills that target the multiple dimensions of patients' problems. A strong yet flexible clinical reasoning framework will allow clinicians to: evolve their practice in response to new knowledge; critically appraise emerging evidence for its applicability to their skills, practice environment and patient populations; contribute to the growth and advancement of the physiotherapy profession.

KEYWORDS

adaptive	impairment
autonomic	inductive
biomedical	interactive reasoning
biopsychosocial theory	interpretive
black flags	knowledge
blue flags	learning
central sensitization	maladaptive
central pain	management
client centred	metacognition
clinical expertise	model
clinical reasoning	motor
clinical reasoning process	motor control
clinical reasoning	narrative reasoning
strategies	neuroendocrine
clinical question	neuroimmune
cognition	nociceptive
collaborative reasoning	pain mechanisms
contraindications	pain science
contributing factors	pathobiological mechanisms
deductive	pattern recognition
diagnosis	peripheral neurogenic
diagnostic reasoning	positivist
dialectical reasoning	precautions
disability	procedural reasoning
empirico-analytical	predictive reasoning
ethical problem-solving	prognosis
ethical reasoning	psychosocial
evidence based health	spondylolisthesis
care (EBHC)	tacit
evidence based medicine	teaching (reasoning about
(EBM)	teaching)
fear-avoidance	therapeutic exercise
functional limitation	tissue mechanisms
hypothesis categories	qualitative
hypothetico-deductive	quantitative
reasoning	yellow flags

References

Agan D 1987 Intuitive knowing as a dimension of nursing. Advances in Nursing Science 10: 63–70

Barrows H S, Tamblyn R M 1980 Problem based learning: an approach to medical education. Springer, New York, pp 40, 45

Beeston S, Simons H 1996 Physiotherapy practice: practitioners' perspectives. Physiotherapy Theory and Practice 12: 231–242

Benner P, Tanner C 1987 Clinical judgement: how expert nurses use intuition. American Journal of Nursing 87: 23–31

Benner P, Tanner C, Chelsa C 1992 Gaining a differentiated clinical world in critical care nursing. Advanced Nursing Science 14: 13–28

Binkley J 2000 Against the myth of evidence-based practice. Journal of Orthopaedic and Sports Physical Therapy 30(2): 98–99

Butler D S 2000 The sensitive nervous system. NOI Group Publications, Adelaide, pp 130–151

Christensen N, Jones M A, Carr J 2002 Clinical reasoning in orthopedic manual therapy. In: Grant R (ed) Physical therapy of the cervical and thoracic spine, 3rd edn, Churchill Livingstone, New York, ch 6

Cibulka M T, Aslin K 2001 How to use evidence-based practice to distinguish between three different patients with low back pain. Journal of Orthopaedic and Sports Physical Therapy 31(12): 678–695

Crepeau E B 1991 Achieving intersubjective understanding: examples from an occupational therapy treatment session. American Journal of Occupational Therapy 45: 1016–1025

DiFabio R P 1999 Myth of evidence-based practice. Journal of Orthopaedic and Sports Physical Therapy 29(11): 632–634

DiFabio R P 2000 What is 'evidence'? Journal of Orthopaedic and Sports Physical Therapy 30(2): 52–55

Edwards I 1995 Cooperative decision making between patient and therapist (Fig. 2). In: Jones M Clinical reasoning and pain. Manual Therapy 1(1): 17–24

Edwards I 2000 Clinical reasoning in three different fields of physiotherapy: a qualitative case study approach. PhD thesis, University of South Australia, Adelaide, South Australia

Elstein A S, Shulman L S, Sprafka S S 1978 Medical problem solving. Harvard University Press, Cambridge

Embrey D G, Guthrie M R, White O R et al 1996 Clinical decision making by experienced and inexperienced pediatric physical therapists for children with diplegic cerebral palsy. Physical Therapy 76: 20–33

Evidence-Based Medicine Working Group 1992 Evidence-based medicine: a new approach to teaching the practice of medicine. Journal of the American Medical Association 268: 2420–2425

Fleming M H 1991 The therapist with the three track mind. American Journal of Occupational Therapy 45: 1007–1014

Fleming M H, Mattingly C 2000 Action and narrative: two dynamics of clinical reasoning. In: Higgs J, Jones M (eds) Clinical reasoning in the health professions. Butterworth Heinemann, Oxford, p 55

Fritz J 2001 Invited commentary. In: Cibulka M T, Aslin K How to use evidence-based practice to distinguish between three different patients with low back pain. Journal of Orthopaedic and Sports Physical Therapy 31(12): 689–692

Gifford L S 1998a Output mechanisms. In: Gifford L S (ed) Topical Issues in Pain. 1: Whiplash: science and management. Fear-avoidance beliefs and behaviour. CNS Press, Falmouth, pp 81–92

Gifford L S 1998b The 'central' mechanisms. In: Gifford L S (ed) Topical Issues in Pain. 1: Whiplash: science and management. Fear-avoidance beliefs and behaviour. CNS Press, Falmouth, pp 67–80

Gifford L S 1998c The mature organism model. In: Gifford L S (ed) Topical Issues in Pain. 1: Whiplash: science and management. Fear-avoidance beliefs and behaviour. CNS Press, Falmouth, pp 45–56

Gifford L S 1998d Tissue and input related mechanisms. In: Gifford L S (ed) Topical Issues in Pain. 1: Whiplash: science and management. Fear-avoidance beliefs and behaviour. CNS Press, Falmouth, pp 57–66

Gifford L S 2001 Perspectives on the biopsychosocial model. 1: Some issues that need to be accepted? Touch, the Journal of the Organisation of Chartered Physiotherapists in Private Practice, 97: 3–9

Gifford L S, Butler D S 1997 The integration of pain sciences into clinical practice. Journal of Hand Therapy 10: 86–95

Gogia P P 1992 The biology of wound healing. Ostomy 38(9): 12–22

Guide to Physical Therapist Practice, 2nd edn. 2001 Physical Therapy 81: 9–744

Guyatt G, Haynes B, Jaeschke R et al 2002 Introduction: the philosophy of evidence-based medicine. In: Guyatt G, Drummond R (eds) Users' guides to the medical literature: a manual for evidence-based clinical practice. Evidence-Based Medicine Working Group. AMA Press, Chicago, pp 3–12

Hagedorn R 1996 Clinical decision making in familiar cases: a model of the process and implications for practice. British Journal of Occupational Therapy 59: 217–222

Hardy M 1989 The biology of scar formation. Physical Therapy 69: 1014–1024

Higgs J, Hunt A 1999 Rethinking the beginning practitioner: introducing the 'interactional professional'. In: Higgs J, Edwards H (eds) Educating beginning practitioners. Butterworth Heinemann, Oxford, pp 10–18

Higgs J, Jones M 2000 Clinical reasoning in the health professions. In: Higgs J, Jones M (eds) Clinical reasoning in the health professions. Butterworth Heinemann, Oxford, pp 3–14

Higgs J, Titchen A 1995 The nature, generation, and verification of knowledge. Physiotherapy 81: 521–530

Higgs J, Titchen A 1998 Research and knowledge. Physiotherapy 84: 72–80

Higgs J, Burn A, Jones M 2001 Integrating clinical reasoning and evidence-based practice. AACN Clinical Issues: 12(4): 482–490

Jensen G M, Shepard K F, Hack L M 1990 The novice versus the experienced clinician: insights into the work of the physical therapist. Physical Therapy 70: 314–323

Jensen G M, Shepard K F, Hack L M 1992 Attribute dimensions that distinguish master and novice physical therapy clinicians in orthopedic settings. Physical Therapy 72: 711–722

Jensen G M, Gwyer J, Hack L M et al 1999 Expertise in physical therapy practice. Butterworth Heinemann, Boston

Jones M A 1992 Clinical reasoning in manual therapy. Physical Therapy 72: 875–884

Jones M A 1994 Clinical reasoning process in manipulative therapy. In: Boyling J D, Palastanga N (eds) Grieve's Modern Manual Therapy, 2nd edn. Churchill Livingstone, Edinburgh, pp 471–489

Jones M 1995 Clinical reasoning and pain. Manual Therapy 1(1): 17–24

Jones M, Higgs J 2000 Will evidence-based practice take the reasoning out of practice? In: Higgs J, Jones M (eds) Clinical reasoning in the health professions. Butterworth Heinemann, Oxford, pp 307–315

Jones M, Rivett D (eds) 2004 Clinical reasoning in manual therapy. Elsevier, Oxford

Jones M, Jensen G, Edwards I 2000 Clinical reasoning in physiotherapy. In: Higgs J, Jones M (eds) Clinical reasoning in the health professions. Butterworth Heinemann, Oxford, pp 117–127

Jones M A, Edwards I, Gifford L 2002 Conceptual models for implementing biopsychosocial theory in clinical practice. Manual Therapy 7(1): 2–9

Koes B W, Hoving J L 1998 The value of the randomized clinical trial in the field of physiotherapy. Manual Therapy 3(4): 179–186

Maher C, Latimer J, Refshauge K 1999 Prescription of activity for low back pain: what works? Australian Journal of Physiotherapy 45: 121–132

Main C J, Burton A K 2000 Economic and occupational influences on pain and disability. In: Main C J, Spanswick C C (eds) Pain management: an interdisciplinary approach. Churchill Livingstone, Edinburgh, pp 63–88

Main C J, Watson P J 1999 Psychological aspects of pain. Manual Therapy 4(4): 203–215

Main C J, Spanswick C C, Watson P J 1999 The nature of disability. In: Main C J, Spanswick C C (eds) Pain management: an interdisciplinary approach. Churchill Livingstone, Edinburgh, pp 89–106

Mattingly C 1991 The narrative nature of clinical reasoning. American Journal of Occupational Therapy 45: 998–1005

Mezirow J 1991 Transformative dimensions of adult learning. Jossey-Bass, San Francisco

Moller H, Sundin A, Hedlund R 2000 Symptoms, signs, and functional disability in adult spondylolisthesis. Spine 25(6): 683–689

Moore A, Petty N 2001 Evidence-based practice: getting a grip and finding a balance. Manual Therapy 6(4): 195–196

O'Sullivan P B, Twomey L T, Allison G T 1997 Evaluation of specific stabilizing exercise in the treatment of chronic low back pain with radiologic diagnosis of spondylolysis or spondylolisthesis. Spine 22(24): 2959–2967

Parry A 2001 Research and professional craft knowledge. In: Higgs J, Titchen A (eds) Practice knowledge and expertise in the health professions. Butterworth Heinemann, Oxford, pp 199–206

Patel V L, Groen G J 1986 Knowledge-based solution strategies in medical reasoning. Cognitive Science 10: 91–116

Payton O D 1985 Clinical reasoning process in physical therapy. Physical Therapy 65: 924–928

Rew L, Barrow E M 1987 Intuition: a neglected hallmark of nursing knowledge. Advances in Nursing Science 10: 49–62

Richardson C, Jull G, Hodges P et al 1999 Therapeutic exercise for spinal segmental stabilization in low back pain: scientific basis and clinical approach. Churchill Livingstone, Edinburgh

Ritchie J E 1999 Using qualitative research to enhance the evidence-based practice of health care providers. Australian Journal of Physiotherapy 45: 251–256

Rivett D, Higgs J 1997 Hypothesis generation in the clinical reasoning behavior of manual therapists. Journal of Physical Therapy Education 11(1): 40–45

Rothstein J M, Echternach J L 1986 Hypothesis-oriented algorithm for clinicians: a method for evaluation and treatment planning. Physical Therapy 66: 1388–1394

Sackett D L, Straus S E, Richardson W S et al 2000 Evidence-based medicine: how to practice and teach EBM, 2nd edn. Churchill Livingstone, Edinburgh, pp 1–27, 129–131

Thomas-Edding D 1987 Clinical problem solving in physical therapy and its implications for curriculum development. Proceedings of the Tenth International Congress of the World Confederation of Physical Therapy, Sydney, pp 100–104

Tulder M W van, Malmivaara A, Esmail R et al 2002 Exercise therapy for low back pain. Cochrane Review. In: Cochrane Library, Issue 1, Update Software, Oxford

Waddell G, Main C 1998 A new clinical model of low-back pain and disability. In: Waddell G (ed) The back pain revolution. Churchill Livingstone, Edinburgh, pp 223–240

Watson P 2000 Psychosocial predictors of outcome from low back pain. In: Gifford L (ed) Topical Issues in Pain. 2: Biopsychosocial assessment and management. Relationships and pain. CNS Press, Falmouth, pp 85–109

Watson P, Kendall N 2000 Assessing psychosocial yellow flags. In: Gifford L (ed) Topical Issues in Pain. 2: Biopsychosocial assessment and management. Relationships and pain. CNS Press, Falmouth, pp 111–129

Chapter 28

The integration of validity theory into clinical reasoning: a beneficial process?

A. M. Downing, D. G. Hunter

INTRODUCTION

Central to manual therapy practice lies the process of clinical reasoning. Higgs & Jones (2000) view this reasoning fundamentally as 'the thinking and decision-making processes associated with clinical practice'. Although there is debate between the proponents of various reasoning models (Barrows & Feltovich 1987), clinical reasoning involves formulating assumptions out of which inferences, decisions and actions are taken, and today's spectre of evidence based practice (EBP) encourages all clinicians to ensure that these assumptions and actions are made using the best available evidence (Sackett et al 1996). EBP champions strong scientific evidence as the best evidence due to its objectivity; subjective evidence is deemed less acceptable. Philosophical debate persists around the integration of EBP and medicine (Greenhalgh & Worrall 1997, Tonelli 1999), yet data generation via the 'scientific method' in clinical reasoning is, for many, intuitively compelling as it is seen to confer credibility on the clinician's assumptions and ensuing actions.

The credibility of the decision making ingredients of clinical reasoning relates to the concept of validity. This may be generally interpreted as judgement of the authenticity of inferences, decisions and subsequent actions. In attempting to satisfy the efficacious scrutiny that manual therapy practice now endures, explicitly heeding the concept of validity is likely to feature highly in our defence. But to what extent can the concept of validity truly become assimilated into our clinical reasoning? And how might it dovetail with and enhance clinical reasoning in practice?

This chapter elucidates the meaning of validity and explores the methodological difficulties that confound the process of validating inferences and actions. Drawing on aspects of validity from the research domain, it explores the notion that explicitly integrating validity into clinical reasoning may facilitate the development of a robust foundation for the credibility of modern manual therapy.

VALIDITY

It has been argued that 'validity has so many connotations . . . that its specificity of meaning has been lost' (Feinstein 1985). Indeed, the notion of validity permeates many disciplines, with its definition and form altering slightly in each case. Despite this variability, validity relates to issues of credibility, soundness and authenticity of an action or inference within a particular context. It is important to note that validity addresses the relationship between a concept or measurement and an indicator or purpose. Therefore a slump test, for example, cannot alone be valid; its validity can only be judged when applied for a particular purpose.

In science, measurement validity is typically defined conceptually in relation to two individual, yet allied, dimensions known as relevancy and reliability (Safrit 1981). These dimensions are relevant to the process of clinical reasoning. Relevancy refers to the ability of test scores to measure accurately, under specified conditions, what they are supposed to measure (Safrit 1981), whereas reliability relates to the notion of freedom from measurement error and to the consistency of scores over repeated testing (Safrit 1981). To claim that an action or inference is valid, the claimant must be able to demonstrate evidence for both relevancy and reliability.

While a claim of validity requires necessary and sufficient levels of both reliability and relevancy, a measurement that is reliable but not relevant cannot be valid. For example, in the assessment of subacromial impingement a therapist may produce reliable positive results from the use of the Hawkins–Kennedy impingement test (Hawkins & Hobeika 1983) and claim that the positive test indicates subacromial impingement. However, the low specificity of this test indicates that a positive result has little meaning (Calis et al 2000). Hence the therapist's claim would only be substantiated by reliable not relevant evidence, and reliability does not presuppose validity.

Superficially, the suggestion that therapists should imbibe the notion of validity and its connotations of credibility into clinical reasoning is hard to reject. Indeed many might claim that this notion is already being addressed through EBP, which has been defined as 'the conscientious and judicious use of current best evidence in making the care of individual patients' (Sackett et al 1996). In this definition, 'best' infers valid evidence and as such the EBP movement attempts to validate clinical practice. However, the influence of EBP appears to be focused on validating the treatment component of clinical reasoning by providing hierarchies of evidence of clinical effectiveness (Moore et al 1995). It appears to have had less influence on addressing the equally important issues of data collection and analysis in clinical reasoning (Delitto & Snyder-Mackler 1995), and on integrating qualitative issues into the process (Greenhalgh & Worrall 1997). Indeed, with incomplete categorization and classification of clinical features, how can the clinician decide which clinical trials to integrate into the clinical reasoning process?

Unlike in some branches of mathematics, within the health sciences the quantification of validity is rarely a binary decision; inferences or actions can be valid to a degree or from a particular perspective. For example, in managing a patient the clinician may have several valid treatment options but chooses one because its use appears more valid than the others for a particular patient at that time. As the patient's presentation changes the validity of the current management programme may decrease while that of others increases. In the context of clinical reasoning, therefore, there has to exist the notion of graded validity. Here the clinician rates the credibility of an action or inference on some sort of scale, but does so with the acceptance that rarely will the statement of 100% certainty be defendable.

In terms of clinical testing with diagnostic validity, it has been argued that appraisal of the validity level (including sensitivity, specificity, positive predictive value and negative predictive value) can be helped somewhat by following suitable appraisal guidelines (Greenhalgh 1997, Stratford 2001). However, across the whole gamut of clinical reasoning, the grading of validity at each step in the process becomes enormously complex. The notion of graded validity introduces the problem of just how to implement it. Ironically this will require reliable and relevant criteria that are sensitive enough to discriminate between high and low levels of validity; a valid measurement tool to validate validity at each step in reasoning!

In summary, validity relates to the authenticity of an inference or action and addressing the notion of validity in clinical reasoning is likely to enhance the credibility of clinical practice. In practice there are many complex issues that require rigorous scrutiny and definition before the validating process can be conducted with confidence. While these problems are considerable, developing the skill of defending reasoning behind action cannot be ignored. The clinician may develop proficiency in this process by reflecting upon analogies drawn from the explicit integration of validity theory from the research paradigm.

THE INTEGRATION OF VALIDITY THEORY INTO CLINICAL REASONING

The authors consider the process of clinical reasoning to consist of four fundamental stages: data acquisition; analysis; action; and re-evaluation with possible further action. During clinical reasoning, the clinician accumulates data through the subjective and objective components of the assessment. Data are then prioritized by being passed through a cognitive filter, a process influenced by propositional and non-propositional factors (Higgs & Jones 2000). When sufficient evidence has been amassed to reach an action threshold, an intervention is made. At any stage of this process the clinician may be challenged over the validity of the inferences or actions taken. Validity theory from the research domain may be helpful in constructing suitable arguments to some of these challenges.

RELIABILITY ISSUES

Reliability deals with the capability of a measurement instrument, index or data collection system to produce reproducible results and it forms a necessary, but not sufficient, component of any validity claim. Different strands of reliability are referred to at length in the research literature and they may be classified as follows:

Instrument reliability

An instrument can be defined as an implement, tool or device designed for delicate work or measurement (Penguin English Dictionary 2002). Manual therapy practice employs measurement tools such as clinical tests, visuopalpatory exploration, movement diagrams, observation and subjective questions. In evaluating the reliability of the instrument, the clinician should consider elements relating to the accuracy, precision and stability which allow comment on one aspect of reliability: freedom from measurement error.

Accuracy

Accuracy concerns a result which reflects the true value of the observation being measured (Griffith 1995). If, for example, the clinician uses the navicular drop test as a predictor of overpronation based upon a critical reading of >15 mm of navicular tuberosity drop during weight bearing (Brody 1982), the accuracy of finding a repeatable point on the navicular tuberosity is critical to this process. Palpation as a measurement tool may not be able to yield sufficient accuracy for the subsequent measurement to reflect the true value (Downing & Coales 2001).

Precision

This refers to the degree to which the measurements vary about the mean measurement of a parameter (Nester 2000) or the refinement in measurement. It relates to the size of the intervals on the measurement scale (Griffith 1995) such as decimal points in the temporal measurement of fast movement analysis. In the preceding example, a crude protocol yielding a large variation in a point location on the navicular tuberosity about the mean value would suggest that the measurement protocol lacks precision. However, a refinement to the protocol has been shown to provide reasonably high precision (Downing & Coales 2001).

Stability

This refers to the ability of an 'instrument' or system to maintain accuracy and precision between different tests (Nester 2000). Recently, van der Wurff et al (2000) evaluated the reliability of clinical tests of the sacroiliac joint and suggested there was little evidence to support acceptance of such mobility tests into clinical practice. Studies into this area are hampered, however, by the low stability of the measurements, which are affected by anatomical variation and artefacts of movement from the hip and lumbar spine (Paris 1992).

Sensitivity and specificity

Sensitivity is the ability of a measurement or test to identify positive cases of the observation of interest (Griffith 1995). Specificity is the ability of the measurement or test to exclude negative cases of the observation of interest (Griffith 1995). The sensitivity of the hands is critical in manual therapy and good reliability of palpation has been cited (Downey et al 1999). However, some authors have challenged the clinician's ability to detect subtle motion reliably (Walker 1992) and the area remains controversial. Sensitivity is important in the application of diagnostic tests and clinical tests are rarely expected to demonstrate 100% accuracy. The goal therefore becomes the characterization of the nature of errors in the clinical test (Kassirer 1989).

In this, the notions of test sensitivity and test specificity become important. As sensitivity relates to the ability of the test to identify a condition when present (Sackett et al 1992), a test with high sensitivity is useful for excluding a condition when it is negative, as there are few false positive results. In contrast, specificity relates to the ability of a test to recognize when the condition is absent (Sackett et al 1992). A test, with high specificity, therefore, is useful for ruling in the condition when positive, as there are few false positive results. The acronyms 'SnNout' and 'SpPin' have been developed to help clarify these terms: SnNout refers to high sensitivity [Sn] and a negative result [N] helping to rule out [out] the condition; SpPin refers to high specificity [Sp] and a positive result [P] being useful for ruling in [in] the condition (Sackett et al 1992). Rarely do clinical tests possess excellent sensitivity and specificity. In the diagnosis of subacromial impingement, for example, the painful arc sign is claimed to have low sensitivity (33%) (Calis et al 2000) but high specificity (81%) (Calis et al 2000). Therefore a clinician who makes the inference that a positive painful arc sign indicates subacromial impingement can claim validity for their statement on the basis of a specificity level of 81%. However, the clinician inferring that the absence of the painful arc implies no subacromial impingement may be making an invalid statement as the low sensitivity indicates that little meaning can be drawn from a negative test.

Subject, patient or therapist reliability

This refers to how subject, patient or therapist responses may randomly change from time to time. Mood, motivation, fatigue, memory fluctuations and previous exposure to the test or treatment procedure itself are some of the factors which may powerfully undermine the reliability of subject and therapist responses.

In conclusion, a high level of validity cannot be claimed unless reliability can be established and addressing this, therefore, forms an important component of credible practice. However, reliability alone is not sufficient as the clinician may reliably be incorrect, therefore, greater credibility in defending clinical arguments may be obtained by addressing the issue of validity more directly.

VALIDITY ISSUES

In the research domain, validity issues are typically addressed under a number of different headings.

Internal and external validity

There are two distinct viewpoints on validity which need addressing: internal and external validity (Bailey 1997a, 1997b). Internal validity refers to the confidence that can be placed on the evidence that a particular experimental treatment produced the observed experimental effects. In the clinical setting, this relates to the validity of the inferences made on the basis of treating a single patient or group of patients. The treatment may be perceived to be valid from the patient's perspective but the absence of a control group means it is difficult to make a valid claim that any change in symptoms was caused by the treatment intervention. External validity encapsulates the extent to which findings can be generalized to other settings and populations. Clinically, this relates to the difficulty of generalizing from single cases to the wider patient population and also to the difficulty in integrating the results of research into the management of an individual patient.

External and internal validity are linked in the research paradigm in that external validity is only possible if there is internal validity; however, internal validity may exist without external validity. It is often the case in research that good internal validity, achieved by controlling variables and extraneous factors, results in reduced external validity and generalizability. For example, the controlled environment of the randomized controlled trial (RCT) may produce conclusions which are internally valid; however, the controlled environment may not suitably mimic the clinical situation for valid inferences to be transferred from the research to the clinical setting.

This issue strikes at the heart of the difficulties in substantiating the effectiveness of clinical practice. Given a single patient, no control group and the absence of the opportunity to apply single case study method, the clinician cannot validate the claim that the treatment was the cause of the patient's improvement and therefore cannot claim internal validity regarding the treatment effect. Consequently, there can be no claim of external validity regarding generalization of this treatment approach to other patients. Does this, however, completely invalidate the process? While the RCT is seen to have strong internal validity, its external validity is limited to an average effect on the patients in the trial. Add to this the difficulty of measuring physiological, physical, cognitive and emotional

consequences of clinical intervention, and the complexity of validating clinical actions becomes apparent. In acknowledging this complexity, any comfort that may be drawn from the RCT may be spurious considering the arguable inadequacy of this method in validating many aspects of manual therapy practice. Even guidelines, soundly based upon meta-analyses, may result in good *average* outcomes. These are accepted by politicians and healthcare managers but, as Grimley Evans (1995) questions, could some patients actually be harmed by such mandatory guidelines? Moore & Petty (2001) elaborate this point by implying that there is a temptation to ignore other evidence lower down the evidentiary ladder, but which may be potentially useful in the management of each unique patient.

Types of measurement validity

Measurement validity is addressed widely in the research literature and is typically classified as follows:

Face validity (logical validity)

Sim & Arnell (1993) view face validity as the extent to which a test or assessment appears to measure what it purports to measure. It is a fairly elementary form of validity but concerns the recipient's view of what is happening, and hence is largely a subjective process of validation (George et al 2000). An assessment or treatment may lose face validity if it includes a number of items that appear to the patient to have little or no relevance. Consider, for example, the patient's perception when presenting with lateral elbow pain and receiving treatment to the cervical spine. The patient's thoughts on the validity of the treatment ('Why would the therapist be treating my neck?') may adversely affect the outcome due to poor face validity. The raising of face validity by explanation and justification may enhance patient compliance and face validity in clinical reasoning.

Content validity

This deals with whether the content measured by an instrument or process truly reflects the whole range of elements it is intending to cover. Sim & Arnell (1993) suggest that it is necessary to define the 'domain of content' of what is being measured and then to decide whether the whole domain is adequately assessed by the instrument. For example, with musculoskeletal examination, content validity would be high if it included exploration of all cued biological sources of the dysfunction (connective tissues, joints, muscles, neural tissue, etc.), together with an evaluation of the psychosocial domain, and poor if only a painful muscle were examined.

Construct validity

Many human characteristics are not directly observable, being hypothetical constructs such as, for example, anxiety and pain. Construct validity refers to the extent to which an instrument measures the construct it was intended to measure and to the accumulated evidence that a test performs as expected when measuring an underlying trait or concept (Feldman et al 1990). It is usually established by relating the test results to some other behaviour pattern (Thomas & Nelson 1990). Many of the constructs associated with manual therapy practice are poorly defined, for example pain, stiffness, discomfort and indeed manual therapy itself. In clinical practice, are the most highly validated tools being used in areas where construct validity is the issue at stake?

Criterion validity

This is typically considered from a number of different angles: concurrent, predictive and prescriptive validity. They all have common elements in that they all deal with correctness and with a comparison to some other criterion.

Concurrent validity

This concerns a quantitative measure of the association between an instrument's measurement and a suitable external measure which is deemed to be an accepted criterion or 'gold standard'. An example of good concurrent validity was reported by Rowe et al (2001) following their study comparing flexible electro-goniometric readings with data from a video motion analysis system. The good concurrent validity suggested that a therapist could justify using the cheaper and more widely available flexible electro-goniometer with the knowledge that the outcome measure is valid as compared to the 'gold standard'.

Predictive validity

This concerns the relationship between an instrument's measurement and a later outcome measure. In the management of low back pain there are a number of prospective cohort studies which identify risk factors for chronicity (Burton & Tillotson 1991, Burton et al 1995, Klenerman et al 1995). As such, they are claimed to have predictive validity, illustrated through their use in the support for the UK Clinical Standards Advisory Group's guidelines for the management of acute back pain (Waddell et al 1996).

Prescriptive validity

This is a form of criterion based validity in which the inferred interpretation of a measurement or clinical feature determines the kind of therapeutic intervention a patient is to receive. In clinical practice, a set of measurements which together generate a 'clinical picture' may be deemed to have high or low prescriptive validity. For example, the McKenzie mechanical diagnosis system claims prescriptive validity on the basis of examination techniques that categorize patients with spinal problems and then prescribes effective interventions (Battie et al 1994). However, the prescriptive validity of this approach has been questioned (Cherkin et al 1998, Riddle & Rothstein 1993).

It should be noted that the prescriptive validity of clinical features is often poorly validated by reference to pathoanatomy. For example, the inference that a lumbar lateral shift indicates a lumbar disc herniation (Charnley 1951) is poorly supported in its prescriptive validity, since its diagnostic accuracy in this capacity is poor (Porter & Miller 1986). However, the sign may still possess high clinical prescriptive validity regarding treatment outcomes, in that identification and correction of the shift may provide superior outcomes compared to other treatment approaches. This is an area which still needs further illumination.

Subjective validity

The experimental paradigm of research strives for objectivity in measurement. In reality, clinical practice is drenched with subjectivity and to eliminate this would be akin to the removal of humanity. But there are acknowledged difficulties in quantifiably measuring parameters to validate subjective information. Within research, the qualitative paradigm uses various methods to validate or authenticate subjective data collection, one being 'triangulation'. Here, evidence is gathered from a variety of different and independent sources and integrated. For example, in the clinical setting observations from physicians, clinical psychologists and manual therapists may be united with the patient's view to generate a more valid and rounded conclusion. Another research approach is to use questions and observations that are guided by what the informants feel is relevant and important for the researcher to know. Data analysis is shared with the informants to check if it 'feels right'. Clinically, the patient's words may be carefully rephrased by the therapist and checked to identify if the therapist's understanding fits with what the patient really intended to say. Qualitative research and clinical data collection do not always attempt to provide numerical evidence of validity; the only real issue is does the researcher or clinician really see what he really thinks he sees? Further information on this area can be obtained from authors such as Bailey (1997b).

This review of validity in clinical reasoning via analogies from the research paradigm may be useful to clinicians in the defence of some of the statements and actions made in practice. However, readers are reminded that so much of the clinician/patient interaction is illusive to 'scientific measurement' and therefore turning to science to bestow credibility on these vague yet essential parameters currently yields sparse rewards. The questions therefore are: can we identify and measure these illusive components, and, if so, how can we validate them?

DISCUSSION

In the research community, researchers live with the concept of validity, considering how they can establish and claim validity at each step of the research process. But, to what extent is it possible to address these issues so meticulously in clinical reasoning?

In order to facilitate the inclusion of such issues in clinical reasoning, perhaps the use of a simple validity evaluation system to train and enhance reasoning through the promotion of overt attention to validity would be helpful (Fig. 28.1)? This system would be akin to the use of movement diagrams as a learning tool (Maitland 1986), to become an internalized process with the development of expertise. To employ this system, the clinician makes an inference or an action and rates its authenticity and credibility on a validity scale. The clinician places a horizontal mark on the vertical line between zero and 100 to indicate how valid they feel that their inference or action is. Then they define the type and level of evidence used to authenticate their validity score.

The proposed system is simplistic in its current form, but the inclusion of this idea into clinical reasoning may promote discussion of the criteria used to authenticate claims for a validity level; through this process the system will be adapted and improved. Although undoubtedly complex and challenging, such debate may deepen the process of clinical reasoning and facilitate the clinician's ability to defend their claims. It is also hoped that the use of the system at different stages of clinical reasoning will help to redress the balance of validity issues, currently stacked towards treatment effectiveness.

To illustrate some of the issues which may occur in using this system, consider the following example. Clinician A performs an anterior draw test of the knee and infers that the patient has a grade 2 anterior cruciate ligament tear. The clinician rates the validity of this inference on the scale at 60%. The evidence presented to validate this statement is that clinician A is an expert in this area. Clinician B carries out the same procedure and comes to the same conclusion, rating the validity at 60%, but has well conducted research to substantiate the 60% value. The level of evidence may be perceived to be higher for clinician B than for clinician A. Is clinician B's statement therefore more valid since it is possible to authenticate the claim to a higher degree in the evidentiary hierarchy? If they both turn out to be correct, as evidenced at arthroscopy, is one clinician's judgement more valid than the other?

Clinician B turned to science and EBP to claim validity. Clinician A authenticated the inference with intuition, expert opinion and resulting pragmatic efficacy. Does this make the inference and decision less valid? Such a notion of pragmatic efficacy (Kapchuk et al 1996, Schwartz & Lellouch 1967) sits surprisingly well with the outcome orientated trends in research and practice. This may offer some degree of validity for a pragmatic reasoning perspective in problem solving among expert clinicians. Yet it seems that the epistemology of EBP categorizes expert opinion as the lowest form of evidence, superseded even by methodologically flawed clinical research evidence (Tonelli 1999). Does this argue invalidity of that expert opinion which is based upon primary experience? Philosophers and scientists have, for centuries, dismissed the validity of primary experience as unable to provide meaningful chance for the discovery of truth and wisdom (Reed 1996). Yet commonly in clinical practice patient data are acquired and interpretations considered, sifted and a 'best fit is judged of past experiences with the current patient presentations' (Brookfield 2000). Subjectivity has always been and always will be a necessary component of clinical reasoning, but tension exists between this notion and the objectivity sought by EBP. For example, clinician A's evidence, based on experience, could unwittingly devalue the reasoning process. As Brookfield (2000) states, 'a self-confirming cycle often develops whereby our uncritically accepted assumptions shape clinical actions, which then serve only to confirm the truth of these assumptions'. Validity at this point becomes central to any discussion of 'are we really doing what we think we are doing?'

A fundamental question exists: is it the case that clinician B's reasoning process, dominated by EBP, is therefore 'better', more valid and an exemplar? Philosophical, theoretical and practical objections to EBP have been raised (Feinstein & Horwitz 1997). However, we would suggest, along with Herbert et al (2001), that if objective evidence is combined with but does not dominate other clinical evidence, EBP can contribute strength to patient care and the systematic use of valid arguments in its defence.

This scenario leads into the question of weighting arguments and of the validity of expertise, experience and intuition. Clinical reasoning theory acknowledges differences of approach. Normative theories (Refshauge 1995) assume that there are optimal answers and may incorporate probability theory to help arrive at the optimal solution. Decision making theories, however, emphasize the use of knowledge and experience and the thinking process. If, for the moment, we have difficulty characterizing the reasoning process, at least the discipline of addressing validity at different stages, perhaps using a validity evaluation system, could help to optimize the situation.

Clearly, the integration of validity issues from the research paradigm is not straightforward. Validity probably needs to be viewed in a broader manner, perhaps as more of an epistemological concept supporting the quest for best practice through clinical reasoning. The place for expert opinion remains debatable. It seems that expert opinion does not overtly embrace the traditional canons of validity and reliability required in support of evidence. Is it possible then, as Tonelli (1999) suggests, that the proponents of evi-

Validity Scale	Evidence	Level of Evidence
100		
0		

Figure 28.1 Validity evaluation system.
*Key: 0 = the inference or action is invalid; 100 = the inference or action is 100% valid.

dence based practice have erred by defining expert opinion as a type of 'evidence' for clinical decision making, one quickly supplanted by the evidence derived from clinical studies as this becomes available? Or is it that expert opinion is a 'separate, complex type of knowledge' (Tonelli 1999) with a value of its own? Could manual therapists identify with Tonelli (1999) in *valuing* the expert opinion of masters in manual therapy, in the help it provides to overcome an epistemic gap that exists between the results of clinical research and the care of individual patients? Tonelli (1999) suggests a view that expert opinion may be the highest form of clinical experience and judgement, and needs to be seen as integral to the multifaceted medical knowledge that underpins patient care. Is there, therefore, a degree of logical face and content validity in expert opinion which is justifiable?

CONCLUSION

A number of issues relating to validity and its close relation, reliability, have been explored. Fundamental issues affecting manual therapy practice are these: are our inferences valid and are we doing what we say we are doing? There seem to be different strands of validity when the research paradigm is examined, and these may usefully be applied to the practice context in an effort to heighten our critical awareness of truly doing what we believe we are doing or not. This has legal and ethical relevance in manual therapy practice. The validity of expert opinion has been aired and some questions raised. For the moment, manual therapy practice is influenced by the EBP movement which, despite its imperfections, has potentially a great value for us and for our patients. Perhaps, however, there is scope for a balancing of thought over the validity of EBP, the validity of expert opinion, the validity of our reasoning processes and an acknowledgement that not all epistemologies can ever stand up to scientific scrutiny. Validity theory may help us get to grips with the balancing act.

KEYWORDS

validity   clinical reasoning
reliability

References

Bailey D M 1997a Quantitative research designs. In: Research for the health professional: a practical guide, 2nd edn. F A Davis, Philadelphia, pp 70–72

Bailey D M 1997b Qualitative research designs. In: Research for the health professional: a practical guide, 2nd edn. F A Davis, Philadelphia, pp 146–150

Barrows H S, Feltovich P J 1987 The clinical reasoning process. Medical Education 21: 86–91

Battie M C, Cherkin D C, Dunn R et al 1994 Managing low back pain: attitudes and treatment preferences of physical therapists. Physical Therapy 74: 219–226

Brody D M 1982 Techniques in the evaluation and treatment of the injured runner. Orthopedic Clinics of North America 13(3): 541–558

Brookfield S 2000 Clinical reasoning and generic thinking skills. In: Higgs J, Jones M (eds) Clinical reasoning in the health professions, 2nd edn. Butterworth Heinemann, Oxford, ch 7, pp 62–67

Burton A K, Tillotson K M 1991 Prediction of the clinical course of low-back trouble using multivariable models. Spine 16: 7–14

Burton A K, Tillotson M, Main M et al 1995 Psychosocial predictors of outcome in acute and subchronic low back trouble. Spine 20: 722–772

Calis M, Akgun K, Birante M et al 2000 Diagnostic value of clinical diagnostic tests in sub acromial impingement syndrome Annals of Rheumatic Disease 59: 44–47

Charnley J 1951 Orthopedic signs in the diagnosis of disc protrusion. Lancet 1: 186–192

Cherkin D C, Deyo R A, Battie M et al 1998 A comparison of physical therapy, chiropractic manipulation, and provision of an educational booklet for the treatment of patients with low back pain. New England Journal of Medicine 339: 1021–1029

Delitto A, Snyder-Mackler L 1995 The diagnostic process: examples in orthopaedic physical therapy. Physical Therapy 75: 203–211

Downey B J, Taylor N F, Niere K R 1999 Manipulative physiotherapists can reliably palpate nominated lumbar spinal levels. Manual Therapy 4(3): 151–156

Downing A M, Coales P J 2001 The intratester reliability of finding a precise point on the navicular tuberosity for use in foot measurements. Book of Abstracts of the sixth Annual Congress of the European College of Sport Science, Cologne, p 367

Feinstein A R 1985 Clinical epidemiology. Saunders, Philadelphia, p 58

Feinstein A R, Horwitz A I 1997 Problems in the 'evidence' of 'evidence-based medicine'. American Journal of Medicine 103: 529–535

Feldman A B, Hailey S M, Coryell J 1990 Concurrent and construct validity of the Pediatric Evaluation of Disability Inventory. Physical Therapy 70: 602–610

George K, Batterham A, Sullivan I 2000 Validity in clinical research: a review of the concepts and definitions. Physical Therapy in Sport 1: 19–27

Gimley Evans J 1995 Evidence-based and evidence-biased medicine. Age and Ageing 24: 461–463

Greenhalgh T 1997 How to read a paper: the basics of evidence-based medicine. BMJ Publishing, London, pp 101–110

Greenhalgh T, Worrall J G 1997 From EBM to CSM: the evolution of context sensitive medicine? Journal of Evaluation in Clinical Practice 3(2): 105–108

Griffith C J 1995 Clinical measurement. In: Merriman LM, Tollafield D R (eds) Assessment of the lower limb. Churchill Livingstone, Edinburgh, pp 35–50

Hawkins R J, Hobeika P E 1983 Impingement syndrome in the athletic shoulder. Clinics in Sports Medicine 2(2): 391–405

Herbert R D, Sherrington C, Maher C, Moseley A 2001 Evidence-based practice: imperfect but necessary. Physiotherapy Theory and Practice 17: 201–211

Higgs J, Jones M 2000 Clinical reasoning in the health professions. In: Higgs J, Jones M (eds) Clinical reasoning in the health professions, 2nd edn. Butterworth Heinemann, Oxford, pp 3–14

Kapchuk T J, Edwards R A, Eisenberg D M 1996 Complementary medicine: efficacy beyond the placebo effect. In: Ernst E (ed) Complementary medicine: an objective appraisal. Butterworth Heinemann, Oxford

Kassirer J P 1989 Our stubborn quest for diagnostic certainty: a cause of excessive testing. New England Journal of Medicine 320: 1489–1491

Klenerman L, Slade P D, Stanley I M et al 1995 The prediction of chronicity in patients with an acute attack of low back pain in a general practice setting. Spine 20: 478–484

Maitland G D 1986 Movement diagram theory and compiling a movement diagram. In: Vertebral manipulation, 5th edn. Butterworths, London, appx 1, pp 351–364

Moore A, McQuay H, Gray J A M (eds) 1995 Evidence-based everything. Bandolier 1(12): 1

Moore A, Petty N 2001 Evidence-based practice: getting a grip and finding a balance. Manual Therapy 6(4): 195–196

Nester C J 2000 Pragmatic approach to the effect of camera arrangement on the performance of a motion analysis system. Journal of Human Movement Studies 39: 265–276

Paris S V 1992 Differential diagnosis of sacroiliac joints from lumbar spine dysfunction. In: Vleeming A et al (eds) Course proceedings for the First Interdisciplinary World Congress on Low back Pain and its Relation to the Sacroiliac Joint, San Diego, California, pp 313–329

Penguin English Dictionary 2002 Penguin Group, London, p 460

Porter R W, Miller C G 1986 Back pain and trunk list. Spine 11: 596–600

Reed E 1996 The necessity of experience. Yale University Press, New Haven

Refshauge K M 1995 Theoretical basis underlying clinical decisions: clinical reasoning in physiotherapy. In: Refshauge K, Gass E (eds) Musculoskeletal physiotherapy, clinical science and practice. Butterworth Heinemann, Oxford, pp 6–44

Riddle D L, Rothstein J M 1993 Intertester reliability of McKenzie's classification of the syndrome types present in patients with low back pain. Spine 18: 1333–1344

Rowe P J, Myles C M, Hillmann S J, Hazlewood M E 2001 Validation of flexible electrogoniometry as a measure of joint kinematics. Physiotherapy 87(9): 479–488

Sackett D, Haynes R B, Guyatt G H, Tugwell P 1992 Clinical epidemiology: a basic science for clinical medicine, 2nd edn. Little, Brown, Boston, Massachusetts

Sackett D L, Rosenberg W M, Gray J A, Haynes R B, Richardson W S 1996 Evidence based medicine: what it is and what it isn't. BMJ 312(7023): 71–72

Safrit M J 1981 Evaluation in physical education, 2nd edn. Prentice-Hall, Englewood Cliffs, New Jersey

Schwartz D, Lellouch J 1967 Explanatory and pragmatic attitudes in therapeutical trials. Journal of Chronic Diseases 20(8): 637–648

Sim J, Arnell P 1993 Measurement validity in physical therapy research. Physical Therapy 73(2): 102–115

Stratford P W 2001 Applying the results from diagnostic accuracy studies to enhance clinical decision-making. Physiotherapy Theory and Practice 17: 153–160

Thomas J R, Nelson J K 1990 Research methods in physical activity, 2nd edn. Human Kinetics, Champaign, Illinois

Tonelli M R 1999 In defense of expert opinion. Academic Medicine 74(11): 1187–1192

Van der Wurff P, Hagmeijer R H M, Meyne W 2000 Clinical tests of the sacroiliac joint: a systematic methodological review. Part 1: Reliability. Manual Therapy 5(1): 30–36

Waddell G, Feder G, McIntosh A et al 1996 Low back pain evidence review. Royal College of General Practitioners, London

Walker J M 1992 The sacroiliac joint: a critical review. Physical Therapy 72(12): 903–916.

Chapter 29

Management of mechanosensitivity of the nervous system in spinal pain syndromes

T. M. Hall, R. L. Elvey

INTRODUCTION

In the management of neuromusculoskeletal disorders arising from the spine, identification of specific diagnostic subgroups should be of significant importance. Patients classified into distinct subgroups, having common readily identifiable disorders, can then be prescribed appropriate treatment strategies. It appears logical that specific treatment designed for a distinct category of pain will have a more favourable outcome when compared to a generic approach, and the literature appears to support this (Jull & Moore 2000, O'Sullivan et al 1997a, 1997b).

For most manual therapists, a significant aspect of the examination procedure is to identify any possible physical cause or the structural origin of the patient's pain. It is accepted that a primary lesion in the peripheral nervous system can cause persistent pain and other sensations (Quintner & Bove 2001) and that neural tissue syndromes are a significant subgroup of spinal pain disorders (Abenhaim et al 2000, Spitzer, 1987), but they can be difficult to define.

In general when considering pain of neural tissue origin, musculoskeletal medicine usually considers nerve compression resulting in pain and axonal conduction block. This occurs in the more readily diagnosable forms of peripheral neuropathies such as nerve root compression and peripheral nerve entrapments but these are a relatively rare occurrence in general clinical practice (Bogduk 1997, Drye & Zachazewski 1996).

In comparison, a far more common clinical presentation is pain arising from neural tissues of the spine that projects to a limb in the absence of detectable peripheral neurological deficit (Hall & Elvey 1999, Sampath et al 1999). There is evidence that increased neural tissue mechanosensitivity occurs in many patients who present with this kind of disorder (Allison et al 2002, Selvaratnam et al 1994). In chronic cervicobrachial pain, increased neural tissue mechanosensitivity has been shown to be the dominant feature in up to one third of cases (Allison et al 2002, Hall et al 1997). Similar proportions were found in subjects with low back and leg pain (Beyerlein et al 2001). Therefore, it is apparent that neural tissue mechanosensitization is a significant factor which should be a routine consideration in the clinical examination.

The pathological basis for increased neural tissue mechanosensitivity remains controversial (Ochoa 1997, Sorkin et al 1997, Willis 1997). Of particular interest is the involvement of sensory mechanisms of neural tissue, the nervi nervorum (Bove & Light 1997). Several studies have demonstrated the presence of nervi nervorum in the connective tissues layers of peripheral nerve trunks as well as the dorsal root ganglion (Bove & Light 1997, Hromada 1963, Shantha & Evans 1972, Thomas et al 1993), a subset of which have features of nociceptive afferents (Sauer et al 1999). Sensitization of the nervi nervorum afferent pathways appears to be the likely cause for the underlying disorder of neural tissue mechanosensitization (Quintner & Bove 2001). However, recently it has been suggested that immune activation near peripheral nerves may have a greater role in creating pain of neural origin than was previously recognised (Chacur et al 2001, Eliav et al 1999) and this may be the explanation for neural tissue mechanosensitization rather than the nervi nervorum.

At present there are no scientific tests that can readily identify neural tissue pain disorders. In these disorders tests for axonal conduction block have limited sensitivity, specificity and positive predictive value (Dvorak 1996). However, with the improvement of magnetic resonance neurography and diagnostic ultrasound, there appears to be hope in the future for the examination of neural tissue (Hough et al 2000, Maravilla & Bowen 1998). For the present the detection of increased neural tissue mechanosensitivity is based on a comprehensive clinical examination.

Although clinical examination and treatment of the peripheral nervous system in disorders of the neuromusculoskeletal system is not new (Madison Taylor 1909, Marshall 1883) the development of this concept in recent years can be attributed to Elvey (1979, 1986) and Butler (1991).

This chapter will present the scientific evidence underlying the concept of neural tissue mechanosensitivity. A comprehensive examination procedure will be outlined to determine whether neural tissue sensitization is the dominant feature in a particular presentation and, where indicated, strategies for management will be presented.

NEURAL TISSUE MECHANOSENSITIZATION

This chapter considers neural syndromes related to the spine, and the most important structures in relation to this are the nerve roots that form an anatomically unique region with characteristics of both the central and peripheral nervous system. Topographically they may be considered to be part of the central nervous system due to their location in the centre of the spine and their close connection to the spinal cord. However, functionally the nerve roots are more similar to peripheral nerves (Olmarker et al 1997).

The ventral and dorsal nerve rootlets originate in the spinal cord and terminate at the level of the dorsal root ganglion by joining to become a mixed spinal nerve. Distal to this point the nerve roots divide into their branches: the ventral and dorsal rami, and exit the intervertebral foramen (Giles 1997). The spinal nerves and peripheral nerve trunks are covered by protective epineurial connective tissue called the epineurium, perineurium and endoneurium. The dura mater and other meninges protect more proximal neural structures (Sunderland 1991). The nerve roots, both ventral and dorsal, as well as the dorsal root ganglion and spinal nerves, are innervated by the nervi nervorum whose functions are varied but include nociception (Bove & Light 1995a, 1995b, Giles 1997, Hasue 1993, Hromada 1963, Janig & Koltzenburg 1991, Thomas et al 1993).

Pain is defined as 'an unpleasant sensory and emotional experience associated with actual or potential tissue damage, or described in terms of such damage' (Merskey & Bogduk 1994). This definition highlights the fact that pain has both physiological and psychological factors and both are important (Unruh et al 2002). The physiological mechanisms underlying pain perception are becoming better understood and there are excellent texts to help the reader understand this complex but clinically significant area (Srinivasa et al 1999, Wright 1999, 2002). It is apparent that there are important changes to both the central and peripheral nervous system which modify a normally quiescent system requiring strong, intense, potentially damaging stimulation before it becomes activated to one where relatively innocuous stimuli activate the system and trigger pain perception (Wright 1999).

Pain has been classified into two types, nociceptive or neuropathic. However, there may be a combination of both (Elliot 1994). Nociceptive pain is that which arises from chemically or mechanically induced impulses from non-neural tissues (Bogduk 1997, Elliot 1994). Neuropathic pain is that which arises from neural structures (Elliot 1994). This type of pain is perceived in cutaneous tissues that may be distant from the pathologic neural tissue. Pain arising from stimulation of the nervi nervorum does not appear to have been classified into either a nociceptive or a neuropathic category. Although physiologically it is nociceptive, we consider pain resulting from stimulation of the nervi nervorum to be included in the neuropathic classification.

The term peripheral neuropathic pain has been suggested to incorporate the varied symptoms in those patients in whom pain is due to pathological changes or dysfunction in neural tissue distal to the dorsal horn (Devor & Rappaport 1990). These structures include peripheral nerve trunks, nerve roots as well as dorsal and ventral rami.

Two types of neuropathic pain following peripheral nerve injury have been recognized: 'dysaesthetic pain' and 'nerve trunk pain' (Asbury & Fields 1984). Dysaesthetic pain is perceived in the distribution of a sensory nerve and is thought to be due to activity in damaged axons (Asbury & Fields 1984). This pain has characteristic features which include: abnormal sensations, frequently having a burning or electrical quality; pain felt in the region of the sensory deficit; pain with a paroxysmal brief shooting or stabbing component; and the presence of allodynia (Devor 1991, Devor & Seltzer, 1999, Fields 1987). Allodynia is the production of pain by a mechanical stimulus that would not normally be painful (Merskey & Bogduk 1994).

In contrast nerve trunk pain has been attributed to increased activity in sensitized nociceptors within nerve connective tissues (Asbury & Fields 1984). This kind of pain is said to follow the course of the nerve trunk. It is commonly described as deep and aching, familiar, and made worse with movement, nerve stretch or palpation (Asbury & Fields 1984). Nerve trunk pain is interchangeable with increased neural tissue mechanosensitization.

The nervi nervorum form a sporadic plexus in all the connective tissues of a peripheral nerve trunk. They have predominantly 'free' endings and are capable of mechanoreception (Hromada 1963, Thomas et al 1993). Electrophysiological studies have demonstrated that at least some of the nervi nervorum afferents have a nociceptive function for they respond to noxious mechanical, chemical and thermal stimuli (Bove & Light 1995b). Most nervi nervorum studied by Bove & Light (1995a) were sensitive to excess longitudinal stretch of the entire nerve they innervated, as well as to local stretch in any direction and to focal pressure. They did not respond to stretch within normal ranges of motion. This evidence is supported by clinical studies that show under normal circumstances nerve trunks are insensitive to non-noxious mechanical stimuli (Hall & Quintner 1996, Kuslich et al 1991).

Recent evidence has shown that the nervi nervorum contain neuropeptides including substance P and calcitonin gene related peptide, indicating a role in neurogenic vasodilation (Bove & Light 1997, Sauer et al 1999, Zochodne 1993). It has been suggested that local nerve inflammation is mediated by the nervi nervorum, especially in cases with no intrafascicular axonal damage (Bove & Light 1997). In keeping with this, it has been postulated that the spread of mechanosensitivity along the length of the nerve trunk distant to the local area of pathology is mediated through neurogenic inflammation via the nervi nervorum whose branches extend for relatively long distances (Quintner 1998, Quintner & Bove 2001). The entire nerve trunk then behaves as a sensitized nociceptor, generating impulses in response to minor mechanical stimuli (Devor 1989).

The mechanism of neurogenic inflammation may help to explain mechanical allodynia of structurally normal nerve trunks, where the pathology is more proximal in the nerve root. An alternative explanation is that non-nociceptive input from the presumed nerve trunk mechanoreceptors is being processed abnormally within the central nervous system (Hall & Quintner 1996). This is probably the result of a sustained afferent nociceptive barrage from the site of nerve damage (Sugimoto et al 1989), a pathological process termed central sensitization (Woolf 1991).

Neural tissue mechanosensitization is a form of mechanical allodynia, which is closely related to the phenomenon of hyperalgesia, an exaggerated or increased response to a noxious stimulus. The process whereby the nociceptive system can be up-regulated to cause these phenomena is dependent upon changes to both central and peripheral sensitization (Wright 2002). Peripheral mechanisms alone cannot explain the process whereby neural tissue becomes sensitive to mechanical stimuli.

Epidemiologically, nerve root compression is an infrequent occurrence in low back disorders, yet it is a commonly cited form of neuropathic disorder that usually results from intervertebral disc herniation but also is commonly caused by age related changes (Bogduk 1997, Epstein et al 1973). Animal models of chronic nerve compression were first carried out by Bennett & Xie (1988) and showed features consistent with neuropathic pain including mechanical allodynia. Although pain is not a necessary feature of nerve root compression (MacNab 1972, Rydevik & Garfin 1989, Wiesel et al 1984), radicular pain can occur in the presence of chronic compression of the nerve root (Bogduk 1997, Winkelstein et al 2002). Under these circumstances there may be minimal evidence of neural tissue mechanosensitivity on tests such as straight leg raise (SLR) (Amundsen et al 1995, Rydevik & Garfin 1989) but there should be clinical, radiological and probably electrodiagnostic evidence of neurological deficit.

Alternatively radicular pain, even when severe, may present where axonal conduction is normal but the nerve trunk is highly mechanically sensitized. In this case clinical, neurological and electrodiagnostic tests may be normal suggesting a lack of nerve root compression. What appears to be the significant factor in radicular pain is the development of inflammation (Olmarker & Rydevik 1991), sensitization of the nervi nervorum and mechanical allodynia of peripheral nerve trunks. It has been suggested that intervertebral disc tissue (Franson et al 1992, Gertzbein 1977, Marshall et al 1977, Saal et al 1990), perhaps following injury or degenerative changes, may cause an autoimmune inflammatory tissue reaction of the nerve roots (Bobechko & Hirsch 1965, Olmarker et al 1993, Spiliopoulou et al 1994). The results of one study suggest a correlation between limited range of SLR and inflammatory cell occurrence in disc herniations (Gronblad & Virri 1997). Recently a role for the immune system in minor neuropathic pain disorders has been proposed (Bennett 2000). In this model macrophages and immunocytes at the site of minor nerve trauma induce inflammatory and immune reactions, although there is very limited damage to axons (Eliav et al 1999). Experiments on animal models have shown that immune reactions induce changes consistent with a neuritis (Chacur et al 2001). An inflammatory/immune model of sciatica, rather than a compressive model, would better explain the efficacy of epidural injections of corticosteroids, local anaesthetics and saline that have been shown to relieve the pain of sciatica and improve range of SLR (Falconer et al 1948, Olmarker & Rydevik 1991, Rogers et al 1992).

The nervi nervorum appear to be prime candidates for mediating increased neural tissue mechanosensitization (Quintner & Bove 2001). However, their role is still controversial and much further work is required to explain the mechanisms of chronic pain associated with peripheral neuropathic pain.

CLINICAL EXAMINATION

The purpose of the clinical examination is firstly to identify the patient's subjective complaint so that an appropriately planned physical examination can be carried out with due respect to the nature of the presenting disorder. The subjective examination also serves to identify factors that may guide management. The use of 'red' and 'yellow' flags helps to screen for contraindications to manual therapy and provides information related to patient outcome and prognosis. While red flags are used to diagnose serious disease such as cancer, yellow flags refer to psychosocial factors that increase the risk of developing or perpetuating disability associated with pain (Maher et al 2000).

In the clinical experience of the authors, serious disease processes can be associated with neural tissue syndromes. Classic examples include diabetic neuropathy and space occupying lesions such as Pancoast's tumour. Features of the subjective examination will help to identify specific patients at risk. Maher et al (2000) compiled a list of red flags outlining possible risk factors for serious lumbar spine pathology. It is beholden upon all primary contact practitioners to acquaint themselves with this type of information.

Psychosocial issues affect to a varying degree all patients with chronic pain but are particularly relevant to disorders of neural tissue sensitization. Frequently, the patient has to deal with the challenge of long-term severe pain, physical impairment and disability. Failure to respond to treatment may be a reflection of psychosocial factors rather than poorly directed management.

At the completion of the subjective examination the clinician should have developed a diagnostic hypothesis, through clinical reasoning, regarding the structural origin of the patient's pain and whether neural structures are involved. Significant features guiding this decision include area and quality of pain and the presence of associated symptoms. For instance, in the lumbar spine, somatic referred pain arising from the zygapophysial joints is commonly perceived in the lumbar and gluteal regions and proximal thigh (Fukui et al 1997, Mooney & Robertson 1976).

By way of contrast, pain that traverses the entire length of the limb, along a narrow band, is said to most likely involve neural structures (Bogduk 1997), although the evidence for this is based on a single pain provocation study (Smyth & Wright 1958). Others have also suggested that pain from the lumbar spine radiating below the knee is likely to involve neural compromise (Austen 1991, McCulloch

& Waddell 1980). In contrast it has been shown that the lumbar disc is capable of referring pain into the entire length of the limb and the extent of radiation is related to the intensity of disc stimulus (O'Neill et al 2002).

As previously mentioned, Asbury & Fields (1984) proposed that pain of nerve trunk origin and axonal compromise have distinctive features which set them apart. The presence of any altered sensation is said to be strongly suggestive of nerve compromise. However, other conditions, including vascular disorders and perhaps altered afferent input from somatic structures, may also cause paraesthesia (Refshauge & Gass 1995).

Based upon the experience of the authors as well as others experience, pain arising from nerve trunk mechanosensitization does not always fit a typical ordered description (Gifford 2001). Pain and paraesthesia that accompany radiculopathy are not well localized anatomically (Slipman et al 1998), due to different nerve roots having a similar dermatomal distribution. In a large series of patients with cervical radiculopathy, only half had pain following a typical discrete dermatomal pattern (Henderson et al 1983). The remainder presented with diffuse non-dermatomally distributed pain. A number of other studies have shown that the location of pain and paraesthesia is not a good predictor of the presence of nerve root compression (Austen 1991, Dalton & Jull 1989, Rankine et al 1998).

One subjective feature that may be of diagnostic benefit is the presence of spontaneous pain. It is well known that damaged axons form ectopic pacemaker sites that are highly mechanically sensitive and capable of spontaneous and self-sustaining impulse generation (Devor & Seltzer 1999), even at rest. This feature may help to differentiate neural tissue disorders related to increased mechanosensitization involving the nervi nervorum from those neuropathic disorders involving damaged axons and the presence of ectopic pacemaker sites. In the experience of the authors, disorders of nerve mechanosensitization, which would appear to involve the nervi nervorum, do not present with spontaneous pain as a common feature. Pain is related to specific aggravating activities or postures that would mechanically stimulate and provoke a pain response from sensitized nervi nervorum.

As is always the case, information from the subjective examination should be interpreted with caution and within the context of the complete clinical evaluation. The combination of local pain, somatic referred pain and neurogenic pain makes planning the scope and range of the physical examination more challenging for the clinician who must evaluate the disorder to determine which aspect predominates.

Physical evaluation of neural tissue follows the same principles used in examination of any other structure in the body. For example, a clinical presentation of tennis elbow, or lateral epicondylalgia, requires a number of physical examination tests correlating with each other before a diagnosis can be made. Such tests would include pain provocation by isometric muscle contraction, muscle stretch and palpation. These physical tests provide mechanical stimuli to the injured tissue and so are provocative tests seeking a subjective pain response. By way of differential diagnosis it would be important to examine for referred symptoms from remote areas (Gunn 1980, Lee 1986). In the absence of remote structure involvement it would be possible to classify the disorder as lateral epicondylalgia. However, it is apparent that no test in isolation is sufficient to provide a consistent accurate diagnosis.

To determine the degree to which increased neural tissue mechanosensitization is involved in a presenting disorder, clinical reasoning must be employed, which is similar to, but more sophisticated than that used for lateral epicondylalgia. A number of very specific correlating signs must be present and it is not possible to say that a single test such as SLR is positive or negative in the diagnosis of lumbosacral nerve root pathology. Indeed investigation of discriminative validity for the SLR test has found it to have high sensitivity but low specificity (Fahrni 1966, Hudgins 1975, McNab 1971, van den Hoogen et al 1995), the reason being that the mechanical stress of SLR is not isolated to neural structures. SLR induces an almost immediate posterior rotation of the pelvis upon lifting the leg from the horizontal (Fahlgren Grampo et al 1991) and many structures in the posterior thigh, pelvis and lumbar spine will be mechanically involved (Kleyhans & Terrett 1986). The example of SLR highlights the fact that individual tests cannot be interpreted in isolation to formulate pathological diagnoses (Boland 1995).

Physical signs of neural tissue involvement

Elvey & Hall (1997) have presented a series of criteria required to be present in the physical examination before a diagnosis of increased neural tissue mechanosensitivity can be determined:

1. antalgic posture
2. active movement dysfunction
3. passive movement dysfunction, which correlates directly with the degree of active movement dysfunction
4. adverse responses to neural tissue provocation tests, which relate specifically and anatomically to 2 and 3
5. mechanical allodynia in response to palpation of specific nerve trunks, which relates specifically and anatomically to 2, 3 and 4
6. evidence of a local cause for the neural tissue mechanosensitization disorder, which relates specifically and anatomically to 4 and 5.

To date there are no studies that have investigated the reliability, sensitivity, specificity or diagnostic validity of this systematic examination. Sensitivity, specificity and validity are difficult to investigate, as there are no gold standard tests available to enable a comparison.

Under normal circumstances, the entire nervous system is well adapted to allow the change in length associated with movement and positional change (Breig 1978, Elvey 1986, Goddard & Reid 1965, McLellan & Swash 1976, Troup 1986). Normal peripheral nerve trunks and nerve roots are painless to non-noxious mechanical stimuli (Hall & Quintner 1996, Howe et al 1977, Kuslich et al 1991, Smyth & Wright 1958). In contrast it has been recorded that inflamed neural tissue is highly sensitive to mild mechanical provocation (Kuslich et al 1991, Smyth & Wright 1958) and hence movement of the sensitized neural tissue will generate nociceptive responses. Under these circumstances even the most basic activities of daily living can become unbearable in the presence of increased neural tissue mechanosensitization.

If the disorder is severe enough, neural tissue becomes non-compliant to movement, be it induced actively by the patient or passively by the therapist. Restriction of movement is probably caused in part by pain and part by protective muscle contraction (Elvey 1992, Hall et al 1998). Muscular responses to mechanical provocative stress of neural tissue have been recorded by electromyography, in both animal and in vivo human experiments (Balster & Jull 1997, Hall & Quintner 1996, Hall et al 1995, Hu et al 1993, 1995, Monsivais et al 1995). This muscular response is an important aspect of the physical examination that can provide useful feedback with respect to mechanosensitive neural structures.

The clinician can use a sound knowledge of neural, peripheral joint and spinal anatomy to apply selective stress to individual nerve trunks as part of the physical examination. Using a combination of pain and muscular responses the clinician can then begin to identify the affected neural structures to formulate a specific diagnosis pertaining to the spinal or peripheral neural structures involved.

Posture

Posture or alignment is the first aspect of the physical examination and may be the first clinical consideration of a neural tissue mechanosensitization disorder. Formal assessment of alignment is carried out with the patient standing, sitting or lying, based on the subjective complaint. Abnormal alignment is a common finding in patients presenting with musculoskeletal disorders (Sahrmann 2002). However, abnormal alignment is not necessarily related to impaired muscle system balance (Sahrmann 2002). Rather, abnormal alignment can be a protective response of the muscle system to increased mechanosensitivity of the neural system (Hall & Elvey 2001). When the disorder is severe enough, the adopted antalgic position is one that would shorten the anatomical distance over which the sensitized neural tissue courses (Hall & Elvey 2001). Guarded postures to avoid movement of sensitized neural tissue have been demonstrated in an animal model (Laird & Bennett 1993). Hu et al (1993, 1995) showed that the application of a small fibre irritant to cervical neuromeningeal tissues resulted in an increased EMG activity in the upper trapezius and jaw muscles. Monsivais et al (1995) showed EMG activity in scalenes associated with pressure on the ipsilateral median and ulnar nerve in goats. Such tonic muscle activity in humans is likely to result in changes to spinal and shoulder girdle alignment (Fig. 29.1). This is a common clinical finding in those patients that present with neck and shoulder pain where neural tissue mechanosensitization is a dominant feature.

The posture subconsciously adopted, for example, to relieve provocation on a mechanosensitive C6 nerve root is any combination of shoulder girdle elevation, shoulder adduction and medial rotation, cervical spine ipsilateral lateral flexion and elbow flexion.

Active movement

Assessment of active movement is a routine part of the physical examination whatever the type and stage of the disorder. During active movement peripheral nerve trunks glide and slide in relation to surrounding structures. For example during shoulder abduction, a movement of the brachial plexus of 15.3 mm has been observed at the shoulder (Wilgis & Murphy 1986) and a distal displacement of 4 mm observed at the C5 spinal nerve level (Elvey 1979). When neural tissue is sensitized such movement is frequently pain provocative.

Active movement assessment is helpful in neural tissue evaluation because it is a physical parameter of impairment undertaken by the patient rather than a passive test undertaken by the therapist. However, it is important to note that there is poor correlation between movement limitation and functional status (Waddell et al 1992). Nevertheless it is a useful reassessment tool that can quantify the change within and between treatment techniques.

In the majority of less painful disorders, active movement dysfunction may be the first aspect of the physical examination that provides evidence for involvement of the neural system. The clinician should inquire about symptom reproduction as well as observe range and quality of movement. Poor quality of movement may present as excessive concurrent movement in the joints proximal and distal to the joint being evaluated. For instance, Figure 29.2 demonstrates active shoulder abduction. The model simulates typical changes to the movement of abduction when associated with increased neural tissue mechanosensitization involving the upper trunk of the brachial plexus. The range of abduction is limited and there is excessive and compensatory movement of the scapula into elevation together with flexion of the elbow and lateral flexion of the neck to the same side. Cervical lateral flexion and rotation normally occur during unilateral arm elevation (Lee 1986) but this movement is excessive in this example. This type of compensatory movement must be differentiated from poor muscle function related to a muscle balance disorder (Mottram 1997). Attempts to reposition the scapula and the cervical spine, and so improve dynamic control, would have a negative effect on the patient's disorder.

With an understanding of applied anatomy the clinician can examine active movements in various ways to support the clinical hypotheses of a neural tissue mechanosensitiza-

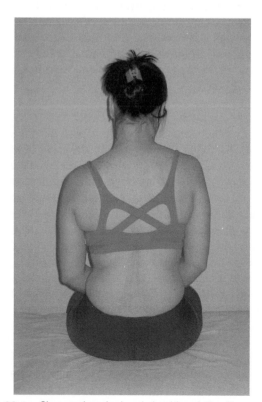

Figure 29.1 Changes in spinal and shoulder girdle alignment.

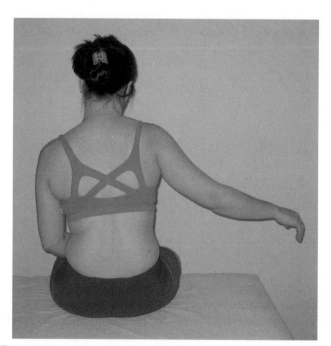

Figure 29.2 Active shoulder abduction.

tion disorder. In the upper quarter various active movements will be affected depending on the particular nerve tract involved. Shoulder abduction and contralateral lateral flexion of the cervical spine will increase the mechanical stress on the brachial plexus and associated neural tissue tracts (Elvey 1979, Ginn 1988, Reid 1987). These movements are the most commonly affected in disorders of the brachial plexus and should form part of a screening process for patients presenting with upper limb pain. Typically abduction is significantly more limited and more painful compared to all other movements of the shoulder. Likewise cervical contralateral lateral flexion is the most restricted movement of the neck.

The clinician can differentiate between local pathology and neural tissue mechanosensitization by repeating the limited or painful movement with the addition of neural sensitizing manoeuvres. For example, wrist extension will place greater provocation on the upper quarter neural tissue via the median nerve (Kleinrensink et al 1995, Lewis et al 1998). If local shoulder structures were the cause of pain the addition of wrist extension would have no effect on the pain provoked during abduction and range of movement would be no more limited than when compared to the same movement repeated on the unaffected side. It is essential to compare sides for there is tremendous variation in flexibility of the peripheral nervous system in both the upper and lower quarter (Troup 1986, Yaxley & Jull 1991). In some normal individuals the addition of wrist extension may completely change the active range of motion.

When adding neural sensitizing manoeuvres to active movement, it is important to make sure that the active movement is repeated in a consistent fashion. When the neural system is sensitized, a typical response is for involuntary compensatory movement at an adjacent joint to relieve the additional stress. For instance great care must be taken to avoid changing the position of the shoulder girdle complex when adding cervical contralateral lateral flexion during active shoulder abduction. A typical response, when upper quarter neural tissue is sensitized, is elevation of the shoulder girdle; preventing elevation will further limit range of abduction. Further useful information is provided from what the clinician feels when preventing compensatory motion. The clinician should be able to detect protective muscle responses. In this example, trapezius muscle would act to elevate the shoulder girdle and scalenes side flex the neck. Trapezius and scalene muscle activity has been associated with provocation of upper limb neural tissues (Balster & Jull 1997, Hu et al 1993, 1995, Monsivais et al 1995).

In the lower quarter lumbar flexion, with hip flexion, knee extension and ankle dorsiflexion are provocative to the sciatic nerve, its terminal branches and the L4–S3 nerve roots (Breig & Troup 1979, Goddard & Reid 1965, Lew et al 1994). If pain is provoked or range of movement is limited on active lumbar flexion in standing, it is possible to use a similar clinical reasoning process to differentiate between pain arising from lumbar somatic structures and pain from neural tissues. The ankle is pre-positioned in dorsiflexion or the cervical spine in flexion and the painful or limited movement is repeated (Hall & Elvey 1999). Should neural tissue be involved, the response to active lumbar flexion would be more pain and further limitation in the range of movement.

The most commonly seen active movement disorders have been discussed but the same thought processes can be applied to other presentations. For example, signs of increased neural tissue mechanosensitivity can be found in some sufferers of cervical headache (Jull 1997). There are fascial connections between the upper cervical dura and the deep suboccipital extensors (Hack et al 1995) and the dura attaches to the posterior cranial fossa and the back of the body of the C2 vertebra. Hence, upper cervical flexion becomes a key movement in the evaluation of cervical headache (Jull 1997). When this movement is limited actively, then repeating the movement with the patient in long sitting can screen for sensitization of the upper cervical neural structures (Fig. 29.3).

Passive movement dysfunction

Neural tissue tracts must comply to active movement in the same way as they do with passive movement (Millesi et al 1995). In other words there should be consistent limitation of range and degree of pain provocation by passive spine and limb movements as the same movements undertaken actively. If a patient presents with 40 degrees of active shoulder abduction, limited by pain provoked from sensitized neural structures, then passively, with the shoulder girdle in the same position, the range should be the same even when

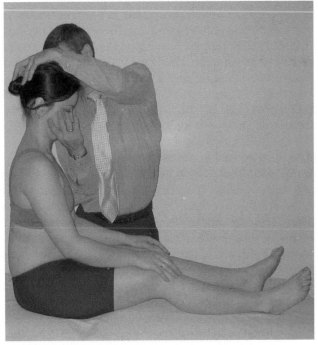

Figure 29.3 Screening for sensitization of the upper cervical structures.

tested in a supine position. Discrepancies in active and passive range suggest that neural tissue involvement is low in the list of hypotheses for that particular disorder.

In addition to the assessment of total range and quality of movement the clinician must evaluate any change in the feel through range of articular passive movement which is perceived as change in the nature and quality of resistance (Jull & Bullock 1987). This enables the clinician to corroborate the patient's report of pain.

Two common passive movement procedures in the upper and lower limb are the 'quadrant position' of flexion–adduction of the hip and the 'quadrant position' of abduction–lateral rotation of the shoulder (Maitland 1991). Maitland (1991) suggested that when all other movements are pain-free, these movements can be restricted and painful when compared to the opposite joint. Hence, they are used to detect the presence of joint dysfunction in more minor disorders. However, these quadrant positions not only stress the joint structures, they also stress peripheral nerve structures (Breig & Troup 1979, Elvey & Hall 1997). In the example of the quadrant test of the hip, the sciatic nerve lies posterior and lateral to the axis of motion of hip flexion–adduction so this movement will be provocative to the sciatic nerve and hence the L4–S2 nerve roots. Consequently, pain provoked by flexion–adduction of the hip may be due to stress placed on neural structures rather than the hip joint. A determination of possible neural tissue involvement can be made by performing the same movement with the lumbar spine laterally flexed away from the side of pain, or with the knee slightly more extended. Both of these manoeuvres should not influence responses to the quadrant test if the joint is involved but would if neural tissue mechanosensitization were.

In the quadrant position of the shoulder (Maitland 1991) the humeral head has an upward fulcrum effect on the overlying neurovascular bundle in the region of the axilla (Elvey 1979). Therefore, it is possible to use this test as a test not only of the shoulder but also of the compliance of the neurovascular tissues to the quadrant position (Hall & Elvey 1999). A similar thought process used for the hip quadrant test can be used to differentiate pain provoked from neural and non-neural structures.

Adverse responses to neural tissue provocation tests
Neural tissue provocation tests (NTPT) have been increasingly incorporated into clinical practice (Milidonis et al 1997) since the pioneering work of Elvey (1979) and Butler (1991). Unfortunately, the early terminology used in describing these tests – 'brachial plexus tension test' and 'adverse mechanical tension' – did little to further the acceptance, understanding or credibility of the physical treatment of neurogenic pain (Elvey 1998). This kind of terminology placed too much emphasis on the mechanical aspects of the tests and subsequent treatment and too little on the physiological responses (Coppieters 2001). A more appropriate term is neural tissue provocation tests (Hall & Elvey 1999) as they are passive tests applied in a manner to

selectively stress different neural tissues in order to assess their sensitivity to mechanical provocation. Lamentably, acceptance of such terminology is slow (Di Fabio 2001b).

A variety of tests have been described that have been shown to mechanically provoke various components of the neural system. The most common of these provocative manoeuvres is the single leg raise (SLR) test (Goddard & Reid 1965). Others include the slump test (Louis 1981), the femoral nerve stress test (Sugiura et al 1979), the passive neck flexion test (Yuan et al 1998), the median nerve stress test (Kleinrensink et al 1995) and the 'brachial plexus tension test' (Elvey 1985). There has been little research investigating the diagnostic validity of such tests (Di Fabio 2001a). However, this is not surprising, considering the complexity of the peripheral nervous system. The SLR test has been shown to have poor validity but only in reference to disc prolapse (van den Hoogen et al 1995) whereas the upper limb neural tissue provocation tests were shown to discriminate between referred and local sources of upper limb pain (Selvaratnam et al 1994).

The basic premise behind such tests is that selective mechanical stress is applied to neural structures, yet it is obvious that many structures are stressed during the test procedures (Kleynhans & Terrett 1986, Moses & Carman 1996). However, using a combination of limb and spine movements it is possible to move and bias mechanical stress to neural structures (Elvey 1979, Kleinrensink et al 1995, Lewis et al 1998, McLellan & Swash 1976, Selvaratnam et al 1988, 1989, Shacklock & Wilkinson 2001). The ability to isolate neural structures is an important issue in structural differentiation and towards making a diagnosis. Again it is important to reiterate that the thrust of this chapter has been that these tests form part of an integrated approach based on a comprehensive subjective and physical examination protocol.

In the clinical setting a flexible approach to examination must be taken. The clinician must formulate appropriate test techniques according to the presentation of each patient with a unique array of signs and symptoms. For instance, in 'frozen shoulder' only limited range of shoulder abduction can be achieved. For these patients it would be impossible to assess for the presence of increased neural tissue mechanosensitivity using a standard test technique.

A methodological approach to neural tissue provocation tests for the upper quarter has been documented (Elvey & Hall 1997, Hall & Elvey 1999). This approach offers guidelines for examination allowing for test technique to be tailored to the severity of a particular pain disorder. The suggested approach incorporates provocative manoeuvres directed to the median, radial and ulnar nerve trunks utilizing movement of the elbow or cervical spine (Elvey & Hall 1997).

Figure 29.4 illustrates an example of test technique using movement of the wrist with the arm and neck in a provocative position for the median nerve trunk. In this example abduction is grossly limited, positioning the shoulder in 90 degrees of abduction and external rotation would not be

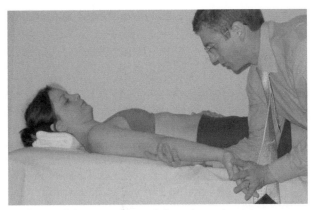

Figure 29.4 Using movement of the wrist and arm in a provocative position.

appropriate, so movement of the wrist is used with the arm positioned short of the limited range of shoulder abduction. The more examination procedures there are to verify examination findings the more certain the clinician can be of a diagnosis. Therefore, by way of confirmation, it is important to apply provocative manoeuvres from 'proximal to distal' as well as 'distal to proximal' (Elvey & Hall 1997). An example of a 'proximal to distal' test is shown in Figure 29.5. Both test procedures should reveal consistent findings in terms of pain provocation and limitation of range of movement.

Neural tissue provocation tests are passive movements carried out by the clinician. Three factors must be considered during such passive movement tests: pain provocation and joint range as it is influenced by resistance to passive motion.

Pain provocation is expected if neural tissue mechanosensitization is considered a dominant feature of the presenting complaint. Ideally the presenting pain complaint should be reproduced during the provocative test technique. In clinical practice this is often unrealistic and it is more common to evoke pain in the area of symptoms experienced by the patient.

Normal responses to various neural tissue pain provocation tests have been documented (Coppieters et al 2001, Kenneally et al 1988, Yaxley & Jull 1991). These studies indicate significant symptom variability between subjects (Coppieters et al 2001). Hence, pain provocation consistent with the area of symptoms is more important than a comparison with expected normal responses (van der Heide et al 2000). Also important is pain provocation by stressing the neural system distant to the site of symptoms, for instance, shoulder pain induced by passive wrist extension with the arm in a position of 60 degrees of abduction, just short of the point in range at which active movement was limited. This test position would be more suited to a patient with severe shoulder limitation and would be entirely inappropriate for a patient with minor end-range restriction.

The second and least important factor is *range of motion*. There is enormous normal variability in measured range during neural tissue provocation tests (Coppieters et al 2001, Troup 1986). This challenges the suggestion of the use of an absolute norm to define impairment and forces the therapist to determine whether the encountered limitation in range is relevant to the individual patient (Coppieters et al 2001). In the past clinicians have compared the affected and unaffected side for range and normal responses (Butler 2000, van der Heide et al 2001). However, recent evidence (Sterling et al 2002) suggests that in patients with chronic post-traumatic neck disorders, there are generalized hyperalgesic responses to neural tissue provocation tests irrespective of the presence of limb pain or clinical signs of specific nerve tissue mechanosensitivity. Hence, comparison between sides may be valid when examining subjects with non-traumatic disorders but not in the presence of altered central pain processing and the tests must be interpreted in the light of information gained from the whole examination.

The third and most important factor is *resistance through range*, which is the examiner's subjective evaluation of compliance of the tissues under examination. Resistance is a clinical observation that is not easily quantifiable. A more correct and scientific meaning for resistance is stiffness (Watson 1994). The examiner must appreciate changes in resistance, which in the case of the SLR test has been shown to be a reflection of changes in muscle tone or activity rather than an increase in stiffness of the lengthening soft tissues (Hall et al 1998). Increased muscle activity is a reflection of increased mechanosensitivity of the neural tissue being tested (Elvey 1988, Hall et al 1998, Quintner 1989). In the lower limb, the onset of protective muscle activity has been shown to coincide with the report of onset of pain (Hall et al 1995) in subjects with mechanosensitive neural tissue and much later at the painful limit of range in normal subjects (Goeken & Hof 1991a, 1991b, 1993). Hence, protective muscle activity can serve to distinguish normal from mechanosensitive neural tissue. In the upper limb the situation is not so clear (Nagy 1999, van der Heide et al 2000, 2001) and further studies are needed.

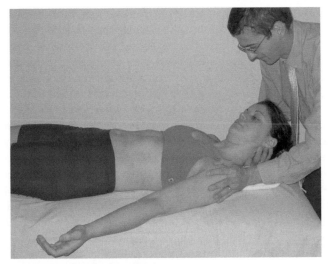

Figure 29.5 Proximal to distal test.

In the lower quarter, for a disorder involving the lumbar spine, provocative manoeuvres directed to the sciatic, femoral and obturator nerve trunks are required and have been well described (Butler 2000). The use of sensitizing manoeuvres is a necessary part of each test. For the SLR test these would include ankle dorsiflexion, medial hip rotation and hip adduction, which have all been shown to increase the mechanical provocation on the sciatic nerve tract (Breig & Troup 1979, O'Connell 1951). Although cervical spine flexion has also been shown to move and tension lumbar nerve roots (O'Connell 1951), the clinical use of cervical spine flexion as a sensitizing manoeuvre for SLR has been shown to be questionable (Hall et al 1995).

The slump test (Maitland 1979) is an important examination procedure when examining lower quarter pain disorders. This test may be performed as described by Maitland (1979) with the patient sitting on the edge of the examination table, or if the patient cannot tolerate this position, in side lying (Hall et al 1993). In the side lying position Hall et al (1993) demonstrated that changing lumbosacral (L5/S1) spine posture from flexion to extension has a significant sensitizing effect on SLR, presumably by increasing provocation on the lumbosacral trunk and the L4 and L5 nerve root. The procedure is shown in Figure 29.6 and can be used in the differential diagnosis of lower lumbar and sacral nerve root disorders.

Comparison cannot be made directly between range of SLR and range of knee extension during the slump test (Butler 2000). The biomechanics of both tests are quite different: in the slump test the spine is flexed and during SLR the whole spine is extended, at least initially.

Mechanical allodynia in response to palpation of specific nerve trunks

Palpation of peripheral neural structures is a necessary part of the neural tissue physical examination protocol. If neural tissue mechanosensitization is felt to be a dominant feature of a patient's presenting complaint then when the involved neural structures are palpated there should be a significant pain response.

It is well known that normal peripheral nerve trunks and nerve roots are painless to non-noxious mechanical stimuli (Hall & Quintner 1996, Howe et al 1977, Kuslich et al 1991, Smyth & Wright 1958). By contrast it has been recorded that inflamed nerve roots are exquisitely sensitive to mild mechanical provocation (Kuslich et al 1991, Smyth & Wright 1958). Similarly, Dyck (1987) reported that the entire extent of the sciatic nerve trunk is invariably tender when a lumbosacral nerve root is traumatized. Comparable findings have been reported in cervical radiculopathy (Hall & Quintner 1996).

The spread of mechanosensitivity along the length of the nerve trunk following proximal nerve trauma and inflammation has been reported elsewhere (Devor & Rappaport 1990) and has been interpreted as reflecting mechanosensitivity of regenerating axon sprouts freely growing, or arrested in disseminated microneuromas. An alternative construct suggests that the spread of sensitization is due to nervi nervorum mediated neurogenic inflammation (Bove & Light 1997, Quintner 1998, Sauer et al 1999).

Activation of the nervi nervorum in response to nerve insult is likely to result in neuropeptide release leading to intraneural oedema. This oedema, particularly within the epineurium, can spread longitudinally as peripheral nerves and spinal nerve roots at the level of the intervertebral foramen have a very poor lymphatic drainage (Sunderland 1991). The endoneurium and epineurium act as closed compartments (Rydevik et al 1984) that become distorted by fluid pressure (Lundborg et al 1983) and so cause further sensitization of the nervi nervorum. The spread of inflammatory mediators within the oedema along the course of the nerve may also act to expand the area of sensitization of the nervi nervorum. Consequently, the entire length of the peripheral nerve trunk becomes sensitive to mild non-noxious palpation. Clinical experience indicates that the closer to the site of initial tissue insult the greater the degree of pain provocation on palpation.

Palpation of peripheral nerve trunks is a skill that involves a high level of anatomical knowledge and must be undertaken with great care. When sensitized, peripheral nerve trunks can be exquisitely tender to very gentle palpation. Overzealous palpation may further compromise damaged and sensitized nerves and exacerbate symptoms for days or even weeks. Compressive forces alter blood flow to the nerve, sustained slight pressure on the outside of a nerve leads to external hyperemia, oedema and demyelination of some axons for up to 28 days (Bove & Light 1997). Extraneural pressure of only 20–30 mmHg compromises intraneural blood supply, impairs axoplasmic flow and reduces nerve function (Rempel et al 1999). Hence, when nerves are palpated directly over hard tissue, such as bone, there is a risk of iatrogenic neuropraxia unless the clinician takes due care.

As well as pain, protective muscle responses have also been demonstrated in response to nerve trunk palpation

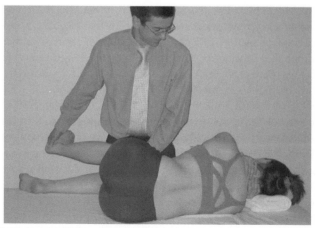

Figure 29.6 Differential diagnosis of lower lumbar or sacral nerve root disorders.

and are an indicator of abnormal neural tissue mechano-sensitivity (Hall & Quintner 1996). Mild non-noxious pressure should be applied to the nerve trunks on the uninvolved side first in order to allow the patient to make a comparison. In some instances palpation can be made directly over the nerve trunk, which can be identified as a distinct structure. In other locations nerve trunks must be palpated through muscle, or they are so closely associated with vascular tissues that it is less easy to identify the nerve as a structure. When this is the case, broad-based pressure is applied in the area of the nerve trunk and the response is compared to the uninvolved side.

Many nerves can be readily palpated but in the clinical context of cervical and lumbosacral pain syndromes the most relevant and commonly palpated include the following:

- spinal nerves as they exit from the gutters of the transverse processes of C4–6
- upper and middle trunk of the brachial plexus
- greater and lesser occipital nerves
- neurovascular bundle of the brachial plexus underlying the tendon of pectoralis minor
- neurovascular bundle in the axilla incorporating the axillary artery and vein together with the median, radial and ulnar nerves
- median, radial, ulnar, axillary, suprascapular and dorsal scapular nerves.

In the lower quarter the following neural structures can be examined:

- sciatic nerve in the gluteal region
- tibial, common peroneal (fibular) and femoral nerves.

By way of verifying that a particular spinal neural level is sensitized, the clinician is advised to examine a number of different peripheral nerve sites pertaining to that particular nerve root level. As well, by way of confirmation, peripheral nerve trunks not involved should be palpated for a normal response. For example, if a C6 nerve root sensitization disorder were suspected based on the previous examination then all peripheral nerve trunks with C6 contribution are expected to be abnormally sensitive to palpation. These include the upper trunk of the brachial plexus as well as the median, radial, suprascapular and axillary nerves. Palpation of the middle trunk of the brachial plexus as well as the ulnar and dorsal scapular nerves should not be pain-provocative as they have no contribution from C6.

Anomalous anatomy of neural structures is common (Bogduk 1997, Tanaka et al 2000). Chotigavanich & Sawangnatra (1992) found a 30% incidence of anomalies of the lumbar and sacral nerve roots. Irregular neural anatomy should be considered if the patient's features do not fit an ordered pattern of segmental involvement.

Evidence of a local area of pathology

At this point in the examination it should be very clear to the clinician whether a disorder has features of neural tis-

sue mechanosensitization. Once this has been established it is important to identify where the process originated. In most cases it will be possible to ascertain a defined local cause for the pathology and in many instances there is a specific spinal segmental level involved. When a local cause of pathology cannot be identified this should start to ring alarm bells. Many central and peripheral nervous system disorders present to physical examination with all the features discussed. This does not mean that they can all be treated with neural tissue treatment techniques. It is quite possible for other conditions such as diabetic mononeuropathy, Guillain–Barré, multiple sclerosis or tumour induced radiculopathy to give rise to many or all of the features discussed so far (Burger & Lindeque 1994, Naftulin et al 1993, Ramirez-Lassepas et al 1992, Wasserstrom et al 1982). Therefore, it is essential that the clinician must determine a cause for the neural tissue mechanosensitization disorder.

A typical example of a local pathology causing all the previously discussed features of neural tissue mechanosensitization is a lower lumbar disc pathology which will often result in radicular leg pain and a specific lumbar spine motion segment dysfunction. Saal et al (1990) speculate that nerve root inflammation (and subsequent mechanosensitization) results from the escape of highly inflamogenic material into the vicinity of the lumbar nerve root. Hence, there is a genuine basis for a very painful mechanically sensitive disorder where spinal imaging procedures may be unhelpful in determining a diagnosis. However, a thorough clinical examination should reveal features of neural tissue mechanosensitization at a specific lumbar nerve root together with a local area of pathology at the level where the disc is leaking inflammatory mediators.

Examination procedures for a local cause of pathology in the spine include palpation and passive segmental mobility tests (Maitland 1986). These tests have been shown to be highly sensitive and specific for detecting the involved lumbar segmental level (Phillips & Twomey 1996).

An important aspect in the evaluation of neural tissue disorders is the assessment of neurological function. Knowledge of the functional status of the central and peripheral nervous system is required before application of any form of treatment techniques aimed at neural structures. When abnormal neurological function is detected this should have a significant influence on treatment prescription and will be discussed in more detail later.

In the clinical setting, the neurological examination is the only means of determining whether there is abnormal axonal conduction. The neurological examination incorporates both subjective enquiry as well as physical tests of nerve function.

Following the subjective examination the clinician must be able to map on a body chart the specific type and area of symptoms including paraesthesias and sensory loss. These areas can then be compared with typical dermatomal and myotomal maps while considering that this information alone is insufficient to determine the specific spinal segmental level of involvement or the presence of nerve root compression (Rankine et al 1998, Slipman et al, 1998).

Physical neurological examination draws on an assessment of skin sensation, tendon reflexes, manual muscle strength and upper motoneuron function.

Skin sensation is commonly tested by light touch and pin-prick, as these sensations are carried by large diameter group II afferent fibres to the dorsal column. These large diameter fibres are particularly vulnerable to compression, therefore altered conduction in large diameter group II afferents may be the first indicator of nerve compression (Refshauge & Gass 1995). Areas of altered sensation are compared with dermatomal maps to determine the segmental level of involvement (Dvorak 1998).

Muscles are tested for maximum voluntary isometric contraction that is determined by maximal resistance to breaking point when the muscle 'gives'. However, in many pain disorders evaluation of neurogenic muscle weakness is not possible because of pain inhibition. In that case, other neurological tests must be interpreted for the presence of abnormal function.

Many different types of reflexes have been described. However, tendon reflexes are most commonly used in determining the presence of nerve root compromise. Tendon reflexes can be tested from C3 to T1 and from L2 to S1 using knowledge of neuromuscular anatomy.

The purpose of examination of upper motor neuron function is to identify contraindications to manual therapy treatment. Such tests include, among others, the Babinski reflex, clonus and tendon reflexes. Note that hyper-reflexia may follow general changes to central nervous system sensitivity and does not necessarily indicate an upper motor neuron lesion.

Although a number of studies have examined the reliability and diagnostic validity of the neurological examination in the diagnosis of radiculopathy, its value is still not well established (Viikari-Juntura 1987, Viikari-Juntura et al 1989, Wainner & Gill 2000). Vroomen et al (2000) and Viikari-Juntura et al (1989) examined inter-observer reliability and showed that agreement was best achieved by incorporating the subjective history together with the physical examination findings. Kappas values for agreement were good for decreased muscle strength and sensory loss (0.57–0.82) but intermediate for reflex changes (0.42–0.53) (Vroomen et al 2000). Likewise diagnostic validity has been shown to increase with pooling of information from all aspects of the neurological examination (van den Hoogen et al 1995, Yoss et al 1999).

Other ways of examining nerve function include electrodiagnostic tests (Dvorak 1998). These are invasive procedures that are more specific to the evaluation of motor or sensory conduction loss (Haldeman 1984); they have no use in detecting increased neural tissue mechanosensitivity and distress the patient, both physically and psychologically. Other more recently introduced diagnostic tests such as

magnetic resonance neurography and diagnostic ultrasound have enabled the visualization of peripheral neural structures (Aagaard et al 1998, Dailey et al 1996, Dilley et al 2001, Greening et al 2001, Loewy 2001, Maravilla & Bowen 1998). These tests show promise for the future since they permit the imaging of peripheral nervous system pathology and are non-invasive; however, they are still in their infancy.

When considering the information gathered from the physical examination it is important to note that the severity and nature of physical signs of increased neural tissue mechanosensitization are consistent and in step with the severity of the subjective complaint. Minor signs of increased neural tissue mechanosensitivity in a clinical presentation of severe sciatica would not be consistent with a diagnosis of neural tissue mechanosensitization and the primary source of the pain should be sought elsewhere.

We propose that the above scheme of examination is effective in determining the presence of increased neural tissue mechanosensitivity and the presence of nerve trunk pain. To date, to our knowledge, only two studies have used this examination protocol to determine the incidence of nerve trunk pain in a particular disorder (Hall et al 1997, Nagy 1999). In these studies, one third of subjects with chronic spinal related limb pain were found to have neural tissue mechanosensitization as the dominant physical examination feature. Many more studies are needed to determine the sensitivity, specificity and validity of this test protocol.

TREATMENT

In this chapter a distinction has been made between two types of peripheral neural pain: pain due to damaged axons and pain due to increased mechanosensitization of peripheral nerve trunks without damage to axons. This distinction is important with respect to the provision of treatment and prognosis. The authors recognize that mechanosensitization can be a feature of some neuropathic disorders but these conditions are rare in clinical practice and have distinctive features that set them apart. These include, among others, a history of nerve trauma, spontaneous pain, neurological deficit and evidence of central sensitization based on the subjective and physical examination (Butler 2000).

Recently, the authors were involved in assessing subjects with chronic cervicobrachial pain for inclusion into two treatment trials (Allison et al 2002, Hall et al 1997). Nearly 200 subjects were evaluated using the protocol presented in this chapter. Of those examined by the authors, 33% had increased neural tissue mechanosensitization as the dominant physical examination feature in the absence of clinically detected neurological dysfunction. In contrast, less than 3% had a true radicular disorder with evidence of neurological dysfunction. In these subjects neural tissue mechanosensitization was an inconsistent and minor finding.

Our observation of the high prevalence of neck/arm pain in the absence of nerve root compression is supported in the literature (Sampath et al 1999). As well, in the lumbar spine, it appears that nerve root compression disorders secondary to intervertebral disc prolapse are rare with only about 1–3% of the back pain population identified with this disorder (Bogduk 1997, Cavanaugh & Weinstein 1994). Yet low back related leg symptoms occur in 14–25% of those with back problems (Cavanaugh & Weinstein 1994, Laslett et al 1991).

Under normal circumstances peripheral nerve trunks are protected from the effects of nerve stretch and compression (Sunderland 1990). However, severe conduction loss may occur at strains as low as 6% (Kwan et al 1992). As the fasciculi are stretched, their cross-sectional area is reduced, the intra-fascicular pressure is increased, nerve fibres are compressed, and the intra-fascicular microcirculation is compromised (Sunderland 1990). An 8% elongation of a defined nerve segment results in impaired venular flow and at 10–15% elongation there is complete arrest of all blood flow in the nerve (Lundborg & Rydevik 1973, Ogato & Naito 1986). In an acute or chronic neurogenic pain disorder, it is likely that the microcirculation within the nerve is already abnormal and therefore minimal increase in length of the nerve will lead to further circulatory compromise, reduced nerve function and pain. For these reasons it is unwise to treat a damaged, compressed or oedematous nerve root or peripheral nerve trunk with neural stretching techniques.

The treatment of increased neural tissue mechanosensitization involves the use of passive movement techniques, but because of the high probability of compromising the already dysfunctional nerve, 'lengthening' or stretching techniques are contraindicated in all but the most minor disorders where pain is not a dominant feature. We advocate the use of gentle, controlled oscillatory passive movements of the anatomical structures surrounding the affected neural tissues at the site of involvement. At no time should pain or other symptoms be evoked by the technique. Treatment can be progressed by using passive movement techniques in a similar manner but involving movement of the surrounding anatomic tissues or structures and the affected neural tissues together in an oscillatory movement (Elvey 1986). These techniques have been described in other texts (Elvey & Hall, 1997, Hall & Elvey 2001).

The following example is the type of treatment approach taken for the common clinical presentation of a C6 mechanosensitization disorder. Passive contralateral lateral glide of the C5/C6 motion segment is carried out with the affected arm in a non-provocative position (Fig. 29.7). The passive movement is dependent on the severity, irritability and nature of the disorder. If the arm is positioned too aggressively, little lateral glide movement will be achieved, and the patient's disorder aggravated. If the arm is positioned too much out of neural provocation then the patient's disorder will not improve. Over subsequent treatment sessions, as the patient's condition improves and

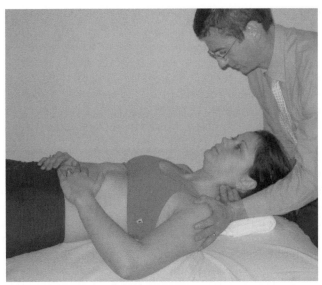

Figure 29.7 Passive contralateral glide of the C5/C6 motion segment with the arm in a non-provocative position.

there are demonstrable changes to subjective features as well as physical impairments, then the treatment technique can be advanced with the arm in progressively more provocative positions.

At a later point in treatment, a home exercise programme should be incorporated which is an adjunct to the treatment provided by the clinician. Active home exercise should only be introduced once consistent beneficial effects of manual therapy treatment have been demonstrated.

For neural tissue mechanosensitization disorders arising from the lumbar spine a similar approach has been described (Hall & Elvey 2001). Lateral glide is not possible; instead a modified lateral flexion manoeuvre is performed with the affected leg in a position which falls just short of neural provocation. Treatment is progressed in a similar fashion to the cervical techniques and patient self-management introduced when appropriate.

The immediate effects of this type of treatment approach have been demonstrated (Coppieters et al 2003, Vicenzino et al 1996). Vicenzino et al (1996, 1998) examined the effects of the technique described above, C5/C6 contralateral lateral glide with the arm positioned to affect the radial nerve, in a group with lateral epicondylalgia. Their study was a randomized, placebo controlled, double blind, repeated measures design. Significant improvements were found in pain measures, responses to neural tissue provocation tests and pain-free grip strength. Coppieters et al (2003) conducted a similar randomized controlled trial to investigate the immediate effects of the same cervical lateral glide technique in a group of sufferers with chronic cervicobrachial pain. Subjects were selected according to the protocol described in this chapter. There were significant improvements of both ranges of motion and pain measures.

Long-term benefits of the treatment approach outlined have also been demonstrated in chronic cervicobrachial pain (Allison et al 2002, Cowell & Phillips 2002, Hall et al 1997). Hall et al (1997), in a case controlled study, selected subjects according to the protocol outlined and showed significant improvements in pain and functional capacity as well as cervical spine and shoulder girdle mobility after a 4-week treatment period utilizing this concept of management. Improvements were maintained at follow-up 3 months later. Similarly, Allison et al (2002) used a single blind randomized controlled trial to compare traditional manual therapy, specific neural tissue mobilization techniques described in this chapter and no treatment in sufferers of cervicobrachial pain. Unfortunately, the sample size was small (n = 30) and although both intervention groups showed significant improvement over controls in pain and functional disability measures, there were no significant differences following treatment between the two intervention groups. However, the specific neural mobilization group demonstrated strong trends towards greater improvement in pain measures. Perhaps a larger sample size would have increased the trend to significance.

Numerous studies have investigated the efficacy of other neural tissue mobilization techniques and have shown beneficial effects (Anderson & Tichenor 1994, Cowell & Phillips 2002, Dreschler et al 1997, George 2000, Kaye & Mason 1989, Kornberg & Lew 1989, Sweeney & Harms 1996, Weirich et al 1999, Zvulun 1998).

Improvement following specific techniques aimed at addressing increased neural tissue mechanosensitivity has been explained in part by changes to physiology of the nerve root complex (Elvey 1986) and changes in pain processing (Vicenzino et al 1998). Likewise the beneficial effects of manipulative therapy have also been explained as due to restoration of normal biomechanics and physiological function of the articular motion segment (Greenham 1996, Haldeman 1994, Jull 1997). If pain from mechanosensitive neural structures limits normal movement of the spine then passive mobilization applied judicially can help to restore normal function to the point when the patient can move for themselves and continue a more active rehabilitation process.

It is important to discuss the limitations of the approach taken in this chapter. A case study recently presented in a discussion of evidence based practice (Cibulka & Aslin

2001) demonstrates how blanket approaches to treatment of patients with apparent pain of nerve origin without consideration of pathobiological mechanisms is, at best, ineffective and at worst, dangerous. The subject in this case had features of acute lumbar nerve root compression but was given a 'sciatic nerve stretching technique' (Cibulka & Aslin 2001). Six sessions of treatment failed to change the patient's symptoms, functional status or signs of physical impairment. This is hardly surprising when one considers the effect sciatic nerve stretching would have on an inflamed, compressed dysfunctional nerve root. This patient exemplifies the kind of situation where neural tissue mobilization techniques have no place, principally acute and subacute nerve root compression.

Neuropathic disorders in general should be assessed with great care. They may have features consistent with mechanosensitization due to ectopic or abnormal impulse generating sites along the course of the damaged nerve (Devor & Seltzer 1999). However, they may also have features of central sensitization and axonal conduction block, in which case it would be inappropriate to treat since even the gentlest movement can trigger pain and feed into the central sensitization state (McMahon & Koltzenburg 1990). A typical example is a patient who presents with neck/shoulder/arm pain 6 months after falling from a bike onto the acromion, forcing contralateral lateral flexion of the neck and depression of the scapula. On physical examination there are features of neural tissue mechanosensitization, sensory neurological dysfunction involving multiple segmental levels and widespread allodynia in the upper limb and neck. Other features of central sensitization are also found. For this patient the neural mobilization techniques described in this chapter are not indicated.

This chapter has outlined an approach to the management of neural tissue mechanosensitization disorders of the spine. The topic is complex, still evolving and requires very careful consideration in clinical practice.

KEYWORDS

| neural tissue mechanosensitization | manual therapy |
| neural tissue provocation test |

References

Aagaard B D, Maravilla K R, Kliot M 1998 MR neurography: MR imaging of peripheral nerves. Magnetic Resonance Imaging Clinics of North America 6(1): 179–194

Abenhaim L, Rossignol M, Valat J et al 2000 The role of activity in the therapeutic management of back pain: report of the International Paris Task Force on Back Pain. Spine 25(4): 1S–33S

Allison G T, Nagy B M, Hall T M 2002 A randomised clinical trial of manual therapy for cervico-brachial pain syndrome: a pilot study. Manual Therapy 7: 95–102

Amundsen T, Weber H, Lilleas F, Nordal H J, Abdelnoor M, Magnaes B 1995 Lumbar spinal stenosis: Clinical and radiological features. Spine 20(10): 1178–1186

Anderson M, Tichenor C J 1994 A patient with de Quervain's tenosynovitis: a case report using an Australian approach to manual therapy. Physiotherapy 74: 314–326

Asbury A, Fields H 1984 Pain due to peripheral nerve damage: an hypothesis. Neurology 34: 1587–1590

Austen R 1991 The distribution and characteristics of lumbar–lower limb symptoms in subjects with and without a neurological deficit. Proceedings of Manipulative Physiotherapists Association of Australia Seventh Biennial Conference, New South Wales pp 252–257

Balster S, Jull G 1997 Upper trapezius muscle activity during the brachial plexus tension test in asymptomatic subjects. Manual Therapy 2(3): 144–149

Bennett G J 2000 A neuroimmune interaction in painful peripheral neuropathy. Clinical Journal of Pain 16(3 Suppl): S139–143

Bennett G J, Xie Y K 1988 A peripheral mononeuropathy in rat that produced disorders of pain and sensation like those in man. Pain 33: 87–107

Beyerlein C, Hansson U, Odemark M, Sainsbury D, Teck Lim H 2001 Efficacy of the Mulligan traction straight leg raise technique on range of motion in patients with low back pain. In: Proceedings of the International Federation of Orthopaedic Manipulative Therapists, Capetown, South Africa

Bobechko W P, Hirsch C 1965 Auto-immune response to nucleus pulposus in the rabbit. Journal of Bone and Joint Surgery 47B: 574–580

Bogduk N 1997 Clinical anatomy of the lumbar spine and sacrum, 3rd edn. Churchill Livingstone, Melbourne

Boland R 1995 Tension tests. In: Refshauge K, Gass E (eds) Musculoskeletal physiotherapy: clinical science and practice. Butterworth Heinemann, Oxford

Bove G M, Light A R 1995a Calcitonin gene-related peptide and peripherin immunoreactivity in nerve sheaths. Somatosensory and Motor Responses 12: 49–57

Bove G M, Light A R 1995b Unmyelinated nociceptors of rat paraspinal tissues. Journal of Neurophysiology 73: 1752–1762

Bove G, Light A 1997 The nervi nervorum: missing link for neuropathic pain? Pain Forum 6(3): 181–190

Breig A 1978 Adverse mechanical tension in the central nervous system: relief by functional neurosurgery. Almquist and Wiksell, Stockholm

Breig A, Troup J 1979 Biomechanical considerations of the straight-leg-raising test. Spine 4(3): 242–250

Burger E L, Lindeque B G 1994 Sacral and non-spinal tumours presenting as backache. Acta Orthopaedica Scandinavica 65(3): 344–346

Butler D 1991 Mobilisation of the nervous system. Churchill Livingstone, Melbourne

Butler D 2000 The sensitive nervous system. Noi Group Publications, Adelaide

Cavanaugh J M, Weinstein J N 1994 Low back pain: epidemiology, anatomy and neurophysiology. In: Wall P D, Melzack R (eds) The textbook of pain, 3rd edn. Churchill Livingstone, Edinburgh

Chacur M, Milligan E D, Gazda L S, Armstrong C, Wang H, Tracey K J, Maier S F, Watkins L R 2001 A new model of sciatic inflammatory neuritis (SIN): induction of unilateral and bilateral mechanical allodynia following acute unilateral peri-sciatic immune activation in rats. Pain 94(3): 231–244

Chotigavanich C, Sawangnatra S 1992 Anomalies of the lumbosacral nerve roots: an anatomic investigation. Clinical Orthopaedics and Related Research 278: 46–50

Cibulka M T, Aslin K 2001 How to use evidence-based practice to distinguish between three different patients with low back pain. Journal of Orthopaedic and Sports Physical Therapy 31(12): 678–695

Coppieters M W 2001 In defense of neural mobilisation. Journal of Orthopaedic and Sports Physical Therapy 31(9): 520

Coppieters M W, Stappaerts K H, Everaert D G, Staes F F 2001 Addition of test components during neurodynamic testing: effect on range of motion and sensory responses. Journal of Orthopaedic and Sports Physical Therapy 31(5): 226–237

Coppieters M, Stappaerts K, Wouters L, Janssens K 2003 The immediate effects of a cervical lateral glide treatment technique in patients with neurogenic cervicobrachial pain. Journal of Orthopaedic and Sports Physical Therapy 33(7): 369–378

Cowell I M, Phillips D R 2002 Effectiveness of manipulative physiotherapy for the treatment of a neurogenic cervicobrachial pain syndrome: a single case study – experimental design. Manual Therapy 7(1): 31–38

Dailey T, Goodkin R, Filler A, Maravilla K 1996 Magnetic resonance neurography for cervical radiculopathy: a preliminary report. Neurosurgery 38(30): 488–492

Dalton P A, Jull G A 1989 The distribution and characteristics of neck-arm pain in patients with and without a neurological deficit. Australian Journal of Physiotherapy 35: 3–8

Devor M 1989 The pathophysiology of damaged peripheral nerves. In: Wall P Melzack R (eds) Textbook of pain, 2nd edn. Churchill Livingstone, Edinburgh, pp 63–81

Devor M 1991 Neuropathic pain and injured nerve: peripheral mechanisms. British Medical Bulletin 47(3): 619–630

Devor M, Rappaport H 1990 Pain and pathophysiology of damaged nerve. In: Fields H L (ed) Pain syndromes in neurology. Butterworth Heinemann, Oxford, pp 47–83

Devor M, Seltzer Z 1999 Pathophysiology of damaged nerves in relation to chronic pain. In: Wall P D, Melzack R (eds) The textbook of pain, 4th edn. Churchill Livingstone, Edinburgh, pp 129–164

Di Fabio R P 2001a Neural tension, neurodynamics, and neural mobilisation. Journal of Orthopaedic and Sports Physical Therapy 31(9): 522

Di Fabio R P 2001b Neural mobilisation: the impossible. Journal of Orthopaedic and Sports Physical Therapy 31(5): 224–225

Dilley A, Greening J, Lynn B, Leary R, Morris V 2001 The use of cross-correlation analysis between high-frequency ultrasound images to measure longitudinal median nerve movement. Ultrasound in Medicine and Biology 27(9): 1211–1218

Dreschler W I, Knarr J F, Snyder-Mackler L 1997 A comparison of two treatment regimens for lateral epicondylitis. Journal of Sport Rehabilitation 6: 226–234

Drye C, Zachazewski J 1996 Peripheral nerve injuries. In: Zachazewski J, Magee D, Quillen W (eds) Athletic injuries and rehabilitation. WB Saunders, Philadelphia, pp 441–462

Dvorak J 1996 Neurophysiologic tests in diagnosis of nerve root compression caused by disc herniation. Spine 21(24S): 39S–44S

Dvorak J 1998 Epidemiology, physical examination and neurodiagnostics. Spine 22(24): 2663–2673

Dyck P 1987 Sciatic pain. In: Watkins R G, Collis J S (eds) Lumbar discectomy and laminectomy. Rockville, Aspen, pp 5–14

Eliav E, Herzberg U, Ruda M A, Bennett G J 1999 Neuropathic pain from an experimental neuritis of the rat sciatic nerve. Pain 83(2): 169–182

Elliot K 1994 Taxonomy and mechanisms of neuropathic pain. Seminars in Neurology 14(3): 195–205

Elvey R 1979 Brachial plexus tension tests and the pathoanatomical origin of arm pain. In: Idczak R (ed) Aspects of manipulative therapy. Lincoln Institute of Health Sciences, Melbourne, pp 105–110

Elvey R 1985 Brachial plexus tension tests and the pathoanatomical origin of arm pain. In: Glasgow E F, Twomey L T, Scull E R, Kleynhans A M, Idczak R M (eds) Aspects of manipulative therapy, 2nd edn. Churchill Livingstone, Melbourne, pp 116–122

Elvey R 1986 Treatment of arm pain associated with abnormal brachial plexus tension. Australian Journal of Physiotherapy 32: 225–230

Elvey R L 1988 The clinical relevance of signs of adverse brachial plexus tension. Proceedings of the International Federation of Orthopaedic Manipulative Therapists, Cambridge

Elvey R 1992 Nerve tension signs. In: Paris S (ed) Proceedings of the Fifth International Conference of the International Federation of Manipulative Therapists. International Federation of Manipulative Therapists, Vail, p 85

Elvey R 1998 Commentary: treatment of arm pain associated with abnormal brachial plexus tension. In: Maher C (ed) Adverse neural tension revisited. Australian Physiotherapy Association, Melbourne, 13–17

Elvey R, Hall T 1997 Neural tissue evaluation and treatment. In: Donatelli R (ed) Physical therapy of the shoulder, 3rd edn. Churchill Livingstone, New York, pp 131–152

Epstein J, Epstein B, Levine L, Carras R, Rosenthall A, Sumner P 1973 Lumbar nerve root compression at the intervertebral foramina caused by arthritis of the posterior facet. Journal of Neurosurgery 39: 362–369

Fahlgren Grampo J, Reynolds H, Vorro J, Beal M 1991 3-D motion of the pelvis during passive leg lifting. In: Anderson P, Hobart D, Danoff J (eds) Electromyographical kinesiology. Elsevier, Amsterdam, pp 119–122

Fahrni W H 1966 Observations on straight-leg-raising with special reference to nerve root adhesions. Canadian Journal of Surgery 9: 44–48

Falconer M A, McGeorge M, Begg A C 1948 Observations on the cause and mechanism of symptom-production in sciatica and low-back pain. Journal of Neurology, Neurosurgery and Psychiatry 11: 13–26

Fields H 1987 Pain. McGraw Hill, New York

Franson R C, Saal J S, Saal J A 1992 Human disc phospholipase A2 is inflammatory. Spine 17: S129–S132

Fukui S, Ohseto K, Shiotani M, Ohno K, Karasawa H, Naganuma Y 1997 Distribution of referred pain from the lumbar zygapophyseal joints and dorsal rami. Clinical Journal of Pain 13: 303–307

George S Z 2000 Differential diagnosis and treatment for a patient with lower extremity symptoms. Journal of Orthopaedic and Sports Physical Therapy 30(8): 468–472

Gertzbein S D 1977 Degenerative disc disease of the lumbar spine: immunological implications. Clinical Orthopaedics and Related Research 279: 101–109

Gifford L 2001 Acute low cervical nerve root conditions: symptom presentations and pathobiological reasoning. Manual Therapy 6(2): 106–115

Giles L G 1997 Innervation of spinal structures. In: Giles L G, Singer K P (eds) Clinical anatomy and management of low back pain. Butterworth Heinemann, Oxford

Ginn K 1988 An investigation of tension development in upper limb soft tissues during the upper limb tension test. Proceedings of the International Federation of Orthopaedic Manipulative Therapist's Conference, Cambridge, England, pp 25–26

Goddard M, Reid J 1965 Movements induced by straight leg raising in the lumbo-sacral roots, nerves and plexus and in the intrapelvic section of the sciatic nerve. Journal of Neurology, Neurosurgery and Psychiatry 28: 12–18

Goeken L N, Hof L 1991a Instrumental straight leg raising: a new approach to Lasegues test. Archives of Physical Medicine and Rehabilitation 72: 959–966

Goeken L N, Hof L 1991b Instrumental straight leg raising: results in healthy subjects. Archives of Physical Medicine and Rehabilitation 72: 194–203

Goeken L N, Hof L 1993 Instrumental straight leg raising: results in healthy subjects. Archives of Physical Medicine and Rehabilitation 74: 194–203

Greenham P E 1996 Principles of manual medicine. Lippincott, Williams and Wilkins, Philadephia

Greening J, Lynn B, Leary R, Warren L, O'Higgins P, Hall-Craggs M 2001 The use of ultrasound imaging to demonstrate reduced movement of the median nerve during wrist flexion in patients with non-specific arm pain. Journal of Hand Surgery 26(5): 401–406

Gronblad M, Virri J 1997 Nerves, neuropeptides and inflammation in spinal tissues: mechanisms of back pain. In: Giles L G, Singer K P (eds) Clinical anatomy and management of low back pain. Butterworth Heinemann, Oxford

Gunn C C 1980 Prespondylosis and some pain syndromes following denervation supersensitivity. Spine 5: 2

Hack G D, Koritzer R T, Robinson W L, Hallgren R C, Greenman P E 1995 Anatomic relation between the rectus capitis posterior minor muscle and the dura mater. Spine 20: 2484–2486

Haldeman S 1984 The electrodiagnostic evaluation of nerve root function. Spine 9: 42–47

Haldeman S 1994 Manipulation and massage for the relief of back pain. In: Wall P, Melzack R (eds) Textbook of pain, 3rd edn. Churchill Livingstone, Edinburgh, pp 1251–1262

Hall T, Elvey R 1999 Nerve trunk pain: physical diagnosis and treatment. Manual Therapy 4: 63–73

Hall T, Elvey R 2001 Evaluation and treatment of neural tissue pain disorders. In: Donatelli R A, Wooden M J (eds) Orthopaedic physical therapy, 3rd edn. Churchill Livingstone, Philadelphia

Hall T, Quintner J 1996 Responses to mechanical stimulation of the upper limb in painful cervical radiculopathy. Australian Journal of Physiotherapy 42(4): 277–285

Hall T, Hepburn M, Elvey R 1993 The effect of lumbosacral postures on the modified SLR test. Physiotherapy 79: 566–570

Hall T, Zusman M, Elvey R 1995 Manually detected impediments during the SLR test. In: Jull G (ed) Manipulative Physiotherapists Association of Australia, Ninth Biennial Conference, Manipulative Physiotherapists Association of Australia, Gold Coast, Queensland, pp 48–53

Hall T, Elvey R, Davies N, Dutton L, Moog M 1997 Efficacy of manipulative physiotherapy for the treatment of cervicobrachial pain. Tenth Biennial Conference of the Manipulative Physiotherapists Association of Australia, Manipulative Physiotherapists Association of Australia, Melbourne, pp 73–74

Hall T, Zusman M, Elvey R L 1998 Adverse mechanical tension in the nervous system? Analysis of straight leg raise. Manual Therapy 3(3): 140–146

Hasue M 1993 Pain and the nerve root: an interdisciplinary approach. Spine 18(4): 2053–2058

Henderson C, Hennessy R, Shuey H 1983 Posterior lateral foraminotomy for an exclusive operative technique for cervical radiculopathy: a review of 846 consecutively operated cases. Journal of Neurosurgery 13: 504–512

Hough A D, Moore A P, Jones M P 2000 Measuring longitudinal nerve motion using ultrasonography. 5(3): 173–180

Howe J, Loeser J, Calvin W 1977 Mechanosensitivity of dorsal root ganglia and chronically injured axons: a physiological basis for the radicular pain of nerve root compression. Pain 3: 25–41

Hromada J 1963 On the nerve supply of the connective tissue of some peripheral nervous system components. Acta Anatomica 55: 343–351

Hu J, Yu X, Vernon H, Sessle B 1993 Excitatory effects on neck and jaw muscle activity of inflammatory irritant applied to cervical paraspinal tissues. Pain 55: 243–250

Hu J, Vernon H, Tatourian I 1995 Changes in neck electromyography associated with meningeal noxious stimulation. Journal of Manipulative and Physiological Therapeutics 18: 577–581

Hudgins W R 1975 The crossed straight leg raise test. New England Journal of Medicine 297: 1127

Janig W, Koltzenburg M 1991 Receptive properties of pial afferents. Pain 45: 77–85

Jull G 1997 Management of cervical headache. Manual Therapy 2(4): 182–190

Jull G, Bullock M 1987 A motion profile of the lumbar spine in an ageing population assessed by manual examination. Physiotherapy Practice 3: 70–81

Jull G, Moore A 2000 Evidence based practices: the need for research directions. Manual Therapy 5(3): 131

Kaye S, Mason E 1989 Clinical implications of the upper limb tension test. Physiotherapy 75(12): 750–752

Kenneally M, Rubenach H, Elvey R 1988 The upper limb tension test: the SLR test of the arm. In: Grant R (ed) Physical therapy of the cervical and thoracic spine. Churchill Livingstone, New York

Kleinrensink G, Stoeckart R, Vleeming A, Sjniders C, Mulder P 1995 Mechanical tension in the median nerve: the effects of joint positions. Clinical Biomechanics 10(5): 240–244

Kleynhans A, Terrett A 1986 The prevention of complications from spinal manipulative therapy. In: Glasgow E F, Twomey L T (eds) Aspects of manipulative therapy. Churchill Livingstone, Melbourne, pp 171–174

Kornberg C, Lew P 1989 The effect of stretching neural structures on grade one hamstring injuries. Journal of Orthopaedic and Sports Physical Therapy 19: 481–487

Kuslich S, Ulstrom C, Cam J 1991 The tissue origin of low back pain and sciatica: a report of pain responses to tissue stimulation during operations on the lumbar spine using local anaesthesia. Orthopaedic Clinics of North America 22(2): 181–187

Kwan M, Wall E, Massie J, Garfin S 1992 Strain, stress and stretch of peripheral nerve: rabbit experiments in vitro and in vivo. Acta Orthopaedica Scandinavica 63(3): 267–272

Laird J, Bennett G 1993 An electrophysiological study of dorsal horn neurons in the spinal cord of rats with an experimental peripheral neuropathy. Journal of Neurophysiology 69(6): 2072–2085

Laslett M, Crothers C, Beattie P, Cregten L, Moses A 1991 The frequency and incidence of low back pain/sciatica in an urban population. New Zealand Medical Journal 104: 424–426

Lee D 1986 Tennis elbow. Journal of Orthopaedic and Sports Physical Therapy 8: 134–142

Lew P, Morrow C, Lew A 1994 The effect of neck and leg flexion and their sequence on the lumbar spinal cord: implications in low back pain and sciatica. Spine 19(21): 2421–2425

Lewis J, Ramot R, Green A 1998 Changes in mechanical tension in the median nerve: possible implications for the upper limb tension test. Physiotherapy 84(6): 254–261

Loewy J 2001 Ultrasonography and magnetic resonance imaging of abnormalities of the peripheral nerves. Canadian Association Radiology Journal 52(5): 292–301

Louis R 1981 Vertebroradicular and vertebromedullar dynamics. Anatomia Clinica 3: 1–11

Lundborg G, Rydevik B 1973 Effects of stretching the tibial nerve of the rabbit: a preliminary study of the intraneural circulation and the barrier function of the perineurium. Journal of Bone and Joint Surgery 55B(2): 390–401

Lundborg G, Myers R, Powell H 1983 Nerve compression injury and increased endoneurial fluid pressure: a 'miniature compartment syndrome'. Journal of Neurology, Neurosurgery and Psychiatry 46: 1119–1124

McCulloch J, Waddell G 1980 Variation of the lumbosacral myotomes with bony segmental anomalies. Journal of Bone and Joint Surgery 62B: 475–480

McLellan D, Swash M 1976 Longitudinal sliding of the median nerve during movements of the upper limb. Journal of Neurology, Neurosurgery and Psychiatry 39: 566–570

McMahon S, Koltzenburg M 1990 The changing role of primary afferent neurones in pain. Pain 43: 269–272

McNab I 1971 Negative disc exploration: an analysis of the causes of nerve-root involvement in sixty-eight patients. Journal of Bone and Joint Surgery 53A: 891–903

MacNab I 1972 The mechanism of spondylogenic pain. In: Hirsch C, Zotterman Y (eds) Cervical pain. Pergamon Press, New York, pp 89–95

Madison Taylor J 1909 Treatment of occupation neuroses and neuritis in the arms. Journal of the American Medical Association 53(3): 198–200

Maher C, Latimer J, Refshauge K 2000 Atlas of clinical tests and measures for low back pain. Australian Physiotherapy Association, Melbourne

Maitland G 1979 Negative disc exploration: positive canal signs. Australian Journal of Physiotherapy 25(3): 129–133

Maitland G 1986 Vertebral manipulation, 5th edn. Butterworths, London

Maitland G 1991. Peripheral manipulation, 3rd edn. Butterworth Heinemann, London

Maravilla K R, Bowen B C 1998 Imaging of the peripheral nervous system: evaluation of peripheral neuropathy and plexopathy. American Journal of Neuroradiology 19: 1011–1023

Marshall J 1883 Nerve stretching for the relief or cure of pain. British Medical Journal 15: 1173–1179

Marshall L L, Trethewie E R, Curtain C C 1977 Chemical radiculitis: a clinical, physiological and immunological study. Clinical Orthopaedics and Related Research 129: 61–67

Merskey H, Bogduk N 1994 Classification of chronic pain: definitions of chronic pain syndromes and definitions of pain terms, 2nd edn. International Association for the Study of Pain, Seattle

Milidonis M K, Ritter R C, Sweeney M A, Godges J J, Knapp J, Antonucci E 1997 Practical analysis survey: revalidation of advanced clinical practice in orthopaedic physical therapy. Journal of Orthopaedic and Sports Physical Therapy 25: 163–170

Millesi H, Zoch G, Riehsner R 1995 Mechanical properties of peripheral nerves. Clinical Orthopaedics and Related Research 314: 76–83

Monsivais J J, Yang Sun, Rajashekhar T P 1995 The scalene reflex: relationship between increased median or ulnar nerve pressure and scalene muscle activity. Journal of Reconstructive Microsurgery 11(4): 271–275

Mooney V, Robertson J 1976 The facet syndrome. Clinical Orthopaedics and Related Research 115: 149–156

Moses A, Carman J 1996 Anatomy of the cervical spine: implications for the upper limb tension test. Australian Journal of Physiotherapy 42: 31–35

Mottram S L 1997 Dynamic stability of the scapula. Manual Therapy 2: 123–131

Naftulin S, Fast A, Thomas M 1993 Diabetic lumbar radiculopathy: sciatica without disc herniation. Spine 18(16): 2419–2422

Nagy B 1999 A randomised placebo controlled clinical trial of the effects of specific manipulative therapy treatment in cervicobrachial pain syndrome. MSc thesis, Curtin University of Technology, Perth

Ochoa J L 1997 Valid versus redundant links in the theory for 'neuropathic pains'. Pain Forum 6(3): 196–198

O'Connell J E 1951 Protrusions of the lumbar intervertebral disc. Journal of Bone and Joint Surgery 33B(1): 8–17

Ogato K, Naito M 1986 Blood flow of peripheral nerves: effects of dissection, stretching and compression. Journal of Hand Surgery 11: 10

Olmarker K, Rydevik B 1991 Pathophysiology of sciatica. Orthopaedic Clinics of North America 22(2): 223–234

Olmarker K, Rydevik B, Nordberg C 1993 Autologous nucleus pulposus induces neurophysiologic and histologic changes in porcine cauda equina nerve roots. Spine 18: 1425–1432

Olmarker K, Kikuchi S, Rydevik B 1997 Anatomy and physiology of spinal nerve roots and the results of compression and irritation: In: Giles L G, Singer K P (eds) Clinical anatomy and management of low back pain. Butterworth Heinemann, Oxford

O'Neill C, Kurgansky E, Derby R, Ryan P 2002 Disc stimulation and patterns of referred pain. Spine 27(24): 2776–2781.

O'Sullivan P, Twomey L, Allison G 1997a Evaluation of specific stabilising exercises in the treatment of chronic low back pain with radiologic diagnosis of spondylosis or spondylolisthesis. Spine 22: 2959–2967

O'Sullivan P, Twomey L, Allison G 1997b Specific stabilising exercise in the treatment of chronic low back pain with a clinical and radiological diagnosis of lumbar segmental 'instability'. In: Manipulative Physiotherapists Association of Australia Tenth Biennial Conference, Melbourne, pp 139–140

Phillips D R, Twomey L T 1996 A comparison of manual diagnosis with a diagnosis established by a uni-level lumbar spinal block procedure. Manual Therapy 2: 82–87

Quintner J 1989 A study of upper limb pain and paraesthesiae following neck injury in motor vehicle accidents: assessment of the brachial plexus test of Elvey. British Journal of Rheumatology 28: 528–533

Quintner J 1998 Peripheral neuropathic pain: a rediscovered clinical entity. Annual General Meeting of the Australian Pain Society, Australian Pain Society, Hobart

Quintner J L, Bove G 2001 From neuralgia to peripheral neuropathic pain: evolution of a concept. Regional Anaesthesia and Pain Medicine 26: 368–372

Ramirez-Lassepas M, Tulloch J W, Quinones M R, Snyder B D 1992 Acute radicular pain as a presenting symptom in multiple sclerosis. Archives of Neurology 49: 255–258

Rankine J, Fortune D, Hutchinson C, Hughes D, Main C 1998 Pain drawings in the assessment of nerve root compression: a comparative study with lumbar spine magnetic resonance imaging. Spine 23(15): 1668–1676

Reid S 1987 The measurement of tension changes in the brachial plexus. In: Dalziel B, Snowsill J (eds) Proceedings of the Fifth Biennial Conference of the Manipulative Therapists Association of Australia, Melbourne, pp 79–90

Refshauge K, Gass E 1995 The neurological examination. In: Refshauge K, Gass E (eds) Musculoskeletal physiotherapy: clinical science and practice. Butterworth Heinemann, Oxford

Rempel D, Dahlin L, Lundborg G 1999 Pathophysiology of nerve compression syndromes: response of peripheral nerves to loading. Journal of Bone and Joint Surgery 81A: 1600–1610

Rogers P, Nash T, Schiller D, Norman J 1992 Epidural steroids for sciatica. Pain Clinic 5(2): 67–72

Rydevik B, Garfin S 1989 Spinal nerve root compression. In: Szabo R (ed) Nerve root compression syndromes: diagnosis and treatment. Slack, New Jersey, pp 247–261

Rydevik B, Brown M, Lundborg G 1984 Pathoanatomy and pathophysiology of nerve root compression. Spine 9(1): 7–15

Saal J S, Fransone R C, Dobrow R et al 1990 High levels of inflammatory phospholipase A2 activity in lumbar disc herniations. Spine 15: 674–678

Sahrmann S 2002 Diagnosis and treatment of movement impairment syndromes. Mosby, St Louis

Sampath P, Bendebba M, Davis J D, Ducker T 1999 Outcome in patients with cervical radiculopathy: prospective, multicentre study with independent clinical review. Spine 24(6): 591–597

Sauer S K, Bove G M, Averbeck B, Reeh P W 1999 Rat peripheral nerve components release calcitonin gene-related peptide and prostaglandin E2 in response to noxious stimuli: evidence that the nervi nervorum are nociceptors. Neuroscience 92: 319–325

Selvaratnam P J, Glasgow E F, Matyas T A 1988 The strain at the nerve roots of the brachial plexus. Journal of Anatomy 161: 260

Selvaratnam P J, Glasgow E F, Matyas T A 1989 Differential strain produced by the brachial plexus tension test on C5 to T1 nerve roots. Proceedings of Manipulative Therapists Association of Australia Sixth Biennial Conference, Adelaide, pp 167–172

Selvaratnam P J, Matyas T A, Glasgow E F 1994 Noninvasive discrimination of brachial plexus involvement in upper limb pain. Spine 19(1): 26–33

Shacklock M, Wilkinson M 2001 Can nerves be moved specifically. Proceedings of Musculoskeletal Physiotherapists Association of Australia, Twelfth Biennial Conference, Adelaide, pp 46–49

Shantha T R, Evans J A 1972 The relationship of epidural anaesthesia to neuromembranes and arachnoid villa. Anesthesiology 37: 543–557

Slipman C W, Plastaras C T, Pamlitier R A, Huston C W, Sterenfeld E B 1998 Symptom provocation of fluoroscopically guided cervical nerve root stimulation: are dynatomal maps identical to dermatomal maps? Spine 23(20): 2235–2242

Smyth M, Wright V 1958 Sciatica and the intervertebral disc: an experimental study. Journal of Bone and Joint Surgery 40A: 1401–1418

Sorkin L S, Wagner R, Myers R R 1997 Role of the nervi nervorum in neuropathic pain: innocent until proven guilty. Pain Forum 6(3): 191–192

Spiliopoulou I, Korovessis P, Konstantinou D, Dimitracopoulos G 1994 IgG and IgM concentration in the prolapsed human intervertebral disc and sciatica etiology. Spine 19(12): 1320–1323

Spitzer W 1987 Scientific approach to the assessment and management of activity-related spinal disorders: a monograph for clinicians. Report of the Quebec Task Force on Spinal Disorders. Spine 12: 9–54

Srinivasa N R, Meyer R A, Ringkamp M, Campbell J N 1999 Peripheral neural mechanisms of nociception. In: Wall P D, Melzack R (eds) The textbook of pain, 4th edn. Churchill Livingstone, Edinburgh, pp 11–57

Sterling M, Treleaven J, Jull G 2002 Responses to a clinical test of mechanical provocation of nerve tissue in whiplash associated disorder. Manual Therapy 7(2): 89–94

Sugimoto T, Bennett G, Kajanda K 1989 Strychnine-induced transynaptic degeneration of dorsal horn neurons in rats with an experimental neuropathy. Neuroscience Letters 98: 139–143

Sugiura K, Yoshida T, Katoh S, Mimatsu M 1979 A study on tension signs in lumbar disc hernia. International Orthopaedics 3: 225–228

Sunderland S 1990 The anatomy and physiology of nerve injury. Muscle and Nerve 13: 771–784

Sunderland S 1991 Nerve injuries and their repair. Churchill Livingstone, Edinburgh

Sweeney J, Harms A 1996 Persistent mechanical allodynia following injury of the hand: treatment through mobilisation of the nervous system. Journal of Hand Therapy 9: 328–338

Tanaka N, Fujimoto Y, An H S, Ikuta Y, Yasuda M 2000 The anatomic relation among the nerve roots, intervertebral foramina and intervertebral discs of the cervical spine. Spine 25(3): 286–290

Thomas P, Berthold C, Ochoa J 1993 Microscopic anatomy of the peripheral nervous system. In: Dyck P, Thomas P (eds) Peripheral neuropathy, 3rd edn. WB Saunders, Philadelphia, vol 1, pp 28–91

Troup J 1986 Biomechanics of the lumbar spinal canal. Clinical Biomechanics 1: 31–43

Unruh A M, Strong J, Wright A 2002 Introduction to pain. In: Strong J, Unruh A M, Wright A, Baxter G D Pain: a textbook for therapists. Churchill Livingstone, Edinburgh

van den Hoogen H M, Koes B W, van Eijk J, Bouter L M 1995 On the accuracy of history, physical examination, erythrocyte sedimentation rate in diagnosing low back pain in general practice: a criteria-based review of the literature. Spine 20(3): 318–327

van der Heide B, Allison G T, Zusman M 2000 Pain and muscular responses to a neural tissue provocation test in patients with cervical radiculopathy. Proceedings of the Seventh Scientific Conference of the International Federation of Orthopaedic Manipulative Therapists, Perth, Western Australia

van der Heide B, Allison G T, Zusman M 2001 Pain and muscular responses to a neural tissue provocation test in the upper limb. Manual Therapy 6(3): 154–162

Vicenzino B, Collins D, Wright A 1996 The initial effects of a cervical spine manipulative physiotherapy treatment on the pain and dysfunction of lateral epicondylitis. Pain 68: 69–74

Vicenzino B, Collins D, Benson H, Wright A 1998 An investigation of the interrelationship between manipulative therapy-induced hypoalgesia and sympathoexcitation. Journal of Manipulative and Physiological Therapeutics 21(7): 448–453

Viikari-Juntura E 1987 Interexaminer reliability of observations in physical examinations of the neck. Physical Therapy 67: 1526–1532

Viikari-Juntura E, Porras M, Laasonen E M 1989 Validity of clinical tests in the diagnosis of root compression in cervical disc disease. Spine 14: 253–257

Vroomen P C, de Krom M C, Knottnerus J A 2000 Consistency of history taking and physical examination in patients with suspected lumbar nerve root involvement. Spine 25(1): 91–97

Waddell G, Somerville D, Henderson I, Newton M 1992 Objective clinical evaluation of physical impairment in chronic low back pain. Spine 17: 617–628

Wainner R S, Gill H 2000 Diagnosis and nonoperative management of cervical radiculopathy. Journal of Orthopaedic and Sports Physical Therapy 30: 728–744

Wasserstrom W R, Glass J P, Posner J B 1982 Diagnosis and treatment of leptomeningeal metastases from solid tumours. Cancer 49: 759–772

Watson N 1994 What is stiffness. Journal of Hand Therapy 1: 147–149

Weirich S D, Golberman R H, Best S A et al 1999 Rehabilitation after subcutaneous transposition of the ulnar nerve: immediate versus delayed mobilisation. Journal of Shoulder and Elbow Surgery 7: 244–249

Wiesel S, Tsourmas N, Feffer H, Citrin C, Patronas N 1984 A study of computer-assisted tomography. 1: The incidence of positive CAT scans in an asymptomatic group of patients. Spine 9: 549–551

Wilgis E F, Murphy R 1986 The significance of longitudinal excursion in peripheral nerves. Hand Clinics 2: 761–766

Willis D W 1997 An alternative mechanism for neuropathic pain. Pain Forum 6(3): 193–195

Winkelstein B A, Weinstein J N, DeLeo J A 2002 The role of mechanical deformation in lumbar radiculopathy: an in vivo model. Spine 27(1): 27–33

Woolf C 1991 Generation of acute pain: central mechanisms. British Medical Bulletin 47: 523–533

Wright A 1999 Recent concepts in the neurophysiology of pain. Manual Therapy 4(4): 196–202

Wright A 2002 Neuropathic pain. In: Strong J, Unruh A M, Wright A, Baxter G D Pain: a textbook for therapists. Churchill Livingstone, Edinburgh

Yaxley G, Jull G 1991 A modified upper limb tension test: an investigation of responses in normal subjects. Australian Journal of Physiotherapy 37: 143–152

Yoss R E, Corbin K B, MacCarty C S, Love J G 1999 Significance of symptoms and signs in localization of involved roots in cervical disc protrusion. Neurology 7: 673–683

Yuan Q, Dougherty L, Margulies S 1998 In vivo human cervical spinal cord deformation and displacement in flexion. Spine 23(15): 1677–1683

Zochodne D 1993 Epineural peptides: a role in neuropathic pain. Canadian Journal of Neurological Sciences 20: 69–72

Zvulun I 1998 Mobilizing the nervous system in cervical cord compression. Manual Therapy 3(1): 42–47

Chapter 30

The use of taping for pain relief in the management of spinal pain

J. McConnell

INTRODUCTION

Spinal pain, particularly nerve root pain, can be extremely disabling for a patient. Treatment usually alleviates symptoms but the treatment effect can be short lived with the symptoms often returning with a vengeance. Chronic symptoms may even be exacerbated with treatment, as long-term adaptive changes in the soft tissues can be difficult to alter. Equally, unravelling the cause of the pain can be a challenge for the clinician, since the source of the symptoms can be quite remote from the site of pain. Additionally, there may be confounding problems of hyper/hypomobility in the surrounding soft tissues making response to treatment less predictable. If clinicians can minimize treatment exacerbations and prolong treatment effectiveness then they can expedite a patient's recovery from low back pain.

WHAT IS PAIN?

Pain has been defined as an unpleasant sensory or emotional experience associated with actual or potential tissue damage (nociception) (Bogduk 1993). Pain involves the patient's reaction to the nociception, so it is very much an individual experience with a learned component. Pain can become memorized because pain mechanisms are not fixed (hard wired) but are plastic (soft wired) (Shacklock 1999). Through neuroplasticity, hyperalgesia can be learned and unlearned, from both tissue based and environmental afferent inputs (Hall & Quintner 1995, Shacklock 1999). Management of chronic pain must therefore address the psychosocial as well as the contributing physical factors (Feuerstein & Beattie 1995, Maras et al 2000, Wheeler 1995, Zusman 1998). Sometimes, however, when a patient has 'failed to respond to treatment' we are quick to label the patient's problem as a psychological or a 'centrally maintained' pain, when in fact it may be our treatment that has failed. Centrally maintained pain (central sensitivity) occurs when non-noxious stimuli and movements cause an inappropriate and persistent pain response (Butler 2000).

A persistent driver from the periphery set up from the original injury seems to cause the central sensitivity (Butler 2000, Coderre et al 1993). The driver may be one or a combination of any of the following:

1. Unsettled inflammation in the periphery, dorsal horn or dorsal root ganglion.
2. Unremitting dorsal root ganglion discharge.
3. Changes in the A fibre phenotype with possible re-sprouting of the fibres in the lamina 2 in the dorsal horn. This occurs when C fibres die back from lamina 2, allowing A fibre sprouting.
4. Supraspinal influences including maladaptive beliefs, fears and attitudes (Butler 2000). Motor performance may also be affected by changes in attentional demands, whereby people with chronic pain perform poorly in tasks demanding attention (Eccleston 1994, Kewman et al 1991) and are less able to focus away from pain (Dufton 1989).

RATIONALE FOR THE DEVELOPMENT OF MUSCULOSKELETAL PROBLEMS

In 1996 Dye proposed the concept of tissue homeostasis of the knee to help explain when an individual would be susceptible to knee pain. This concept can be generalized to any musculoskeletal condition if the amount or frequency of loading is too great for the underlying structures. The system then is no longer in balance, so the individual is outside their envelope of function (Fig. 30.1), having reached a particular threshold which is unique to that individual. For example, an Olympic weight lifter can usually lift over three times his body weight without injury, whereas an office worker may not be able to lift much more than his own body weight before he incurs an injury. A labourer may be able to move 50 × 20 kg boxes in a day and remain injury free, but if he moves 52 boxes that may take him over his threshold and result in tissue breakdown and pain. Breaching the threshold causes a complex biological cascade of trauma and repair which is manifested clinically as pain and swelling, further diminishing the patient's envelope of function, so that activities that initially were not painful for a patient become painful (Dye 1996, Novacheck 1997, Schacle et al 1999). For example, before the onset of back pain, a patient could carry five shopping bags from the supermarket and lift them into the car, but now, after the onset of back pain, can only lift one small grocery bag into the car and has difficulty manoeuvring the supermarket trolley without exacerbating the pain.

Dye (1996) has described four factors that are pertinent to determining the size of the envelope of function: anatomical, kinematic, physiological and treatment factors. The anatomical factors involve the morphology, structural integrity and biomechanical characteristics of tissue. The kinematic factors, which are enhanced by training, include the dynamic control of the joint involving proprioceptive

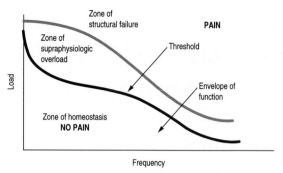

Figure 30.1 Homeostasis of the musculoskeletal system. Adapted from Dye 1996.

sensory output, cerebral and cerebellar sequencing of motor units, spinal reflex mechanisms, muscle strength and motor control. The physiological factors involve the genetically determined mechanisms of molecular and cellular homeostasis that determine the quality and rate of repair of damaged tissues. Treatment factors include the type of rehabilitation or surgery received. The therapist can have a positive influence on the patient's envelope of function by minimizing the aggravation of the inflamed tissue and can even increase the patient's threshold of function by improving the control of the mobile segments, the flexibility of the stiff segments and the overall muscle strength.

UNLOADING PAINFUL STRUCTURES

The concept of minimizing the aggravation of inflamed tissue is central to all interventions in orthopaedics. Clinicians have a number of weapons in their armoury, such as anti-inflammatory medication, topical creams, ice, electrotherapy modalities, acupuncture and tape, to attack pain and reduce inflammation. With acute low back pain, the therapist can augment treatment by supporting, or in some cases almost splinting, the lumbar spine with tape. The rigid support minimizes movement in the lumbar spine. The direction of tape is primarily determined by the symptom response, but to some extent on the desired movement restriction. Generally tape is applied in the direction of the symptoms at the symptomatic level (Fig. 30.2). If the spine is to be maintained in a neutral position, two diagonal pieces of tape are used in conjunction with the tape described above, commencing at the iliac crest on each side and pulling over to the opposite ilium (mid-buttocks region – Fig. 30.3). This configuration of tape will keep the spine from flexing and extending. If a bias is sought for the sacroiliac (SI) joint then closing down of the joint can be achieved if both diagonal tapes are commenced on the painful side. The first tape commences on the iliac crest pulling towards the opposite ilium with the second commencing on the ilium on the same side coursing up to the opposite iliac crest (Fig. 30.4). These tapes should cross over the symptomatic SI joint. If opening the SI joint is required both tapes start on the side opposite the symptomatic SI to open and support the joint. Symptom reduction signifies

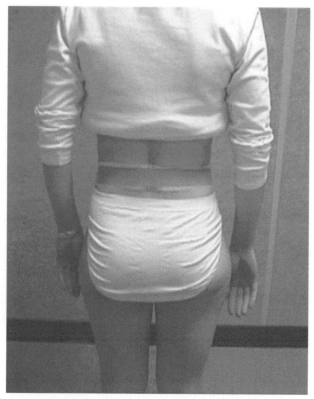

Figure 30.2 Tape to stabilize an unstable segment. Tape usually in direction of pain.

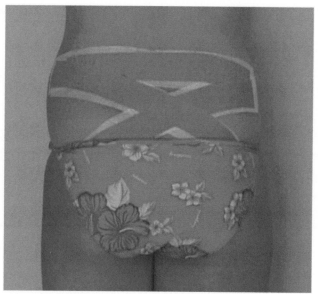

Figure 30.4 To close down the right sacroiliac joint, tape at L5/S1 level from asymptomatic to symptomatic side, then tape from right iliac crest to opposite buttock and finally from inferior part of right ilium to left iliac crest.

taping success, so tape can be extremely useful in allowing an environment for healing by unloading the painful structures and restricting excessive motion.

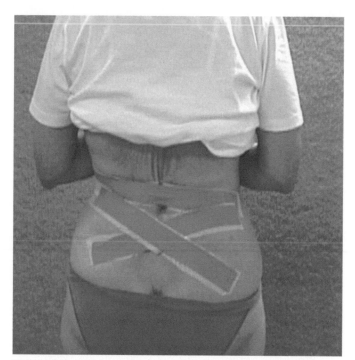

Figure 30.3 Tape to minimize movement in the lumbar spine. This is particularly useful for acute low back pain.

However, chronic pain can be less amenable to treatment as symptoms are often increased by the very treatment that is designed to diminish them. For example, the patient with chronic back and leg pain who can only flex to his knees is given a slump stretch as part of his treatment but the pain is increased, so there is an adverse reaction to treatment. The patient then is reluctant to have further treatment, limits his movement even more, becomes stiffer and has increases in pain (McConnell 2000). Key to the success of management of this patient is to unload the inflamed soft tissues so that the clinician can address the issues of lack of flexibility and poor dynamic control. The principle of unloading is based on the premise that inflamed soft tissue does not respond well to stretch (Gresalmer & McConnell 1998, McConnell 2000). For example, if a patient presents with a sprained lateral ligament of the ankle, applying an inversion stress to the ankle will exacerbate the pain, whereas an eversion stress will decrease the symptoms. The same principle applies for patients with an inflamed nerve root, producing leg pain. The inflamed tissue needs to be shortened or unloaded. Tape can be used to unload (shorten) the inflamed neural tissue, which will in turn decrease the pain. Tape can be used for both acute and chronic nerve root conditions.

Initially the buttock is unloaded, which should decrease the proximal symptoms but may increase the distal symptoms (Fig. 30.5). The distal symptoms will decrease once the tissues are unloaded down the leg, with tape placed on the upper and lower leg. A diagonal strip of tape is placed mid-thigh over the appropriate dermatome (posterior thigh for S1, lateral aspect of the thigh for L5 and so forth – Fig. 30.6). The soft tissues are lifted

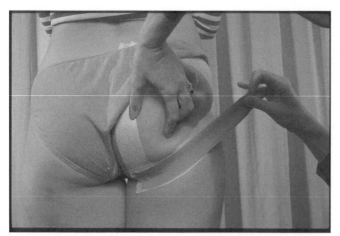

Figure 30.5 Unloading the buttock to decrease leg symptoms. The tape must be sculptured into the gluteal fold.

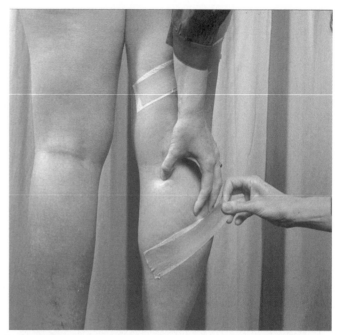

Figure 30.7 Unloading the calf to further decrease sacroiliac symptoms.

up towards the buttock. The direction of the tape is dependent on symptom response; if there is a local increase in symptoms then the direction of the diagonal should be reversed. Another diagonal piece of tape is commenced mid-calf/shin (following the dermatome), again lifting the skin towards the buttock (Fig. 30.7). If there is still some pain, pins and needles or numbness on the foot, the navicular may need to be lifted to further unload the soft tissue (Fig. 30.8). The patient should experience an immediate 50% decrease in symptoms. If the symptoms are unchanged, then the soft tissue may not have been unloaded sufficiently or the tape was placed in the wrong direction. The tape is kept on for a week before it is

renewed and usually only needs two or three applications before the symptoms have settled sufficiently.

EFFECT OF TAPE

The effect of tape on pain, particularly patellofemoral pain, has been fairly well established in the literature, although there has been a dearth of studies examining the effect of tape in the management of lumbar spine pain (Bockrath et al 1993, Cerny 1995, Conway et al 1992, Cowan et al 2002a, Cushnaghan et al 1994, Gilleard et al 1998, Powers et al 1997).

The reason patellar taping has been widely accepted as clinically useful in managing patients with patellofemoral symptoms is its capacity to reduce anterior knee pain and allow a functional rehabilitation program of the knee to

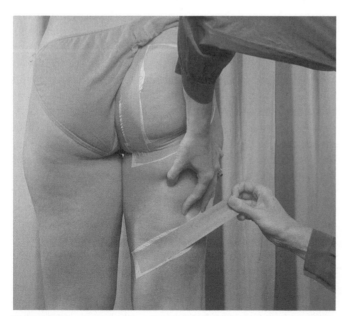

Figure 30.6 For sacroiliac distribution of pain, the posterior thigh is taped, with the skin being lifted to the buttock. If the proximal symptoms worsen, the tape diagonal should be reversed.

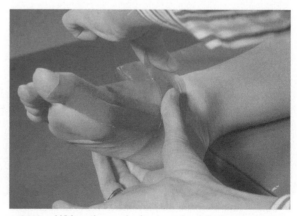

Figure 30.8 Lifting the navicular to unload foot symptoms.

proceed. Thus, taping techniques can be viewed as a successful and safe method to help create the internal biomechanical environment, which results in the restoration of tissue homeostasis and associated resolution of pain. (Dye 1999).

The mechanism causing the tape induced pain reduction in patellofemoral sufferers is still debated in the literature. However, it has been found that patellar taping: causes an earlier activation of the vastus medialis oblique (VMO) relative to the vastus lateralis (VL) on stair ascent and descent; improves shock absorption during weight bearing; and increases quadriceps muscle torque (Conway et al 1992, Cowan et al 2002a, Gilleard et al 1998, Handfield & Kramer 2000, Powers et al 1997).

However, as far as the effect of the unloading tape is concerned, the mechanism is yet to be investigated. It could inhibit an overactive hamstrings muscle, which is a protective response to mechanical provocation of neural tissue (Hall & Quintner 1995). Tobin & Robinson (2000) found that firm taping across the muscle belly of vastus lateralis (VL) of asymptomatic individuals significantly decreased the VL activity during stair descent, so taping across the hamstrings and gastrocnemius bellies could diminish the protective response of these muscles when the neural tissue is provoked. Unloading tape could have some effect on changing the pull or orientation of the fascia. Traction to the gluteus maximus and biceps femoris muscles in vitro has been found to cause displacement of the posterior layer of the thoracolumbar fascia (Vleeming et al 1995), so tape may decrease this displacement by shortening the muscles. Alternatively, the effect could be proprioceptive, affecting the gating mechanism of pain (Garnett & Stephens 1981, Jenner & Stephens 1982). 'The goal of any treatment program should be to achieve maximal painless joint function as safely and predictably as possible' (Dye 1999). Unloading tape enables the patient to be treated without an increase in symptoms so, in the long term, treatment is more efficacious. The therapist is then able to address the issues of lack of flexibility and poor control without exacerbating the symptoms.

MANAGING RECALCITRANT CHRONIC LOW BACK AND LEG PAIN

When managing low back pain, the clinician may need to change the treatment focus, so the treatment is not just directed at the involved segment but addresses the contributory factors. Patients with chronic back and leg pain often complain of increasing pain not only with prolonged sitting, but also with walking and occasionally even standing. It has been observed clinically that a large number of low back pain sufferers have internally rotated femurs. It is postulated that the internal femoral rotation reduces the available hip extension and external rotation range. This causes an increase in the rotation required in the lumbar spine when the patient walks. The normal ranges of pelvic move-

ments during gait are 4 degrees of lateral tilt, 10 degrees of rotation and 7 degrees of anteroposterior tilt (Perry 1992). The internal rotation in the hip also causes tightness in the iliotibial band and diminished activity in the gluteus medius posterior fibres, so the pelvis exhibits dynamic instability and the amount of trunk side flexion increases (McConnell 2000, 2002a).

The lack of control around the pelvis further increases the movement of an already mobile lumbar spine segment. It has been established that excessive movement, particularly in rotation, is a contributory factor to disc injury and the torsional forces may irrevocably damage fibres of the annulus fibrosus (Farfan et al 1970, Kelsey et al 1984). Therefore, an excessive amount of movement about the lumbar spine because of limited hip movement and control in combination with poor abdominal support seems to be a significant factor in the development of low back pain. In a recent study (Karol et al 2000) examining the long-term effect of hip arthrodesis on gait in adolescents all subjects showed excessive motion in the joint above and below the arthrodesis, that is, the ipsilateral knee and the lumbar spine. The authors hypothesized that this led to the high incidence of low back pain in these individuals (Karol et al 2000). Further evidence of the interrelationship of hip muscle control and lumbar spine function has surfaced recently when it was found that hip muscle imbalance was predictive of the development of low back pain in female athletes (Nadler et al 2001). It has been estimated that if an individual walks for about 80 minutes in a day, then each limb will go through 2500 stance and swing cycles per day, which equates to 1 million cycles per year (Dananberg 1997). By age 30 then, each limb has performed almost 30 million cycles so if there is any asymmetry in the system there will be a greater propensity for tissue overload (resulting in a loss of tissue homeostasis) and hence pain.

Lumbopelvic movement is further increased during gait if adequate shock absorption has not occurred at the knee or the foot, or if dorsiflexion of the great toe is inadequate at push off, reducing the available ankle range of plantarflexion and hip extension (Dananberg 1997). Initial shock absorption occurs with knee flexion of 10–15 degrees because the foot is supinated when the heel first strikes the ground (Perry 1992). As soon as the heel hits the ground, the foot rapidly pronates and the lower leg internally rotates. If the knee is hyperextended or the subtalar joint is stiff, there will be increased rotation and/or lateral tilting of the pelvis, which will manifest as excessive motion in the spine. This excessive lumbar spine movement is further aggravated during forward leaning in sitting, as individuals with low back pain use more lumbar spine movement in this position than individuals with no low back pain, indicating an increase in relative spinal flexibility in these individuals (Hamilton & Richardson 1998).

It has been postulated that the sacroiliac (SI) joint also has a role in the control of locomotion and body posture (Indahl et al 1999). Indahl and colleagues (1999) have found that stimulation of the porcine SI joint capsule elicited activity in the multifidus muscle, whereas stimulation of the anterior aspect of the joint elicited responses in quadratus lumborum and gluteus maximus. Interestingly, it has been found that the activity of the gluteus maximus is shorter in duration in back pain patients during trunk flexion and extension than in controls. Dysfunction in the SI joint, therefore, may also contribute to the poorer activation of the gluteus maximus in low back pain individuals. The gluteus maximus can be facilitated by shortening the muscle with tape, as shown in Figure 30.5. The tape not only unloads inflamed tissue but also seems to improve gluteal activation. Taping the patella such that the VMO is shortened has been found to cause an earlier onset of VMO relative to VL whereas placebo taping make no difference to the firing pattern (Cowan et al 2002b), so it makes sense that shortening the gluteus maximus muscle with tape would also change the firing pattern. Certainly, patients report increased stability and improved balance when the buttock is taped. It could be said then that the SI joint has a role in the activation of spinal and gluteal muscles, which helps control locomotion and body posture as well as providing stability on a segmental level in the lumbar spine (Indahl et al 1999).

Increased lumbar spine mobility is often accompanied by poor segmental muscle recruitment/control (Hodges & Richardson 1996, Richardson et al 1999). A variety of strategies are used to control spinal stability at different levels. The deep intrinsic muscles of the spine are recruited to control translation and rotation at the intervertebral level, enabling spine stiffening, while the long multisegmental muscles prevent buckling of the spine (Bergmark 1989). However, in low back pain sufferers changes in the recruitment pattern of the local muscles of the trunk have been found, compromising intervertebral stability (Hodges & Richardson 1996, King et al 1988, Wilder et al 1996). In contrast, a delayed offset of activity when a load is released from the trunk has been found in the global muscles such as the oblique abdominals and erector spinae, possibly indicating an attempt by these superficial muscles to compensate for poor deep muscle function (Radebold et al 2000). It has not yet been established whether the muscle control problem causes the back pain or whether the back pain triggers the muscle control problem (Hodges 2000).

TREATMENT

Treatment should therefore be directed at increasing hip and thoracic spine mobility as well as improving the stability of the relevant lumbar segments. The anterior hip structures, particularly the adductor muscles, will be tight. Tightness in the adductor longus and brevis accentuates further flexion and internal rotation of the hip, and the only adductor with an extension and external rotation moment is the posterior fibres of the adductor magnus (Basmajian & De Luca 1985). However, if the hip remains flexed the

adductor magnus is more likely to assist internal rotation of the hip, causing further anterior hip tightness (Williams & Warwick 1980).

Palpation of the adductor longus tendon can often be painful and may reproduce posterior buttock pain. If palpation of the adductor tendon is extremely painful, stretching the tight anterior structures will be difficult unless a sustained pressure is applied to the tendon to alleviate the trigger point. The patient can then improve anterior hip flexibility by lying prone (the hip is externally rotated and the knee flexed in a figure of four position) and elongating the thigh in an attempt to flatten the hip (Fig. 30.9). Ideally, in the figure of four position the pelvis should be flat on the table. Usually the hip on the painful side is higher off the plinth than that on the non-painful side. As the patient's pain decreases, the distance from the anterior superior iliac spine (ASIS) to the plinth also decreases.

Many patients with chronic low back pain have associated stiffness in the thoracic spine. The thoracic spine is inherently stiff as it is constrained by the ribs and possesses long spinous processes. If the thoracic spine is stiff, there will be increased movement demands on the areas above and below, such as the lumbar, cervical and shoulder regions. Increasing the mobility of the thoracic spine and surrounding soft tissue structures will allow a more even distribution of load through the spine during movement. To optimize treatment effectiveness in the chronic situation, mobilization of the thoracic spine can be performed in sitting. This allows the therapist not only to increase segmental thoracic mobility, but also to elongate tight neural and fascial tissue both inferiorly and superiorly. Recent evidence has suggested that the posterior layer of the lumbar fascia may be implicated as the symptom producing structure causing lumbar pain in the slump position (Barker & Briggs 1999). Elongation of the neural and fascial tissues may be achieved by adding a straight leg raise or by stretching the arms out onto the plinth with the palms facing up to put the latissimus dorsi muscle on stretch (Fig. 30.10). Vleeming and co-workers (1995) found that displacement of the posterior thoracolumbar fascia also occurs when a superior muscle such as the latissimus dorsi is

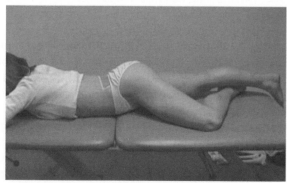

Figure 30.9 Elongating stiff anterior hip structures.

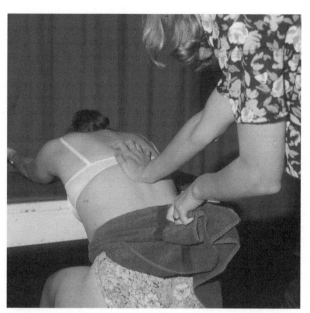

Figure 30.10 Mobilizing a stiff thoracic spine in sitting with latissimus dorsi on stretch. The lumbar spine is stabilized with the towel.

tractioned. Mobilization in the sitting position is contraindicated, however, if there is an acute lumbar disc problem.

At the same time as increasing the mobility of adjacent areas, the therapist needs to commence stability work on the unstable areas. The compensatory mobility (instability) in the lumbar spine can be examined using accessory or physiological movements. This increased movement is often in a non-physiological direction. If the palpation is being performed in prone and the patient has an increased lumbar lordosis, the segment may actually feel stiff unless the spine has been placed in a neutral position prior to commencing palpation. Thus the starting position of the joint is critical in the decision making process as a different treatment will be given if it has been deemed that the lumbar spine is stiff rather than mobile. A good example of how the starting position makes a difference in the diagnosis and hence in the management of a condition is the acutely injured knee. When the posterior cruciate is ruptured, although there is an increased anterior draw, the therapist examines the resting position of the tibia before deciding that the increased anterior movement was a consequence of the starting position rather than a pathological increase in movement. If the anterior cruciate had been ruptured hamstrings activation would be emphasized in rehabilitation whereas with a posterior cruciate rupture quadriceps activity is needed to pull the tibia forward. So, if a lumbar spine example of spondylolithesis were considered, a postero-anterior mobilization of the segment in prone would actually exacerbate the symptoms even though the segment felt stiff in this position. A flexion or anteroposterior movement is a more appropriate mobilization direction in treatment, although stabilizing the segment rather than mobilizing would be a more desirable treatment option.

Spinal stability requires the interaction of three systems: passive (the vertebrae, ligaments, fascia and discs), active (the muscles acting on the spine) and neural (central nervous system and nerves controlling the muscles) (Panjabi 1992). The most vulnerable area of the spine (the neutral zone) occurs around the neutral position of a spinal segment, where little resistance is offered by the passive structures (Panjabi 1992). If decreased passive stability occurs, the active and neural systems can compensate by providing dynamic stability to the spine. Stability around the neutral zone can be increased by muscle activity of as little as 1–3% (Cholewicki et al 1997). Segmental stability training involves muscle control of the multifidus, transversus abdominis and the posterior fibres of the gluteus medius. The therapist must carefully supervise specific exercises for these muscles so the appropriate muscles are recruited during the exercise. If there has been habitual disuse of the muscles activation will be difficult. Feedback to the patient must be precise to achieve the desired outcome (Sale 1987).

A recent study by Cowan and colleagues (2002a) found that 6 weeks of one session per week of physiotherapy treatment, where emphasis was placed on specific muscle training of the VMO using a dual channel biofeedback, changed the onset timing of VMO relative to VL during stair stepping and postural perturbation tasks in patients with patellofemoral pain. At baseline in both the placebo and treatment groups, the VMO came on significantly later than the VL. Following treatment, there was no change in muscle onset timing of the placebo group, but in the physiotherapy group the onset of VMO and VL occurred simultaneously during concentric activity and the VMO actually preceded VL during eccentric activity. Precise training of the transversus abdominis and multifidus has been adequately described in the literature (Comerford & Mottram 2001, O'Sullivan 2000, Richardson et al 1999). The training should simulate movement in terms of anatomical movement pattern, velocity, type and force of contraction. Thus, with training, the neuromuscular system will tend to become better at generating tension for actions that resemble the muscle actions employed in training but not necessarily for actions that are dissimilar to those used in training (Herbert 1993, Sale & MacDougall 1981).

As the multifidus, transversus abdominis and gluteus medius muscles all have a stabilizing function, endurance training should be emphasized in treatment. Decreased activity of the obliques and transversus abdominis has been reported when subjects perform rapid ballistic sit-up exercises (Richardson et al 1991). Thus, exercises should be performed in a slow, controlled fashion. The number of repetitions performed by the patient at a training session will depend upon the onset of muscle fatigue. The long-term aim is to increase the number of repetitions before the onset of fatigue. Patients should be taught to recognize fatigue so that they do not train through fatigue and risk exacerbating their symptoms. Muscle training to control mobile segments dynamically may take many months to achieve. Comerford & Mottram (2001) have described a three-stage model for training local trunk muscles. The training process may be enhanced by the addition of firm tape across the lumbar mobile segment, minimizing the amount of movement and enhancing the proprioceptive input to the stabilizing muscles as shown in Figure 30.2. It has been found that taping is effective in preventing ankle sprains and improving proprioception in the ankle (Robbins et al 1995, Verhagen et al 2000) as well as preventing the lateral shift of the patella that occurs with exercise (Larsen et al 1995), so there could be a similar proprioceptive effect on an unstable segment in the spine.

Pelvic stability training should not be overlooked, as poor pelvic control can undermine the progress of the muscle training of the spine. If possible, gluteus medius training should be performed in weight bearing, simulating the stance phase of gait (Fig. 30.11). This can be done with the patient standing with the foot and hip of the exercising leg parallel to the wall and the knee slightly flexed. The other knee is flexed to 60 degrees and is resting on the wall for balance. The patient externally rotates the standing knee without moving the hips or the feet. This contraction is held for 15 seconds and should be repeated often to effect an automatic change in the motor programme. If the patient experiences pain or has poor 'core' stability then a more sta-

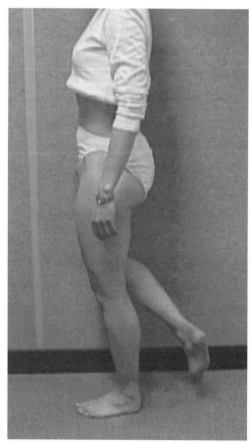

Figure 30.11 Training the gluteals in weight bearing.

ble position such as side lying or prone should be chosen initially. However, as muscle training is very specific to limb position, a return to functional positions should occur as soon as possible.

While therapists need to emphasize stability in treatment, they also need to examine where the patient is shock absorbing during weight-bearing activities to ensure that most of the load is being dissipated by the lower limb. A small amount of knee flexion (soft knees) during walking may need to be practised, with eccentric quadriceps control incorporated into the treatment. Shock absorption can also be improved by mobilizing a stiff subtalar joint, everting the calcaneum to increase eversion. The mobilization position should simulate the foot position at heel strike. This can be achieved by having the patient in side lying with the talocrural joint in a close-packed position and the tibia stabilized. The therapist then glides the calcaneum laterally. A small increase here can have significant effects up the kinetic chain. If there is a problem with push-off the first metatarsophalangeal joint may need to be mobilized and the mid-foot position stabilized by training the tibialis posterior muscle to minimize the possibility of compensatory lumbar spine movement.

During the mid-stance in gait the foot should be slightly supinated so the base of the first metatarsal is higher than the cuboid; this allows the peroneus longus to work more efficiently, increasing the stability of the first metatarsal complex for push-off (Root et al 1977). If the foot remains pronated at mid-stance activation of the peroneus longus causes the first metatarsal to drop. Consequently, not only is there an unstable push-off, but there is also a decrease in the dorsiflexion range of the great toe facilitating a medial heel whip, which in turn increases pelvic instability and internal rotation of the hip. This excess movement will put added stress on the lumbar spine. The therapist can therefore train the supinators of the foot to improve the efficiency of push-off. The position of training is in mid-stance. The patient is instructed to lift the arch while keeping the first metatarsal head on the floor and then pushing the first metatarsal and great toe into the floor (McConnell 2002b). If the patient is unable to keep the first metatarsophalangeal joint on the ground when the arch is lifted, then the foot deformity is too large to correct with training alone and orthotics may be necessary to control the excessive pronation (McConnell 2002b).

CONCLUSION

Management of chronic low back and leg pain requires a multifactorial approach. Low back pain can be difficult to treat as the clinician not only has to identify the underlying causative factors to restore homeostasis to the system, but also has to ensure that the treatment does not unnecessarily exacerbate the symptoms. The inflamed soft tissue needs to be unloaded so the symptoms are not increased when there is an attempt, in treatment, to gain range. Flexibility is required in the anterior hip structures and thoracic spine, while at the mobile lumbar segment(s) and pelvis, stability is required. The aim of treatment is to increase the active control of the passively unstable and associated areas so the patient is operating with an increased envelope of function, which will minimize symptom recurrences. The training must be simple, requiring minimal equipment so it is readily accessible to the individual and can be practised frequently. For long-term treatment success, the stabilizing muscles need an endurance programme so they can become fatigue resistant. There is also a need in the management of chronic pain problems in general for therapists to review patients every 6 or 12 months to ensure patients still know how to manage their symptoms as chronic problems are never cured, only managed.

KEYWORDS	
chronic pain	muscle control
unloading	hip flexibility
tape	

References

Barker P J, Briggs C A 1999 Attachments of the posterior layer of lumbar fascia. Spine 24(17): 1757–1764.

Basmajian J, De Luca C 1985 Muscles alive, 5th edn. Williams and Wilkins, Baltimore.

Bergmark A 1989 Stability of the lumbar spine: a study in mechanical engineering. Acta Orthopaedica Scandinavica Supplementum 230: 1–54

Bockrath K, Wooden C, Worrell T, Ingersoll C, Farr J 1993 Effects of patella taping on patella position and perceived pain. Medicine and Science in Sports and Exercise 25(9): 989–992

Bogduk N 1993 The anatomy and physiology of nociception. In: Crosbie J, McConnell J (eds) Key issues in musculoskeletal physiotherapy. Butterworth Heinemann, Oxford

Butler D 2000 The sensitive nervous system. Noigroup, Australia

Cerny K 1995 Vastus medialis oblique/vastus lateralis muscle activity ratios for selected exercises in persons with and without patellofemoral pain syndrome. Physical Therapy 75(8): 672–683

Cholewicki J, Panjabi M M, Khachatryan A 1997 Stabilizing function of trunk flexor-extensor muscles around a neutral spine posture. Spine 22(19): 2207–2212

Coderre T J, Katz J, Vaccarino A L, Melzack R 1993 Contribution of central neuroplasticity to pathological pain: review of clinical and experimental evidence. Pain 52(3): 259–285

Comerford M J, Mottram S L 2001 Functional stability re-training: principles and strategies for managing mechanical dysfunction. Manual Therapy 6(1): 3–14

Conway A, Malone T, Conway P 1992 Patellar alignment/tracking alteration: effect on force output and perceived pain. Isokinetics and Exercise Science 2(1): 9–17

Cowan S, Bennell K, Crossley K, Hodges P, McConnell J 2002a Physical therapy alters recruitment of the vash in patellofemoral pain syndrome. Medicine and Science in Sport and Exercise 34(12): 1879–1885.

Cowan S, Bennell K, Hodges P 2002b Therapeutic taping alters recruitment of the vash in patellofemoral pain syndrome. Clinical Journal of Sports Medicine 12(6): 339–347

Cushnaghan J, McCarthy R, Dieppe P 1994 The effect of taping the patella on pain in the osteoarthritic patient. BMJ (308): 753–755

Dananberg H 1997 Lower back pain as a gait related repetitive motion injury. In: Vleeming A, Mooney V, Dorman T, Snijders C, Stoeckart R (eds) Movement and stability and low back pain: the essential role of the pelvis. Churchill Livingstone, Edinburgh

Dufton B D 1989 Cognitive failure and chronic pain. International Journal of Psychiatry in Medicine 19(3): 291–297

Dye S 1996 The knee as a biologic transmission with an envelope of function: a theory. Clinical Orthopaedics and Related Research (325): 10–18

Dye S 1999 Invited commentary. Journal of Orthopaedic and Sports Physical Therapy 29: 386–387

Eccleston C 1994 Chronic pain and attention: a cognitive approach. British Journal of Clinical Psychology 33(4): 535–547

Farfan H F, Cossette J W, Robertson G H, Wells R V, Kraus H 1970 The effects of torsion on lumbar intervertebral joints: the role of torsion in the production of disc degeneration. Journal of Bone and Joint Surgery 52A: 468–497

Feuerstein M, Beattie P 1995 Biobehavioral factors affecting pain and disability in low back pain: mechanisms and assessment. Physical Therapy 75(4): 267–280

Garnett R, Stephens J A 1981 Changes in recruitment threshold of motor units produced by cutaneous stimulation in man. Journal of Physiology 311: 463–473

Gilleard W, McConnell J, Parsons D 1998 The effect of patellar taping on the onset of vastus medialis obliquus and vastus lateralis muscle activity in persons with patellofemoral pain. Physical Therapy 78(1): 25–32

Gresalmer R, McConnell J 1998 The patella: a team approach. Aspen Publishers. Gaithersburg, Maryland

Hall T, Quintner J 1995 Mechanically evoked EMG responses in peripheral neuropathic pain: a single case study. Proceedings of the Ninth Biennial Conference of the Manipulative Physiotherapists Association of Australia, Gold Coast, pp 38–41

Hamilton C, Richardson C 1998 Active control of the neutral lumbopelvic posture: a comparison of low back pain and non-low back pain subjects. In: Vleeming A, Mooney V, Tilsher H, Dorman T, Snijders C (eds) Proceedings of the Third Interdisciplinary World Congress on Low Back and Pelvic Pain, Vienna, Austria.

Handfield T, Kramer J 2000 Effect of McConnell taping on perceived pain and knee extensor torques during isokinetic exercise performed by patients with patellofemoral pain syndrome. Physiotherapy Canada Winter: 39–44

Herbert R 1993 Human strength adaptations: implications for therapy. In: Crosbie J, McConnell J (eds) Key issues in musculoskeletal physiotherapy. Butterworth Heinemann, Oxford

Hodges P W 2000 The role of the motor system in spinal pain: implications for rehabilitation of the athlete following lower back pain. Journal of Science and Medicine in Sport 3(3): 243–253

Hodges P, Richardson C 1996 Inefficient muscular stabilization of the lumbar spine associated with low back pain: a motor control evaluation of transversus abdominis. Spine 21(22): 2640–2650

Indahl A, Kaigle A M, Reikeras O, Holm S H 1999 Sacroiliac joint involvement in activation of the porcine spinal and gluteal musculature. Journal of Spinal Disorders 12(4): 325–330

Jenner J R, Stephens J A 1982 Cutaneous reflex responses and their central nervous system pathways studied in man. Journal of Physiology 333: 405–419

Karol L A, Halliday S E, Gourineni P 2000 Gait and function after intra-articular arthrodesis of the hip in adolescents. Journal of Bone and Joint Surgery 82(4): 561–569

Kelsey J L, Githens P B, White A A 1984 An epidemiological study of lifting and twisting on the job and the risk for acute prolapsed lumbar intervertebral disc. Journal of Orthopaedic Research 2: 61–66

Kewman D G, Vaishampayan N, Zald D, Han B 1991 Cognitive impairment in musculoskeletal pain patients. International Journal of Psychiatry in Medicine 21(3): 253–262

King J C, Lehmkuhl D L, French J, Dimitrijevic M 1988 Dynamic postural reflexes: comparison in normal subjects and patients with chronic low back pain. Current Concepts in Rehabilitation Medicine 4: 7–11

Larsen B, Andreasen E, Urfer A, Mickleson M R, Newhouse K E 1995 Patellar taping: a radiographic examination of the medial glide technique. American Journal of Sports Medicine 23: 465–471

McConnell J 2000 A novel approach to pain relief pre-therapeutic exercise. Journal of Science and Medicine in Sport 3(3): 325–334

McConnell J 2002a Recalcitrant chronic low back and leg pain: a new theory and different approach to management. Manual Therapy 7(4): 183–192

McConnell J 2002b The physical therapist's approach to patellofemoral disorders. In: Fithian D (ed) Injuries to the extensor mechanism of the knee. Clinics in Sports Medicine 21(3): 363–387

Marras W S, Davis K G, Heaney C A, Maronitis A B, Allread W G 2000 The influence of psychosocial stress, gender, and personality on mechanical loading of the lumbar spine. Spine 25: 3045–3054

Nadler S F, Malanga G A, Feinberg J H, Prybicien M, Stitik T P, DePrince M 2001 Relationship between hip muscle imbalance and occurrence of low back pain in collegiate athletes: a prospective study. American Journal of Physical Medicine and Rehabilitation 80(8): 572–577

Novacheck T F 1997 The biomechanics of running and sprinting. In : Guten G N (ed) Running injuries. WB Saunders, Philadelphia, pp 4–19

O'Sullivan P B 2000 Lumbar segmental 'instability': clinical presentation and specific stabilizing exercise management. Manual Therapy; 5(1): 2–12

Panjabi M 1992 The stabilizing system of the spine. II: Neutral zone and instability hypothesis. Journal of Spinal Disorders 5(4): 390–396; discussion, 397

Perry J 1992 Gait analysis. McGraw-Hill, New York

Powers C, Landel R, Sosnick T et al 1997 The effects of patellar taping on stride characteristics and joint motion in subjects with patellofemoral pain. Journal of Orthopaedic and Sports Physical Therapy 26(6): 286–291

Radebold A, Cholewicki J, Panjabi M M, Patel T C 2000. Muscle response pattern to sudden trunk loading in healthy individuals and in patients with chronic low back pain. Spine 25(8): 947–954

Richardson C, Jull G, Wohlfahrt D 1991 Ballistic exercise: can it undermine the protective stability role of the lumbar musculature? Proceedings of the Manipulative Physiotherapists Association of Australia, Seventh Biennial Conference, New South Wales, Australia

Richardson C A, Jull G A, Hodges P W, Hides J A 1999 Therapeutic exercise for spinal segmental stabilisation in low back pain: scientific basis and clinical approach. Churchill Livingstone, Edinburgh

Robbins S, Waked E, Rappel R 1995 Ankle taping improves proprioception before and after exercise in young men. British Journal of Sports Medicine 29(4): 242–247

Root M, Orien W, Weed J 1977 Clinical biomechanics. Clinical Biomechanics Corp, Los Angeles, vol 2

Sale D 1987 Influence of exercise and training on motor unit activation. Exercise and Sports Science Review 5: 95–151

Sale D, MacDougall D 1981 Specificity of strength training: a review for coach and athlete. Canadian Journal of Applied Sports Sciences 6(2): 87–92

Schache A G, Bennell K L, Blanch P D, Wrigley T V 1999 The coordinated movement of the lumbo-pelvic hip complex during running : a literature review. Gait and Posture 10(1): 30–47

Shacklock M 1999 Central pain mechanisms: a new horizon in manual therapy. Australian Journal of Physiotherapy 45(2): 83–92

Tobin S, Robinson G 2000 The effect of McConnell's vastus lateralis inhibition taping technique on vastus lateralis and vastus medialis activity. Physiotherapy 86: 174–183

Verhagen E A, van Mechelen W, de Vente W 2000 The effect of preventive measures on the incidence of ankle sprains. Clinical Journal of Sport Medicine 10(4): 291–296

Vleeming A, Pool-Goudzwaard A L, Stoeckart R, van Wingerden J P, Snijders C J 1995 The posterior layer of the thoracolumbar fascia: its function in load transfer from spine to legs. Spine. 20: 753–758

Wheeler A 1995 Diagnosis and management of low back pain and sciatica. American Family Physician 52(5): 133–141

Wilder D G, Aleksiev A R, Magnusson M L, Pope M H, Spratt K F, Goel V K 1996 Muscular response to sudden load: a tool to evaluate fatigue and rehabilitation. Spine 21(22): 2628–2639

Williams P, Warwick R 1980 Gray's Anatomy, 36th edn. Churchill Livingstone, London

Zusman M 1998 Structure-oriented beliefs and disability due to back pain. Australian Journal of Physiotherapy 44: 13–20

Chapter **31**

The rationale for a motor control programme for the treatment of spinal muscle dysfunction

C. A. Richardson, J. A. Hides

INTRODUCTION

Therapeutic exercise for low back pain has traditionally focused on programmes for enhancing cardiovascular fitness as well as trunk muscle strength and endurance. More recently, exercises which address changing motor control strategies in back pain patients have been recommended by many health professionals involved in treating low back pain. One motor control method, a segmental stabilization model, was described in a text by Richardson et al (1999) and was based on considerable research which focused on the function and dysfunction of the deep muscles of the lumbopelvic region. Further research has been completed in many different associated areas and the result is an extension of this motor control model. The updated segmental stabilization model focuses not only on the function of the deep muscles to support individual joints of the lumbar spine but also on their function as part of a larger antigravity system of muscles which ensures joint protection while transferring load safely and efficiently through the lumbopelvic region. An expanded therapeutic exercise model, proprioceptive antigravity training, incorporates this additional load transfer function of the antigravity muscles. In essence, such training consists of the initial activation of the deep muscle system to 'stiffen' the joints in preparation for weight bearing, followed by the integration of the deep, local muscle system into full weight bearing function through progressive antigravity exercise, with the emphasis on slowly increasing proprioceptive load cues.

While the updated segmental stabilization exercise model is closely associated with the management of musculoskeletal conditions of all limb joints, this chapter will focus on providing the rationale for the model in relationship to management of low back and pelvic pain.

THE RATIONALE FOR THE PROPRIOCEPTIVE ANTIGRAVITY TRAINING MODEL FOR THE PREVENTION AND TREATMENT OF LOW BACK PAIN

A historical perspective

A new type of stabilization exercise for the management of low back pain was developed by physiotherapists at the University of Queensland in the early 1990s. It placed a new focus on exercise to relieve pain through activation of the deep muscles transversus abdominis and multifidus in back pain patients (Richardson & Jull 1995). This approach was different to other stabilization exercise programmes designed for low back pain as it had a focus on segmental (or individual joint) stabilization. The emphasis was on changing the neural control of the muscles which were directly related to the stabilization and protection of the joints of the lumbopelvic region prior to focusing on functional patterns involving the whole body (Richardson et al 1999).

The segmental stabilization model of exercise has been modified and extended. This has been possible through involvement in space research, which has given new insights into the relationship between synergistic muscle function, gravity and joint loading. The model now includes muscle support for each joint in the kinetic chain for the integrated function of weight bearing through the spine, pelvis and lower limbs. However, the essence of the programme remains with the segmental stabilization (deep muscle support) concept, but it is its role in weight bearing, rather than movement, which is highlighted.

The segmental stabilization model of exercise

For the development of this part of the model, it is necessary to first differentiate the synergists into local and global muscle categories, where 'local' refers to smaller, deeper muscles which are closely related to the stability of a joint but do not produce joint torque and 'global' refers to the large superficial muscles which generate joint torque and are responsible for movement.

Muscle dysfunction of the local system of the lumbopelvic region

The research which led to an emphasis on the deep local muscles and the segmental stabilization concept involved new experimental models which allowed, for the first time, dysfunction of the local muscles to be assessed and quantified. For the deep lumbar muscles this was achieved by the identification of dysfunction in the lumbar multifidus by Hides et al in 1994 using real-time ultrasound, and dysfunction of the deep abdominal muscle transversus abdominis by Hodges & Richardson in 1996 using a trunk perturbation model with fine wire EMG to assess the recruitment patterns of the deep muscles.

Multifidus had long been recognized as an important muscle in the stabilization and protection of the lumbar spine (Goel et al 1993, Quint et al 1998, Wilke et al 1995). Hides et al (1996) demonstrated a segmental loss of cross-sectional area in the lumbar multifidus in acute first episode low back pain and went on to explain this loss of muscle cross-sectional area as indicative of segmental muscle reflex inhibition (for recent review see Hides &

Richardson 2002) which did not resolve on resumption of normal activity and relief of the low back pain.

These findings influenced the segmental stabilization model substantially as Hides and colleagues went on to demonstrate, through clinical research, that patients who learned to reactivate their multifidus through specific exercise techniques, with the aid of real-time ultrasound feedback, not only corrected the loss of cross-sectional area (CSA) but 3 years later had significantly fewer recurrences than the control group who had medical management alone (Hides et al 2001). Through this clinical research it was also discovered that the deep and superficial parts of multifidus were functionally different and it was the deep part which was the problem in patients with low back pain (Hides 1996). This was recently verified by Moseley et al (2002) who used fine wire EMG to determine the function of the two separate parts of the muscle. Recent evidence has demonstrated that problems in multifidus also occur in chronic low back pain. The CSA of the multifidus is selectively decreased in chronic LBP patients when compared with controls (Danneels et al 2000). Cross-sectional areas of the multifidus, lumbar erector spinae and psoas were obtained. Only the multifidus at the lowest lumbar level was statistically smaller in LBP patients than in controls.

In comparison to multifidus, there were few biomechanical research studies which addressed the function of transversus abdominis. Initial studies of Cresswell et al (1992) demonstrated that the transversus abdominis remained active during repetitive trunk flexion and extension, while the global trunk muscles switched on and off depending on the direction of movement. A further study investigated the response of the transversus abdominis to perturbations, and showed that the response of the transversus abdominis was of short latency (Cresswell et al 1994). Hodges & Richardson (1996) also studied the response of the transversus abdominis to perturbation, this time induced by movement of a limb in response to a stimulus. The results indicated that the transversus abdominis was activated in a feedforward manner (prior to the deltoid in upper limb movements), and this response was unrelated to the direction of movement (Hodges & Richardson 1997). This reaction was in contrast to that of the superficial muscles, which reacted to the direction of limb movement. This study suggested that the transversus abdominis has a separate control mechanism and that its function was likely joint stabilization. Further studies were conducted into the possible mechanism of this muscle in relation to the stabilization of the spine. Hodges et al (1997) also demonstrated that the response of the transversus abdominis was associated with a change in intra-abdominal pressure and that the diaphragm also reacted in a feedforward manner. Recent studies have also shown co-activation of the transversus abdominis and the pelvic floor muscles, in particular the pubococcygeus (Sapsford et al 2001).

Biomechanical models which are aligned to the segmental stabilization model

These concepts, which formed the initial versions of the segmental stabilization model, were supported by two pioneering studies of the time in the area of biomechanics. The main researcher who shaped the direction of the exercise model was Manohar Panjabi.

In 1992, Panjabi introduced an innovative biomechanical model dealing with the function of the spinal stabilization system. The model incorporated a passive subsystem, an active subsystem and a control subsystem (Fig. 31.1). The passive subsystem included the osseous and articular structures and the spinal ligaments. The active subsystem referred to the spinal muscles, which are under the control of the neural control subsystem to provide spinal stability. An important feature of the model that has influenced the development of the motor control programme was the hypothesis that one system was capable of compensating for another in the case of pathology, pain or injury. For example, it was hypothesized that injury to the passive system could be compensated for by the muscle system. This gave a rationale for why specifically directed exercise aimed at enhancing joint stability could be effective in relieving joint pain.

In addition, Bergmark, in 1989, had suggested, based on his biomechanical model, that the skeletal muscle system could be broadly divided into two separate systems, the local and global muscle systems. Using Bergmark's classification, the local muscle system included deep muscles and the deep portions of some muscles which have their origin or insertion on the lumbar vertebrae. These local muscles, it was argued, controlled the stiffness and intervertebral relationship of the spinal segments. In contrast, the global muscle system, encompassing the large, more superficial muscles of the trunk, was responsible for moving the spine and transferring load directly between the thoracic cage and pelvis.

These biomechanical models encouraged researchers to look more closely at the function of the local muscle system in relation to the development and treatment of musculoskeletal injuries such as mechanical low back pain. The new direction for our research has been based on some new biomechanical models which explain the close link between the segmental stabilization model of exercise and safe and efficient weight-bearing function.

The segmental stabilization model of exercise for weight bearing

The local muscle system has been implicated in providing the stiffness of the joints of the lumbopelvic region for both movement and weight-bearing function. Evidence based treatment of the local muscle system (Hides et al 1996, 2001, O'Sullivan et al 1997) has demonstrated that the exercise which is effective in the management of low back pain involves teaching patients to form a dynamic muscle 'corset' involving contraction of transversus abdominis and multifidus. We believe that this corset system offers support to the region due to the close relationship between the muscles, transversus abdominis and multifidus, with the fascial system (and joint structures) of the lumbar spine and pelvis. It is our contention that it is this deep, dynamic muscular corset which provides the basic support of the skeleton for weight bearing.

The deep muscular corset

One of the most important aspects of the local muscle function (and dysfunction) is the relationship between transversus abdominis, multifidus and the deep fascial system which surrounds the lumbopelvic region. Transversus abdominis, with its insertion to the thoracolumbar fascia posteriorly and the abdominal fascia anteriorly, appears to exert its effect on spinal stability through the fascial system. Our research is demonstrating that dysfunction in this musculofascial system is closely related to the presence of low back pain.

The importance of the concept of the deep muscle corset for the support of the lumbopelvic region has come through the clinical use of real-time ultrasound (Hides et al 1998) and our current research, involving the use of magnetic resonance imaging (MRI). These imaging techniques have allowed the deep musculofascial system to be viewed in its normal and dysfunctional state.

In selected pain-free individuals, a muscular corset is formed automatically in response to a simple instruction to pull in the lower abdomen (without spinal movement occurring). Figure 31.2 gives a diagrammatic interpretation, taken from MRI data, of the deep musculofascial corset which is formed with this instruction. This deep muscle contraction, involving symmetrical muscle shortening of each side of transversus abdominis, does not occur in response to drawing in the abdominal wall in patients with low back pain.

Similarly, the multifidus is also capable of contributing to the changing tension in the thoracolumbar fascia. The influence of the multifidus and the lumbar erector spinae on the thoracolumbar fascia was investigated by Gracovetsky et al (1977) using a mathematical model. It was proposed in the

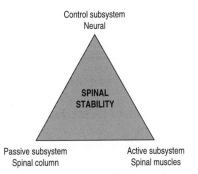

Figure 31.1 The three subsystems which contribute to active spinal stabilization. Reproduced from Richardson et al 1999.

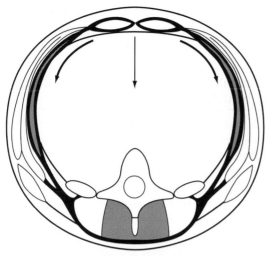

Figure 31.2 A diagrammatic representation of the 'deep muscle corset'. Reproduced from Richardson et al 1999.

hydraulic amplifier mechanism that contraction of the muscles exerts a pushing force on the fascia, thus tensioning it and increasing the stiffness of the spine. Exercises to improve segmental stabilization involve increasing local muscle activation to tension the fascia, often with the assistance of real-time ultrasound to assess and train deep muscle control (Richardson et al 1999). In order to develop and explain the role of the deep, dynamic muscle corset in relation to weight bearing, it is important to review the biomechanical models that have been devised in relation to weight bearing through the spine as well as weight bearing through the pelvis.

The function of transversus abdominis and multifidus: providing joint stiffness for weight bearing through the lumbar spine

The studies of Keifer et al (1997, 1998) addressed the issue of integration between local and global muscles and emphasized the importance of the relationship between spinal curves, spinal loading and muscle recruitment. The studies used a finite element model (passive osseoligamentous spine) with optimization of the muscles (active and passive components of muscle force). In the first study, Keifer et al (1997) loaded the spine without the muscles using compressive axial forces. They demonstrated that the thoracolumbar spine translates into hypermobility under axial loads which are less than physiological loads (indicated by displacement of the T1 vertebra). Addition of local and global muscles into the model increased the ability of the spine to withstand compressive forces without buckling. Pelvic rotation (anterior tilt) stiffened the spine, and only 2 degrees of anterior rotation allowed the spine to carry axial compression of up to 400 newtons, with only 7 mm of anterior displacement of T1. There was less anterior displacement of T1 with local and global muscles incorporated into the model than with global muscles alone,

highlighting the importance of integration of the two muscle systems.

In the second study, Keifer et al (1998) investigated the synergy of the spine in neutral positions. Using the same model, they displaced T1 40 mm anteriorly and 20 mm posteriorly. Results demonstrated that for very small displacements, the global muscles and passive structures are sufficient to stabilize the spine. However, the system is far more efficient with inclusion of the local muscles. Activation of the local muscles decreased muscle forces in the global system, provided stiffness, increased stability and increased compression. Considering the contribution of the local muscles, 80% was provided by multifidus, with some contribution by iliocostalis. Another finding was that the position of the thoracolumbar junction was important. If T12 was held back, then the upper lumbar spine was forced into flexion and the synergy was disturbed. This had a resultant marked effect on the distribution of intersegmental rotations, and lessened the capacity of the passive system to carry sagittal moments.

This model of spinal loading has resulted in the increased emphasis on the importance of the neutral spine position for weight bearing, as well as its importance as an optimal position for the integration of the local and global muscle function.

The function of transversus abdominis and the deep pelvic muscles: providing joint stiffness for weight bearing through the pelvis

The biomechanical aspects of weight bearing in the lumbopelvic region have been extensively researched by Snijders and colleagues (1995). They developed models to explain how the pelvis and the sacroiliac joints can resist shear from the force of gravity as well as resisting the extremely high forces developed by the skeletal muscles which have large attachments to the pelvis. The model predicts that the action of the transverse fibres of pelvic muscles such as transversus abdominis, ischiococcygeus and piriformis can stiffen the sacroiliac joints (i.e. force closure) and stabilizes the pelvis for weight bearing (this is similar to the effects of a belt around the pelvis). Thus a key function of these transverse muscles for the pelvis is likely to be the control of weight bearing through the lumbopelvic region (Fig. 31.3).

Our recent study demonstrated that the biomechanical effect of an independent contraction of transversus abdominis and lumbar multifidus (elicited through instructing the subjects to pull in the abdomen without moving the spine) on the laxity of the sacroiliac joints (Richardson et al 2002). Sacroiliac joint laxity was measured using Doppler imaging of vibrations. A specific contraction of the transversus abdominis and multifidus (confirmed using real-time ultrasound and electromyography) increased stiffness (or decreased laxity) of the sacroiliac joints to a greater degree than a higher level 'bracing' contraction involving all the muscles of the abdominal wall. These results confirm

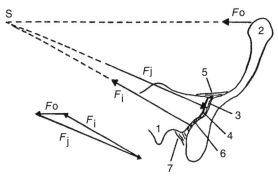

Figure 31.3 The transverse muscle force which compresses the sacroiliac joint surfaces to help prevent shearing due to vertical (weight-bearing) force (F). Reproduced from Snijders et al 1995.

the biomechanical model of the mechanics of the sacroiliac joint by Snijders et al (1995), which proposed that the transversely oriented muscles such as transversus abdominis are well suited for a role of increasing the stiffness of the sacroiliac joints for weight bearing but that the superficial abdominals are not as efficient. This study has provided some initial evidence of how the transversus abdominis can directly help to stabilize and control the pelvis for weight bearing and also explains how specific activation of the deep local muscles could exert an effect on pain and pathology of the sacroiliac joints.

Poor patterns of weight bearing

The study by Richardson et al (2002) also demonstrated that a 'bracing co-contraction' pattern involving global muscle contraction of all of the abdominals and erector spinae was less efficient in producing stiffness of the sacroiliac joints than the deep corset action. Interestingly there is some evidence that such co-contraction patterns are associated with low back pain. An important study which has investigated recruitment of global muscles in LBP patients was conducted by Radebold et al (2000). In this study, a quick release method in four directions of isometric trunk exertions was used to study muscle response patterns in LBP patients and matched controls. Subjects were placed in a semi-seated position in an apparatus that fixated the pelvis. They performed isometric exertions of the trunk, the resisted force was suddenly released, and the muscles measured using electromyography (EMG). Reaction time was compared between the two groups. Results showed that controls quickly shut off the agonistic muscles and switched on the antagonists. In contrast, LBP patients exhibited a pattern of co-contraction, with agonists remaining active while the antagonists switched on. This may have been a compensation mechanism to support the lumbar spine.

Another study has also indicated that global muscles are used more in back pain patients. Ng et al (2002) demonstrated higher activation levels and decreased fatigability of the right external oblique muscles in chronic LBP patients, suggesting that the global muscles may be used to compen-

sate for poor segmental stability. As suggested by Keifer et al (1997, 1998) and Richardson et al (2002), increasing global muscle activity may not be the most efficient strategy for stabilization of the lumbopelvic region, especially in weight bearing.

Thus the segmental stabilization model for weight bearing focuses on exercises for the deep muscle system and also addresses the increased activity of the global system. Specific exercise techniques involve retraining the contractions of the local muscle system combined with methods to decrease the recruitment of the global muscles. Details of these techniques have been described in detail in the text by Richardson et al (1999).

The antigravity muscle system for high load function

To explain the further development of this weight bearing, antigravity model of exercise, it is necessary to first differentiate the synergists into local and global muscle subgroups of mono-articular and multi-articular categories. 'Mono-articular' refers to muscles which span a single joint (or one area of the spine) and are capable of generating high joint torque as well as controlling a single joint position. The second category, the 'multi-joint/multi-function' muscles, is the antithesis of this group. These muscles cross over more than one joint (or one area of the spine), are usually more superficial, perform multiple functions at multiple joints and are more aligned to efficient movement rather than joint protection and stability. It will be argued that the local and mono-articular muscles work together to form an efficient 'antigravity' system with the multijoint/multifunction muscles aligned to a movement role with minimal contribution to the opposition of the force of gravity in weight-bearing positions. This gravity related hypothesis has been developed through research using models of de-loading or microgravity environments where gravity has been minimized or eliminated.

Change in the recruitment of the antigravity muscle system with de-loading of the skeleton

The gravity related hypothesis has been developed from studying the recruitment patterns and muscle physiology changes occurring with de-loading of the skeleton.

A de-loading model was designed (in a non-weight-bearing prone position) to study the muscle synergists of the knee during fast (phasic) lower leg movement where feedback from gravitational load cues was minimized (Richardson & Bullock 1986). A specifically positioned spring (Fig. 31.4) calibrated to the weight of the individual's lower leg, was used to de-load the muscle system.

Muscle recruitment patterns were investigated through studying changes in levels of muscle activation (total EMG for three movement cycles) in slow, medium and fast speeds of lower leg movement. High-speed repetitive movement is known to be pre-programmed and not to rely on sensory

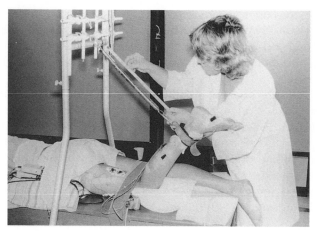

Figure 31.4 The exercise model used a spring attachment to minimize the effect of gravity on the lower leg. Reproduced from Richardson et al 1999.

feedback. Thus this de-loading model not only reduced gravitational load via a spring, it also resulted in reduced proprioceptive feedback due to the nature of the task.

The results proved to be very significant. The multijoint muscles, rectus femoris and hamstrings contracted in a phasic pattern with the movement and increased their activation levels significantly with increases in speed. The local muscle, vastus medialis oblique, as well as the mono-articular muscle, vastus lateralis, did not increase their activation levels over the increasing speeds. This finding highlighted their antigravity role, rather than a movement role as demonstrated in the multijoint muscles. In addition, in 90% of cases the vastus medialis oblique, and in 45% of cases the vastus lateralis demonstrated a tonic, continuous response to the phasic lower leg movement. This would seem to indicate that these muscles do not respond to movement cues but rather require proprioceptive feedback, including gravitational load cues for their recruitment into functional movement.

The knee musculature has been extensively investigated in space (microgravity) research in both animal and human studies. Similar recruitment patterns are demonstrated when gravitational load cues are absent. While marked atrophy of the non-weight-bearing vastus medialis (local) and weight-bearing vastus lateralis (mono-articular) occurs, there is no change in the size of the multijoint hamstrings and rectus femoris (see Richardson 2002 for review). This would further support the hypothesis that multijoint muscles are closely linked to movement but not gravitational load, while the local and mono-articular have antigravity roles and respond to gravitational and load cues. These issues, as they relate to the lumbopelvic region, have become the focus of our research direction in relation to the expanded exercise concept of proprioceptive antigravity training.

We believe that research into the problems which develop from de-loading the skeleton has important implications for the way exercise is used to promote the functional integration of the local, mono-articular and multijoint muscle systems. Long-term de-loading of the skeleton, which occurs when gravitational load is removed, results in predicted, consistent patterns of neuroplasticity of the nervous system. These patterns consist of an increase in recruitment of muscles designed for movement and a reduced recruitment in the muscles involved in the control of gravitational load. Thus integration of the local muscle system must occur in weight bearing where the antigravity muscles work together to protect joints from injury. Weight bearing (closed chain) exercise is the key to rehabilitation as the multijoint (movement) muscles are not required in exercise completed in weight-bearing postures with lower limb joints flexed. The design of the weight-bearing exercise has been streamlined by the previously described biomechanical models which have linked gravitational load, the pelvis and spinal posture with muscle function.

Widening perspectives for segmental stabilization to a more functional proprioceptive antigravity training model

The segmental stabilization model has now been further refined and evolved through new information in the areas of motor control and biomechanics related to weight bearing. This overall gravity focus has led to the proprioceptive antigravity training model. Most importantly, in the area of motor control, muscle recruitment patterns have been investigated in relation to the influence of gravity. It is gravitational physiology research, including research into the motor control problems which develop from de-loading the skeleton, which is forming the foundation for the development of exercise strategies used to promote the functional integration of the local and global muscle systems. The muscle recruitment patterns are closely linked to two biomechanical weight-bearing models, addressing both the pelvis and the spine, which explain how the body deals best with gravitational forces in a weight-bearing exercise method which minimizes the more active multijoint (movement) muscle system. Thus research in both biomechanics and motor control are influencing the evolution of the training programme.

As explained in previous sections, there are several important changes in direction for rehabilitation which have been based on the described rationale for the weight-bearing, antigravity model of exercise. Activating the 'corset action' of the deep local muscle system is considered essential to increase stiffness of both the lumbar spine and pelvis in preparation for weight bearing. In this regard, it is the neutral spine, most particularly the lumbar lordosis, which is important for training weight-bearing function. For the integration of the antigravity system (i.e. local and one-joint muscles) into function, the most important aspect of training is to increase the sensory load cues in weight bearing or simulated weight bearing, while ensuring that the local and one-joint muscles are responding to gravitational (sensory) load cues and there is minimal contraction of the multijoint/multifunction muscles during the training.

Our new research stream is currently being developed through microgravity research, which will allow us to further understand the function and dysfunction of the lumbopelvic muscle synergists in relation to de-loading (as well as to injury and pain). More importantly, our continued research is investigating the most efficient exercise countermeasures for the motor control problems in the antigravity musculature.

KEYWORDS

low back pain	weight-bearing exercise
motor control dysfunction	antigravity muscle function
rehabilitation	unloading skeleton

References

Bergmark A 1989 Stability of the lumbar spine: a study in mechanical engineering. Acta Orthopaedica Scandinavica 230(Suppl): 20–24

Cresswell A G, Grundstrom A, Thorstensson A 1992 Observations on intra-abdominal pressures and patterns of abdominal intra-muscular activity in man. Acta Physiologica Scandinavica 144: 409–418

Cresswell A G, Oddson L, Thorstensson A 1994 The influence of sudden perturbations on trunk muscle activity and intra-abdominal pressure while standing. Experimental Brain Research 98: 336–341

Daneels L A, Vanderstraeten G G, Cambier D C, Witvrouw E E, Cuyper H J 2000 CT imaging of trunk muscles in chronic low back pain patients and healthy control subjects. European Spine Journal 9: 266–272

Goel V K, Kong W, Han J S, Weinstein D O, Gilbertson L G 1993 A combined finite element and optimization of lumbar spine mechanics with and without muscles. Spine 18: 1531–1541

Gracovetsky S, Farfan H F, Lamy C 1977 A mathematical model of the lumbar spine using an optimal system to control muscles and ligaments. Orthopedic Clinics of North America 8: 135–153

Hides J A 1996 Multifidus muscle recovery in acute low back pain patients. PhD Thesis, University of Queensland, Australia

Hides J A, Richardson C A 2002 Exercise and pain. In: Strong J, Unruh A M, Wright A, Baxter G D (eds) Pain: a textbook for therapists. Churchill Livingstone, Edinburgh

Hides J A, Stokes M J, Saide M, Jull G A, Cooper D H 1994 Evidence of lumbar multifidus muscle wasting ipsilateral to symptoms in patients with acute/subacute low back pain. Spine 19(2): 165–172

Hides J A, Richardson C A, Jull G A 1996 Multifidus muscle recovery is not automatic following resolution of acute first episode low back pain. Spine 21(23): 2763–2769

Hides J A, Richardson C A, Jull G A 1998 Use of real-time ultrasound imaging for feedback in rehabilitation. Manual Therapy 3(3): 125–131

Hides J A, Jull G A, Richardson C A 2001 Long-term effects of specific stabilizing exercises for first episode low back pain. Spine 26(11): E243–E248

Hodges P W, Richardson C A 1996 Inefficient muscular stabilisation of the lumbar spine associated with low back pain: a motor control evaluation of transversus abdominis. Spine 21(22): 2640–2650

Hodges P W, Richardson C A 1997 Feedforward contraction of the transversus abdominis is not influenced by the direction of arm movement. Experimental Brain Research 114: 362–370

Hodges P W, Butler J E, McKenzie D, Gandevia S C 1997 Contraction of the human diaphragm during postural adjustments. Journal of Physiology 505: 239–548

Keifer A, Shirazi-Adl A, Parnianpour M 1997 Stability of the human spine in neutral postures. European Spine Journal 6: 45–53

Keifer A, Shirazi-Adl A, Parnianpour M 1998 Synergy of the human spine in neutral postures. European Spine Journal 7: 471–479

Moseley G L, Hodges P W, Gandevia S C 2002 Deep and superficial fibres of multifidus are differentially active during voluntary arm movements. Spine 27: E29

Ng J K-F, Richardson C A, Parnianpour M, Kippers V 2002 Fatigue related changes in torque output and electromyographic parameters in trunk muscles during isometric axial rotation exertion: an investigation in patients with back pain and in healthy subjects. Spine 27(6): 637–646

O'Sullivan P B, Twomey L T, Allison G T 1997 Evaluation of specific stabilizing exercise in the treatment of chronic low back pain with radiologic diagnosis of spondylolysis or spondylolisthesis. Spine 22: 2959–2967

Panjabi M 1992 The stabilising system of the spine. I: Function, dysfunction, adaptation and enhancement. Journal of Spinal Disorders 5: 383–389

Quint U, Wilke H J, Shirazi-Adl A, Parnianpour M, Loer F, Claes L E 1998 Importance of the intersegmental trunk muscles for the stability of the lumbar spine: a biomechanical study in vitro. Spine 23: 1937–1945

Radebold A, Cholewicki J, Panjabi M, Patel T 2000 Muscle response pattern to sudden trunk loading in healthy individuals and in patients with chronic low back pain. Spine 25: 947–954

Richardson C A 2002 The health of the human skeletal system for weight bearing against gravity: the role of deloading the musculo-skeletal system in the development of musculo-skeletal injury. Journal of Gravitational Physiology 9(1): P7–10

Richardson C, Bullock M I 1986 Changes in muscle activity during fast, alternating flexion-extension movements of the knee. Scandinavian Journal of Rehabilitation Medicine 18: 51–58

Richardson C, Jull G 1995 Muscle control–pain control. What exercises would you prescribe? Manual Therapy 1: 2–10

Richardson C, Jull G, Hodges P, Hides J 1999 Therapeutic exercise for spinal segmental stabilization in low back pain: scientific basis and clinical approach. Churchill Livingstone, Edinburgh

Richardson C A, Snijders C J, Hides J A, Damen L, Pas M S, Storm J 2002 The relationship between the transversely oriented abdominal muscles, sacroiliac joint mechanics and low back pain. Spine 27(4): 399–405

Sapsford R R, Hodges P W, Richardson C A, Cooper D H, Markwell S J, Jull G A 2001 Co-activation of the abdominal and pelvic floor muscles during voluntary exercise. Neurophysiology and Urodynamics 20: 31–42

Snijders C J, Vleeming A, Stoekart R, Mens J M A, Kleinrensink G J 1995 Biomechanical modeling of sacro-iliac joint stability in different postures. Spine. State of the Art Reviews. Hanley and Belfus, Philadelphia

Wilke H J, Wolf S, Claes L E, Arand M, Wiesend A 1995 Stability increase of the lumbar spine with different muscles groups: a biomechanical in vitro study. Spine 20: 192–198

Chapter 32

A therapeutic exercise approach for cervical disorders

G. A. Jull, D. Falla, J. Treleaven, M. Sterling, S. O'Leary

INTRODUCTION

The flexible cervical column has multiple simultaneous functions. It allows three-dimensional head movements and distributes load from the weight of the head and the upper limbs while maintaining mechanical stability of the head–neck system at any given orientation. The muscle system of the neck is intimately related to reflex systems associated with stabilization of the head and the eyes, vestibular function and proprioceptive systems that serve not only local needs in the neck but also needs for general postural orientation and stability (Dutia 1991, Keshner 1990, Winters & Peles 1990). Therefore the cervical spine presents a multisegmental, multimuscle complex which is required to switch its control operations between intrinsic kinetic and mechanical demands, proprioception and reflex demands associated with postural stability, head stabilization and eye movement control and still achieve an appropriate coordinated response.

The complexity of the cervical sensory–motor system challenges clinicians and researchers to understand and identify the changes that may occur in the system with pain, injury and pathology and to develop suitable rehabilitation programmes. Progress is being made. Recent research is beginning to increase our understanding of how the muscle system may be disturbed in its provision of stability and support and how disturbances in the sensory–motor system may contribute to the myriad of symptoms that can present in patients with cervical disorders, ranging from pain, dizziness/unsteadiness to difficulties swallowing (Heikkilä & Astrom 1996, Sjaastad et al 1998, Treleaven et al 2003). While more will be learned in coming years, current knowledge is directing therapeutic exercise into a multifaceted programme of specific exercises.

This chapter will focus on the clinical application of the exercise programme. In the clinical environment, various elements of exercise are used in an integrated manner to address the impairments revealed in the clinical evaluation of the individual patient. For convenience of presentation this chapter is divided into two sections. The first section will present the exercise components for restoration of muscle function for joint support and control. The second section of the chapter will introduce exercise approaches to address problems in the sensory–motor system that may underlie symptoms such as dizziness and unsteadiness, including kinaesthetic sense, ocular motor function and balance. As Heikkilä & Astrom (1996) observed, treatment of neck disorders has often focused on neck strength and mobility. The wealth of neck receptors suggests that therapeutic exercises that provide proprioceptive information and include dynamic function of the head and neck region should have a major emphasis in rehabilitation programmes.

IMPAIRMENT IN MUSCLE CONTROL AND SUPPORT OF THE CERVICAL SPINE

It is estimated that the osseoligamentous system contributes 20% to the mechanical stability of the cervical spine while 80% is provided by the surrounding neck musculature (Panjabi et al 1998). The role of the ligaments in stabilization occurs mainly at end of range postures (Harms-Ringdahl et al 1986) while muscles supply dynamic support in activities around the neutral and mid-range postures. Considering that most functional daily tasks are performed in and around mid-range postures, the muscles controlling the cervical spine are subject to constant external and internal forces. In the presence of injury or pathology that may jeopardize the integrity of the ligamentous system, the role of the muscular system becomes even greater. This highlights the importance of appropriate rehabilitation of the muscle system when the articular system is compromised.

Considerable biomechanical, physiological and clinical research in both the cervical and lumbar regions has been undertaken which supports Bergmark's (1989) model for a functional division between the deep and more superficial muscles in their relative contributions to spinal support and control. Simplified, the more superficial multisegmental muscles have the responsibility for maintaining equilibrium of external forces so that the load transmitted to the spinal segments can be controlled efficiently by the deep intersegmental muscle system. Mayoux-Benhamou et al (1997) describe the deep longus colli and dorsal neck muscles as a muscle sleeve which surrounds the cervical column to support the cervical spinal segments in functional movements. In a computer model, Winters & Peles (1990) showed regions of local segmental instability if only the large more superficial muscles of the neck were simulated to produce movement, particularly in near upright or neutral postures. Deep muscle activity was required in synergy with superficial muscle activity to stiffen or stabilize the cervical segments, especially in functional mid-ranges.

There is a loss of strength and endurance in the neck muscles in patients with chronic neck pain (Silverman et al 1991, Vernon et al 1992, Watson & Trott, 1993). However, addressing strength alone in research and exercise programmes may oversimplify the problems in the neuromuscular system associated with neck pain. Consideration of the functional division of the muscle system has directed research to investigate muscle activation patterns in the deep and superficial neck muscles and their supporting role in neck pain patients (Jull 2000, Jull et al 1999). In addition, research is demonstrating that there are disturbances in what may be termed coordination within the cervical and cervicoscapular muscle synergies in simple functional tasks in neck pain patients (Bansevicius & Sjaastad 1996, Falla et al 2004a, Nederhand et al 2000, 2003). Aberrant patterns of muscle activation may overload cervical structures and disturb muscle function for joint stabilization.

Impairment in the cervical muscles

Our particular interest has been in trying to identify and define any problems in the neck flexor synergy. This was in recognition of the deep neck flexor muscles' vital role in supporting the cervical segments and the cervical curve (Conley et al 1995, Mayoux-Benhamou et al 1997, 1994) as well as clinical theory and evidence of impairment in these muscles in neck pain patients (Janda 1994, Watson & Trott 1993). We developed the craniocervical flexion muscle test (C-CFT) (Jull 2000, Jull et al 1999), a low load task that is the anatomical action of the deep longus capitis and colli muscles. The test is performed in crook lying, and requires the person to perform a head nod action (craniocervical flexion) in incremental stages of increasing range and hold each position for 5–10 seconds. Performance is guided by feedback from a pressure sensor which is positioned suboccipitally to monitor the flattening of the cervical lordosis which occurs with the contraction of longus colli (Mayoux-Benhamou et al 1994, 1997). The patient performs the head nod action and attempts to target five incremental pressure targets (increment: 2 mmHg) from a baseline level of 20 mmHg. As could be predicted anatomically, a strong linear relationship has been demonstrated between activity in the longus capitis and longus colli muscles and the progressive stages of the test (Falla et al 2003b). Several controlled studies have been performed on populations of patients with idiopathic neck pain or neck pain following a whiplash injury. These studies have shown that people with neck pain perform poorly in the test compared to control subjects. In a series of studies on the C-CFT, it has been shown that: activity of the deep neck flexors (EMG signal amplitude) is less in neck pain patients (Falla et al 2004b); neck pain patients demonstrate higher levels of superficial neck flexor (sternocleidomastoid and the anterior scalene muscles) activity (Falla et al 2004b, Jull et al 2004, Sterling et al 2003); neck pain patients have a tendency to retract the head in substitution (Falla et al 2004b) for the progressive sagittal rotation of the head demonstrated by asymptomatic subjects (Falla et al 2003a); and neck pain patients are less able to hold the target levels of craniocervical flexion (Jull 2000, Jull et al 2002).

Thus our research has demonstrated that neck pain patients have a disturbance in the neck flexor synergy, where impairment in the deep muscles, important for segmental control and support, appears to be compensated for by increased activity in the superficial muscles (an altered movement pattern of craniocervical flexion) and loss of ability to hold a low level contraction. Of relevance to rehabilitation, the impairment in the neck flexor synergy is independent of the insidious or traumatic origin of neck pain (Jull et al 2004), occurs early in the history of onset of neck pain (Sterling et al 2004) and does not resolve automatically with lessening or resolution of symptoms (Jull et al 2002, Sterling et al 2003).

The emphasis on the neck flexor synergy in our clinical research does not imply a lack of importance or interest in the neck extensor synergy or the co-activation of the flexors and extensors for support of the cervical joints. Conley et al (1995) quantified shifts in signal relaxation times of T2-weighted magnetic resonance images in an in vivo analysis of neck muscle function after direction-specific exercises performed in lying. They demonstrated that in contrast to the superficial extensor muscles (semispinalis capitis and splenius capitis), the multifidus and semispinalis cervicis had a high T2 index before exercise, suggesting an important postural function for these muscles. Furthermore, when the relative activity of all muscles was calculated across all movements, the results revealed what can be described as a flexor and extensor co-contraction, a muscle pattern to enhance joint stiffness. This occurred mainly in the longus capitis and colli muscles ventrally and the multifidus, semispinalis cervicis and splenius capitis muscles dorsally. Low levels of muscle activity were registered in movements in which the muscles were antagonists, that is, in extension and flexion respectively. This supports Mayoux-Benhamou et al's (1997) concept that the longus colli and dorsal neck muscles form a muscle sleeve to support the cervical spinal segments in functional movements and signifies the importance of the re-education of this deep muscle co-contraction in rehabilitation. In relation to the integrity of this muscle sleeve, in

addition to the impairment identified in the deep neck flexors, pathological change has been demonstrated in the deep suboccipital muscles of subjects with chronic upper cervical dysfunction, which would compromise their function. Atrophy and fatty infiltration in the deep suboccipital muscles have been identified in patients with chronic neck pain using magnetic resonance imaging (Andrey et al 1998, Hallgren et al 1994, McPartland et al 1997). Our study using ultrasound imaging also demonstrated reduced cross-sectional areas of the rectus capitis posterior major and the semispinalis cervicis but not the more superficial longissimus capitis in patients with cervicogenic headache (Amiri et al, unpublished data). Research is currently underway to better understand the coordination between the deeper and more superficial neck extensor muscles in motor control experiments using normal and neck pain subjects.

Impairment in the axio-scapular-girdle muscles

Impairment in the axio-scapular-girdle muscles has been linked clinically to cervical pain syndromes (Behrsin & Maguire 1986, Janda 1994, Mottram 1997). Coordinated scapular muscle activity (particularly the contribution of such muscles as the serratus anterior and the tripartite trapezius) is important for the maintenance of scapular orientation and control in posture and for the correct transference of loads from upper limb function to the axial skeleton (Johnson et al 1994, Ludewig et al 1996, Lukasiewicz et al 1999, McQuade et al 1998). Poor function within the axio-scapular-girdle muscle synergy can change load distribution to the axial skeleton. Increased activity in muscles such as the levator scapulae with its suspension from the upper four cervical segments may adversely increase vertical compressive loads on cervical joints (Behrsin & Maguire 1986).

There have been several studies, which have shown altered activity levels in the axio-scapular-girdle muscles in patients with neck pain during low load functional activities. Bansevicius et al (1996) investigated the influence of mental load on muscle activity in patients with neck pain and headache and demonstrated that the stress of the activity increased the level of non-voluntary muscle activity in the upper trapezius muscle. Nederhand et al (2000, 2002, 2003) demonstrated greater co-activation of the upper trapezius muscles in chronic neck pain patients during a unilateral low load repetitive upper limb task. Using a similar task model, Falla et al (2004a) also demonstrated greater activation of the sternocleidomastoid and anterior scalene muscles when compared to asymptomatic control subjects, which might be a functional correlate of performance in the C-CFT. More recently, Nederhand et al (2003) found decreased activity in the upper trapezius in the low load task in patients with an acute whiplash injury. Overall there appears to be an altered pattern of muscle activation during performance of functional tasks, which may represent an altered strategy to minimize activation of painful muscles or compensate for inhibited muscles. Increased activity in the form of a decreased ability of neck pain patients to relax the superficial neck muscles after neck (Barton & Hayes 1996) and shoulder flexion activities (Fredin et al 1997) has likewise been demonstrated in patients with chronic neck pain of idiopathic and post trauma (whiplash) origins respectively.

Nederhand et al (2002, 2003) suggested that psychological factors such as fear-avoidance beliefs are likely a cause of the altered muscle activity. However, our recent investigation has shown that motor changes (including increased superficial muscle activity) seen in both acute and chronic whiplash occur independently to the patient's fear of movement/reinjury (Sterling et al 2003). These findings support those of George et al (2001), who showed that the relationship between fear avoidance beliefs and disability in cervical spine pain might be weaker than that for lumbar pain. These muscle reactions in the cervical and axioscapular muscles likely reflect underlying physiological disturbances in motor function. Such changes have the potential to impact on patterns of muscle coordination of the cervical region, compromise joint stability, cause unnecessary loading on cervical structures and thus provoke pain. The challenge for researchers and clinicians alike is to transfer this knowledge to the clinical setting and the individual patient and to test the muscle system in a manner clinically that might detect the impairment. Similarly, the most appropriate exercise regimes must be developed to address these problems. An assessment and exercise approach is presented which has proven to be effective in achieving lasting pain relief in patients with chronic neck pain and headache (Jull et al 2002).

THE CLINICAL EXAMINATION OF THE CERVICAL MUSCLE SYSTEM

The nature of the impairment in the cervical and cervicobrachial muscle systems indicates the need for careful and precise movement analysis and muscle testing to appreciate and accurately define the problem. Information about the muscle system can be gained from the observation of postural form and the examination of active cervical and arm movements as well as from more formal muscle tests.

The tests, which form part of the initial assessment of the patient during the first consultation, can be described as tests of muscle coordination and control. The tests are low load and results are usually not flawed by factors such as pain inhibition. In line with the deficits that have been found in neck pain patients, the tests assess the patient's ability to cognitively perform and hold a low level contraction of the deep cervical and shoulder girdle postural muscles to reflect their functional supportive role as well as their pattern of activity in function. They include the following, in an order that may be used in a usual assessment of a patient with a musculoskeletal disorder:

- Muscle control in posture
  – pattern of postural correction to an upright 'neutral' posture
  – orientation of the scapulae in the upright 'neutral' posture.
- Analysis of movement patterns
  – pattern of active cervical extension and return to the upright posture
  – pattern of scapular muscle activity and control with arm movement.
- Specific muscle tests
  – craniocervical flexion test (pattern of activation and holding capacity)
  – scapular retraction/depression test (pattern of activation and holding capacity).
- Tests of muscle length of the axio-scapular-girdle muscles.

Muscle control in posture

Pattern of postural correction to an upright 'neutral' posture

The patient is asked to assume an upright neutral postural position from a relaxed sitting position. The clinician can gain an idea of which muscle strategy the patient is using to support the natural spinal curves. A good pattern would have the pelvis being brought into an upright neutral position with the formation of a low lumbar lordosis (lumbar multifidus) rather than with thoracolumbar extension (thoracopelvic extensors). The position of the thoracic and cervical curves as well as the craniocervical posture is then observed. These often assume a satisfactory position with correction of the lumbopelvic region.

Orientation of the scapulae in the upright neutral posture

Initial indications of scapular muscle impairment can be gained from an analysis of scapular position in association with muscle bulk/tone of the axio-scapular-girdle muscles both anteriorly and posteriorly in a standing or sitting posture (Janda 1994, Mottram 1997). Ideally the resting scapulae should sit such that the superior angle lies level with the T2 or T3 spinous process, the root of the spine of the scapula level with the T3 or T4 spinous process, and the inferior angle level with the T7–9 spinous process (Sobush et al 1996). These bony landmarks may be palpated. The scapula should also sit approximately 30 degrees anterior to the frontal plane, in slight upward rotation and with the medial border and inferior angle flat against the chest wall. The scapula is maintained in this position by the balanced synergy of scapular muscle co-activation and the orientation of the clavicle, which is its only connection with the axial skeleton. Common 'abnormal' postural positions of the scapula include a downwardly rotated and protracted scapula (Mottram 1997, Sahrmann 2002), which is often associated with a dominant action of levator scapulae and an increased resting length of upper trapezius. Conversely the scapula may appear slightly elevated. While the upper portion of trapezius may be involved in this postural position, the clinician should check if the position is protective and associated with neural tissue mechanosensitivity.

In the presence of an abnormally orientated scapula the therapist should manually facilitate it to the optimal position and test the ability of the patient to actively maintain this position. Patients are then asked to relax and reposition the scapula themselves. The clinician should observe what muscle strategy they automatically use to achieve this position.

Analysis of movement patterns

Opportunities present to observe movement and patterns of muscle use throughout the entire assessment of the neck pain patient. There are two particular movements which give indications of the functional use of key muscles for joint support and control of the cervicoscapular region:

Pattern of active cervical extension and return to the upright position

The test of active control of extension assesses the ability of the craniocervical flexor muscles to eccentrically control the centre of gravity of the head into a position behind the frontal plane of the shoulders, before returning the head to the upright position with a concentric contraction of the same muscles.

Neutral to extension

The sternocleidomastoid is a flexor of the lower cervical spine and an extensor of the upper cervical spine. During extension, the flexor moment arms of sternocleidomastoid and anterior scalene muscles reduce and in extreme extension are less than 25% of their value in neutral (Vasavada et al 1998). The extensor moment arm of the sternocleidomastoid increases the further the head goes into extension (Vasavada et al 1998), making it incapable of eccentrically controlling extension of the upper cervical region. The anterior scalene muscles too cannot control the head and upper cervical segments (Moore & Dalley 1999). This leaves the hyoid muscle group and the deep cervical flexors to eccentrically control cervical extension. The hyoid group have no control of cervical segments. The deep cervical flexors with their extensive longitudinal intersegmental attachments from the upper thoracic spine to the skull are best suited to control extension. In the presence of poor eccentric control of the deep neck flexors, two characteristic patterns of movement are evident:

- The patient is unwilling to allow the centre of gravity of the head to move posteriorly behind the frontal plane of the shoulders, thus minimizing the effects of gravity. There is a dominant upper cervical spine extension pattern with minimal, if any, movement of the head posteriorly (Fig. 32.1). This can be mistaken for a good cervical extension effort particularly when an individual has significant range of upper cervical extension. When the

movement is corrected so that the head moves backwards in extension, loss of control as described below is evident.

- The head moves backwards but the flexor muscles cannot control the effects of gravity/head weight. The head reaches a point of extension and then appears to drop or translate backwards, loading the osteoligamentous structures. This is often quite uncomfortable and, when control is poor, the patient often wishes to return immediately to the upright position, occasionally with help of their hands. Patients may describe a feeling of loss of control as if 'my head was going to fall off the back of my shoulders'.

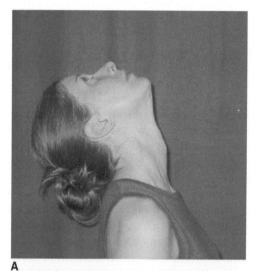

A

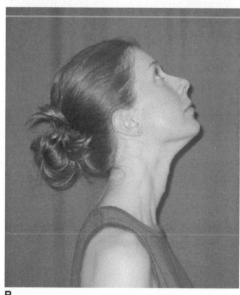

B

Figure 32.1 A: A good pattern of full cervical extension. B: A poor pattern of cervical extension. The patient is unwilling to allow the centre of gravity of the head to move posteriorly behind the frontal plane of the shoulders and performs predominantly upper cervical spine extension.

Extension to neutral

The return from a fully extended position to a neutral upright position demands a coordinated concentric contraction of the craniocervical flexors. The dominant poor pattern is initiation of the movement from extension with the sternocleidomastoid and anterior scalene muscles resulting in lower cervical flexion but not upper and craniocervical flexion. In this poor pattern, recovery from the craniocervical extension element is the last, rather than a leading element of the movement.

Pattern of scapular muscle activity and control with arm movement

There are two aspects of scapular muscle function to analyse in the neck pain patient. The first is muscle activity with arm function without significant arm elevation and the second is the analysis of scapular movement with arm elevation.

Research examining activity of the upper trapezius (Falla et al 2004a, Nederhand et al 2000, 2002, 2003), sternocleidomastoid and anterior scalene muscles (Falla et al 2004a) during a repetitive unilateral low load functional task simulating writing has demonstrated, variously, patterns of increased and decreased activity in the upper trapezius in the neck pain patients and increased activity in the sternocleidomastoid and anterior scalene muscles. The pattern of activity was evident within 10 seconds of commencement of the task (Falla et al 2004a). Whether such activity can be observed visually in a clinical assessment is unknown, but the research draws the clinician's attention to observing the patient's pattern of muscle use in such tasks. Concurrently, the patient's ability to maintain the scapula in the starting position, avoiding downward rotation, protraction, or excessive elevation can be analysed. Activity in the levator scapulae has not been researched to date in such experiments and this is a muscle which, clinically, has been observed to be dysfunctional in neck pain patients.

In the second test, appropriate and controlled scapular rotation is sought throughout arm raising and lowering. Elevation of the arm past 60 degrees should be accompanied by external rotation of the scapula ensuring that the glenoid fossa is appropriately positioned facing superiorly. Excessive elevation of the scapula, often associated with overactivity of the levator scapulae muscle, can be a compensatory strategy for poor synergistic activity of the tripartite trapezius and serratus anterior muscle to externally rotate the scapula. With its attachment to the upper four cervical vertebrae, overactivity of levator scapulae may place detrimental mechanical strain on the cervical spine.

Specific muscle tests

The craniocervical flexion test (C-CFT)

The craniocervical flexion test will be described in some detail. It is a newer test and has evolved since original descriptions (Jull 1994) as more understanding has been gained from research and its clinical application with patients. While in the

research setting surface EMG has been used to quantify the activity in the deep and superficial muscles, the techniques used especially for the deep neck flexors are not applicable clinically[1]. Rather, the skills of the clinician in movement and muscle analysis are employed. The findings of our research offer guidelines for the clinician in using the C-CFT, namely, the therapist must: carefully observe for the correct rotation action of craniocervical flexion and identify any substitutions; monitor the contribution from the superficial flexors in all stages of the test (observation, palpation); and determine how well the patient can hold the craniocervical flexion positions in each progressive stage of the test.

The C-CFT is performed in two stages. Stage 1 is an analysis of the craniocervical flexion movement pattern in performing the five incremental stages of the test. Stage 2 tests the holding capacity of the deep neck flexors in those stages of the test that the patient can achieve with the correct movement pattern.

For the test, the starting position is supine crook lying (Fig. 32.2). The patient may automatically assume the desired mid-range neutral position of the craniocervical region where the line of the forehead and chin are in a horizontal plane and an imaginary line extending from the tragus and bisecting the neck longitudinally is parallel to the plinth. There are two deviations from this desired posture. Firstly, the head may be in a slightly extended position. This should alert the clinician to consider at least three possibili-

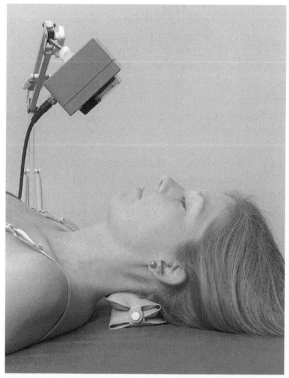

Figure 32.2   The starting position for craniocervical flexion test with the head and neck resting in a mid-range neutral position.

[1]Electrodes are inbuilt into a nasopharyngeal catheter, inserted through the nose and suctioned onto the oropharyngeal wall (Falla et al 2003b).

ties in interpretation. It may result from the shape of the thoracic or cervicothoracic curves (kyphosis). Layers of towel are placed under the head to position the craniocervical region in a mid-range neutral position. Occasionally it is necessary to place a few layers of towel behind the neck to partially fill the space between the neck and testing surface, for placement of the pressure cuff. The craniocervical region could be in an extended position, reflecting some lack of range due to shortened craniocervical extensor muscles or upper cervical joint hypomobility. These usually have insufficient impact to delay testing. However, the slightly extended position or restriction of craniocervical flexion may be protective of mechanosensitive neural tissues. If this is the case the C-CFT may be provocative of these neural tissues and in these circumstances testing and retraining may be delayed. Indications of mechanosensitive neural tissue are gained if passive upper cervical flexion produces head or neck pain and range can be altered in a repeated test with the upper or lower limbs in a neurally pre-tensioned position (Jull 1997). In such cases, initial treatment should aim to resolve the neural tissue mechanosensitivity.

The second positional anomaly is that the craniocervical region is resting in a position of flexion. This is often associated with increased tone in the anterior scalene muscles flexing the middle and lower cervical regions, which could reflect their habitual overactivity to compensate for impairment in the longus colli. Overactivity of the scalene muscles may also reflect overuse in a poor upper chest breathing pattern. However, it may be a clinical sign reflecting impairment in, or loss of kinaesthetic acuity in, the deep cervical extensors which may accompany the changes that have been observed in, at least, the cervical suboccipital extensors (Andrey et al 1998, Hallgren et al 1994, McPartland et al 1997). In such cases, the patient must learn the more neutral, resting mid-position as part of the retraining process.

Once the craniocervical region is placed in a mid-range neutral position, the pressure sensor (Stabilizer, Chattanooga Inc, USA) is folded in three, fastened and placed behind the neck such that it abuts the occiput. It is inflated until the pressure is stabilized on the baseline of 20 mmHg, a volume sufficient to fill the space between the back of the neck and the testing surface without pushing the neck into a lordosis. The patient is taught the correct movement without any feedback from the pressure sensor. The test is one of precision and control, rather than a test of strength. A good analogy to use in teaching is to describe the craniocervical flexion movement as 'gently nod your head as though you were saying "yes" '. It is not a head lift or head retraction action.

Stage 1: Analysis of the craniocervical flexion movement pattern

In the first stage of the test, the patient attempts to nod their head to reach each of the five stages of incremental craniocervical flexion, with a few seconds rest between each stage. They are guided by the feedback from the pressure sensor to sequentially target each progressive 2 mmHg increment from the baseline of 20 mmHg to the final target of 30 mmHg. The clinician analyses the patient's attempt and observes the pattern of the craniocervical movement as well as the activity in the superficial flexors (sternocleidomastoid, hyoid and anterior scalene muscles). Research on asymptomatic subjects, indicates that there should be a pattern of progressively increasing craniocervical flexion with each stage of the test (Falla et al 2003a). As measured in research and observed clinically, the most common substitution used by neck pain patients is incorporation of a head and neck retraction action rather than the rotation action of craniocervical flexion to reach the pressure targets. This is observed as a decreasing range of craniocervical flexion with increasing pressure targets, rather than an increasing range. The other variance is an overuse of the sternocleidomastoid, hyoid or scalene muscles to perform the tasks. While some progressively increasing activity will be observed (or palpated) in the superficial flexors, it should not be dominant (Falla et al 2004b, Jull 2000, Jull et al 2004). This may or may not be associated with a retraction action. The clinician notes and records the level of the task that can be achieved with the correct movement pattern and without dominant activity of the superficial flexors.

Stage 2: Testing the holding capacity of the deep neck flexors

The test of the holding capacity assesses the target level that the patient can hold steadily for 10 seconds without resorting to a retraction action, without the obvious use of the superficial neck flexors and without a quick, jerky craniocervical flexion movement. The test is begun at the first level, 22 mmHg, and progressed to each target pressure separately. Usually three or four 10-second repetitions at each pressure target are sufficient to inform the clinician of the patient's abilities at that level. The pressure level at which the patient reverts to a substitution strategy is noted and the test ceased. In the therapeutics, the patient will begin endurance training on the pressure level that they can achieve with an appropriate pattern and with control. This is often at the lowest level of 22 mmHg.

It should be noted that if the analysis of the craniocervical flexion movement has revealed a poor pattern, even at the lowest levels of the test, the test of holding capacity of the deep neck flexors should be delayed. The first priority is to re-educate a correct pattern of craniocervical flexion. There is little to be gained from testing the holding capacity of the incorrect muscle action.

Scapular retraction/depression test

The scapular retraction/depression test is a modification of the grade 3 standard muscle test for the lower and middle trapezius. The patient is positioned in prone with the arm by the side to lessen load. In the test, the scapula is gently lifted into position on the chest wall (Fig. 32.3) and

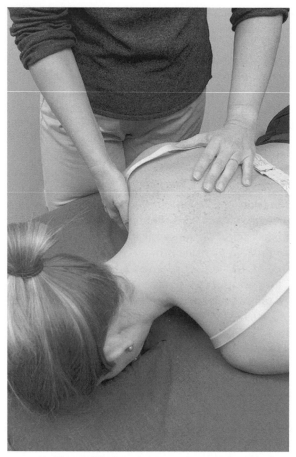

Figure 32.3 The modified grade 3 scapular retraction/depression test.

the patient is asked to gently hold the position. The clinician observes for inappropriate movement or loss of position of the scapula indicating the inability of the middle and lower trapezius to hold the position in this low load task. Elevation of the scapula may indicate incorrect use of levator scapulae. Scapular retraction that is associated with some downward rotation of the scapula may indicate overactivity of the rhomboid muscles. Adduction and extension of the arm must be avoided with this basic test as it indicates substitution with the latissimus dorsi muscle, which can grossly mask poor performance of the scapular muscles. An inability of the patient to maintain the medial border of the scapula on the chest wall (resulting in scapular winging) may indicate poor synergy of the serratus anterior muscle.

The clinician tests the patient's ability to hold the scapular position and their ability to then reposition the scapula themselves. Up to 10 repetitions of 10-second holding contractions is used to test the capacity of this coordinated scapular muscle action. If the clinician finds it difficult to passively position the scapula on the chest wall they should test the length of the anterior shoulder girdle muscles, particularly the pectoralis minor muscle.

Tests of muscle length

Tests of muscle length have been described in detail in other texts to which the reader is referred (Evjenth & Hamberg 1984, Janda 1994). Muscle tightness has been determined in neck pain patients using clinical tests (Jull et al 1999, Treleaven et al 1994), although the prevalence of a moderate degree of tightness was not high. What has to be investigated more closely in future research is the relationship between the increased activity observed in functional tasks with EMG studies and the results of clinical tests of muscle length. Such information would more accurately direct assessment and rehabilitation approaches.

THE EXERCISE APPROACH

The exercise approach is in essence a motor relearning programme where there is an emphasis initially on training the coordination and holding capacities of specific neck flexor and extensor muscles and shoulder girdle muscles as well as retraining their action in functional postures and tasks. It is believed that retraining the coordination of the muscle system is fundamental in the rehabilitation process.

The assessment of the muscle system and the programme of exercises are commenced from the first treatment. Exercises are low load and pain free, and are effective in assisting the patient to achieve pain relief (Jull et al 2002). The components of the programme are integrated but for ease of description, each component and its progression will be described separately and a suggested integrated sequence will be presented at the conclusion of the chapter.

Retraining the cervical muscles

Flexors of the craniocervical spine
Re-education of the craniocervical flexion movement
It is often observed that patients with neck pain have problems in performing the C-CFT. A first essential element of the exercise programme is the re-eduction of the correct craniocervical movement. The patient must be able to perform craniocervical flexion correctly before any testing or training is undertaken to improve the holding capacity of the deep muscles. Table 32.1 outlines some of the common faults that occur with the movement and suggestions for strategies that can be used to correct them. Most patients will achieve a correct movement with a few days of practice. An emphasis on precision and control is essential.

Training the holding capacity of the deep neck flexors
Training the holding capacity of the deep neck flexors is commenced as soon as the patient can perform the craniocervical flexion movement correctly. The pressure biofeedback is used to guide training. Without this feedback, it is difficult for the therapist or patient to know if the contraction is being maintained. The feedback is motivational for patient compliance and allows the therapist to gain some quantification of improvement to guide progression of the

Table 32.1   Common faults in performance of the craniocervical flexion test and suggestions for correction

Common faults	Correction
The patient performs a neck retraction movement rather than the rotation action of craniocervical flexion	Teach the patient to initiate the movement with their eyes. Look down with the eyes and follow with a slow and controlled chin nod. Look up to the ceiling with the eyes only and follow with the chin to resume the neutral position Emphasize the sliding of the occiput on the bed to achieve the pure craniocervical flexion. Therapist may guide the movement with fingers placed on either side of the patient's head
The pressure change is achieved using excessive superficial muscle activity	Palpate the sternocleidomastoid and scalene muscles during the test, to give the patient an awareness of the superficial muscle contraction. Limit the range of craniocervical flexion to the point just short of palpating the dominant superficial muscle activity. Teach the patient self palpation and an awareness of the correct action EMG biofeedback may also be beneficial while the patient practices a slow and controlled craniocervical flexion
The patient rests in a position of flexion, with associated tension in the scalene muscles	Re-educate the awareness of the neutral position by focusing eyes to the ceiling above the head, lifting the chin and palpating the relaxation in the scalenes Relaxation training may be required in cases of anxiety Diaphragmatic breathing training can help to relax respiratory accessory muscles
There is evident jaw clenching and use of the jaw muscles	Instruct the patient in the relaxed position of the mandible – the anterior one third of the tongue on the roof of the mouth, lips together, teeth apart
The patient is holding their breath	Instruct in relaxed nasal breathing while performing the exercise
The patient performs the action quickly and often overshoots the target pressure. This is a common substitution strategy	Reteach the craniocervical flexion action and emphasize that the movement should be slow and controlled

exercise. Training is commenced at the pressure level that the patient has been assessed to be able to achieve and hold steadily with a good pattern, without dominant use or substitution by the superficial flexor muscles, which the patient can monitor by palpation of the muscles. This is often at the lowest levels of the test (22 or 24 mmHg). The movement is facilitated with eye movement into the flexion direction and emphasis is always on precision and control. Any fast or jerky movements are discouraged as they often mask inadequacies in the deep neck flexors. Some patients who have a poor pattern of craniocervical flexion revert to this pattern when given the feedback to train holding capacity. In training holding capacity with the feedback, such patients should first focus on the action of craniocervical flexion and then look at the pressure dial and maintain the pressure level that they have achieved. In all circumstances, training should be short of fatigue, so that an incorrect pattern is not encouraged.

The patient should practice the exercise at least twice daily, for example before rising in the morning and when retiring at night, so that exercise is not too intrusive on their daily activities. For each pressure level, the holding time is built up to 10 seconds and 10 repetitions are performed. At this point, the exercise is progressed to train holding capacity at the next pressure level. Various studies have shown that asymptomatic subjects can achieve an increase in pressure to at least 26 mmHg and can hold the pressure steady for 10 seconds with 10 repetitions (Jull 2000, Jull et al 1999). Some more ideal performances successfully target and hold the levels of 28 to 30 mmHg. The aim for neck pain patients is to train the muscles towards an optimal performance and most neck pain patients are capable of achieving these higher levels (Jull et al 2002). The time taken to achieve these levels is variable but can usually be achieved in 4–6 weeks, although some patients with more difficult conditions may require concerted effort for up to 10–12 weeks. Patients may benefit by using the pressure biofeedback for home practice. It assists in the learning process and in attaining the correct perception of the contraction. Patients can be successfully 'weaned' from the visual feedback once they have gained the correct perception of the exercise.

Retraining cervical spine extension in upright postures

Once the patient shows improvement in deep cervical flexor activation in training the craniocervical action in supine lying, the cervical flexion patterning is progressed to the sitting or standing position. The exercise is a controlled eccentric action of the flexors into cervical extension followed by a concentric action of these muscles to return the head to neutral from the extended position. The patient initiates cervical extension with a chin lift and extends the neck slowly and within a range that is pain-free and able to be controlled. It is helpful to initiate the motion by asking the patient to raise their eyes towards the ceiling and to continue the movement by trying to look further along the ceiling until the end of their comfortable range. This instruction encourages the patient to allow the weight of the head to move backwards and accept the challenge of gravity. If correct instruction is not given before commencing the exercise some patients will try to control the movement by retracting the head on the neck, which is an incorrect pattern. The return to the upright position must be initiated by craniocervical flexion, rather than a dominant action of sternocleidomastoid, which encourages extension in the upper cervical region. The exercise is progressed in two ways. Firstly, the range to which the head is moved into extension is gradually increased as control is improved. Secondly, isometric holds through range are added to the exercise in the sitting position. To perform this latter exercise, the patient extends the neck to predetermined positions in range that are able to be controlled and are pain-free, and then initiates the craniocervical flexion action as if to return to the upright posture and holds the position for 5 seconds before returning to the upright position. The exercise re-educates the cervical flexion synergy through functional ranges of extension. These exercises are potentially high load and should be progressed with care.

Extensors of the craniocervical spine

To train the coordination of the deep and superficial extensors of the cervical and craniocervical spines, the patient practises eccentric control into flexion followed by concentric control back to the neutral position. These exercises can at first be performed in sitting and progressed to the four-point kneeling and/or prone on elbows positions. These exercises are incorporated with re-education of the scapular muscles in these positions. Patients are instructed to flex the head and neck slowly, controlling the speed against gravity, and to return to the neutral position without excessive chin poke to avoid excessive craniocervical extension. Excessive craniocervical extension may signal dominance by superficial extensors such as semispinalis capitis. Manual facilitation of this motion is helpful. When performed in four-point kneeling or prone on elbows, the patient is asked to begin and finish the movement with their eyes focused directly at their hands as this helps avoid excessive craniocervical extension.

The exercise in four-point kneeling is progressed by performing alternating small ranges of craniocervical extension and flexion while maintaining the cervical spine in a neutral position. The aim is to encourage the deep cervical extensors such as semispinalis cervicis and multifidus to maintain a neutral cervical spine (without the dominant action of semispinalis capitis) while the craniocervical extensors perform fine eccentric and concentric contractions as well as holding contractions. Small ranges of head rotation (no greater then 40 degrees) can also be performed such that the movement is a pure spin of the head on the neck. The aim is to encourage the obliquely orientated suboccipital and craniocervical extensor muscles to contribute to the motion rather than the dominant pattern of larger muscles such as splenius capitis and cervicis. These exercises aim to retrain the coordinated action of the deep craniocervical muscles, which have been demonstrated to be impaired in chronic cervical spine conditions (Andrey et al 1998, Hallgren et al 1994, McPartland et al 1997).

Co-contraction of the neck flexors and extensors

Co-contraction of the neck flexor and extensor muscles, in their action as a muscle sleeve (Mayoux-Benhamou et al 1997), occurs during movements of the neck (Conley et al 1995). Co-contraction exercises are added once the patient can achieve the correct postural correction with the appropriate action of the deep and supporting muscles. The co-contraction is facilitated with rotation. The exercise is performed by the patient, using self-resisted isometric rotation in either supine, or in a correct upright sitting posture (Fig. 32.4). Ensure that the patient performs the occipital lift in the correct postural position to pre-facilitate the activation of the longus colli before adding the gentle resistance. Instruct the patient to look into the palm of the hand providing the resistance as a facilitating procedure. The patient performs the alternating rhythmic stabilization exercise with an emphasis on slow onset and slow release holding contractions, using resistance to match about a 10–20% effort. This exercise can easily be incorporated into a daily work routine.

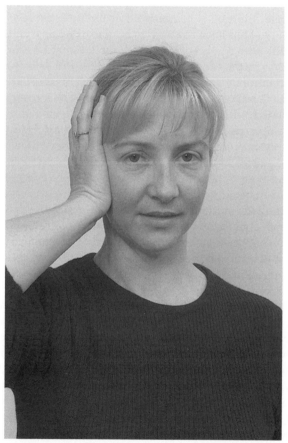

Figure 32.4 The co-contraction is facilitated using self-resisted isometric rotation in a correct upright sitting posture.

Retraining the strength of the superficial and deep flexor synergy

A final element of training addresses the strength and endurance deficits in the neck flexor synergy that have been identified in neck pain patients (Barton & Hayes 1996, Vernon et al 1992, Watson & Trott 1993). Gravity and head load provide the resistance. Care must be taken that this high load exercise is not introduced too early, as it may be provocative of symptoms. The head lift must be preceded with craniocervical flexion followed by cervical flexion to just lift the head from the bed. During the holding contraction, the craniocervical flexion position must be maintained to ensure an appropriate interaction of the deep and superficial flexors. If a head lift is too high a resistance in the first instance, the exercise can be graded so that the patient attempts to lift 25% of their head weight without their head leaving the bed, progressing to 50% head weight and so forth. Strength training to higher levels may not be necessary for the majority of patients. It must be noted that progression to strength training should not be undertaken before the problems in the interaction between the deep and superficial muscles have been addressed. Otherwise, the exercise risks retraining and perpetuating the imbalance between these muscle layers.

Retraining the scapular muscles

Retraining scapular orientation in posture

Regaining control of scapular orientation can be a challenging clinical skill due to the small changes of scapular position that are often required and the difficulty for the patient to visualize scapular motion or to palpate specific muscle contraction or overactivity. It is important initially that the patient has a feel for the correct motion. Initial retraining may need to exaggerate the movement required before fine-tuning the desired contraction intensity. Emphasis should also be placed on relaxation of unwanted muscle activity.

One of the more commonly observed postural faults is the protracted and downwardly rotated position of the scapula. A correction strategy is to move the coracoid upwards and the acromion backwards, which results in a slight retraction and external rotation of the scapula. The aim is to facilitate the coordinated action of all parts of trapezius and serratus anterior, allowing lower trapezius to slightly depress the medial border of the scapula, consequently lengthening (and relaxing) the levator scapulae. This can be taught to the patient by having them place their opposite hand along the line of pectoralis minor with the index finger on the coracoid process. They move the coracoid process away from the fingertip along the line of the hand (Mottram 1997). Emphasis is placed on the subtlety of the movement. If the downward rotation is excessive, the patient may need to be taught to slightly elevate the acromion to facilitate further upward rotation of the scapula. To encourage the contribution of serratus anterior, the patient can be asked to maintain the corrected scapular position while gently pushing onto their thigh or desktop with their hand. The contribution of serratus anterior helps to position the scapular in external rotation and maintain it against the thorax.

Another scapular positional fault is the protracted and elevated scapula. Care must be taken that this is not a posture adopted to protect mechanosensitive neural tissues. If this is the case, the mechanosensitivity of the neural tissues needs to be addressed before scapular retraining is commenced to avoid aggravation of symptoms. Once mechanosensitivity of nerve tissue has decreased, the residual position of the scapula is assessed and corrected as required. If excessive scapular elevation remains, patients are trained to gently draw the scapulae inwards and downwards to specifically activate the middle and lower portions of the trapezius.

Once the patient learns correct scapular orientation, they are encouraged to repeat the correction and maintain the position regularly through the day so that it becomes a habit. The use of memory joggers is essential. Taping to facilitate position may be a helpful tool.

Precision is required in rehabilitating the scapular synergy within the postural exercise. Common faults in attempts of scapular correction include: overcorrection and excessive muscle usage; poor isolation and substitution strategies; fixing the scapula to the humerus which encourages scapular motion by the scapulohumeral rather than the scapulothoracic muscles. The clinician must also ensure that the patient is not performing thoracic extension as a substitution for scapulothoracic movement.

Training the endurance capacity of the scapular stabilizers

Once the optimal scapular position, direction and intensity of the scapular muscle contraction have been learned, the patient trains to improve the tonic endurance capacity of the synergistic muscle contraction. Repeated repetitions of 10-second holds of the corrected scapular position will encourage early endurance retraining. The endurance of the middle and lower trapezius muscles can be improved by performing exercise in prone against the effects of gravity. The exercise is performed as described for the scapular retraction/depression test. Initial training may need to be commenced in side lying with later progression to the prone position if the patient finds the correct movement difficult. It may also necessitate repeated manual facilitation from the therapist.

Retraining scapular control with arm movement and load

The control of scapular orientation in posture can be progressed by the addition of small range arm movements. This is considered important when activities such as the operation of a mouse at a computer is a pain aggravating factor. The patient is encouraged to maintain their newly learned scapular position while performing small range (60 degrees and less) humeral elevation and/or rotation, or while performing the previously aggravating activity such as mouse operation. The exercise can be progressed with the addition of speed and repetitions, with the emphasis on endurance and the maintenance of correct scapular orientation.

The scapular muscles can be further challenged with the use of closed chain exercises. This may initially be achieved in sitting with the patient's hands on their thighs or table with elbows slightly bent. The scapulae are set in the correct position and the patient applies pressure through the heel of the hand to attempt to disturb the corrected position of the scapula. The position is maintained for a sustained period (10 seconds) and repeated several times. Similarly, the patient may apply gentle pressure to the wall while maintaining scapular position in standing with varying degrees of flexion of the arm. Closed chain exercise can be advanced to include body weight in positions such as four-point kneeling and prone on elbows with rhythmic weight shift, and prone on elbows with gentle controlled scapular protraction and retraction incorporating practice of neutral scapular positioning. In this exercise, the patient first relaxes and allows their chest to 'sink' between their shoulder blades. By pushing through their hands, serratus anterior is used to draw the chest up between the shoulder blades. The position is held for at least 10 seconds, and repeated 10 times. At the same time, the therapist ensures that the spine as a whole, and the craniocervical region in particular, is in a mid-position, to capitalize on the position to train the holding capacity of the neck extensors. If this position is too difficult for the patient to control, performing the same task in standing leaning against a wall can reduce the level of the exercise. For progression of the exercise, the patient trains in a prone on elbows position (Fig. 32.5).

Re-education of posture

Re-education of control of posture begins from the first treatment. Frequent correction to an upright neutral postural position serves two functions. It ensures a regular reduction of adverse loads on the cervical joints induced by poor spinal, cervical and scapular postures. Most importantly, it trains the deep and postural stabilizing muscles in their functional postural supporting role. While formal training of the holding capacity of the deep neck flexors and scapular muscles occurs twice per day, their activation and holding ability is trained as part of postural correction repeatedly throughout the day, the emphasis being a change in postural habit.

Postural position is trained in sitting and is corrected from the pelvis. The patient trains to correct posture by first drawing their pelvis up to an upright neutral position with the formation of a low lumbar lordosis and activation of the lumbar multifidus. The clinician must ensure that the upright posture is achieved by correct positioning of the lumbopelvic region, not with thoracolumbar extension. If further correction of thoracic posture is required, this may be achieved via a subtle sternal lift. The second aspect of re-education of postural position is correction of scapular

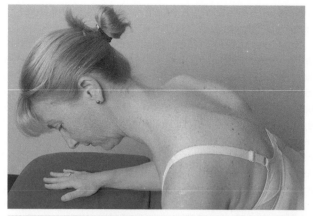
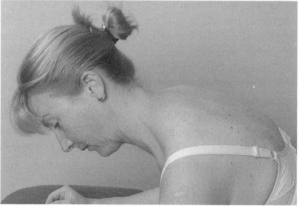

Figure 32.5   Training the holding capacity of scapular stabilizing muscles in four-point kneeling with the focus on serratus anterior. The patient practices both eccentric (A) and concentric (B) control, as well as holding capacity. Note the head and neck are held in a neutral position to train the cervical extensor holding capacity.

position. This aspect was addressed under the previous section on the scapula.

A final element of the postural exercise is to ask the patient to add a gentle 'occipital lift' (imagine lifting the occiput 1 mm off the atlas). This action of gentle lengthening has been shown to activate the longus colli (Fountain et al 1966). This element is added once the patient has mastered the correction of pelvic and scapular position.

Workplace training

Harms-Ringdahl et al (1986) have demonstrated that extreme positions of the cervical spine do occur in sitting work postures. As with usual patient management, correction of work station layouts and work practices are essential components of overall management. It is notable that much of the upper limb activity in the more sedentary occupations of the modern day workforce is performed under more open chain conditions (for example computer use). There is evidence that patients with neck pain have abnormal patterns of activation of the upper trapezius and superficial flexor muscles during such upper limb tasks (Falla et al 2004a, Nederhand et al 2000, 2002, 2003). Therefore training should incorporate postural correction exercises and active maintenance of scapular position while typing, writing or performing other light activities with the hands. Maintenance of a correct scapular position with appropriate muscle coordination as described previously has the added benefit of inducing reciprocal relaxation in muscles such as levator scapulae, which reduces the muscular pain in the area. These exercises are incorporated in daily work practices and are repeated frequently during the day. They are a progression of the postural control exercises introduced in the initial treatment.

Scapular control in association with control of cervicothoracic postural position is also trained for functional activities such as lifting and carrying. All principles of lifting, shifting and carrying taught to the low back patient are applicable to patients with neck disorders. Following any correction of techniques, activities should be progressed, as normal, from light loads to loads appropriate to the patient's activities of daily living and work requirements.

Self-management programme

As described throughout this text, exercises are provided for the patient to continue in a home programme. Success can only be achieved with the patient being an active participant. The clinician has a responsibility to educate, encourage and gain patient compliance. This can be achieved if the patient understands fully the consequence of poor muscle control, the adverse loads that are placed on cervical structures through inappropriate patterns of muscle use and the vulnerability of cervical structures to strain with inadequate muscle support. The consequence is neck pain. The evidence indicates that neck pain can be reduced in the long term with the exercise programme (Jull et al 2002) and this feature must be 'sold' to the patient.

Thus, thorough and effective education is a vital aspect of patient management. A feature of the active stabilization programme is that the self-management component is not inordinately time-consuming. Formal exercises for the re-education of the neck flexor synergy and scapular muscles are performed twice per day and take only about 10 minutes to perform. The need for precision and accuracy in performance must be stressed. Other components of the programme are performed within normal work or daily activities, and should become part of normal working routines. This is a time-efficient and preferable home exercise strategy. Cues are required to remind the patient to assume the upright neutral posture, unloading the spinal structures by activating the deep and postural stability muscles. These memory triggers should be actions or situations occurring frequently during the day, for example: answering the telephone, while stationary in a car, travelling on public transport, during advertisements on television.

PROPRIOCEPTIVE RETRAINING

After pain, dizziness and unsteadiness are the most common symptoms reported by patients with chronic whiplash associated disorders (Treleaven et al 2003) and symptoms of dizziness or light-headedness are not infrequently associated with cervicogenic headache (Sjaastad et al 1998). Such disturbances may often be ascribed to altered afferent input from the cervical mechanoreceptors. Mechanoreceptors located in the cervical joints and muscles are an important component of afferent information from the proprioceptive system to the postural control system. The deep neck muscles in particular have a vast density of muscle spindles (Bakker & Richmond 1982, Boyd-Clark et al 2002, Kulkarni et al 2001). Proprioceptive reflexes of the neck, the cervicoocular reflex (COR), the cervicocolic reflex (CCR) and the tonic neck reflex (TNR) originate from these cervical afferents and influence ocular control as well as vestibular and proprioceptive integration (Bolton 1998, Peterson et al 1985).

The importance of cervical proprioceptive information to the control of posture, spatial orientation and coordination of the eyes and head has been emphasized from results of experimental studies and studies of patients with neck pain (Bolton et al 1998, Peterson et al 1985). It has been shown that local anaesthetic injected into the deep tissues of the neck produces unsteadiness, ataxia and a tendency to fall in humans (DeJong & DeJong 1977). Alterations in eye movement control and standing balance have also been demonstrated when vibration was applied to neck muscles (Kavounoudias et al 1999, Lennerstrand et al 1996). Manifestations of disturbance to postural control were also evident in studies of patients with both idiopathic and traumatic origins of neck pain where deficits in cervical joint reposition error, standing balance and eye movement control have been demonstrated (Heikkilä & Astrom 1996, Karlberg et al 1995a, 1995b, 1996a, Revel et al 1991, Tjell & Rosenhall 1998, Tjell et al 2003, Treleaven et al 2003, 2004).

Direct damage or functional impairment of the cervical afferents is thought to be responsible for these changes in postural control (Heikkilä & Astrom 1996). Morphological changes in the muscles, such as fatty infiltration and changes in muscle fibre type, have been seen that may influence the proprioceptive capabilities of the muscle (Andrey et al 1998, McPartland et al 1997, Uhlig et al 1995). The influence of pain and inflammatory mediators on muscle spindle afferents as well as disturbances to the central modulation of proprioceptive information may also contribute to disturbed postural control (Ro & Capra 2001, Wenngren et al 1998).

THE CLINICAL EXAMINATION OF POSTURAL CONTROL DISTURBANCES

The clinical examination of postural control disturbances encompasses three main elements, assessment of joint position error, balance and eye movement control.

Joint position error

Cervical joint position error is considered to primarily reflect afferent input from the neck joint and muscle receptors. A commonly used measure is the person's ability to relocate the natural head posture while vision is occluded (Revel et al 1991). The joint position error is the angular difference between the starting and resumed natural head postures. Greater cervical joint position errors have been shown in patients with idiopathic neck pain and with both acute and persistent whiplash associated disorders (Heikkilä & Astrom 1996, Heikkilä & Wengren 1998, Revel et al 1991, Sterling et al 2004, Treleaven et al 2003). Furthermore, it has been shown that whiplash patients who complain of dizziness or unsteadiness have greater deficits in joint position error than those who do not report these symptoms, suggesting that the complaint of dizziness may be due to a mismatch of abnormal information from the cervical spine with normal information from the vestibular and visual systems (Treleaven et al 2003).

In a research environment, very accurate movement measurement systems are often used in assessment of joint position error, and these are not available in the clinical setting (Fig. 32.6). Although moderate deficits can be determined visually in a clinical assessment, as little as 3–4 degree errors can indicate a deficit in cervical joint position sense (Treleaven et al 2003) and such ranges may be difficult to judge visually. Simple, inexpensive objective measures can be made in the clinical setting to avoid inaccurate assessment of joint position errors. For example, as demonstrated by Revel et al (1991), a small laser pointer mounted onto a lightweight headband can be used. The laser light projects the starting position of natural head posture onto a wall (90 cm away) and this is marked. The movements of extension and rotation are usually tested. The difference, in centimetres, between starting and final positions is measured. Alternatively, a gravity dependent goniometer can be used (Loudon et al 1997). Other signs which can be observed clinically which may indicate problems in kinaesthetic sense include: jerky movements, uncertainty and/or searching for the initial position, overshooting the initial position, reproduction of dizziness and/or a noticeable difference between movement patterns performed with the eyes closed compared to eyes open.

Balance

Deficits in standing balance have been demonstrated in persons with persistent neck pain of both idiopathic and traumatic origins (Alund et al 1993, Dieterich et al 1993, Karlberg et al 1995b, 1996b, McPartland et al 1997, Treleaven et al 2004). This evidence indicates that this factor should be routinely assessed in patients with neck disorders.

The standard sensory organization test is often used in research to measure a person's ability to maintain equilibrium while systematically changing the sensory selection process by altering the environmental information available to the somatosensory and/or visual inputs (Shumway-Cook & Horak 1986). True dynamic posturography uses either instantaneous movements of a platform, or surrounding visual environment, or both. Shumway-Cook & Horak (1986) developed the clinical test for sensory interaction in balance. It is an alternative to using a moveable force plate and moveable surrounds, as the latter equipment is not always readily available in a clinical setting. The test regime is well suited for adoption in the examination of the cervical spine patient.

In the clinical examination of standing balance, the neck pain patient can be progressed through tasks which progressively challenge the postural control system by altering foot position, visual input and the supporting surface. Balance in comfortable and subsequently narrow stance can be assessed with the patient standing on a firm and then a soft surface such as a piece of 10 cm dense foam. The tests should be performed with both eyes open and closed. It is reasonable to expect that a person can maintain stability for up to 30 seconds in each test (Treleaven et al 2004). For increasing challenge, the patient can be tested in tandem and then single leg stance on a firm surface with eyes open and closed. The relationship between postural stability tests and more dynamic and functional tasks has not

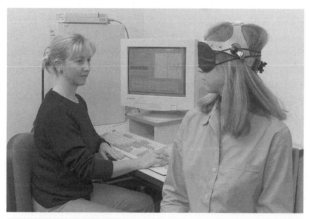

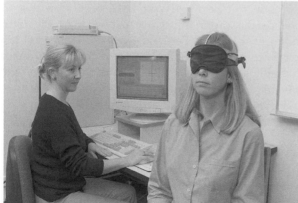

Figure 32.6 The measurement of joint position error in a laboratory setting from rotation (A) to the natural head posture (B).

been investigated in patients with neck disorders. However, it is not unreasonable to suggest that clinicians consider dynamic tests such as reach and step and external perturbations, as performed with neurological or aged patients, for their neck pain patients, especially those complaining of dizziness or unsteadiness.

Tests of eye movement control

Disturbances in eye movement control have been demonstrated in patients with chronic neck pain (Tjell & Rosenhall 1998, Tjell et al 2003). Control of eye movement has been investigated with the smooth pursuit neck torsion test. In this test, eye movement control is measured with the patient facing straight ahead and then with the neck torsioned, that is, the trunk and neck rotated beneath the stationary head. Although patients with vestibular disorders and central nervous system dysfunction overall may have greater deficits in eye movement control than patients with neck dysfunction, unlike the neck pain patients, they do not demonstrate any greater loss of eye movement control with the neck in the torsioned position (Tjell & Rosenhall 1998, Tjell et al 2003). The greater loss of eye movement control of the neck pain patients, particularly those with chronic whiplash associated disorders, implies a cervical cause of this eye movement disturbance. Oculomotor assessment involves tests of eye follow, gaze stability and eye–head coordination. They are usually performed with the patient in a sitting position but can be tested initially in supine lying if necessary.

Eye follow

The patient keeps the head still and follows a moving target with the eyes: from side to side, up and down, progressing to an H pattern. The clinician monitors the patient's ability to follow the target and notes any jerky eye movements (saccadic movements) and reproduction of symptoms such as dizziness, unsteadiness or nausea. The trunk is rotated (up to 45 degrees neck torsion) or to a point just short of pain and the test repeated. Any difference in eye follow is noted.

Gaze stability

Gaze stability is assessed by asking the patient to keep the eyes focused on a fixed point while the head is moved actively or passively (by the clinician) in all directions. Relevant findings are an inability to maintain focus or reproduction of symptoms such as dizziness.

Eye and head coordination

Eye/head coordination is assessed with the following tests:

- The patient rotates the eyes and head to the same side. Left and right sides are tested.
- The eyes move first to a target. The patient then turns the head ensuring the eyes are kept focused on the target.
- The eyes move first and then the head to look between two targets placed either horizontally or vertically, maintaining focus between the two points (two-point focus).

- The eyes and head are rotated to the opposite side, left and right.

The starting position, speed and focus points can be altered to increase the challenge on the oculomotor system. Relevant findings are an inability to complete the tasks and/or any symptom reproduction.

THE EXERCISE APPROACH

Specific management of disordered postural control is warranted in neck pain patients demonstrating such disturbances. There have been a few small preliminary studies that have examined efficacy of various treatments. Manual therapy and acupuncture were shown to gain some improvement in joint position error and the complaint of dizziness in subjects with whiplash associated disorders, while stretching and topically applied anti-inflammatory gel had no effect (Heikkilä et al 2000, Rogers 1997). One study of acupuncture showed improved balance responses in patients with whiplash associated disorders (Fattori et al 1996).

Revel et al (1994) conducted a randomized controlled trial in subjects with neck pain using a programme which consisted mainly of eye, head coupling exercises. The 8-week programme (two supervised sessions per week of 30–40 minutes duration) consisted of exercises that emphasized gaze stability, eye–head coordination and head on trunk relocation practice. The results showed not only an improvement in joint position error but also improvements in range of motion, neck pain, drug intake and perceived disability. No other treatments were used in conjunction with the programme. More recently, Humphreys & Irgens (2002) demonstrated an improvement in joint position error in subjects who performed home exercises of eye, head and arm coordination. Two studies have included eye, head coupling and coordination exercises as part of a multimodal approach to neck pain. Improvements in joint position error, neck pain and disability were observed in those patients undertaking the programme as compared to the control group (Heikkilä & Astrom 1996, Provinciali et al 1996).

Given the current knowledge of the nature of the changes in postural control in neck pain and the results of studies to date, a combination of therapy aimed at improving muscle function, decreasing pain and inflammation, and exercises aimed to improve cervical joint position error, eye–head coordination, gaze stability and balance would appear ideal for subjects with neck pain, especially those patients complaining of dizziness or light-headedness. However, more extensive research is needed to determine the most effective methods of management of postural control disturbances in patients with neck pain. The following specific exercise regime is offered on knowledge and evidence available to date. Exercises should be performed two to three times per day, gradually increasing the degree of difficulty and time of the activity. As disturbances in postural control (in this case increased joint position errors) have been shown to occur in some patients very soon after symptom onset (Sterling et al 2003, 2004), early introduction of these exercises may be optimal.

Retraining exercises

The elements of the exercise programme are introduced at the clinically assessed level of impairment. The tasks can be introduced early into the rehabilitation programme and should be performed such that they do not produce pain. They may be conducted to the point of onset of dizziness but should not aggravate these symptoms for prolonged periods of time.

Relocation practice

The patient practises relocating the head back to the natural head posture and to predetermined positions in range. All active movements of the cervical spine (flexion, extension, rotation and lateral flexion) are used. The patient may practise first with the eyes open and then with eyes closed. The patient may line up their natural head posture with a point on the wall, and check their accuracy on return. The exercise can be made more precise with use, for example, of a pencil torch attached to a headband. This is a simple method for home use and improves the precision of the exercise.

Balance

The starting level for balance retraining will depend on which tests the patient failed in the clinical assessment. This could be narrow base stance, tandem stance or one-foot stance. The conditions for training progress from eyes open, eyes closed to different supporting surfaces, for example standing on foam or an unstable surface.

Patients practise the exercise at home, gradually increasing the time of maintaining stability until they can maintain the position for at least 30 seconds. Challenges to the system can be increased with the addition of relocation practice or oculomotor exercises to the balance exercise, introducing more functional tasks such as reach, stepping and progressing to work on the limits of stability with external perturbations.

Oculomotor exercises

The exercises are progressed through several stages, commencing with eye movement with the head stationary and progressing to movements of the head with visual fixation on a target (Revel et al 1994). Although the exercises appear simple, as mentioned previously they can be quite provocative of symptoms, including pain and dizziness. While exercises may be practised to the point of onset of dizziness they should not be provocative of pain. Exercises may need to be commenced in standing for some patients and then progressed to sitting and standing positions.

- *Eye follow with a stationary head.* The patient's eyes follow a target moving side to side and up and down (Fig. 32.7). As a progression, the eye follow exercises can be per-

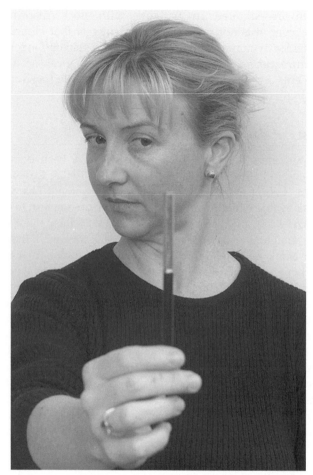

Figure 32.7   Training oculomotor control, the patient follows a moving target with the eyes.

formed with the trunk in a prerotated position (up to 45 degrees) akin to the principle of the smooth pursuit neck torsion test (Tjell & Rosenhall 1998). As a further progression, the speed of eye follow can be increased or saccadic movements of the object can be introduced at randomized eye positions.

- *Eye/head coordination.* The exercises for eye/head coordination are performed in the sitting or standing positions. They commence with rotating the eyes and head to the same side, in both left and right directions. Subsequently, the patient practises leading with the eyes first to a target and then the head, ensuring the eyes keep focused on the target. As a further progression, the eyes are moved first, then the head, to look between two targets positioned horizontally or vertically. Finally the patient practises rotating the eyes and head to the opposite side in both the left and right directions.

Any stage of the eye/head coordination exercises can be progressed by: increasing the speed and range of movements, adding busy patterns (e.g. stripes or checks) to the background of the visual target or making the target a word to keep in focus rather than just a spot. Consideration could also be given to performing the activities while sitting on an unstable surface such as a therapy ball or wobble board or standing with feet on an unstable base of support, for example tandem stance or while walking.

- *Gaze fixation with head movement.* These exercises may be commenced in a supine lying position and the head movement may be passive or active. For example, training may commence with the clinician performing slow passive neck movements while the patient fixes their gaze on a point on the ceiling. This may be progressed to a sitting or standing position with the patient visually fixing on a target while moving the head through all active movement directions. The clinician can also passively move the trunk while the patient maintains gaze on a target. Any task may be progressed by restricting peripheral vision. Other strategies which can be used to progress these exercises include: increasing the speed and range of movements, adding busy patterns (e.g. stripes or checks) to the background of the visual target, making the target a word to keep in focus rather than just a spot and changing the patient's position.

INTEGRATION OF EXERCISE

The evidence suggests that a multimodal programme inclusive of exercise is more efficacious than any single modality alone for the management of cervical disorders (Gross et al 2002). Thus the active stabilization programme is a key element of management in a rehabilitation programme also inclusive of education and assurance, pain management (manipulative therapy, electrophysical agents), encouragement of normal activity and active movement performed without adverse stresses, proprioceptive retraining (encompassing eye–head coordination and postural stability) (Heikkilä & Astrom 1996, Revel et al 1994) and ergonomic strategies for activities of daily living and work.

The progressive exercise plan for active stabilization training can be summarized as follows:

- Train the pattern of craniocervical flexion and the holding capacity of the deep cervical flexors and scapular supporting muscles.
- Formal training in non-weight bearing twice per day.
- Train the spinal and scapular postural supporting muscles by repeatedly activating the muscles in a postural correction exercise. This should be performed on average every 15 minutes during the day. Cues are required to help the patient develop the action as a lifestyle habit.
- Add exercises for proprioceptive retraining encompassing eye–head coordination and postural stability.
- Add co-contraction exercises in an upright neutral postural position using a low level self-applied rotatory resistance to facilitate the co-contraction of the deep cervical flexors and extensors, that is, rehabilitate the deep 'muscle sleeve' to support the cervical segments.

- Retrain cervical movement patterns in four-point kneeling, sitting or standing. Train isometric holds of the neck flexors through progressive ranges of extension.
- Retrain scapular muscle control in four-point kneeling, with arm movements, and with load relevant to functional tasks.
- Progress proprioceptive training with higher level coordination and balance tasks.
- High load endurance training for the neck flexors using progressive head weight in a head lift action, ensuring that the upper cervical flexion position is controlled.
- Further strengthening and endurance exercise as required by the individual patient.

Evaluation

The effectiveness of management is monitored throughout the programme. Essential are the patient centred outcomes such as level of neck pain (visual analogue scale, VAS), and functional performance (e.g. functional VAS, formalized neck pain questionnaires). Measures of physical impairments, for example craniocervical flexion test, cervical range of movement, are important to the clinician to assess the effectiveness of the exercise strategies and to guide treatment progression. While clinicians may experiment with different exercise strategies to train the deep supporting muscles, it is essential that they constantly retest the muscles with a formal test to ensure the exercise method is achieving the desired outcome.

The rate of improvement, not unexpectedly, is variable between patients. As was revealed in the clinical trial with patients with neck pain and headache (Jull et al 2002), good outcomes were achieved with 4–6 weeks of training for many patients; however, other patients require longer times to achieve maximum outcomes. Constant re-evaluation is the key. It is not known whether patients need to continue exercises indefinitely. Until musculoskeletal physiotherapists have better knowledge about this issue patients should be encouraged to incorporate activation of the deep and postural supporting muscles in the postural correction exercise in routine daily activities as a preventative measure.

CONCLUSION

Contemporary evidence is indicating that exercise is a key element of effective management programmes for the cervical region. Research has demonstrated impairments in the muscles vital for control of the cervical segments and the cervical curve. This chapter has presented an exercise approach which has been designed to address these impairments directly. Its efficacy has been proven in a clinical trial of patients with neck pain and headache and further clinical trials with other neck disorders are underway. The case for addressing the impairments in the muscle system with specific exercise has been well illustrated in research that has revealed that the problems in muscle control do not automatically reverse even if there has been a lessening of pain and resumption of normal activities (Jull et al 2002, Sterling et al 2003). A challenge that has not been met with previous management strategies is the prevention of chronic or recurrent episodes of neck pain. Future research and monitoring in clinical practice will determine if the approach of precise training directed at restoration of muscle control and active stabilization can meet this challenge.

KEYWORDS	
therapeutic exercise	stabilization training
cervical spine	cervical kinaesthetic
muscle control	training

References

Alund M, Ledin T, Odkvist L, Larsson S E 1993 Dynamic posturography among patients with common neck disorders: a study of 15 cases with suspected cervical vertigo. Journal of Vestibular Research Equilibrium and Orientation 3: 383–389

Andrey M T, Hallgren R C, Greenman P E, Rechtien J J 1998 Neurogenic atrophy of suboccipital muscles after a cervical injury. American Journal of Physical Medicine and Rehabilitation 77: 545–549

Bakker D A, Richmond F J 1982 Muscle spindle complexes in muscles around upper cervical vertebrae in the cat. Journal of Neurophysiology 48: 62–74

Bansevicius D, Sjaastad O 1996 Cervicogenic headache: the influence of mental load on pain level and EMG of shoulder-neck and facial muscles. Headache 36: 372–378

Barton P M, Hayes K C 1996 Neck flexor muscle strength, efficiency, and relaxation times in normal subjects and subjects with unilateral neck pain and headache. Archives of Physical Medicine and Rehabilitation 77: 680–687

Behrsin J F, Maguire K 1986 Levator scapulae action during shoulder movement: a possible mechanism of shoulder pain of cervical origin. Australian Journal of Physiotherapy 32: 101–106

Bergmark A 1989 Stability of the lumbar spine: a study in mechanical engineering. Acta Orthopaedica Scandinavica 230(Suppl.): 20–24

Bolton P S 1998 The somatosensory system of the neck and its effects on the central nervous system. Journal of Manipulative and Physiological Therapeutics 21: 553–563

Boyd-Clark L, Briggs C, Galea M 2002 Muscle spindle distribution, morphology, and density in longus colli and multifidus muscle of the cervical spine. Spine 27: 694–701

Conley M S, Meyer R A, Bloomberg J J, Feeback D C, Dudley G A 1995 Noninvasive analysis of human neck muscle function. Spine 20: 2505–2512

DeJong P I V M, DeJong J M B V 1977 Ataxia and nystagmus induced by injection of local anaesthetics in the neck. Annals of Neurology 1977: 240–246

Dieterich M, Pollmann W, Pfaffenrath V 1993 Cervicogenic headache: electronystagmography, perception of verticality and posturography in patients before and after C2-blockade. Cephalalgia 13: 285–288

Dutia M B 1991 The muscles and joints of the neck: their specialisation and role in head movement. Progress in Neurobiology 37: 165–178

Evjenth O, Hamberg J 1984. Muscle stretching in manual therapy. Alfta Rehab Forlag, Alfta

Falla D, Campbell C, Fagan A, Thompson D, Jull G 2003a The relationship between upper cervical flexion range of motion and pressure change during the cranio-cervical flexion test. Manual Therapy 8: 92–96

Falla D, Jull G, Dall'Alba P, Rainoldi A, Merletti R 2003b An electromyographic analysis of the deep cervical flexor muscles in the performance of cranio-cervical flexion. Physical Therapy 83: 899–906

Falla D, Bilenkij G, Jull G 2004a Chronic neck pain patients demonstrate altered patterns of muscle activation during performance of a functional upper limb task. Spine (in press)

Falla D, Jull G, Hodges P 2004b Neck pain patients demonstrate reduced activity of the deep neck flexor muscles during performance of the craniocervical flexion test. Spine (In press)

Fattori B, Borsari C, Vannucci G et al 1996 Acupuncture treatment for balance disorders following whiplash injury. Acupuncture and Electro-Therapeutics Research 21: 207–217

Fountain F P, Minear W L, Allison P D 1966 Function of longus colli and longissimus cervicis muscles in man. Archives of Physical Medicine and Rehabilitation 47: 665–669

Fredin Y, Elert J, Britschgi N, Nyberg V, Vaher A, Gerdle B 1997 A decreased ability to relax between repetitive contractions in patients with chronic symptoms after trauma of the neck. Journal of Musculoskeletal Pain 5: 55–70

George S, Fritz J, Erhard R 2001 A comparison of fear-avoidance beliefs in patients with lumbar spine pain and cervical spine pain. Spine 26: 2139–2145

Gross A, Kay T, Hondras M et al 2002 Manual therapy for mechanical neck disorders. Manual Therapy 7: 131–149

Hallgren R C, Greenman P E, Rechtien J J 1994 Atrophy of suboccipital muscles in patients with chronic pain: a pilot study. Journal of American Osteopathic Association 94: 1032–1038

Harms-Ringdahl K, Ekholm J, Schuldt K, Nemeth G, Arborelius VP 1986 Load moments and myoelectric activity when the cervical spine is held in full flexion and extension. Ergonomics 29: 1539–1552

Heikkilä H V, Astrom P-G 1996 Cervicocephalic kinesthetic sensibility in patients with whiplash injury. Scandinavian Journal of Rehabilitation Medicine 28: 133–138

Heikkilä H, Wengren B 1998 Cervicocephalic kinesthetic sensibility, active range of cervical motion, and ocular function in patients with whiplash injury. Archives of Physical Medicine and Rehabilitation 79: 1089–1094

Heikkilä H, Johansson M, Wenngren B 2000 Effect of acupuncture, cervical manipulation and NSAID therapy on dizziness and impaired head repositioning of suspected cervical origin: a pilot study. Manual Therapy 5: 151–157

Humphreys B, Irgens P 2002 The effect of a rehabilitation exercise program on head repositioning accuracy and reported levels of pain in chronic neck pain subjects. Journal of Whiplash and Related Disorders 1: 99–112

Janda V 1994 Muscles and motor control in cervicogenic disorders: assessment and management. In: Grant R (ed) Physical therapy of the cervical and thoracic spine. Churchill Livingstone, New York, pp 195–216

Johnson G, Bogduk N, Nowitzke A, House D 1994 Anatomy and actions of the trapezius muscle. Clinical Biomechanics 9: 44–50

Jull G 1994 Headaches of cervical origin. In: Grant R (ed) Physical therapy of the cervical and thoracic spine. Churchill Livingstone, New York, pp 261–285

Jull G A 1997 The management of cervicogenic headache. Manual Therapy 2: 182–190

Jull G A 2000 Deep cervical neck flexor dysfunction in whiplash. Journal of Musculoskeletal Pain 8(1/2): 143–154

Jull G, Barrett C, Magee R, Ho P 1999 Further characterisation of muscle dysfunction in cervical headache. Cephalalgia 19: 179–185

Jull G, Trott P, Potter H et al 2002 A randomized controlled trial of exercise and manipulative therapy for cervicogenic headache. Spine 7: 1835–1843

Jull G, Kristjansson E, Dall'Alba P 2004 Impairment in the cervical flexors: a comparison of whiplash and insidious onset neck pain patients. Manual Therapy 9: 89–94

Karlberg M, Persson L, Magnusson M 1995a Impaired postural control in patients with cervico-brachial pain. Acta Oto-Laryngologica 520(2): 440–442

Karlberg M, Persson L, Magnusson M 1995b Reduced postural control in patients with chronic cervicobrachial pain syndrome. Gait and Posture 3: 241–249

Karlberg M, Johansson R, Magnusson M, Fransson P A 1996a Dizziness of suspected cervical origin distinguished by posturographic assessment of human postural dynamics. Journal of Vestibular Research, Equilibrium and Orientation 6: 37–47

Karlberg M, Magnusson M, Malmstrom E M, Melander A, Moritz U 1996b Postural and symptomatic improvement after physiotherapy in patients with dizziness of suspected cervical origin. Archives of Physical Medicine and Rehabilitation 77: 874–882

Kavounoudias A, Gilhodes J C, Roll R, Roll J P 1999 From balance regulation to body orientation: two goals for muscle proprioceptive information processing? Experimental Brain Research 124: 80–88

Keshner E A 1990 Controlling stability of a complex movement system. Physical Therapy 70: 844–854

Kulkarni V, Chandy M, Babu K 2001 Quantitative study of muscle spindles in suboccipital muscles of human foetuses. Neurology India 49: 355–359

Lennerstrand G, Han Y, Velay J L 1996 Properties of eye movements induced by activation of neck muscle proprioceptors. Graefes Archive for Clinical and Experimental Ophthalmology 234: 703–709

Loudon J K, Ruhl M, Field E 1997 Ability to reproduce head position after whiplash injury. Spine 22: 865–868

Ludewig P, Cook T M, Nawoczenski D M 1996 Three-dimensional scapular orientation and muscle activity at selected positions of humeral elevation. Journal of Orthopaedic and Sports Physical Therapy 24: 57–65

Lukasiewicz A, McClure P, Michener L, Pratt N, Sennett B 1999 Comparison of 3-dimensional scapular position and orientation between subjects with and without shoulder impingement. Journal of Orthopaedic and Sports Physical Therapy 29: 574–586

McPartland J M, Brodeur R R, Hallgren R C 1997 Chronic neck pain, standing balance, and suboccipital muscle atrophy: a pilot study. Journal of Manipulative and Physiological Therapeutics 20: 24–29

McQuade K J, Dawson J D, Smidt G L 1998 Scapulothoracic muscle fatigue associated with alterations in scapulohumeral rhythm kinematics during maximum resistive shoulder elevation. Journal of Orthopaedic and Sports Physical Therapy 28: 74–80

Mayoux-Benhamou M A, Revel M, Vallee C, Roudier R, Barbet J P, Bargy F 1994 Longus colli has a postural function on cervical curvature. Surgical Radiologic Anatomy 16: 367–371

Mayoux-Benhamou M A, Revel M, Vallee C 1997 Selective electromyography of dorsal neck muscles in humans. Experimental Brain Research 113: 353–360

Moore K L, Dalley A F 1999 Clinically orientated anatomy, 4th edn. Lippincott, Williams and Wilkins, Philadelphia

Mottram S 1997 Dynamic stability of the scapula. Manual Therapy 2: 123–131

Nederhand M J, Ijerman M J, Hermens H J, Baten C T, Zivold G 2000 Cervical muscle dysfunction in chronic whiplash associated disorder grade 11 (WAD-11). Spine 25: 1939–1943

Nederhand M J, Hermens H J, Ijerman M J, Turk D C, Zivold G 2002. Chronic neck pain disability due to an acute whiplash injury. Pain 102: 63–71

Nederhand M J, Hermens H J, Ijerman M J, Turk D C, Zivold G 2003 Cervical muscle dysfunction in chronic whiplash-associated disorder grade 2: the relevance of the trauma. Spine 27: 1056–1061

Panjabi M M, Cholewicki J, Nibu K, Grauer J, Babat L B, Dvorak J 1998 Critical load of the human cervical spine: an in vitro experimental study. Clinical Biomechanics 13: 11–17

Provinciala L, Baroni M, Illuminati L, Ceravolo M G 1996 Postural and symptomatic improvement after physiotherapy in patients with dizziness of suspected cervical origin. Scandinavian Journal of Rehabilitation Medicine 77: 874–882

Peterson B W, Goldberg J, Bilotto G, Fuller J H 1985 Cervicocollic reflex: its dynamic properties and interaction with vestibular reflexes. Journal of Neurophysiology 54: 90–109

Revel M, Andre-Deshays C, Minguet M 1991 Cervicocephalic kinesthetic sensibility in patients with cervical pain. Archives of Physical Medicine and Rehabilitation 72: 288–291

Revel M, Minguet M, Gergoy P, Vaillant J, Manuel J L 1994 Changes in cervicocephalic kinesthesia after a proprioceptive rehabilitation program in patients with neck pain: a randomized controlled study. Archives of Physical and Medical Rehabilitation 75: 895–899

Ro J, Capra N 2001 Modulation of jaw muscle spindle afferent activity following intramuscular injections with hypertonic saline. Pain 92: 117–127

Rogers R G 1997 The effects of spinal manipulation on cervical kinesthesia in patients with chronic neck pain: a pilot study. Journal of Manipulative and Physiological Therapeutics 20: 80–85

Sahrmann S A 2002 Diagnosis and treatment of movement impairment syndromes. Mosby, St Louis

Shumway-Cook A, Horak F 1986 Assessing the influence of sensory integration on balance. Physical Therapy 66: 1548–1550

Silverman J, Rodriquez A, Agre J 1991 Quantitative cervical flexor training in healthy subjects and in subjects with mechanical neck pain. Archives of Physical Medicine and Rehabilitation 72: 679

Sjaastad O, Fredsriksen T A, Pfaffenrath V 1998 Cervicogenic headache: diagnostic criteria. Headache 38: 442–445

Sobush D C, Simoneau G G, Dietz K E, Levene J A, Grossman R E, Smith W B 1996 The Lennie test for measuring scapular position in healthy young adult females: a reliability and validity study. Journal of Orthopaedic and Sports Physical Therapy 23: 39–50

Sterling M, Jull G, Vicenzino B, Kenardy J, Darnell R 2003 Development of motor system dysfunction following whiplash injury. Pain 103: 65–73

Sterling M, Jull G, Vicenzino B, Kenardy J 2004 Characterisation of acute whiplash associated disorders. Spine 29: 182–188

Tjell C, Rosenhall U 1998 Smooth pursuit neck torsion test: a specific test for cervical dizziness. American Journal of Otology 19: 76–81

Tjell C, Tenenbaum A, Sandstrom S 2003 Smooth pursuit neck torsion test: a specific test for WAD. Journal of Whiplash and Related Disorders 1: 9–24

Treleaven J, Jull G, Atkinson L 1994 Cervical musculoskeletal dysfunction in post-concussional headache. Cephalalgia 14: 273–279

Treleaven J, Jull G, Sterling M 2003a Dizziness and unsteadiness following whiplash injury: characteristic features and relationship to cervical joint position error. Journal of Rehabilitative Medicine 34: 1–8

Treleaven J, Jull G, LowChoy N 2004 Standing balance in chronic whiplash associated disorders: comparison of subjects with and without dizziness. (Submitted for publication)

Uhlig Y, Weber B R, Grob D, Muntener M 1995 Fiber composition and fiber transformations in neck muscles of patients with dysfunction of the cervical spine. Journal of Orthopaedic Research 13: 240–249

Vasavada A N, Li S, Delp S L 1998 Influence of muscle morphology and moment arms on moment-generating capacity of human neck muscles. Spine 23: 412–422

Vernon H T, Aker P, Aramenko M, Battershill D, Alepin A, Penner T 1992 Evaluation of neck muscle strength with a modified sphygmomanometer dynamometer: reliability and validity. Journal of Manipulative and Physiological Therapeutics 15: 343–349

Watson D H, Trott P H 1993 Cervical headache: an investigation of natural head posture and upper cervical flexor muscle performance. Cephalalgia 13: 272–284

Wenngren B, Pedersen J, Sjolander P, Bergenheim M, Johansson H 1998 Bradykinin and muscle stretch alter contralateral cat neck muscle spindle output. Neuroscience Research 32: 119–129

Winters J M, Peles J D 1990 Neck muscle activity and 3-D head kinematics during quasi-static and dynamic tracking movements. In: Winters J M, Woo S L Y (eds). Multiple muscle systems: biomechanics and movement organization. Springer-Verlag, New York, pp 461–480

Chapter **33**

A contemporary approach to manual therapy

R. L. Elvey, P. B. O'Sullivan

INTRODUCTION

Manual therapy within an evidence based framework is under threat and struggling for relevance. In our opinion the reason for this is twofold: firstly, manual therapy has largely developed from a culture of signs and symptoms resulting in the inappropriate application of intervention for many disorders. Secondly, there has traditionally been a lack of consideration given to diagnostics and in particular classification of disorders both in clinical practice and evidence based research. This has led to a lack of recognition that a complaint of 'pain' is only one part of a disorder which is complex and involves far more than the expressed complaint. These factors have led manual therapy into its current crisis.

DEFINING MANUAL THERAPY

'Manual therapy' as a term is selected for use in this chapter in preference to 'musculoskeletal physiotherapy', both for historical reasons and because of its integral relationship to manual medicine. Manual therapy is favoured over 'manipulative therapy', which also has a historical background, because of the narrow scope of practice the word 'manipulation' implies. Manual therapy on the other hand, as it applies to this chapter, has a sufficient scope of practice to enable its ethical use in disorders where the characteristics of the disorder may be a combination of organic and non-organic features. In other words, the scope of manual therapy, again as it applies to this chapter, embraces a great deal more than the physical treatment of articulations and musculoskeletal tissues by manipulation and mobilization. It involves the evaluation of a disorder and, on the basis of this evaluation, prescribing an intervention for the disorder rather than administering treatment based simply on signs and symptoms.

While manual therapy fulfils a valuable and important role in health care its scope is naturally limited. With some exceptions, it is apparent that clinical practice, education and the academic pursuit of evidence for the efficacy of manual therapy have either not recognized, or have ignored, the limitations of manual therapy. An impression is gained that in many instances this has led to inappropriate manual therapy clinical practice, inappropriate education and inappropriate methodologies for research into manual therapy treatments. As a result of this, as might be anticipated, there is a certain degree of lack of acceptance of the efficacy of manual therapy beyond its practitioners and educators. This chapter therefore endeavours to promote manual therapy as very valuable to health care when it is instigated and provided in appropriate circumstances. In this manner the limitations of manual therapy can be recognized and at the same time it can be accepted that clinical practice or research protocols for intervention studies based solely upon signs and symptoms or a complaint of a regional area of pain are inappropriate.

The indications and limitations of manual therapy therefore must centre upon the evaluation of a disorder. Integral to this evaluation is the need to define the term 'disorder'. In defining the term the scope of manual therapy practice can then be determined accordingly. McKenzie (1981) made a notable contribution to manual therapy and health care when he stressed the need for physical intervention for mechanical spinal pain to be based upon a classification system. While this comment is obviously fundamental to manual therapy practice and manual therapy research, its importance appears to have gone unnoticed to a large extent by clinical practitioners, educators and researchers, as is evidenced by the common practice of prescribing treatment simply on a signs and symptoms basis, education consisting of countless isolated 'techniques of treatment' and research based on a complaint of 'mechanical' spinal pain. These approaches all fail to appreciate the limitations of manual therapy and the multidimensional nature of the disorders that require intervention. The opinion is held that the value of manual therapy to health care will never be realized if the limitations of manual therapy and the reasons for its limitations continue to remain unrecognized in this way.

The means towards a recognition and an acceptance of the limitations of manual therapy by practitioners and researchers alike must be through the acceptance of the fact that individuals suffering from a non-specific musculoskeletal disorder of pain do not make up a homogenous group. This simply means that while some non-specific musculoskeletal disorders of pain may be amenable to manual therapy intervention, others are not. Those disorders which are not amenable to manual therapy intervention should not be pursued in clinical practice with manual therapy treatment nor should they be included in manual therapy research in order to determine the efficacy of manual therapy. It would appear that the only avenue to demonstrate manual therapy efficacy is in the promotion of a disorder classification system. This would allow specific manual therapy intervention to be tested for its effect on a specific disorder, and selected for the intervention based on

a classification system. At the same time it would be folly and lead to a trivialization of manual therapy if future research focuses on single approaches to intervention used in isolation.

In order to be selective with respect to manual therapy intervention, disorder selection criteria must be paramount. Manual therapy intervention based purely upon signs and symptoms ignores the multitude of factors which constitute a disorder. Patient selection appropriate for intervention is therefore lacking. Diagnostics rather than signs and symptoms should be considered in gaining an understanding of the nature of a disorder. Diagnostics, in the sense in which it is used in this chapter, embraces a disorder diagnosis, a disorder classification and a disorder stage. It is considered that the future acceptance of manual therapy in the healthcare system rests with the promotion of diagnostics where intervention is based upon a system incorporating a diagnosis, a classification and a stage, which allows for the limitations of intervention to be recognized before it is commenced. By means of diagnostics the many features which constitute a disorder can be recognized and, within an acceptable scope of manual therapy practice, intervention may be determined as being either indicated or contraindicated. The emphasis on diagnostics in this chapter is intended to present a contemporary balance to manual therapy practice. It allows for recognition of the value of manual therapy as well as its limitations. While this applies equally in both acute and chronic disorders, it is of utmost importance in chronic disorders where the disorder may be dominated by non-organic morbidity such as psychosocial features.

The scope of manual therapy practice must be broad enough to encompass various forms of treatment and management. The scope of treatment and management must be suited to manual therapy intervention for disorders from an immediate acute phase to a late chronic phase. The scope must be sufficiently wide to deal with organic morbidity and its effects. It must also be capable of recognizing and dealing with non-organic effects providing they are in context with the organic nature of the disorder. A contemporary balance to manual therapy practice as it is portrayed in this chapter is therefore reliant upon a scope of practice which goes well beyond a focus on isolated 'techniques' such as manipulation, mobilization, stabilization, etc. The nature of the disorder, a broad scope of practice and a rationale for the benefits of manual therapy are fundamental to the indications for manual therapy. The indications for manual therapy are fundamental to clinical practice, education, research and evidence based practice.

Summary

This chapter promotes responsible manual therapy practice by emphasizing:

- An acknowledgement that the practice of manual therapy has limitations.

- The requirement to define the term disorder and to determine the nature of a disorder.
- The use of diagnostics in the determination of the nature of a disorder.
- The prescription of manual therapy intervention according to the diagnosis, classification and stage of a disorder.
- A requirement to define a sufficient scope of manual therapy practice to enable it to provide the potential for an effective outcome when a disorder is suitable for manual therapy intervention – that is, when it is indicated.
- The presentation of a rationale for the potential effectiveness of manual therapy intervention for a disorder when it is suitable for manual therapy intervention – that is, a premise for what manual therapy does and how it works.
- The recognition of the indications for manual therapy and, as a direct consequence, the contraindications.
- A reasoned opinion concerning evidence based practice and manual therapy.

DEFINING DISORDER

Disorder is a term used in this chapter to embrace and acknowledge all of the cumulative features of anomaly resulting from some type of presumed initial tissue pathology. These features of a disorder are either 'morbid' or they are 'effects'. Various combinations of features which are morbid in nature or in the form of effects will constitute a disorder. In some disorders the morbid nature of the disorder may predominate while in others the effects might dominate.

Morbidity

Morbid means pertaining to unwholesome, unhealthy, disease or illness. Morbidity is the condition of being morbid. Morbidity may be physical or psychological.

- *Physical morbidity* refers to an underlying physical state of anatomical tissue pathology. For example, ruptured elements of a ligament related to an ankle sprain constitutes tissue pathology, or a disc protrusion resulting from an injury constitutes tissue pathology in a case of low back pain. Physical morbidity is also referred to as organic morbidity. 'Red flags' is the clinical term used to indicate the presence of physical features of a disorder which may indicate a serious level of morbidity. For example, evidence of multilevel lumbar nerve root signs is regarded as a red flag for a disorder involving the cauda equina (Waddell 1996).
- *Psychological morbidity* refers to an underlying emotional state which might be regarded as psychiatric in nature. As such, it constitutes an 'illness'. For example, psychological morbidity might rarely result from an ankle sprain and, less rarely, might be associated with chronic low back pain. Psychological morbidity is also referred to as non-organic morbidity and is usually the result of excessive psychological and/or social effects (see below). 'Yellow flags' is the clinical term used to indicate the presence of psychological features of a disorder which may indicate morbidity (Linton 2000). For example, evidence of abnormal pain behaviour may be regarded as a yellow flag for a disorder classification of psychosocial.

Effects

Effects are an outcome or the consequences of an underlying disturbance. They may be physical or psychological. Any disorder involving pain and disability has associated effects, which are both physical and psychological

- *Physical effects* refers to the physical outcome, which is associated with an underlying physical state. For example, an inability to weight bear following an ankle sprain is a physical effect, or an impairment of lumbar flexion due to low back pain is a physical effect. These effects are also referred to as organic effects.
- *Psychological effects* refers to an experience of pleasantness or unpleasantness associated with an underlying emotional state. A psychological effect in the context of physical medicine and manual therapy is unpleasant and constitutes various forms of suffering. For example, fear-avoidance, abnormal illness behaviour or psychosocial features will accompany an ankle sprain to some degree and commonly chronic low back pain to a larger degree. These effects are also referred to as non-organic effects. When the non-organic effects are excessive or dominant they are referred to as morbid in nature. The term 'yellow flags' applies to psychological effects when they are prominent in a disorder.

By defining a disorder in this manner it acknowledges the fact that a complaint of pain is accompanied by wide-ranging features which are both organic and non-organic in nature. With respect to manual therapy this means a careful evaluation is required in order to differentiate between organic and non-organic features and to determine any dominance of either organic or non-organic features. The reason for this lies in whether manual therapy intervention is indicated or contraindicated and, if it is indicated, what form of intervention is appropriate.

For example, in the case of an acute ankle sprain there would generally be a dominance of organic morbidity and organic effects. Non-organic effects would be present but within the context of the acute ankle sprain, and would constitute the normal suffering expected in the acute stage. The same situation might also apply to a case of low back pain resulting from tissue sprain. In both cases intervention would focus on the organic morbidity and organic effects. That is, intervention would focus on the physical state. Should the non-organic effects begin to dominate, as might happen with non-early resolution of either the ankle sprain or the low back pain, intervention would have to focus on the non-organic effects of the disorder while continuing to act on the organic morbidity and effects. That is, intervention would focus on the psychological state but continue to deal with the physical state. In the event of the non-organic effects becoming excessive and morbid in nature, intervention would necessarily focus entirely on the psychological state.

Effective manual therapy evaluation has to consider suffering and the proposed intervention must have the capacity to deal with suffering. If a disorder is interpreted in terms of the relative contribution to it of organic features or non-organic features, appropriate intervention for that disorder can be prescribed. On the other hand, if a disorder is regarded simplistically as the patient's complaint, inappropriate treatment may result. The term disorder is therefore defined in this text in order to advance the indications for manual therapy and in order to demonstrate the limitations and scope of manual therapy.

Summary

- Responsible manual therapy practice and research is dependent upon the determination of the nature of a disorder.
- The nature of a disorder is a complex mix of organic and non-organic features and is therefore based on a biopsychosocial model.
- It is necessary to identify the nature of a disorder in terms of the dominance of organic or non-organic features. In other words the balance of biological, psychological and social features.
- The non-organic features of a disorder must be a result of, and within the context of, the organic features of a disorder for manual therapy to be indicated.
- Manual therapy is not indicated if the non-organic effects are largely out of context with the organic features or if they become morbid in nature.
- It is considered that should the organic features of a disorder successfully resolve with manual therapy, when it is indicated, the non-organic features will resolve as a consequence.
- Individual clinicians may acquire additional academic qualifications to allow a scope of manual therapy practice which enables them to intervene in the presence of excessive non-organic effects or even morbidity.

DIAGNOSTICS IN MANUAL THERAPY

Diagnostics determines the disorder and the nature of the disorder. Diagnostics consists of a diagnosis, a classification and a stage. These three features are used to determine the nature of a disorder. The diagnosis and classification refer to the disorder in biopsychosocial terms. Subsequently this permits a clinical interpretation of the relationships of organic and non-organic features of the disorder, their dom-

inance and their relative context within the disorder. For example, two presentations of a complaint of chronic low back pain may have a similar traumatic history of onset with the same diagnosis. However, the resultant non-organic effects and hence the individual suffering associated with the complaint of low back pain may be quite different in the two examples. In one example an individual might continue to be fully occupied with their suffering within the context of the organic morbidity, the complaint of pain and the associated impairments. The suffering remains as an associated effect. However, in another example, the non-organic effects may be in the nature of abnormal suffering. This abnormal suffering may prevent any meaningful activity. In this case the suffering may be regarded as a morbid state rather than an associated effect. The non-organic nature of the disorder would appear to overwhelm its organic nature. While the two examples have a similar physical cause for the complaint of low back pain resulting in the same diagnosis, they are totally different disorders. There is therefore a requirement to classify them individually. In the first example the complaint is pain and impairment without evidence of dominant non-organic morbidity. The disorder classification would therefore be one of a physical nature, such as movement impairment or dysfunction with non-organic features in context with the disorder. However, in the second example, while there is a complaint of pain, the suffering is foremost. It is the dominating feature of the disorder and hence the disorder classification would be non-organic morbidity or psychosocial. The classification of the two disorders has therefore provided indications or contraindications for manual therapy.

The disorder stage is used to indicate the time-frame of the disorder, whether it is or is not resolving, and the stability of the disorder. By due consideration of these features of the stage of a disorder an indication can be gained as to the indications and contraindications for manual therapy and the type of manual therapy intervention which would be appropriate for that particular stage. These same features allow for predictions with respect to the prognosis of a disorder.

Summary

- Diagnostics embraces a disorder diagnosis, classification and stage.
- Diagnostics assists in determining the nature of a disorder.
- A disorder diagnosis is determined as a result of the complete evaluation and investigation relating to an individual complaint.
- A disorder classification is determined as a result of the evaluation of the features which dominate the disorder.
- A disorder stage represents in an indication of various features of the disorder at a point in time.
- An indication for manual therapy is dependent upon diagnostics.

SCOPE OF MANUAL THERAPY PRACTICE

In order for manual therapy to be portrayed and accepted as having a valuable role in health care its scope of practice must be defined. All too often manual therapy is portrayed in such narrow terms that its credibility within health care is questionable. Largely, this has been due to the proponents of manual therapy presenting it as a 'passive' system consisting of countless 'techniques of treatment' and giving a rationale for its effect which does not take into account the complexity of the disorder. Consequently, evidence that any technique has any long-term beneficial effects on a disorder is lacking. These two issues invite questions concerning the credibility of manual therapy.

The scope of manual therapy practice is integral to what manual therapy is intended to do and how it works. Obviously these questions depend upon the nature of a disorder. Disorders are many and varied and therefore for manual therapy to have a role in health care it must have sufficient scope of practice to accomodate this variation. A consideration of the variety of disorders of the musculoskeletal system presenting in an outpatient department gives an indication as to the requirements for a scope of manual therapy practice, if it is to be effective. Additional to this, when consideration is given to the various stages of those presenting disorders, an indication of the scope of manual therapy required to deal with them is further realized. Techniques of treatment used in isolation are insufficient to influence the various disorders and various disorder stages of the musculoskeletal system to recovery.

Manual therapy practice must be of sufficient scope to allow for an effective outcome or recovery of the disorder. This scope must take into consideration a number of factors. These could be listed as requirements for prevention of further tissue damage or injury, pain relief, restoration of localized homeostasis, restoration of specific function and restoration of general function. Integral to these factors are all of the requirements of manual therapy practice associated with the non-organic effects of the presenting disorder. Manual therapy, when portrayed only as a 'hands on' technique based practice of health care, could not possibly bring about an appropriate outcome when consideration is given to all these requirements. Furthermore, many of the requirements could not be considered in terms of requiring 'treatment'. Rather they would be considered more appropriately in terms of requiring 'management'. Manual therapy should therefore be considered as offering 'treatment' or 'management' or more commonly a combination of the two. This will be referred to in general terms in this chapter as *intervention*.

Treatment is regarded as specific intervention performed by the clinician. The aim of treatment is to have a favourable influence on the local environment involving the organic morbidity or pathology of the disorder. The pathology of the disorder is regarded as a local environment of increased tissue sensitivity and lowered tissue

mechanosensitivity thresholds. An example of treatment is mobilization, which may be passive or active in its administration.

Management is either a specific or general intervention performed by the patient under the direction or on prescription by the clinician. Management has a much greater range than treatment. Management deals with strategies for the prevention of further tissue strain, damage or injury, the maintenance of restoration of general function and prevention of the recurrence of the disorder. Management utilizes a cognitive behavioural framework, which also takes into account and impacts on the non-organic aspects of a disorder.

Strategies of management would naturally accompany procedures of treatment at all stages of a disorder. However, treatment may not accompany management. For example, in the early stages of an acute disorder, management alone may be preferable; in an acute and subacute stage a combination of treatment and management may be indicated; and in chronic stages treatment would be less indicated while management would always be indicated. In the event of treatment being indicated for a chronic disorder, it would always be in conjunction with management.

By defining treatment and management in this manner, the scope of manual therapy is sufficiently broadened to give it more clinical application and hence credibility. For example, where non-organic effects dominate a disorder, the scope of practice of manual therapy may justify management. Management in this sense must be cognitive behavioural in nature and may incorporate a functional restoration programme. In this sense, a functional restoration programme would only be an adjunct to a more central intervention based on dealing with the non-organic dominance of the disorder. As a result of this intervention the credibility of manual therapy would be preserved.

Summary

- A scope of manual therapy practice is defined in order to promote appropriate guidelines for the use of manual therapy and to give it credibility.
- The scope of manual therapy practice consists of procedures of treatment and strategies of management.
- Intervention is a term used to embrace all or any manual therapy procedures of treatment or strategies of management or combinations of both.
- Treatment is passive. It is specifically directed towards the local environment involving the pathology of the disorder.
- Management is an action or activity performed by the patient under the direction of the clinician.

A RATIONALE OF MANUAL THERAPY CAN FAVOURABLY INFLUENCE A DISORDER

The terms disorder, diagnostics and scope of practice have been discussed because of their combined importance to the provision of manual therapy. Of importance also is how manual therapy might achieve a favourable outcome. This is fundamental to clinical practice, education and academic research. What manual therapy does and how it works is an essential question. It is no longer acceptable for proponents of manual therapy to present 'techniques of treatment' without also answering this fundamental question. It is also no longer acceptable for techniques of treatment to be deemed effective 'because they work' or because of 'patient satisfaction'. These statements are ambiguous and become meaningless as outcome measures for manual therapy effectiveness.

This chapter presents a premise for the questions 'what does manual therapy do' and 'how does it work' which may essentially appear simplistic. However, it is this simplicity upon which it relies for acceptance. In order to discuss what manual therapy does or how it works the scope of manual therapy practice has had to be discussed first, for it is the scope of manual therapy practice which is integral to what manual therapy does and how it works The discussion on the scope of practice highlighted the fact that manual therapy is not an accumulation of 'techniques'. Manual therapy is not, for example, manipulation, mobilization or stabilization, as these modalities utilized in isolation cannot be effective interventions in dealing with the complexity of a disorder. Manual therapy is much more than the use of isolated techniques and it is much more than the use of a combination of techniques. Therefore to search for a reason as to how a technique of manipulation, or mobilization or even stabilization works or, more precisely, how they favourably affect pain appears to be a meaningless exercise when consideration is given to the complex multidimensional nature of a disorder.

Pain is sensory and personal – it is an unpleasant experience. Pain is a feature of a disorder. Suffering and numerous other effects of the disorder accompany the pain of a disorder. Physical impairment, dysfunction and disability accompany the pain of a disorder. A disorder cannot be created in research methodology with the use of 'normal' subjects. 'Techniques of treatment' may produce central nervous system, peripheral nervous system and sympathetic nervous system effects either in normal subjects or in subjects with a complaint of pain or dysfunction. However, this cannot be extrapolated into considering that those same 'techniques of treatment' have the capacity to resolve a disorder. The opinion is put that single 'techniques of treatment' used in isolation are not capable of favourably influencing a disorder to recovery. Given the fact that the nature of a disorder is multifactorial, a range of interventions must be available. This range must incorporate both treatment where indicated and management. When incrementally incorporated it must have the cumulative capacity to reverse the pathology of a disorder and the effects of a disorder in part or in full, leading to a partial or full recovery.

Rather than manual therapy providing a technique which has some special effect of pain relief or modulation

of muscle activity, the view is held that manual therapy intervention simply stimulates, activates or promotes innate mechanisms leading towards recovery. These mechanisms are the normal mechanisms which would operate under normal or optimal conditions. The premise for the benefits of manual therapy treatment is that it replicates the effects of localized physical function, when localized physical function has been adversely affected by the pathology of the disorder. The effects of localized physical function are regarded as physiological functions. These are the physiological functions which accompany localized and general musculoskeletal function and movement. In turn it is considered that enhancing physiological function leads to the stimulation and enhancement of biological functions. These effects, considered to be at a cellular level, are integral to tissue repair and remodelling. As tissue repair and remodelling progress, pain is controlled due to a decrease in tissue sensitization and an increase in tissue mechanosensitivity thresholds. The view is held that stimulation of physiological and biological functions leads to a normalization of the local environment and the return to local homeostasis in the region of pathology. Homeostasis refers to physiological stabilization at a cellular level. It is the stabilization of the organism resulting from the return to normal of the physiological functions at a local cellular level. This is what occurs through the various stages of tissue response to injury leading to repair, remodelling and recovery. Treatment stimulates, activates or promotes this process.

The premise for the benefits of manual therapy management is that it will enhance, promote and stabilize normal physiological function. Management is required when physiological function is present but affected to some degree. The difference from treatment here is that with the requirement for treatment, the local or regional movement is impaired. When management is required in isolation, local or regional movement is present but is aberrant in some manner. Aberrant movement may be in the form of faulty movement patterns or segmental hypermobility resulting in clinical instability. Management in this case provides the means of enhancing physiological function leading to the prevention of repetitive tissue stress and strain associated with the aberrant movement, and in this manner the control of pain. In other examples, management might be prescribed with consideration more for nonorganic effects than aberrant movement, such as functional restoration or reduction of muscle guarding associated with excessive fear of movement.

As opposed to management, the need for treatment is dependent upon the patient's inability to effectively move a local area or region. Treatment is intended to replicate the effects of movement and hence local function. A lack of effective local or regional movement reflects an underlying absence of local function. Passive treatment is required only when the patient cannot move effectively, or, in other words, when there is impairment. If a patient is able to incrementally overcome a movement impairment there should be no need for passive treatment. The use of passive treatment is simply to stimulate physiological function, which would normally be a direct result of restoration of active movement.

With regard to the obvious question of how manual therapy treatment or management reduces pain, the premise is again simple. It is suggested that pain is controlled and reduces as a natural consequence of the enhancement of physiological and biological function and a return towards homeostasis. As homeostasis of the local environment is reached tissue sensitization reduces, mechanosensitivity thresholds increase and pain reduction is regarded as a natural consequence. This is no different to the experience of any individual who has sprained their ankle. Pain reduces as function is restored. Function is restored as a consequence of a natural process. When this process is hampered or requires enhancement external assistance is instigated.

With regard to the next logical question of how manual therapy results in the resolution of non-organic effects, the premise is given that as pain control is gained, these effects resolve accordingly. Suffering which accompanies pain will resolve with pain control, on the proviso that the suffering is within the context of the organic pathology.

The use of treatment and management and their effects can be considered when continuous passive motion is utilized in the rehabilitation of a disorder involving the knee. It is accepted that an inability actively to move the knee due to pain appears to have a deleterious effect on recovery. Passive movement is instigated only because of an inability to move the knee actively or adequately due to pain. Passive movement leads to increased mobility and the ability to move actively, more adequately. As active movement improves and is restored, pain control is a natural consequence. A natural consequence of this is a resolution of suffering. The passive movement has been used only and solely to replicate the effects of unavailable or inadequate active movement – nothing more, nothing less. With the improvement and restoration of active movement, passive movement becomes redundant. Passive movement has not been a 'technique' of treatment directly inducing pain control. Rather it has served the purpose of re-establishing normal physiological and biological function and hence promoting active movement and related pain control. Passive movement was a treatment, whereas management would involve long-term rehabilitation.

While a focus has been placed upon tissue pathology or organic morbidity, it is acknowledged that a disorder is much more complex than tissue pathology. Also it is acknowledged that the experience of pain is much more than nociception associated with peripheral tissue pathology. This is taken into account in the discussion on a disorder where a disorder represents much more than pathology. However, regardless of the scope of manual therapy, when a disorder is suited to manual therapy treatment it must have as its basis a peripheral process of pathology. Furthermore, this peripheral pathology must be the feature which dominates the disorder. For a disorder to be suited to manual therapy intervention the wider effects of the disorder, including the non-organic effects such as suffering and any complaint of pain, must continue to be driven by a physical pathology. Again taking as an example the rehabilitation of a disorder involving the knee, continuous passive motion is used because the patient is unable to move the knee effectively. This is generally a direct consequence of pain. Pain in this case is associated with local pathology in the form of abnormal increased tissue sensitivity and decreased tissue mechanosensitivity thresholds. It is tissue sensitivity which prevents active movement. Any applied treatment must influence the abnormal tissue sensitivity and decreased tissue mechanosensitivity thresholds. With sufficient pharmacological pain control the abnormal tissue sensitivity is favourably influenced, tissue mechanosensitivity thresholds are increased and the patient can move the knee more readily. Physical treatment must likewise have the same effect. If, on the other hand, an individual is unable or unwilling to move the knee for non-organic reasons rather than because of pain, pharmacology for pain control in isolation would be an inappropriate treatment. For the same reason physical treatment would also be inappropriate.

For physical treatment to be indicated there must be some feature of a disorder to which it can be directed in an appropriate way. This would be the physical pathology of the disorder. On the other hand, as previously explained, management strategies may well be appropriate in the resolution of a disorder involving the knee when active movement was impaired as a consequence of non-organic effects.

With regard to the above, it must be understood that all manual therapy intervention, whether treatment or management should be carried out within a cognitive behavioural framework.

Summary

- Treatment provides the stimulus towards normalization of physiological and hence biological function.
- Physiological and biological functions are the effects of active movement and localized function.
- Treatment replicates these effects in the absence of active movement and localized function.
- Physiological and biological function promotes homeostasis.
- Treatment produces an effect at a cellular level.
- Management allows the stabilization of physiological and hence biological functions resulting in the stabilization of homeostasis.
- Pain control is dependent upon a reduction in abnormal tissue sensitivity and increased tissue mechanosensitivity thresholds.
- Tissue sensitivity is reduced and tissue mechanosensitivity thresholds are increased as a natural consequence of a return or stabilization of physiological and biological

functions and as a consequence of a return to, or stabilization of, homeostasis.

- The non-organic effects of a disorder will favourably resolve as pain is controlled, provided they remain within the context of the pathology of the disorder.
- It is considered that when the non-organic effects of a disorder have become morbid in nature the disorder will not be favourably influenced simply by the control of pain.
- For a disorder where the non-organic effects have become morbid in nature, or when they are overwhelming, manual therapy treatment does not have the capability to change the nature of the disorder. However, in certain circumstances, management may be indicated, if the aim is to promote functional restoration in conjunction with the primary intervention for the non-organic effects.
- Manual therapy intervention, whether treatment or management, must be carried out within a cognitive behavioural framework.

INDICATIONS AND CONTRAINDICATIONS OF MANUAL THERAPY

Manual therapy cannot be considered a panacea, nor should it be considered indicated for all disorders of the neuro-musculo-skeletal system which have commonly been referred to as 'mechanical' in nature. It has been stated previously that manual therapy has limitations. These limitations may preclude manual therapy for many disorders commonly referred to as 'non-specific spinal pain', 'simple neck or back pain' or 'mechanical spinal pain'. The limitations of manual therapy would most certainly preclude its use in many disorders where physical 'techniques of treatment' would commonly be instigated based upon the signs and symptoms of the disorder. And yet many such disorders might be considered to be 'mechanical'. The contribution of manual therapy towards health care is governed by the ability of manual therapy intervention to favourably influence a disorder towards recovery. When manual therapy intervention does not have this capability it is not indicated. If it is not indicated it is contraindicated. At the same time, under certain circumstances manual therapy management may be indicated when it does not have the capacity to favourably influence the disorder providing it has another role.

Throughout this chapter, manual therapy is associated with a disorder rather than a patient complaint. A disorder has been defined in a manner which embraces much more than the patient's complaint. A complaint of spinal pain is frequently regarded in terms of 'non-specific spinal pain', 'simple neck or back pain' or 'mechanical neck or back pain'. These terms simply mean serious or specific pathology has been ruled out as a cause of the pain. The terms do not give sufficient recognition to the accompanying effects of a complaint of pain. As such, there is the common implication that

physical treatment is automatically indicated. This is not the case. The ability of manual therapy to favourably influence a disorder towards recovery cannot be judged unless the nature of the disorder is fully understood. A disorder should not be defined simply as 'non-specific spinal pain', 'simple neck or back pain' or 'mechanical neck or back pain'. This ignores the nature and wider ramifications of the disorder resulting in spinal pain. Without recognizing the total disorder, appropriate intervention cannot be prescribed. Manual therapy is not indicated for neck or back pain simply by ruling out serious or specific pathology

In the determination of the indications for manual therapy there is one basic consideration. This consideration is based upon a rationale as to how manual therapy works and whether it has the potential to favourably influence the disorder. This consideration is the fundamental reason why it is so important to present a rationale for the potential effects and benefits of manual therapy. With respect to this, two case examples of low back pain have previously been given where in one case, manual therapy was indicated and in the other it was contraindicated. Both cases had the same diagnosis; however, the classifications were different. In the first case classification involved movement dysfunction while in the second case the classification was psychosocial. In this case it was stated therefore that manual therapy was contraindicated. Why? Simply because it was not indicated. Why was it not indicated? Because manual therapy, in offering physical intervention, would not provide the means towards recovery.

By considering the appropriateness for manual therapy in keeping with the diagnosis, classification and stage of a disorder the indications and contraindications become readily apparent. There should be no requirement to list specific diagnoses under contraindications for manual therapy. In order to determine the contraindications to manual therapy a simple question should be asked, namely what potential does manual therapy have, to favourably influence the particular disorder. For example, malignancy, fractures, osteoporosis, osteomyelitis, tuberculosis, aortic aneurysm, cauda equina syndrome, etc. are disorder diagnoses frequently cited as contraindications for manual therapy. Clearly, in these examples and in many more frequently cited manual therapy has nothing to offer. It is not even a consideration. Medical intervention is indicated and manual therapy as a 'treatment' for the condition is naturally contraindicated for two reasons: firstly, it has nothing to offer and secondly, another form of intervention does.

In considering indications and contraindications for manual therapy a clear distinction is required between treatment and management. This has been previously stated. While a (compression) fracture of the thoracic spine is a contraindication for manual therapy treatment, it does not necessarily contraindicate manual therapy management. This could take the form of management of the patient. It would not relate directly to the fracture but to the effects of the fracture. For example this might involve various strategies such as posture control, activity modification and functional exercise. At all times the intention of manual therapy is really the question as to whether it is indicated or contraindicated. This generally is based upon clinical reasoning but it is in the main common sense. Does the disorder diagnosis, classification and stage provide an indication for treatment or management or a combination of the two? For example, common sense suggests that treatment in the form of a manipulation procedure is contraindicated for a disorder diagnosis of spondylolisthesis and that management strategies of motor control intervention are indicated. Segmental hypomobility associated with a painful impairment of movement would indicate procedures of treatment as the prime intervention, with strategies of management, such as specific exercise, being prescribed in order to enhance and maintain the effects of the treatment.

Finally there is a need to consider any contraindications for procedures of treatment or strategies of management resulting from a feature unrelated to the disorder such as co-morbidity or due to other opinions. Potential vertebrobasilar arterial insufficiency, for example, automatically contraindicates certain procedures of treatment, even though that treatment may be indicated as an intervention for the disorder.

If manual therapy has the potential to favourably influence a disorder towards recovery it is indicated, providing another form of intervention is not more suitable. If manual therapy is not indicated it is contraindicated. Manual therapy treatment procedures or management strategies which might be indicated become contraindicated if there is any potential for causing harm.

Indications

The indications for manual therapy intervention are based upon the following questions:

- Is the nature of the patient complaint suitable for manual therapy?
- In general, is the apparent nature of the disorder suitable for manual therapy?
- Is the disorder diagnosis suitable for manual therapy? Does it involve physical or organic pathology which might be favourably influenced by manual therapy?
- Is the disorder classification suitable for manual therapy? Does it involve the presence of organic features which dominate over any non-organic features and which might be favourably influenced by manual therapy?
- Is the disorder stage suitable for manual therapy?
- Have all considerations been given and appropriate evaluations been carried out to ensure that the proposed intervention does not have the potential to cause harm?
- Is the patient compliant with the proposed intervention?
- Does the proposed intervention satisfy the intent of the patient referral?
- Has informed consent for manual therapy intervention been obtained?

Contraindications

The contraindications for manual therapy intervention are when:

- Any other form of intervention is more appropriate.
- The nature of the patient is unsuited for manual therapy.
- The nature of the disorder in terms of the diagnosis, classification and stage is unsuited for manual therapy.
- There are any unrelated features to the disorder, or co-morbidity, which mean that manual therapy or certain interventions are contraindicated.
- The intent of the patient referral is not satisfied by the proposed intervention.
- The patient is likely to have any type of adverse reaction to manual therapy.
- Any form of harm may result.
- Informed consent has not been obtained.
- The patient is affected by alcohol or illicit drugs.

EVIDENCE BASED PRACTICE IN MANUAL THERAPY

Manual therapy rates poorly when documented evidence for treatment efficacy is examined. There is significant debate regarding the efficacy of manual therapy treatment for acute low back pain (Maher et al 1999), and little evidence for the efficacy of manual therapy treatment for chronic low back pain (Koes et al 1996). While the reasons for this should be obvious they appear to be overlooked in the academic appraisal of manual therapy. The more obvious reasons can be listed:

- It appears that there is a general lack of consideration that a group of individuals with a complaint of non-specific mechanical neck or low back pain is not a homogeneous group.
- There is a general lack of consideration that a complaint of neck or back pain is only a feature of a disorder. In itself pain is not a disorder.
- There is a general lack of appreciation that a reduction in pain does not necessarily result in a resolution of the disorder.
- There appears to be a necessity to continually search for a physical 'technique' or 'protocol' which will favourably influence pain.
- There appears to be continuous clamour for supremacy in the physical treatment of the spine by different professional groups.
- There is a lack of appreciation that manual therapy has a scope of practice which includes many interventions and that these interventions must be utilized systematically and incrementally towards the resolution of a disorder.
- There appears to be a lack of appreciation that disorders are different even though there may be a superficial pattern or sameness and complaint of pain.

Evidence based practice is determined as a result of systematic reviews and meta-analyses of randomized controlled trials. The vast majority of randomized controlled trials which are subject to scrutiny for evidence based practice involve 'techniques' of treatment used in isolation in non-specific patient populations. This is erroneously regarded as research into manual therapy. Techniques of treatment used in isolation do not represent manual therapy and research into their individual effectiveness does not in our opinion represent research into manual therapy.

There are a number of randomized controlled trials which have investigated 'treatment protocols' such as that proposed by McKenzie (1981). Studies compare the effectiveness of such protocols to manipulation (Cherkin et al 1998). 'Techniques of treatment' are taken out of the context of manual therapy and are used academically in a manner which demonstrates a lack of appreciation of the distinction between a complaint of pain and a disorder. The 'McKenzie protocol' is a physical approach to the alleviation of spinal pain. It is in fact manual therapy. The appreciation of this fact is lacking, with the conclusion that 'while there is evidence for the benefits of the McKenzie protocol for the treatment of low back pain there isn't for manual therapy' (McKenzie 2000). This is a contradiction in terms.

It appears futile to continue the pursuit for efficacy of mobilization, manipulation or any other technique of treatment when used in isolation to intervene in a disorder. In fact to refer to these isolated techniques as manual therapy is misleading and incorrect. However when a 'protocol' for intervention has the scope to deal with a specific disorder it should show a favourable outcome. The scope of practice which is suitable for an acute disorder is not necessarily suitable for a chronic disorder and vice versa. A broad scope of practice which is suitable for both acute and chronic disorders is required.

A disorder which evolves as a result of an ankle sprain is a good example to cite when discussing the evidence based practice of manual therapy for a complaint of spinal pain. It appears well accepted that an ankle sprain may be quite different in different individuals. That is, the disorder, which has as its genesis an injury resulting in a sprain of an ankle, is different in different individuals. This is dependent upon organic and non-organic factors and consideration is given to the following:

- While most ankle sprains resolve without chronicity some continue on to become chronic.
- While an ankle sprain mostly does not result in abnormal non-organic effects it is possible that it may do so.
- While most ankle sprains do not result in long-term movement impairment some do.
- While most ankle sprains do not result in instability some do.
- In the immediate acute stage there is generally no requirement to specify the pathology providing fractures, a dislocation or subluxation is excluded.

- While a sprained ankle may be a diagnostic term, it leads to a disorder which is a wider manifestation of the ankle injury.
- There is a general consensus that management is required and treatment may be required.
- Management is prescribed according to the requirements of a particular disorder involving an ankle sprain.
- Treatment is prescribed according to the necessity to promote a resolution of the pathology of the disorder, that is, the tissues involved in the injury.
- Management and treatment progress from rest, non-weight bearing, partial weight bearing, active treatment with mobilization exercise, active rehabilitation with graded functional exercise and graded activity eventually leading to a return to normal activity.
- Management and treatment are intended to prevent further tissue damage and to provide the optimum environment for the natural resolution of the ankle sprain.
- When the individual is incapable of performing adequate active movement, passive treatment is instigated as a means of replicating the effects of the unavailable active movement.
- There may be a requirement for specific treatment according to individual differences associated with the pathology of the disorder and management associated with particular differences associated with the disorder in general.
- Resultant instability requires specific management.
- When suffering is a feature of the disorder it may require management.
- Non-organic effects and occasionally non-organic morbidity of the disorder may be the main concern and require specific management.
- Generally individuals will seek advice and treatment following an ankle sprain.
- There is a necessity for healthcare providers to cater for the requirements of an individual following an ankle sprain.
- There may be no associated effects of any consequence resulting from an ankle sprain and in this case the disorder is the ankle sprain. The disorder may resolve naturally without the need for any form of treatment or management prescription.
- When an ankle sprain leads to more complex associated effects and hence a more complex disorder the requirement for treatment or management might be more extensive, resolution may be more difficult and in some cases there may never be a satisfactory resolution.

Randomized controlled trials into the efficacy of manual therapy for spinal pain exclude subjects for whom physical treatments would be contraindicated. This leaves a treatment group considered to have non-specific 'mechanical' spinal pain or simple neck or back pain. Mostly, but not always, individuals with this category of neck or low back pain can identify the onset as being related to a physical event. It could therefore be suggested that a tissue sprain or strain has occurred. A sprained ankle is a tissue sprain and therefore a common approach to intervention should be indicated in this situation, as it should be in that of a tissue sprain relating to spinal pain.

This chapter challenges the evidence which is given as to the efficacy of manual therapy in the treatment of spinal pain. It is considered manual therapy has not been adequately researched. If a study is to be undertaken into the efficacy of manual therapy towards the resolution of a disorder of spinal pain, the methodology has to be suitable to intervene in the disorder. It has to be of broad enough scope to allow treatment and management of various types according to the classification and stage of a disorder. It also has to allow for the individual differences in the manner in which disorders associated with the complaint of spinal pain will present. Developing a methodology in keeping with these requirements would appear academically very difficult to control, due to the many variables in the presentation of disorders and therefore in the many variations of intervention required towards their resolution.

The position held is that when pain of spinal origin is suitable for manual therapy the intervention prescribed should take into account a common sense approach which relies upon defining the disorder associated with the pain and providing optimal circumstances leading towards its natural resolution. There is ample clinical evidence in support of this approach. Finally, the scope of intervention where treatment and management are defined differently is essential to the recognition of the potential efficacy of manual therapy. This may seem unnecessary to many and in addition the two terms are commonly used interchangeably in health care. However, it is essential to present them differently in order to understand the need for different interventions and different strategies for different disorders and for different stages of those disorders.

IMPORTANCE OF DIAGNOSTICS TO MANUAL THERAPY

Three generic presentations of disorders involving an ankle sprain demonstrate the importance of diagnostics. These presentations are used in order to illustrate the broad indications and contraindications for manual therapy in selected disorders of musculoskeletal and specifically spinal pain.

Acute ankle sprain
The first disorder involving an acute ankle sprain is represented by a dominance of organic features with associated non-organic features (Fig. 33.1). The non-organic features are considered normal and within the context of the initiating event or injury, within the context of the organic features and of the disorder.

Organic features:

- Morbidity – ligamentous and other soft tissue pathology resulting in increased tissue sensitivity and lowered tissue mechanosensitivity thresholds.

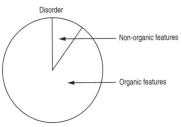

Figure 33.1   The complaint of acute ankle pain following a sprain.

- Effects – limited active movement or movement impairment, inability to ambulate, disability and inability to participate.

Non-organic features:

- Effects – pain: directly related to the organic morbidity and induced by inflammatory and mechanical stimuli. Complaint of pain severity in context with the event or injury. Suffering: directly related to pain and the organic effects.

Manual therapy intervention indicated:

- Management – prescribed graded rest in order to prevent further tissue harm and mechanical induced stimuli. Strategies to stabilize the immediate effects of the injury.
- Management in the form of active mobilization to overcome movement impairment.
- Management in the form of active rehabilitation which would include ankle proprioception, motor control, coordination and strength, to overcome disability.
- General patient functional rehabilitation aimed at a return to normal participation.

As the disorder progressed normally to resolution and the individual returned to normal participation it would be presumed all non-organic effects would likewise resolve.

When an event or injury leading to a sprain of the low back results in a complaint of acute low back pain, the intervention should be no different in principle to the example given above for a disorder involving an acute ankle sprain, providing the same balance of organic features to non-organic features existed in the disorder.

Subacute to chronic ankle sprain
Case examples of two disorders involving subacute to chronic ankle sprains are presented (Figs 33.2A and 33.2B). The disorder in A is represented by a dominance of organic features, with associated non-organic features in context with the disorder, where in case B the non-organic features are considered excessive and abnormal.

Organic features:

- Morbidity – possibly due to a lack of full repair and remodelling with ligamentous and other soft tissue pathology remaining to some extent. In A continuing increased tissue sensitivity and lowered tissue mechanosensitivity thresholds are observed but to a lesser extent than in an acute stage. In B abnormally

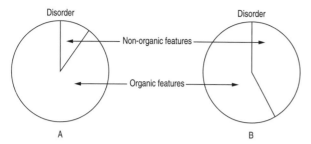

Figure 33.2 Case examples of two disorders involving subacute to chronic ankle sprains. The disorder in A is represented by a dominance of organic features, with associated non-organic features. In case B the non-organic features are excessive and abnormal.

lowered mechanosensitivity thresholds (high levels of tissue sensitization) are noted.

- Effects – in A limited active movement to some degree resulting in some physical impairment, inability to function fully, minor disability, inability to participate fully. In B limitation in range of movement with high levels of functional impairment and disability noted.

Non-organic features:

- Effects – pain A: directly related to the continuing organic morbidity and induced by mechanical stimuli. Less severe than in an acute stage. B: directly related to the continuing organic morbidity and induced by mechanical stimuli but exaggerated.

Suffering: A: related to a degree of pain and the organic effects of the disorder, more so related to an inability to participate fully. B: abnormal and excessive, related to fear avoidance. Severe disability and an inability to participate to a large degree.

Manual therapy intervention indicated:

- A and B: treatment aimed at the movement impairment complemented with management consisting of active mobilization to restore full mobility.
- A and B: management with active rehabilitation to include ankle proprioception, motor control, coordination and strength.
- B: management with a primary emphasis on cognitive coping strategies aimed at reducing the level of the non-organic effects of suffering and disability to a more normal expected level.
- A and B: general patient functional rehabilitation aimed at a return to full participation.

In case B an essential form of intervention is management for the non-organic features. In both cases the non-organic features should resolve with successful intervention leading to full or an acceptable level of participation.

For a complaint of subacute or chronic low back pain following the non-resolution of an acute episode due to an event or injury leading to a sprain, intervention for the resultant disorder should reflect the same process as that given in these two case examples of ankle sprain.

Chronic ankle sprain with dominant non-organic effects

This case example is of a disorder involving a chronic ankle sprain, represented by a dominance of non-organic features which appear totally out of context with the history and the presentation of the resultant disorder (Fig. 33.3).

Non-organic features:

- Morbidity – possible evidence of psychiatric disturbance.
- Effects – gross suffering consisting of fear-avoidance, abnormal illness behaviour, marked disability and inability to participate.

Organic features:

- Morbidity –?? may be some evidence of lack of full repair.
- Effects – ?? unable to ambulate effectively, this may be due to non-resolved morbidity but more likely a result of the non-organic features.

Manual therapy intervention would be inappropriate as the primary intervention and is therefore contraindicated. However, a case could be presented for functional exercise as an addition to appropriate psychosocial intervention. Functional exercise, if undertaken, could not be considered as having a primary role towards the resolution of the disorder. It would be instigated to improve or maintain the physical function of the individual with the disorder. That is, the manual therapy 'provision of exercise' would not be prescribed for the primary management of the disorder.

With a 'sprain' of the low back resulting in a chronic low back pain disorder where the non-organic features dominate, manual therapy would not be indicated. The comment regarding functional exercise, given in the case example of a chronic ankle sprain, would apply also to a disorder involving chronic low back pain, when the non-organic features were excessive and abnormal.

DIAGNOSTICS AND CHRONIC LOW BACK PAIN

Manual therapists commonly classify patients purely on the basis of signs and symptoms such as the presence of spinal pain, movement impairment or motor control dysfunction, without determining the underlying basis of the

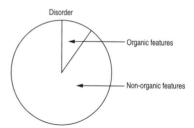

Figure 33.3 Case example of a disorder involving chronic ankle sprain. The disorder is represented in this case by a dominance of non-organic features totally out of context with the history and the resultant disorder.

disorder. This frequently leads to inappropriate or prescriptive applications of treatment or management of these disorders, resulting in poor outcomes. All disorders involving pain of the lumbopelvic region result in reflex motor control changes with associated movement or control impairments. The mere presence of these impairments does not imply that they represent the underlying basis for the disorder, or that correcting these impairments will resolve the disorder.

Classification systems must consider the variety of pathological processes and bio-psycho-social factors involved in all disorders that result in spinal pain. Some of these disorders are amenable to manual therapy and some are not. It is critical for the manual therapist to classify disorders involving pain on the basis of the history and the clinical presentation of the disorder while taking into consideration medical investigations and imaging as well as tissue pathology, to determine if manual therapy is indicated. If manual therapy is indicated, the disorder classification and staging determines what specific approach to treatment and/or management is necessary to facilitate the resolution of the disorder.

Disorders of the lumbopelvic region can be sub-classified into three broad groups from a manual therapy intervention perspective. The first group involves disorders involving spinal pain that are associated with movement impairment and motor control dysfunction as a protective or guarding response to the underlying disorder. Attempts to correct the movement impairment or normalize the faulty motor patterns in these disorders frequently results in exacerbation of pain (Fig. 33.4). The second group of disorders are characterized by an underlying primary psychiatric or psychosocial basis for the disorder associated with pain, movement impairment and motor control dysfunction. In this group manual therapy intervention in isolation is likely to be ineffective (Fig. 33.5). There appears to be a third group of subjects who present with disorders where either their movement impairment or control impairments maintain or contribute to their pain state (Fig. 33.6). There may be a component of non-organic signs associated with these disorders but they do not dominate the disorder. These patients appear very amenable to specifically directed manual therapy intervention, based on a cognitive behavioural model, to either control or resolve the disorder. The following case studies highlight the importance of diagnostics for the appropriate application of manual therapy interventions in lumbopelvic pain disorders.

The examples given in Figures 33.4 to 33.6 and in the following case studies are not exhaustive but are presented to document the importance of determining a disorder diagnosis, classification and stage to ascertain the indications and contraindications for manual therapy.

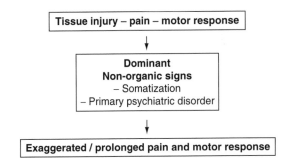

Figure 33.5 Disorder of the lumbopelvic region: underlying primary psychiatric or psychological basis for pain.

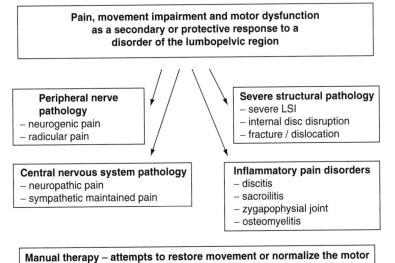

Figure 33.4 Disorder of the lumbopelvic region: spinal pain guarding or protecting underlying disorder.

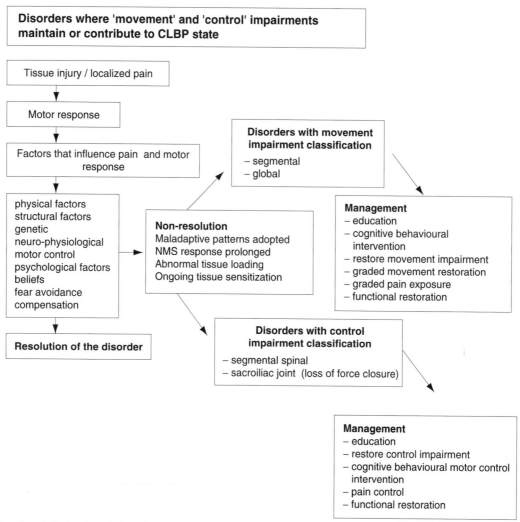

Figure 33.6   Disorder of the lumbopelvic region: movement impairment or control impairments maintaining or contributing to pain state.

CASE STUDY 1

A 28-year-old man reports a 2-year history of disabling left-sided chronic low back pain. The history involved a flexion/rotation lifting injury while working in the garden. He reported that, following relaxing on the sofa that evening, his back became painful and stiff. The next morning he found it very difficult to weight bear and reported a spinal deformity with his spine in a flexed and laterally deviated posture to the left. He reported severe pain when attempting to 'straighten his back'. He consulted a doctor and was instructed to rest for a few days; however, due to work commitments he continued with his sedentary desk work which involved sitting for long periods of time. After 3 weeks (while taking pain relieving medication) he was still unable to stand straight without deviation. He consulted his doctor again and was prescribed NSAIDs and was told to take some time off work and rest. After 3 weeks of resting he reported some improvement in the pain, was able to stand more erect, but was still laterally deviated. He then consulted a physiotherapist who prescribed a stabilizing exercise routine in conjunction with real-time ultrasound with a graduated progression into Pilates. He reported minimal improvement over a 4-month period and reported pain when activating his transversus abdominis and lumbar multifidus muscles.

He reported that his symptoms were exacerbated by assuming any upright postures such as standing and walking, as well as by spinal movements of backward and left side bending. Flexion movements of the spine were pain-free. He reported he was concerned that he could not stand without an obvious lateral deviation of his trunk in relation to his pelvis and that attempts to correct this provoked pain. Because of this he reported that he avoided performing movements and activities that provoked his pain due to fear of further exacerbation of the disorder. He was working full time.

Physical examination
Observation

An obvious lateral shift was noted in standing with the thoracolumbar spine markedly deviated to the right

In sitting the patient leaned to the right side

AROM	Flexion – full range of motion with some lateral deviation to the right noted
	Extension – 10° of backward bending with obvious lateral deviation of the thoracolumbar spine to the right and the report of pain
	Right side bending – full and pain-free
	Left side bending – markedly restricted and painful
	Lateral shift of the thoracolumbar spine to the left was restricted and painful
	Repeated movement into impairment reduced pain and increased movement
CM	Marked restriction and pain with left side bending and extension
Neuro	normal
Motion palpation	L4/L5 – hypomobile especially in extension, left side bending and left rotation
	Provocation palpation of L4 and L5 centrally and over the left L4/L5 facet joint – reproduced pain
SIJ	NAD
SLR	NAD
Slump test	NAD

Motor control

1. Functional movement tests. Gait, single leg stand, sit to stand and squat were associated with obvious lateral deviation of the thoracolumbar spine to the right
2. Specific muscle tests. Inability to isolate the activation of the pelvic floor or transverse abdominal muscles without further bracing whole abdominal wall, back muscles and breath holding with reports of pain. Attempts at activating lumbar multifidus in prone revealed an inability to activate on the left

Investigations	MRI 2000 – NAD
Diagnosis	L4/L5 back strain
Classification	Movement impairment disorder (segmental) – L4/L5 left lateral shift
Stage	Chronic – stable
Manual therapy indicated?	Yes
Treatment?	Yes – mobilization L4/L5 in combined movement of left rotation/left side bending and extension
Management?	Yes – mobilization exercises to restore lateral shift and extension

movement impairments. Once spinal mobility has been restored patient given postural advice, taught to activate postural stabilizing muscles in upright postures and return to normal function

Outcome – excellent

The disorder diagnosis of *back sprain* is based upon the history, the clinical presentation, normal findings on medical imaging and the absence of a specific diagnosis. The disorder classification of this patient as a *movement impairment disorder (segmental)* is based on the non-resolution of a back strain that has left the patient with a specific and consistent movement impairment at a segmental level. The stage of the disorder is *chronic* and stable. The patient reports a mechanical basis to his pain disorder with consistent and repeatable active movement, functional movement, passive movement and pain provocation signs that relate to an impairment of movement at the L4/L5 spinal segment. This patient avoids provoking pain by not moving into the movement impairment due to perception that he will cause further injury and provocation. The basis of this pain disorder is a loss of normal physiological tissue compliance due to avoidant behaviour, resulting in abnormal tissue strain and loading, tissue sensitization and pain. Secondary motor inhibition and muscle dysfunction are sequelae of this disorder.

Intervention is based on a cognitive behavioural framework. Treatment of the disorder logically focuses on the restoration of normal tissue compliance in the impaired movement direction, with passive and active movement techniques. This is combined with management strategies with graded active movement encouraged into the new found range and the restoration of functional movement capacity. The patient must be assured that the pain provoked is not dangerous or damaging, but is directed to restore normal spinal function. As the movement impairment is restored the disorder resolves. Direct motor control intervention with these disorders is not indicated unless the restoration of normal tissue compliance is first achieved.

CASE STUDY 2

A 30-year-old man reports a 2-year history of severe and disabling chronic low back pain. History involved a flexion/rotation lifting injury while working in a mine. He reported that he was instructed to continue to work without a rest although he was in severe pain. He further reported that he was able to work only if he consciously dynamically splinted his spine. He continued working for 1 month, after which he was laid off work with severe and disabling low back pain. He had not returned to work since this time.

He reported undergoing various interventions which gave him short-term relief. These included physiotherapy dynamic stabilization exercises, facet joint injections, TENS, massage, psychological and medical intervention. All rehabilitation programmes markedly exacerbated his symptoms. His condition worsened with time.

He reported that his symptoms were exacerbated by any exertion, forward bending activities and extension activities such as standing, walking, swimming. He reported a constant tension in his back that he could not relieve. He was told that his problem was in his head and he should live with it. He was depressed, very anxious, fearful and highly disabled. He reported suffering from an anxiety disorder prior to his injury.

Physical examination

Observation	Generalized increase in lumbar lordosis
	Observable hypertonicity of the lumbar erector spinae and abdominal wall
	Laboured breathing was noted
	Standing and sitting postures were accented with very erect and rigid posture of the lumbar spine
AROM	Flexion – 30° in forward bending – it was noted that this was achieved with hip flexion while the thoracolumbar spine was held in lordosis with the report of pain
	Extension – 10° of backward bending achieved with hip extension with the lumbar spine held rigid and the report of pain
	Right and left side bending – were also rigid and limited in motion
	Repeated movement into flexion and extension further increased muscle guarding and pain
Neuro	Normal
Palpation	Motion palpation L5–L1 flexion, extension, (L) & (R) rotation – hypomobile
	Provocation palpation of L4 and L5 (central) – reproduced pain
	Palpation of the back and abdominal wall muscles revealed very high tone and an inability to relax the muscles
SLR	NAD
Slump test	NAD – trunk flexion limited

Motor control

1. Functional movement tests. All movements were limited with associated rigid spinal motion and breath holding. Forward bending, reaching, sit to stand and squat were associated with splinting of the lumbar spine

in lordosis and reports of pain. When the patient was encouraged to flex the spine, breath holding and support with his hands was noted. Relaxation of the spinal posture into slump sitting and relaxation of the abdominal wall, use of diaphragm breathing reduced back pain
2. Specific movement tests. Inability to initiate posterior or anterior pelvic tilt, with the thorax rigid on the pelvis. Supine, side lying and four-point kneeling – splinting of the abdominal wall and apical breathing was noted at rest
3. Specific muscle tests. Inability to isolate the activation of the pelvic floor or transverse abdominal muscles without further bracing whole abdominal wall, back muscles and breath holding. Inability to perform relaxed belly breathing. Short hip flexors in Thomas test position.

Investigations	Plain X-ray – NAD
	MRI 2000 – NAD, healthy lumbar multifidus was noted
Diagnosis	Severe back strain
Classification	Movement impairment (global) – muscle guarding disorder
	Non-organic signs also present although not dominant
Stage	Chronic – stable
Manual therapy indicated?	Yes – in conjunction with psychological intervention
Treatment?	Yes – inhibitory deep soft tissue massage and stretching of trunk and hip muscles
Management?	Yes – motor control management to reduce trunk muscle tone, focus on encouraging relaxed posture and normal movement patterns without muscle guarding, incorporating muscle stretching and mobilization exercises to restore movement

Outcome – excellent

The disorder diagnosis of *back sprain* was based upon the history, the clinical presentation, normal findings on medical imaging and the absence of a specific diagnosis. The classification of this patient as a *movement impairment (global) – muscle guarding disorder,* is based on the non-resolution of a back strain that is associated with an exaggerated and prolonged reflex muscle guarding response of the trunk muscles, leading to a multidirectional *movement* impairment disorder of the lumbar spine. The stage of the disorder is chronic and stable. The patient presents with multidirectional movement impairment of the thoracolumbar spine with associated pain and observable trunk muscle co-contraction and guarding. This movement impairment is consistent in all active, functional and passive movement tests. The patient is anxious and fearful of movement. He perceives that spinal movement may damage his spine further, continually 'protects' his spine and is unable to relax his trunk muscles.

This exaggerated protective reaction to pain manifests itself in high levels of co-contraction of the abdominal wall, diaphragm (associated with breath holding or apical breathing) and back muscles with generation of high levels of intra-abdominal pressure, resulting in excessive spinal compression and multidirectional restriction of spinal movement. This chronic abnormal spinal loading results in further sensitization of nociceptive tissue promoting the maintenance of the pain disorder. Both organic signs and non-organic signs are present in this disorder. These pain disorders commonly coexist with underlying anxiety disorders and high levels of fear-avoidance behaviour.

Manual therapy intervention for this disorder is based on a cognitive behavioural framework. It is critical to give the patient reassurance that the spine is not damaged and that relaxation of the trunk muscles and normalization of movement patterns will reduce the stress on their spine and decrease pain. This process involves averting the patient's focus from their pain to reduce the muscle guarding protective responses they have adopted. This can be facilitated by treatment strategies such as soft tissue massage, inhibitory muscle stretching, postural relaxation, relaxed diaphragm breathing and regular low level aerobic exercise. As the reduction in trunk muscle co-activation occurs, so too does the movement impairment and pain levels due to the normalization of physiological movement and tissue loading. Management of the disorder involves gradually encouraging the adoption of normal patterns of functional movement and cognitive strategies to reduce the protective focus for the back pain disorder. Psychological intervention may also be necessary if there is a dominating coexisting anxiety disorder. Passive treatment intervention in isolation is contraindicated in this disorder due to its non-organic features. Stabilizing exercises and resistance training are contraindicated in the early intervention of these disorders, as this will cause further facilitation of trunk muscle co-contraction, resulting in exacerbation of the disorder.

CASE STUDY 3

A 45-year-old woman reports a 7-year history of chronic low back pain. It began insidiously while she was working as a nurse. She reported that it was exacerbated by repetitive sustained forward bending postures she had to perform during her work duties. She was initially investigated with plain X-rays, with no abnormality detected. She underwent numerous treatment interventions which gave her only short-term relief. Her condition worsened with time and she had to cease her work as a nurse and entered administration work. She was again investigated with plain X-rays and again no abnormality was detected. Her disorder progressed further, resulting in severe low back pain and high levels of disability. She underwent a CT and MRI scan 6½ years after the onset of her low back pain. On this occasion it was apparent that she had developed a degenerative spondylolisthesis at L4/L5. There was no trauma in the intervening time between investigations. At this time she underwent pain management, with facet joint injections, followed by rhyzotomy at L4/L5 which did not afford her long-term relief. A dynamic stabilization exercise intervention exacerbated her pain condition. She then underwent a discogram, which identified disc disruption at L3/L4, L4/L5 and L5/S1, with pain provocation at L4/L5. She was referred for surgical opinion and was given the option of a multilevel fusion.

She reported that her symptoms were exacerbated by any sustained and repeated forward bending and extension activities such as standing, walking, swimming or overhead work such as hanging out washing. She reported 'clunking' of her back when performing these activities and relief of her symptoms with sustained flexion exercises such as supine knees to chest and slumped sitting.

Physical examination

Observation	Generalized increase in lumbar lordosis with a notable step of the spinous process at L4/L5
	Observable hypertrophy of the lumbar erector spinae
	Standing and sitting postures were accented with very erect hyperextended posture of the lumbar spine
AROM	Flexion – in forward bending it was noted that she maintained hyperlordosis until mid-range of motion where she experienced pain, then she flexed to full range with no pain at the end of range. On mid-range return to neutral she again hyperextended her spine and this was associated with central pain at L4/L5
	Extension – 30° of backward bending with the onset of pain. Hinging at L4/L5 and a 'clunking' sound was noted. There was no posterior pelvic rotation associated with this movement
	Right and left side bending – low back pain and a 'clunking' sound was noted
	Repeated movement into extension increased back pain while repeated flexion (knees to chest in supine lying) reduced back pain
Neuro	Normal

PPIVM L4/L5 – hypermobile with crepitius	Provocation palpation of L4/L5 central and Z Jt – very painful
Neural tissue provocation tests	NAD

Motor control

1. Functional movement tests. Forward bending, reaching, sit to stand and squat were associated with hyperlordotic posturing of the lumbar spine and pain. When the patient was encouraged to flex the spine this was associated with a painful arc at mid-range. Breath holding and use of the hands to support the trunk were also observed during load transfer

2. Specific movement tests. Inability to initiate posterior pelvic rotation in standing with a tendency to flex hips. Supine – ASLR was associated with the sensation and pain and heaviness with splinting of the abdominal wall and hyperextension of the spine. No relief was reported with pelvic compression. Supine – attempts to initiate posterior pelvic rotation were associated with hyperextension of the spine and splinting of the abdominal wall. Prone – hip extension and knee flexion were associated with hyperextension of the lumbar spine and pain. Four-point kneeling – rest position was hyperlordosis with an inability to initiate posterior pelvic rotation. Tests of spinal kinaesthesia revealed an inability to reposition the spine in neutral positions and a tendency to overextend the spine into extension

3. Specific muscle testing. Inability to isolate the activation of the pelvic floor or transverse abdominal muscles without hyperextending the lumbar spine, bracing whole abdominal wall and breath holding. Inability to activate lumbar multifidus at L4/L5 within a neutral spine position in co-contraction with the transverse abdominal muscles

Investigations	Plain X-rays (1993) – NAD MRI 1999 – degenerative spondylolisthesis at L4/L5, with obliteration of the facet joints. It was noted that at L4/L5 there was significant atrophy and fat infiltration within the lumbar multifidus. Hypertrophy of the erector spinae was noted Discogram – multilevel disc disruption (pain positive L4/L5)
Diagnosis	L4/L5 degenerative spondylolisthesis
Classification	L4/L5 control impairment disorder. Segmental instability – active extension pattern
Stage	Chronic – stable
Manual therapy indicated?	Yes
Treatment?	No
Management?	Yes – motor control management to inhibit dominant erector spinae and dynamically stabilize the L4/L5 within the neutral zone of motion

Outcome – excellent

The disorder diagnosis of *degenerative spondylolisthesis at L4/L5* was based upon the history and clinical presentation correlating with the radiological investigations. The disorder classification of *control impairment disorder – segmental instability* (active extension pattern) was based on the non-resolution of a repeated back strain with associated motor control deficits that has resulted in a control impairment of the spinal motion segment. The stage of the disorder is chronic and stable. The patient reports a mechanical basis to her pain disorder with pain related to extension activities, loading of the spine in extension and through range pain when she moves into and out of forward bending. She does not have a movement impairment, but rather she presents with an impairment in the control of the spinal segment with resulting pain. This is confirmed by active and passive movement tests, which confirm segmental hypermobility at L4/L5. Motor dysfunction present (a loss of neutral zone control of the L4/L5 spinal motion segment and a dominant extensor motor pattern) results in repetitive extension strain of pain sensitive tissue with maintenance of the pain state. The presence of non-organic signs is in keeping with the disorder.

Intervention of this disorder is based on a cognitive behavioural framework. The patient is educated that they have adopted a maladaptive motor control pattern that exposes the symptomatic segment to abnormal and repetitive extension strain – which in turn maintains the pain state. Management focuses on enhancing the dynamic control to the L4/L5 spinal segment by means of motor control intervention in order to reduce the extension strain to the spinal segment and in turn pain. The critical difference to this approach is that the patient is taught to control previously aggravating postures and movements, in a pain-free and functional manner. Enhancing the dynamic control of the motion segment aims to reduce the repeated stress of pain sensitive tissue resulting in symptomatic improvement of the disorder.

Passive manual therapy treatment is not indicated as an intervention for this disorder.

CASE STUDY 4

A 22-year-old man reports a 2-year history of chronic low back pain. He first developed back pain following a head-on motor vehicle accident 2 years ago in which he lost control of his car and hit a wall. At this time he had been working as a mechanic. He reported that he returned to work after a week, but his back pain became exacerbated and he was laid off after 3 months. Light duties as a mechanic failed due to increasing back pain. His complaint was of low back pain with radiation into the buttocks. He also reported that he had developed mid-thoracic spine pain 3 months after the initial injury. He reported that his low back pain was aggravated with any sustained and repeated spinal flexion activities such as bending, lifting (especially with load) and sitting. He reported that he avoided all such activities as they exacerbated his back pain and only lifted with a straight back. Extension activities and postures relieved his low back pain but increased his thoracic spine pain. He reported chiropractic manipulation had given short-term benefit but had not changed the disabling nature of the disorder. General trunk strengthening and stabilizing exercise rehabilitation had also been ineffective.

Plain X-ray and MRI scan revealed no structural abnormality. He had been out of work now for 21 months. He was depressed due to the nature of his disability and was fearful he would not be able to return to work. He was also limited in his ability to socialize with his friends. He walked every day for fitness and continued with his stabilizing exercise training. He had been told he might have to learn to live with his problem.

Physical examination

Observation	Loss of lower lumbar lordosis (L5/S1) with a lordosis in the thoracolumbar spine observed in sitting and standing
	Atrophy of the lumbar multifidus at L5/S1
	Increased tone in thoracolumbar erector spinae and upper abdominal wall
AROM	Flexion – in forward bending it was noted that he initiated forward bending in the lower lumbar spine, while maintaining the thoracolumbar spine in lordosis. He then flexed to full range with pain at the end of range
	Extension – 30° of backward bending with the onset of thoracic spine pain. Minimal extension was observed at L5/S1, with a tendency to extend in the thoracolumbar spine
	Right and left side bending full ROM and pain free
	Repeated spinal flexion increased his low back pain

CM	Lumbar spine – flexion/side bending right and left increased low back pain
	Thoracic spine – extension left and right side bending increased thoracic pain
Neuro	Normal
PPIVM L5/S1 – hypermobile	Provocation palpation of L5/S1 central and Z Jt left – painful with radiation into buttocks. Central T6/T7 painful
Neural provocation tests	NAD

Motor control

1. Functional movement tests. Forward bending, reaching, lifting, sit to stand and squat were associated with increased flexion at L5/S1, posterior pelvic rotation and a tendency to lordosis in the thoracolumbar spine above L5/S1.
2. Specific movement tests. Inability to initiate anterior pelvic tilt and extend the lower lumbar spine in standing and sitting, with a tendency to extend the thoracolumbar spine above L5/S1. Supine – attempts to initiate anterior pelvic tilt were associated with hyperextension of the thoracic spine. Four-point kneeling – rest position was posterior pelvic tilt, lower lumbar flexion with thoracolumbar spine lordosis. Tests of spinal kinaesthesia revealed an inability to reposition the spine in neutral positions and a tendency to overflex the lower lumbar spine and posterior tilt the pelvis
3. Specific muscle tests. Inability to isolate the activation of the pelvic floor or transverse abdominal muscles without posterior pelvic rotation and flexion the lower lumbar spine, with bracing of the upper abdominal wall. Inability to activate lumbar multifidus at L5/S1 within posterior pelvic rotation and flexion of L5/S1

Investigations	Plain X-rays / MRI 2003 – NAD
Diagnosis	L5/S1 back strain
Classification	L5/S1 control impairment disorder – flexion pattern
Stage	Chronic – stable
Manual therapy indicated?	Yes
Treatment?	No
Management?	Yes – motor control management to dynamically control L5/S1 within the neutral zone of motion

Outcome – excellent

The disorder diagnosis was based upon the history, the clinical presentation, the normal imaging and the absence of a specific diagnosis. The classification of a *control impairment disorder* (segmental flexion pattern) is based on the non-resolution of a back strain with associated motor control deficits that has resulted in a *control impairment* of the spinal motion segment into flexion. The stage of the disorder is chronic and stable.

The patient reports a mechanical basis to his pain disorder with pain related to flexion activities and loading of the spine. Repeated and sustained movements into flexion exacerbate the pain and extension activities relieve it. He has no movement impairment at L5/S1 into flexion, but rather presents with an impairment in the control of the L5/S1 spinal segment in this direction. This is confirmed by active and passive movement tests, which confirm segmental hypermobility at L5/S1 and a loss of motor control of this segment into flexion observed in the functional, specific movement and specific muscle tests. The loss of dynamic control at L5/S1 results in repetitive end-range strain and loading of this segment into flexion, resulting in maintenance of the pain state. The thoracic spine pain presumably arose secondary to compensatory extension of the thoracolumbar spine to compensate for the deficit in segmental control of lordosis at L5/S1. The patient presents with a maladaptive movement based pain disorder that resulted in ongoing repetitive strain of the L5/S1 into flexion during all forward bending activities and postures with resultant ongoing pain. The presence of non-organic signs was in keeping with the disorder.

Intervention in this disorder is based on a cognitive behavioural framework. The patient is educated that he has adopted a maladaptive movement disorder that exposes the symptomatic segment to abnormal and repetitive strain into flexion, which in turn maintains the pain state. Management focuses on enhancing the dynamic control of L5/S1 by means of motor control intervention in order to reduce the repeated flexion strain to L5/S1 and in turn reduce pain. The prime focus in this case is to reduce the flexion strain at L5/S1 in a functionally specific manner with relaxation of the thoracolumbar spine and control of segmental lordosis at L5/S1. Previously aggravating postures and movements into forward bending are targeted and trained so that the patient can perform them in a *pain-free* manner. Enhancing the dynamic control of the motion segment aims to reduce the repeated stress of pain sensitive tissue resulting in symptomatic improvement of the disorder and functional restoration.

Passive manual therapy treatment is not indicated as an intervention for this disorder.

CASE STUDY 5

A 45-year-old woman reports a 4-year history of right sided chronic buttock pain. It began following a motor vehicle accident in which her vehicle was hit from behind and forced her right foot on the brake on impact. She reported that her buttock pain was exacerbated by weight-bearing activities such as sitting, standing and walking. She tended to avoid weight bearing on the right buttock when sitting and right leg when standing. She was initially investigated with plain X-ray radiology with no abnormality detected. She underwent various physiotherapy treatment interventions which only gave her short-term relief.

Her condition worsened with time and she gradually became severely disabled. She was referred for pain management and psychological intervention. Little improvement was noted. A gym based programme and exercise intervention exacerbated her pain condition. She was told that her pain was of psychological origin and that she had to manage it.

Physical examination

Observation	Loss of lower lumbar lordosis
	Observable atrophy of the lumbar multifidus and right gluteal muscle
	During standing and sitting postures avoidance of right weight bearing was noted
	Antalgic gait was noted with difficulty in right side weight bearing and a loss of right hip extension
AROM	Flexion – full pain-free range
	Extension – some stiffness but minimal pain
	Right and left side bending – full pain-free range
	Repeated movement – NAD
Neuro	Normal
Motion palpation	L5/S1 extension – hypomobile without pain provocation
	SIJ provocation stress tests – positive shear, distraction, sacral spring and PA tests (right sided)
ASLR	Positive on the right with abdominal bracing and breath holding associated with sensation of heaviness
	Normalized with pelvic compression
SLR	NAD
Slump test	NAD

Motor control

1. Functional movement tests. Single leg stand – anterior shift of pelvis relative to thorax and unstable stance, absence of gluteal activation. Sit-to-stand and squat – weight shift to left leg noted. Manual pelvic compression and a SIJ joint belt relieve loading pain
2. Specific movement tests. Supine – ASLR was associated with splinting of the abdominal wall and breath

holding with the sensation of extreme heaviness. Pelvic compression normalized this. Supine – attempt to initiate anterior rotation of the pelvis was associated with hyperextension of the thoracolumbar spine and an inability to rotate the pelvis. Prone – hip extension – lack of gluteal activation was noted with associated heaviness. Pelvic compression normalized this and gluteal activation was noted

3. Specific muscle tests. Inability to isolate the activation of the pelvic floor or transverse abdominal muscles – bracing whole abdominal wall and breath holding was noted. Inability to activate LM at L5/S1 within a neutral spine position in co-contraction with the transverse abdominal muscles

Investigations	MRI 2001 – NAD It was noted that at L5/S1 there was significant atrophy and fat infiltration within the lumbar multifidus
Diagnosis	Right SIJ strain
Classification	Control impairment disorder – loss of force closure of right SIJ
Stage	Chronic – stable
Manual therapy indicated?	Yes
Treatment?	No
Management?	Yes – motor control management directed at the pelvic floor, transverse abdominal wall, lumbar multifidus and gluteal muscles to increase force closure of the SI joint

Outcome – excellent

The disorder diagnosis is based upon the history, clinical presentation and absence of a specific diagnosis. The disorder classification of *control impairment – loss of force closure of the right SIJ joint* is based upon: the history of a shear strain injury to the SIJ joint and surrounding ligaments; pain located directly over the SIJ joint; pain associated with weight-bearing postures and activities of right leg loading; spinal movement being full and pain-free; a positive ASLR normalized with pelvic compression; the relief of loading pain with a SIJ joint belt; the presence of positive SIJ joint provocation tests and dysfunction of muscles responsible for the provision of force closure to the SIJ joint. The stage of the disorder is chronic and stable.

These findings support the presence of a disorder of the right SIJ joint with associated motor control dysfunction resulting in a loss of adequate force closure or compression of the right SIJ joint complex. This results in excessive and repeated strain being placed through the pain sensitive supporting ligamentous structures of the SIJ joint, with resultant maintenance of pain.

Intervention in this disorder is based on a cognitive behavioural framework. Management logically focuses on a motor control intervention directed at the functional activation of the key force closure muscles of the right SIJ joint to enhance the dynamic stability to the joint. This involves the specific facilitation of the pelvic floor, transverse abdominal wall, lumbar multifidus and gluteal muscles, and integration of their activation into functional postures and activities in order to reduce and control pain by decreasing strain over the sensitized tissue. This in turn results in a reduction in functional impairments. Passive manual therapy treatment intervention in isolation is not indicated in the intervention of this disorder.

CASE STUDY 6

A 32-year-old man reports a 12-month history of severe and disabling chronic low back pain. History involved a minor flexion injury while working on a factory site. He went off work and reported that for the first 6 weeks he rested his back and was advised to avoid doing anything that increased his pain. His pain did not go away. He has not returned to work since this time.

He reported severe and disabling back pain. He reported undergoing various and multiple treatment interventions which gave him no long-term relief. These included physiotherapy (mobilization and stabilizing exercises), facet joint injections, massage and medical intervention. All general rehabilitation programmes he reported, markedly exacerbated his symptoms. He reported that his condition worsened with time. He reported dissatisfaction with all medical advice.

He reported that any exertion and activity exacerbated his symptoms. This included forward bending and extension activities such as standing, walking and swimming. He reported an inability to carry out any activities and that his pain is 10/10 in intensity and that nothing relieves his pain apart from rest. He does no exercise as he reports it makes him worse. He was on a sickness benefit. He is a smoker and reports that he does not believe he will return to work or get better as his back is 'stuffed'. He has family problems and financial problems. He drinks heavily. He has a history of psychological problems.

Physical examination

Observation	Generalized increase in lumbar lordosis Observable hypertonicity of the lumbar erector spinae muscles Standing and sitting postures were accented with very extended and rigid posture of the lumbar spine with a hesitancy to move
AROM	Flexion – 20° in forward bending was noted; he maintained his spine in lordosis and reported the onset of pain

	Extension – 10° of backward bending with the reported onset of pain
	Right and left side bending – were also rigid and limited in motion
	All movements associated with grimacing, exaggerated use of hands and breath holding and sighing
Neuro	Normal
Palpation	Motion palpation could not be carried out due to voluntary muscle guarding
	Provocation palpation – L1–5 and surrounding soft tissues–reportedly reproduced pain
	SIJ joint stress tests positive
	ASLR positive – with associated breath holding and abdominal bracing and the sensation of heaviness – not relieved with pelvic compression
Hip screen	Muscle guarding prohibited hip flexion with arching of back and grimacing even though at least 90° hip flexion was noted in sitting
SLR	Muscle guarding prohibited hip flexion and knee extension
Slump test	Trunk flexion limited – but knee extension was full

Motor control

1. Functional movement tests. All movements were limited with associated rigid spinal motion and difficulty in moving, grimacing, breath holding and groaning. It was noted that there was a discrepancy between the patient's functional capacity on undressing and when conversing compared to apparent severe disability when asked to perform specific functional and passive movement tests. For example, when asked to sit-stand without the use of hands he indicated that this was not possible. Attempts to do so were associated with grimacing, breath holding and laboured breathing
2. Specific movement tests. Inability to initiate posterior or anterior pelvic rotation due to muscle guarding. Inability to perform simple trunk and lower limb movement tasks such as rolling, flexing knee to chest etc.
3. Specific muscle tests. Inability to isolate the activation of the pelvic floor and transverse abdominal muscles without further bracing whole abdominal wall, back muscles and breath holding

Investigations	MRI 2000 – NAD, healthy lumbar multifidus was noted
Diagnosis	Minor back strain
Classification	Psychosocial

Stage	Chronic – progressive
Manual therapy indicated?	No
Treatment?	No
Management?	No

The disorder diagnosis was based upon a history of injury, results of medical imaging and lack of specific diagnosis. The disorder classification of *psychosocial* was based on the overwhelming dominance of non-organic signs. These signs are marked by a minor back strain which resulted in a sequelae of pain and disability totally out of context with the initial injury. Features supporting this classification are the report of 10/10 widespread pain, high levels of fear-avoidance behaviour, extremely high levels of functional disability, the absence of structural pathology, exaggerated limitation of active and functional movements, facial grimacing, inconsistency in functional capacity and the complete lack of consistent clinical findings of an organic nature. Disorder stage is chronic and progressive, as the deterioration of the disorder is ongoing.

Evaluation of these complex disorders must recognize the dominance of non-organic signs within the physical presentation. Functional rehabilitation may be undertaken but should only be done so in conjunction with appropriate management for a psychosocial classification intervention. In the event of functional rehabilitation being undertaken it could not be considered as a 'treatment' of the disorder. Manual therapy treatment, motor control and stabilizing exercise management is not indicated in the primary intervention of these pain disorders.

CONCLUSION

In this chapter a contemporary approach to manual therapy has been presented which is based upon the reflective considerations of the authors. The approach emphasizes the requirement to define the scope of manual therapy in context with the complexities of a disorder. A disorder has been defined as representing an accumulation of organic and non-organic features. A disorder is therefore more than the patient's complaint. This understanding provides considerations for manual therapy intervention whereby it is required to operate at a bio-psycho-social level. Diagnostics must therefore underpin manual therapy intervention. The scope of manual therapy practice has been defined and a rationale as to how manual therapy works has been presented. The scope of practice presented implies that manual therapy has the capacity to operate at a biopsychosocial level, to both treat and/or manage a disorder if indicated. The rationale as to how manual therapy works provides its indications and an understanding of its limitations. Research into the efficacy of manual therapy must take into account careful disorder selection, the indications and the limitations of manual therapy. With regard to the above, it must be understood that all manual therapy intervention, whether treatment, management or a combination of both, should be carried out within a cognitive behavioural framework.

KEYWORDS

diagnosis	low back pain
classification	intervention
disorder	evidence based practice

References

Cherkin D, Deyo R, Battie M, et al 1998 A comparison of physical therapy, chiropractic manipulation, and provision of an educational booklet for the treatment of patients with low back pain. New England Journal of Medicine 339: 1021–1029

Koes B, Asendelft W, van der Heijden G, et al 1996 Spinal manipulation for low back pain: an updated systematic review of randomised clinical trials. Spine 21: 2860–2873

Linton S 2000 A review of psychological risk factors in back and neck pain. Spine 25: 1148–1156

Maher C, Latimer J, Refshauge K, 1999 Prescription of activity for low back pain: what works? Australian Journal of Physiotherapy 45: 121–132

McKenzie R 1981 The lumbar spine, mechanical diagnosis and treatment. Spinal Publications, Waikanae, New Zealand

McKenzie R 2000 Mechanical diagnosis and therapy for disorders of the low back. In: Twomey L, Taylor J (eds) Physical therapy for the low back. Churchill Livingstone, New York, pp 141–166

Waddell G 1996 Low back pain: a twentieth century health care enigma. Spine 21: 2820–2825

Chapter **34**

The management of pelvic joint pain and dysfunction

D. G. Lee, A. Vleeming

INTRODUCTION

Over the past decade there has been considerable attention and debate about the sacroiliac joint (SIJ) and the role the pelvis plays in low back and pelvic pain. Through multidisciplinary discussion and research, a consensus is arising as to the causes and treatment of pelvic joint pain and dysfunction. This chapter presents the principles of an integrated approach to the management of pelvic joint pain and dysfunction which comes from anatomical and biomechanical studies of the pelvis, as well as from the clinical experience of treating patients with lumbopelvic pain. This approach addresses why the pelvis is painful and no longer able to sustain and transfer loads, as opposed to one which seeks to identify pain-generating structures.

Several studies have sought to understand pelvic function. The anatomical research on the SIJ and the connections between it and the lumbopelvic muscles (Snijders et al 1993a, Vleeming et al 1990a, 1990b, 1995b, 1996) led to conclusions regarding the form and force closure of joints. The timing of specific muscle activation (Hodges 1997, Hodges & Richardson 1997) and the pattern of muscular co-contraction (or lack thereof) in patients with low back pain (Danneels et al 2000, Hides et al 1994, 1996, Hodges & Richardson 1996) further enhanced the force closure theory and suggested a crucial role for motor control. Based on this knowledge, functional tests for the pelvis were developed (Buyruk et al 1995a, 1995b, 1999, Lee 2004, Mens et al 1999, 2001) and treatment protocols were established (Lee 2004). Clinically, it was soon apparent that the patient's emotional state could significantly influence the outcome.

The integrated approach presented in this chapter (Lee & Vleeming 1998) has four components (Fig. 34.1). Three are physical:

- form closure (structure)
- force closure (forces produced by myofascial action)
- motor control (specific timing of muscle action/inaction during loading)

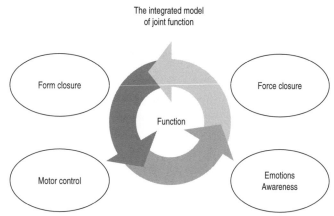

Figure 34.1 The four components of the integrated model of function.

and one is psychological:

- emotions.

The proposal is that joint mechanics can be influenced by multiple factors including articular, neuromuscular and emotional factors. The management of pelvic joint pain and dysfunction requires attention to all these elements.

FUNCTION OF THE PELVIS

Managing dysfunction requires an understanding of function. A primary function of the pelvis is to transfer the loads generated by body weight and gravity during standing, walking and sitting (Snijders et al 1993a, 1993b). How well this load is managed dictates how efficient function will be. Stability is a term often used to describe effective load transfer. According to Panjabi (1992) stability is achieved when the passive, active and control systems work together. Snijders and Vleeming (Snijder et al 1993a, 1993b) believe that the passive, active and control systems produce approximation of the joint surfaces, essential if stability is to be ensured. The amount of approximation required is variable and difficult to quantify since it is essentially dependent on an individual's structure (form closure) and the forces they need to control (force closure). The term 'adequate' has been used (Lee & Vleeming 1998) to describe how much approximation is necessary and reflects the non-quantitative aspect of this measure. Essentially, it means 'not too much and not too little'; in other words, just enough to suit the existing situation. Consequently, the ability to effectively transfer load through the pelvis is dynamic and depends on:

1. Optimal function of the bones, joints and ligaments (form closure or joint congruency) (Vleeming et al 1990a, 1990b).
2. Optimal function of the muscles and fascia (force closure) (Richardson et al 1999, Vleeming et al 1995b).
3. Appropriate neural function (motor control, emotional state) (Bo & Stien 1994, Hodges 1997, Hodges &

Gandevia 2000, Hodges & Richardson 1997, Holstege et al 1996).

FORM CLOSURE: MOBILITY AND STABILITY OF THE SACROILIAC JOINT

The term 'form closure' was coined by Vleeming & Snijders (Snijders et al 1993a, 1993b, Vleeming et al 1990a, 1990b) and is used to describe how the joint's structure, orientation and shape contribute to stability. All joints have a variable amount of form closure and the individual's inherent anatomy will dictate how much additional force (force closure) is needed to ensure stabilization when loads are increased. How does the 'form' of the SIJ contribute to stability? The SIJ transfers large loads and its shape is adapted to this task. The articular surfaces are relatively flat and this helps to transfer compression forces and bending moments (Snijders et al 1993a, 1993b, Vleeming et al 1990a, 1990b). However, a relatively flat joint is theoretically more vulnerable to shear forces. The SIJ is anatomically protected from shear in three ways. First, the sacrum is wedge-shaped in both the anteroposterior and vertical planes and thus is stabilized by the innominates. The auricular surface of the SIJ comprises two or three sacral segments and each is oriented differently (Solonen 1957). Secondly, in contrast to other synovial joints, the articular cartilage is not smooth but irregular, especially on the ilium (Bowen & Cassidy 1981, Sashin 1930). Thirdly, a frontal dissection through the SIJ reveals cartilage covered bony extensions protruding into the joint (Vleeming et al 1990a), the ridges and grooves. They seem irregular, but are in fact complementary. All three factors enhance stabilization of the joint when compression is applied to the pelvis.

For many decades, it was thought that the SIJ was immobile due to the close fitting nature of the articular surfaces. Research has now shown that mobility of the SIJ is not only possible (Egund et al 1978, Lavignolle et al 1983, Sturesson et al 1989, 2000), but essential for shock absorption during weight-bearing activities. It has also been shown (Vleeming et al 1992) that the SIJ normally retains its mobility with age. The quantity of motion available at this joint has been investigated (Jacob & Kissling 1995, Sturesson et al 1989, 2000) with highly sophisticated imaging and motion analysis techniques and the results reflect the wide anatomical variance. It is known that the angular motion available at the SIJ is small (Sturesson et al 1989, 2000) and that this motion couples with linear translation (Sturesson et al 1989).

This research has answered the question 'does the SIJ move and if so how much?' It moves a small amount and the amplitude varies between individuals. Can we palpate this motion? To date, no manual diagnostic tests have shown reliability for determining how much an individual's SIJ is moving in either symptomatic or asymptomatic subjects (Carmichael 1987, Dreyfuss et al 1994, 1996, Herzog et al 1989, Laslett & Williams 1994). Given the wide individual variation and the limited potential range of motion, it is no wonder we have not been able to demonstrate reliability with manual testing when amplitude is considered. And yet, how can a diagnosis of SIJ hypomobility or SIJ hypermobility/instability be made, and management therefore specified, without clinically reliable passive motion tests of SIJ mobility? Subsequent research has helped to clarify this dilemma.

Buyruk et al (1995a) established that the Doppler imaging system could be used to measure stiffness (or laxity) of the SIJ. This research has recently been repeated and verified by Richardson et al (2002). Buyruk et al (1995b, 1997, 1999) used this method to measure SIJ stiffness in subjects with and without pelvic pain and noted a high degree of individual variance. Within the same subject, the asymptomatic individual demonstrated similar values for both SIJs, whereas the symptomatic individual demonstrated different stiffness values for the left and right SIJ. In other words, asymmetry of stiffness between sides correlated with the symptomatic individual. In keeping with this research, the emphasis of manual motion testing should therefore focus less on how much the SIJ is moving and more on the symmetry, or asymmetry, of the motion palpated. Form closure analysis (see below for specific test description) requires a comparison of the symmetry of stiffness of the right and left SIJs. A clinical reasoning approach, which considers all of the findings from the examination, is required to determine if the amplitude of motion is less or more than optimal for that individual.

FORCE CLOSURE: COMPRESSION AND STABILITY OF THE PELVIS

If the articular surfaces of the sacrum and the innominate were constantly and completely compressed, mobility would not be possible. However, compression during loading is variable (Sturesson et al 2000) and therefore motion is possible and stabilization required. This is achieved by increasing compression across the joint surface at the moment of loading (force closure). The amount of force closure required depends on the individual's form closure and the magnitude of the load. The anatomical structures responsible for force closure are the ligaments, muscles and fascia.

For every joint, there is a position called the close-packed or self-locked position in which there is maximum congruence of the articular surfaces and maximum tension of the major ligaments. In this position, the joint is under significant compression and the ability to resist shear forces is enhanced by the tension of the passive structures and increased friction between the articular surfaces (Snijders et al 1993a, 1993b, Vleeming et al 1990b). For the SIJ, this position is nutation of the sacrum or posterior rotation of the innominate (van Wingerden et al 1993, Vleeming et al 1989a, 1989b). Studies have shown (Egund et al 1978, Lavignolle et al 1983) that sacral nutation occurs bilaterally whenever the lumbopelvic spine is loaded. The amount of sacral nutation varies with the magnitude of the load. Full sacral nutation

(self-bracing or close packing) occurs during forward and backward bending of the trunk (Sturesson et al 2000).

Counternutation of the sacrum (anterior rotation of the innominate) is thought to be a relatively less stable position for the SIJ. The long dorsal ligament becomes taut during this motion; however, the other major ligaments (sacrotuberous, sacrospinous and interosseus) are less tensed (Vleeming et al 1996).

Function would be significantly compromised if joints could only be stable in the close-packed position. Stability for load transfer is required throughout the entire range of motion and this is provided by the active, or neuro-myofascial, system. Currently, two different muscle systems can be identified functionally – a local system and a global system (Bergmark 1989, Comerford & Mottram 2001, Richardson et al 1999). The local system pertains to those muscles essential for segmental or intrapelvic stabilization (Richardson et al 1999, 2002, Vleeming et al 1995a, 1995b) while the global system appears to be more responsible for regional stabilization (between the thorax and pelvis or pelvis and legs) (Bergmark 1989, Comerford & Mottram 2001) and motion.

With respect to the lumbopelvic region, the local system consists of the muscles of the pelvic floor, the transversus abdominis, the diaphragm and the multifidus. The global system consists of several muscle slings that are anatomically and functionally related.

The role of the local muscle system

The function of the local muscles is to increase stiffness such that the system is stabilized in preparation for the addition of external loads. With respect to the pelvis, it achieves this through several mechanisms, which include:

- increasing the intra-abdominal pressure (Hodges & Gandevia 2000)
- increasing the tension of the thoracodorsal fascia (Vleeming et al 1995a, Willard 1997) and/or
- increasing the articular stiffness (Richardson et al 2002).

Research has shown (Bo & Stien 1994, Constantinou & Govan 1982, Hodges 1997, Hodges & Gandevia 2000, Moseley et al 2002, Sapsford et al 2001) that the local muscle system is anticipatory when functioning optimally. In other words, these muscles work at low levels at all times and increase their action *before* any further loading or motion occurs.

Hodges & Richardson (1996, 1997) have shown that transversus abdominis is an anticipatory muscle for stabilization of the low back and pelvis and is recruited prior to the initiation of any movement of the upper or lower extremity. Although it does not cross the SIJ directly, it has an impact on stiffness of the pelvis (Richardson et al 2002) through, in part, its direct pull on the large attachment to the middle layer and the deep lamina of the posterior layer of the thoracodorsal fascia (Barker & Briggs 1999). Richardson et al (2002) propose that contraction of the transversus abdominis produces a force which acts on the ilia perpendicular to the sagittal plane (i.e. approximates the ilia anteriorly). They also propose that the 'mechanical action of a pelvic belt in front of the abdominal wall at the level of the transversus abdominis corresponds with the action of this muscle'. At this time, the specific direction of force produced by contraction of transversus abdominis has not been validated through research but this hypothesis has been developed clinically as a means for diagnosis and exercise prescription (see ASLR below).

In a study of patients with chronic low back pain, a timing delay was found in which transversus abdominis failed to anticipate the initiation of arm and/or leg motion (Hodges & Richardson 1997). Delayed activation of transversus abdominis means that the thoracodorsal fascia is not pretensed and the pelvis is therefore not stiffened (compressed) in preparation for external loading. Therefore, it is potentially vulnerable to the loss of intrinsic stability.

Moseley et al (2002) have shown that the deep fibres of the multifidus muscle are also anticipatory for stabilization of the lumbar region and are recruited prior to the initiation of any movement of the upper extremity. In contrast, the superficial fibres of the multifidus muscle were shown to be direction dependent. In the pelvis, this muscle is contained between the dorsal aspect of the sacrum and the deep layers of the thoracodorsal fascia. When the deep fibres of the multifidus contract, the muscle can be felt to broaden or swell (Fig. 34.2). As the deep fibres of multifidus broaden, it 'pumps up' the thoracodorsal fascia much like blowing air into a balloon (Gracovetsky 1990, Vleeming et al 1995a). Using the Doppler imaging system, Richardson et al (2002) noted that a co-contraction of multifidus and transversus abdominis increased the stiffness of the SIJ. These authors state that 'Under gravitational load, it is the transversely oriented muscles that must act to compress the sacrum between the ilia and maintain stability of the SIJ'. Although multifidus is not oriented transversely, its contraction tenses the thoracodorsal fascia and we believe that it is this structure which imparts compression to the posterior pelvis. This has yet to be scientifically verified; however, this hypothesis has been developed clinically as a means for diagnosis and exercise prescription (see ASLR below).

Hides et al (1994), O'Sullivan (2000) and Danneels et al (2000) have studied the response of multifidus in low back and pelvic pain patients and note that multifidus becomes inhibited and reduced in size in these individuals. The normal 'pump-up' effect of multifidus on the thoracodorsal fascia, and therefore its ability to compress the pelvis, is lost when the size or function of this muscle is impaired. Rehabilitation requires both retraining (Hides et al 1996, O'Sullivan et al 1997) and hypertrophy of the muscle (Danneels et al 2001) for the restoration of proper force closure of the lumbopelvic region. Together, multifidus and transversus abdominis form a corset of support for the lumbopelvic region. The 'roof and floor' of this canister are

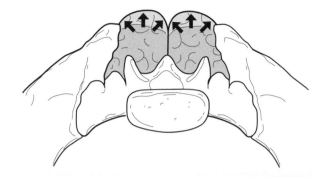

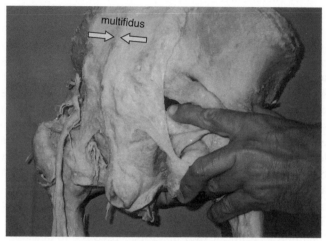

Figure 34.2 A: When multifidus contracts it broadens. Reproduced with permission from Lee 2001. B: The broadening of multifidus tenses the thoracodorsal fascia which approximates the posterior pelvis.

supported by the muscles of the pelvic floor and the respiratory diaphragm.

The muscles of the pelvic floor play a critical role both in stabilization of the pelvic girdle and in the maintenance of urinary and faecal continence (Ashton-Miller et al 2001, Bo & Stein 1994, Constantinou & Govan 1982, Sapsford et al 2001). Constantinou & Govan (1982) measured the intraurethral and intrabladder pressures in healthy continent women during coughing and Valsalva manoeuvre (bearing down) and found that during a cough the intra-urethral pressure increases approximately 250 ms before any pressure increase is detected in the bladder. This suggests an anticipatory reflex. The increase in urethral pressure occurred simultaneously with the increase in bladder pressure during a Valsalva. Constantinou & Govan suggest that the timing difference in pressure generation within the urethra and bladder during a cough versus a Valsalva may be due to the contraction of the pelvic floor during a cough and relaxation of the pelvic floor during a Valsalva.

Sapsford et al (2001) investigated the co-activation pattern of the pelvic floor and the abdominals via needle EMG for the abdominals and surface EMG for the pelvic floor. In two subjects, fine-wire needle EMG was used to detect activation of the right pubococcygeus through the lateral vaginal wall. They found that the abdominals contract in response to a pelvic floor contraction command and that the pelvic floor contracts in response to both a 'hollowing' and 'bracing' abdominal command. The results from this research suggest that the pelvic floor can be facilitated by co-activating the abdominals and vice versa.

When the local muscle system is functioning optimally, it applies compression to the pelvis (Richardson et al 2002) and thus stabilizes the SIJs, augmenting the form closure and helping to prevent excessive shearing of the SIJs. The pelvis is then prepared to 'accept' additional load from outside the pelvis from the global muscle system.

The role of the global muscle system

In the past, four slings of muscle systems which stabilize the pelvis regionally (between the thorax and legs) have been described (Snijders et al 1995, Vleeming et al 1995a, 1995b). The posterior oblique sling contains connections between the latissimus dorsi and the gluteus maximus through the thoracodorsal fascia. The anterior oblique sling contains connections between the external oblique, the anterior abdominal fascia and the contralateral internal oblique abdominal muscle and adductors of the thigh. The longitudinal sling connects the peroneii, the biceps femoris, sacrotuberous ligament, deep lamina of the thoracodorsal fascia and the erector spinae. The lateral sling contains the primary stabilizers for the hip joint, namely the gluteus medius/minimus, tensor fascia lata and the contralateral adductors of the thigh. These muscle slings were initially classified to gain a better understanding of how local and global stability of the pelvis could be achieved by specific muscles. It is now recognized that although individual muscles are important for regional stabilization as well as for mobility, it is critical to understand how they connect and function together. A muscle contraction produces a force that spreads beyond the origin and insertion of the active muscle. This force is transmitted to other muscles, tendons, fasciae, ligaments, capsules and bones that lie both in series and in parallel to the active muscle. In this manner, forces are produced quite distant from the origin of the initial muscle contraction. These integrated muscle systems produce slings of forces that assist in the transfer of load. Van Wingerden et al (2001) used the Doppler imaging system to analyse the effect of contraction of the biceps femoris, erector spinae, gluteus maximus and latissimus dorsi on compression of the SIJ. None of these muscles directly crosses the SIJ yet each was found to effect compression (increase stiffness) of the SIJ.

The global system of muscles is essentially an integrated sling system comprising several muscles which produces forces. A muscle may participate in more than one sling and the slings may overlap and interconnect depending on the task being demanded. The hypothesis is that the slings have no beginning or end but rather connect to assist in the transference of forces. It is possible

that the slings are all part of one interconnected myofascial system and the particular sling (anterior oblique, posterior oblique, lateral, longitudinal) which is identified during any motion is merely due to the activation of selective parts of the whole sling.

The identification and treatment of a specific muscle dysfunction (weakness, inappropriate recruitment, tightness) is important when restoring global stabilization and mobility (between the thorax and pelvis or between the pelvis and legs) and for understanding why parts of a sling may be inextensible (tight) or too flexible (lacking in support).

MOTOR CONTROL

Motor control pertains to patterning of muscle activation (Comerford & Mottram 2001, Danneels et al 2001, O'Sullivan et al 1997, Richardson et al 1999) or, in other words, the timing of specific muscle action and inaction. Efficient movement requires coordinated muscle action such that stability is ensured while motion is controlled and not restrained. With respect to the lumbopelvic region, it is the coordinated action between the local and global muscle systems that ensures stability without rigidity of posture and without episodes of collapse. Exercises which focus on sequencing muscle activation are necessary for restoring motor control (Lee 2001, 2004).

EMOTIONS AND BODY AWARENESS

Emotional states can play a significant role in human function, including the function of the neuro-musculo-skeletal system. Many chronic pelvic pain patients present with traumatizing life experiences in addition to their functional complaints. Several of these patients adopt motor patterns indicative of defensive posturing which suggest a negative past experience. A negative emotional state leads to further stress. Stress is a normal response intended to energize our system for quick fight and flight reactions. When this response is sustained, high levels of adrenaline (epinephrine) and cortisol remain in the system (Holstege et al 1996), in part due to circulating stress related neuropeptides (Sapolsky & Spencer 1997, Sapolsky et al 1997) which are released in anticipation of defensive or offensive behaviour.

Emotional states (fight, flight or freeze reactions) are physically expressed through muscle action and when sustained, influence basic muscle tone and patterning (Holstege et al 1996). If the muscles of the pelvis become hypertonic, this state will increase compression of the SIJs (Richardson et al 2002, van Wingerden et al 2001).

It is important to understand the patient's emotional state since the detrimental motor pattern can often only be changed by affecting the emotional state. Sometimes it can be as simple as restoring hope through education and awareness of the underlying mechanical problem. At other times, professional cognitive behavioural therapy is required to retrain more positive thought patterns.

A basic requirement for cognitive and physical learning is focused, or attentive, training – in other words not being absent-minded. Teaching an individual to be 'mindful' or aware of what is happening in their body during times of physical and/or emotional loading can reduce sustained, unnecessary muscle tone and therefore joint compression (Murphy 1992).

THE CLINICAL DIAGNOSIS

Impaired pelvic function can be defined as an inability to effectively transfer forces through the pelvis. To reach this diagnosis, specific functional tests that analyse the ability of the pelvis to transfer load are required. To understand the precise cause for the impairment, specific tests that examine form closure, force closure, motor control and the impact of negative emotional states are required.

Functional tests of load transfer through the pelvis

Forward bending in standing

This test examines the ability of the pelvis to tolerate both vertical and horizontal shear forces and control forward sagittal rotation during forward bending of the trunk. When the leg lengths are equal, the sacrum should nutate bilaterally relative to the innominates and remain nutated throughout the forward bending motion as the pelvic girdle flexes symmetrically at the hip joints (Sturesson et al 1989, 2000). Asymmetry of motion of the innominates during forward bending is a positive finding; however, it is *not* indicative of any specific dysfunction of the SIJ since many articular and myofascial problems can be causal.

One leg standing with contralateral hip flexion

This test examines the ability of the patient to transfer load through one lower extremity, retain their balance and flex the contralateral hip. During this task, the sacrum should nutate relative to the innominate on both the weight-bearing and non-weight-bearing side (Hungerford et al 2001, Sturesson et al 2000). The load should be transferred to one leg smoothly with minimal adjustments of the lower extremity and the pelvis should remain in its original coronal and transverse plane.

Sturesson et al (2000) have challenged the clinical relevance of any motion analysis between the innominate and the sacrum on the non-weight-bearing side during this test. Using radiostereometric analysis, the range of motion of the SIJ in women with suspected hypermobility was measured. Minimal motion (0.2 degrees) actually occurred on the non-weight-bearing (apparently hypermobile) side. Secondary overactivation of the local muscle system can effectively compress the SIJ and make a hypermobile joint appear hypomobile on active movement testing. Therefore, this test should not be used to determine mobility of the SIJ. Hungerford et al (2001), using a similar analysis system,

investigated the pattern of innominate motion in both healthy (asymptomatic and functionally normal) and dysfunctional (symptomatic with signs of failed load transfer) groups. They found that in the healthy subjects, the innominate rotated posteriorly relative to the sacrum on both the weight-bearing and non-weight-bearing sides during this test. In the dysfunctional group, they found that the innominate tended to rotate anteriorly relative to the sacrum on the weight-bearing side. This research suggests that the pattern of innominate motion may be a more relevant finding from this test and one which evaluates effective, or failed, load transfer.

Once a diagnosis of pelvic impairment has been made, specific tests to determine the cause are required. These tests examine the articular and the neuromyofascial system and are essential for the determining subsequent management.

Tests for form closure

The following tests examine the form closure of the SIJ and its ability to resist horizontal and vertical translation forces (shear) that are applied passively to the non-weight-bearing joint (Lee 2004). The patient is supine with the hips and knees flexed and supported over a bolster. Since muscle activation can compress the SIJ (Richardson et al 2002, van Wingerden et al 2001), it is essential that the patient is completely relaxed during this test. The sacral sulcus is palpated just medial to the posterior superior iliac spine (PSIS) with the long and ring fingers to monitor translation between the innominate and the sacrum. An anteroposterior force is applied to the innominate with the other hand in a variety of directions to determine the plane of the SIJ. Once the plane of the joint has been established, the stiffness for anteroposterior translation of the SIJ is compared bilaterally. To test the ability of the pelvic girdle to resist vertical translation, a superior/inferior pressure is applied to the innominate through the distal end of the femur or through the ischial tuberosity. The symmetry of stiffness is compared between the left and right sides. Optimally, symmetry should be present. Asymmetry indicates that a different amount of compression exists across the left and right SIJ.

Tests for force closure and motor control

The active straight leg raise (ASLR) test (Mens et al 1997, 1999, 2001) can be used to identify non-optimal stabilization of the pelvic girdle. The supine patient is asked to lift their extended leg off of the table and to note any effort difference between the left and right leg (does one leg seem heavier or harder to lift?). The strategy used to stabilize the lumbopelvic region during this task is observed. The leg should flex at the hip joint and the pelvis should not rotate, side bend, flex or extend relative to the lumbar spine. The ribcage should not draw in excessively (overactivation of the external oblique muscles), nor should the lower ribs flare out excessively (overactivation of the internal oblique muscles) or the abdomen bulge (breath holding – Valsalva). The provocation of any pelvic pain is also noted at this time. The pelvis is then compressed passively (Fig. 34.3). The ASLR is repeated and any change in effort and/or pain is noted. The location of the compression can be varied to simulate the force which would be produced by optimal function of the local muscle system. Although still a hypothesis, clinically it appears that compression of the anterior pelvis (at the level of the anterior superior iliac spine (ASIS) simulates the force produced by contraction of lower fibres of transversus abdominis and compression of the posterior pelvis (at the level of the PSIS) simulates that of the sacral multifidus. This test is very useful for individual exercise prescription. If anterior compression of the pelvis facilitates elevation of the leg, then a training programme for isolation, timing and strength should be instituted for transversus abdominis. If posterior compression of the pelvis facilitates elevation of the leg, then a similar programme for the deep fibres of multifidus should be given.

Test for the integrity of the active force closure mechanism

When the active force closure mechanism is effective, co-contraction of the muscles of the local muscle system should compress the SIJ (Richardson et al 2002), thereby increasing its stiffness. To test the status of the active force closure mechanism, the patient is first instructed to recruit the local muscle system (transversus abdominis, multifidus and pelvic floor). This instruction may take a few sessions to master. Once the patient is able to sustain a tonic co-con-

traction of local muscle system, the effect of this contraction on the stiffness of the SIJ is assessed by repeating the form closure tests. The SIJ stiffness should increase and no relative motion between the innominate and sacrum should be felt. This means that an adequate amount of compression of the SIJ has occurred and the force closure mechanism is effective. If the local muscle system is contracting appropriately and has no effect on the stiffness of the SIJ, then the active force closure mechanism is ineffective for controlling shear. This is a poor prognostic sign for successful rehabilitation with exercise.

A biomechanical diagnosis can now be made regarding the mobility of the SIJ, the stability of the SIJ, and the ability of the pelvic girdle to transfer load.

THE MANAGEMENT OF PELVIC DYSFUNCTION

Motion of the SIJ can either be restricted (too much compression) or poorly controlled (too little compression). The next section will describe some common clinical presentations for dysfunction of the SIJ and the protocol for clinical management.

Excessive compression of the sacroiliac joint

Excessive compression of the SIJ can be the end-result of inflammatory pathology such as ankylosing spondylitis or due to fibrosis of the capsule secondary to trauma. These are true articular causes of excessive compression of the SIJ. The joint can also be compressed by overactivation of certain lumbopelvic muscles. When an individual habitually uses the piriformis, ischiococcygeus and the erector spinae as a strategy for stabilization, the constant activation of these muscles can excessively compress the SIJ. In both instances (articular or myofascial), the stiffness of the SIJ is increased and the following are found on clinical examination:

1. Forward bending in standing – consistently asymmetrical on repeated testing.
2. One leg standing – no difficulty standing on one leg; the pattern of motion on the weight-bearing leg is often dysfunctional. The innominate may be anteriorly rotated at the onset of the test and remain so throughout the test, or the innominate may anteriorly rotate as load is transferred to the supporting leg.
3. Form closure – there is asymmetric stiffness of both anteroposterior and vertical translation and the compressed or fibrotic side has reduced motion. The stiff joint has a hard, solid end-feel of motion whereas the myofascially compressed joint has a softer end-feel which gives slightly under sustained pressure.

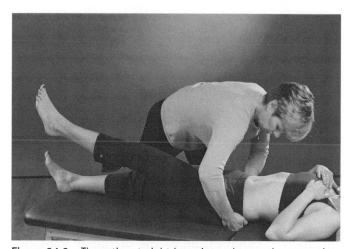

Figure 34.3 The active straight leg raise and manual compression. ©Diane G. Lee Physiotherapist Corp., with permission.

4. ASLR – reveals poor pelvic position control, often associated with a dysfunctional motor control strategy for lumbopelvic stabilization. Adding more compression to the pelvis rarely facilitates elevation of the leg since the pelvis is already overly compressed.

A fused SIJ cannot be mobilized with manual therapy techniques; however, the fibrosed joint is easily mobilized in one or two treatments when specific, localized, passive techniques are used (Fig. 34.4) (Lee 2004). Manual therapy is an essential part of the treatment for this individual. The SIJ which is excessively compressed due to imbalances in the local/global muscle systems requires a more comprehensive treatment protocol. While manual therapy techniques such as passive mobilization, muscle energy, pressure-stretch and/or strain–counterstrain may assist in relieving the compression, the impaired pattern is likely to recur unless the motor control strategy for stabilization is addressed. This individual requires an emphasis on exercise and education rather than manual therapy for long-term results.

Excessive compression of the sacroiliac joint with an underlying instability

When a force is applied to the SIJ sufficient to attenuate the articular ligaments (fall on the buttocks or a lift/twist injury), the muscles will respond to prevent dislocation and further trauma to the joint. The resulting spasm may fix the joint in an abnormal resting position and marked asymmetry of the pelvic girdle (innominate and/or sacrum) can be present. This is an unstable joint under excessive compression. It commonly occurs unilaterally and presents with the following findings on examination:

1. Forward bend in standing – consistently asymmetrical on repeated testing.

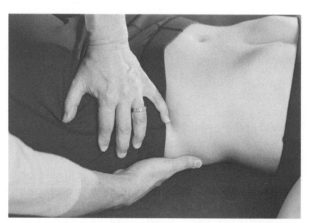

Figure 34.4 Passive mobilization of the right sacroiliac joint. In this illustration, the sacrum is fixed posteriorly with the therapist's right hand and the right innominate is mobilized into posterior rotation with a sustained grade 4+ hold via the left hand. ©Diane G. Lee Physiotherapist Corp., with permission.

2. One leg standing – significant difficulty standing on the dysfunctional side and the patient is often reluctant to do so.
3. Form closure – there is asymmetrical stiffness of both anteroposterior and vertical translation. The joint is excessively compressed (fixated) such that no joint play is palpable. The underlying instability is not evident on the form closure tests until the compression has been reduced. Positional testing defines the actual lesion (superior fixation of the innominate, anterior/posterior sacral shear lesion (Lee 2004)).
4. ASLR – reveals poor pelvic position control and frequently an inability to lift the leg at all. There is no improvement in function when passive compression is applied to the pelvis, and in fact this may make the ASLR worse. After the articular compression has been reduced, the ASLR should improve when compression is applied manually to the pelvis. This is an impairment of both form and force closure in that the relationship between the articular surfaces has been disturbed and the muscle response is excessive.

Treatment of this individual which focuses on exercise without first addressing the 'posture', 'position', 'alignment' of the pelvis tends to be ineffective and commonly increases symptoms. Conversely, if treatment only includes manual therapy (mobilization, manipulation or muscle energy) for correction of 'posture', 'position', 'alignment', relief tends to be temporary and dependence on the healthcare practitioner providing the manual correction is common. This impairment requires a combination of manual therapy, exercise and education for a successful outcome.

The initial treatment is a specific distraction manipulation (Hartman 1997, Lee 1999) of the affected SIJ to reduce the articular compression (Fig. 34.5) and restore the symmetrical resting position of the pelvis. Subsequently, the form closure tests will reveal a decrease in stiffness of the affected SIJ compared to the opposite side. Treatment now requires the restoration of the active force closure mechanism with an individually prescribed exercise programme.

Once the local muscle system has been trained (Lee 1999, 2001, Richardson & Jull 1995, Richardson et al 1999), the efficacy of the active force closure mechanism (ability to control shear of the SIJ) can be evaluated. If translation of the SIJ can be controlled via contraction of the local muscle system, then a good clinical outcome can be predicted. If translation (either anteroposterior or vertical) is still possible while the local system is contracting properly, then the force closure mechanism is not able to control shear of the SIJ. This is the indication for prolotherapy (Dorman 1994).

Insufficient compression of the sacroiliac joint

This pelvic impairment arises when there is either inadequate or inappropriate motor control such that there is

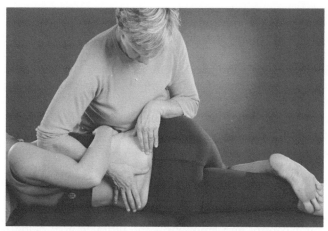

Figure 34.5 Specific distraction manipulation for the left sacroiliac joint. The direction of the manipulative thrust is such that internal rotation of the innominate relative to the sacrum is induced. This force produces distraction of the posterior aspect of the SIJ. It is critical that L5–S1 be stabilized during the thrust since this segment does not tolerate axial rotation well. ©Diane G. Lee Physiotherapist Corp., with permission.

insufficient compression of the SIJ during movement and loading (Fig. 34.6). The patient often complains of sensations of giving way or a lack of trust when loading through the involved extremity. The following findings are noted on clinical examination:

1. Forward bend test in standing – inconsistently asymmetrical on repeated testing.
2. One leg standing – may or may not present with difficulty standing on either leg; the pattern of motion on the weight-bearing leg is often dysfunctional (anterior rotation).

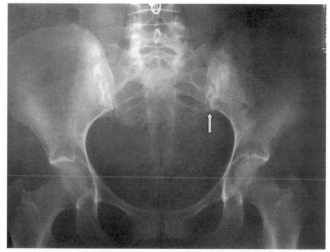

Figure 34.6 Note the larger gap between the articular surfaces of the left sacroiliac joint (arrow) compared to the right. A diagnosis cannot be made from an X-ray alone. When the clinical history and complete objective examination was considered, it was apparent that this was due to insufficient compression of the left hemipelvis.

3. Form closure – there is symmetrical stiffness with a normal capsular end-feel.
4. ASLR – reveals poor pelvic position control, often associated with a dysfunctional motor control strategy for lumbopelvic stabilization. Function may improve (decreased effort to lift the leg) when passive compression is applied to the anterior and/or posterior aspect of the pelvis.

Treatment of this pelvic impairment requires the restoration of the active force closure mechanism with specific exercises that isolate and then train the muscles required for stabilization followed by a programme which addresses regional motor control (control between the thorax and pelvis or pelvis and legs). The ASLR coupled with compression assists in determining where to begin stabilization training. The reader is referred to other sources for detailed descriptions of this exercise instruction (Lee 2001, 2004, Richardson & Jull 1995, Richardson et al 1999).

In the meantime, the temporary application of a sacroiliac belt can be used to augment the force closure mechanism. The Com-pressor (Fig. 34.7) is a specific pelvic compression belt that allows both the location (bilateral

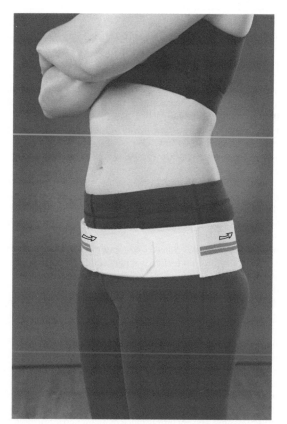

Figure 34.7 The Com-pressor allows both the location and the amount of compression to be customized through the use of removable elastic Com-pressor bands. Reproduced with permission from D. Lee and OPTP – Orthopaedic Physical Therapy Products, Plymouth, USA.

anterior, bilateral posterior, unilateral anterior and unilateral posterior) and the amount of compression to be customized through the use of removable elastic compression bands. The ASLR is used to determine the placement of the bands.

TREATING THE EMOTIONAL COMPONENT

The patient's emotional state can maintain a detrimental motor pattern and prevent a successful outcome. As physical therapists, we are in the perfect position to address the patient's emotional state. Anxiety regarding their current physical status and the future can be relieved with an explanation of the possible causal factors. Restoring hope by providing a scientific treatment plan is often motivational and helps to build trust. When positive changes in function occur, the treatment plan is reinforced and this builds commitment. In the end, it is our job to teach people to accept responsibility for their health through education and motivation.

CONCLUSION

It has long been recognized that physical factors impact joint motion. The model presented here suggests that joint mechanics are influenced by multiple factors, some intrinsic to the joint itself others produced by muscle action which in turn is influenced by the emotional state. This chapter has briefly outlined the assessment findings and the principles for management of the articular (form closure) and muscular (force closure and motor control) factors which impact function of the SIJ and consequently the ability of the pelvic girdle to transfer load. The effective management of pelvic pain and dysfunction requires attention to all four components – form closure, force closure, motor control and emotions – the ultimate goal being to guide patients towards a healthier way to live in their body.

KEYWORDS

pelvic girdle pain	sacroiliac joint
low back pain	

References

Ashton-Miller J A, Howard D, DeLancey J O L 2001 The functional anatomy of the female pelvic floor and stress continence control system. Scandinavian Journal of Urology and Nephrology Supplementum 207: 1–7; discussion, 106–125

Avery A, O'Sullivan P, McCallum M 2001 Evidence of pelvic floor muscle dysfunction in subjects with chronic sacro-iliac joint pain dysfunction. In: Proceedings of the 7th Scientific Conference of IFOMT, Perth, Australia, pp 35–38

Barker P J, Briggs C A 1999 Attachments of the posterior layer of the lumbar fascia. Spine 24(17): 1757–1764

Bergmark A 1989 Stability of the lumbar spine: a study in mechanical engineering. Acta Orthopaedica Scandinavica 230(60): 20–24

Bo K, Stein R 1994 Needle EMG registration of striated urethral wall and pelvic floor muscle activity patterns during cough, valsalva, abdominal, hip adductor, and gluteal muscles contractions in nulliparous healthy females. Neurourology and Urodynamics 13: 35–41

Bowen V, Cassidy J D 1981 Macroscopic and microscopic anatomy of the sacroiliac joint from embryonic life until the eighth decade. Spine 6: 620–628

Buyruk H M, Stam H J, Snijders C J, Vleeming A, Laméris J S, Holland W P J 1995a The use of colour doppler imaging for the assessment of sacroiliac joint stiffness: a study on embalmed human pelvises. European Journal of Radiology 21: 112–116

Buyruk H M, Snijders C J, Vleeming A, Laméris J S, Holland W P J, Stam H J 1995b The measurements of sacroiliac joint stiffness with colour doppler imaging: a study on healthy subjects. European Journal of Radiology 21: 117–121

Buyruk H M, Stam H J, Snijders C J, Vleeming A, Laméris J S, Holland W P J 1997 Measurement of sacroiliac joint stiffness with color doppler imaging and the importance of asymmetric stiffness in sacroiliac pathology. In: Vleeming A, Mooney V, Dorman T, Snijders C, Stoeckart R (eds) Movement, stability and low back pain. Churchill Livingstone, Edinburgh, pp 297–307

Buyruk H M, Stam H J, Snijders C J, Laméris J S, Holland W P J, Stijnen W P 1999 Measurement of sacroiliac joint stiffness in peripartum

pelvic pain patients with doppler imaging of vibrations (DIV). European Journal of Obstetrics, Gynecology, and Reproductive Biology 83(2): 159–163

Carmichael J P 1987 Inter- and intra-examiner reliability of palpation for sacroiliac joint dysfunction. Journal of Manipulative and Physiological Therapeutics 10(4): 164–171

Comerford M J, Mottram S L 2001 Movement and stability dysfunction: contemporary developments. Manual Therapy 6(1): 15

Constantinou C E, Govan D E 1982 Spatial distribution and timing of transmitted and reflexly generated urethral pressures in healthy women. Journal of Urology 127: 964–969

Danneels L A, Vanderstraeten G G, Cambier D C, Witvrouw E E, De Cuyper H J 2000 CT imaging of trunk muscles in chronic low back pain patients and healthy control subjects. European Spine 9(4): 266–272

Danneels L A, Vanderstraeten G, Cambier D, Witvrouw E, Raes H, de Cuyper H 2001 A randomized clinical trial of three rehabilitation programs for the lumbar multifidus in patients with chronic low back pain. In: Proceedings from the Fourth Interdisciplinary World Congress on Low Back and Pelvic Pain, Montreal, Canada, pp 219–220

Dorman T 1994 Failure of self bracing at the sacroiliac joint: the slipping clutch syndrome. Journal of Orthopaedic Medicine 16: 49–51

Dreyfuss P, Dreyer S, Griffin J, Hoffman J, Walsh N 1994 Positive sacroiliac screening tests in asymptomatic adults. Spine 19: 1138–1143

Dreyfuss P, Michaelsen M, Pauza D, McLarty J, Bogduk N 1996 The value of history and physical examination in diagnosing sacroiliac joint pain. Spine 21: 2594–2602

Egund N, Olsson T H, Schmid H 1978 Movements in the sacro-iliac joints demonstrated with roentgen stereophotogrammetry. Acta Radiologica 19: 833–846

Gracovetsky S 1990 Musculoskeletal function of the spine. In: Winters J M, Woo S L Y (eds) Multiple muscle systems: biomechanics and movement organization. Springer Verlag, New York

Hartman L 1997 Handbook of osteopathic technique, 3rd edn. Chapman and Hall, London

Herzog W, Read L, Conway P J W, Shaw L D, McEwen M C 1989 Reliability of motion palpation procedures to detect sacroiliac joint fixations. Journal Manipulative and Physiological Therapeutics 12(2): 86–92

Hides J A, Stokes M J, Saide M, Jull G A, Cooper D H 1994 Evidence of lumbar multifidus muscles wasting ipsilateral to symptoms in patients with acute/subacute low back pain. Spine 19(2): 165–177

Hides J A, Richardson C A, Jull G A 1996 Multifidus recovery is not automatic following resolution of acute first episode low back pain. Spine 21(23): 2763–2769

Hodges P W 1997 Feedforward contraction of transversus abdominis is not influenced by the direction of arm movement. Experimental Brain Research 114: 362–370

Hodges P W, Gandevia S C 2000 Changes in intra-abdominal pressure during postural and respiratory activation of the human diaphragm. Journal of Applied Physiology 89: 967–976

Hodges P W, Richardson C A 1996 Inefficient muscular stabilization of the lumbar spine associated with low back pain: a motor control evaluation of transversus abdominis. Spine 21(22): 2640–2650

Hodges P W, Richardson C A 1997 Contraction of the abdominal muscles associated with movement of the lower limb. Physical Therapy 77: 132–144

Holstege G, Bandler R, Saper C B 1996 The emotional motor system. Elsevier, Amsterdam

Hungerford B, Gilleard W, Lee D 2001 Alteration of sacroiliac joint motion patterns in subjects with pelvic motion asymmetry. In: Proceedings from the Fourth World Interdisciplinary Congress on Low Back and Pelvic Pain, Montreal, Canada, pp 263–268

Jacob H A C, Kissling R O 1995 The mobility of the sacroiliac joints in healthy volunteers between 20 and 50 years of age. Clinical Biomechanics 10(7): 352–361

Laslett M, Williams W 1994 The reliability of selected pain provocation tests for sacroiliac joint pathology. Spine 19(11): 1243–1249

Lavignolle B, Vital J M, Senegas J et al 1983 An approach to the functional anatomy of the sacroiliac joints in vivo. Anatomica Clinica 5:169–176

Lee D G 2001 Imagery for core stabilization. Diane G. Lee Physiotherapist Corporation Publisher, Delta, Canada

Lee D G 2004 The pelvic girdle, 3rd edn. Churchill Livingstone, Edinburgh

Lee D G, Vleeming A 1998 Impaired load transfer through the pelvic girdle: a new model of altered neutral zone function. In: Proceedings from the Third Interdisciplinary World Congress on Low Back and Pelvic Pain, Vienna, Austria, pp 76–82

Mens J M A, Vleeming A, Snijders C J, Stam H J 1997 Active straight leg raising test: a clinical approach to the load transfer function of the pelvic girdle. In: Vleeming A, Mooney V, Dorman T, Snijders C, Stoeckart R (eds) Movement, stability and low back pain. Churchill Livingstone, Edinburgh, pp 425–431

Mens J M A, Vleeming A, Snijders C J, Stam H J, Ginai A Z 1999 The active straight leg raising test and mobility of the pelvic joints. European Spine 8: 468–473

Mens J M A, Vleeming A, Snijders C J, Koes B J, Stam H J 2001 Reliability and validity of the active straight leg raise test in posterior pelvic pain since pregnancy. Spine 26(10): 1167–1171

Moseley G L, Hodges P W, Gandevia S C 2002 Deep and superficial fibers of the lumbar multifidus muscle are differentially active during voluntary arm movements. Spine 27(2): E29–E36

Murphy M 1992 The future of the body: explorations into the further evolution of human nature. Tarcher Putnam, New York

O'Sullivan P 2000 Lumbar segmental instability: diagnosis and specific exercise management. In: Proceedings of the Seventh Scientific Conference of the International Federation of Orthopaedic Manipulative Therapists (IFOMT), Perth, Australia, p 46

O'Sullivan P, Twomey L, Allison G 1997. Evaluation of specific stabilising exercise in the treatment of chronic low back pain with radiological diagnosis of spondylolysis and spondylolisthesis. Spine 15(24): 2959–2967

Panjabi M M 1992 The stabilizing system of the spine. I: Function, dysfunction, adaptation, and enhancement. Journal of Spinal Disorders 5(4): 383–389

Richardson C A, Jull G A 1995 Muscle control – pain control. What exercises would you prescribe? Manual Therapy 1: 2–10

Richardson C A, Jull G A, Hodges P W, Hides J A 1999 Therapeutic exercise for spinal segmental stabilization in low back pain: scientific basis and clinical approach. Churchill Livingstone, Edinburgh

Richardson C A, Snijders C J, Hides J A, Damen L, Pas M S, Storm J 2002 The relationship between the transversely oriented abdominal muscles, sacroiliac joint mechanics and low back pain. Spine 27(4): 399–405

Sapolsky R M, Spencer E M 1997 Insulin growth factor 1 is suppressed in socially subordinate male baboons. American Journal of Physiology 273(4/2): 1346–1351

Sapolsky R M, Alberts R C, Altmann J 1997 Hypercortisolism associated with social subordinance isolation among wild baboons. Archives General Psychiatry 54(12): 1137–1143

Sapsford R R, Hodges P W, Richardson C A, Cooper D H, Markwell S J, Jull G A 2001 Co-activation of the abdominal and pelvic floor muscles during voluntary exercises. Neurourology and Urodynamics 20: 31–42

Sashin D 1930 A critical analysis of the anatomy and the pathologic changes of the sacro-iliac joints. Journal of Bone and Joint Surgery 12: 891–910

Snijders C J, Vleeming A, Stoeckart R 1993a Transfer of lumbosacral load to iliac bones and legs. 1: Biomechanics of self-bracing of the sacroiliac joints and its significance for treatment and exercise. Clinical Biomechanics 8: 285–294

Snijders C J, Vleeming A, Stoeckart R 1993b Transfer of lumbosacral load to iliac bones and legs. 2: Loading of the sacroiliac joints when lifting in a stooped posture. Clinical Biomechanics 8: 295–301

Snijders C J, Slagter A H E, Strik R van, Vleeming A, Stoeckart R, Stam H J 1995 Why leg-crossing? The influence of common postures on abdominal muscle activity. Spine 20(18): 1989–1993

Solonen K A 1957 The sacro-iliac joint in the light of anatomical roentgenological and clinical studies. Acta Orthopaedica Scandinavica 26(Suppl.): 9–116

Sturesson B, Selvik G, Uden A 1989 Movements of the sacroiliac joints: a roentgen stereophotogrammetric analysis. Spine 14(2): 162–165

Sturesson B, Uden A, Vleeming A 2000 A radiostereometric analysis of movements of the sacroiliac joints during the standing hip flexion test. Spine 25(3): 364–368

Van Wingerden J P, Vleeming A, Snijders C J, Stoeckart R 1993 A functional-anatomical approach to the spine-pelvis mechanism: interaction between the biceps femoris muscle and the sacrotuberous ligament. European Spine Journal 2: 140–144

Van Wingerden J P, Vleeming A, Buyruk H M, Raissadat K 2001 Muscular contribution to force closure: sacroiliac joint stabilization in vivo. In: Proceedings from the Fourth Interdisciplinary World Congress on Low Back and Pelvic Pain, Montreal, Canada

Vleeming A, Stoeckart R, Snijders C J 1989a The sacrotuberous ligament: a conceptual approach to its dynamic role in stabilizing the sacroiliac joint. Clinical Biomechanics 4: 201–203

Vleeming A, van Wingerden J P, Snijders C J, Stoeckart R, Stijnen T 1989b Load application to the sacrotuberous ligament: influences on sacroiliac joint mechanics. Clinical Biomechanics 4: 204–209

Vleeming A, Stoeckart R, Volkers A C W, Snijders C J 1990a Relation between form and function in the sacroiliac joint. 1: Clinical anatomical aspects. Spine 15(2): 130–132

Vleeming A, Volkers A C W, Snijders C J, Stoeckart R 1990b Relation between form and function in the sacroiliac joint. 2: Biomechanical aspects. Spine 15(2): 133–136

Vleeming A, van Wingerden J P, Dijkstra P F, Stoeckart R, Snijders C J, Stijnen T 1992 Mobility in the SI-joints in old people: a kinematic and radiologic study. Clinical Biomechanics 7: 170–176

Vleeming A, Pool-Goudzwaard A L, Stoeckart R, van Wingerden J P, Snijders C J 1995a The posterior layer of the thoracolumbar fascia: its function in load transfer from spine to legs. Spine 20: 753–758

Vleeming A, Snijders C J, Stoeckart R, Mens J M A 1995b A new light on low back pain. In: Proceedings from the Second Interdisciplinary World Congress on Low Back Pain, San Diego, California, pp 149–168

Vleeming A, Pool-Goudzwaard A L, Hammudoghlu D, Stoeckart R, Snijders C J, Mens J M A 1996 The function of the long dorsal sacroiliac ligament: its implication for understanding low back pain. Spine 21(5): 556–562

Willard 1997

Willard F H 1997 The muscular, ligamentous and neural structure of the low back and its relation to back pain. In: Vleeming A, Mooney V, Dorman T, Snijders C, Stoeckart R (eds) Movement, stability and low back pain. Churchill Livingstone, Edinburgh, pp 3–35

Chapter **35**

Pelvic floor dysfunction in low back and sacroiliac dysfunction

R. Sapsford, S. Kelley

INTRODUCTION

This chapter aims to heighten the awareness of musculoskeletal physiotherapists to the possibility of pelvic floor (PF) problems in their patients with low back pain (LBP) and sacroiliac (SIJ) dysfunction. It provides details of the pelvic floor muscles, their function and dysfunction, and the evidence connecting this dysfunction with LBP. Hypotheses are proposed as to the mechanisms of the associated dysfunctions. Discreet questioning regarding PF problems may be facilitated during explanations to patients about the muscles of the abdominal capsule. If problems are admitted, referral for further management may be indicated. Management strategies for combined low back and PF problems are discussed.

CO-MORBIDITY OF LOW BACK PAIN, SACROILIAC AND PELVIC FLOOR DYSFUNCTION

Pelvic floor disorders are very common in the community. In a survey of 3010 subjects in a representative population survey, 46.2% of women and 11.1% of men acknowledged some form of major PF dysfunction at the time of the study (McLennan et al 2000). The co-morbidity of PF dysfunction and LBP/SIJ pain is rarely investigated, but is well recognized in cauda equina syndrome.

Cauda equina syndrome

Musculoskeletal physiotherapists are trained to recognise the cauda equina (CE) syndrome. The nerve roots of the CE provide the sensory and motor innervation of most of the lower extremities, the PF and the urethral and anal sphincters. CE syndrome occurs with single or double-level compression of the lumbosacral nerve roots located in the dural sac. The symptoms include low back pain, saddle anaesthesia, bilateral sciatica, sexual dysfunction, motor weakness of the lower extremities and bladder and bowel dysfunction (Orendacova et al 2001).

Multiple aetiology can cause the CE syndrome and includes ischaemic insults, inflammatory conditions, spinal arachnoiditis, infections, herniated lumbosacral discs, spinal stenosis and spinal neoplasms (Orendacova et al 2001). The incidence of lower urinary tract dysfunction as a result of disc prolapse is approximately 20% (Chancellor 1998). Disc herniation may disturb the bladder emptying reflex either by directly compressing the nerve roots or by indirectly disturbing the activity in the sacral micturition reflex centre (S2–4) when the pathways from the supraspinal regulation centres are affected (Eriksen et al 1988).

Specifically, the bowel and bladder symptoms include urinary retention, saddle anaesthesia, reduced anal sphincter tone and possibly constipation (Eriksen et al 1988). Urinary retention occurs due to an acontractile bladder as the detrusor contraction is under parasympathetic control. Urodynamic studies in CE patients demonstrate 'areflexia' of the bladder in approximately one quarter of the cases (Bartolin et al 1998). In milder degrees of compression there is sometimes difficulty initiating voiding or incomplete emptying of the bladder (Duthie 1996). Urinary frequency and nocturia are also signs of CE syndrome (Susset et al 1982) and probably result from the partial emptying at each void.

If CE is suspected by the physiotherapist any form of mobilization or manipulation is contraindicated (Maitland 2001). The patient should be referred immediately to a medical specialist as this syndrome is best managed by surgical decompression (Hanley et al 1996). However, complete recovery of bladder function does not necessarily occur (Chang et al 2000, Yamanishi et al 2002) and electrical stimulation of the PF has been shown to help these patients (Eriksen et al 1988).

Some patients may present with subclinical CE that is only aggravated by positions such as lumbar extension (Dyck et al 1977). Therefore it is important for the therapist to closely question patients on any mechanical links to their bowel and bladder symptoms and also the timing of onset of symptoms. Additionally the therapist needs to be aware of patient sensitivities when conducting a subjective examination involving bladder and bowel dysfunction, as some patients are reluctant to admit to such symptoms.

Low back pain and the pelvic floor

Some patients with LBP may also present with bladder symptoms but do not have any signs of CE compression on radiographic examination (Sprangfort 1989). Patients may mention episodes of stress incontinence, and these are often disregarded by the therapist. Recent surveys have highlighted the coexistence of LBP and PF dysfunction. Seim et al (2000) surveyed 4034 women aged from 40 to 42 years, who were involved in a cardiovascular screening programme and found 7.7% had a current or past history of urinary incontinence. A connection between connective tissue changes and stress urinary incontinence (SUI) with bladder neck prolapse (Sayer et al 1990) prompted a further investigation of musculoskeletal disorders in these women. Of the incontinent group 53.5% had LBP and 10.1% had a pelvic joint syndrome, whereas in the continent group the incidence of LBP and pelvic joint syndrome was 22.3% and 2.1% respectively. In some patients with LBP there are anecdotal reports that as their spinal stability improves with rehabilitation, the urinary incontinence decreases.

Eisenstein et al (1994) also investigated the link between urinary symptoms and severe LBP. In his clinical practice, only 16 cases out of 5000 were identified who had urinary dysfunction and LBP, without any definable pathology in either system. The 16 patients were noted to have frequency, urge urinary incontinence, perineal anaesthesia, normal anal sphincter tone and LBP. Of these 16 patients 12 underwent surgery (spinal fusion in 11 and total hip replacement in one) and four were awaiting surgery. Surgery reduced the LBP in the large majority and as an unexpected result the urinary incontinence also improved. Eisenstein (1994) and his colleagues simply suggested that the low back pain caused bladder symptoms. They went on to suggest that pain neuropeptides influenced the parasympathetic discharge at S2–4 resulting in detrusor contraction or bladder neck relaxation. Alternatively the pudendal nerve (S2–4) may also have been affected by parasympathetic outflow and that could have explained the reduced sensation in the perineum experienced by these patients.

In another questionnaire with 86 respondents (Pool-Goudzwaard & Stoeckart 2000) 38 were found to suffer from LBP with three also reporting PF pain. Pelvic joint pain was reported by 25 of the 86 respondents, with 20 of these reporting PF pain. In some patients stabilizing exercises increased the PF dysfunction, in particular SUI, coccygodynia and anal incontinence. The authors considered that these symptoms were due to a hypertonic PF, and recommended that care must be taken to relax the PF before initiating stabilization exercise programmes (Pool-Goudzwaard & Stoeckart 2000).

Sacroiliac joint dysfunction and the pelvic floor

The coexistence of PF dysfunction and LBP/SIJ dysfunction does not occur exclusively in females. While there are variations in the more superficial pelvic floor muscle (PFM) layers between the genders this does not alter the overall pain patterns. Devreese et al (2000) presented a case report documenting the importance of differentiating between testicular pain caused by prostatitis and caused by LBP/SIJ dysfunction. The patient was found to have pathology in the prostate, which was treated by antibiotics, as well as in the low back and SIJ. Initially manual therapy and PF exercise improved the low back and low abdominal pain and resolved the incontinence and erection problems. A few months later these complaints returned. Recurrent prostatitis was treated with prostatic resection. A subsequent recurrence of all the other painful symptoms was resolved by pelvic floor retraining. This allowed the patient to return to his former active lifestyle. It has also been observed that men with lumbosacral radiculopathy may have their urinary retention symptoms attributed to bladder outlet obstruction secondary to benign prostatic hyperplasia. Then follows unnecessary transurethral resection of the prostate (TURP) when the real cause is central disc protrusion (Chancellor 1998).

Some recent investigations have focused on the link between PF control and pelvic stability (Avery et al 2000, O'Sullivan et al 2002). Avery et al (2000) investigated the function of the PFM in subjects with chronic SIJ pain with a positive active straight leg raise (ASLR) test that was eased with pelvic compression. The subjects were matched with controls. Real-time ultrasound (US), using a suprapubic approach, monitored the PF movement, using the bladder neck as a reference point. The ASLR test and cognitive PFM activation in those with SIJ pain resulted in caudal movement of the bladder which was greatly reduced with manual compression of the pelvis. These findings differed significantly from those found in control subjects in whom the PF position either did not change or was elevated during the different manoeuvres. Avery (Avery et al 2000) hypothesized that dysfunction of the PFM caused a deficit in the stability of the SIJ.

O'Sullivan et al (2002) investigated the respiratory patterns and calculated minute volume as well as monitoring the descent of the PFM (real-time US) in patients with SIJ dysfunction versus controls, during the ASLR test. Patients with SIJ pain had decreased diaphragmatic excursion and increased PF descent during the ASLR test when compared with controls. Manual compression through the ilia increased the stability of the pelvis and reversed the differences between the patient group and controls. O'Sullivan et al (2001) extended this study by retraining elevation of the PF in co-contraction with the deep abdominals and lumbar multifidus, using real-time US for visual feedback. The training period was 10 weeks and progressed from non-weight-bearing to weight-bearing positions. Normalization of diaphragmatic and PF excursion occurred during the ASLR following muscle retraining. Urinary symptoms also improved. The authors hypothesized that the dysfunctional PFM action may have affected the force closure mechanism of the SIJ in these cases.

Sacroiliac joint dysfunction has also been linked to urinary frequency and urgency in a case study presented by Dangaria (1998). Urodynamic investigation of bladder function and MRI of the lumbar spine were normal. Non-steroidal anti-inflammatory drugs and back strengthening exercises did not alter either the LBP or urinary symptoms. SIJ manipulation was performed for the treatment of LBP and unexpectedly relieved the urinary symptoms. The author believed that the combination of problems could be attributed to the same segmental nerve supply.

Pelvic floor dysfunction and low back pain

Self-reports of LBP among gynaecological patients are non-specific. There is not any evidence in the literature of assessment or management of the pain. It seems that the condition is attributed to the gynaecological pathology and is assumed to resolve once surgery has alleviated the urogenital defect.

Koppe et al (1984) performed a long-term follow-up (7–13 years) of women following surgical repair of genital prolapse. The results indicated that low back pain had recurred in 29% of the patients, whereas it was present in 53.5% preoperatively. Prolapses also recurred, but whether recurrence of back pain and prolapse were in the same patients was not detailed. There were no data on back pain history prior to prolapse or in the intervening years.

LBP has also been noted in women in whom SUI recurred some years after surgery (Kjolhede & Ryden 1997). These women were compared with a group presenting with a similar primary condition prior to surgery. The group with recurrence complained of more 'lumbago and sciatica' than the primary group (66% compared with 38%), and were less able to develop a palpable PFM contraction (56% compared with 83%). The authors considered that the LBP might have contributed to neurological disturbance of the PFM and this may have influenced the surgical outcome.

PELVIC FLOOR MUSCLES: THEIR FUNCTION AND DYSFUNCTION

This review of PFM function and associated problems is included to help musculoskeletal physiotherapists increase their understanding of this area, and enable more accurate interpretation of symptoms reported by their patients.

Pelvic floor muscle function

The PF is a musculoskeletal unit with active, passive and neural systems of control (Panjabi 1992). The function of the PFM complex is to support the pelvic organs against gravity at rest and with light, heavy and sudden loading, and to contribute to intra-abdominal pressure (IAP). It contributes to urinary and faecal continence and releases for elimination from bladder and bowel. Details of the muscles are provided in Table 35.1. See also Figure 35.1.

There is a high proportion of slow twitch fibres in the PFM, which reflects their function (Gilpin et al 1989). During normal function, the PFM show tonic activity at rest in supine, increasing in sitting and standing (Vereeken et al 1975). The muscle recruitment increases with effort, and the strength developed depends on the demands placed upon the muscle by the increasing IAP. Though resting tonic PFM activity is expected in normal subjects, in some nulliparous women who could cognitively contract the muscles pubococcygeal tonic activity was absent at rest during testing, though a phasic response to demand occurred (Deindl et al 1993).

Table 35.1 The pelvic floor muscles in the female

Layers	Muscles	Attachments	Function
Superficial NB gender variations occur	Bulbospongiosus Ischiocavernosus Sup. transverse perinei External anal sphincter	Perineal body to clitoris Ischial tub. to clitoris Ischial tub. to perineal body Coccyx to perineal body	Sexual arousal Sexual arousal Perineal stability Anal continence
Intermediate NB gender variations occur	Intrinsic urethral sphincter Compressor urethrae Urethrovaginal sphincter	Intramural urethra Ischiopubic ramus to urethra Urethra to perineal body	Resting urethral pressure and rapid urethral closure before ↑ IAP
Deep (levator ani) (see Fig. 35.1)	Puborectalis	U-shaped muscle from pubic bone around anorectal junction	Anal continence

	Pubococcygeus (PC)	Pubic bone and arcuate line to
		  tip of coccyx
			Compresses and supports vagina and
			  rectum

	Iliococcygeus	Arcuate line and ischial spine to sides of coccyx	Rectal support

	(Ischio)coccygeus	Ischial spine and sacrospinous
		  ligament[a] to sides of lower
		  sacral segments
			Rectal support and
			  counternutation SIJ

[a]The sacrospinous ligament, from which (ischio)coccygeus arises, runs from the ischial spine to the lateral margins of the sacrum and coccyx and rests on the anterior aspect of the sacrotuberous ligament. Their fibres intermingle. The fibres of gluteus maximus, piriformis and, in some subjects, biceps femoris often have direct attachments to the sacrotuberous ligament. It has been hypothesized that these muscles, interacting with the sacrotuberous ligament, influence the movement at the SIJ (Vleeming et al 1989).
  Key: SIJ = sacroiliac joint; IAP = intra-abdominal pressure; ischial tub. = ischial tuberosity.

The PFM form the base of the abdominal capsule and along with transversus abdominis (TrA), multifidus and the diaphragm they contribute to the stability of the lumbosacral region (Fig. 35.2). A contraction in one of these muscles elicits a contractile response in other muscles of the group in normal subjects. Thus with a voluntary contraction of the PFM a contraction can be palpated in TrA and lumbar multifidus. There is no direct mechanical link between the

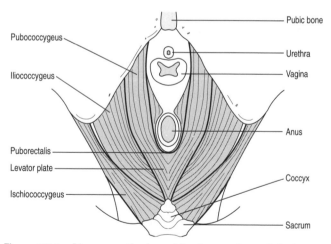

Figure 35.1 Diagrammatic view of the four sections of the levator ani viewed from the pelvic surface. Puborectalis forms a U-shaped sling which is incorporated into and functions with the external anal sphincter; pubococcygeus, the principal component, supports and compresses the vagina and rectum and fuses posteriorly to form the levator plate between the anorectal junction and the coccyx; iliococcygeus fuses with pubococcygeus into the levator plate which supports the upper vagina and the rectum; ischiococcygeus provides further rectal support. Reproduced from Sapsford 2001 with permission of the Chartered Society of Physiotherapy, UK.

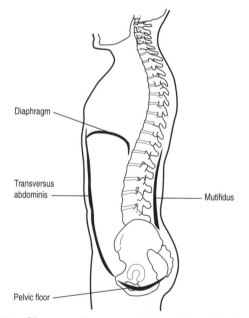

Figure 35.2 Diagrammatic representation of the abdominopelvic cavity surrounded by the local muscle system which contributes to respiration, spinal stability, intra-abdominal pressure and continence. Reproduced with permission of C. P. Sapsford.

PF and abdominal muscles, though there is some embryological evidence of a developmental continuum of rectus abdominis and puborectalis (Power 1948). The co-activation is attributed to motor control. Scientific evidence for this, demonstrated in cats, focuses on motor neuronal pathways from the nucleus retroambiguous to the lumbosacral cord. The motor neuronal pathways project densely to both the abdominal wall and PF neurones (S2–4) (Vanderhorst & Holstege 1997) and it is likely that similar pathways occur in man (G. Holstege, personal communication, 1998).

Micturition occurs without an increase in IAP and requires relaxation of the abdominal and PFM prior to the contraction of the bladder (detrusor muscle). When bowel emptying proceeds effortlessly, in response to demand, the anus relaxes and the rectum expels contents with its intrinsic contractions. If evacuation requires effort the rectum needs more muscular support against the IAP. This is provided by pubo/ilio/ischiococcygeus. However, if these muscles are not recruited appropriately and straining occurs, fascial stretch and neurological damage can develop over time.

Co-activation of the abdominal capsule

It is only recently that co-activation of the abdominal muscles and PFM, as part of abdominal capsule function, has been recognized. In an EMG study on normal subjects, cognitive isometric contractions of the abdominal muscles resulted in increased EMG activity in pubococcygeus and the external anal sphincter (EAS) (Sapsford & Hodges 2001). This activity increased as the abdominal effort increased. When the abdominal isometric hold was very gentle, simulating a TrA contraction, there was a definite but small increase in EMG activity in pubococcygeus and EAS. The reverse action has also been shown. TrA, the obliquus internus and obliquus externus abdominis were active during a voluntary maximal PFM contraction (Neumann & Gill 2002, Sapsford et al 2001).

The position of the lumbar spine (flexion, extension or neutral) during the PFM contraction varied the proportion of each abdominal muscle recruited. However, when the subject was asked to contract the PF gently, TrA was the principal muscle recruited irrespective of the spinal position.

Research in normal subjects has demonstrated that a PF contraction occurs prior to rapid arm movement and before the contraction of deltoid (Hodges et al 2002). When the arm was moved rapidly and repeatedly, pubococcygeus and EAS muscles were active tonically with phasic bursts with each movement. No research to date has attempted to measure the recruitment timing in those with PF dysfunction.

From biomechanical principles, tasks that increase IAP result in diaphragmatic and PFM co-contraction. In respiration in lying, if the diaphragm does not increase the IAP there is no reason for the PFM to be activated above their resting tone. Respiration in standing occurs against a background of increased abdominal and PFM tonic activity. A strong co-contraction of the abdominal and PF muscles occurs in forced expiration.

Types and causes of pelvic floor dysfunction

Many problems of PF function can be attributed to disturbances of tonic activity and the timing of muscle recruitment. Insufficient muscle strength and power, partial neuropathy, obesity, menopause and ageing all contribute to the plethora of PF problems. There are many forms of PF dysfunction and these are listed in Table 35.2.

Vaginal deliveries are considered the predominant initiating factor in PF dysfunction with 80% of women showing evidence of denervation and reinnervation of pubococcygeus after the first vaginal delivery (Allen et al 1990). Occult anal sphincter tears to either the internal anal sphincter or EAS or both occur in 35% of women having a first vaginal delivery (Sultan et al 1993). There is also evidence of neurological damage to the EAS after vaginal delivery (Snooks et al 1984, Sultan et al 1994). Contributing factors during the delivery are prolonged second stage of labour, forceps delivery and, in some studies, babies larger than 4000 g. The first delivery has the greatest impact (McLennan et al 2000, Viktrup 2002). Women having elective caesarean sections have been noted to have normal PF function following delivery (Allen et al 1990, Snooks et al 1984, Sultan et al 1994, Viktrup et al 1992) but do not necessarily avoid PF dysfunction in the longer term (McLennan et al 2000, Viktrup 2002). Disruption of muscle activation has been demonstrated in some women with SUI. Pubococcygeal tonic activity was deficient, and there was asymmetrical recruitment and paradoxical inhibition during effort despite the ability to activate the muscle voluntarily (Deindl et al 1994).

It is important to be aware of the contribution of fascial and ligamentous laxity to dysfunction. Most parous women who have delivered babies vaginally demonstrate some laxity of passive tissues and the vaginal wall in comparison with nulliparous females. Further stretch to these passive structures occurs with heavy lifting without muscular support and regular straining to empty the bowel (Spence-Jones et al 1994). Regular straining has been implicated in uterovaginal prolapse, while women who demonstrate joint hypermobility are at greater risk of prolapse (Norton et al 1995).

A PROPOSAL FOR THE BASIS OF CO-MORBIDITY

The authors have considered the role of the three systems of control that Panjabi (1992) proposed to explain this co-morbidity. Panjabi developed his model of three interacting systems – active, passive and neural – to explain lumbar spine stability and instability, but the same principles can be applied to the PF musculoskeletal unit as well. There is an overlap in the three systems, with one system being able to compensate to a certain degree for the insufficiency in the other systems. This may help the understanding of problems in the PF as well as the lumbosacral region and

Table 35.2 Pelvic floor dysfunction

Type	Symptoms	Causes
Urinary		
Increased daytime frequency	More than 5–6 voids a day – increases with age	Poor bladder inhibition/poor PF support contributes to all
Nocturia	Waking from sleep to void. Voiding >1× at night, >2× over 70 years – a problem	
Urgency	Inability to defer voiding	Bladder (detrusor) overactivity
Urge urinary incontinence	Larger loss with strong urge to void	Bladder overactivity
Stress urinary incontinence	Spot loss with sudden increase in IAP	PFM timing, strength deficits, fascial laxity
Voiding dysfunction	Slow or intermittent urine flow – incomplete bladder emptying – urinary tract infections	Non-relaxation of urethral sphincter mechanism[a]
Pelvic organ prolapse (Vaginal wall descent) Anterior (bladder) Posterior (rectum) Apical (cervix + uterus)	These three often present with suprapubic and/or vaginal dragging/discomfort/a vaginal lump – worse with lifting, bending, squatting, prolonged standing and at end of the day	Straining to evacuate, poor PF support against ↑ gravity and IAP.
Anorectal		
Obstructed defaecation	Regular straining, sense of incomplete emptying	Poor rectal support/non relaxation of anal sphincter
Anal incontinence	Includes flatus, liquid and solid matter	Vaginal delivery – sphincter tears, neuropathy
Perineal/perianal pain	Levator ani spasm – levator syndrome	Overactive abdominals can contribute to overactive PF
	Excessive extensibility of perineal structures termed descending perineum syndrome	Pudendal nerve stretch is responsible for pain

[a]Non relaxation of the urethral sphincter mechanism can result from poor relaxation of the abdominal wall, and has been demonstrated in young girls who perch on the toilet seat, using trunk muscles to provide stability (Wennergren et al 1991).
Key: PF = pelvic floor; IAP = intra-abdominal pressure; PFM = pelvic floor muscle.

provide a management approach for each problem. We believe motor control dysfunction is a contributing factor to the co-morbidity described in this chapter. Evidence can be found if the three systems are examined.

The active system

It has been proven that LBP and SIJ pain affect the normal functioning of different components of the abdominal muscle capsule. Hides et al (1994) demonstrated that a decrease in lumbar multifidus cross-sectional area occurred with first episode LBP. Hodges & Richardson (1996) showed that the recruitment of TrA was disturbed in patients with LBP. Avery et al (2000) and O'Sullivan et al (2002) found that there was decreased PFM activation in patients with SIJ instability and pain. While pain inhibition is probably the initial cause of disruption of muscle function, disturbances in motor control of these muscle components could well be the basis for ongoing co-morbidity of the LBP, SIJ and PF problems.

O'Sullivan et al (2001) were able to demonstrate that muscle rehabilitation of the PF in co-contraction with the deep abdominal and multifidus muscles alleviated SIJ instability and pain in their patients. As a result diaphragmatic activity was normalized during the ASLR test and symptoms of PF dysfunction were improved. The contribution of TrA to SIJ stability has been demonstrated by Richardson et al (2002), who successfully linked the activation of TrA to increasing joint stiffness of the SIJ. The hypothesis by Avery et al (2000) that SIJ pain during the ASLR test was due to PFM dysfunction may not have considered the whole picture. Manual compression of the pelvis might change the passive system and allow better recruitment of the active system (PFM) in patients with SIJ pain (Avery et al 2000). It could be questioned whether the effect was due to relief of pain, with its associated muscle inhibition, or whether it was due to generation of a lower IAP. Increases in IAP and trunk stability both involve diaphragmatic, abdominal and PFM activity. O'Sullivan et al (2002) commented that diaphragmatic excursion was reduced during the ASLR test in SIJ pain. Perhaps the patients were recruiting all of their IAP generating muscles in the effort to raise the limb and the increased IAP depressed the PF. In those patients who could isolate the activation of TrA, yet could not maintain the PF position on ASLR (Avery et al 2000), TrA may not have had adequate holding ability for the time taken and the load added to do the ASLR test. Alternatively, the attempted movement may have triggered pain that inhibited the muscle activity. To obtain an accurate picture of the mechanisms involved in the findings of Avery and O'Sullivan, it would be necessary to monitor all the muscle components as well as IAP.

An increase in PF pain has been observed in some LBP patients when stabilizing exercises were commenced (Pool-Goudzwaard & Stoeckart 2000). The authors suggested that the pain was associated with hypertonicity of the PFM, in particular pubococcygeus. They recommended that care must be taken to relax the PFM before commencing stabilization exercises. However, this suggestion could be questioned. In the study neither EMG nor real-time US was used to monitor which abdominal muscles were active during the exercises. Global abdominal muscle activity and poor respiratory patterns occur frequently among patients with LBP (Richardson et al 1999). Increasing global abdominal activity increases PFM activity and conscious relaxation of the abdominal muscles has been shown to decrease resting pubococcygeal EMG activity (Sapsford & Hodges 2001). Thus the patients developing an increase in PF pain during stabilizing exercises may have been recruiting the global abdominal muscles instead of low level local muscle (TrA) activity, or they may not have relaxed the global muscles before commencing the stabilization programme. A similar mechanism of global abdominal muscle overactivity may apply in other cases of perineal and perianal pain, even if not associated with significant LBP.

The passive system

While the previous section considered the active system in the control of SIJ, factors related to the passive system also need to be considered. It is impossible for therapists to restore the integrity of passive structures of the pelvic floor. Surgery is the only means by which this system can be improved. Decreases in LBP have been noted in patients who undergo vaginal repairs (Koppe et al 1984). That the LBP resolved after the repair may indicate that the PF passive system contributes to spinal stability, or that the supported tissue allows better functioning of the active system. However, it is possible that these women followed advice to decrease the level of stress by avoiding heavy physical activity in order to prevent a recurrence of the prolapse.

Passive compression through the ilia has been found to reduce pain and improve the function of the active system (Avery et al 2000, O'Sullivan et al 2002). Maintenance of manual compression during function would be difficult. The only means therapists have to do this is by the prescription of SIJ belts. There is little research available on the efficacy of these belts in pregnant women; however, they appear to reduce pain and allow improved function. It has

been suggested that these belts could increase proprioception and muscle activity and thus force closure around the SIJ. However, research has demonstrated that a narrow, non-elastic belt with a tension of 50 newtons, positioned just above the greater trochanter in human pelvis and spine preparations, significantly restricted rotational movement at the SIJs (Vleeming et al 1992). In living subjects a similarly placed belt was found to decrease muscle activity in obliquus internus abdominis by reducing the load of gravity through the SIJs (Snijders et al 1998). Thus these belts are considered to improve form closure. In addition, advice on correct movement patterns that minimize passive stretch of the SIJ appears to be clinically beneficial.

Marked laxity of the PF passive system, which frequently occurs in SUI and vaginal prolapse, requires a stronger active system to maintain PF stability. It has been observed clinically that a sudden rise in IAP, as in a cough, results in a sense of vaginal opening or bulging (PF descent) in a number of parous women. This descent also occurs in SUI (Wijma et al 1991) and is more noticeable when the abdominal wall is relaxed. Yet when stability muscles function automatically, or are recruited appropriately, often with a changed postural position, a PF contraction can be felt during a cough.

Pubococcygeus supports the vagina, which in turn supports the urethra and the bladder base, and PFM tonic activity has an inhibitory effect on bladder activity (Mahony et al 1977). If this support is deficient then a sense of urgency and more frequent voiding are likely to occur. Urinary urgency and frequency were the symptoms reported by Eisenstein et al (1994) and Dangaria (1998) in their patients with LBP and with SIJ dysfunction. Eisenstein's patients reported improved urinary control after successful surgery (spinal fusion and total hip replacement) and a decrease in their pain. In one patient where the spinal fusion was not successful spinal pain persisted and so did the urinary symptoms. Hodges & Richardson (1996) showed that TrA altered its action from tonic to phasic activity in patients with low back pain, and it is likely that a similar effect occurs in the PFM. Clinically, urinary urgency and urge urinary incontinence, but not SUI, have been reported by a patient with confirmed SIJ instability and pain. It would seem that the periurethral sphincter mechanism was recruited phasically, but the PFM lost their tonic action. One explanation for these symptoms focuses on the motor control of TrA and the PFM. It has been observed clinically that rehabilitation of tonic activity in TrA, and hence in PFM, decreases symptoms of frequency and urge. This also seems to restore the recruitment timing for urethral closure prior to the increased IAP during a cough.

In cases of a recurrence of SUI some years after initial surgery, more 'lumbago and sciatica' occurred and there was a decreased ability to activate the PFM compared to women who had not yet had surgery (Kjolhede & Ryden 1997). Passive support achieved by the initial surgery was frequently intact, leaving deficits in the active or neural systems as possible reasons for the recurrence.

The neural system

The findings of Seim et al (2000) of a higher prevalence of LBP and pelvic pain in women with urinary incontinence might also be explained on the basis of motor control of TrA and the PFM. The types of urinary incontinence were not defined. Neither was there any indication of whether the musculoskeletal problems or urinary incontinence came first. Many women have a history of back pain, and perhaps the disturbances in motor control at that time contribute to changes in PFM function. Urinary incontinence often commences many years after pregnancy and vaginal delivery. Conversely disturbances in neural control systems associated with partial neuropathy, pain and swelling following vaginal delivery will disturb the sensory feedback from the muscle spindles and consequent efferent activity to the muscles. Women who have had a prolonged second stage of labour frequently report that they are unable to feel

their PF in the immediate postpartum period. Return of awareness may take several days. It can be questioned whether this disturbance in function could affect the rest of the stability muscles. There have been clinical observations supporting this hypothesis in women 3–4 months postpartum. In these patients, palpation of asymmetrical pubococcygeal muscle activity was accompanied by a same side deficit in the deep abdominal muscle recruitment during the PFM activation.

TREATMENT STRATEGIES FOR CO-MORBIDITY

The treatment of co-morbidity problems presented in the flow chart (Fig. 35.3) is based upon the rehabilitation model developed for retraining motor control by Richardson and colleagues (Richardson et al 1999). It commences with stability work and progresses to antigravity and functional activities.

While this treatment plan can be applied to all patients within the co-morbidity group, it is important to understand that incorrect muscle activation can worsen lumbosacral

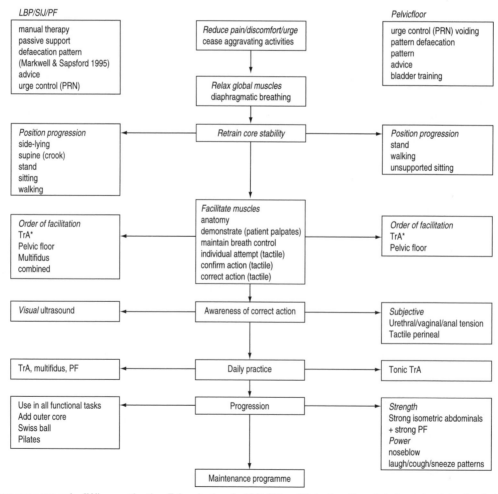

Figure 35.3 Treatment protocols. *When activating TrA, whether in LBP, SIJ or PF dysfunction, it is important to check that co-activaion is occuring within the PFM group. It is necessary to ask the patient for subjective feedback about the sensation of gentle tensioning around urethra/vagina/perineum/anus. If they feel that the vagina opens or bulges this indicates that the PFM are not activated correctly.

and PF problems. For example, if the superficial rather than the deep fibres of multifidus are recruited, LBP may worsen as a result of the increased anterior pelvic tilt. Additionally overactivity of the abdominal oblique muscles during specific TrA retraining may increase IAP and aggravate vaginal prolapse. Very specific instructions, meticulous monitoring and correction of performance, and detailed progressions are required for a successful outcome.

CONCLUSION

The precipitating factor for the different types of co-morbidity discussed in this chapter is generally an insult to the passive lumbo/sacral/pelvic structure. A minor insult may have major effects if the passive system is compromised by the hormonal changes of pregnancy. Consequent pain inhibition, reflex inhibition and disruption of timing of muscle recruitment due to disturbances in motor control involve the neural and active systems.

Why some patients develop a PF co-morbidity is open to conjecture. It is likely that there is some latent pathology within the abdominal capsular system that only becomes apparent once the motor control has been disturbed. This

may include partial PF neuropathy, PF fascial extensibility (prolapse and perineal descent) and abdominal muscle weakness or overactivity. Pregnancy, vaginal delivery and regular defaecation straining can cause these. Increases in IAP without appropriate PFM recruitment compound the problem.

The authors believe that the deep muscle system can be used to compensate for the passive dysfunction by improving motor control. The timing of PF, TrA and deep lumbar multifidus is the key factor in the prevention and treatment of ongoing LBP, SIJ dysfunction and PF dysfunction.

Some of the ideas presented in this chapter aim to challenge current thinking and hopefully will provide stimulus for further research.

KEYWORDS

pelvic floor dysfunction
low back pain
sacroiliac joint dysfunction
co-morbidity
treatment protocols

References

Allen R E, Hosker G L, Smith A R B et al 1990 Pelvic floor damage and childbirth: a neurophysiological study. British Journal of Obstetrics and Gynaecology 97: 770–779

Avery A F, O'Sullivan P B, McCallum M J 2000 Evidence of pelvic floor muscle dysfunction in subjects with chronic sacro-iliac joint pain syndrome. In: Proceedings of the Seventh Scientific Conference of the International Federation of Orthopaedic Manipulative Therapists (IFOMT) Perth, Australia, abstract 39

Bartolin Z, Gilja I, Bedalon G et al 1998 Bladder function in patients with lumbar intervertebral disc protrusion. Journal of Urology 159: 969–971

Chancellor M B 1998 Bladder dysfunction with neurological disease. Continuum: Lifelong Learning in Neurology 4(4): 105–107

Chang H S, Nakagawa H, Mizuno J 2000 Lumbar herniated disc presenting with cauda equina syndrome: long-term follow-up of four cases. Surgical Neurology 53(2): 100–104

Dangaria T R 1998 A case report of sacroiliac joint dysfunction with urinary symptoms. Manual Therapy 3(4): 220–221

Deindl F M, Vodusek D B, Hesse U et al 1993 Activity patterns of pubococcygeal muscles in nulliparous continent women. British Journal of Urology 72: 46–51

Deindl F M, Vodusek D B, Hesse U et al 1994 Pelvic floor activity patterns: comparison of nulliparous continent and parous urinary stress incontinent women: a kinesiological EMG study. British Journal of Urology 73: 413–417

Devreese A, Dankaerts W, Staes F et al 2000 Can testicular pain be related to low back/sacroiliac junction dysfunction? In: Proceedings of the Seventh Scientific Conference of the International Federation of Orthopaedic Manipulative Therapists (IFOMT) Perth, Australia, abstract 115

Duthie R 1996 Affections of the spine. In: Duthie R, Bentley G (eds) Mercer's Orthopaedic surgery, 9th edn. Arnold, London, p 956

Dyck P, Pheasant H C, Doyle J B 1977 Intermittent cauda equina compression syndrome: its recognition and treatment. Spine 2(1): 75–81

Eisenstein S M, Engelbrecht D J, El Masry W S 1994 Low back pain and urinary incontinence. Spine 19: 1148–1152

Eriksen B C, Sand T, Sjaastad O 1988 Detrusor hyporeflexia after anterior sciatic syndrome: Effect of short term maximal electrostimulation. Neurourology and Urodynamics 7: 501–506

Gilpin S A, Gosling J A, Smith A R B at al 1989 The pathogenesis of genitourinary prolapse and stress incontinence of urine: a histological and histochemical study. British Journal of Obstetrics and Gynaecology 96: 15–23

Hanley E, Delamarter R, McCulloch J et al 1996 Surgical indications and techniques. In: Weisel S W, Weinstein J N, Herkowitz H et al (eds) The lumbar spine, 2nd edn. W B Saunders, Philadelphia, pp 492–523

Hides J A, Stokes M J, Saide M et al 1994 Evidence of lumbar multifidus muscle wasting ipsilateral to symptoms in patients with acute/subacute low back pain. Spine 19: 165–172

Hodges P W, Richardson C A 1996 Inefficient muscular stabilization of the lumbar spine associated with low back pain. Spine 21: 2640–2650

Hodges P W, Sapsford R, Pengel L 2002 Feedforward activity of the pelvic floor muscles precedes rapid upper limb movements. Australian Physiotherapy Association Conference, Sydney, abstract 21

Kjolhede P, Ryden G 1997 Clinical and urodynamic characteristics of women with recurrent urinary incontinence after Burch colposuspension. Acta Obstetrica Gynecologica Scandinavica 76: 461–467

Koppe A, Koppius P W, Lens-van-Rijn J M et al 1984 A vaginal approach to the treatment of genital prolapse. European Journal of Obstetrics, Gynecology and Reproductive Biology 16: 359–364

MacLennan A H, Taylor A W, Wilson D H et al 2000 The prevalence of pelvic floor disorders and their relationship to gender, age, parity and mode of delivery. British Journal of Obstetrics and Gynaecology 107: 1460–1470

Mahony D T, Laferte R O, Blais D J 1977 Integral storage and voiding reflexes. Urology 9: 95–106

Maitland G D 2001 Vertebral manipulation, 6th edn. Butterworth Heinemann, London

Markwell S, Sapsford R 1995 Physiotherapy management of obstructed defaecation. Australian Journal of Physiotherapy 41: 279–283

Neumann P, Gill V 2002 Pelvic floor and abdominal muscle interaction: EMG activity and intra-abdominal pressure. International Urogynecology Journal 13: 125–132

Norton P A, Baker J E, Sharp H C et al 1995 Genitourinary prolapse and joint hypermobility in women. Obstetrics and Gynecology 85: 225–228

Orendacova J, Cizkova D, Kafka J et al 2001 Cauda equina syndrome. Progress in Neurobiology 64(6): 613–637

O'Sullivan P B, Beales D J, Avery A F 2001 Normalisation of aberrant motor patterns in subjects with sacroiliac joint pain following a motor relearning intervention: a multiple subject case study investigating the ASLR test. In: Fourth Interdisciplinary World Congress on Low Back and Pelvic Pain, Montreal, pp 178–179

O'Sullivan P B, Beales D J, Beetham J A et al 2002 Alterations of motor control in subjects with sacroiliac joint pain during the active straight leg raise test. Spine 27: E1–E8

Panjabi M M 1992 The stabilizing system of the spine. 1: Function, dysfunction, adaptation and enhancement. Journal of Spinal Disorders 5: 383–389

Pool-Goudzwaard A, Stoeckart R 2000 The need for assessment of the pelvic floor in patients with low back pain and pelvic pain before using stabilizing exercises. In: Proceedings of the Seventh Scientific Conference of the International Federation of Orthopaedic Manipulative Therapists (IFOMT), Perth, Australia, abstract 83

Power R M H 1948 Embryological development of the levator ani muscle. American Journal of Obstetrics and Gynecology 55: 367–381

Richardson C, Jull G, Hodges P, Hides J 1999 Therapeutic exercise for spinal segmental stabilization in low back pain. Churchill Livingstone, Edinburgh

Richardson C, Snijders C, Hides J et al 2002 The relation between the transversus abdominis muscles, sacroiliac joint mechanics, and low back pain. Spine 27(4): 399–405

Sapsford R 2001 The pelvic floor: a clinical model for function and rehabilitation. Physiotherapy 87: 620–630

Sapsford R R, Hodges P W 2001 Contraction of the pelvic floor muscles during abdominal maneuvers. Archives of Physical Medicine and Rehabilitation 82: 1081–1088

Sapsford R R, Hodges P W, Richardson C A et al 2001 Co-activation of the abdominal and pelvic floor muscles during voluntary exercises. Neurourology and Urodynamics 20: 31–42

Sayer T R, Dixon J S, Hosker G L et al 1990 A study of paraurethral connective tissue in women with stress incontinence of urine. Neurourology and Urodynamics 9: 319–320

Seim A, Morkved S, Schei B 2000 Musculoskeletal disorders among women with urinary incontinence. International Continence Society Conference, Finland, abstract 171

Snijders C J, Ribbers M T L M, de Bakker H V et al 1998 EMG recordings of abdominal and back muscles in various standing postures: validation of a biomechanical model on sacroiliac joint stability. Journal of Electromyography and Kinesiology 8: 205–214

Snooks S J, Setchell M, Swash M et al 1984 Injury to innervation of pelvic floor sphincter musculature in childbirth. Lancet 2(8402): 546–550

Spence-Jones C, Kamm M A, Henry M M et al 1994 Bowel dysfunction: a pathogenic factor in uterovaginal prolapse and urinary stress incontinence. British Journal of Obstetrics and Gynaecology 101: 147–152

Sprangfort E 1989 Disc surgery. In: Wall P, Melzack R (eds) Textbook of pain, 2nd edn. Churchill Livingstone, Edinburgh, pp 795–802

Sultan A H, Kamm M A, Hudson C N et al 1993 Anal sphincter disruption during vaginal delivery. New England Journal of Medicine 329: 1905–1911

Sultan A H, Kamm M A, Hudson C N 1994 Pudendal nerve damage during labour: a prospective study before and after childbirth. British Journal of Obstetrics and Gynaecology 101: 22–28

Susset J, Peters N, Cohen S et al 1982 Early detection of neurogenic bladder dysfunction caused by protruding lumbar disc. Urology 20(4): 461–463

Vanderhorst V G, Holstege G 1997 Nucleus retroambiguous projections to lumbosacral motoneuronal cell groups in the male cat. Journal of Comparative Neurology 382: 77–88

Vereeken R L, Derluyn J, Verduyn H 1975 Electromyography of the perineal striated muscles during cystometry. Urology International 30: 92–98

Viktrup L 2002 The risk of urinary tract symptoms five years after first delivery. Neurourology and Urodynamics 21: 2–29

Viktrup L, Lose G, Rolff M et al 1992 The symptom of stress incontinence caused by pregnancy or delivery in primiparas. Obstetrics and Gynecology 79: 945–949

Vleeming A, Stoeckart R, Snijders C J 1989 The sacrotuberous ligament: a conceptual approach to its dynamic role in stabilizing the sacroiliac joint. Clinical Biomechanics 4: 201–203

Vleeming A, Buyruk H M, Stoeckart R et al 1992 An integrated therapy for peripatum pelvic instability: a study of the biomechanical effect of pelvic belts. American Journal of Obstetrics and Gynecology 166: 1243–1247

Wennergren H M, Ogerg B E, Sandstedt P 1991 The importance of leg support for relaxation of the pelvic floor muscles. Scandinavian Journal of Urology and Nephrology 25: 205–221

Wijma J, Tinga D J, Visser G H A 1991 Perineal ultrasonography in women with stress incontinence and controls: the role of the pelvic floor muscles. Gynecologic and Obstetric Investigation 32: 176–179

Yamanishi T, Yuki T, Yasuda K et al 2002 The urodynamics evaluation of surgical outcome in patients with urinary retention due to central lumbar disc prolapse. Neurourology and Urodynamics 21: 425

Chapter **36**

Vascular syndromes presenting as pain of spinal origin

A. J. Taylor, R. Kerry

VASCULAR PAIN SYNDROMES: ARE THEY MISDIAGNOSED AS PAIN OF SPINAL ORIGIN?

Seldom in modern medicine do we encounter new conditions which alter the thinking behind our approach to the diagnosis and management of patients. The recent emergence of previously little known vascular conditions as a cause of local or peripheral pain syndromes in young adults has added a new facet to the clinical reasoning and diagnostic process in physical therapy.

History

Arterial disease is seldom reported in patients under the age of 40 years (Sise et al 1989) and so is rarely considered when dealing with young patients. Abraham et al (1997b) asserted that 'the wide variety of musculo-tendinous or skeletal problems affecting young athletes has probably contributed to an underestimation of the importance of lower extremity arterial disease'. External iliac artery endofibrosis (EIAE) was first described in the medical literature as recently as 1984 (Walder et al 1984). At the time it was little known and thought to be a rare condition causing stenosis or narrowing of the major artery to the lower limb. Since then its discovery has 'revolutionized' the approach to the diagnosis of leg pain (Abraham et al 1997b). The emergence of EIAE and the research into it has provided the springboard for an increased awareness of vascular syndromes.

The 'revolution', while gaining ground in the world of sports medicine, has been slow to permeate manual therapy. Indeed, physicians in Europe have been critical of medical practitioners and manual therapists alike for their poor recognition and management of lower and upper limb vascular conditions which are thought to have led to considerable delays in diagnosis (Abraham et al 1997a, Schep et al 1999).

There is growing awareness within manual therapy of the concept that altered haemodynamics within blood vessels can lead to the pathogenesis of a host of pain syndromes which are known to mimic neuro-musculo-skeletal

(NMS) conditions. Although initial descriptions seemed confined to athletes (Rousselet et al 1990), case reports in sedentary subjects indicate that many of the biomechanical principles and aetiological factors involved apply equally to the rest of the population (Sise et al 1989).

Clinical Reasoning

In all but the most extreme of cases, the clinical presentation of vascular conditions can be misleading. This is especially so if the clinician over-attends to one particular set of therapeutic models. The hypothetico-deductive reasoning process (Barrows & Feltovitch 1987, Jones 1994) facilitates and encourages early recognition of patterns. Pattern recognition has more recently been demonstrated as a trait of the expert clinician (King & Bithell 1998). One significant purpose of early pattern recognition is to identify pathologies which may not benefit from attention within a pathokinesiological model, or which may even be made worse by inappropriate intervention. An early tenet of the Maitland concept was to first ask oneself if harm could be done by proceeding further (Maitland 1986). More urgently, the early identification of certain pathologies might avoid the serious consequences of a delayed diagnosis. Grieve has recognized the desperate significance of the rapidly growing responsibilities of physiotherapists as our roles evolve into first contact and extended scope practitioners (Grieve 1994). He spoke of the importance of recognizing non-musculoskeletal conditions, which should 'promptly be directed elsewhere for the best chance of skilled detection and proper help'. Grieve continued in this work to present a number of systemic, neoplastic and visceral conditions, which 'masquerade' as musculoskeletal complaints.

This chapter introduces a number of vascular conditions of the lower and upper quadrants. Such conditions may present as neuromusculoskeletal complaints of supposed spinal origin. It is the authors' concern that these pathologies possess patterns close to more common neuromusculoskeletal complaints due to their relationship to movement and exertion. Furthermore, if these conditions fail to receive the proper help, the problem can become limb- and life-threatening. Thus, failure to recognize these conditions in the early stages may lead to serious sequelae for the patient and therapist alike. Current research is presented and the implications for manual therapists of lower and upper limb vascular syndromes are discussed. While the described conditions are considered rare, there is some debate as to whether they are in fact under-diagnosed and therefore under-reported (Levien & Veller 1999). Each condition is worthy of inclusion in the differential diagnosis and clinical reasoning process of all manual therapists. Case studies are used where appropriate to illustrate typical presentation patterns.

COMMON PRESENTATIONS OF LOWER LIMB VASCULAR INSUFFICIENCY: RECOGNITION AND CLINICAL REASONING

External iliac artery endofibrosis (EIAE)

In the mid- to late 1980s when it first became apparent, EIAE was described by the French as 'une étrange panne de jambe [a strange failure in the leg]'. This was largely because of its ability to mimic lumbar referral patterns and therefore elude accurate diagnosis. A number of case studies relate to long periods of misdiagnosis characterized by failed physical therapy and medical interventions (Taylor & George 2001a). EIAE is a typical example of mild to moderate arterial occlusion which affects young active patients and for that very reason often evades detection until its late stages.

CASE STUDY 1

A 32-year-old racing cyclist presented with a 5-year history of intermittent (initially) left lower limb (non-dermatomal) pain affecting the buttock, anterolateral thigh, calf and foot with a feeling of paraesthesia and numbness in the middle three toes. Symptoms had worsened and were described as a dull ache particularly noticeable when standing and worsened by walking, cycling and driving in particular. Specialist examination had resulted in a diagnosis of 'transient lumbar referred pain'. Magnetic resonance imaging (MRI) in lying had revealed no abnormality of the lumbar spine. Over the 5-year period the patient had undergone a host of manual therapy interventions including spinal mobilization/manipulation, rehabilitation for 'muscle imbalance' and various pain-relieving modalities including electrotherapy and acupuncture.

Standard physical therapy NMS examination was entirely normal. Further clinical examination revealed a reduced femoral pulse and absent distal pulses. The patient was referred for vascular examination. A treadmill exercise test proved positive at 40 metres. Arteriogram revealed a short complete occlusion of the external iliac artery and surgery (endarterectomy) was performed to restore normal blood flow to the limb (Fig. 36.1) (Taylor et al 1997). The described case is just one of many that illustrate that young apparently fit individuals may be subject to vascular flow issues, which present as and are mistaken for pain of spinal origin.

EIAE is an example of intrinsic trauma to vessel walls and is characterized by asymmetrical fibrous intimal thickening of the external iliac artery (Fig. 36.2). Endofibrotic lesions have also been reported on the common iliac artery (Chevalier et al 1994). The resulting narrowing leads to vascular flow problems in the affected lower limb. The symptoms are described variously as pain, weakness or 'cramping' and are generally experienced in the thigh but may extend to the calf. A subjective feeling of swollen thigh

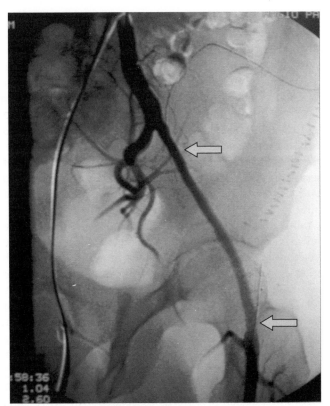

Figure 36.1   Post surgery arteriogram showing restoration of flow to the lower limb in a 32-year-old athlete using a saphenous vein graft (arrows). Reproduced with permission from Taylor et al 1997.

is often described (Beck 1995). Symptoms become apparent at times of effort or exercise due to inadequate oxygenation of tissue at times of high demand. Cyclists commonly describe a loss of force or 'riding with one leg' (P. Boyd, personal communication, 1997). Advanced cases may manifest as standing, walking or sitting pain (Taylor et al 1997).

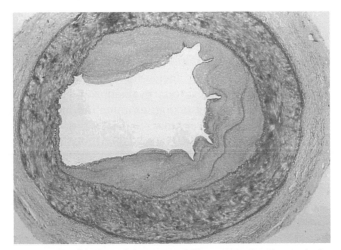

Figure 36.2   Section of the external iliac artery showing typical asymmetrical thickening of the artery at the site of haemodynamic stress. Courtesy of P. Abraham, Angers, France.

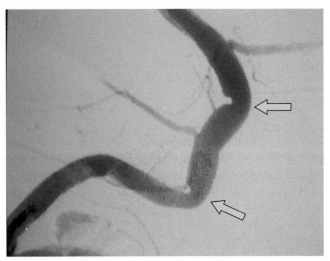

Figure 36.3   Arterial kinking (arrows) clearly demonstrated in the external iliac artery during hip flexion.

The problem is thought to be related to altered haemodynamics within vessels at times of high demand (Rousselet et al 1990). This is thought to be related to looping or kinking of the vessels during acute hip or trunk flexion (Fig. 36.3) and repeated movement exercise such as cycling, speed skating and fell running (Gallegos et al 1989, Schep et al 1999). The abnormal looping is hypothesized to lead to 'jet lesions' within the artery at times of high demand resulting in intrinsic microtrauma and fibrotic thickening of the endothelium (Chevalier et al 1991, Rousselet et al 1990). Extrinsic trauma due to falls or direct injury to vessels have also been cited in the literature (Roth & Boyd 1999) as possible aetiological factors. These cases are often associated with local thrombus formation leading to advanced stenosis or complete occlusion (Taylor et al 1997).

Such cases may visit physical therapists complaining of leg symptoms, fatigue, numbness, paraesthesia and poor athletic performance. The age of the patient, absence of true comparable physical signs and concomitant failure to examine the vascular system (either at all or adequately) may lead therapists to trial techniques for perceived referred pain or muscle imbalances. Some patients report being routed down the biopsychosocial pathway (P. Boyd, personal communication, 1997). Fortunately there are a number of simple clinical vascular examination methods commonly used in medicine which can be incorporated into the physical therapy examination to aid differential diagnosis and reduce the propensity for error and unnecessary prolonged treatment or mismanagement in suspected cases.

Current research advocates specific clinical examination with a strong emphasis on history and behaviour of symptoms. If detailed NMS examination is normal but the index of suspicion of an arterial lesion is high then clinical testing involving pulse palpation, hand-held Doppler ultrasound assessment of the lower limb superficial pulses and resting ankle to brachial pressure index (ABPI) may reveal advanced cases. However, mild or moderate endofibrotic arterial lesions in young patients have a perfectly normal vascular examination at rest (Abraham et al 2001). Furthermore, conventional walking treadmill tests may not provide the biomechanical conditions necessary to reveal the lesion (Ouriel 1995). Maximal exercise testing specific to the activity or sport has been advocated as a valid clinical test with an 85% sensitivity value for the identification of arterial flow problems in the lower limb (Chevalier et al 1991). These specific validated clinical tests are covered in the section on exercise testing in this chapter.

As EIAE is a recent discovery there is currently no long-term follow-up of surgical cases. Intervention has to be considered very carefully in young patients. The use of angioplasty is reported to be of short-term benefit in endofibrotic lesions (Wijesinghe et al 2001) and considered to have a high risk for arterial rupture by some authors (Abraham et al 1997a). Artificial stenting or prosthetic grafting of the artery is reported to fail at this anatomical site, especially in athletes (Batt et al 1984). A great deal depends on the degree of impairment and the effect on the patient's activities of daily living. As the disease is known to affect professional or Olympic level sports participants, premature retirement from a sport which provides them with a living may be a daunting option.

Surgical options include extravascular release in mild cases (Schep et al 1999) or endofibrosectomy with vein grafting and shortening of the artery (Chevalier et al 1991). A number of patients have chosen to modify their activity levels and refused surgery on the grounds that the risks outweigh the potential benefits. Unfortunately, as few cases have so far been confirmed in the UK, diagnostic imaging and surgical expertise (relating to the young athletic population) has not had the chance to develop to the same degree as in Europe, where many cases have now been successfully treated. Some UK based sufferers have therefore sought diagnostic and surgical assistance in Europe.

The emergence of EIAE and the research into it has heightened the awareness of the medical profession as a whole to vascular issues affecting the young (<40 years) population. Physical therapists can play a major role in the screening of patients referred with non-specific lower limb pain and thereby prevent unnecessary delays in diagnosis. This chapter goes on to describe three of the more common presentations of lower limb pain which, for the unwary, may be mistaken for and treated as pain of spinal origin.

Aortic stenosis, low back pain and 'referred pain'

Cyriax (1975) considered aortic, common iliac and external/internal iliac arterial stenoses as rare but potential sources of low back, buttock and lower limb pain. Arterial stenosis is known to lead to ischaemia in the tissues distal to the lesion (Ouriel 1995). However, Kauppila et al (1997), in a study based on radiographic findings and interviews,

suggested that there may be a link between atherosclerotic calcification in the posterior wall of the aorta and lumbar disc degeneration resulting in local back pain. As the posterior wall of the aorta is the source of the feeding arteries of the lumbar spine the authors hypothesized that ischaemia of the lumbar spine may be a factor in disc degeneration. This linked in with further work by the same author (Kauppila & Tallroth 1993, Kauppila et al 1997) where studies based on post mortem aortogram findings suggested that atherosclerotic narrowing of the lumbar and middle sacral arteries correlated with disc space narrowing or endplate sclerosis and historical complaints of chronic low back pain.

Yabuki et al (1999) took this concept a stage further when they used the term 'vascular backache' following a report of two cases of chronic low back pain and intermittent claudication symptoms which were significantly improved after vascular reconstructive surgery for atherosclerosis of the aorta and iliac vessels. They put forward the hypothesis that one factor leading to low back pain might be varying degrees of ischaemia of the extensor muscles of the lumbar spine and described various pathomechanisms by which this could take place. Wohlgemuth et al (1999) described a form of ischaemia of the lumbosacral plexus leading to 'pelvic' or buttock symptoms associated with lower limb muscle weakness and loss of reflexes after walking or exercise. They differentiated this from classical lower limb peripheral claudication and spinal stenosis. Their cases were characterized by high-grade atherosclerotic stenosis of the abdominal aorta and internal iliac artery, which was hypothesized as a possible cause of temporary ischaemia of the lumbosacral plexus at times of lower limb demand for extra blood flow. While many of these theories are in their infancy and require further study, they illustrate the potential intimate link between vascularity and common pain syndromes. Indeed, they will come as little surprise to those who consider that circulation and adequate perfusion of tissues are integral to the normal function and patency of NMS structures.

As, increasingly, atherosclerosis (Sise et al 1989) and other vascular disorders (see EIAE) are seen to affect younger subjects, the importance of adequate vascular assessment is highlighted. Increasingly manual therapists may need to incorporate arterial evaluation and circulatory issues into their history taking, examination and clinical reasoning processes. Recent case studies by physical therapists (Laslett 2000, Taylor & George 2001a) relating to arterial flow and resulting pain syndromes issues illustrate the increasing awareness of vascular issues within the profession. Laslett's (2000) description of aortic stenosis is an excellent example of clear clinical reasoning and eloquently describes a typical presentation and initial misdiagnosis of arterial stenosis. The difficulty the author encountered convincing both the GP and specialists involved in the case of an arterial lesion is by no means unusual. Fortunately, practical advances in clinical assessment applicable to physical therapy assessment (see clinical testing) should in future facilitate this process by providing sound objective science based data.

CASE STUDY 2

A 41-year-old woman was referred complaining of bilateral buttock pain experienced when walking upstairs or pushing her children in a pram. The referring orthopaedic consultant had requested physical therapy assessment of the lumbar spine and hips and appropriate treatment. The patient reported previous episodes of mild low back pain, but was currently asymptomatic and demonstrated full lumbar range of movement. Segmental palpation of the lumbar spine revealed local stiffness without referral. Sacroiliac tests were considered normal. Hip joint range of motion was full and there were no demonstrable muscle balance issues. The patient was able to reproduce her pain by walking up the stairs in the clinic three times. Palpation of distal pulses post stair walking revealed barely palpable posterior tibial and dorsalis pedis pulses. Resting ankle to brachial pressure index performed in the clinic was lowered (left 0.76, right 0.69 – see Table 36.1, p 529), indicating reduced arterial flow to the lower limbs bilaterally. The patient was referred for vascular assessment and found to have a positive treadmill test. Subsequent arteriogram revealed a significant aortic stenosis and the patient underwent successful angioplasty.

Aortic stenosis may occur as a result of atherosclerosis or due to underlying congenital defects in the descending aorta known as coarctation, which may coexist with associated heart abnormalities such as mitral valve defects (Warnes et al 1996). While aortic coarctation is usually discovered in childhood, it is not uncommon for it to go undiagnosed until early adulthood (Annett et al 2000). The therapist should be wary of bilateral non-specific buttock/pelvic/lower limb symptoms including paraesthesia and sensory or motor deficits which do not tie in with history or NMS examination. Further detailed questioning may be required to ascertain underlying lifestyle risk factors or family history of arterial or circulatory disease. Specific details of symptom behaviour, colour or temperature changes and exercise-induced components may all contribute to the clinical reasoning process and steer the clinician down the right path. Above all, reproduction of symptoms in the clinic by simple exercise testing (see clinical testing) may provide further clues as to the vascular nature (or otherwise) of the symptoms.

Adductor canal syndrome

The concept of trauma or injury to blood vessels is rarely covered in physical therapy texts. However, blood vessels may suffer trauma, injury or insult in much the same way as other soft tissue and nerves. While the tough external coat (tunica adventitia) is only usually breached by acute trauma, damage to the intimal layer may occur over time due to extrinsic compression or microtrauma caused by biomechanical factors (Vlychou et al 2001).

Adductor canal syndrome (ACS) is an example of extrinsic chronic biomechanical trauma to a blood vessel. It leads to stenosis or occlusion of the femoral artery in the aponeurotic tunnel (Hunter's canal) in the middle third of the thigh (Fig. 36.4). The condition is thought to be due to the scissor-like action of adductor magnus and vastus medialis and is usually associated with anatomical abnormality (tight fascial slips) combined with muscle or tendon hypertrophy (Balaji & De Weese 1981).

The condition is rare but has been reported in athletes, skiers, runners and sedentary subjects (Balaji & De Weese 1981). Mild cases experience intermittent muscle pains/cramps with varying degrees of paraesthesia distal to the lesion (i.e. calf/foot/toes). For this reason mild cases may logically be mistaken for nerve entrapment. However, much like the previous descriptions, the clinical examination will not be consistent with a NMS lesion and further examination may reveal reduced distal pulses or reduced ABPI at rest (see clinical testing). ACS is known to progress rapidly if thrombus forms at the occluded vessel. At this stage the diagnosis becomes more straightforward as the patient presents with typical claudication symptoms.

Acute cases should be referred immediately for vascular assessment. Delays in recognition may be serious. Irreversible damage to the limb may occur if the condition progresses rapidly (usually in association with thrombus). Arteriogram or MRA will confirm diagnosis and differentiate it from popliteal artery entrapment. Surgery involves

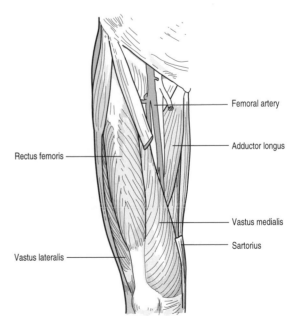

Figure 36.4 Femoral artery occlusion in the adductor canal (Hunter's canal).

exploration and repair of the affected portion of artery using endarterectomy with a saphenous vein patch or saphenous vein bypass.

Popliteal artery entrapment (PAES)

PAES is another classical presentation of extrinsic mechanical trauma to blood vessels which is known to affect young adults and adolescents (Stager & Clement 1999). The condition is often associated with paraesthesia in the calf or foot and perceived weakness of the ankle during exercise. It is these factors combined with the transient nature of the symptoms and the patient's age which may lead to delays in diagnosis in the early stages. Trials of treatments for 'nerve entrapments' or other musculoskeletal issues are not uncommon in the literature (Bradshaw 2000).

Progressive stenosis of the popliteal artery is thought to occur as a result of mechanical trauma related to abnormal relationships between the popliteal artery and surrounding myofascial structures (Stager & Clement 1999). Various anomalies are reported relating to the popliteal vessels and the medial head of gastrocnemius or the popliteus muscle (Fig. 36.5) (Levien & Veller 1999). As it is increasingly recognized, it is becoming a significant cause of transient bi/unilateral calf or tendo Achillis pain in young athletes (Touliopolous & Hershman 1999).

In the early stages discomfort tends to occur at specific levels of activity such as sprinting or running/walking on slopes/hills. Symptoms are eased by reducing the intensity of the activity. In more advanced cases the patient may need to stop exercising to gain relief. Examination at rest is usually normal. Pulse palpation after exercise may be diminished at the posterior tibial and dorsalis pedis sites. This may be affected by provocative manoeuvres such as full active plantarflexion or passive dorsiflexion with the knee held in hyperextension.

Again it is important to reproduce symptoms in the clinic. A simple clinical test is to ask the patient to hop on the spot until symptoms are reproduced and follow this by pulse palpation with or without provocative manoeuvres. Ideally the exercise should replicate the biomechanical conditions experienced by the patient – the runner complaining of pain on slopes, for example, should be tested on an inclined treadmill. Loss of pulses, reduced systolic pressure on the affected leg or a significantly lowered ABPI post exercise compared to the normal limb raises the suspicion of an arterial cause for the pain (see clinical testing).

CASE STUDY 3

A 35-year-old physical therapist and regular runner complained of mild intermittent right-sided calf/foot discomfort and paraesthesia of the toes associated with running up slopes. As she suffered concomitant low back pain she had put her symptoms down to 'sciatica'. Various manual therapy interventions by her colleagues had failed to bring a resolution of her symptoms. Spinal range of motion and neural mobility were normal. However, the lower lumbar spine was tender and stiff on segmental palpation but without referral of symptoms. After further questioning with regard to the nature of the symptoms the patient was asked to perform a hopping test. After 90 seconds hopping the familiar symptoms were produced strongly and she was unable to continue. Post exercise pulse palpation with the ankle in forced active plantarflexion revealed barely palpable posterior tibial and dorsalis pedis pulses. Despite the strong suggestion of an arterial cause for her pain the subject chose not to go on for further investigation at that stage. Definitive diagnosis in this case therefore remained unproven.

If the index of suspicion for arterial impingement is high, referral to a vascular specialist is recommended with a detailed letter (referenced if necessary) listing clinical findings. Ultrasonography using continuous wave Doppler may reveal a change in flow or pulse loss during forced active plantarflexion or passive dorsiflexion. The results may be misleading, however, as pulse disappearance has been noted in normal asymptomatic subjects (McDonald et al 1980). Duplex flow studies (ultrasound) allow visualization of the artery walls with simultaneous monitoring of arterial flow (Schep et al 2001a). This may reveal the lesion with the use of provocative manoeuvres. Standard arteriogram or MRA will usually confirm the site of the lesion and differentiate it from adductor canal syndrome.

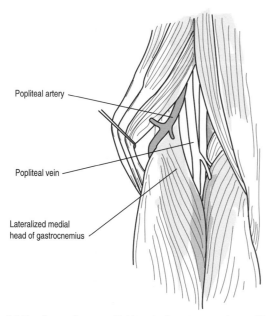

Popliteal artery

Popliteal vein

Lateralized medial head of gastrocnemius

Figure 36.5 Anomalous medial head of gastrocnemius affecting the popliteal artery. This figure demonstrates one of at least 15 different anatomical anomalies around the popliteal artery which may cause vascular leg pain.

As PAES is thought to be progressive and due to regular trauma to the artery, an increase in vascular occlusion is expected over time together with a heightened risk of aneurysm or embolization. Surgery involves exploration and decompression and may require simple release of fascial or musculotendinous slips in cases of functional entrapment. Thrombectomy or endarterectomy and saphenous vein grafting may be required in advanced cases (Levien & Veller 1999).

COMMON PRESENTATIONS OF CERVICAL AND UPPER LIMB VASCULAR CONDITIONS: RECOGNITION AND CLINICAL REASONING

Pain and altered sensation around the cervical spine, supraclavicular fossa, chest, upper arm, forearm and hand are common in conditions diagnosed and treated by manual therapists as cervicothoracic neuromusculoskeletal dysfunction. These pain patterns and sites can also be suggestive of arguably less well-understood vascular conditions originating from vascular structures within the upper quadrant. Literature suggests that vascular conditions of the upper quadrant can be the subject of inaccurate diagnosis or recognition when the patient seeks the attention of the manual therapist (see, for example, Arko et al 2001, Nuber et al 1990, Wilson et al 1994).

The anterior cervical vascular system

Cervical arteries have been the focus of attention for manual therapists for some time. The main anatomical area of attention has been the posterior vascular system, consisting of the vertebrobasilar arteries. This is an important focus in respect of not only high velocity manipulations but also other forms of manual therapy for the cervical spine. Recent thinking in this area suggests a conflict with the once commonly held view that serious accident following manipulation is a rare and unusual event (Mann & Refshauge 2001). The fact that the majority of incidents are not reported due to medico-legal restrictions skews the true picture of the prevalence and incidence of treatment induced complications. Thus important research attention in this area grows.

Much attention is given to the issue of vertebrobasilar insufficiency in this text (see Chs 19 and 37). The present chapter focuses its attention on the arguably less well-understood and appreciated anterior cervical vascular system. Clinically, this pertains to the subclavian and carotid arteries (Fig. 36.6). The following section provides an overview of vascular conditions of the anterior cervical system, which mimic more commonly seen musculoskeletal conditions. Additionally, knowledge of such pathologies must be included in the manual therapist's knowledge base as their presence may impact upon the clinical decisions and treatment options.

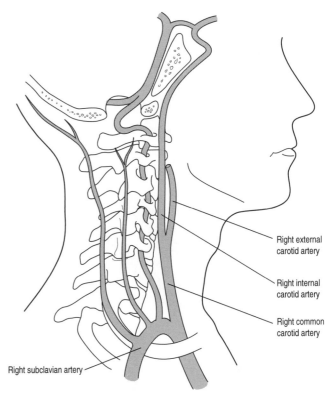

Figure 36.6   Anterior cervical system showing the simplified anatomical course of the right subclavian and carotid arteries.

Right external carotid artery

Right internal carotid artery

Right common carotid artery

Right subclavian artery

Carotid artery pathology

The carotid system includes the common, external and internal carotid arteries. The bifurcation of the internal and external arteries is a clinically important site due to the nature of haemodynamics around this area (Berman et al 1994, Biller 2000). Carotid artery pathology may be a result of vascular disease, most commonly atherosclerosis (Bath & Kennedy 2000, Carolei et al 1995), dissection following direct trauma (Carr et al 1996, Windfuhr 2001), spontaneous dissection (Duyff et al 1997, McCarron et al 2000), or dissection following cervical manipulation (Beatty 1977, Hufnagel et al 1999). Aneurysm dissection has also been the result of other activities including mild physical effort, vomiting, prolonged telephone use, 'headbang' dancing, coughing, and sneezing (Zetterling et al 2000, personal clinical experience).

Aneurysm dissection most commonly affects the internal carotid artery. Internal carotid artery dissection accounts for about one fifth of strokes in young adults, compared to about 2.5% of strokes in older people (Blunt & Galton 1997). Although extracranial dissections have a slightly better prognosis than intracranial dissections (Hart & Easton 1985), extracranial dissections are more prevalent and the consequences are still very serious, with stroke and death being the most common.

Arterial dissection is the result of blood tracking into the vessel wall through an intimal tear (Fig. 36.7). The line of

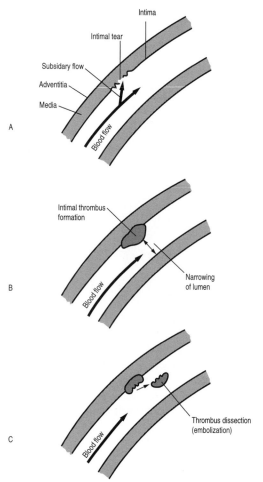

Figure 36.7 Mechanism of thrombus dissection following tear to the arterial intima. A: Intimal tear induced by injury, altered haemodynamics or disease allows inflow of blood into subintimal space from main bloodstream. B: Eventual subintimal thrombus formation. C: Thrombus dissection induced by injury, altered haemodynamics or time.

tracking may be subintimal resulting in luminal narrowing or occlusion (Blunt & Galton 1997). Alternatively, subadventitial penetration may result in aneurysmal or pseudo-aneurysmal dilation (Zetterling et al 2000) potentiating the risk of haemorrhage and thromboembolic event. This process may be the result of vessel wall damage, but the risk and seriousness of the event is increased in the presence of atherosclerotic changes. Furthermore, atherosclerosis has been described as an inflammatory process caused by injury (Ross 1999). The risk of dissection is also increased in patients with fibromuscular disease, smokers, hypertension and hypercoagulable states.

The implications of carotid artery pathology for the manual therapist are twofold: firstly, the risk of causing carotid artery dissection and other complications in the presence of atherosclerotic disease as a result of manual therapy treatment techniques (manipulation and traction being the two

most obvious) should be considered in clinical decision making. Secondly, the differential diagnosis of carotid disease with many other cervicocranial neuromusculoskeletal conditions is difficult, and the consequences of misdiagnosis are dire.

Commonly, carotid pathology can present as unilateral neck pain, facial pain and headache/migraine. Pain can be described as aching, throbbing, stabbing or pulsating and it is related to physical exertion and cervical movement. The headaches may be sudden in onset and of a 'thunderclap' nature. Pulsatile tinnitus is also an observed clinical feature (Mohyuddin 2000). Typically pain precedes neurological features by a time period ranging from hours to weeks (Silbert et al 1995). This period represents a window of diagnostic confusion for the physician and the manual therapist, and diagnoses of migraine, cervicogenic neck pain and temporomandibular joint dysfunction are not uncommon. When neurological deficit and symptoms are present, the diagnostic field widens and the manual therapist may be more cautious of other pathologies. However, even in the presence of obvious neurology, misdiagnosis is possible. The manual therapist should therefore be aware of any description of unilateral headache/retro-orbital pain associated with physical exertion and cervical motion. Signs of unilateral facial palsy, ptosis or miotic pupil are suggestive of carotid pathology and indicative of Horner's or Raeder's syndrome.

Further specific carotid artery testing for the manual therapist is limited to palpation, auscultation and the use of hand-held Doppler ultrasound in an attempt to assess the quality of the carotid pulses (see below). However, as is the case in many vascular conditions, it is the history and the quality and specificity of questioning which is important. Referral for further investigation (angiography, MRI/MRA, colour duplex Doppler ultrasound) can be made on the basis of a sound history alone. Thus, the manual therapist should consider special questioning directed towards establishing a clear picture of the patient's cardiovascular history and that of their family. The awareness of hyperlipidaemia, hypercholesterolaemia, hypertension, homocysteine state affecting plasma concentration, diabetes mellitus, and recent infections should be paramount. Knowledge of the social and dietary habits of the patient will also inform clinical decisions.

CASE STUDY 4

A 62-year-old woman was referred for physiotherapy by her general practitioner with intermittent unilateral neck and upper arm pain. The pain was described as dull and aching and an ipsilateral temporal headache was associated. Symptoms were worsened by activity of the upper quadrant and with excessive walking. Symptoms took about a day to settle. The physiotherapist found unilateral cervical facet dysfunction in the mid and upper cervical spine, which would account for the symptoms.

Appropriate intervertebral passive movement techniques were undertaken and when these did not help mechanical traction was attempted. Over the course of treatment symptoms worsened and the patient complained of nausea associated with the headaches. A clinical review encompassing a vascular knowledge base revealed that the patient also suffered claudication-type leg pain, suggesting underlying arterial pathology. Palpation of the carotid arteries revealed an ipsilateral pulsatile nature at the carotid bifurcation. The patient was referred for assessment by the vascular consultant who listed her for emergency carotid endarterectomy. The painful episodes had been transient ischaemic attacks.

Subclavian–axillary syndromes

The relatively recent evolutionary assumption of an upright posture has allowed and facilitated greater mobility of the upper limb. However, structural adaptations have failed to keep pace with these changes in evolutionary function of the arm (Ouriel 1998). As a result, a variety of vascular as well as neuromusculoskeletal problems have developed which result in pain, swelling and sensory–motor dysfunction of the upper limb. Subclavian–axillary vascular pathologies occur at varying sites along this system, can affect the arterial or the venous structures, can have endogenous or exogenous factors, and can be the result of inter- or extravascular compromise.

The thoracic outlet is a well-recognized anatomical region where such problems occur, and no doubt thoracic outlet syndrome (TOS) is a collection of clinical patterns with which most physiotherapists will be familiar. Compression of the neurovascular structures as they exit between the musculotendinous and bony boundaries is responsible for many neurological, venous and arterial symptoms.

TOS has been accused of being both under-diagnosed (Roos 1999) and over-diagnosed (Wilbourn 1999a). However, what is certain is that TOS is a prevalent clinical phenomenon, albeit in varied form. Vascular components of TOS presentations are suggested to have a lower incidence than neurological TOS (Hood et al 1997, Wilbourn 1999b). However, it is far from clear as to what degree a vascular component exists in presentations of possible multi-aetiology. It is the opinion of the authors that the term 'thoracic outlet syndrome' is non-specific and unhelpful when exploring the characteristics and signs of upper quadrant dysfunction.

It is therefore suggested that aetiologies be broken down into the particular components so that a better reasoned and more informed judgement as to the further assessment and management of the patient can be made. The following are presentations of some of the more common vascular conditions affecting the subclavian–axillary system.

Paget–Schroetter syndrome

Paget–Schroetter syndrome is a deep vein thrombosis of the subclavian–axillary venous system, affecting the subclavian more commonly than the axillary vein. Due to a high level of misdiagnosis, the true incidence of Paget–Schroetter is unknown; however, it may account for about 3–7% of all deep vein thromboses. The risk of pulmonary embolism from Paget–Schroetter is around 12%. Paget–Schroetter syndrome refers to the primary form of subclavian–axillary vein thrombosis and is also commonly referred to as effort vein thrombosis or effort thrombosis (Rutherford 1998, Zell et al 2001). This syndrome was first described following cases reported in 1875 by Sir James Paget and later, in 1899, by Leopold von Schroetter (Hurlbert & Rutherford 1995). Since this time, Paget–Schroetter syndrome has been the subject of much attention and contention with regard to recognition and management.

The typical clinical presentation of Paget–Schroetter syndrome is characterized by the youthfulness and healthiness of the patient. Males present three times more commonly than females, and the dominant arm is affected approximately 70% of the time (Rutherford 1998). The average patient is in their late 20s to early 30s although ages ranging from 17 to 59 years have been described (Brochner et al 1989). The patient most commonly complains of a quick insidious onset of arm pain with the possibility of associated supraclavicular fossa and ipsilateral neck pain. The onset may also be related to over-activity of the arm (e.g. in athletics, manual work) (Shovman et al 1997), unusual positioning (Taira et al 2001), or upper quadrant trauma (Butsch 1983, Zell et al 2000). The usual aetiology of Paget–Schroetter syndrome is in keeping with the time-honoured triad of Virchow, suggesting that stasis, vessel wall damage and a hypercoagulable state must exist in order for the development of a thrombus to occur (Fig. 36.8). A thorough history taking considering past and family medical history with focused special questions is therefore required. The correlation to a hypercoagulable state has been documented with case and research reports (Aquino & Barone 1989, Earle & Lloyd 1989, Hingorani et al 2000, Leebeek et al 2001, Sayinalp et al 1999). Other risk factors include 'traditional' thoracic outlet syndrome factors such as cervical rib, anomalous first rib, hypertrophy of anterior scalene, subclavius or pectoralis minor as well as endogenous factors such as activated protein C resistance and anticardiolipin antibodies (Ellis 2000).

Swelling of the arm is a common manifestation, and can indeed be the sole presentation (Skerker & Flandry 1992). More often though, pain and swelling accompany one another. Stasis dermatitis or ulceration are rare in upper extremity venous events due to the relatively lower gravitational state (Rutherford 1998). As Paget–Schroetter is a condition of venous obstruction, pain and swelling are a result of muscular activity needed to increase venous pressure in order to meet the venous outflow (for a limited time via collateral circulation) which is required to match arterial

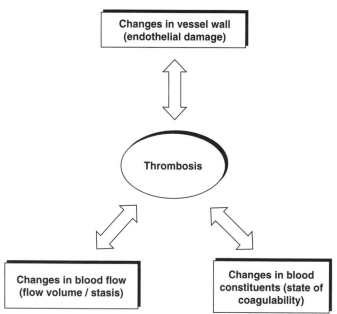

Figure 36.8 Virchow's triad – the aetiology of thrombosis.

inflow. Pain and distal dysthaesia are related to repetitive activity of the upper limb. Other symptoms may include peripheral cyanosis. If pulmonary embolization has developed then there may be a description of shortness of breath, pleuritic chest pain, haemoptysis and non-productive cough.

On examination oedema, cyanosis and superficial vein distension around the supraclavicular fossa and chest wall might be noticed. Distal pulses are not affected, although some abnormality and discomfort around the supraclavicular pulse may be found. Signs and symptoms need to be recorded in relation to exertion of the upper extremity during the examination. The signs and symptoms associated with Paget–Schroetter syndrome may mimic patterns more commonly associated with adverse neural mechanics, and indeed neurodynamic testing may well be positive in this condition given the association with the subclavian vascular structure around the brachial plexus. A working diagnosis of reflex sympathetic dystrophy or shoulder–hand syndrome might also be inaccurately given.

CASE STUDY 5

The case of a young female rounders player represents a typical presentation of Paget–Schroetter syndrome. The 19-year-old player presents with right (dominant) cervical, supraclavicular fossa and glenohumeral pain described as a constant ache and 'restlessness'. In addition there is an intermittent increase in the ache related to activity of her arm and neck. She has previously been seen by two physiotherapists, the first one diagnosing a glenohumeral instability, the second suggesting altered neurodynamics due to the constant nature and the association between neck and arm movement. An examina-

tion considering a haemodynamic knowledge base would have revealed that the patient was taking oral contraceptives (offering a hypercoagulable state) and suggested that the repetitive nature of hitting the ball during rounders might produce vessel wall injury, thereby meeting two out of the three criteria of Virchow's triad. Further investigation (chest X-ray) revealed the presence of a cervical rib thus meeting the third criterion, constriction induced stasis. Photoplethysmography and colour Duplex ultrasound imaging revealed the presence of a thrombosis in the right subclavian vein. Treatment consisted of anticoagulation therapy together with stopping oral contraceptives, and symptoms quickly resolved. Physiotherapy intervention was appropriate at this point (i.e. after beginning anticoagulation therapy) to address the movement dysfunction components.

Subclavian–axillary arterial occlusion

Occlusive lesions of the subclavian and axillary arteries may be misinterpreted as more familiar cervicogenic, neurogenic or glenohumeral dysfunctions. As suggested above, ipsilateral neck, supraclavicular fossa and arm pain is seldom considered to have a vascular origin, especially in the younger population. Orthopaedic attention is given to these complaints utilizing and expanding our rich neuromusculoskeletal knowledge base, while vascular conditions are regarded as the province of the older population with obvious circulatory pathology (Nuber et al 1990). However, recent attention has been paid to cervicobrachial problems of arterial origin in the young, healthy worker and athlete, thereby expanding the haemodynamic knowledge base (Arko et al 2001).

Arterial occlusion in the subclavian–axillary region may be of an external or internal aetiology. External occlusion involves compression of the artery from the surrounding musculoskeletal structures. Within the region of the thoracic outlet the muscular structures which can cause compression are the anterior scalene, subclavius and pectoralis minor (Palmer et al 1991). Hypertrophy or more subtle muscle imbalance dysfunctions can result in the occlusion of distal blood flow and create local and peripheral altered haemodynamics (McCarthy et al 1989). Bony structures include the costoclavicular space where the clavicle crosses over the first rib, the presence of a cervical rib or an anomalous first rib (Durham et al 1995). Occlusion via these mechanisms can be a result of repetitive upper quadrant activity or direct trauma.

The presence of atherosclerosis accounts for one of the internal mechanisms producing arterial occlusion. In contrast to the external iliac artery, endofibrosis of the subclavian or axillary arteries has not been described in the literature. The clinical implication from this for the physiotherapist is to appreciate not only the medical history of the patient but also the more subtle markers concerning family history, lifestyle and dietary patterns which may place the patient in a high risk group for atherosclerosis. The natural sequela of arterial occlusion is aneurysm development leading to a possible thromboembolic event, coronary or cranial accident, intractable arm pain, gangrene and amputation (Arko et al 2001, Hood et al 1997, McCarthy et al 1989). The clinical presentation for arterial occlusion at this anatomical region mimics various neuromusculoskeletal conditions including: ulnar nerve injury, glenohumeral pathology, cervical dysfunction, tennis elbow, localized hand pathology and non-vascular TOS. Typically, unilateral supraclavicular fossa and arm pain, with the possibility of associated neck pain due to the biomechanical and movement dysfunctions around the area, form the clinical pattern. A description of distal symptoms, including weakness, fatigue, coldness and neurological dysthaesia, is common. In the young, healthy patient with early occlusion signs the presence of gangrenous fingers would be unlikely, although these signs are present in late stage pathology. A typical Raynaud's type intolerance to cold would also alert the clinician to an arterial cause.

Clinical examination of the arterial signs might reveal reduced or absent distal pulses during positional change, therefore classic thoracic outlet tests (Adson's, Allen's, Halstead's manoeuvre, Roos's EAST test, etc.) could be positive. However, negative positional tests do not exclude an arterial cause as the exertional component may be more significant than the positional in some cases. Examination of the digits might reveal a prolonged capillary refill time in different positions/levels of exertion together with some cooling of the extremity. A supra- or infra-clavicular pulsatile mass may be present on palpation, or a visible or palpable cervical rib would indicate occlusive factors (Green 1998). A bruit may be produced with abduction of the arm if there is not one present at rest (Green 1998).

CASE STUDY 6

A 22-year-old violin player had suffered left-sided cervical, supraclavicular fossa, arm and ulnar border forearm/hand pain for 2 years. Repeated physiotherapy sessions over this period involved mobilization of the left C4/C5 and C5/C6 intervertebral motion segments (based on accurate passive motion examination), neurodynamic treatment, pain relieving modalities, and exercise – all reasonable approaches based on examination findings. No significant progress, however, had been made. Clinical vascular assessment revealed reduced systolic left brachial pressure after 20 minutes violin playing. Reduced left radial and ulnar pulses post playing were also recorded together with a prolonged distal capillary refill time. Positional contrast angiography revealed occlusion of the left subclavian artery, possibly from surrounding soft tissue (anterior scalenus). Prophylactic antithrombolytic therapy together with manual therapy aimed at appropriate soft tissue release and repositioning during violin playing produced rapid

improvement in symptoms and vascular objective markers. If no improvement had been made this patient could have become a candidate for scalenectomy.

SPECIFIC CLINICAL TESTS FOR LOWER AND UPPER LIMB VASCULAR INSUFFICIENCY

The intent of this section is not to describe medical tests which are used in the investigation of vascular disease. Rather, a number of practical observations and tests are presented which the manual therapist can include in their day-to-day clinical practice. These procedures may inform the clinician of the presence or absence of a vascular component to the patient's complaint at an early stage in the differential diagnostic process.

General observation

The clinician should be aware of observable signs that may indicate significant vascular disease. Local pallor or cyanosis is more easily detectable in light-skinned individuals. Pallor (blanching) reflects decreased oxyhaemoglobin levels and is indicative of occlusive disease. Elevation of the lower or upper extremity should be checked initially for signs of positional pallor. Peripheral cyanosis (a bluish hue) reflects increased deoxygenated haemoglobin levels and can result from diminished perfusion, possibly from arterial vasoconstriction. Foot/ankle or hand oedema at rest or superficial venous dilation is indicative of venous obstruction. Corneal arcus or xanthelasmas (yellowish raised skin changes) around both eyes are associated with hyperlipidaemia and hypercholesterolaemia. Staining of the fingers may be a more accurate indicator of tobacco consumption than the history suggests. Obesity, state of mental awareness and attitude may also reflect underlying cerebrovascular states.

Hand and digital examination

The purpose of hand and digit examination in the upper limb is to assess subtle markers of possible arterial or venous compromise. Obvious non-pitting hand oedema suggests venous obstruction and is common in subclavian–axillary venous thrombosis and shoulder–hand syndromes. Peripheral cyanosis may be associated with these conditions and observation of finger ends and nail bases may reveal characteristic skin mottling.

Blanching of the hand, finger ends or nail beds is associated with subclavian–axillary arterial occlusion. The nails can be squeezed and tested for capillary refill timings. Normal refill results in an immediate return of colour to the nail beds. This test should be performed in different positions of the upper extremity and neck as well as pre and post exertion via functional demonstration in the clinic. Comparisons can be made with the non-symptomatic limb.

Digital pulses are unlikely to be detected with palpation and the use of hand-held Doppler can assist in the examination of the hand and fingers. Further examination of the nails can reveal deformities which are characteristic of prolonged oxygen deprivation. Two common nail deformities are koilonychia ('spoon nail') and clubbing. Koilonychia can be associated with peripheral arterial abnormalities such as Raynaud's disease, but can also be associated with many other non-vascular events and is therefore not diagnostic. Clubbing is indicative of long-standing venous compromise and the nail beds feel soft to the touch with a thickened, hard nail displaying a curved tip.

Pulse palpation

In an article relating to vascular disease in young adults Sise et al (1989) cited an average 2-year delay in diagnosis. The authors described the delay in referral as 'alarming' and stated that 93% of the patients in their series could have been diagnosed by 'simple examination of peripheral pulses'. Pulse palpation has become one of physical therapy's lost arts. As manual therapy has 'progressed' many of the basic skills on which the profession was founded have been gradually eroded. Pulse palpation falls into that category and as it is not generally taught at undergraduate level (I. Rutherford, personal communication, 2002) it is seldom practised or used routinely in NMS assessment. It is the authors' experience both from research (Taylor & George 2001b) and clinical experience that there are many apparent spinal and lower/upper limb conditions which have a vascular component to them and therefore require the clinician's expertise in pulse palpation as a basic skill.

Pulse palpation, like all hands-on skills, is a learned technique. It is commonly used before surgery to assess limb perfusion. The practised professional can assess presence, strength, quality and changes of pulses throughout the body. The skilled clinician may learn to detect changes in quality of the carotid pulses, for example, indicating possible stenosis. In many of the conditions described in this chapter pulse palpation is often perfectly normal at rest. However, because arterial flow and therefore pulses may be reduced at times of high demand or during arterial impingement, it becomes a particularly useful tool. Therefore exercise or provocative clinical tests (see EIAE and PAES) are advised in conjunction with pulse palpation in suspected cases. It is useful to note, however, that the dorsalis pedis pulse is absent in 10% of the normal population (Barnhorst et al 1968).

Stethoscope auscultation

Abnormalities found on palpation should be followed by stethoscope auscultation for bruits. A bruit is a low-pitched blowing sound which may indicate abnormal turbulence. The bell of the stethoscope is used and the artery is auscultated at various points along its path. The clinician should be aware of normal variations in pulse quality as well as observer error in pulse examination.

Hand–held doppler ultrasound

Ultrasound has been described as the most important advance in vascular diagnosis since the introduction of angiography (Faris et al 1992). The use of ultrasound assessment has achieved some prominence in physical therapy with the work into vertebral artery flow issues (Johnson et al 2000; see also Chs 19 and 37). Ultrasound in vascular assessment ranges from simple hand-held devices like the 'pencil' Doppler to sophisticated colour duplex spectral analysis. The manual therapist can utilize the benefits of audible hand-held Doppler units. Hand-held Doppler is used for two purposes: firstly, to detect pulses which are difficult to palpate (e.g. weak pulses or digital pulses). Secondly, to assess the quality of the pulse waveform, which may indicate disease. The hand-held Doppler unit may be used in conjunction with a sphygmomanometer to assess systolic blood pressure.

Pencil Doppler ultrasound is commonly used in medicine to assess peripheral pulses and arterial flow. Transducer probes with frequencies between 4 and 10 mHz are selected according to the depth of structure to be assessed. Qualitative waveform analysis of healthy arteries reveals a triphasic (three phases) waveform (Fig. 36.9) which comprises a rapid forward systolic flow, a short period of rapid reversed flow and then a low speed forward flow in late diastole (Donnelly et al 2000). Abnormal biphasic and monophasic waveforms are indicative of arterial disease. As with pulse palpation, Doppler assessment may be used in conjunction with either exercise or provocative manoeuvres such as forced active ankle plantar flexion in PAES.

Doppler ultrasound may be used for accurate blood pressure measurement at both the upper and lower limb (Fig. 36.10). This allows calculation of ankle to brachial

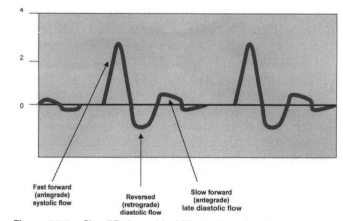

Fast forward
(antegrade)
systolic flow

Reversed
(retrograde)
diastolic flow

Slow forward
(antegrade)
late diastolic flow

Figure 36.9 Simplified graphical illustration of a triphasic waveform. The waveform from a Doppler is audible or can be visualized via software. A normal (non-pathological) waveform possesses the three components shown.

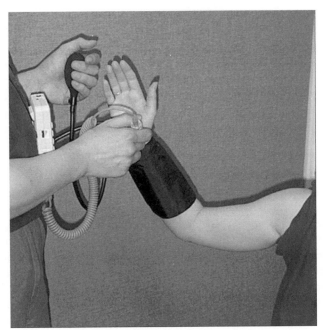

Figure 36.10 Hand-held Doppler ultrasound being used with a manual sphygmommanometer to take systolic pressure of the upper limb.

Table 36.1 Normal resting values for the ankle to brachial pressure index (ABPI)

Lower ABPI value	Upper ABPI value	Disease severity
1.00	1.2	Normal
0.75	0.9	Moderate disease
0.5	0.75	Severe disease
<0.5		Limb threatening

pressure index (see ABPI testing), which is used in medicine to assess for lower limb vascular insufficiency.

Blood pressure measurement

Measurement of lower and upper extremity blood pressure should be routine manual therapy practice in the suspicion of vascular disease (Marston 1992). Chiropractors and osteopaths use basic clinical vascular assessment such as pulse palpation and brachial blood pressures routinely. It has been reported that differences of between 30 and 50 mmHg between arms indicates upper extremity peripheral arterial insufficiency (e.g. in cases of subclavian–axillary or peripheral branch occlusion). The clinician may use either an automated unit, or manual sphygmomanometer, as in Figure 36.10.

In the lower limb blood pressure is taken at the ankle. In the upper quadrant the manual therapist should be concerned with measurement for brachial, wrist and digital pressures. Depending on the hypotheses being tested, measurements should be taken bilaterally, pre and post exertion (functional demonstration), or in different positions of the extremity. Reduced systolic measurements will be found in the presence of obstructive disease. Increases in systolic pressure are indicative of systemic atherosclerotic disease without obstruction (Table 36.1).

Resting ankle to brachial pressure index (ABPI)

The patient should rest supine for 20 minutes prior to blood pressure measurement. Testing requires the use of a sphyg-

momanometer and hand-held Doppler or automatic blood pressure monitor.

Method
- Systolic brachial pressure Left and Right – use highest value
- Systolic ankle pressure at posterior tibial and dorsalis pedis – use highest value

$$\text{Ankle to brachial pressure index} = \frac{\text{Ankle systolic BP}}{\text{Brachial systolic BP}}$$

Lower Limb Exercise Testing

A number of protocols for lower limb testing have been put forward involving treadmills and ergometer cycling (Arko et al 2001). However, because there may be biomechanical factors involved in the aetiology of the presenting condition, the exercise of choice should reflect this and achieve maximal blood flow through the suspected lesion. The use of treadmill testing, for example, has been criticized by some authors (Abraham et al 2001). Testing a rower or a cyclist on a treadmill may not replicate the conditions under which the symptoms occur and may provide false negative results. For that reason the test should be activity-specific and aimed to reproduce the symptoms as strongly as the patient experiences them during activity (Fig. 36.11).

Incremental ergometer cycling is the test of choice for EIAE in cyclists and the subject rides to reproduction of symptoms or volitional exhaustion. On completion of the test the subject transfers immediately to the couch where ankle and brachial systolic pressures are repeated within the first minute post exercise. Chevalier et al (1991) suggested an ABPI cut-off point of 0.5 post maximal exercise; however, this was modified in 2001 to 0.66 at the first minute of recovery (Abraham et al 2001). If history/examination and maximal exercise testing are indicative of an arterial lesion according to the above criteria the patient should be referred on for further arterial investigation. This may involve ultrasound imaging of the vessels, colour flow Doppler assessment of flow rates within the artery or ultimately arteriogram/MRA (Schep et al 2001b). Unfortunately, as none of these tests, including arteriography, have a 100% sensitivity for diagnosis, some ambiguity may still remain. Therefore, ultimately only angioscopy or

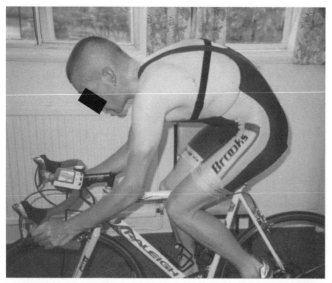

Figure 36.11 Acute hip and trunk flexion combined with maximal effort in the functional position reproduces the biomechanical factors leading to altered haemodynamics in the external iliac artery.

surgery will confirm the presence of an endofibrotic lesion. Surgery is only usually considered when three of four investigations (history, examination, ultrasound scanning, arteriography) are considered abnormal (Abraham et al 2001, Schep et al 1999).

In essence, what this section introduces is a series of simple scientific clinical examination and differential diagnostic principles which may be applied to patients suspected of vascular syndromes. The tests are basic and based on the very principles on which our profession was founded, namely the consideration and restoration of blood flow to tissues. However, contemporary literature and clinical observation suggest that these skills have become a lost art within physical therapy. It is hoped that the literature presented provides enough information to allow the clinician to begin to consider and reintroduce vascular hypotheses into their reasoning processes.

CONCLUSION

As our neuro-musculo-skeletal knowledge base continues to develop, it is important that our awareness and under-

standing of other somatic systems is not neglected. It seems rather odd to consider the NMS system divorced from its blood supply. However, because the vascular system forms a minuscule part of undergraduate and postgraduate education there is a misapprehension within manual therapy that vascular disease is a 'medical' issue and therefore of little consequence to day-to-day practice. As a consequence manual therapists have been implicated as being instrumental in delaying diagnosis and initiating inappropriate management of patients.

This chapter has demonstrated that a variety of vascular pathologies in both core and peripheral structures can, and invariably do, mimic painful conditions usually associated with NMS spinal dysfunction. The similarity in presentation is largely due to the relationship which the vascular syndromes have to movement and exertion, making differential diagnosis a cognitive and physical challenge. Consequently, both the assessment of conditions and the application of treatment techniques and modalities require some consideration of the vascular system. The extending diagnostic role of the manual therapist puts us in a position where early identification of conditions outside of our usual scope of knowledge is a desperate necessity. In the case of vascular conditions, this is of utmost urgency given the severe and unfortunate consequences of delayed diagnosis.

This new thinking not only expands the knowledge base but also opens up a whole new area for research within physical therapy. Further development of this area with regard to the fundamentals of haemodynamic concepts related to underlying conditions, applied modalities and resulting responses to treatment can only lead to an advancement of the profession. Above all, a combination of finely tuned clinical reasoning and appropriate testing will allow manual therapists to quickly and safely sift out those patients who require a 'different' approach to treatment or management.

KEYWORDS	
differential diagnosis	exercise testing
clinical reasoning	endofibrosis
arterial disease	artherosclerosis
vascular examination	

References

Abraham P, Saumet J L, Chevalier J M 1997a External iliac artery endofibrosis in athletes. Sports Medicine 24(4): 221–226

Abraham P, Chevalier J M, Leftherios G, Saumet J L 1997b Lower extremity arterial disease in sports. American Journal of Sports Medicine 25(4): 581–584

Abraham P, Chevalier J M, Saumet J L 1997c External iliac artery endofibrosis: a 40 year course. Journal of Sports Medicine and Physical Fitness 37: 297–300

Abraham P, Bickert S, Vielle B et al 2001 Pressure measurements at rest and after heavy exercise to detect moderate arterial lesions in athletes. Journal of Vascular Surgery 33(4): 721–727

Annett P, Hardman D, Fricker P 2000 Coarctation of the abdominal aorta as a presentation of the fatigued athlete. Clinical Journal of Sport Medicine 10(3): 201–203

Aquino B C, Barone E J 1989 'Effort' thrombosis of the axillary and subclavian vein associated with cervical rib and oral contraceptives in a young woman athlete. American Board of Family Practitioners 2(3): 208–211

Arko F R, Harris E J, Zarins C K et al 2001 Vascular complications in high performance athletes. Journal of Vascular Surgery 33: 935–942

Balaji M R, De Weese J A 1981 Adductor canal outlet syndrome. Journal of the American Medical Association 245: 167–170

Barnhorst D A, Sutton-Tyrell K, Rutan G H 1968 Prevalence of congenitally absent pedal pulse. New England Journal of Medicine 278: 264–265

Barrows H S, Feltovich P J 1987 The clinical reasoning process. Medical Education 21: 86–91

Bath P M W, Kennedy R L 2000 Acute stroke. In: Donnelly R, London N J M (eds) ABC of arterial and vascular disease. BMJ Books, London, pp 13–16

Batt M, King M, Guidoin R 1984 Mechanical fatigue of an arterial prosthesis. Presse Medicale 13(33): 1997–2000

Beatty R A 1977 Dissecting hematoma of the internal carotid artery following chiropractic cervical manipulation. Journal of Trauma 17(3): 248–249

Beck F 1995 L'endofibrose arterielle: formes typiques et atypiques. Thesis, Université Claude Bernard, Lyon, dissertation no 49

Berman S C, Bernhard V M, Erly W K, McIntyre K E, Erdoes L S, Hunter G C 1994 Critical carotid artery stenosis: diagnosis, timing of surgery, and outcome. Journal of Vascular Surgery 20(4): 499–510

Biller J 2000 When to operate in carotid artery disease. American Family Physician 61(1): 400–406

Blunt S B, Galton C 1997 Cervical carotid or vertebral dissection: an underdiagnosed cause of stroke in the young. British Medical Journal 314(7076): 243

Bradshaw C 2000 Exercise related lower leg pain: vascular. Medicine and Science in Sports and Exercise 32: S34–S36

Brochner G, Rojas M, Armas A J et al 1989 Axillary-subclavian venous thrombosis. Journal of Cardiovascular Surgery 30(1): 108–111

Butsch J L 1983 Subclavian thrombosis following hockey injuries. American Journal of Sports Medicine 11(6): 448–450

Carolei A, Marini C, Nencicni P et al 1995 Prevalence and outcome of symptomatic carotid lesions in young adults. British Medical Journal 310: 1363–1366

Carr S, Troop B, Hurley J et al 1996 Blunt trauma carotid injury: mild symptoms may disguise serious trouble. Physician and Sportsmedicine 24(2): Online. Available: http://www.physsportsmed.com/isssues/feb_96/troop.htm [accessed 30 Nov 1999]

Chevalier J M, Hoste P, Bouvat E 1991 L'endofibrose arterielle du sportif de haut niveau: formes inhabituelles. Journal of Traumatology in Sport 8: 176–181

Chevalier J M, Beck F, Megret A 1994 Endofibrose arterielle du sportif. In: Kieffer E, Godeau P (eds) Actualités de chirurgie vasculaire: maladies arterielles non athersclereuses de l'adulte. AERCV, Paris, pp 455–466

Cyriax J 1975 Textbook of orthopaedic medicine, 6th edn. Baillière Tindall, London, vol 1

Donnelly R, Hinwood D, London N J M 2000 Non-invasive methods of arterial and venous assessment. In: Donnelly R, London N J M (eds) ABC of arterial and venous disease. BMJ Books, London, ch 1

Durham J R, Yao J S T, Pearce W H et al 1995 Arterial injuries in the thoracic outlet syndrome. Journal of Vascular Surgery 21(1): 57–70

Duyff R F, Snijders C J, Vanneste J A 1997 Spontaneous bilateral internal carotid artery dissection and migraines: a potential diagnostic delay. Headache 37(2): 109–112

Earle K A, Lloyd M H 1989 Paget–Schroetter syndrome in a patient on the contraceptive pill. New York State Journal of Medicine 89(5): 293

Ellis M 2000 Risk factors and management of patients with upper limb deep vein thrombosis. Chest 117(1): 43–46

Faris I B, McCollum P, Mantese V et al 1992 Investigation of the patient with atheroma. In: Bell P R F, Jamieson C W, Ruckley C V (eds.) Surgical management of vascular disease. WB Saunders, London, pp 131–196

Gallegos C R R, Studley J G N, Hamer D B 1989 External iliac artery occlusion: another complication of long distance running? European Journal of Vascular Surgery 4: 195–196

Green R M 1998 Vascular manifestations of the thoracic outlet syndrome. Seminars in Vascular Surgery 11(2): 67–76

Grieve G P 1994 The masqueraders. In: Boyling J D, Palastanga N (eds) Grieve's Modern Manual Therapy. 2nd edn. Churchill Livingstone, London

Hart R G, Easton J D 1985 Dissections. Stroke 16: 925–927

Hingorani A, Ascher E, Yorkovich M et al 2000 Upper extremity deep vein thrombosis: an underecognised manifestation of a hypercoaguable state. Annals of Vascular Surgery 14(5): 421–426

Hood D B, Kuehne J, Yellin A E, Weaver F A 1997 Vascular complications of thoracic outlet syndrome. American Surgeon 63(10): 913–917

Hufnagel A, Hammers A, Scholne P W, Bohm K D, Leonhardt G 1999 Stroke following chiropractic manipulation of the cervical spine. Journal of Neurology 246(8): 683–688

Hurlbert S N, Rutherford R B 1995 Primary subclavian-axillary vein thrombosis. Annals of Vascular Surgery 9: 217–223

Jones M 1994 Clinical reasoning process in manipulative therapy In: Boyling J D, Palastanga N (eds) Grieve's Modern Manual Therapy, 2nd edn. Churchill Livingstone, London

Kauppila L I, Tallroth K 1993 Post mortem angiographic findings for arteries supplying the lumbar spine: their relationship to low back symptoms. Journal of Spinal Disorders 6(2): 124–129

Kauppila L I, McLindon T, Evans S et al 1997 Disc degeneration/back pain and calcification of the abdominal aorta. Spine 22: 1642–1647

King C A, Bithell C 1998 Expertise in diagnostic reasoning: a comparative study. British Journal of Therapy and Rehabilitation 5: 78–87

Laslett M 2000 Bilateral buttock pain caused by aortic stenosis: a case report of claudication of the buttock. Manual Therapy 5(4): 227–233

Leebeek F W, Stanhouders N A, van Stein D et al 2001 Hypercoaguable states in upper-extremity deep vein thrombosis. American Journal of Hemotology 67(1): 15–19

Levien L J, Veller M G 1999 Popliteal artery entrapment syndrome: more common than previously recognised. Journal of Vascular Surgery 30(4): 587–598

McCarron M O, Metcalfe R A, Muir K W 2000 Facial nerve palsy secondary to internal carotid artery dissection. European Journal of Neurology 7: 723–725

McCarthy W J, Yao J S T, Schafer M F et al 1989 Upper extremity arterial injury in athletes. Journal of Vascular Surgery 9(2): 317–327

McDonald P T, Easterbrook J A, Rich N M 1980 Popliteal artery entrapment syndrome: clinical non invasive and angiographic diagnosis. American Journal of Surgery 139: 318–325

Maitland G D 1986 Vertebral manipulation, 5th edn. Butterworth Heinemann, Oxford

Mann T, Refshauge K M 2001 Causes of complications from cervical spine manipulation. Australian Journal of Physiotherapy 47: 255–266

Marston A 1992 Clinical examination of the patient with atheroma. In: Bell P R F, Jamieson C W, Ruckley C V (eds) Surgical management of vascular disease. W B Saunders, London

Mohyuddin A 2000 Indirect carotid cavernous fistula presenting as pulsatile tinnitus. Journal of Laryngology and Otology 114: 788–789

Nuber G W, McCarthy W J, Yao J S T et al 1990 Arterial abnormalities of the shoulder in athletes. American Journal of Sports Medicine 18(5): 514–519

Ouriel K 1995 Lower extremity vascular problems. W B Saunders, Philadelphia

Ouriel K 1998 Upper extremity vascular problems: overview. Seminars in Vascular Surgery 11(2): 53

Palmer J B, Uematus S, Jankel W R et al 1991 A cellist with arm pain: thermal asymmetry in scalenus anticus syndrome. Archives of Physical Medicine and Rehabilitation 72(3): 237–242

Roos D B 1999 Thoracic outlet syndrome is underdiagnosed. Muscle and Nerve 22(1): 126–129

Ross R 1999 Atherosclerosis: an inflammatory disease. New England Journal of Medicine 340(2): 115–125

Roth J W, Boyd C R 1999 Recreational bicycling and injury to the external iliac artery. American Surgery 65(5): 460–463

Rousselet M C, Saint-Andre J P, L'Hoste P 1990 Stenotic intimal thickening of the external iliac artery in competition cyclists. Human Pathology 21: 524–529

Rutherford R B 1998 Primary subclavian-axillary vein thrombosis: the relative roles of thrombolysis, percutaneous angioplasty, stents and surgery. Seminars in Vascular Surgery 11(2): 91–95

Sayinalp N, Ozcebe O I, Kirazli S et al 1999 Paget–Schroetter syndrome associated with FV:Q506 and prothrombin 20210A: a case report. Angiology 50(8): 689–692

Schep G, Bender M H M, Kaandorp D et al 1999 Flow limitations in the iliac arteries in endurance athletes: current knowledge and directions for the future. International Journal of Sportsmedicine 20: 421–428

Schep G, Bender M H, Schmikli S L 2001a Colour Doppler used to detect kinking and intravascular lesions in the iliac artery in endurance athletes with claudication. 14(2–3): 129–140

Schep G, Kaandorp D W, Bender M H et al 2001b magnetic resonance angiography used to detect kinking in the iliac arteries in endurance athletes with claudication. Physiological Measurement 22(3): 475–487

Shovman O, George J, Shoenfeld Y 1997 Primary subclavian vein thrombosis after intensive physical exertion. Harefuah 133(12): 610–612

Silbert P L, Mokri B, Schievink W I 1995 Headache and neck pain in spontaneous internal carotid and vertebral artery dissections. Neurology 45: 1517–1522

Sise M J, Shackford S R, Rowley S R 1989 Claudication in young adults: a frequently delayed diagnosis. Journal of Vascular Surgery 10: 68–74

Skerker R S, Flandry F C 1992 Case presentation: painless arm swelling in a high school football player. Medical Science and Sports Exercise 24(11): 1185–1189

Stager A, Clement D 1999 Popliteal artery entrapment syndrome. Sports Medicine (Auckland, New Zealand) 28(1): 61–70

Taira N, Mano M, Asano H et al 2001 Primary subclavian venous thrombosis which developed after sleeping with the arm in an outstretched position: report of a case. Surgery Today 31(4): 333–335

Taylor A J, George K P 2001a Exercise induced leg pain in young athletes misdiagnosed as pain of musculoskeletal origin. Manual Therapy 6(1): 48–52

Taylor A J, George K P 2001b Ankle to brachial pressure index in normal subjects and trained cyclists with exercise induced leg pain. Medicine and Science in Sports and Exercise 33(11): 1862–1867

Taylor A J, Tennant W G, Batt M et al 1997 Traumatic occlusion of the external iliac artery in a racing cyclist: a cause of ill defined leg pain. British Journal of Sports Medicine 31: 155–156

Touliopolous S, Hershman E B 1999 Lower leg pain: diagnosis and treatment of compartment syndrome and other pain syndromes of the lower leg. Sports Medicine (Auckland, New Zealand) 27(3): 193–204

Vlychou M, Spanomichos G, Chatziioannou A et al 2001 Embolisation of a traumatic aneurysm of the posterior circumflex humeral artery in a volleyball player. British Journal of Sports Medicine 35: 137

Walder J, Mosimann F, Van Melle G 1984 A presentation of endofibrosis of the iliac artery in two racing cyclists. Helvetia Chirugie Acta 51: 793–795

Warnes C A, Fuster V, McGoon M D 1996 Coarctation of the aorta. In: Guiliani E R, Gersch J, McGoon M D, Hayes D L, Schaff H V (eds) Mayo Clinic practice of cardiology, 3rd edn. Mosby, St Louis

Wijesinghe L D, Coughlin P A, Robertson I 2001 Cyclist's iliac syndrome: temporary relief by balloon angioplasty. British Journal of Sports Medicine 35(1): 70–71

Wilbourn A J 1999a Thoracic outlet syndrome is overdiagnosed. Muscle and Nerve 22(1): 130–136

Wilbourm A J 1999b Thoracic outlet syndromes. Neurologic Clinics 17(3): 447–497

Wilson S, Selvaratnam P, Briggs C 1994 Strain at the subclavian artery during the upper limb tension test. Australian Journal of Physiotherapy 40(4): 243–248

Windfuhr J P 2001 Aneurysm of the internal carotid artery following soft tissue penetration injury. International Journal of Pediatric Otorhinolaryngology 61(2): 155–159

Wohlgemuth A, Rottach K G, Stoehr M 1999 Intermittant claudication due to ischaemia of the lumbosacral plexus. Journal of Neurology and Neurosurgery Psychiatry 67: 793–795

Yabuki S, Kikuchi S, Midorikawa H, Hoshino S 1999 Vascular backache and consideration of its pathomechanisms: report of two cases. Journal of Spinal Disorders 12(2): 162–167

Zell L, Scheffler P, Marschall F et al 2000 Paget–Schroetter syndrome caused by wrestling. Sportverletz Sportschaden 14(1): 31–34

Zell L, Kindermann W, Marschall F et al 2001 Paget–Schroetter syndrome in sports activities: case study and literature review. Angiology 52(5): 337–342

Zetterling M, Carlstrom C, Konrad P 2000 Internal carotid artery dissection. Acta Neurologica Scandinavica 101: 1–7

Chapter 37

Adverse effects of cervical manipulative therapy

D. A. Rivett

TYPES OF ADVERSE EFFECTS OF CSM

The earliest documented case of complication following cervical spine manipulation (CSM), a fracture and dislocation of the atlas, was published almost a century ago (Roberts 1907). Subsequent case reports and retrospective surveys of health practitioners have provided evidence that CSM can produce a variety of serious adverse effects, some of which may be fatal (Box 37.1) (Assendelft et al 1996, Di Fabio 1999, Dvorák & Orelli 1985, Dvorák et al 1993, Gorman 1978, Grieve 1994, Gross et al 1996, Hurwitz et al 1996, Jaskoviak 1980, Livingston 1971, Michaeli 1993, Patijn 1991, Schmitt 1991, Sédat et al 2002, Sivakumaran & Wilsher 1995, Terrett 1987a). Manipulative complications have most frequently been attributed to chiropractic intervention, although it should be borne in mind that chiropractors perform the overwhelming majority of manipulations (Assendelft et al 1996, Di Fabio 1999, Jaskoviak 1980, Michaeli 1993).

Lee et al (1995) described the results of a survey of neurologists in California, USA. The neurologists were asked to document any neurological complications resulting from chiropractic spinal manipulation they had witnessed in the preceding 2 years. The 177 respondents reported 102 complications in total. Of these 91 (89%) were related to CSM, including 56 cases of stroke (53 in the vertebral artery (VA) distribution, three in the carotid distribution), 13 cases of myelopathy and 22 cases of radiculopathy. However, the number of manipulations performed over this period and the proportion of these which were applied to the cervical spine was not ascertained. Nevertheless, the number of serious complications found in this study alone approximates the total number of case reports described in the English language literature (Hurwitz et al 1996). In a survey of South African physiotherapists, Michaeli (1991, 1993) also found that the majority (92%) of manipulative complications involved CSM, although only approximately one-third of spinal manipulations involved the cervical spine.

Rivett & Milburn (1997) investigated the types of complication resulting from spinal manipulative therapy in

Box 37.1   Types of serious complications attributed to cervical spine manipulation

- Cerebrovascular accident as a result of injury to the vertebrobasilar arterial system or occasionally the internal carotid artery or posterior inferior cerebellar artery
- Transient symptoms or signs potentially attributable to vertebrobasilar insufficiency, such as dizziness or vertigo, nausea, vomiting, balance deficits, loss of consciousness and blurring of vision
- Cervical disc herniation
- Radiculopathy
- Myelopathy
- Vertebral fracture
- Vertebral dislocation
- Diaphragmatic paralysis
- Tracheal rupture
- Severe or markedly increased neck pain, arm pain or headache
- Rupture of a venous sinus of the posterior fossa
- Cardiac arrest
- Anterior spinal artery occlusion
- Musculoskeletal strain/sprain
- Cranial nerve lesions

New Zealand and which manipulative professions were held responsible for any such unfavourable outcomes. Medical specialists likely to encounter the consequences of serious complications of spinal manipulative therapy (neurologists, neurosurgeons, orthopaedic surgeons and vascular surgeons) were surveyed regarding cases of spinal manipulative complication personally encountered in the previous 5 years. Of the 146 respondents (63.5% response rate), 23 reported 42 specific cases of complication. Over half of the incidents (23 cases) were attributed to chiropractic treatment, with a further one third (14 cases) attributed to physiotherapy. Osteopathic (three cases) and medical intervention (two cases) accounted for the remaining complications. Twenty-six adverse effects (62%) resulted from treatment of the cervical spine and included 14 cerebrovascular accidents (CVA), seven radiculopathies, three disc prolapses and two cases of increased pain. No deaths were reported, but unresolved outcomes ranged from sensory deficits to hemiparesis.

The findings of Rivett & Milburn (1997) indicate that all professions utilizing manipulation are at risk of causing serious complications with spinal manipulative therapy, especially of the cervical spine and the extracranial arteries. In particular, 10 of the 14 incidents attributed to physiotherapy resulted from cervical spine manipulative treatment, including two cases of CVA. This is of interest as there have been very few case reports in the literature describing complications in which manipulative physio-

therapy to the neck was implicated (Fritz et al 1984, Grant 1988, Michaeli 1993, Parkin et al 1978, Patijn 1991, Rivett & Milburn 1996). In a review of 118 cases of adverse responses to manual therapy of the cervical spine, physiotherapy treatment is not specifically described, although it could be included in some of the 19 'other/unknown therapist' cases cited (Hurwitz et al 1996). This suggests that serious complications of manipulative physiotherapy of the cervical spine may be substantially more common than the case reports in the medical literature indicate.

The number and type of serious physiotherapeutic complications reported by Rivett & Milburn (1997) is somewhat similar to those found by Michaeli (1993) in his survey of South African physiotherapists. On the other hand, there were no cases of CVA reported in a survey of members of the Manipulative Physiotherapists Association of Australia (Grimmer 1998), although 94% of an unspecified number of adverse responses to cervical spine manipulative physiotherapy procedures were related to vertebrobasilar insufficiency (VBI), and 16% of patients required medical attention. Nevertheless, the results of these three studies probably represent an underestimation of the true number of complications as a result of modest response rates and the retrospective nature of the surveys (with associated recall bias), even accounting for the possibility of some cases occurring spontaneously and being incorrectly attributed to manipulative therapy.

It is clear from the literature that instances of VA injury resulting in stroke constitute the majority of the reported serious complications of CSM (Greenman 1991, Hurwitz et al 1996, Jaskoviak 1980, Rivett & Milburn 1997, Schmitt 1991, Senstad et al 1996a). Indeed, Patijn (1991) calculated that VA injury comprises 65.1% of all manipulative therapy complications reported in the literature. In addition to serious complications, there is also a range of frequent, minor and transient side-effects of CSM, including local discomfort, tiredness, mild headache, altered sensitivity, psychological symptoms and radiating discomfort (Gross et al 1996, Leboeuf-Yde et al 1997, Senstad et al 1996a, 1996b, 1997). It is also clear that CSM carries with it a degree of risk irrespective of whether it is performed by a physiotherapist, chiropractor, osteopath or medical practitioner (Adams & Sim 1998, Lee et al 1995, Michaeli 1993, Patijn 1991, Rivett & Milburn 1997).

CASES OF NEUROVASCULAR COMPLICATION

Several reviews of the literature have documented a growing number of cases of stroke resulting from the application of CSM by members of all the manipulative professions (Box 37.2). Generally, case reports of neurovascular complication implicate manipulative injury of the VA, but occasionally the internal carotid artery (ICA) or another vascular structure is thought to be involved (Greenman 1991, Hurwitz et al 1996, Lee et al 1995, Schmitt 1991). In the majority of published cases (approximately 80%) an

Box 37.2 Reviews of published cases of neurovascular complication

Authors	Cases*	Period	Comments
Jaskoviak (1980)	46	1947–80	
Sherman et al (1987)	52	1947–87	
Terrett (1987a)	107	1934–87	English, French, German, Norwegian literature
Grant (1988)	58	1947–86	English language literature
Patijn (1991)	84	Not stated	
Kunnasmaa & Thiel (1994)	139	Not stated	English, French, German, Scandinavian literature
Terrett (1995)	160	1934–94	English, Chinese, German, French, Scandinavian literature
Assendelft et al (1996)	178	Pre-1993	
Hurwitz et al (1996)	92	Pre-1995	English language literature – vertebrobasilar strokes only
Di Fabio (1999)	177	1925–97	Includes all cervical spine manipulation complications in all languages
Haldeman et al (1999)	115	Pre-1993	English language literature – vertebrobasilar artery dissection/occlusion only

*Some cases are counted in more than one review.

immediate cause and effect relationship is evident, often supported by angiographic data and less frequently by post mortem findings (Bogduk 1994, Corrigan & Maitland 1998, Daneshmend et al 1984, Dunne et al 1987, Frumkin & Baloh 1990, Grant 1988, 1994a, 1994b, Lyness & Wagman 1974, Rivett 1994, Sherman et al 1987). In a few cases the link between CSM and the subsequent CVA is more tenuous, usually because the time interval between the two events potentially permits the occurrence of unrelated pathology such as VA spontaneous dissection (Haldeman et al 1999, Leboeuf-Yde et al 1996, Terrett 1995).

It is generally agreed that published case reports represent only a small fraction of all incidents and that the majority remain unreported (Assendelft et al 1996, Grant 1988, 1994a, 1994b, 1996, Grieve 1994; Leboeuf-Yde et al 1996, Middleditch 1991, Patijn 1991, Robertson 1981). This view is supported by the results of an informal survey of delegates at a meeting of the Stroke Council of the American Heart Association (Robertson 1982), which revealed 360 previously unpublished cases of extracranial arterial injury associated with CSM, most of which were confirmed by arteriography. However, further clinical details of these cases have not been published (Di Fabio 1999, Terrett 1995). In addition, there are iatrogenic strokes reported in newspapers and magazines that have not been documented in the medical literature (Consumers' Institute of New Zealand 1997, Di Fabio 1999, Terrett 1995). Complications of a more minor or transient nature would also likely not be of sufficient importance to warrant publication, but undoubtedly occur more frequently than serious complications (Assendelft et al 1996, Grant 1994a, Michaeli 1991, 1993, Schellhas et al 1980).

For various reasons clinicians involved in cases of manipulative complication may choose not to, or are unable to, report or publish the incident. Factors such as

legal constraints could lead to a considerable under-reporting of the extent of the problem. It is therefore apparent that while published cases provide evidence of a causal link between CSM and extracranial arterial injury, they cannot be used to accurately estimate the incidence rate of stroke. They also frequently lack detail, such as the type of technique used, the spinal segment manipulated and the frequency of treatment (Di Fabio 1999).

Published cases of iatrogenic stroke have been predominantly attributed to CSM performed by chiropractors (Assendelft et al 1996, Di Fabio 1999, Grant 1988, Hurwitz et al 1996, Michaeli 1993), although a few cases are likely to have been incorrectly ascribed to chiropractic intervention (Assendelft et al 1996, Terrett 1995). There are relatively few physiotherapeutic neurovascular incidents described in the literature, with no fatal cases attributed to physiotherapists (Assendelft et al 1996, Di Fabio 1999, Fritz et al 1984, Hurwitz et al 1996, Parkin et al 1978, Patijn 1991). Grant (1994b) identifies only two cases of stroke due to physiotherapeutic CSM, while Terrett (1995) provides new evidence that two of the cases of stroke described by Frisoni & Anzola (1991) as resulting from chiropractic manipulation were actually caused by physiotherapists. Assendelft et al (1996), in a comprehensive review of the literature, found that less than 5% of 142 cases of vertebrobasilar or other cerebral complications in which the practitioner's profession could be identified were attributed to physiotherapy treatment. Furthermore, in a systematic review of complications of CSM (Hurwitz et al 1996) physiotherapy intervention was not specifically stated as the cause of any of the cases.

There are a few studies in which adverse responses to CSM resulting from manipulative physiotherapy have been investigated (Hurley et al 2002, Michaeli 1991, 1993, Rivett & Milburn 1996, 1997, Rivett & Reid 1998). In a retrospective survey of 153 manipulative physiotherapists in South Africa, Michaeli (1991, 1993) failed to document a single stroke from the application of approximately 75 500 cervical manipulations. In a prospective study of adverse responses to CSM performed by manipulative physiotherapists, no neurological complications were reported following nearly 500 procedures (Rivett & Milburn 1996).

Rivett & Milburn (1997), in their survey of medical specialists in New Zealand, reported 14 cases of manipulative stroke during a 5-year period, none of which were fatal but which resulted in permanent disability for seven patients. Nine incidents were attributed to chiropractors, two complications were attributed to osteopaths and one case was considered to result from manipulative treatment applied by a general practitioner. Physiotherapists were held to be responsible for the other two cases of CVA, despite the Australian premanipulative testing protocol (Australian Physiotherapy Association 1988) being an accepted part of clinical practice and physiotherapy education in New Zealand throughout the 5-year reporting period. Interestingly, two of the complications were thought to have resulted from trauma to a carotid artery, with eight strokes in the vertebrobasilar distribution (in four cases the traumatized vessel was not indicated). Rivett & Reid (1998) report two further cases of vertebrobasilar stroke attributed to CSM performed by physiotherapists in New Zealand, and Hurley et al (2002) at least one case of VA injury, supporting the view that physiotherapists are more often responsible than was previously believed.

The initial use of passive joint mobilization and subsequent assessment of the patient's response prior to the application of CSM (high velocity thrust procedures) is commonly advocated (Australian Physiotherapy Association 1988). The underlying assumption, that mobilization is, relatively, a safer procedure, is supported by the findings of Hurwitz et al (1996) who conclude that cervical spine mobilization results in fewer complications than does CSM. However, mobilization is not entirely free of the risk of stroke, with Michaeli (1991, 1993) describing an incident due to vigorous end-range rotary mobilization of the upper cervical spine by a physiotherapist in South Africa. Another 115 transient or minor potential ischaemic complications were also reported following cervical spine mobilization. In a recent survey of Australian manipulative physiotherapists it was found that 27.5% of complications possibly related to VBI were caused by passive mobilization procedures, particularly those involving a rotation component (Grimmer 1998). A similar survey of New Zealand manipulative physiotherapists revealed a case of suspected stroke following a C1–2 mobilization and a transient ischaemic attack following a sustained natural apophyseal glide (SNAG) (Kankamedala et al 2003), despite the application of a premanipulative protocol (Australian Physiotherapy Association 1988).

It is clear that manipulative stroke is an important issue of concern for the physiotherapy profession. It is also clear

that relying on published case reports to determine the risk of neurovascular complication will lead to a marked underestimation of the frequency of these events (Assendelft et al 1996, Rivett & Milburn 1996, Stevinson et al 2001). Nevertheless, case reports provide much of the available information pertaining to the technical factors and the pathologies involved in neurovascular complications.

TECHNICAL FACTORS

Although it is generally recognized that all CSM techniques are associated with an element of risk, it is likely that the hazards can be reduced by the avoidance of certain practices (Box 37.3) (Klougart et al 1996b). The application of multiple manipulations during an individual treatment session probably increases the likelihood of VA injury (Carey 1994, Grant 1994a, 1994b, Grieve 1994, Klougart et al 1996b, Middleditch 1991, Refshauge 1995, Sherman et al 1987). It is recommended that only a single CSM be applied in any one treatment session (Australian Physiotherapy Association 1988, Grant 1994a, 1994b, Michaeli 1991). Repeated manipulations performed over a number of treatment visits can also increase the possibility of complication (Cook & Sanstead 1991, Grieve 1994, Robertson 1982, Sherman et al 1987), perhaps due to cumulative subclinical damage (Di Fabio 1999, Frumkin & Baloh 1990, Grant 1994a). Despite the recommendation to shun manipulation until the response to other forms of manual therapy has been assessed over at least 24 hours (Australian Physiotherapy Association 1988, Grant 1994a, 1994b, Michaeli 1991), there is little evidence that this helps avoid complications (Carey 1995).

The use of non-localized or non-specific manipulative procedures is also considered to increase the risk associated with CSM, and therefore localized, specific techniques are advocated (Adams & Sim 1998, Carey 1995, Grant 1994a, 1994b, Grieve 1994, Michaeli 1991, Middleditch 1991,

---

Box 37.3 Hazardous practices in the performance of cervical spine manipulation

- Multiple manipulations in any one treatment session
- Repeated manipulations over a number of treatment sessions
- Manipulating without having first assessed the effect of mobilization
- Non-specific multisegmental techniques
- Thrusting through large ranges of physiological movement
- Techniques involving upper cervical spine rotation
- Manipulating at end-range cervical spine rotation or extension
- Techniques involving a traction component
- Applying excessive force in the thrust component

Refshauge 1995). Michaeli (1991, 1993) describes 18 cases of transient complications attributed to generalized rotary CSM performed by physiotherapists, and only seven adverse responses following localized manipulation, although the actual incidence rate for each type (local or general) of manipulation was not determined. Similarly, procedures involving large ranges of physiological movement are not recommended (Australian Physiotherapy Association 1988, Corrigan & Maitland 1998, Eder & Tilscher 1990, Grant 1994a, 1994b, Grieve 1991, 1994).

Cervical spine rotation has been implicated in case reports in the literature as being the movement with the greatest risk of causing VA injury during CSM (Bourdillon et al 1992, Di Fabio 1999, Dvorák et al 1991, 1993, Grant 1994a, 1994b, Grieve 1991, 1994, Haynes 1996a, 1996b, Hinse et al 1991, Jaskoviak 1980, Krueger & Okazaki 1980, Michaeli 1991, 1993, Refshauge 1995, Schellhas et al 1980, Shekelle & Coulter 1997). Hurwitz et al (1996) found that 82% of case reports of stroke following CSM describe rotary manipulative procedures. Rotation manipulation involving the atlanto-axial joint is considered particularly hazardous because of the large amount (approximately 45 degrees) of rotation permitted at this segment and the relative fixity of the VA at the C1 and C2 transverse foramina (Bogduk 1994, Corrigan & Maitland 1998, Dumas et al 1996, Dunne et al 1987, Easton & Sherman 1977, Grant 1994b, Grieve 1991, Hinse et al 1991, Michaeli 1991, 1993, Robertson 1981, Roy 1994, Schmitt 1991, Terrett 1987b). Angiographic and pathological findings from patients experiencing VA injury post manipulation confirm the traumatic involvement of the atlanto-axial region of the artery in the majority of cases (Aspinall 1989, Bogduk 1994, Easton & Sherman 1977, Frumkin & Baloh 1990, Grant 1994a, 1994b, 1996, Grieve 1991, 1994, Krueger & Okazaki 1980, Lee et al 1995, Mas et al 1989, Sherman et al 1981, Teasell & Marchuk 1994). Furthermore, cadaveric, angiographic, magnetic resonance angiographic and ultrasonographic studies have demonstrated that cervical rotation can interfere with contralateral VA blood flow at the atlanto-axial level (Brown & Tissington-Tatlow 1963, Dumas et al 1996, Licht et al 1998a, Refshauge 1994, Rivett et al 1999, 2000, Stevens 1991, Tissington-Tatlow & Bammer 1957, Toole & Tucker 1960, Weintraub & Khoury 1995a).

Further support for this assertion is provided by retrospective surveys of chiropractors in Denmark (Klougart et al 1996a, 1996b). The results of these investigations indicated that manipulation of the upper neck was much more frequently associated with cerebrovascular incidents than treatment of the lower neck. Notably, rotation procedures applied to the upper cervical spine were more likely to cause complications than non-rotation techniques used in this region. Similarly, Dvorák & Orelli (1985) found that most adverse reactions indicative of VBI that were reported in a survey of Swiss manual medicine physicians followed manipulation of the upper cervical spine. Indirect evidence of the danger associated with rotary CSM is also provided

by Haynes (1996a) who argues that a decrease in the rate of incidence of manipulative strokes attributed to chiropractors in Perth, Australia, could have resulted from a reduction in use of such techniques. In addition, complications of CSM reported by manipulative physiotherapists in Australia were mainly associated with manoeuvres involving rotation (Grimmer 1998). Because of this growing evidence, manipulation using end-range rotation is generally not recommended, particularly in the upper cervical spine (Assendelft et al 1996, Carey 1995, Di Fabio 1999, Gutmann 1983, Michaud 2002, Terrett 1987a, 1987b).

In contrast, Haldeman et al (1999) found that there was no information about the types of manipulative procedures used in 61% of 115 case reports of vertebrobasilar arterial dissection in the English language literature. In almost all of the other case reports, the technical description of the manipulation was not provided by the practitioner responsible for the ensuing complication, introducing the potential for descriptive error (Haldeman et al 1999, Klougart et al 1996a). It is also possible that rotation is the most frequently applied CSM, and therefore the majority of complications would be expected to occur after rotary manipulation (Di Fabio 1999, Haldeman et al 1999, Rivett & Reid 1998).

Manipulative techniques utilizing traction also probably involve a higher risk of VA injury and are not recommended, particularly those using traction combined with rotation (Australian Physiotherapy Association 1988, Grant 1994a, 1994b, Grieve 1994, Refshauge 1995). At the very least, the addition of traction to rotary manipulative procedures is very unlikely to render them safer as has been previously suggested (Grieve 1991, 1994, Middleditch 1991, Rivett 1994). Research using cadavers and biomechanical models indicates that the addition of traction to cervical spine rotation markedly increases the stress applied to the contralateral VA (Brown & Tissington-Tatlow 1963, Stevens 1991). An extension component to the manipulative technique is also considered inadvisable, as it has been linked to some instances of vertebrobasilar arterial complication (Bourdillon et al 1992, Carey 1995, Dvorák & Orelli 1985, Dvorák et al 1991, 1993, Grant 1994a, 1994b, Grieve 1994, Haldeman et al 1999, Hamann et al 1993, Hinse et al 1991, Jaskoviak 1980, Schellhas et al 1980, Shekelle & Coulter 1997).

The use of minimal force in the execution of high velocity thrust techniques is advocated, and the use of excessive force is regarded as very dangerous (Campbell 1994, Carey 1995, Grant 1994a, Hutchison 1989, Kleynhans & Terrett 1985). It is plausible that the application of unnecessary positional and thrusting forces will increase the likelihood of vascular trauma (Bogduk 1994, Grieve 1993, 1994, Klougart et al 1996b, Krueger & Okazaki 1980, Michaeli 1991, Rivett 1994, Schmitt 1991). Both Grieve (1994) and Bogduk (1994) comment that case reports of manipulative complications frequently stress the excessive force used in the responsible manoeuvre. It has been demonstrated in an animal model that a high velocity thrust applied to the cervical spine can temporarily disrupt VA blood flow, suggesting that the application of minimal force is advisable (Licht et al 1999).

Despite these technical recommendations, an element of risk of vascular trauma remains with all CSM procedures (Aspinall 1989, Campbell 1994, Carey 1995, Grant 1994b, Haldeman et al 1999, Rivett 1994). The consequent neurological insult experienced by the patient is largely dependent upon the pathological processes initiated (Grant 1994b).

VASCULAR PATHOLOGY

Case reports documenting angiographic results, surgical findings and occasionally autopsy evidence provide some information regarding the pathogenesis of stroke following CSM. Importantly, it has been suggested that smaller calibre vessels (such as the VA) may have an increased risk of vascular pathology and blood flow impedance in response to external mechanical stimuli (Haynes 1996b, Macchi et al 1996, Mitchell & McKay 1995).

The atlanto-axial segment of the contralateral VA is most commonly the site of injury with neck manipulation involving rotation (Arnetoli et al 1989, Bogduk 1994, Easton & Sherman 1977, Grant 1987, 1994b, Grieve 1991, 1994, Rothrock et al 1991, Sherman et al 1982, Teasell & Marchuk 1994, Terrett 1987b). A few authors consider that the usual site of injury is at the atlanto-occipital joint, where the artery changes from its vertical course to a horizontal route (Assendelft et al 1996, Fast et al 1987, Frumkin & Baloh 1990, Lee et al 1995, Sinel & Smith 1993). Most commonly a tear of the intima (and perhaps the tunica media) is produced in the endothelial surface of the vessel, followed by blood tracking into the arterial wall leading to dissection (splitting of layers) and formation of a pseudoaneurysm, with subsequent thrombus formation and stenosis (Bogduk 1994, Côté et al 1996, Di Fabio 1999, Easton & Sherman 1977, Frumkin & Baloh 1990, Grant 1994b, Lee et al 1995, Mas et al 1989, Nakamura et al 1991, Patijn 1991, Rivett 1994, Rothrock et al 1991, Roy 1994, Schmitt 1991, Teasell & Marchuk 1994, Terrett 1987b).

Dissection of the VA is often accompanied by ipsilateral posterosuperior neck or occipital head pain, frequently described as sudden, severe and sharp, and which sometimes precedes ischaemic symptoms (Bartels & Flügel 1996, Curt & Dietz 1994, Frumkin & Baloh 1990, Jull 1994, Mas et al 1987, 1989, Norris et al 2000, Schellhas et al 1980, Sturzenneger et al 1993, Tulyapronchote et al 1994). There is no past history of a similar pain (Haldeman et al 2002a, Krespi et al 2002). The cause of the pain is not well understood but is probably due to excitation of nociceptors in the damaged vessel wall (Hinse et al 1991). It may be that the pain of spontaneous or traumatic VA dissection sometimes prompts patients to seek help from a manipulative practitioner, with the subsequent administration of CSM propagating the dissection cephalically or dislodging an

intraluminal thrombosis, leading to stroke (Frumkin & Baloh 1990, Haldeman et al 1999, Hamann et al 1993, Mas et al 1989). Subarachnoid haemorrhage can also occasionally eventuate from dissection (Dunne et al 1987, Teasell & Marchuk 1994, Terenzi & DeFabio 1996). Some authors consider that pre-existing arteriopathy, such as proteoglycan accumulation in the tunica media related to cystic mucoid degeneration, may predispose the VA to dissection (Haldeman et al 1999, Johnson et al 1993, Rivett 1994).

Other pathologies involving trauma of the vascular wall have been described. These include mural perforation with perivascular haemorrhage, intramural haematoma secondary to rupture of the vasa vasorum, and reflex vasospasm following mechanical irritation of the vessel (or the innervating cervical afferent nerves) or in response to sympathetic excitation (Di Fabio 1999, Dunne et al 1987, Fast et al 1987, Fritz et al 1984, Frumkin & Baloh 1990, Grant 1994b, Hurwitz et al 1996, Oostendorp et al 1992a, Parkin et al 1978, Patijn 1991, Rivett 1994, Schellhas et al 1980, Schmitt 1991, Sherman et al 1981, 1987, Sinel & Smith 1993, Teasell & Marchuk 1994, Terrett 1987b). Turbulent blood flow produced by focal luminal narrowing associated with spasm, stretching or external compression of the VA may denude the epithelium, leading to platelet deposition or thrombus formation, and perhaps weaken the vessel wall (Grant 1996, Haynes et al 2002, Mann 1995, Mann & Refshauge 2001, Schellhas et al 1980, Symons & Westaway 2001). Mechanical irritation of the endothelium may also cause the release of vasoconstrictive substances that initiate VA spasm and consequent thrombosis (Grant 1996, Mann 1995). However, the role of vasospasm in vertebrobasilar complications is controversial. Notably, both Bogduk (1994) and Jull (1994) discount the theory, termed posterior cervical sympathetic syndrome of Barré–Lieou, that mechanical irritation of the vertebral nerve can provoke spasm and alter VA blood flow, largely because of the lack of supportive anatomical evidence. In addition, both authors note the finding that VA flow in the monkey is not responsive to direct stimulation of the cervical sympathetic system (Bogduk et al 1981).

Neurological insult often results from anterograde propagation of thrombosis or dissection causing obstruction of the posterior inferior cerebellar or basilar arteries, or from artery-to-artery embolism to distal branches (Frumkin & Baloh 1990, Licht et al 1998b, Mitchell & McKay 1995, Refshauge 1994, Sherman et al 1981, Teasell & Marchuk 1994, Terenzi & DeFabio 1996). Frequently emboli produced by VA pathology travel to the distal basilar artery, particularly at the branches to the posterior cerebral and superior cerebellar arteries, and also to the posterior inferior cerebellar arteries (Budgell & Sato 1997, Caplan et al 1992, Frumkin & Baloh 1990, Middleditch 1991, Simeone & Goldberg 1968). In fact, it is estimated that 80% of all strokes are thromboembolic in origin (Fontenelle et al 1994, Terenzi & DeFabio 1996). While it is theoretically possible that an embolus could dislodge from an arteriosclerotic plaque in the VA following CSM, there is no evidence that this has ever occurred, and the relatively young mean age of patients experiencing neurovascular complication tends to discount this hypothesis as well (Bogduk 1994, Budgell & Sato 1997, Côté et al 1996, Licht et al 1998b).

Most neurological consequences are immediately evident, although a delayed, stuttering or progressive clinical course to infarction is not unusual (Easton & Sherman 1977, Fritz et al 1984, Frumkin & Baloh 1990, Grant 1994a, 1994b, Hurwitz et al 1996, Jaskoviak 1980, Mas et al 1989, Roy 1994, Sherman et al 1982, Teasell & Marchuk 1994, Tulyapronchote et al 1994). In such cases it is likely that the CSM produces subclinical damage to the tunica intima or tunica media, and that progressive or delayed symptoms result from slow propagation of a thrombus or dissection to the posterior inferior cerebellar or basilar artery, or from distal embolism (Auer et al 1994, Frisoni & Anzola 1991, Schellhas et al 1980, Sherman et al 1987). Cases of stroke following previously uneventful manipulation may provide some indirect support for the possibility of cumulative subclinical damage to the intima with repeated neck manipulations (Di Fabio 1999, Frumkin & Baloh 1990, Sherman et al 1987, Weintraub & Khoury 1995b).

NEUROLOGICAL DEFICITS

Vertebrobasilar insufficiency (VBI) occurs when either focal or overall blood volume is reduced to a level producing ischaemia. It is generally thought to require about a 50% reduction (Refshauge 1995, Seidel et al 1999). Symptoms and signs are caused by ischaemia in the neurological structures supplied by the vertebrobasilar system, and will vary depending on the structures affected (Assendelft et al 1996, Bogduk 1994, Grant 1994b). Ischaemia of the brain stem (several vital functions, sensory and motor pathways, and nuclei), occipital cerebral lobes (vision), or the cerebellum (balance) will produce varying responses (Assendelft et al 1996, Sell et al 1994). Notably, the vestibular nuclei receive their blood supply entirely from the branches of the vertebral and basilar arteries, as does the labyrinth to a lesser extent (Bogduk 1994, Grant 1987, Meadows & Magee 1994, Middleditch 1991, Refshauge 1995). Thus, impaired vertebrobasilar flow may result in vestibular dysfunction, most frequently dizziness (Bogduk 1994). The capacity of the collateral circulation is an important factor in determining the degree of neurological insult sustained, particularly the contralateral VA and the ICAs via the posterior communicating arteries (Carney 1981, Dunne et al 1987, Fritz et al 1984, Gass & Refshauge 1995, Hedera et al 1993, Petersen et al 1996, Roy 1994, Sturzenneger et al 1994). The posterior inferior cerebellar artery ipsilateral to the occluded VA may be supplied by retrograde flow from the opposite VA (Maslowski 1960, Miyachi et al 1994, Schwarz et al 1991). Secondary collateral pathways are also important in some cases of VA stenosis, including the ophthalmic, occipital, choroidal and distal branches of the superior cerebellar arteries, as well as the leptomeningeal vessels (Terenzi &

DeFabio 1996). However, the development of these secondary circulatory pathways is generally dependent upon gradual, chronic perfusion deficits more commonly related to cardiovascular disease.

Patijn (1991) reported that of 84 cases of VA injury in the literature, 16 were lethal and 55 resulted in permanent neurological deficit. Terrett (1987a) found that only 11 patients in 107 published neurovascular incidents completely recovered, with 26 deaths reported, and the remainder experiencing a range of deficits of varying severity and nature. Assendelft et al (1996) determined that of 165 vertebrobasilar complications in the literature, 44 completely recovered, 29 died and 86 were left with a residual handicap (six unknown). In a survey of neurologists, it was reported that 86% of patients experiencing manipulative stroke had at least a mild deficit 3 months after the onset of the stroke (Lee et al 1995). Most complications involve unilateral brain stem or cerebellar infarction, but vary considerably in severity (Easton & Sherman 1977, Hurwitz et al 1996, Mas et al 1989, Parkin et al 1978, Roy 1994, Sherman et al 1981). Less frequently, upper spinal cord infarction (anterior spinal artery occlusion) or occipital lobe infarction (posterior cerebral artery occlusion) is reported (Daneshmend et al 1984, Easton & Sherman 1977, Fritz et al 1984, Mas et al 1989, Sherman et al 1981, Tulyapronchote et al 1994). Case reports tend to document the more severe complications, such as Wallenberg's syndrome (dorsolateral medullary infarction resulting from posterior inferior cerebellar artery or VA occlusion), 'locked in' syndrome (essentially complete paralysis and muteness following basilar artery obstruction with infarction of the ventral pons), quadriplegia and sudden death (Dunne et al 1987, Greenman 1991, Hurwitz et al 1996, Lyness & Wagman 1974, Povlsen et al 1987, Refshauge 1995, Roy 1994, Schellhas et al 1980, Terrett 1987b).

ICA INJURY

While it is clear the VA is at risk of injury during CSM, there are cases of manipulative stroke that indicate the internal carotid artery (ICA) is also vulnerable, but to a much lesser extent (Gross et al 1996, Haldeman et al 2002b, Hart & Easton 1983, Hurwitz et al 1996, Parwar et al 2001, Robertson 1982). Beatty (1977) reports on a case of hemispheric stroke as a result of a dissecting intramural haematoma of the ICA. Peters et al (1995) describe a fatal case of dissection and subsequent thrombosis of the ICA following chiropractic manipulation. Jumper & Horton (1996) attribute a case of central retinal artery occlusion to the dislodging of an embolus from an atherosclerotic plaque in the ICA by manipulation. Furthermore, the survey of neurologists by Lee et al (1995) revealed that 5% of strokes following CSM were in the carotid distribution and the survey by Rivett & Milburn (1997) found two such cases of stroke.

Toole & Tucker (1960) demonstrated in cadavers that flow in the ICA could be impeded by neck rotation, usually involving the ipsilateral vessel. Faris et al (1963) describe a case of ICA occlusion during rotation using angiography. More recently, Refshauge (1994) demonstrated a significant change in ICA blood flow velocity in healthy volunteers at both 45 degrees and full contralateral rotation using duplex ultrasonography. Rivett et al (1999) also showed ICA flow velocity changes in end-range positions involving rotation and extension on ultrasound examination, although these were much less marked than for the VA. These findings, however, are in contrast to those of Licht et al (2002) who reported no difference in ICA blood flow velocity measured with colour duplex sonography in different head positions in nine patients with positive premanipulative test results.

Refshauge (1994) considers that the ICA may normally be constricted between several layers of muscle that are stretched on contralateral rotation. In addition, it has been suggested that CSM may cause an intimal tear of the ICA by stretching or compression of the vessel against the transverse processes of the upper cervical vertebrae, notably the ipsilateral lateral mass of the atlas and the transverse process of the axis, during contralateral rotation and hyperextension (Arnetoli et al 1989, Beatty 1977, Boldrey et al 1956, Haneline & Croft 2003, Lee et al 1995, Terrett 1987b). Nevertheless, a causal link between CSM and ICA injury is disputed by some authors, who consider there are no biologically plausible mechanisms (Dabbs & Lauretti 1995, Haneline & Croft 2003).

RISK OF VERTEBROBASILAR STROKE

The determination of the rate of incidence of neurovascular complication following CSM is of importance in considering the question of the costs versus the benefits of the procedure. In particular, the issue of risk is critically linked to that of informed consent and the collaborative therapist–patient clinical reasoning process (Delany 1996, Haswell 1996, Jones & Rivett 2004).

Using only case reports documented in the literature, Hosek et al (1981) estimate that there are approximately three manipulative strokes each year, suggesting that it is a rare adverse effect. This estimate is almost certainly flawed as it is extremely unlikely that all neurovascular complications are published (Assendelft et al 1996, Di Fabio 1999, Grant 1987, 1994b, 1996, Grieve 1991, 1994, Mas et al 1989, Nakamura et al 1991, Oostendorp et al 1992b, Patijn 1991, Robertson 1981, 1982, Teasell & Marchuk 1994). In fact, it is generally agreed that the actual incidence rate of stroke complicating CSM is unknown (Carey 1993, Côté et al 1996, Di Fabio 1999, Ernst 1997, Grant 1994a, Haldeman 1996, Haynes 1994, Leboeuf-Yde et al 1996, Lee et al 1995, 1996, Michaeli 1991, 1993, Oostendorp et al 1992b, Patijn 1991, Roy 1994, Shekelle & Coulter 1997, Teasell & Marchuk 1994, Terrett 1987a).

Nevertheless, there have been a growing number of reports that have attempted to ascertain the incidence rate, or risk of, severe neurovascular complication arising from CSM (Box 37.4). The uncertainty about the risk involved is reflected in the wide range of proposed incidence rates, varying from approximately one stroke per 77 000 manipulations to one in over 5 million. Gross et al (1996) conclude that present estimates are fraught with inherent methodological biases and are not based on sound data. It is widely recognized that a large-scale, prospective epidemiological study of this problem is required and that

Box 37.4 Various estimates of the risk of stroke following neck manipulation

Authors	Profession	Incidence rate	Source
Jaskoviak (1980)	Chiropractic	<1 per 5 million manipulations	Clinic records; no strokes recorded
Hosek et al (1981)	Chiropractic	1 per 1 million manipulations	Published case reports
Gutmann (1983)	Chiropractic	1 per 400 000 high neck manipulations	Published case reports
Dvorák & Orelli (1985)	Medicine	1 per 383 750 manipulations	Survey manual medicine physicians
Carey (1993)	Chiropractic	1 per 3 846 153 manipulations	Insurance records
Dvorák et al (1993)	Medicine	<1 per 150 450 manipulations	Survey manual medicine physicians; no strokes recorded
Haynes (1994)	Chiropractic	<1 per 200 000 manipulations	Survey chiropractors and neurologists; clinic records
Dabbs & Lauretti (1995)	Chiropractic	<1 per 2 million manipulations	Insurance records
Lee et al (1995)/ Dabbs & Lauretti (1995)	Chiropractic	1 per 500 000 manipulations	Survey neurologists
Klougart et al (1996a)	Chiropractic	1 per 1 320 000 manipulations	Survey chiropractors
Rivett & Milburn (1997)/ Rivett & Reid (1998)	Physiotherapy	1 per 163 371 manipulations	Insurance records and survey medical specialists
Rothwell et al (2001)	Chiropractic	1.3 per 100 000 patients < 45 years	Population based nested case control study

present estimates are unreliable (Carey 1993, Côté et al 1996, Dabbs & Lauretti 1995, Di Fabio 1999, Dvorák et al 1991, Haldeman et al 1999, Haynes 1994, Hurwitz et al 1996, Leboeuf-Yde et al 1996). Notably, no serious complications have been reported in clinical trials evaluating the efficacy of manipulative therapy of the cervical spine, although some patients may have dropped out because of adverse effects and the total sample size is small (Gross et al 2002, Hurwitz et al 1996, Shekelle & Coulter 1997).

Case reports have described instances in which the patient has died as a result of neurovascular complication following CSM. However, the sensational nature of these incidents suggests that they are likely to be over-represented in the literature (Dabbs & Lauretti 1995). Reviews of case reports vary in their mortality rates from 15 to 24% (Assendelft et al 1996, Di Fabio 1999, Hurwitz et al 1996, Patijn 1991, Sherman et al 1987, Terrett 1987a). In contrast, Lee et al (1995) found only one death in 56 cases of stroke (2% mortality rate) ascribed to chiropractic CSM. Dabbs & Lauretti (1995) propose that there is one death per 400 000 patients treated with a course of neck manipulation. On the other hand, minor and transient neurovascular incidents occur much more frequently (Di Fabio 1999, Grant 1987, Grieve 1994, Michaeli 1991, Oostendorp et al 1992b, Senstad et al 1996a, 1996b, Sinel & Smith 1993). Klougart et al (1996b) used data from two surveys of chiropractors to determine that transient cerebrovascular incidents, including paralysis, ataxia and loss of consciousness, occurred once per 120 000 manipulations.

Some authors argue that it is unrealistic to consider the risk of manipulative stroke in relation to the nil risk of no treatment (Carey 1993, Dabbs & Lauretti 1995, Gross et al 1996, Hurwitz et al 1996, Nilsson 1996, Raskind & North 1990, Rivett 1995). Because patients have sought intervention in order to gain relief from their symptoms, it is more appropriate to compare the estimated risk of CSM with that of an alternative, common conservative treatment for musculoskeletal disorders of the cervical spine, for example nonsteroidal anti-inflammatory drugs (NSAIDs). It has been calculated by Fries (1992) that approximately one in 220 patients consuming NSAIDs for musculoskeletal disorders (excluding rheumatological diseases) will be hospitalized for gastrointestinal complications and one patient in 2200 will die from an adverse reaction. Dabbs & Lauretti (1995) contend that NSAIDs are 100 to 400 times more likely to lead to hospitalization or death than is CSM. It should be noted that the exact complication rate for CSM may actually be higher than the rate upon which these findings are based.

Most studies that have attempted to estimate the risk of neurovascular complication have been limited by the use of retrospective study designs with inherent recall bias (Assendelft et al 1996, Di Fabio 1999, Lachenbruch et al 1992, Rivett 1995). An underestimation of the incidence rate is possible as respondents may forget the less severe and more chronologically distant events (Lachenbruch et al 1992, Leboeuf-Yde et al 1996), although this is unlikely in

the case of manipulative stroke because of its infrequency and seriousness. A further confounding factor is intentional non-reporting of incidents because of legal or other reasons. The clinician may also fail to recognize signs and symptoms of induced vertebrobasilar ischaemia or may not ask the patient about their presence. While an immediate reaction following the application of CSM strongly indicates a causal mechanism, the cause and effect relationship becomes less distinct with the passage of time. Sherman et al (1981) found that in 22 of 43 cases there was progressive brain infarction or a delay in onset of neurological symptoms, ranging from a few minutes to several days. Underreporting of incidents may therefore occur as the temporal connection between CSM and neurological insult is overlooked (Haynes 1994, Lee et al 1996, Nakamura et al 1991, Roy 1994), as it also may when patients who experience an adverse reaction are unable or unwilling to notify the responsible practitioner.

Conversely, it is possible that some strokes may be wrongfully attributed to manipulation leading to an overestimation of the event rate. Interestingly, Leboeuf-Yde et al (1996), in raising the possibility of over-reporting, discuss three cases of stroke from natural causes that could have easily been mistakenly ascribed to CSM. They argue that even a short latency period may be potentially deceptive in cases where the vascular injury was initiated by a prior activity or movement involving the neck (e.g. painting the ceiling) and in which the application of manipulation was coincidental.

Most retrospective surveys are also limited by low response rates (non-respondent bias) and a failure to determine the validity of the survey tool (Haldeman 1996, Klougart et al 1996b). In addition, problems in accurately determining the denominator (or number of neck manipulations performed) have been identified (Campbell 1994, Hurwitz et al 1996, Klougart et al 1996a, Leboeuf-Yde et al 1996). To overcome these problems, Senstad et al (1997) conducted a prospective study in which they reported no serious neurovascular incidents following approximately 1555 applications of chiropractic spinal manipulative therapy to the cervical spine. In a similar but smaller prospective investigation of complications of chiropractic manipulation, Leboeuf-Yde et al (1997) also did not find any serious ischaemic reactions. Nevertheless, the probable infrequency of this complication renders prospective research practically difficult (Klougart et al 1996a, 1997, Rivett & Milburn 1996).

RISK FOR PHYSIOTHERAPY

Most studies have investigated complications of chiropractic and medical manipulation and the generalizability of their results to manipulative physiotherapy is questionable (Di Fabio 1999, Rivett & Milburn 1996, Rivett & Reid 1998). There are very few studies which have investigated the incidence rate of CVAs attributed to CSM applied by physiotherapists.

Michaeli (1991, 1993) surveyed 88 physiotherapists in South Africa who had completed a 100-hour course in manipulative therapy and who used CSM regarding their experience with complications. Although no serious neurovascular complications were reported from an estimated 75 500 manipulations, a total of 48 other complications were described, many possibly related to VBI. These included 14 cases of nausea or vomiting, 12 instances of dizziness, 10 cases of severe headache, three instances each of blurred vision and nystagmus and one occurrence of loss of consciousness. This equates to a risk of approximately one minor or transient adverse response in every 1756 manipulations.

Using a prospective study design, Rivett & Milburn (1996) conducted a pilot investigation of the incidence rate of complications resulting from physiotherapeutic CSM in New Zealand. Nine physiotherapists with postgraduate qualifications in manipulative physiotherapy and who clinically used neck manipulation participated in the study. No ischaemic complications were reported but the rate of complication (for a single incident of exacerbated neck pain) per manipulation was 0.21%, or one adverse effect for every 476 manipulations. The incidence rate per patient was 0.42%, or one in 238. An estimate of the risk of stroke for physiotherapeutic CSM was subsequently calculated by Rivett & Reid (1998). Based on government insurance and workforce records and the results of two surveys (Rivett & Milburn 1996, 1997), they propose an approximate incidence rate of one CVA for every 163 371 neck manipulations.

In contrast to the results of Rivett & Reid (1998), there were no strokes reported in a 1997 survey of manipulative complications experienced by Australian manipulative physiotherapists (Grimmer 1998). Some doubt is cast on the accuracy of this finding, however, by the revelation of two cases of major vertebrobasilar complication in Australia between 1988 and 1995 (Grant 1996). Grimmer (1998) reports a figure of one minor transient adverse effect indicative of VBI for every 50 000 cervical manipulations.

PREDISPOSING FACTORS FOR MANIPULATIVE STROKE

Whatever the rate of incidence of stroke following CSM, the potentially devastating outcome means it is important to identify any clinical factors that may contribute to increased risk. An understanding of these factors may assist in premanipulatively screening for higher risk patients unsuitable for this procedure.

In the majority of cases of documented manipulative stroke a predisposing factor in the patient's clinical presentation has not been able to be identified (Dunne et al 1987, Haldeman et al 2002b, Jaskoviak 1980, Meadows 1992, Oostendorp 1988, Schmitt 1991, Sherman et al 1982, Teasell & Marchuk 1994, Terrett 1987a, 1987b). None the less, Kunnasmaa & Thiel (1994) reviewed 139 cases of cerebrovascular complications resulting from CSM and identified an associated predisposing condition or risk factor in

approximately half (53%) of the cases. Corrigan & Maitland (1998) argue that the abnormalities identified by Kunnasmaa & Thiel (1994) do not necessarily indicate any causal relationship.

Atherosclerosis and Osteoarthritis

Although frequently cited as predisposing conditions (Corrigan & Maitland 1998, Dvorák & Orelli 1985, Grieve 1994, Kleynhans & Terrett 1985, Lewit 1992, Livingston 1971, Sturzenegger et al 1994, Teasell & Marchuk 1994, Thiel 1991), there is little evidence to suggest that either osteoarthritic or atherosclerotic changes are important risk factors based on the reported case studies (Assendelft et al 1996, Di Fabio 1999, Grant 1994b, 1996, Hamann et al 1993, Kleynhans & Terrett 1985, Krueger & Okazaki 1980, Lyness & Wagman 1974, Patijn 1991, Schmitt 1991, Shekelle & Coulter 1997, Teasell & Marchuk 1994, Terrett 1987b). It is unlikely that age-related factors such as these are particularly relevant considering that the average age of neurovascular complication is consistently reported as being between 35 and 40 years (Assendelft et al 1996, Bogduk 1994, Di Fabio 1999, Grant 1994a, 1994b, 1996, Grieve 1994, Jaskoviak 1980, Kleynhans & Terrett 1985, Lee et al 1995, Patijn 1991, Schmitt 1991, Sherman et al 1981, Teasell & Marchuk 1994, Terrett 1987a). Although most cases involve patients between 30 and 45 years of age, it does not follow that people in this age range are especially at risk (Haldeman et al 1999, Schmitt 1991, Terrett 1987a). Notably, Terrett (1987a) demonstrates that the age distribution of patients attending chiropractic clinics closely parallels that of 107 cases of neurovascular complication following CSM.

In contrast, Patijn (1991) found that the average age of patients suffering adverse neurological reactions was considerably lower than the mean age of the patient population at his clinic. Furthermore, it has been suggested that minor degenerative changes of the cervical spine which accompany ageing might afford the VA some protection by limiting the extent the neck can be rotated (Grant 1994a). There also does not appear to be any obvious gender bias (Easton & Sherman 1977, Ernst 2002, Haldeman et al 1999, Patijn 1991, Terrett 1987b), although a few authors report a slightly higher number of female cases (Assendelft et al 1996, Jaskoviak 1980, Klougart et al 1996b, Mas et al 1989).

Despite the lack of direct evidence, it is theoretically possible that atherosclerosis could play a predisposing role in the pathogenesis of stroke consequent to CSM (Bogduk 1994, Miller & Burton 1974, Patijn 1991, Teasell & Marchuk 1994). An artery with sclerotic changes is more susceptible to mechanical irritation and intimal layer injury (Jaskoviak 1980, Lewit 1992). Mitchell (2002) reports that 42% of 362 VAs were moderately diseased in the vulnerable third part, although the age of the cadavers examined likely differs to that of the population undergoing CSM. Moreover, the basilar artery and vessels contributing to the collateral circulation are frequently affected by atherosclerosis, increasing the risk of infarction after CSM (Aspinall 1989, Bogduk 1994, Keggi et al 1966).

Some authors propose that patients be screened for risk factors for atherosclerosis and cardiovascular disease, including smoking, hypertension, oral contraception, diabetes, migraine and a family history of stroke (Aspinall 1989, Carey 1995, Combs & Triano 1997, Corrigan & Maitland 1998, Haldeman et al 1999, Jaskoviak 1980, Kleynhans & Terrett 1985, Mas et al 1987). Cardiovascular disease was present in 14% of cases reviewed by Kunnasmaa & Thiel (1994), although a causal relationship was not established and no comparative data were provided. Other reviews indicate that the prevalence of risk factors for cardiovascular disease in published case reports was consistent with or lower than the prevalence in the general population (Haldeman et al 1999, Hurwitz et al 1996, Terrett 1987b). However, there is some evidence from case reports indicating that it would be inadvisable to manipulate a patient with a history suggestive of transient ischaemic attacks (Carey 1995, Dunne et al 1987, Mestan 1999, Rivett 1994, Rivett & Reid 1998).

Similarly, cervical spine osteoarthritis is commonly promulgated as a predisposing condition for manipulative stroke. It has been demonstrated that laterally projecting osteophytes related to the neurocentral joints (and to a lesser degree the zygapophysial joints) may encroach on the VA as it ascends through the C4 to C6 transverse foramina, causing the VA to be displaced anterolaterally and its

Dvorák & Dvorák 1990, Kleynhans & Terrett 1985, Krueger & Okazaki 1980, Kunnasmaa & Thiel 1994, Sturzenegger et al 1994, Terrett 1987b, Thiel 1991, Tissington-Tatlow & Bammer 1957). It has also been proposed that cervical disc degeneration and zygapophysial joint subluxation can cause the spine to shorten and oblige the VAs to become more tortuous in their course, increasing the likelihood of lumen narrowing from kinking of the vessel (Aspinall 1989, Kleynhans & Terrett 1985, Teasell & Marchuk 1994).

However Grant (1994b) reported that in 23 of 26 cases where cervical spine X-rays were taken after a neurovascular complication, only normal findings or minor degenerative changes were exhibited. Similarly, Patijn (1991) found degenerative changes on X-ray in only nine of 59 cases of VA injury following CSM, but these were just slight changes and no osteophytes were reported. Kunnasmaa & Thiel (1994) also report that only 5% of cases of manipulative stroke demonstrate evidence of degenerative changes in the cervical spine. Importantly, there are no cases in the literature of VA injury associated with CSM in which osteoarthritic changes were considered to be causative (Bogduk 1994, Terrett 1987b).

Anatomical Anomalies

A variety of anatomical features have been frequently nominated as factors contributing to iatrogenic stroke, despite a complete lack of evidence to this effect (Bogduk 1994, Refshauge 1995, Terrett 1987b). Surgical case reports have occasionally described compression of the first part of the VA at the level of the sixth vertebra by the longus colli and scalenus anterior and medius muscles during contralateral rotation of the cervical spine, particularly where there is an anomalous VA origin or course (Aspinall 1989, Bogduk 1994, Husni & Storer 1967, Husni et al 1966, Keggi et al 1966, Kunnasmaa & Thiel 1994, Refshauge 1995, Terrett 1987b, Thiel 1991). In particular, an anomalous VA origin from the posterior aspect of the subclavian artery has been reported as causing vessel kinking during neck rotation (Bogduk 1994, Hardin & Poser 1963, Husni et al 1966, Keggi et al 1966, Powers et al 1961). The artery may also be constricted by bands of cervical fascia in its first part (Aspinall 1989, Bogduk 1994, Hardin & Poser 1963, Kunnasmaa & Thiel 1994, Refshauge 1995, Terrett 1987b).

In the high cervical spine, the obliquus capitis inferior and the intertransversarii muscles have been infrequently implicated in cases of intermittent compression of the atlanto-axial portion of the VA on rotation (Aspinall 1989, Keggi et al 1966, Schellhas et al 1980, Terrett 1987b). A dense fibrous tissue ring that surrounds the VA as it enters the atlanto-occipital membrane may also distort the vessel during movement (Kunnasmaa & Thiel 1994, Thiel 1991). Finally, congenital craniovertebral bony anomalies have been proposed as predisposing features in the absence of any evidence, notably aplasia of the odontoid process and

stressing of the VA (Aspinall 1989, Bogduk 1994, Jaskoviak 1980, Keggi et al 1966, Kleynhans & Terrett 1985, Lewit 1992, Miller & Burton 1974, Sturzenegger et al 1994). Interestingly though, flow disturbances in maximal rotation have been shown in the presence of an underdeveloped atlanto-axial arterial loop and an atlanto-axial angle of opening exceeding 35 degrees (Dumas et al 1996).

It is considered that the adequacy of the collateral blood flow is an important factor in the development of neurological insult following VA trauma, especially the competence of the alternate VA and the circle of Willis (Arnetoli et al 1989, Grant 1994b, Hutchison 1989, Lyness & Wagman 1974, Schmitt 1991, Sturzenegger et al 1994, Teasell & Marchuk 1994). Anomalies in the vertebrobasilar system are extremely common and satisfactory cerebral perfusion is normally maintained by forming competent collateral circulation (Grieve 1994, Refshauge 1995). Potential contributory congenital anomalies of vertebrobasilar arterial structure were reported in 22% of 139 cases by Kunnasmaa & Thiel (1994). Other authors have cited congenital variation and disease in the collateral circulation as contributing factors in cases of iatrogenic stroke (Bogduk 1994, Grant 1994b, Grieve 1994, Keggi et al 1966, Lyness & Wagman 1974, Teasell & Marchuk 1994).

Asymmetries in VA diameter are common, with individuals able to function normally with a hypoplastic artery or with one that terminates in the posterior inferior cerebellar artery without connecting to the basilar artery (Arnetoli et al 1989, Aspinall 1989, Dan 1976, Grant 1994b, Lyness & Wagman 1974, Mestan 1999, Oostendorp 1988, Terrett 1987b, Thiel et al 1994). Problems may arise, though, if the dominant artery is occluded following CSM, particularly if other collateral pathways are inadequate to maintain hindbrain perfusion because of anomaly or disease (Bogduk 1994, Dumas et al 1996, Hedera et al 1993, Husni & Storer 1967, Husni et al 1966, Jaskoviak 1980, Pásztor 1978, Sherman et al 1981, Sturzenegger et al 1994). For example, if the posterior communicating artery is hypoplastic, this may disrupt collateral flow from the anterior circulation (Carney 1981, Cook & Sanstead 1991, Husni et al 1966, Pásztor 1978, Schellhas et al 1980, Sturzenegger et al 1994). However, Teasell & Marchuk (1994) and Krueger & Okazaki (1980) argue that the angiographic findings in case reports of manipulative complication indicate an absence of marked vascular asymmetry in the majority of patients.

Previous Trauma

There is pathological evidence indicating that previous cervical spine trauma may subclinically damage the vessel wall, predisposing the artery to further injury when subjected to the subsequent stress of manipulation, notably intimal disruption (Auer et al 1994, Carey 1995, Easton & Sherman 1977, Frumkin & Baloh 1990, Haldeman et al 1999, Keggi et al 1966, Kleynhans & Terrett 1985, Mann & Refshauge 2001, Patijn 1991, Rivett 1994, Tulyapronchote et al 1994). Kunnasmaa & Thiel (1994) report that 9% of 139 cases had sustained previous trauma to the neck, but no comparative data are provided for patients without complication. Trauma may also cause instability of the cervical spine, with excessive motion potentially stressing the VA at the extremes of range (Aspinall 1989, Gutmann 1983, Klougart et al 1996b). However, Patijn (1991), in a review of 84 cases of VA injury, found no evidence of excessive segmental mobility, and Kunnasmaa & Thiel (1994) found only five cases.

Arteriopathies

The forces sustained by the VA during CSM have been measured in cadavers as being approximately one-ninth that required for mechanical failure (Symons et al 2002). It follows that a pre-existing arteriopathy of an ill-defined nature may contribute to some VA injuries by predisposing

the vascular bed to rupture or thrombus (Frumkin & Baloh 1990, Haldeman et al 1999, Johnson et al 1993, Kleynhans & Terrett 1985, Peters et al 1995, Rivett 1994). The presence of such pathology may mean that forces which a healthy artery could readily withstand lead to traumatic damage of the intima and perhaps the media, precipitating a dissection, thrombosis or haematoma. Evidence is difficult to acquire because of the infrequency of the complication and the associated low mortality rate (Lee et al 1995). What evidence there is suggests that fibromuscular dysplasia is rarely a contributing factor (Frumkin & Baloh 1990, Haldeman et al 1999, Mas et al 1987, Rivett 1994).

The average age of patients experiencing spontaneous VA dissection is comparable to that of patients suffering neurovascular complications (Haldeman et al 1999, 2002b, Norris et al 2000, Schmitt 1991). It is possible that a VA undergoing spontaneous dissection may unknowingly be further damaged by CSM (Mas et al 1989). Many patients with a spontaneous vertebrobasilar arterial dissection in progress initially report symptoms of acute neck pain and headache, perhaps prompting them to seek manipulative therapy which may precipitate a vascular occlusion or dislodge a thrombus (Haldeman et al 1999, Hamann et al 1993, Krueger & Okazaki 1980, Mas et al 1989). The patient may also present with what seems to be a migraine, but which is actually a slowly dissecting VA with associated transient ischaemic attacks (Di Fabio 1999, Haldeman et al 1999, Mas et al 1987, Rivett 1994). There is bilateral involvement in 50% of cases of spontaneous VA dissection, supporting the proposal of a predisposing arteriopathy (Hinse et al 1991), possibly an ultrastructural connective tissue abnormality of a genetic nature (Brandt et al 1996, Rubinstein & Haldeman 2001).

CONCLUSION

At present it is difficult, if not impossible, to detect the patient at risk of vertebrobasilar arterial dissection with CSM (Haldeman et al 1999, 2002b). It appears that in most cases of neurovascular complication no predisposing condition or risk factor can be identified (Kunnasmaa & Thiel 1994, Teasell & Marchuk 1994).

KEYWORDS	
cervical spine	complications
manipulation	risk

References

Adams G, Sim J 1998 A survey of UK manual therapists' practice of and attitudes towards manipulation and its complications. Physiotherapy Research International 3: 206–227

Arnetoli G, Amadori A, Stefani P, Nuzzaci G 1989 Sonography of vertebral arteries in De Kleyn's position in subjects and in patients

with vertebrobasilar transient ischemic attacks. Angiology 40: 716–720

Aspinall W 1989 Clinical testing for cervical mechanical disorders which produce ischemic vertigo. Journal of Orthopaedic and Sports Physical Therapy 11: 176–182

Assendelft W J J, Bouter L M, Knipschild P G 1996 Complications of spinal manipulation: a comprehensive review of the literature. Journal of Family Practice 42: 475–480

Auer R N, Krcek J, Butt J C 1994 Delayed symptoms and death after minor head trauma with occult vertebral artery injury. Journal of Neurology, Neurosurgery, and Psychiatry 57: 500–502

Australian Physiotherapy Association 1988 Protocol for pre-manipulative testing of the cervical spine. Australian Journal of Physiotherapy 34: 97–100

Bartels E, Flügel K A 1996 Evaluation of extracranial vertebral artery dissection with duplex color-flow imaging. Stroke 27: 290–295

Beatty R A 1977 Dissecting hematoma of the internal carotid artery following chiropractic cervical manipulation. Journal of Trauma 17: 248–249

Bogduk N 1994 Cervical causes of headache and dizziness. In: Boyling J D, Palastanga N (eds) Grieve's Modern Manual Therapy, the Vertebral Column, 2nd edn. Churchill Livingstone, Edinburgh, pp 317–331

Bogduk N, Lambert G, Duckworth J W 1981 The anatomy and physiology of the vertebral nerve in relation to cervical migraine. Cephalalgia 1: 1–14

Boldrey E, Maass L, Miller E R 1956 The role of atlantoid compression in the etiology of internal carotid thrombosis. Journal of Neurosurgery 13: 127–139

Bourdillon J F, Day E A, Bookhout M R 1992 Spinal manipulation, 5th edn. Butterworth Heinemann, Oxford

Brandt T, Orberk E, Hausser I, Muller-Kuppers M, Lamprecht I A, Hacke W 1996 Ultrastructural abberations of connective tissue components in patients with spontaneous cervicocerebral artery dissections. Neurology 46: 193–194

Brown B S J, Tissington-Tatlow W F 1963 Radiographic studies of the vertebral arteries in cadavers. Radiology 81: 80–88

Budgell B S, Sato A 1997 The cervical subluxation and regional cerebral

20: 103–107

Campbell J 1994 The dangers of cervical spine manipulation. Journal of Orthopaedic Medicine 16: 1

Caplan L R, Amarenco P, Rosengart A et al 1992 Embolism from vertebral artery origin occlusive disease. Neurology 42: 1505–1512

Carey P F 1993 A report on the occurrence of cerebral vascular accidents in chiropractic practice. Journal of the Canadian Chiropractic Association 37: 104–106

Carey P F 1994 Cerebral vascular accidents: a report of the occurrences and the true incidence in a five year period in Canada. Journal of Manipulative and Physiological Therapeutics 17: 274

Carey P F 1995 A suggested protocol for the examination and treatment of the cervical spine: managing the risk. Journal of the Canadian Chiropractic Association 39: 35–39

Carney A L 1981 Vertebral artery surgery: historical development, basic concepts of brain hemodynamics, and clinical experience of 102 cases. In: Carney A L, Anderson E M (eds) Advances in Neurology. Diagnosis and treatment of brain ischemia. Raven Press, New York, vol 30, pp 249–282

Combs S B, Triano J J 1997 Symptoms of neck artery compromise: case presentations of risk estimate for treatment. Journal of Manipulative and Physiological Therapeutics 20: 274–278

Consumers' Institute of New Zealand 1997 Non-conventional therapies from arsenic to zinc. Consumer 363: 20–27

Cook J W, Sanstead J K 1991 Wallenberg's syndrome following self-induced manipulation. Neurology 41: 1695–1696

Corrigan B, Maitland G D 1998 Vertebral musculoskeletal disorders. Butterworth Heinemann, Oxford

Côté P, Kreitz B G, Cassidy J D, Thiel H 1996 The validity of the extension-rotation test as a clinical screening procedure before neck manipulation: a secondary analysis. Journal of Manipulative and Physiological Therapeutics 19: 159–164

Curt A, Dietz V 1994 Wallenberg's syndrome with delayed onset after cervical spine fracture: a case report. Journal of Neurology, Neurosurgery, and Psychiatry 57: 868–874

Dabbs V, Lauretti W J 1995 A risk assessment of cervical manipulation vs NSAIDs for the treatment of neck pain. Journal of Manipulative and Physiological Therapeutics 18: 530–536

Dan N G 1976 The management of vertebral artery insufficiency in cervical spondylosis: a modified technique. Australian and New Zealand Journal of Surgery 46: 164–165

Daneshmend T K, Hewer R L, Bradshaw J R 1984 Acute brain stem stroke during neck manipulation. British Medical Journal 288: 189

Delany C 1996 Should I warn the patient first? Australian Journal of Physiotherapy 42: 249–255

Di Fabio R P 1999 Manipulation of the cervical spine: risks and benefits. Physical Therapy 79: 50–65

Dumas J-L, Salama J, Dreyfus P, Thoreux P, Goldlust D, Chevrel J-P 1996 Magnetic resonance angiographic analysis of atlanto-axial rotation: anatomic bases of compression of the vertebral arteries. Surgical and Radiologic Anatomy 18: 303–313

Dunne J W, Conacher G N, Khangure M, Harper C G 1987 Dissecting aneurysms of the vertebral arteries following cervical manipulation: a case report. Journal of Neurology, Neurosurgery, and Psychiatry 50: 349–353

Dvorák J, Dvorák V 1990 Manual medicine diagnostics, 2nd edn. Theme Medical Publishers, New York

Dvorák J, Orelli F V 1985 How dangerous is manipulation to the cervical spine? Case report and results of a survey. Journal of Manual Medicine 2: 1–4

Dvorák J, Baumgartner H, Burn L et al 1991 Consensus and recommendations as to the side-effects and complications of manual therapy of the cervical spine. Journal of Manual Medicine 6: 117–118

Dvorák J, Loustalot D, Baumgartner H, Antinnes J A 1993 Frequency of complications of manipulation of the spine: a survey among the members of the Swiss Medical Society of Manual Medicine.

Easton J D, Sherman D G 1977 Cervical manipulation and stroke. Stroke 8: 594–597

Eder M, Tilscher H 1990 Chiropractic therapy: diagnosis and treatment. Aspen Publishers, Rockville

Ernst E 1997 Complementary medicine: the facts. Physical Therapy Reviews 2: 49–57

Ernst E 2002 Manipulation of the cervical spine: a systematic review of case reports of serious adverse events, 1995–2001. Medical Journal of Australia 176: 376–380

Faris A A, Poser C M, Wilmore D W, Agnew C H 1963 Radiologic evaluation of neck vessels in healthy men. Neurology 13: 386–396

Fast A, Zinicola D F, Marin E L 1987 Vertebral artery damage complicating cervical manipulation. Spine 12: 840–842

Fontenelle L J, Simper S C, Hanson T L 1994 Carotid duplex scan versus angiography in evaluation of carotid artery disease. American Surgeon 60: 864–868

Fries J F 1992 Assessing and understanding patient risk. Scandinavian Journal of Rheumatology 92(Suppl.): 21–24

Frisoni G B, Anzola G P 1991 Vertebrobasilar ischemia after neck motion. Stroke 22: 1452–1460

Fritz V U, Maloon A, Tuch P 1984 Neck manipulation causing stroke: case reports. South African Medical Journal 66: 844–846

Frumkin L R, Baloh R W 1990 Wallenberg's syndrome following neck manipulation. Neurology 40: 611–615

Gass E M, Refshauge K M 1995 The use of information in clinical practice. In: Refshauge K M, Gass E M (eds) Musculoskeletal physiotherapy: clinical science and practice. Butterworth Heinemann, Oxford, pp 182–201

Gorman R F 1978 Cardiac arrest after cervical spine mobilisation. Medical Journal of Australia 2: 169–170

Grant E R 1987 Clinical testing before cervical manipulation: can we recognize the patient at risk? In: Proceedings of the Tenth

International Congress of the World Confederation for Physical Therapy. World Confederation for Physical Therapy, Sydney, pp 192–197

Grant R 1988 Dizziness testing and manipulation of the cervical spine. In: Grant R (ed) Clinics in physical therapy. Physical therapy of the cervical and thoracic spine. Churchill Livingstone, New York, vol 17, pp 111–124

Grant R 1994a Vertebral artery concerns: premanipulative testing of the cervical spine. In: Grant R (ed) Clinics in physical therapy. Physical therapy of the cervical and thoracic spine, 2nd edn. Churchill Livingstone, New York, vol 17, pp 145–165

Grant R 1994b Vertebral artery insufficiency: a clinical protocol for pre-manipulative testing of the cervical spine. In: Boyling J D, Palastanga N (eds) Grieve's Modern Manual Therapy, the Vertebral Column, 2nd edn. Churchill Livingstone, Edinburgh, pp 371–380

Grant R 1996 Vertebral artery testing: the Australian Physiotherapy Association Protocol after 6 years. Manual Therapy 1: 149–153

Greenman P E 1991 Principles of manipulation of the cervical spine. Journal of Manual Medicine 6: 106–113

Grieve G P 1991 Mobilisation of the spine, 5th edn. Churchill Livingstone, Edinburgh

Grieve G P 1993 Scrutinizing tacit assumptions in manual therapy. Journal of Manual and Manipulative Therapy 1: 123–133

Grieve G P 1994 Incidents and accidents of manipulation and allied techniques. In: Boyling J D, Palastanga N (eds) Grieve's Modern Manual Therapy, the Vertebral Column, 2nd edn. Churchill Livingstone, Edinburgh, pp 673–692

Grimmer K 1998 Cervical manipulation: compliance with, and attitudes to, the current Australian Physiotherapy Association protocol for pre-manipulative testing of the cervical spine. Incidence of complications. Centre for Physiotherapy Research, University of South Australia, Adelaide

Gross A R, Aker P D, Quartly C 1996 Manual therapy in the treatment of neck pain. In: Lane N E, Wolfe F (eds) Rheumatic disease clinics of North America. Musculoskeletal medicine. W B Saunders, Philadelphia, vol 22, pp 579–598

Gross A R, Kay T M, Kennedy C et al 2002 Clinical practice guideline on the use of manipulation or mobilization in the treatment of adults with mechanical neck disorders. Manual Therapy 7: 193–205

Gutmann G 1983 Injuries to the vertebral artery caused by manual therapy. Manuelle Medizin 21: 2–14

Haldeman S 1996 Chiropractic complications [Letter]. Neurology 46: 885

Haldeman S, Kohlbeck F J, McGregor M 1999 Risk factors and precipitating neck movements causing vertebrobasilar artery dissection after cervical trauma and spinal manipulation. Spine 24: 785–794

Haldeman S, Kohlbeck F J, McGregor M 2002a Stroke, cerebral artery dissection, and cervical spine manipulation therapy. Journal of Neurology 249: 1098–1104

Haldeman S, Kohlbeck F J, McGregor M 2002b Unpredictability of cerebrovascular ischemia associated with cervical spine manipulation therapy. Spine 27: 49–55

Hamann G F, Felber S, Schimrigk K 1993 Cervicocephalic artery dissections and chiropractic manipulations. Lancet 342: 114

Haneline M T, Croft A C 2003 Internal carotid artery dissection following chiropractic manipulation: clinical features and mechanisms of injury. Journal of the American Chiropractic Association 40: 20–24

Hardin C A, Poser C M 1963 Rotational obstruction of the vertebral artery due to redundancy and extraluminal cervical fascial bands. Annals of Surgery 158: 133–137

Hart R, Easton J 1983 Dissection of cervical and cerebral arteries. Neurological Clinics 1: 155–182

Haswell K 1996 Informed choice and consent for cervical spine manipulation. Australian Journal of Physiotherapy 42: 149–155

Haynes M J 1994 Stroke following cervical manipulation in Perth. Chiropractic Journal of Australia 24: 42–46

Haynes M J 1996a Cervical spine adjustments by Perth chiropractors and post-manipulation stroke: has a change occurred? Chiropractic Journal of Australia 26: 43–46

Haynes M J 1996b Doppler studies comparing the effects of cervical rotation and lateral flexion on vertebral artery blood flow. Journal of Manipulative and Physiological Therapeutics 19: 378–384

Haynes M J, Cala L A, Melsom A, Mastaglia F L, Milne N, McGeachie J K 2002 Vertebral arteries and cervical rotation: modeling and magnetic resonance angiography studies. Journal of Manipulative and Physiological Therapeutics 25: 370–383

Hedera P, Bujdáková J, Traubner P 1993 Blood flow velocities in basilar artery during rotation of the head. Acta Neurologica Scandinavica 88: 229–233

Hinse P, Thie A, Lachenmayer L 1991 Dissection of the extra-cranial vertebral artery: report of four cases and review of the literature. Journal of Neurology, Neurosurgery, and Psychiatry 54: 863–869

Hosek R S, Schram S B, Silverman H, Myers J B, Williams S E 1981 Cervical manipulation [Letter]. Journal of the American Medical Association 245: 922

Hurley L, Yardley K, Gross A R, Hendry L, McLaughlin L 2002 A survey to examine attitudes and patterns of practice of physiotherapists who perform cervical spine manipulation. Manual Therapy 7: 10–18

Hurwitz E L, Aker P D, Adams A H, Meeker W C, Shekelle P G 1996 Manipulation and mobilization of the cervical spine: a systematic review of the literature. Spine 21: 1746–1760

Husni E A, Storer J 1967 The syndrome of mechanical occlusion of the vertebral artery: further observations. Angiology 18: 106–116

Husni E A, Bell H S, Storer J 1966 Mechanical occlusion of the vertebral artery: a new clinical concept. Journal of the American Medical Association 196: 101–104

Hutchison M S 1989 An investigation of premanipulative dizziness testing. In: Jones H M, Jones M A, Milde M R (eds) Proceedings of the Sixth Biennial Conference of the Manipulative Therapists Association of Australia. Manipulative Therapists Association of Australia, Adelaide, pp 104–112

Jaskoviak P A 1980 Complications arising from manipulation of the cervical spine. Journal of Manipulative and Physiological Therapeutics 3: 213–219

Johnson C P, Lawler W, Burns J 1993 Use of histomorphometry in the assessment of fatal vertebral artery dissection. Journal of Clinical Pathology 46: 1000–1003

Jones M A, Rivett D A 2004 Introduction to clinical reasoning. In: Jones M A, Rivett D A (eds) Clinical reasoning for manual therapists. Butterworth Heinemann, Edinburgh, pp 3–24

Jull G A 1994 Cervical headache: a review. In: Boyling J D, Palastanga N (eds) Grieve's Modern Manual Therapy, the Vertebral Column, 2nd edn. Churchill Livingstone, Edinburgh, pp 333–347

Jumper J M, Horton J C 1996 Central retinal artery occlusion after manipulation of the neck by a chiropractor. American Journal of Ophthalmology 121: 321–322

Kankamedala R, Hing W, Reid D 2003 Vertebrobasilar insufficiency: the use of pre-manipulative guidelines in New Zealand. Report of results of the survey of NZMPA members. New Zealand Manipulative Physiotherapists Association, Wellington

Keggi K J, Granger D P, Southwick W O 1966 Vertebral artery insufficiency secondary to trauma and osteoarthritis of the cervical spine. Yale Journal of Biology and Medicine 38: 471–478

Kleynhans A M, Terrett A G J 1985 The prevention of complications from spinal manipulative therapy. In: Glasgow E F, Twomey L T, Scull E R, Kleynhans A M, Idczak R M (eds) Aspects of manipulative therapy. Churchill Livingstone, Melbourne, pp 161–175

Klougart N, Leboeuf-Yde C, Rasmusssen L R 1996a Safety in chiropractic practice. I: The occurrence of cerebrovascular accidents after manipulation to the neck in Denmark from 1978–1988. Journal of Manipulative and Physiological Therapeutics 19: 371–377

Klougart N, Leboeuf-Yde C, Rasmussen L R 1996b Safety in chiropractic practice. II: Treatment to the upper neck and the rate of cerebrovascular incidents. Journal of Manipulative and Physiological Therapeutics 19: 563–569

Klougart N, Rasmussen L R, Leboeuf-Yde C 1997 Safety in chiropractic practice. II: Treatment to the upper neck and the rate of cerebrovascular incidents [Letter]. Journal of Manipulative and Physiological Therapeutics 20: 566–567

Krespi Y, Gurol M E, Coban O, Tuncay R, Bahar S 2002 Vertebral artery dissection presenting with isolated neck pain. Journal of Neuroimaging 12: 179–182

Krueger B R, Okazaki H 1980 Vertebral-basilar distribution infarction following chiropractic cervical manipulation. Mayo Clinic Proceedings 55: 322–332

Kunnasmaa K T T, Thiel H W 1994 Vertebral artery syndrome: a review of the literature. Journal of Orthopaedic Medicine 16: 17–20

Lachenbruch P A, Reinsch S, MacRae P G, Tobis J S 1992 Adjusting for recall bias with the proportional hazards model. In: van Bemmel J H, McCray A T (eds) Yearbook of medical informatics 1992. Advances in an interdisciplinary science. IMIA, USA, pp 469–471

Leboeuf-Yde C, Rasmussen L R, Klougart N 1996 The risk of over-reporting spinal manipulative therapy-induced injuries: a description of some cases that failed to burden the statistics. Journal of Manipulative and Physiological Therapeutics 19: 536–538

Leboeuf-Yde C, Hennius B, Rudberg E, Leufvenmark P, Thunman M 1997 Side effects of chiropractic treatment: a prospective study. Journal of Manipulative and Physiological Therapeutics 20: 511–515

Lee K P, Carlini W G, McCormick G F, Albers G W 1995 Neurologic complications following chiropractic manipulation: a survey of California neurologists. Neurology 45: 1213–1215

Lee P, Carlini W, McCormick G, Albers G W 1996 Chiropractic complications [Letter]. Neurology 46: 886–887

Lewit K 1992 Clinical picture and diagnosis of vertebral artery insufficiency. Journal of Manual Medicine 6: 190–193

Licht P B, Christensen H W, Højgaard P, Høilund-Carlsen P F 1998a Triplex ultrasound of vertebral artery flow during cervical rotation. Journal of Manipulative and Physiological Therapeutics 21: 27–31

Licht P B, Christensen H W, Højgaard P, Marving J 1998b Vertebral artery flow and spinal manipulation: a randomized, controlled and observer-blinded study. Journal of Manipulative and Physiological Therapeutics 21: 141–144

Licht P B, Christensen H W, Svendsen P, Høilund-Carlsen P F 1999 Vertebral artery flow and cervical manipulation: an experimental study. Journal of Manipulative and Physiological Therapeutics 22: 431–435

Licht P B, Christensen H W, Høilund-Carlsen P F 2002 Carotid artery blood flow during premanipulative testing. Journal of Manipulative and Physiological Therapeutics 25: 568–572

Livingston M C P 1971 Spinal manipulation causing injury: a three-year study. Clinical Orthopaedics and Related Research 81: 82–86

Lyness S S, Wagman A D 1974 Neurological deficit following cervical manipulation. Surgical Neurology 2: 121–124

Macchi C, Giannelli F, Cecchi F et al 1996 The inner diameter of human intracranial vertebral artery by color doppler method. Italian Journal of Anatomy and Embryology 101: 81–87

Mann T W 1995 Mechanisms of non-traumatic vertebral artery injury from manipulation of the cervical spine: implications for the Australian Physiotherapy Association Protocol for Pre-manipulative Testing. In: Proceedings of the Ninth Biennial Conference of the Manipulative Physiotherapists Association of Australia. Manipulative Physiotherapists Association of Australia, Gold Coast, pp 97–98

Mann T, Refshauge K M 2001 Causes of complications from cervical spine manipulation. Australian Journal of Physiotherapy 47: 255–266

Mas J-L, Bousser M G, Hasboun D, Laplane D 1987 Extracranial vertebral artery dissections: a review of 13 cases. Stroke 18: 1037–1047

Mas J-L, Henin D, Bousser M G, Chain F, Hauw J J 1989 Dissecting aneurysm of the vertebral artery and cervical manipulation: a case review with autopsy. Neurology 39: 512–515

Maslowski H A 1960 The role of the vertebral artery. Journal of Neurology, Neurosurgery, and Psychiatry 23: 355

Meadows J 1992 Safety considerations in vertebral artery testing. In: Proceedings of the Fifth International Conference of the International Federation of Orthopaedic Manipulative Therapists. International Federation of Orthopaedic Manipulative Therapists, Vail, p 124

Meadows J T S, Magee D J 1994 An overview of dizziness and vertigo for the orthopaedic manual therapist. In: Boyling J D, Palastanga N (eds) Grieve's Modern Manual Therapy, the Vertebral Column, 2nd edn. Churchill Livingstone, Edinburgh, pp 381–390

Mestan M A 1999 Posterior fossa ischemia and bilateral vertebral artery hypoplasia. Journal of Manipulative and Physiological Therapeutics 22: 245–249

Michaeli A 1991 Dizziness testing of the cervical spine: can complications of manipulations be prevented? Physiotherapy Theory and Practice 7: 243–250

Michaeli A 1993 Reported occurrence and nature of complications following manipulative physiotherapy in South Africa. Australian Journal of Physiotherapy 39: 309–315

Michaud T C 2002 Uneventful upper cervical manipulation in the presence of a damaged vertebral artery. Journal of Manipulative and Physiological Therapeutics 25: 472–483

Middleditch A 1991 The cervical spine: safe in our hands? In: Proceedings of the Eleventh International Congress of the World Confederation For Physical Therapy. World Confederation For Physical Therapy, London, book 3, pp 1779–1781

Miller R G, Burton R 1974 Stroke following chiropractic manipulation of the spine. Journal of the American Medical Association 229: 189–190

Mitchell J 2002 Vertebral artery atherosclerosis: a risk factor in the use of manipulative therapy? Physiotherapy Research International 7: 122–135

Mitchell J, McKay A 1995 Comparison of left and right vertebral artery intra-cranial diameters. Anatomical Record 242: 350–354

Miyachi S, Okamura K, Watanabe M, Inoue N, Nagatani T, Takagi T 1994 Cerebellar stroke due to vertebral artery occlusion after cervical spine trauma: two case reports. Spine 19: 83–88

Nakamura C T, Lau J M, Polk N O, Popper J S 1991 Vertebral artery dissection caused by chiropractic manipulation. Journal of Vascular Surgery 14: 122–124

Nilsson N 1996 A risk assessment of spinal manipulation vs. NSAIDs for the treatment of neck pain [Letter]. Journal of Manipulative and Physiological Therapeutics 19: 220

Norris J W, Beletsky V, Nadareishvili Z G 2000 Sudden neck movement and cervical artery dissection. Canadian Medical Association Journal 163: 38–40

Oostendorp R A B 1988 Vertebrobasilar insufficiency. In: Proceedings of the Fourth International Conference of the International Federation of Orthopaedic Manipulative Therapists. International Federation of Orthopaedic Manipulative Therapists, Cambridge, pp 42–44

Oostendorp R A B, van Eupen A A J M, Elvers J W H 1992a Aspects of sympathetic nervous system regulation in patients with cervicogenic vertigo: 20 years-experience. In: Proceedings of the Fifth International Conference of the International Federation of Orthopaedic Manipulative Therapists. International Federation of Orthopaedic Manipulative Therapists, Vail, pp 132–134

Oostendorp R A B, Hagenaars L H A, Fischer A J E M, Keyser A, Oosterveld W J, Pool J J M 1992b Dutch standard for 'cervicogenic dizziness'. In: Proceedings of the Fifth International Conference of the International Federation of Orthopaedic Manipulative Therapists. International Federation of Orthopaedic Manipulative Therapists, Vail, pp 128–129

Parkin P J, Wallis W E, Wilson J L 1978 Vertebral artery occlusion following manipulation of the neck. New Zealand Medical Journal 88: 441–443

Parwar B L, Fawzi A A, Arnold A C, Schwartz S D 2001 Horner's syndrome and dissection of the internal carotid artery after chiropractic manipulation of the neck. American Journal of Ophthalmology 131: 523–524

Pásztor E 1978 Decompression of vertebral artery in cases of cervical spondylosis. Surgical Neurology 9: 371–377

Patijn J 1991 Complications in manual medicine: a review of the literature. Journal of Manual Medicine 6: 89–92

Peters M, Bohl J, Thömke F et al 1995 Dissection of the internal carotid artery after chiropractic manipulation of the neck. Neurology 45: 2284–2286

Petersen B, von Maravic M, Zeller J A, Walker M L, Kömpf D, Kessler C 1996 Basilar artery blood flow during head rotation in vertebrobasilar ischemia. Acta Neurologica Scandinavica 94: 294–301

Povlsen U J, Kjaer L, Arlien-Søborg P 1987 Locked-in syndrome following cervical manipulation. Acta Neurologica Scandinavica 76: 486–488

Powers S R, Drislane T M, Nevins S 1961 Intermittent vertebral artery compression: a new syndrome. Surgery 49: 257–264

Raskind R, North C M 1990 Vertebral artery injuries following chiropractic cervical spine manipulation: case reports. Angiology 41: 445–452

Refshauge K M 1994 Rotation: a valid premanipulative dizziness test? Does it predict safe manipulation? Journal of Manipulative and Physiological Therapeutics 17: 15–19

Refshauge K M 1995 Testing adequacy of cerebral blood flow (vertebral artery testing). In: Refshauge K M, Gass E M (eds) Musculoskeletal physiotherapy: clinical science and practice. Butterworth Heinemann, Oxford, pp 125–131

Rivett D A 1995 Neurovascular compromise complicating cervical spine manipulation: what is the risk? Journal of Manual and Manipulative Therapy 3: 144–151

Rivett D A, Milburn P 1996 A prospective study of complications of cervical spine manipulation. Journal of Manual and Manipulative Therapy 4: 166–170

Rivett D A, Milburn P 1997 Complications arising from spinal manipulative therapy in New Zealand. Physiotherapy 83: 626–632

Rivett D A, Reid D 1998 Risk of stroke for cervical spine manipulation in New Zealand. New Zealand Journal of Physiotherapy 26: 14–17

Rivett D A, Sharples K J, Milburn P D 1999 Effect of pre-manipulative tests on vertebral artery and internal carotid artery blood flow: a pilot study. Journal of Manipulative and Physiological Therapeutics 22: 368–375

Rivett D, Sharples K, Milburn P 2000 Vertebral artery blood flow during pre-manipulative testing of the cervical spine. In: Singer K P (ed) Proceedings of the International Federation of Orthopaedic and Manipulative Therapists Conference. International Federation of Orthopaedic and Manipulative Therapists, Perth, pp 387–390

Rivett H M 1994 Cervical manipulation: confronting the spectre of the vertebral artery syndrome. Journal of Orthopaedic Medicine 16: 12–16

Roberts J B 1907 Fracture dislocation of the atlas without symptoms of spinal cord injury. Annals of Surgery 45: 632–635

Robertson J T 1981 Neck manipulation as a cause of stroke. Stroke 12: 1

Robertson J T 1982 Neck manipulation as a cause of stroke [Letter]. Stroke 13: 260–261

Rothrock J F, Hesselink J R, Teacher T M 1991 Vertebral artery occlusion and stroke from cervical self-manipulation. Neurology 41: 1696–1697

Rothwell D M, Bondy S J, Williams J I 2001 Chiropractic manipulation and stroke: a population-based case-control study. Stroke 32: 1054–1060

Roy G 1994 The vertebral artery. Journal of Manual and Manipulative Therapy 2: 28–31

Rubinstein S M, Haldeman S 2001 Cervical manipulation to a patient with a history of traumatically induced dissection of the internal

carotid artery: a case report and review of the literature on recurrent dissections. Journal of Manipulative and Physiological Therapeutics 24: 520–525

Schellhas K P, Latchaw R E, Wendling L R, Gold L H A 1980 Vertebrobasilar injuries following cervical manipulation. Journal of the American Medical Association 244: 1450–1453

Schmitt H P 1991 Anatomical structure of the cervical spine with reference to the pathology of manipulation complications. Journal of Manual Medicine 6: 93–101

Schwarz N, Buchinger W, Gaudernak T, Russe F, Zechner W 1991 Injuries to the cervical spine causing vertebral artery trauma: case reports. Journal of Trauma 31: 127–133

Sédat J, Dib M, Mahagne M H, Lonjon M, Paquis P 2002 Stroke after chiropractic manipulation as a result of extracranial postero-inferior cerebellar artery dissection. Journal of Manipulative and Physiological Therapeutics 25: 588–590

Seidel E, Eicke B M, Tetterborn B, Krummenauer F 1999 Reference values for vertebral artery flow volume by duplex sonography in young and elderly adults. Stroke 30: 2692–2696

Sell J J, Rael J R, Orrison W W 1994 Rotational vertebrobasilar insufficiency as a component of thoracic outlet syndrome resulting in transient blindness. Journal of Neurosurgery 81: 617–619

Senstad O, Leboeuf-Yde C, Borchgrevink C 1996a Predictors of side effects to spinal manipulative therapy. Journal of Manipulative and Physiological Therapeutics 19: 441–445

Senstad O, Leboeuf-Yde C, Borchgrevink C 1996b Side-effects of chiropractic spinal manipulation: types, frequency, discomfort and course. Scandinavian Journal of Primary Health Care 14: 50–53

Senstad O, Leboeuf-Yde C, Borchgrevink C 1997 Frequency and characteristics of side effects of spinal manipulative therapy. Spine 22: 435–441

Shekelle P G, Coulter I 1997 Cervical spine manipulation: summary report of a systematic review of the literature and a multidisciplinary expert panel. Journal of Spinal Disorders 10: 223–228

Sherman D G, Hart R G, Easton J D 1981 Abrupt change in head position and cerebral infarction. Stroke 12: 2–6

Sherman D G, Easton J D, Hart R G 1982 Neck manipulation as a cause of stroke. Stroke 13: 260

Sherman M R, Smialek J E, Zane W E 1987 Pathogenesis of vertebral artery occlusion following cervical spine manipulation. Archives of Pathology and Laboratory Medicine 111: 851–853

Simeone F A, Goldberg H I 1968 Thrombosis of the vertebral artery from hyperextension injury to the neck: case report. Journal of Neurosurgery 29: 540–544

Sinel M, Smith D 1993 Thalamic infarction secondary to cervical manipulation. Archives of Physical Medicine and Rehabilitation 74: 543–546

Sivakumaran P, Wilsher M 1995 Diaphragmatic palsy and chiropractic manipulation. New Zealand Medical Journal 108: 279–280

Stevens A 1991 Functional Doppler sonography of the vertebral artery and some considerations about manual techniques. Journal of Manual Medicine 6: 102–105

Stevinson C, Honan W, Cooke B, Ernst E 2001 Neurological complications of cervical spine manipulation. Journal of the Royal Society of Medicine 94: 107–110

Sturzenegger M, Mattle H P, Rivoir A, Rihs F, Schmid C 1993 Ultrasound findings in spontaneous extracranial vertebral artery dissection. Stroke 24: 1910–1921

Sturzenneger M, Newell D W, Douville C, Byrd S, Schoonover K 1994 Dynamic transcranial Doppler assessment of positional vertebrobasilar ischemia. Stroke 25: 1776–1783

Symons B P, Westaway M 2001 Virchow's Triad and spinal manipulative therapy of the cervical spine. Journal of the Canadian Chiropractic Association 45: 225–231

Symons B P, Leonard T, Herzog W 2002 Internal forces sustained by the vertebral artery during spinal manipulative therapy. Journal of Manipulative and Physiological Therapeutics 25: 504–510

Teasell R W, Marchuk Y 1994 Vertebro-basilar artery stroke as a complication of cervical manipulation. Critical Reviews in Physical and Rehabilitation Medicine 6: 121–129

Terenzi T J, DeFabio D C 1996 The role of transcranial Doppler sonography in the identification of patients at risk of cerebral and brainstem ischemia. Journal of Manipulative and Physiological Therapeutics 19: 406–414

Terrett A G J 1987a Vascular accidents from cervical spine manipulation: report on 107 cases. Journal of the Australian Chiropractors' Association 17: 15–24

Terrett A G J 1987b Vascular accidents from cervical spine manipulation: the mechanisms. Journal of the Australian Chiropractors' Association 17: 131–144

Terrett A G J 1995 Misuse of the literature by medical authors in discussing spinal manipulative therapy injury. Journal of Manipulative and Physiological Therapeutics 18: 203–210

Thiel H W 1991 Gross morphology and pathoanatomy of the vertebral arteries. Journal of Manipulative and Physiological Therapeutics 14: 133–141

Thiel H W, Wallace K, Donat J, Yong-Hing K 1994 Effect of various head and neck positions on vertebral artery blood flow. Clinical Biomechanics 9: 105–110

Tissington-Tatlow W F, Bammer H G 1957 Syndrome of vertebral artery compression. Neurology 7: 331–340

Toole J F, Tucker S H 1960 Influence of head position upon cerebral circulation. Archives of Neurology 2: 616–623

Tulyapronchote R, Selhorst J B, Malkoff M D, Gomez C R 1994 Delayed sequelae of vertebral artery dissection and occult cervical fractures. Neurology 44: 1397–1399

Weintraub M I, Khoury A 1995a Critical neck position as an independent risk factor for posterior circulation stroke: a magnetic resonance angiographic analysis. Journal of Neuroimaging 5: 16–22

Weintraub M I, Khoury A 1995b Transcranial Doppler assessment of positional vertebrobasilar ischemia. Stroke 26: 330–332

Chapter 38

Managing chronic pain

P. J. Watson

INTRODUCTION

Despite our best efforts and those of our healthcare colleagues, a number of patients will continue to suffer persistent pain. Chronic pain is classically defined as pain lasting more than 12 weeks (Bigos et al 1994, Clinical Standards Advisory Group 1994, Von Korff & Saunders 1996). In the case of low back pain, it is often reported that only a small minority continue to have problems after 4–6 weeks, about 80% having already returned to work (Watson et al 1998a, Waddell 1998). However, this does not mean that the symptoms have completely resolved. Most people return to work but continue to have symptoms and may remain symptomatic for a year or more after an initial episode (Croft et al 1998) but may not consult a practitioner. The fact is that chronic and recurrent pains are common symptoms in the general population, but not everyone continues to seek treatment. Most people only consult a practitioner when the pain starts to limit their activities or interferes with their work (Waddell 1998).

Manual therapy has demonstrated its use in successfully treating specific dysfunctions and symptoms and this volume is a testament to that, but symptom management and rehabilitation is *not* the same thing. Management of dysfunction and symptoms are the means to an end, not the end itself; they are *not* rehabilitation. Successful symptom management is only the starting point of rehabilitation.

The small proportion of people who have a painful episode and who remain disabled by their condition and either continue to consult and/or report significant disability seem particularly resistant to all types of therapy. The poor relationship between pathology, pain reports and disability in these patients requires a broader concept of illness and disability to illuminate the problem and provide a solution.

A BIOPSYCHOSOCIAL MODEL OF ILLNESS

Modern approaches to the management of pain, and not just chronic pain, recognize that the report of pain is multiply determined. The previous labelled line and specificity theories, where sensory dimension and intensity of the pain are a direct reflection of the stimulation of a specific receptor organ and the intensity of the stimulus (often also of damage) it sustains, are indefensible in the light of a modern understanding of nociception and pain. As has been pointed out (Watson 2002):

> pain is not merely the end-product of a transmission of nociceptive impulses from receptor organ to an area of interpretation. It is a dynamic process of integration, perception and interpretation of a wide range of incoming stimuli, some of which are associated with actual or potential harm, and some of which are benign, even though interpreted and described in terms of damage.

The process is dynamic because it changes in response to type and duration of the nociceptive input, previous learned experience, attentional demand, mood and cognitions. This is only the first stage; the report of pain as a sensation, the progress to reduced function and disability is even more complex.

Engel (1962) made one of the first attempts to distinguish disease processes and expressions of illness (illness behaviour) as a psychosocial construct. In this attempt, personal constructs and understanding of disease and the resultant illness behaviour were considered in the light of the individual's interpretation of symptoms and beliefs about disease. The gate control theory developed by Melzack & Wall (1965) proposed that pain was a psychophysiological phenomenon, modulated by competing sensations and psychological factors. The resultant research made the specificity theories untenable. Loeser (1980) adapted Engel's model to explain chronic pain-associated disability in the light of new theories about pain perception and illness behaviour. The biopsychosocial model of pain-associated disability was developed to its present form in a series of papers by Waddell and colleagues and best explained by Waddell in 1987. This was the first time that theory was supported by strong research evidence for the importance of psychosocial variables in the development and maintenance of back pain disability. The most recently refined model is given in Figure 38.1.

Pain, or at least a sensation interpreted as pain, is at the heart of the model, the patient's cognitions about the meaning of pain and beliefs the patient has give an effective response (the suffering component), which is then expressed as illness behaviour in the form of treatment seeking, change in posture, altered movement. Altered posture and movement not only protect the area from further pain to allow recovery from injury, they also communicate the presence of pain to others (Keefe & Dunsmore 1992). All this takes place in a social environment which can help to reinforce the behaviour and, equally important, inculcate and reinforce the beliefs and cognitions which underlie and drive the behaviour.

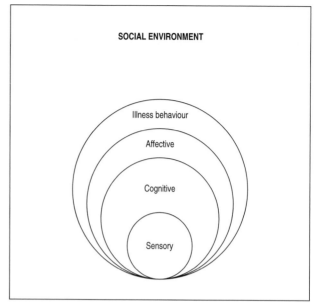

Figure 38.1 A biopsychosocial model of low back pain disability (Waddell 1992).

If we accept the gate control theory then we must accept that treating the (perceived) cause of nociception alone is only one part of the process of managing pain. If we accept the biopsychosocial model of disability then we must try and address more than the sensation of pain alone if we are to prevent disability and return the patient back to their previous levels of activity, or at least encourage them to their best possible function. In those with chronic pain problems, the observed structural abnormality or dysfunction does not adequately predict the accompanying level of disability. The level of disability is more closely related to the individual's beliefs about their condition, how they are currently coping and the level of psychological distress (Linton 2000, Turk et al 1996, Vlaeyen & Linton 2000, Waddell 1987, 1988). If we fail to address these factors we are failing the patient.

ASSESSING AND MANAGING CHRONIC PAIN

Managing the patient with a 'biopsychosocial approach' has become one of those phrases that all students are expected to include in their essays and all authors are required to pay lip service to if they are to be seen to be up to date. At its best, a biopsychosocial approach identifies the non-physical barriers to progress in the individual patient, allows the development of an approach to address these and leads to an improved outcome. At worst, it is a broad-brush, one-size-fits-all approach consisting of general advice, weak reassurance and a few non-specific exercises. A psychosocial approach does not necessarily dictate the treatment approach to the clinician but it will inform one of the framework within which that treatment should be delivered.

A biopsychosocial approach is not the antithesis of the biomedical model, as is sometimes presented; rather, the biomedical model fits within such an approach. It is the over-reliance on the biomedical model, seeing all pain problems purely from a biomedical perspective, which prevents the clinician seeing the whole patient and may lead to sub-optimal treatment, poor patient compliance and poor outcomes. An ability to correctly identify treatable pathology and dysfunction is an essential part of training. It is unethical to ignore important clinical findings and if there is an evidence based approach that can be used to remediate the problem then it should be used. However, once again, with the fear of being repetitious, it is only the starting point of rehabilitation.

Psychosocial assessment

The Clinical Standards Advisory Group (1994), the Royal College of General Practitioners in the UK (1996) and the Accident and Compensation Corporation of New Zealand (Kendall et al 1997) recommended that those not improving following an episode of low back pain should have a psychosocial assessment and a multidisciplinary management approach. However, relatively few patients with chronic pain ever make it to a multidisciplinary clinic (Feuerstein & Zastowny 1996, Smith et al 1996) and these resources are likely to remain scarce. Furthermore, few of these patients need to see a psychologist. A manual therapist or physiotherapist with the appropriate approach and skills should be capable of managing most people with persistent or recurrent pain problems. Pain management programmes are for those who are becoming increasingly distressed and psychologically dysfunctional (Spanswick & Main 2000).

Even though recommendations have been made for the conduct of a psychosocial assessment, only the New Zealand guideline was specific about what this entailed. In *Guidelines to the Assessment of Yellow Flags* (Kendall et al 1997), it was suggested that there were seven areas of concern neatly conceptualised in a mnemonic – ABCDEFW. Although this was initially developed to manage acute low back pain in an occupational setting, there are lessons that can be useful to those working with chronic pain. The areas of concern are as follows:

- **A**ttitudes and beliefs about the causes of pain and the eventual outcome.
- **B**ehaviours – what they are currently doing/not doing because of their pain problem, how they report their pain experience and how this impacts on the others around them.
- **C**ompensation – the role of wages compensation (sickness benefits) and medico-legal claims.
- **D**iagnosis and treatment – previous explanations about the cause of the pain and the treatment indicated and how these interact with the patient's beliefs about back pain and their expectation of their (the patient's) role in treatment.

- **E**motion – the fears and worries which might develop as the pain fails to resolve and the depression that may result from this. Fears that arise from mistaken beliefs about the pain.
- **F**amily – the reinforcing of unhelpful beliefs and behaviours by significant others. Friends and families can be a force for good as well as a barrier to success.
- **W**ork – the physical and psychological demands of work and the opportunity for graded return. The social environment at work and co-workers' perceptions about pain.

Clinicians may find it useful to remember these prompts when assessing patients (see Watson & Kendall 2000). Readers might find it interesting that Main & Watson (2002) have developed from the above a structured interview which has been tested out in a number of clinical environments by physiotherapists and occupational health nurses.

Cognitive variables

No person comes for treatment to an injury or a medical condition without having made some attempt to make sense of the problem themselves, labelling it and giving it meaning. The cognitions the patient may have about their condition might usefully be placed in three areas: specific beliefs about pain and treatment; the nature of cognitive processes; and coping styles/strategies (Main & Watson 1999).

Once a person suffers from a painful condition they make judgements based on previous experience and knowledge, beliefs developed over the years and perception of the importance of the pain. Lazarus & Folkman (1984) have suggested a two-stage appraisal of the cognitive dimensions of a stressful event such as back pain. In the first stage the pain is perceived as a threat. There is a perceived threat of losing something valuable; good health, social status, work, independence for example. The second evaluation relates to the patient's capacity to deal with the event. A perception of a loss of control or distress will arise if the patient's evaluation of the problem is that it is beyond their resources to cope. This is not a static appraisal but dynamic and it changes in the light of new experience and new challenges. The development of distress or depression will negatively influence the appraisal of the problem and this may lead to a reinforcement of the subject's perceived level of disability (Geisser at al 1997, 2000).

Specific beliefs about back pain and treatment

Patients may develop pessimistic or negative beliefs regarding pain and outcome of treatment. This may be based on previous experience with health care or may be based upon the 'folk beliefs' of their own cultural environment. Beliefs about the extent to which pain can be controlled is a powerful determinant of the development of incapacity (Crisson & Keefe, 1988, Main & Waddell 1991).

DeGood & Shutty (1992) suggest that patients develop beliefs about pain in the following areas: aetiology of pain, expectations about diagnoses, expectations about treatments and their (the patient's) role in it and expectations about the outcome of treatment. It is these beliefs, which can colour the individual's response to pain and the role they adopt in the management of their condition.

The way in which patients respond to their illness and whether they seek treatment and the type of treatment they prefer depends upon their 'locus of control'. Broadly, patients have been classified into those with an 'internalized' locus of control, where the individual seeks to manage the problem themselves; those with an externalized locus of control are more likely to rely on healthcare workers to cure their problem. However, locus of control lies on a continuum and patients lie at a point on that continuum. The way in which we manage patients can move them to be more externalized or internalized about their ability to manage pain (Williams & Keefe 1991, Symonds et al 1995). In a recent study on the use of complementary therapies, those who had a more externalized locus of control (believed it was the health professionals' role to cure their problem) were more likely to seek passive treatments. Those who demonstrated an internal locus of control (felt they should assume more control) were more likely to seek self-management techniques (Palinkas et al 2000). Encouraging a passive approach may encourage an externalization of control from the patient to the therapist. Manual therapy alone is (for the patient) a passive treatment, so care must be taken not to foster a passive coping style in the patient.

Fear avoidance beliefs

A factor which has received much recent attention in the development of chronic incapacity is fear of injury and mistaken beliefs about hurting and harm. It is an intuitively appealing concept, as anyone who has an injury will naturally develop at the least a wariness of the activity that caused it. Whether this develops into a fear and avoidance of activity and an increase in reported disability is still open to question because of a relative lack of evidence.

Lethem et al (1983) developed a fear/avoidance model of exaggerated pain perception to help explain the development of disability following an acute onset of pain. They suggested that patients respond to the pain by adopting different styles of coping, which they termed confronters or avoiders. As the names suggest, some people may remain active and use activity and distraction as a strategy to cope with pain whereas others withdraw from activity and use rest as their predominant coping style. At its worse this fear may transfer to simple everyday activities. It is therefore, they suggest, crucial to recognize the role of fear and avoidance as obstacles to rehabilitation following injury.

A number of fear/avoidance measures have been developed and increased scores on these instruments have been associated with increased disability and increased work loss (Waddell et al 1993, 2003, Vlaeyen et al 1995a, 1995b). Waddell et al (1993) demonstrated in a mixed group of subjects from different referral sources that there was a strong relationship between fear about work and activity and both current disability and work loss in the previous year. Using different assessment tools Jensen et al (1994) demonstrated that the belief that activity will lead to increased pain and possibly damage are strongly related to current self-report of function.

Klenerman et al (1995) found in a large group of acute back pain patients that fear avoidance variables could correctly classify 66% of cases with persistent pain and disability at 12 months. Further to this, initial fear avoidance variables explained 25% of the variance for pain and disability at 12 months. These findings are supported by the work of Rose et al (1992, 1995).

Vlaeyen & Linton (2000) give one of the most comprehensive reviews of the literature in this area and have concluded that fear avoidance beliefs are related to the onset and maintenance of disability in musculoskeletal pain. However, most of the studies reviewed specifically focused on fear avoidance and did not examine the possible explanations offered by other variables such as depression, coping and other anxieties not directly related to fear of pain and injury. In this way they have demonstrated that fear avoidance is important in back pain disability but have not established the influence beyond that of other psychological variables. They propose a model in which catastrophization (fearing the worst) and fear of injury predisposes the individual to increased report of pain, avoidance of activity, hypervigilance to bodily sensations and eventually depression and disability. They further suggest that the pain related fear fuels increased disability.

Pain coping styles and strategies

People vary in their range of coping strategies. Brown & Nicassio (1987) distinguished between active (adaptive) and passive (non-adaptive) coping strategies. Active strategies (e.g. taking exercise, ignoring the pain) require the individual to take a degree of responsibility for pain management by either attempting to control pain or attempting to function despite pain. Passive strategies (e.g. resting, relying on medication) either involve withdrawal or the passing on of responsibility for the control of pain to someone else (the clinician).

Rosenstiel & Keefe (1983) identified both positive (or adaptive) and negative (or maladaptive) coping strategies. Use of the negative coping strategies such as passive praying/hoping and catastrophizing (fearing the worst) are suggested as predictive of poor response to treatment. In addition to this, the patient makes an assessment of how well they are able to control the pain and decrease the pain as a result of their coping (the effectiveness of their particular strategy). The evidence for the predictive nature of coping strategies in the acute back pain patient is most clearly demonstrated in the work of Burton et al (1995). For the whole patient group (acute and subchronic) the negative coping strategy of 'praying and hoping' (that the pain will go away) accounted for 23% of the variance. However, in the subchronic group alone, coping strategies did not appear to be important in disability. Klenerman et al (1995) also found that negative coping was associated with poor outcome. It is interesting to note that, although the negative coping strategies were predictive of poor outcome, the positive coping strategies have not been reported to have a significant predictive value.

Psychological distress

Psychological distress is the term that has come to relate to the exaggerated attention to bodily symptoms, anxiety, anger and the development of depression in those who go on to develop chronic incapacity. In this context depression should really be seen as depressed mood rather than a clinical diagnosis and can be anywhere in wide spectrum of emotion ranging from the slightly demoralized or fed-up to the suicidal (Main & Watson 1999). Pain patients certainly often seem to be demoralized or depressed. The similarities between chronic pain patients and depressed patients have led to a vigorous debate about the nature of depression in pain patients.

In the past there had been an assumption that depressed individuals develop pain secondary to their depression. This has been challenged by a number of good studies (von Korff et al 1993, Hassenbring et al 1994, Hansen et al 1995, Averill et al 1996) which suggest that depression is a consequence of rather than an antecedent to back pain. However, whether a patient consults a health professional may be influenced by their current mood (Croft et al 1995, Papageorgiou et al 1997, Thomas et al 1999).

The initial reaction to a painful injury is usually recognized in terms of anxiety, shock and fear rather than depression (Lazarus & Folkman 1984). Gatchel & Gardea (1999) suggest that with the passage of time and the failure of treatment and a patient's coping skills, depression becomes more evident. In this way pain-associated depression is often best viewed as a form of 'learned helplessness'. In the context of the development of chronic pain it is best understood as a psychological consequence of the persistence of pain, the interference with everyday life and its incapacitating effects.

The predictive ability of mood and somatic anxiety has been well documented in a number of studies. Main et al (1992) developed the Distress Risk Assessment Method (DRAM), a combination of two questionnaires, the Modified Zung Depression Questionnaire and the Modified Somatic Perception Questionnaire (Main 1983). Since its publication, this questionnaire has received widespread use because of its specificity for back pain. In a study of those low back pain patients with various lengths of duration it demonstrated that those identified as at risk or distressed had 2.0 to 3.5 times the risk of having the same or worse pain at follow-up. With respect to disability, the at risk group were at 1.9 times greater risk of remaining disabled or getting worse and the distressed groups were at 5.2 times greater risk (Main et al 1992).

These findings have been replicated in other studies in secondary care (Greenough 1993) and primary care (Burton et al 1995).

Pain behaviour

Pain behaviour is defined as 'any and all outputs that a reasonable observer would characterise as pain' (Loeser & Fordyce 1983). This includes reporting of pain, demonstrations of pain, treatment seeking, taking medication, altered social role, 'downtime' and altered habits (for example increased alcohol/tobacco consumption).

Systematic observation of overt pain behaviour has been developed (Keefe & Block 1982, Richards et al 1982). It does seem that high levels of pain behaviour are related to increased self-report of disability (Keefe & Block 1982, Richards et al 1982, Watson & Poulter 1997). Increased demonstration of overt pain behaviours is also influenced by the solicitousness of the spouse or significant other (Main et al 2000). Continued demonstration of pain behaviour may also be reinforced by the demands of the social compensation or medicolegal system (Main & Spanswick 1995, Hadler 1996, 1997).

One of the most commonly used and researched tests with respect to prediction of outcome from back pain are the non-organic signs, often referred to as the 'Waddell' signs (Waddell et al 1980, 1984). These comprise a series of simple examination tests designed to elicit behaviour responses to examination and assist in the identification of illness (pain) behaviour (Main & Waddell 1998). Most of the research performed using these tests has been on outcomes from medical and surgical intervention rather than rehabilitation. Results have demonstrated a link between the presence of non-organic signs and poor outcome (Dzioba & Doxey 1984, Waddell 1987, Atlas et al 1996). The non-organic signs have been demonstrated both to predict (Lancourt & Kettelhut 1992, Ohlund et al 1994, Kummel 1996) and to have no association with return to work (Fritz et al 2000). A similar examination system has now been developed for the cervical spine (Sobel et al 2000). It is better to view these signs as an additional screen in the context of a physical examination for assisting the clinician to identify the need for a more broad assessment to identify psychological distress and fear of injury or harm in the examination. The originators themselves have never suggested that they be used alone as predictive measures or screening tools for outcome (Main & Waddell 1998).

Compensation and socioeconomic factors

The role of socioeconomic factors in the development of disability has engaged much opinion and has generated a lot of debate. Nachemson (1992) related the high levels of back pain related incapacity in Sweden to the generous levels of wages compensation and the relative ease with which disability benefits can be claimed. Changes in the benefits system in Sweden resulting in lower rates of compensation were accompanied by a fall in the claims for incapacity for back pain (Nachemson et al 2000).

Watson et al (1998a) suggested that there was no difference in the return to work rate in Jersey and the UK mainland where the compensation rates were more generous. Most of the evidence for the role of 'wages compensation' in chronic pain absence comes from North America and in particular from the workers' compensation schemes. Some results have demonstrated a relationship between those who are compensated under this system and delayed return to work and increased healthcare costs (Cats-Baril & Frymoer 1991, Rohling et al 1995, Rainville et al 1997, Atlas et al 2000). Others have found no strong association (Volinn et al 1991, Gallagher et al 1995, Hadler et al 1995, Watson & Main 2004). After a review of much of the evidence, Waddell (1998) concludes that there is a relationship between wages compensation, increased work absence, poor surgical outcome and poor rehabilitation outcome from back pain. He identified significant demographic differences between those receiving and not receiving compensation. He adds that most people on wages compensation get better and that it is only one of many social influences and must be seen in that context.

Fishbain et al (1995) reviewed a large series of papers relating to litigation and lump sum compensation claims for chronic pain and could find no evidence that settlement of the claim led to a resolution or improvement in the patient's condition or a return to work. Other workers have found that seeking lump sum compensation claims (medico-legal claims) was related to poor outcome from low back pain and psychological disturbance (greater distress) (Greenough & Fraser 1989, 1992, Greenough 1993). Settlement of these lump sum compensations did not influence employment status or resolution of the psychological disturbance at 1 year or 5-year follow-up. We must not assume that all litigants are likely to have a poor outcome. Once again the influences are many and complex. A return to work may reduce the amount of the final settlement and furthermore, involvement in the medico-legal system may contribute to the general level of psychological distress (Main & Spanswick 1995).

Work

Despite the technological advances in the Western society, the decline of heavy industries and a general reduction in the physical nature of work over the past three decades there are still some occupations that place the employee in a position where their body is subjected to stresses which make them more prone to report back pain symptoms (Halpern 1992). These occupations include builders, forestry workers, nurses and those who operate machinery which results in whole body vibration (Waddell & Burton 2000). There is no evidence that people of different occupations become more disabled than others but perceptions of work do affect whether a person is likely to return to their job after treatment.

Satisfaction with work, relationships between the injured and the employer, the worker's perception of safety in the workplace and the worker's perception of workplace stress, monotony and physical demands of the workplace have all been demonstrated to be influential in workplace absence and the rate of return to work (Bigos et al 1991, Williams et al 1998, Waddell & Burton 2000). Cats-Baril & Frymoer (1991) studied subjects with acute back pain and demonstrated four main areas of risk for long-term work absence: job characteristics, which included work status at the time of onset of pain, past work history and type of occupation, job satisfaction factors, including local retirement policies, wages compensation benefits, perceptions of job safety and employer liability for injury.

Other evidence for the nature of the occupation were identified by Bongers et al (1993). They found that perceived monotony, high physical demand or high workload and time pressure were predictive of the development of musculoskeletal pain and prolonged work absence. In addition, musculoskeletal pain was more prevalent in those who perceived they had low job control and poor support from colleagues was also an important factor.

We can see from this brief overview that the influences of work on the development of incapacity and work loss are many. They depend not only on the physical and ergonomic demands of the work but also on the subject's perception of the intensity of those demands. Workers who perceive their work as monotonous, who believe their employer is uncaring and who perceive a lack of safety in the workplace are more likely to be absent from work and remain absent for longer than those without these perceptions.

Other barriers to successful rehabilitation

Rehabilitation is the raison d'être for physical therapy in musculoskeletal pain. If we fail to get the patient back to what they were doing before they consulted or if we fail to help them achieve their optimum potential then we are selling our patients and ourselves short.

In the first part of this chapter, I outlined briefly the factors in individuals which have been found to affect outcome. The barriers are not all one-sided – we must reflect on our own practice as well. Delays in providing treatments aimed at rehabilitation, restoration of function and return to normal activity are detrimental to successful outcomes (Loeser 1996, Loeser & Sullivan 1997). Frequent reassessments and confusing diagnostic language used to justify a clinician's particular approach does not serve to improve the patient and may actually delay rehabilitation (Loeser & Sullivan 1995, 1997, Hadler 1996).

MANAGEMENT OF CHRONIC PAIN

The objective of managing those with chronic pain were first identified by Turk et al (1983) and remain constant today. They are founded on cognitive behavioural therapy (CBT), which acknowledges that what we know, believe and are told about a disease influences our reaction to it which is seen in how we behave in response. This in no way denies the existence of a disease process and, in an ideal situation, the pathology and the illness behaviour should be managed in parallel. If the pathology is not obvious or not amenable to treatment then the aim is to change the impact of the disease on function – the behaviour. The objectives were originally developed for pain management programmes run chiefly by psychologists. However, we can adapt them to be more relevant to rehabilitation practitioners in general. The objectives of a pain management approach are to (Watson 2003):

- assist patients in altering their belief that their problems are unmanageable and beyond their control
- inform patients about their condition
- assist patients to move from a passive to an active role in the management of their condition
- enable patients to become active problem solvers to help them cope with their pain through the development of effective ways of responding to pain, emotion and the environment
- help patients to monitor thought, emotions and behaviours, and identify how these are influenced by internal and external events
- give patients a feeling of competence in the execution of positive strategies in the management of their condition
- help patients to develop a positive attitude to exercise and personal health management
- help patients to develop a programme of paced activity to reduce the effects of physical deconditioning
- assist patients to develop coping strategies that can be developed once contact with the clinician has ended.

The key components of a CBT approach have been established over the years, mainly in pain management programmes (Turk et al 1983, Bradley 1996, Keefe et al 1996), and consist of education, goal setting, pacing activity, physical exercise and specific skills training (for example relaxation, assertiveness). The skills learned should be practised to generalize the skills into everyday situations and novel situations. Guzman et al (2002) reviewed the CBT approach in low back pain and found that this approach was superior to 'passive' approaches but the improvements were less significant when compared to 'active' (exercise based) approaches. Morley et al (1999) conducted a meta-analysis of 25 studies of behavioural approaches and demonstrated that they were more effective than waiting list controls and more beneficial than other 'active' treatments alone with respect to improvements in pain, pain appraisal and ability to cope with the pain. Van Tulder et al (2000) conducted a systematic review that found that CBT approaches alone were not more effective than multidisciplinary programmes (those combining physiotherapy, education, psychological and medical treatment). It would appear that combining a cognitive behavioural approach with an 'active' management strategy is the most effective way of managing chronic pain conditions. Activity based programmes incorporating CBT techniques have been used by physiotherapists with success and have demonstrated sustained treatment effects when compared to controls (Frost et al 1995, 1998, Klaber Moffett et al 1999).

More specifically, the aims of a physical activity intervention for chronic pain are to (Watson 2000):

- overcome the effects of deconditioning
- challenge and reduce patients' fears of engaging in physical activity
- reduce physical impairment and capitalize on recoverable function
- increase physical activity in a safe and graded manner
- help patients to accept responsibility for increasing their functional capacity
- promote a positive view of physical activity in the self-management of health
- introduce challenging functional activities to rehabilitation.

The cognitive behavioural approach acknowledges that behavioural responses to illness can be influenced by the consequences of those responses, one of the tenets of operant-behavioural theory. For example, if a painful activity is avoided, the resultant short-term reduction in pain reinforces the avoidance behaviour. Equally, if the presence of pain during a task is aversive and observed by the partner, they may suggest taking over that task. If this help is reinforcing, further pain-associated behaviour may elicit further help from the spouse, leading to the relinquishing of several activities over time.

Education

Patients need relevant and understandable information to help them make choices and change behaviour (Ley & Llewelyn 1995, Moseley 2004). Education of patients actually starts at the first consultation. An initial explanation of the possible causes of pain and of the pain management approach with an explicit focus on improving function should give patients information that helps them make an informed decision about participating in treatment, and offer them a credible rationale for engagement. Effective communication is the essence of good education; for a brief review of good practice in patient communication and treatment planning see Price & Leaver (2002).

Education is a cognitive event: the effect of a good education strategy should be a reappraisal of unhelpful beliefs and, eventually, a change in behaviour and application of the new knowledge in novel situations. Practical rehearsal of new information enhances the learning; if the patient is informed that exercise is helpful they should embark on a course of activity to test out and reinforce this with guidance from the clinician, giving correction, evaluation, feedback, explanation and ongoing practice. Public health education in the management of acute back pain appears to have had some success in changing perceptions of back pain (Buchbinder et al 2001). However, some authors (Daltroy et al 1997, Hazard et al 2000) have pointed out that education alone may not be sufficient to effect behavioural change. Daltroy et al (1997) demonstrated in an industrial setting that people who attended regular educations sessions, when compared to those who did not attend, had no fewer injuries or sickness absence over a 5-year study period.

In chronic pain problems education is an integral part of treatments; the effect of education alone, however, may be insufficient to improve those with significant disability. The content of an education programme involves an explanation of the pain condition in those who have a diagnosed condition. Many may not have a clear diagnosis, or the cause of pain may have become obscured by subsequent interventions (operations or neuro-ablative techniques). An explanation of the known physiology of persistent pain in the absence of ongoing damage and the role of altered neuronal sensitivity can be understood by most patients if the clinician takes into account their educational level, previous explanations and underlying beliefs about pain and injury.

A frequently reported phenomenon in those with chronic pain is the fear of pain, the assumption that pain always indicates ongoing damage and the associated reduction in movement – the fear/avoidance model (Lethem et al 1983, Vlaeyen & Linton 2000). Information on separating the link between pain and damage and reassurance that exercise is safe in low back pain appear to be powerful messages in the prevention of low back pain (Symonds et al 1995, Waddell & Burton 2000, Vlaeyen et al 2001).

Education on the beneficial effects of regular exercise is useful in most people attending our clinics. Whether chronic pain patients are physically deconditioned is a moot point. Certainly chronic low back pain patients demonstrate the factors normally associated with lack of physical exercise – increased weight, reduced maximal strength for example – but in a number of studies healthy, sedentary controls have been equally unfit on cardiovascular assessment (Wittink et al 2000).

It is helpful if patients come to realize that increases in symptoms following mild exercise are a normal bodily response in a deconditioned system (or one not accustomed to exercise), or, additionally, part of central hypersensitivity that they can perhaps see as abnormally amplified signals: 'imprinting' of pain in the CNS rather than signals of damage.

Ergonomic influences on pain, including education and advice about safe lifting, working postures and practices for efficiency of movement, should be covered. Although some didactic teaching is unavoidable, education needs to be effective and engaging, so discussion groups and tutorial based education drawing on the experiences of the patient are a useful tool. Rather than offer specific advice and rules, patients should be taught to adopt a problem solving approach to identifying *unhelpful* postures and *inefficient* working positions (note, *damaging* and *dangerous* are not used).

When dealing with chronic pain patients ask yourself the questions: 'What information does this person need to see increasing general activity as a positive way of managing their pain?' 'What can I say that will help them take a more benign view of their pain problem?'

Goal setting and pacing

Gil and colleagues (1988) described pacing as moderate activity–rest cycling. It is a strategy to enable patients to control exacerbations in pain by learning to regulate activity and, once a regime of paced activity is established, to gradually increase their activity level. The converse of this is the 'overactivity–pain–rest' cycle (Gil et al 1988).

Chronic pain patients often report levels of activity that fluctuate dramatically over time. On questioning at initial assessment, they report that they frequently persist at activities until they are prevented from carrying on by the ensuing level of pain. This leads them to rest until the pain subsides or until frustration moves them to action whereupon they then try again until defeated by the increase in pain. Patients may also misattribute the muscle aching and stiffness that are normal after unaccustomed exercise as further injury and damage. Increases in pain following excessive exercise, engendered by post-exertional pain in unfit individuals, can also serve to increase excitation of pain receptors in an already sensitive pain system, presumably through secondary central sensitization (Coderre et al 1993, Mense 1994, Bennett 1996, Wilder-Smith et al 2002).

The purpose of goal setting is to regulate daily activities and to structure an increase in activity through the gradual pacing-up. Activity is paced by time or by the introduction of quotas of exercise interspersed by periods of rest or change in activity (Fordyce 1976, Gil et al 1988, Keefe et al 1996, Johansson et al 1998, Marhold et al 2001).

Goals are set in three separate domains: physical, which relates to the exercise programme patients follow and sets the number of exercises to be performed or the duration of the exercise and the level of difficulty; functional/task, which relates to the achievement of functional tasks of everyday living such as housework or hobbies; and social, where patients are encouraged to set goals relating to the performance of activities in the wider social environment. It is important that goals are personally relevant, interesting, measurable and achievable. Patients will always pursue highly valued goals even in the face of increased symptoms (Affleck et al 2001) so it is important that the patient values the goals. Continued goal attainment will reinforce self-efficacy (Bandura 1977) and lead to a perception of mastery over the task or problem (such as managing to exercise despite the pain). It is therefore important that goals are set which encourage success but are sufficiently challenging to assure progress. The setting of long-term and immediate goals should be a matter of negotiation between the patient and their therapist.

Physical Exercise

Limited physical capacity in chronic pain is due to a myriad of factors (Watson 1999). Tight scar tissue or shortened soft tissues may limit movement so that certain activities become difficult and the patient starts to avoid them. Altered muscle tension, posture and muscle activity in response to an original injury may persist and be reinforced by psychological factors and habit (Main & Watson 1996, Watson et al 1997). Non-specific advice from health professionals to 'take it easy' or avoid 'heavy lifting' could lead to conscious avoidance. Fear is a great motivator of behaviour and pain related fear is associated with the avoidance of activities considered to be threatening or potentially dangerous (Vlaeyen & Linton 2000).

It has already been mentioned that there is a debate as to whether chronic pain patients are deconditioned. Most of the data on cardiovascular fitness seems to suggest that they are not (Wittink et al 2000). This might be more accurately interpreted that most healthy controls are not physically conditioned (Protas 1999). Chronic pain patients do demonstrate other signs of deconditioning in terms of reduced muscle strength performance, reduced range of motion, reduced performance in skilled motor functions and poorer proprioceptive function (Luoto et al 1996, 1999, Radebold et al 2001).

Exercise in the management of chronic pain can be divided into four components: the first three, stretching, strengthening and cardiovascular (aerobic) conditioning exercises, are components of any good exercise session, and the fourth is the practice of feared activities. Weight-resisted strengthening exercises are not contraindicated but should be introduced gradually because of the likely effect of an increase in muscle soreness.

There is no compelling evidence to date that specific exercise has any benefit over general exercise in the management of chronic pain but the consensus of opinion is that aerobic exercise and the promotion of an active lifestyle are beneficial (Faas 1996, Waddell & Burton 2000). This does not mean that specific exercises should not be undertaken where an obvious problem exists (for example obvious unilateral weakness of a painful limb), but it is only part of an activity plan. Concentrating on specific exercises should not divert the clinician from getting the patient back to normal everyday function.

Stretching and range of motion exercises

It has already been stated that chronic pain may have started with an initial injury or condition, or started insidi-

ously with or without coexisting musculoskeletal problems. Although the pain may be widespread there may be areas where the effects are greatest. Stretching exercises need to be general and comprehensive to address the general loss of flexibility, as well as specific to the individual's needs.

Motion only through a restricted range results in limitation of joint range through the shortening of joint soft tissue structures, and an impoverishment of joint nutrition. Motion through complete joint range is required to assist in the nutrition of the cartilage of synovial joints as well as in the maintenance of the length and strength of the joint capsule, ligaments and muscles (Buckwalter 1996).

There is a wide literature on the performance of stretching exercises and the physiological mechanisms will not be discussed here. There are two main schools of thought on stretching technique. These are static/sustained where the muscle is taken to its limit and the stretch is maintained for at least 5–6 seconds, although many authors suggest longer and advocate ballistic stretching where dynamic, rhythmic bouncing exercises are performed at the outer range of the muscle. Exaggerated guarding and increased myotatic stretch reflexes have been identified in those with painful muscles (Coderre et al 1993, Mense 1994). Additionally psychological factors have been demonstrated to be closely associated with abnormal patterns of muscle activity (Watson et al 1997). Such abnormalities of movement could potentially lead to ineffective stretching and, at worst, injury to the muscle, therefore the ballistic stretching technique is inadvisable. Combining the muscle relaxation skills discussed below with stretching will increase the effectiveness of the stretch.

Stretching forms part of the patient's daily routine, especially in warm-up and warm-down sessions. Goal setting will encompass increases in the length of time the stretch is maintained as well as the number of stretches performed. Patients report that introducing regular stretching into daily work and home routines, especially between different activities and after periods of static work (e.g. reading, typing), is extremely helpful.

Aerobic conditioning

The importance of aerobic conditioning in chronic pain is covered elsewhere (Protas 1999, Wittink 1999, Watson 2000). Aerobic exercise should be presented within the goal setting and pacing approaches and patients given information on how it relates to a healthy lifestyle as well as to pain management. Aerobic conditioning has demonstrated improvements in pain distribution, experimental pain testing, depression, physical capacity and self-efficacy (Burckhardt et al 1994, Wigers et al 1996, Haldorsen et al 1998). The reported relationship between improvements in physical capacity/fitness and reductions in self-reported disability is mixed. Some have found no association between physical improvement and reduced disability (Jensen et al

1994, Hildebrandt et al 1997). Where an association is found it has only explained a small amount of the variance for improvement (Burns et al 1998). The contribution of improvement in physical function is so often overshadowed by the importance of changes in psychosocial factors.

It would appear that engagement in activity improves the patient's self-efficacy, their confidence in performing physical activities, and this acts as a mediating variable in changing disability. Physical activity must enable patients to feel a sense of achievement (hence the importance of goal setting). Increasing physical activity without a sense of personally relevant achievement is unlikely to lead to a change in reported function.

Practising feared movements

It seems logical that the way one improves or returns to an activity is to do it and practise until the required performance is achieved. Many 'rehabilitation' approaches do not seem to have understood this, have forgotten it or have been seduced by new 'fix-all' exercise prescriptions. It seems a vague hope that improved function can be brought about by sole adherence to a series of abstract exercises. Few people get pleasure out of exercise for exercise's sake. Waddell (1998) reminds us that active exercise is not the same as active rehabilitation. Specific exercises that are remote from the activities the patient needs to do in daily life are likely to be less effective than specific management. Patients must practise the type of activities they find difficult, and particularly those they are afraid to do.

In a series of single case experiments Vlaeyen et al (2001) have demonstrated that a graded exposure technique where subjects repeatedly practise feared movements can be successful in improving the outcome of treatment over and above the effects of graded non-specific exercise. Subjects were required to identify and grade exercises they were worried about or that they feared would increase their pain or cause damage. These exercises were then practised starting with the least feared and progressing onto the most feared. Feedback on performance was given with positive reinforcement to challenge fears. However, it is not clear if reducing fear of one specific activity generalizes to other feared activities (Crombez et al 2002, Goubert et al 2002). Neither has the research demonstrated that patients will adhere to or become adept at practising feared movements without close supervision. Despite these concerns it would appear logical to include the identification and performance of feared movements in rehabilitation.

Exercise adherence

Most exercise programmes have reported a reduction in exercise adherence following completion (Lewthwaite 1990, Proschaska & Marcus 1994). Wigers and colleagues (1996) found that 73% of patients failed to continue an exer-

cise programme when followed up although 83% felt they would have been better if they had done so.

Continuance with exercise is more likely if the individual finds it interesting and rewarding. Exercising in a gym may not be suitable for all. Some may not have access to such facilities; others may not be motivated by this form of exercise. Developing activities that are patient- and family-orientated and can be integrated into the normal daily routine will help to improve adherence with exercise. Exercise should be part of life not an intrusion into it. Encouraging patients to investigate local swimming or walking groups is one way to foster social links and may lead to improved exercise adherence after contact has finished.

Reducing pain behaviour

Pain behaviours are 'all outputs of the individual that a reasonable observer would characterise as suggesting pain' (Loeser & Fordyce 1983). Most commonly these are verbal complaints, altered posture and movements and deviation from normal behaviour (lying down and/or resting for long periods). Patients are relatively unaware of their demonstration of such behaviour and the effects that it has on other people. Pain behaviours are closely associated not only to pain intensity, but also to fear of pain accompanying activity, low self-efficacy and psychological distress (Keefe & Block 1982, Waddell 1992, Bucklew et al 1994, Watson & Poulter 1997).

The most florid pain behaviour is often demonstrated during exercise sessions. Operant behavioural theories suggest that the physiotherapist should ignore all pain behaviours and recognize only well behaviours and improved function (Fordyce 1976). This may not be as productive as is often claimed. Well behaviours and achievements should be acknowledged, but simply ignoring pain behaviour without explanation can be counterproductive. An explanation by the clinician to the individual or the group that all are attending for a significant pain problem is helpful. The clinician can then acknowledge their difficulties with this chronic pain, but that the focus will be on what is attempted *despite* the pain, rather than responding to demonstrations of pain. The clinician needs to make sure the patient understands that they believe the reality of their pain but, although they might ask them to do things that are uncomfortable, they will never ask the patient to do things that could result in injury.

As mentioned above, family and partners often respond to pain behaviours in a solicitous manner and in doing so unwittingly reinforce the behaviour. This is rarely overt manipulation by patients. Asking patients and partners to identify the behaviours and their responses to them is a useful way of demonstrating the interaction between the expectation of pain, beliefs about pain and their own reactions. Video recording patients during standardized tasks is an established method of recording pain behaviours (Keefe & Block 1982, Watson & Poulter 1997). Patients are often unaware of their pain behaviour so video recording of patients, especially when performing tasks and interacting with others, is a useful way of providing feedback on their pain behaviour. From this discussion we can identify how the behaviour might be counterproductive and how it might be changed (Watson & Parker 2000).

Relaxation

Suffering chronic pain is a stressful experience and patients often report feeling under stress from factors associated with the pain (poor family relations, guilt, anxiety) and have difficulty in truly relaxing despite feeling fatigued. In addition, people who have muscle pain may increase their muscle tension in response to pain, which may also contribute to pain (Flor & Turk 1989, Watson et al 1998b, Watson 2002). To help counter this, relaxation is included in many pain management programmes. There is evidence that relaxation can be effective in managing pain in those individuals who can master the technique (NIH Technology Assessment 1996) although some have pointed out that relaxation is rarely used in isolation from other cognitive techniques so it is difficult to evaluate the effect (Arena & Blanchard 1996).

There are a number of approaches to relaxation: patients may have to try more than one until they find the most effective for them in the various situations where relaxation is necessary. The deep methods relaxed imagery, autogenic relaxation and progressive muscular relaxation are usually done during a period of time set aside for relaxation. The brief methods (diaphragmatic breathing and modified progressive muscular relaxation) are often done during the day when the patient feels themselves becoming tense.

In relaxed imagery relaxation patients imagine a peaceful and relaxing scene. They may choose, for instance, walking through a forest or lying in warm sunshine with the pleasant sounds, scents, feelings and associations that can accompany these activities. The purpose of this is to choose an image that they can access readily and rehearse until they are able to bring the image to mind within a few minutes of beginning the relaxation. Imagery is idiosyncratic and patients have to develop their own strategy with the help of the clinician.

With autogenic relaxation, patients concentrate on a phrase and repeat it quietly to themselves while developing a feeling of calmness. Once again, it is useful if patients develop their own phrases but there are lists of standardized phrases for patients to practise this technique (Blanchard & Andrasik 1985).

Many people will be familiar with progressive muscular relaxation (PMR) in which muscle tension is reduced through tension and relaxation in each of 15 major muscle groups in turn (Jacobsen 1929). Deep diaphragmatic breathing is another very useful technique, and one that is easily incorporated into the techniques above. Many patients with chronic pain breathe rapidly and typically utilize primarily the upper chest during the breathing cycle. Using slow controlled diaphragmatic breathing, patients learn to reduce their breathing rate progressively until they reach a rate of about 6–8 breaths per minute.

Although the effectiveness of relaxation or breathing control as a therapy may be limited in some individuals, it is almost always used as an adjunct to other techniques and it does give patients a sense of control over their body and over their pain. This sense of control is important for giving them a feeling of optimism that they can use and for the development of self-management strategies. For the rehabilitation clinician, a combination of relaxation and stretching might make a more effective combination than stretching alone.

Sleep management

Poor sleep is a very common feature of chronic pain and is implicated in the development and maintenance of muscle tenderness (Wolfe et al 1990, Moldofsky 1993, White et al 1999). Medication may help but is rarely sufficient as poor sleep is a consequence of a combination of factors. Advice on sleep management and good sleep hygiene is important. The success of a sleep programme is evaluated by the use of sleep diaries or standardized questionnaires (for example the Pittsburgh Sleep Quality Index, Buysse et al 1989).

Specific management of insomnia secondary to chronic pain using CBT alone has had some success (Currie et al 2000, 2002) although the improvements that have been reported have been criticized for not being clinically important (NIH Technology Assessment 1996). However, those who improve their sleep demonstrate decreases in distress and pain associated disability (Currie et al 2002).

Sleep hygiene management involves making the patient aware of the habits they have which are not conducive to successful sleep and to try and change them (Buysse & Perlis 1996, Perlis et al 2001). These involve avoiding stimulants (caffeine, smoking, alcohol and some proprietary pain killing or cold remedies), avoiding excessive intake of liquid for some hours before sleep and appropriate timing of analgesic medication. Patients are told to stay in bed only when asleep and to restrict the time in bed if they are not sleeping. They should get up and go to another room and read or perform routine tasks until they feel sleepy then return to bed. They should only use the bed for sleep or sex.

Sleep hygiene and relaxation are combined for best effect but patients must also be taught how to refrain from reacting to intrusive negative or worrying thoughts. In one experiment negative thoughts and rumination about pain and disability were associated with difficulty in getting to sleep (Smith et al 2001), whereas pain report was negatively correlated with the length of time from falling to sleep to reawakening.

Relapse self-management

It is almost inevitable that chronic pain patients will, at some stage, experience a flare-up of pain. According to

Croft et al (1998), two-thirds of people with long-standing back pain continued to have pain a year later, and the other third go on to have intermittent pain. Of those who reported intermittent pain, more than half had a second bout of pain within a year. Nearly 75% of those with a first onset of back pain still reported symptoms a year later. So, it is valuable that chronic pain patients recognize and then prepare for the situations that might make them prone to relapse. Furthermore, patients are just as prey to strains, pulled muscles and injuries as the rest of the population once they become active.

The first approach is to reassure patients that the increase in pain is not a sign of a worsening of the condition or an inevitable decline, but that it is part of the natural variation in the pain pattern as occurs with all chronic diseases. An increase in pain should not be taken by patients as failure or evidence of an inability to manage their own condition. It is a challenge to their self-management not the end of it. Reassurance on these points and getting patients to identify how successful they have been thus far can help 'rescue' patients at this stage. Catastrophizing about the ability to cope and about the future may be an initial reaction to a flare-up of symptoms, which could result in return to a passive coping strategy. It is important this is prevented (Watson & Spanswick 2000).

Relapse may not be entirely caused by an individual physical event. The build up of daily stresses may produce challenges to their daily coping resources and their ability to manage their pain. Differentiating what is a new pain, associated with new pathology, and their usual chronic pain is essential as this will determine the need to consult (Watson & Spanswick 2000). New symptoms indicative of new pathology is not common in chronic simple low back pain but must be investigated accordingly.

Keefe & van Horn (1993) suggest that relapse planning is an essential part of management of chronic pain and should encompass a number of key areas:

- the planning and practising of coping strategies in 'high risk' situations
- identification of early warning signs of relapse (for example fatigue, low mood, pain)
- planning for responding to early signs of relapse
- review of improvement to date ('reality check' on progress so far)
- self-reinforcement for successful coping with relapse.

The development of an 'emergency card' in collaboration with their family and partner can be useful in these situations. This is a written plan of how they will deal with increases in pain and/or new pathology. An emergency strategy should include:

- criteria for further consultation
- short-term medication usage
- review of pacing
- plan to return to normal activities as soon as possible.

This of course cannot cover all eventualities but helps patients to retain a feeling of control. Support from the family or significant others is essential during a relapse when the patient might react more emotionally than logically.

From time to time practitioners may encounter patients who have developed a good self-management strategy, but who turn to the practitioner in times of increased pain for help with symptom management. If any specific treatment is clearly indicated (e.g. manipulation, mobilizations, trigger point therapy) it must be time limited and should be presented to patients as a short-term measure to assist them over the crisis, and to support them in getting back on track with their self-management programme. Symptomatic relief must support self-management not threaten it. Self-management is the primary component of chronic pain management and the management of symptoms, however skilled, is complementary to this.

The management of chronic pain problems is complex and cannot be achieved overnight. We all like to treat patients who get better in a few simple treatments using our hands-on skills. But not all patients will be so uncomplicated. If a person has had pain for many years and is severely incapacitated we will not be able to completely resolve their symptoms very often in a few simple treatments. The contact with the patient needs to be over a longer period of time, although this might not mean more contact sessions, but regular reappraisal of goals and progress with education and guidance over many months. Helping people live well despite their pain is a strange concept for some clinicians to accept, but for a minority of patients complete cure is not yet an option. Helping people to get the most from life takes a different set of skills, which are just as rewarding to use as our more traditional skills as clinicians.

KEYWORDS	
biopsychosocial	fear avoidance
pain management	depression
physical activity	rehabilitation
psychological	pacing
coping strategies	

References

Affleck G, Tennen H, Zautra A, Urrows S, Abeles M, Karoly P 2001 Women's pursuit of personal goals in daily life with fibromyalgia: a value-expectancy analysis. Journal of Consulting and Clinical Psychology 69: 587–596

Arena J G, Blanchard E B 1996 Biofeedback and relaxation therapy for chronic pain disorders. In: Gatchel R J, Turk D C (eds) Psychological approaches to pain management. Guilford Press, New York, pp 179–230

Atlas S J, Deyo R A, Keller R B et al 1996 The Maine lumbar spine study. 2: 1-year outcomes of surgical and non-surgical management of sciatica. Spine 21: 1777–1786

Atlas S J, Keller R B, Robson D, Deyo R A, Singer D E 2000 Surgical and nonsurgical management of lumbar spinal stenosis: four-year outcomes from the Maine lumbar spine study. Spine 25: 556–562

Averill P M, Novy D M, Nelson D V, Berry L A 1996 Correlates of depression in chronic pain patients: a comprehensive examination. Pain 65: 93–100

Bandura A 1977 Self-efficacy: towards a unifying theory of behavioral change. Psychological Review 84: 191–215

Bennett R M 1996 Multidisciplinary group treatment programmes to treat fibromyalgia patients. Rheumatic Disease Clinics of North America 22: 351–367

Bigos S J, Battie M C, Spengler D M et al 1991 A prospective study of work perceptions and psychosocial factors affecting the report of back injury. Spine 16: 1–6

Bigos S, Bower O, Braen G et al 1994 Acute back problems in adults. Clinical practice guideline no. 14. AHCPR publication no. 95-0642. Agency For Health Care Policy And Research, Rockville, Maryland

Blanchard E B, Andrasik F 1985 Management of chronic headache: a psychological approach. Pergamon Press, New York

Bongers P M, de Winter C R, Kompier M A J, Hildebrandt V H 1993 Psychosocial factors at work and musculoskeletal disease. Scandinavian Journal of Work and Environmental Health 19: 297–312

Bradley L A 1996 Cognitive therapy for chronic pain. In: Gatchel R J, Turk D C (eds) Psychological approaches to pain management. Guilford Press, New York, pp 131–147

Brown G K, Nicassio P M 1987 Development of a questionnaire for the assessment of active and passive coping strategies in chronic pain patients. Pain 31: 53–64

Buchbinder R, Jolley D, Wyatt M 2001 Population based intervention to change back pain beliefs and disability: three part evaluation. British Medical Journal 322: 1516–1520

Bucklew S P, Parker J C, Keefe F J 1994 Self-efficacy and pain behavior among subjects with fibromyalgia. Pain 59: 377–384

Buckwalter J A 1996 Effects of early motion on healing of musculoskeletal tissues. Hand Clinics 12: 13–24

Burckhardt C S, Mannerkopi K, Hedenberg L, Bjelle A 1994 A randomised controlled trial of education and physical training for women with fibromyalgia. Journal of Rheumatology 21: 714–720

Burns J W, Johnson B J, Mahoney N, Devine J, Pawl R 1998 Cognitive and physical capacity process variables predict long-term outcome after treatment of chronic pain. Journal Of Consulting and Clinical Psychology 66: 434–439

Burton A K, Tillotson K M, Main C J, Hollis S 1995 Psychological predictors of outcome in acute and sub-chronic low back trouble. Spine 20: 722–728

Buysse D J, Perlis M L 1996 The evaluation and treatment of insomnia. Journal of Psychology and Behavioural Health (March): 80–93

Buysse D J, Reynolds C F, Berman S R, Kupfer D J 1989 The Pittsburgh Sleep Quality Index: a new instrument for psychiatric practice and research. Psychiatry Research. 28: 193–213

Cats-Baril W L, Frymoyer J W 1991 Identifying patients at risk of becoming disabled because of low-back pain: the Vermont Rehabilitation Engineering Center predictive model. Spine 16: 605–607

Clinical Standards Advisory Group 1994 Back pain: report of a CSAG committee on back pain. HMSO, London, pp 1–89

Coderre J T, Katz J, Vaccarino A L, Melzack R 1993 Contribution of central neuroplasticity to pathological pain: review of clinical and experimental evidence. Pain 52: 259–285

Crisson J E, Keefe F J 1988 The relationship of locus of control to pain coping strategies and psychological distress in chronic pain patients. Pain 35: 147–154

Croft P R, Papageorgiou A C, Ferry S, Thomas E, Jayson M I, Silman A J 1995 Psychologic distress and low back pain: evidence from a prospective study in the general population. Spine 20: 2731–2737

Croft P R, Macfarlane G J, Papageorgiou A C, Thomas E, Silman A J 1998 Outcome of low back pain in general practice: a prospective study. British Medical Journal 316: 1356–1359

Crombez G, Vlaeyen J W S, Lysens R, Eccleston C, Vansteenwegen D, Eelen P 2002 Exposure to physical movements in low back pain patients: restricted effects of generalisation. Health Psychology 21(6): 573–578

Currie S R, Wilson K G, Pontefract A M, deLaplante L 2000 Cognitive behavioral treatment of insomnia secondary to chronic pain. Journal of Consulting and Clinical Psychology 68: 407–416

Currie S R, Wilson K G, Curran D 2002 Clinical significance and predictors of treatment response to cognitive behavior therapy for insomnia secondary to chronic pain. Journal of Behavioural Medicine 25: 135–153

Daltroy L H, Iversen M D, Larson M G et al 1997 A controlled trial of an educational program to prevent low back injuries. New England Journal of Medicine 337: 322–328

DeGood D E, Shutty M S 1992 Assessment of pain beliefs, coping and self efficacy. In: Turk D C, Melzack R (eds) Handbook of pain assessment. Guilford Press, New York, p 221

Dzioba R D, Doxey N C 1984 A prospective investigation into the orthopaedic and psychological predictors of outcome of first lumbar surgery following industrial injury. Spine 9: 614–623

Engel G L 1962 Psychological development in health and disease. Saunders, Philadelphia

Faas A 1996 Exercises: which ones are worth trying, for which patients, and when? Spine 21: 2874–2879

Feuerstein M, Zastowny T R 1996 Occupational rehabilitation: multidisciplinary management of work related musculoskeletal pain and disability. In: Gatchel R J, Turk D C (eds) Psychological approaches to pain management. Guilford Press, New York, pp 458–585

Fishbain D A, Rosomoff H L, Cutler R B, Rosomoff R S 1995 Secondary gain concept: a review of the scientific evidence. Clinical Journal of Pain 11: 6–21

Flor H, Turk D C 1989 Psychophysiology of chronic pain: do chronic pain patients exhibit symptom-specific psychophysiological responses? Psychological Bulletin 105: 215–259

Fordyce W E 1976 Behavioural methods for chronic pain and illness. Mosby, St Louis

Fritz J M, Wainner R S, Hicks G E 2000 The use of nonorganic signs and symptoms as a screening tool for return-to-work in patients with acute low back pain. Spine 25: 1925–1931

Frost H, Klaber Moffett J A, Moser J S, Fairbank J C 1995 Randomised controlled trial for evaluation of fitness programme for patients with chronic low back pain. British Medical Journal 310: 151–154

Frost H, Lamb S E, Klaber Moffett J A, Fairbank J C, Moser J S 1998 A fitness programme for patients with chronic low back pain: 2-year follow-up of a randomised controlled trial. Pain 75: 273–279

Gallagher R M, Williams R A, Skelly J, et al 1995 Workers compensation and return to work in low back pain Pain 6: 299–307

Gatchel R J, Gardea M A 1999 Psychosocial issues: their importance in predicting response to treatment and search for compensation. Neurological Clinics of North America 17: 149–166

Geisser M E, Roth R S, Robinson M E 1997 Assessing depression among persons with chronic pain using the centre for epidemiological studies-depression scale and the beck depression inventory: a comparative analysis. Clinical Journal of Pain 13: 163–170

Geisser M E, Roth R S, Theisen M E, Robinson M E, Riley J L 2000 Negative affect, self-report of depressive symptoms and clinical depression: relation to the experience of chronic pain. Clinical Journal of Pain 16: 110–120

Gil K M, Ross S L, Keefe F J 1988 Behavioural treatment of chronic pain: four pain management protocols. In: France R D, Krishnan K R R (eds) Chronic pain. American Psychiatric Press, Washington, pp 317–413

Goubert L, Francken G, Crombez G, Vansteenwegen D, Lysens R 2002 Exposure to physical movement in chronic back pain patients: no evidence for generalization across movements. Behaviour Research and Therapy 40: 415–429

Greenough C G 1993 Recovery from low back pain: 1–5 year follow-up of 287 injury-related cases. Acta Orthopaedica Scandinavica Supplement 254: 1–34

Greenough C G, Fraser R D 1989 The effects of compensation on recovery from low-back injury. Spine 14: 947–955

Greenough C G Fraser R D 1992 Assessment of outcome in patients with low-back pain. Spine 17: 36–41

Guzman J, Esmail R, Karjalainen K, Malmivaara A, Irvin E, Bombardier C 2002 Multidisciplinary biopsychosocial rehabilitation for chronic low back pain. Cochrane Database of Systematic Reviews (1): CD000963

Hadler N M 1996 If you have to prove you are ill, you can't get well. Spine 21: 2397–2400

Hadler N M 1997 Fibromyalgia, chronic fatigue, and other iatrogenic diagnostic algorithms: do some labels escalate illness in vulnerable patients? Postgraduate Medicine 165: 161–162

Hadler N M, Carey T S, Garrett J 1995 The influence of indemnification by workers' compensation insurance on recovery from acute backache: North Carolina back pain project. Spine 20: 2710–2715

Haldorsen E M, Kronholm K, Skouen J S, Ursin H 1998 Multimodal cognitive behavioral treatment of patients sicklisted for musculoskeletal pain: a randomized controlled study. Scandinavian Journal of Rheumatology 27: 16–25

Halpern M 1992 Prevention of low back pain: basic ergonomics in the workplace and the clinic. Bailliere's Clinical Rheumatology 6: 705–730

Hansen F R, Biering-Sorensen F, Schuffel W 1995 Minnesota Multiphasic Personality Inventory in persons with or without low back pain: a 20 years follow up study. Spine 20: 2716–2720

Hassenbring M, Marienfeld G, Kuhlendahl D, Soyka D 1994 Risk factors of chronicity in lumbar disc patients: a prospective investigation of biologic, psychologic and social predictors of therapy outcome. Spine 19: 2759–2765

Hazard R G, Reid S, Haugh L D, McFarlane G 2000 A controlled trial of an educational pamphlet to prevent disability after occupational low back injury. Spine 25: 1419–1423

Hildebrandt J, Pfingsten M, Saur P, Jansen J 1997 Prediction of success from a multidisciplinary treatment program for chronic low back pain. Spine 22: 990–1001

Jacobsen E 1929 Progressive relaxation. University of Chicago Press, Chicago

Jensen M P, Turner J A, Romano J M 1994 Correlates of improvement in multidisciplinary treatment of chronic pain. Journal of Consulting and Clinical Psychology 62: 172–179

Johansson C, Dahl J, Jannert M, Melin L, Andersson G 1998 Effects of a cognitive-behavioral pain-management program. Behaviour Research and Therapy 36: 915–930

Keefe F J, Block A R 1982 Development of an observational methods for assessing pain behaviour in chronic low back pain. Behavior Therapy 13: 363–375

Keefe F J, Dunsmore J 1992 Pain behaviour: concepts and controversies. American Pain Society Journal 1: 92–100

Keefe F J, van Horn Y 1993 Cognitive-behavioural treatment of rheumatoid arthritis: maintaining gains. Arthritis Care and Research 6: 213–222

Keefe F J, Beaupre P M, Gil K M 1996 Group therapy for patients with chronic pain. In: Gatchel R J, Turk D C (eds) Psychological approaches to pain management. Guilford Press, New York

Kendall N A S, Linton S J, Main C J 1997 Guide to assessing psychosocial yellow flags in acute low back pain: risk factors for long-term disability and workloss. Accident Rehabilitation and Compensation Insurance Corporation of New Zealand and the National Health Committee, Ministry of Health. Wellington

Klaber-Moffett J, Torgerson D, Bell-Sayer S, et al 1999 Exercise for low back pain: clinical outcomes, costs and preferences. British Medical Journal 319: 279–283

Klenerman L, Slade P D, Stanley I M, et al 1995 The prediction of chronicity in patients with an acute attack of low back pain in a general practice setting. Spine 20: 478–484

Kummel B M 1996 Nonorganic signs of significance in low back pain. Spine 21: 1077–1081

Lancourt J, Kettelhut M 1992 Predicting return to work for lower back pain patients receiving worker's compensation. Spine 17: 629–640

Lazarus R S, Folkman S 1984 Stress, appraisal and coping, Springer, New York

Lethem J, Slade P D, Troup J D G, Bentley G 1983 Outline of a fear-avoidance model of exaggerated pain perception. Behavioral Research and Therapy 21: 401–408

Lewthwaite R 1990 Motivational considerations in physical therapy involvement. Physical Therapy 70: 808–819

Ley P, Llewelyn S 1995 Improving patients' understanding, recall, satisfaction and compliance. In: Broome A, Llewelyn S (eds) Health psychology: processes and applications. Chapman and Hall, London, pp 75–98

Linton S J 2000 A review of psychological risk factors in back and neck pain. Spine 25: 1148–1156

Loeser J D 1980 Perspective on pain. In: Turner P (ed) Proceedings of the First World Congress on Clinical Pharmacology and Therapeutics. Macmillan, London, pp 316–326

Loeser J D 1996 Mitigating the dangers of pursuing cure. In: Cohen M J M, Campbell J N, (eds). Progress in Pain Management. Pain treatment centers at a crossroads: a practical and conceptual reappraisal. IASP Press, Seattle, vol 7, pp 101–108

Loeser J D, Fordyce W E 1983 Chronic pain. In: Carr J E, Dengerik H A Behavioural science in the practice of medicine. Elsevier, Amsterdam

Loeser J D, Sullivan M 1995 Disability in the chronic low back pain patient may be iatrogenic. Pain Forum 4: 114–121

Loeser J D, Sullivan M 1997 Doctors, diagnosis, and disability: a disastrous diversion. Clinical Orthopaedics and Related Research 336: 61–66

Luoto S, Taimela S, Hurri H, Aalto H, Pyykko I, Alaranta H 1996 Psychomotor speed and postural control in chronic low back pain patients a controlled follow-up study. Spine 21: 2621–2627

Luoto S, Taimela S, Hurri H, Alaranta H 1999 Mechanisms explaining the association between low back trouble and deficits in information processing: a controlled study with follow-up. Spine 24: 255–261

Main C J 1983 The Modified Somatic Perception Questionnaire (MSPQ). Journal of Psychosomatic Research 27: 503–514

Main C J, Spanswick C C 1995 'Functional overlay', and illness behaviour in chronic pain: distress or malingering? Conceptual difficulties in medico-legal assessment of personal injury claims. Journal of Psychosomatic Research 39: 737–753

Main C J, Waddell G 1991 A comparison of cognitive measures in low back pain: statistical structure and clinical validity at initial assessment. Pain 46: 287–298

Main C J, Waddell G 1998 Behavioral responses to examination: a reappraisal of the interpretation of 'nonorganic signs'. Spine 23: 2367–2371

Main C J, Watson P J 1996 Guarded movements: development of chronicity. Journal of Musculoskeletal Pain 4(4): 163–170

Main C J, Watson P J 1999 Psychological aspects of pain. Manual Therapy 4: 203–215

Main C J, Watson P J 2002 The distressed and angry low back pain patient. In: Gifford L (ed) Topical issues in pain. CNS Press, Falmouth, vol 3, part 2, pp 175–200

Main C J, Wood P L, Hollis S, Spanswick C C, Waddell G 1992 The distress and risk assessment method: a simple patient classification to identify distress and evaluate the risk of poor outcome. Spine 22: 42–52

Main C J, Spanswick C C, Watson P J 2000 The nature of disability. In: Main C J, Spanswick C C (eds) Pain management: an interdisciplinary approach. Churchill Livingstone, Edinburgh, pp 89–106

Marhold C, Linton S J, Melin L 2001 A cognitive-behavioral return-to-work program: effects on pain patients with a history of long-term versus short-term sick leave. Pain 91: 155–163

Melzack R, Wall P D 1965 Pain mechanisms: a new theory. Science 150: 971–979

Mense S 1994 Referral of muscle pain: new aspects. American Pain Society Journal 3: 1–9

Moldofsky H 1993 Fibromyalgia, sleep disorder and chronic fatigue syndrome. In: Block G R, Whelen J (eds) Chronic fatigue syndrome. Wiley, Chichester, pp 262–279

Morley S, Eccleston C, Williams A 1999 Systematic review and meta-analysis of randomized controlled trials of cognitive behaviour therapy and behaviour therapy for chronic pain in adults, excluding headache. Pain 80: 1–13

Moseley G L 2004 Evidence of a direct relationship between cognitive and physical change during an education intervention in people with chronic low back pain. European Journal of Pain: 39–45

Nachemson A 1992 Newest knowledge of low back pain: a critical look. Clinical Orthopaedics and Related Research 279: 8–20

Nachemson A, Waddell G, Norlund A I 2000 Epidemiology of neck and low back pain. In: Nachemson A, Jonsson E (eds) Neck and back pain: the scientific evidence of causes, diagnosis and treatment. Lippincott, Williams and Wilkins, New York, pp 165–188

NIH Technology Assessment 1996 Integration of behavioral and relaxation approaches into the treatment of chronic pain and insomnia. NIH Technology Assessment Panel on Integration of Behavioral and Relaxation Approaches into the Treatment of Chronic Pain and Insomnia. Journal of the American Medical Association 276: 313–318

Ohlund C, Lindstrom I, Areskoug B, Eek C, Peterson L E, Nachemson A 1994 Pain behavior in industrial subacute low back pain. I: Reliability: concurrent and predictive validity of pain behavior assessments. Pain 58: 201–209

Palinkas L A, Kabongo M L, San Diego Unified Practice Research in Family Medicine Network 2000 The use of complementary and alternative medicine by primary care patients: a surf net study. Journal of Family Practice 49: 1121–1130

Papageorgiou A C, Macfarlane G J, Thomas E, Croft P R, Jayson M I, Silman A J 1997 Psychosocial factors in the workplace: do they predict new episodes of low back pain? Evidence from the South Manchester Back Pain Study. Spine 22: 1137–1142

Perlis M L, Sharpe M, Smith M T, Greenblatt D, Giles D 2001 Behavioural treatment of insomnia: treatment outcome and the relevance of medical and psychiatric morbidity. Journal of Behavioural Medicine 24: 281–296

Price J, Leaver L 2002 ABC of psychological medicine: beginning treatment. British Medical Journal 325: 33–35

Proschaska J O, Marcus B H 1994 The transtheoretical model: applications to exercise. In: Dishman R K (ed) Advances in exercise adherence. Human Kinetics, New York, pp 161–180

Protas E J 1999 Physical activity and low back pain. In: Max M (ed) Pain 1999: an updated review. IASP Press, Seattle, pp 145–151

Radebold A, Cholewicki J, Polzhofer G K, Greene H S 2001 Impaired postural control of the lumbar spine is associated with delayed muscle response times in patients with chronic idiopathic low back pain. Spine 26: 724–730

Rainville J, Sobel J, Hartigan C, Monlux G, Bean J 1997 Decreasing disability in chronic back pain through aggressive spine rehabilitation. Journal of Rehabilitation Research and Development 34: 383–393

Richards J S, Nepomuceno C, Riles M, Suer Z 1982 Assessing pain behaviour: the UAB pain behavior scale. Pain 12: 393–398

Rohling M L, Binder L M, Langhinrichsen-Rohling J 1995 Money matters: a meta-analytical review of the association between financial compensation and the experience and treatment of chronic pain. Health Psychology 14: 537–547

Rose M J, Klenerman L, Atchison L, Slade P D 1992 An application of the fear avoidance model to three chronic pain problems. Behaviour Research and Therapy 30: 359–365

Rose M J, Reilly J P, Slade P D, Dewey M 1995 A comparative analysis of psychological and physical models of low back pain experience. Physiotherapy 81: 710–716

Rosenstiel A K, Keefe F J 1993 The use of coping strategies in chronic low back pain patients: relationship to patient characteristics and current adjustment. Pain 17: 33–44

Royal College of General Practitioners 1996 Clinical guidelines for the management of acute low back pain. Royal College of General Practitioners, London

Smith B, Chambers W, Smith W 1996 Chronic pain: time for epidemiology. Journal of the Royal Society of Medicine 89: 181–183

Smith M T, Perlis M L, Carmody T P, Smith M S, Giles D E 2001 Presleep cognitions in patients with insomnia secondary to chronic pain. Journal of Behavioral Medicine 24: 93–114

Sobel J B, Sollenberger P, Robinson R, Polatin P B, Gatchel R J 2000 Cervical nonorganic signs: a new clinical tool to assess abnormal illness behavior in neck pain patients: a pilot study. Archives of Physical Medicine and Rehabilitation 81: 170–175

Spanswick C C, Main C J 2000 Clinical decision making. In: Main C J, Spanswick C C (eds) Pain management: an interdisciplinary approach. Churchill Livingstone, Edinburgh, pp 233–254

Symonds T L, Burton A K, Tillotson K M, Main C J 1995 Absence resulting from low back trouble can be reduced by psychosocial intervention at the work place. Spine 20: 2738–2745

Thomas E, Silman A J, Croft P R, Papageorgiou A C, Jayson M I, Macfarlane G J 1999 Predicting who develops chronic low back pain in primary care: a prospective study. British Medical Journal 318: 1662–1667

Turk D C, Michenbaum D H, Genest M 1983 Pain and behavioural medicine: a cognitive behavioural perspective. Guilford Press, New York

Turk D C, Okifuji A, Sinclair J D, Starz T W 1996 Pain, disability, and physical functioning in subgroups of patients with fibromyalgia. Journal of Rheumatology 23: 1255–1262

Van Tulder M W, Ostelo R, Vlaeyen J W S, Linton S J, Morley S J, Assendelft W J J 2000 Behavioural treatments for chronic low back pain. Cochrane Database Systematic Reviews (2): CD000335

Vlaeyen J W S, Linton S J 2000 Fear avoidance and its consequence in chronic musculoskeletal pain: state of the art. Pain 85: 317–332

Vlaeyen J W S, Kole-Snijders A M J, Boeren R G B, van Eek H 1995a Fear of movement/(re)injury in chronic low back pain and its relation to behavioural performance. Pain 62: 363–372

Vlaeyen J W S, Kole-Snijders A M J, Rotteveel A M, Ruesink R, Heuts P H T G 1995b The role of fear of movement/(re)injury in pain disability. Journal of Occupational Rehabilitation 5: 235–252

Vlaeyen J W S, de Jong J, Geilen M, Heuts P H T G, van Breukelen G 2001 Graded exposure in vivo in the treatment of pain related fear: a replicated single case experimental design in four patients with chronic low back pain. Behaviour Research and Therapy 39: 151–166

Volinn E, Van Koevering D, Loeser J D 1991 Back sprain in industry: the role of socioeconomic factors in chronicity. Spine 16: 542–548

Von Korff M, Saunders K 1996 The course of back pain in primary care. Spine 21: 2833–2837

Von Korff M, Le Resche L, Dworkin S F 1993 First onset of common pain symptoms: a prospective study of depression as a risk factor. Pain 55: 251–258

Waddell G 1987 A new clinical model for the treatment of low-back pain. Spine 12: 632–644

Waddell G 1992 Biopsychosocial analysis of low back pain. Bailliere's Clinical Rheumatology 6: 523–557

Waddell G 1998 The back pain revolution. Churchill Livingstone, Edinburgh

Waddell G, Burton A K 2000 Occupational health guidelines for the management of low back pain at work: evidence review. Faculty of Occupational Medicine, London

Waddell G, McCulloch J A, Kummel E, Venner R M 1980 Nonorganic physical signs in low-back pain. Spine 5: 117–125

Waddell G, Main C J, Morris E W, Di Paola M, Gray I C M 1984 Chronic low-back pain, psychologic distress, and illness behaviour. Spine 9: 209–213

Waddell G, Newton M, Henderson I, Somerville D, Main C J 1993 A Fear-Avoidance Beliefs Questionnaire (FABQ) and the role of fear-avoidance beliefs in chronic low back pain and disability. Pain 52: 157–168

Waddell G, Burton A K, Main C J 2003 Screening for risk of a long-term incapacity: a conceptual and scientific review. Royal Society of Medicine Press, London

Watson P J 1999 Non-physiological determinant of physical performance in musculoskeletal pain. In: Max M (ed) Pain 1999: an updated review. IASP Press, Seattle, pp 153–158

Watson P J 2000 The pain management programme: physical activities programme content. In: Main C J, Spanswick C C (eds) Pain management: an interdisciplinary approach. Churchill Livingstone, Edinburgh, pp 285–301

Watson P J 2002 Psychophysiological models of pain. In: Gifford L (ed) Topical issues in pain. CNS Press, Falmouth, vol 4, pp 181–198

Watson P J 2003 Interdisciplinary pain management in fibromyalgia. In: Chaitow L (ed) Fibromyalgia: a practitioner's guide to treatment. Harcourt, Edinburgh, ch 7, pp 129–147

Watson P J, Kendall N A S 2000 Assessing psychosocial yellow flags. In: Gifford L (ed) Topical issues in pain. CNS Press, Falmouth, vol 2, pp 111–130

Watson P J, Main C J 2004 The influence of benefit type on presenting characteristics and outcome from an occupationally orientated rehabilitation programme for unemployed people with chronic low back pain. Physiotherapy 90: 4–11

Watson P J, Parker H 2000 Assessment of pain, disability and physical function in pain management. In: Main C J, Spanswick C C (eds) Pain management: an interdisciplinary approach. Churchill Livingstone, Edinburgh, pp 163–183

Watson P J, Poulter M E 1997 The development of a functional task orientated measure of pain behaviour in chronic low back pain patients. Journal of Back and Musculoskeletal Rehabilitation 9: 57–59

Watson P J, Spanswick C C 2000 Maintenance of change and skill enhancement. In: Main C J, Spanswick C C (eds) Pain management: an interdisciplinary approach. Churchill Livingstone, Edinburgh, pp 321–333

Watson P J, Booker C K, Main C J 1997 Evidence for the role of psychological factors in abnormal paraspinal activity in patients with chronic low back pain. Journal of Musculoskeletal Pain 5: 41–56

Watson P J, Main C J, Waddell G, Gales T F, Purcell Jones G 1998a Medically certified work loss, recurrence and costs of wage compensation for back pain: a follow-up study of the working population of Jersey. British Journal of Rheumatology 37: 82–86

Watson P J, Chen A C N, Booker C K, Main C J, Jones A K P 1998b Differential electromyographic response to experimental cold pressor test in chronic low back pain patients and normal controls. Journal of Musculoskeletal Pain 6: 51–64

White K P, Speechley M, Harth M, Ostbye T 1999 The London fibromyalgia epidemiology study: comparing the demographic and clinical characteristics in 100 random community cases of fibromyalgia versus controls. Journal of Rheumatology 26: 1577–1585

Wigers S H, Stiles T C, Vogel P A 1996 Effects of aerobic exercise versus stress management treatment in fibromyalgia: a 4.5 year prospective study. Scandinavian Journal of Rheumatology 25: 77–86

Wilder-Smith O H G, Tassonyi E, Arendt-Neilsen L 2002 Preoperative back pain is associated with diverse manifestations of central neuroplasticity. Pain 97: 189–194

Williams D A, Keefe F J 1991 Pain beliefs and the use of cognitive-behavioral coping strategies. Pain 46: 185–190

Williams R, Pruitt S, Doctor J et al 1998 The contribution of job satisfaction to the transition from acute to chronic low back pain. Archives of Physical Medicine and Rehabilitation 79: 366–374

Wittink H 1999 Physical fitness, function and physical therapy in patients with pain: clinical measures of aerobic fitness and performance in patients with chronic low back pain. In: Max M (ed) Pain 1999: an updated review. IASP Press, Seattle, pp 137–144

Wittink H, Hoskins Michel T, Wagner A, Sukiennik A, Rogers W 2000 Deconditioning in patients with chronic low back pain: fact or fiction? Spine 25: 2221–2228

Wolfe F, Smythe H A, Yunus M B, et al 1990 The American College of Rheumatology 1990 criteria for the classification of fibromyalgia: report of the multi-centre criteria committee. Arthritis and Rheumatism 33: 160–172

SECTION 5

Establishing the evidence base for manual therapy

Chapter 39

A case for evidence-based practice in manual therapy

A. R. Gross, B. Chesworth, J. Binkley

INTRODUCTION

The term evidence-based practice is commonly used by manual therapists and refers to applying it in our practices. Evidence-based care uses current best evidence in making decisions about the care of individual patients. Clinical judgement informed by and integrated with best evidence from systematic research and professional experience leads to optimal practice. But how do we actually accomplish this? Sackett et al (1997) suggest that five steps are needed:

1. The clinical problem is converted into an answerable question.
2. Best evidence is tracked down efficiently.
3. The validity and usefulness of the evidence is established.
4. The results of this critique are applied to practice.
5. Self-evaluation of performance is reviewed.

A typical clinical case will help us illustrate and implement these points:

CLINICAL SCENARIO

A 24-year-old woman has chronic non-specific mechanical neck pain and reports some dizziness when turning her head. Her primary concern is her decreased function at the computer terminal due to pain. We are called on to assess and treat. The patient asks whether she will recover. We set out to implement some of the current evidence into our practice.

There are at least four areas of concern that we decided to address in this case:

1. The first is diagnosis. This patient reports dizziness. Should we perform the pre-manipulative tests for the cervical spine?
2. The second is prognosis. What is the expected recovery profile for non-specific mechanical neck disorders?
3. The third is efficacy. Will mobilization improve this patient's pain and function?
4. The fourth is measurement. What measurement tools will we use to track this patient's progress?

The four critical appraisal modules below help us resolve these four areas of concern. They depict one step by step approach to applying evidence in practice and arriving at a clinical conclusion. Discussion points will relate to the questions posed in Sackett et al (2000). Detailed methodology and background information can be found on <http://hiru.mcmaster.ca/ebm.htm>, in Sackett et al (2000) and in Streiner & Norman (1995).

DIAGNOSIS: PRE-MANIPULATIVE TESTING

This section concerns the diagnostic assessment using pre-manipulative testing of the cervical spine for signs and symptoms associated with vertebrobasilar insufficiency (VBI).

Step 1: Clinical question

In this patient with chronic non-specific neck disorder, will pre-manipulative testing of the cervical spine for the presence or development of dizziness or other associated symptoms of VBI enable us to identify the patient at risk for serious adverse events such as stroke or death following manipulation, mobilization or end-range neck exercise?

Step 2: The search

Since we are aware of the Australian Physiotherapy Association's clinical guidelines for pre-manipulative procedures for the cervical spine, we decide to search the association's website for further details. We had attended a conference (International Federation of Orthopaedic Manipulative Therapists 2000) where a primary diagnostic paper was presented on symptoms of possible VBI. Articles were selected if data on diagnostic accuracy fitting a 2 × 2 summary table (see Fig. 39.1) could be extracted. From the practice guideline we retrieved two such articles (Côté et al 1996, Rivett et al 1999) and from the conference proceedings one abstract (Rivett et al 2000). To further update our search and target primary research articles on the diagnostic accuracy of VBI tests, we limited our search to the MEDLINE database. We used index terms and text word searching for anatomical terms and disorder terms as well as the search filter ('specificity') from December 1999 to December 2002. We did not discover any new diagnostic papers on MEDLINE.

Step 3A: Are the results of this diagnostic study valid?

There was no independent blind comparison with a reference (gold) standard of diagnosis in any of the studies. The method for blinding the reader of the diagnostic test and reference test was not specified in two studies (Côté et al 1996, Rivett et al 1999) and was definitely not blind in the third (Rivett et al 2000). The absence of an independent and blind comparison with a reference standard in these trials indicates this is level IV evidence (Sackett et al 2000).

The reference standards were various types of Doppler ultrasound. One trial indicated that Doppler ultrasound is a reliable and valid test for blood flow and occlusion of blood flow evaluation (Côté et al 1996). However, one key clinical question remains, namely will this reference standard detect VBI resulting from vertebral artery dissection or occlusion that leads to stroke or death? The notion that occlusion of the vertebral blood flow is a potential marker for such a circumstance is based on theory and may be flawed.

The diagnostic test was not evaluated across a clinical spectrum (the range of patients in whom it would be used in practice) of the disorder/disease. In two case-control studies, the spectrum of the case mix was limited to comparing normal controls versus cases with perceived high practice prevalence of dizziness associated with possible VBI. Practice prevalence refers to the prevalence of the problem in our clinical setting. This case mix with high practice prevalence inflates the sensitivity of the diagnostic test. Sensitivity is the proportion of patients with the disorder who have a positive test result. In the cohort trial (Rivett et al 2000), the case mix appeared to more closely match a typical clinical spectrum. However, the co-morbidity and pathological spectrums were excluded. A clinical spectrum includes typical patients with both positive and negative clinical test responses as well as the presence of other health problems that are commonly confused with the reference disorder (the co-morbidity spectrum) and the presence of pathologies commonly confused with the cases (the pathological spectrum). The study designs used by the three trials were phase I or II. In phase I trials, a diagnostic test is compared in cases of markedly diseased individuals versus healthy controls. In phase II trials, the spectrum of comparison is expanded to include different types of diseased cases versus controls with a wider spectrum of commonly confused disease and health conditions. Future studies would be strengthened by the use of phase III and IV trial designs (Feinstein 1985), where the clinical performance of the test is assessed. This progression of trial design evaluates a test's ability to minimize false positive and false negative findings thereby increasing the test's validity and accuracy.

The reference standard was applied regardless of the test results in two of the three studies. In Rivett et al (1999), four subjects did not undergo Doppler testing due to pain and possible ischaemic symptoms. However, further analysis showed that the missing data did not bias the results.

In conclusion, there are a number of reasons to suspect that the validity of the diagnostic test is low. So we should *STOP HERE*. However, we are curious to see whether the diagnostic study results could influence our treatment decisions so we proceed to the next step.

Step 3B: Are the valid results of this diagnostic study important?

The following calculations are based on somewhat powerful ideas concerning likelihood ratios where the pre-test probability of VBI being present is transformed into the post-test probability. The pre-test probability is what we thought before the diagnostic test: the proportion of patients with VBI in the population at risk at a certain time or period of time. The post-test probability is what we think after applying the diagnostic test: the proportion of patients with a positive neck extension-rotation test who have the disorder VBI. In other words, will this test change our minds about the diagnosis? How will what we thought before doing the test compare to what we think after having done the test? The diagnostic test is dizziness (or other signs or symptoms) during neck extension-rotation, and the reference test is Doppler ultrasound imaging of the

hydrodynamics of blood flow in the vertebral artery and/or internal carotid artery. Diagnostic tests resulting in large changes from pre-test to post-test probabilities are most important to our clinical decision about the diagnosis. For example, a shift from 25% pre-test probability of having VBI to 50% post-test probability of a positive VBI test depicts some increase in our certainty that this patient has the dizziness associated with VBI but still only suggests the odds are about 50:50 that it is due to VBI. We are still uncertain. A shift to 90% post-test probability strongly supports that this test detects VBI. We will therefore not perform manipulation techniques following this testing. Table 39.1 depicts the mathematical definitions of various diagnostic terms and Figure 39.1 illustrates a 2×2 table used to summarize the findings of the diagnostic study. Fortunately, the maths has been made easy by downloading a 'catnip program' from the Sackett et al 2000 website. This program allows us to build our own CAT (critical appraised topic).

Table 39.1 sets out the findings from two of three studies. Sufficient data to fit this 2×2 table were not reported in Rivett et al (1999) so this study was excluded from further analysis. There are a few concepts to keep in mind concerning pre-test probability (prevalence) when applying test results:

- Applying the test to patients who have a low chance of having the disorder for which they are being tested (low pre-test probability or prevalence) will result in an

Table 39.1 Our calculations from the diagnostic studies

Author	Côté et al 1996	Rivett et al 2000
Study setting	Chiropractic clinics, department of neurology	Manual therapy clinics
Target disorder	Decreased vertebrobasilar blood flow	Decreased vertebral artery hydrodynamics
Reference standard	Doppler US imaging of VA (C3–5 level) with neck extended and rotated	Doppler US imaging of VA (C1–2 level) with neck rotated and extended
Diagnostic test	Dizziness associated with neck extension-rotation	Dizziness at end-range neck rotation-extension
Sensitivity = a/(a+c)	0.00	0.10
Specificity = d/(b+d)	0.86	0.39
Likelihood ratio for a positive test = $LR\rho$ = sensitivity/(1-specificity)	0.00	0.16
Likelihood ratio for a negative test = $LR\sigma$ = (1-sensitivity)/specificity	1.16	2.30
Positive predictive value = a/(a+b)	0	0.04
Pre-test probability (prevalence) = (a+c)/(a+b+c+d)	33%	25%
Pre-test odds = prevalence/(1-prevalence)	0.50	0.33
Post-test odds (ρ test) = Pre-test odds (LRρ)	0	0.05
Post-test odds (σ test) = Pre-test odds (LRσ)	0.58	0.76
Post-test probability (ρ test) = Post-test odds/ (post-test odds +1)	0%	5%
Post-test probability (σ test) = Post-test odds/ (post-test odds +1)	36%	43%

Key: values for a, b, c, d: see Figure 39.1.

Figure 39.1 Illustration of a 2 × 2 summary table used to report diagnostic test findings. Key: a: true positive; b: false positive; c: false negative; d: true negative; data in parentheses (x,y): (data from Côté et al 1996, data from Rivett et al 2000).

Diagnostic test:		Reference standard: Doppler ultrasound		
neck extension and rotation		Present	Absent	
	Positive	a (0, 2)	b (4, 49)	a+b
	Negative	c (14, 18)	d (24, 31)	c+d
	Totals	a+c	b+d	a+b+c+d

increased chance of a false positive findings. Even though the pre-test probability or prevalence of having dizziness associated with VBI is noted to be between 25 and 33% in two studies (see Table 39.1), the pre-test probability or prevalence of occluding or dissecting the vertebral artery or internal carotid artery is not known. The probability of occluding or dissecting the vertebral artery resulting in serious adverse events is thought to be extremely low (1 in 20 000) (Hurwitz et al 1996). If the patient is unlikely to have these serious adverse events, doing the diagnostic test for possible symptoms of VBI will not appreciably alter this likelihood. There is a high risk of a false positive conclusion in this circumstance.

- Applying the test to patients who have a high chance of having the disorder for which they are being tested will result in increased false negative findings.

The interpretation of the two studies' findings follows. First, in Côté et al (1996) the test had a somewhat, but not extremely, high specificity. Specificity is the proportion of patients without the target disorder who have a negative test. At first glance, we may think this positive test (dizziness on neck extension-rotation), should generally help rule the presence of VBI in (**SpPin** mnemonic: In the presence of an extremely high **Sp**ecificity, a **P**ositive finding rules **in** the diagnosis). However, the post-test probability of a positive test is 0%, and the post-test probability of a negative test shifts the probability of having the disorder from 33% pre-test to 36% post-test. In other words, the probability of not having the disorder after a negative test shifts downward from 67% pre-test to 64% post-test. So doing this diagnostic test does not help us in detecting the presence of VBI.

Second, in the study by Rivett et al (2000), the post-test probability of a positive test shifts downward from 25% pre-test to 5% post-test, meaning that after doing this test we are less certain that VBI is present. The post-test probability of having VBI after a negative test shifts from 25% pre-test to 43% post-test. That is, the probability of not having the disorder shifts downward from 75% to 67%. Again, our certainty of not having VBI is not appreciably altered, although it is reduced slightly. After doing the test for dizziness (or other signs and symptoms) with neck rotation-extension, we have not made a diagnosis and the test has not produced an important result for our patient. *We have no evidence that this diagnostic test helps to rule VBI in or out.*

Step 4: Can you apply this valid, important evidence about a diagnostic test to caring for your patient?

If the results of the diagnostic study were shown to be important, we would go on, but in this case would be pointless. We do note that the test is affordable, and is done accurately and precisely in our practice setting.

Step 5: Self-evaluation

We have overstepped the process a bit by moving forward and doing calculations and a clinical application even though valid result did not yet exist.

The clinical bottom line

It can be argued that patients at risk of a serious adverse event following manipulation are undetectable in spite of the use of pre-manipulative tests. We may wish to wait until further information from valid and important evidence about pre-manipulative testing becomes available before changing our current practice. Alternatively, we may wish to follow the expert opinion noted in the CPG on pre-manipulative testing until higher level evidence comes available.

PROGNOSIS: NON-SPECIFIC NECK PAIN

In this section, we will base our clinical thoughts on recent systematic reviews (SR) of prognostic factors in patients with non-specific neck pain.

Step 1: Clinical question

What are this 24 year old's chances of complete recovery in terms of pain and function if she suffers from chronic non-specific neck pain?

Step 2: The search

We limited our search of MEDLINE to systematic reviews. We used index keyword terms related to the anatomical area and disorder [exp NECK/ or exp NECK INJURIES/ or exp NECK MUSCLES/ or exp NECK PAIN] and the search filter 'specificity' for prognosis [(PROGNOSIS or SUR-VIVAL ANALYSIS).sh]. One citation (Borghouts et al 1998) was retrieved.

Step 3A: Is the evidence valid?

Was there a representative and well–defined sample of patients at a similar point in the course of the disease?

While patient selection was a notable weakness in the studies evaluated in this SR, we make the following points. It appears that a broad spectrum of patients with mechanical neck pain were studied. The study sample included typical patients who present to clinicians in an outpatient orthopaedic environment (i.e. non-specific neck pain, without a specific underlying systemic cause). Patients with tumours, fractures, infection, inflammatory disease, osteoporosis and motor vehicle trauma were excluded. This is important, since we want to know that our patient 'fits' with the group of patients that generated the results we will cite to our client.

We note the treatment environments from which study subjects were recruited: mainly secondary care settings along with a few occupational care settings and one primary care environment. If we work in primary care this mix of treatment settings would be a concern since the patient samples would not be representative of our caseload. Telling our patient about her prognosis using results from a different patient population would be inaccurate and would misrepresent the current state of knowledge. If, however, we work in a secondary care setting we should worry less about this issue.

Only one study used an inception cohort, meaning prognosis was determined on patients who were at a variety of stages in the course of their neck complaints. This limits our ability to interpret the results fully because changes (for better or worse) that took place before the patient entered the study remain unknown. This makes some reports about prognoses look better or worse than they really are. Since there is no way to determine how this would relate to the prognosis of our patient, this design flaw suggests that conversations about prognosis with our patient should indicate that a range of outcomes are possible, hence the importance of patient compliance and outcome measures in the treatment process.

Was follow–up sufficiently long and complete?

Only 25% of the studies in the SR reported prognosis using follow-up data longer than 12 months. This is important, because we need to think about the time frame over which we are discussing prognosis with our patient. Factors that affect neck status 1 month from the time of treatment may differ from those that affect longer-term outcomes. With our patient, therefore, we should limit our discussion to short-term prognosis. The fact that half of the studies had a loss to follow-up or drop-out rate of less than 10% means that prognostic factors associated with patients who

dropped out of the study are less likely to affect the results of those studies.

Were objective and unbiased outcome criteria used?

The outcomes in the studies cited in this SR were categorized into decreased pain, general improvement, functional improvement and health care utilization. Not all studies reported outcomes in these categories. Most studies did report on decreases in pain and general improvement so we should focus on these outcomes with our patient. The SR findings suggest that about half of patients have a 34% improvement in pain complaints. The results were obtained from a mixture of chronic and acute patients. Although some studies did not report quantitative data, most measurements of pain were obtained using valid and clinically acceptable measures (i.e. visual analogue scale and numeric rating scale). Therefore, we can feel relatively comfortable relating this quantitative information about pain to our patient, especially if we use the same tools in our treatment environment.

We notice that results about general improvement were generated from both patient and therapist ratings. Both of these sources are problematic, since therapists may have inflated their estimates of patient outcome in favour of their treatment intervention and patients could have biased estimates of their status depending on their expectations of treatment. Furthermore, we do not know how general improvement was measured, so it is difficult to relate this concept to measurement tools used in our own clinical practice. Therefore, although half of the patients studied showed a general improvement of 47%, we should be careful how we articulate this to our patient. Once again, the opportunity arises for us to emphasize the importance of outcome measures in the treatment process.

Was adjustment for important extraneous prognostic factors carried out?

Only one study used appropriate statistical techniques to evaluate prognostic factors, making specific comments about prognosis more problematic. Thus, a detailed answer about prognosis is unclear. Once again, we can see the importance of tempering discussions about prognosis with education about the role of clinical outcome measures in the treatment process.

Step 3B: What are the results?

Most studies reported results based on a follow-up period of less than 6 months. Conclusions about prognosis were that:

- there was no association between a 'worse outcome' and 'radiation to arms/neurologic signs'
- there was no association between radiologic findings in the neck and a worse prognosis
- there was an association between a worse prognosis and severity of pain and a history of previous attacks.

However, typical measures of association (such as the odds ratio or relative risk) were not presented. Since none were reported, we cannot tell our patient her chances of achieving a specific outcome within a certain time frame. Since no statistics are given, we have no indication of how precise the reported estimates of prognosis truly are.

Step 4: Will the results help in the care of my patient?

The generalizability of study subjects to our own patient caseload was covered above. For our purposes, we will conclude that, although there were problems with patient selection in the studies cited in the SR, we believe the patients who were studied may have been similar to those seen in our treatment setting.

While no specific treatments were favoured in the SR, no serious adverse outcomes were noted either. Even though we cannot offer much specific detail about short-term or long-term outcomes to our patient, the absence of outcome information provides the ideal background for discussions with our patient about our proposed course of treatment, patient goal setting and treatment evaluation, with validated outcome measures used in our clinic.

Since we can only say that the clinical course will not necessarily follow any specific direction, we should use this opportunity to focus our patient education on the importance of treatment compliance and outcome measurement in determining the value of any specific intervention.

Step 5: Self-evaluation

We could progress to a second literature search that probes in more detail for pertinent articles published after the publication date or the most recently cited article in the SR. Integrating these additional findings into the results of the SR may change our position about prognosis derived from the one SR article.

The clinical bottom line

If our patient did present with more severe complaints of pain and a history of prior attacks of neck pain, we guard our comments about the possibility of a worse outcome with the fact that the prognostic literature is limited. We make this point to our patient to emphasize the importance of the outcome measures we use in our clinic and the critical role she plays with regard to treatment compliance.

EFFICACY: MANUAL THERAPY

In this section, we will limit our discussion to passive mobilizations or mobilizations using various neuromuscular techniques for the cervical spine.

Step 1: Clinical question

We are aware of one evidence based clinical practice guideline (Gross et al 2001, 2002) on the topic of manual therapy. The findings are not conclusive but support the notion of

manual therapies with exercise and some other modalities such as heat, medication and patient education. Mobilizations done alone seemed to be less effective. The search date ends December 1997. We are advanced trained manual therapists who use mobilization routinely. In more recent randomized controlled trials, do mobilizations applied to adults with subacute/chronic non-specific mechanical neck disorders without radicular findings improve their pain, function and return to work? Are patients satisfied with this care?

Step 2: The search

We start up MEDLINE 1995–2002, enter the search filter 'sensitivity' search [(DOUBLE and BLIND:) or PLACEBO:], manual therapy as a key word term [exp PHYSICAL THERAPY/ or exp MANIPULATION, SPINAL/ or exp MANIPULATION, ORTHOPAEDIC/ or exp CHIRO-PRACTIC/ or exp OSTEOPATHIC MEDICINE], and anatomical/disorder terms as text word and keyword terms and find no randomized trials. In our personal files, we have a thesis by Hoving (2001) as well as trials reports (Hoving et al 2002).

Step 3A: Is the evidence valid?

Was the assignment of patient to treatments randomized?

Yes, randomized to one of three intervention groups:

* Manual therapy care: manual therapy, instruction on home exercise, analgesics prescribed at baseline; manual therapist with advanced training utilized specific articular movement techniques (mobilizations) and muscular movement techniques (soft tissue mobilization); one 45-minute session per week over 6 weeks.
* GP care: general practitioner care included analgesics; education regarding ergonomic advice, self-care (heat, home exercise), awaiting spontaneous recovery; two 10-minute follow-up sessions over 6 weeks were optional.
* Physical therapy care: physical therapy and analgesics prescribed at baseline; 10 minutes exercise therapy prescribed by a registered physiotherapist with adjunct treatment including massage, manual traction, heat, interferential, instruction on home exercise.

Randomized permuted blocks of six patients were produced for each stratum, using a computer generated random sequence table.

Was the randomized list concealed?

An administrative research assistant who was not involved in the project performed the randomization according to the previously mentioned randomization scheme. She prepared the concealed randomization by using opaque, sequentially numbered sealed envelopes.

Were all patients who entered the trial accounted for at its conclusion?

Yes. At 1 year MT had 58/60, PT 59/59 and GP 61/64 follow-up.

Were they analysed in the groups to which they were randomized?

Yes. Intention-to-treat analysis was performed.

Were patients and clinicians kept 'blind' as to which treatment was being received?

The patients were blind to the treatment; however, the therapists were not.

Aside from the experimental treatment, were the groups treated equally?

There was substantive crossover in the GP and PT care groups. There was at least one additional treatment during the entire follow-up period for all categories of care: GP 63%, PT 58% and MT 30%. The typical additional treatment in the GP and PT group was referral to MT care. Thus, the long-term benefits are underestimated for MT when compared with GP or PT. Co-intervention patients were allowed to perform exercises at home and to take medication prescribed at baseline or over-the-counter analgesics. A maximum number of visits was set; however, patients did not have to use all the visits if their problem resolved with treatment before the schedule ended.

Were the groups similar at the start of the trial?

Yes. Only minor differences were found between the baseline values of the three groups.

Step 3B: If valid, is this evidence important?

We note that there are at least two outcomes that explore the notion of pain (pain intensity and analgesic use), two that explore activation or function (absenteeism and Neck Disability Index, NDI), and one that assesses patient satisfaction, at least in part (patient perceived recovery six-point ordinal transition scale, ranging from 'much worse'

to 'completely recovered'). Our calculations for dichotomous outcomes are noted in Table 39.2. We were pleased that the 'catnip' program did the calculations for us. Note that for the purposes of this report, the experimental treatment is MT and the control treatment is GP. The most striking finding is that after 7 weeks of treatment we need only treat three patients with mobilizations to make one substantively better (perceived recovery equals full recovery or much improved) and this improvement is maintained for one in seven patients at 1 year follow-up. Additionally, one in four patients in the MT group no longer use analgesics. MT care when compared to GP care prevented one in eight people from missing work. The data for pain were continuous and presented as a standard mean difference (SMD). SMD is a unitless measure reported in standard deviation units with a conversion to a common scale. A positive score indicates decreased pain (i.e. an improvement in the patient's condition). An effect size can be small (0.20), medium (0.50) or large (0.80) (Cohen 1988). Although the average pain intensity was not significantly different at the 1 year follow-up [SMD 0.04 (95%CI fixed: −0.32, 0.40)], there was a clinically meaningful difference after 7 weeks of treatment [SMD 0.31 (95%CI fixed: −0.04, 0.67)], equal to a moderate effect. The gains in clinical terms were 1.0 (95%CI: −1.3, 3.4) NDI units compared to GP care or 6.3 (SD: 6.8) NDI units from baseline compared to GP care with a gain of 5.3 (SD:6.8) NDI units. Function improved in all groups by at least 5–6 NDI points at 7 weeks of treatment and 7–9 NDI points at 1 year follow-up. A four-point change is the minimum clinically important difference (Stratford et al 1999). The MT group had similar improvements compared to the GP group. In summary, there are statistically and clinically important benefits for the MT over GP care in pain, perceived recovery and absenteeism over both the short- and long-term. The benefits are most profound immediately following 7 weeks of MT care. Additionally, in subgroup analysis, MT seemed to help those with a more severe pain rating at baseline. Recall that crossover of treatment by the GP and PT group was substantive after 7 weeks of treatment.

Table 39.2 Our calculations for efficacy of mobilization

Outcome measure	Event rate CER	EER	Relative risk reduction (95%CI)	Absolute risk reduction (95%CI)	Number needed to treat (95%CI)
Use of analgesics @7 w	0.80	0.64	36% (16, 56)	0.29 (0.13, 0.45)	4 (3, 8)
Absenteeism @7 w	0.19	0.13	51% (−1, 100)	0.13 (−0.004, 0.27)	8 (4, 4)
Perceived recovery @7 w	0.66	0.32	51% (26, 76)	0.33 (0.17, 0.50)	3 (2, 6)
@52 w f-u	0.41	0.26	37% (−3%, 77%)	0.15 (−0.01, 0.32)	7 (4, 4)

Key: CER: control event rate; EER: experimental event rate; 95% CI: 95% confidence interval; 7 w: 7 weeks of treatment; 52 w f-u: one year follow-up data; perceived recovery: success equals 'complete recovery' or 'much improved' on a 6-point scale.

Step 4: If valid and important, can you apply this evidence in caring for your patients?

Is your patient so different from those in the trial that its results can't help you?

The adult participants in this trial had subacute/chronic (≥ 2 weeks) neck complaints; the majority in this trial had been experiencing pain for less than 3 months. Some 60–70% had experienced at least one previous episode of neck complaint. The majority of subjects suffered from mechanical neck disorder; however, approximately 25% had radicular findings and at least 50–64% had headache of cervical origin. The NDI mean was 14.5 (minimally disabled). We note that this profile is somewhat similar to the patients in our private practice. The GP approach in our community seems similar to that in the study.

How great would the potential benefit of therapy actually be for your individual patients?

We will consider our patients to have the same rate of recovery as that noted in the Hoving et al 2002 study's control group, GP care. Table 39.2 notes the patient experimental event rate (PEER) and relative risk reduction (RRR) for perceived poor recovery. If the expected rate of recovery in our patient (PEER) is equal to 0.67 at 7 weeks of treatment and 0.41 at the 1-year follow-up, the number needed to treat (NNT) for patients like ours after 7 weeks of treatment is $1/(\text{PEER} \times \text{RRR}) = 1/0.67 \times 0.37 = 4$, and at 1-year follow-up is $1/0.41 \times 0.37 = 7$.

As manual therapists we may see patients who have had standard PT care. Then the numbers shift slightly when we consider our patients to have the same rate of recovery as that noted in the Hoving et al 2002 study's PT group. In this circumstance, we need to treat 7 people to make one substantively better than PT care at 1-year follow-up, and we need to treat six people to make one substantively better after 7 weeks of treatment.

Are the patient's values and preferences satisfied by the regimen and its consequences?

Minor benign short-term adverse reactions were reported. Headache, pain in the upper extremities, tingling in the upper extremities and dizziness all occurred more frequently in the MT group than in the GP or PT group. So considering the gains and minimal risks to the patients, our patient decides she will undergo the MT treatment regime.

Step 5: Self-evaluation

Analysis of continuous data was not available in the 'catnip'. To simplify the analysis, we used an additional program called Revman 4.1 for Cochrane reviews.

The clinical bottom line

The main concern of the patient in the scenario was a loss of function at work due to pain. There are clear benefits to doing mobilizations for reducing pain, reducing analgesic use, reducing absenteeism and maximizing perceived recovery. However, although the benefit in terms of NDI was substantive from baseline for all groups, doing mobilizations alone as a treatment regimen does not seem to improve the NDI self-report score any more than GP or PT care and therefore does not lead to function advantages.

OUTCOME MEASUREMENT FOR CLINICAL SETTING

In this section, we will address the issue of selecting, interpreting and applying measures of progress and outcome in our patients. The following are criteria for selecting an outcome measure:

- Measure is developed using a systematic process of item selection and use appropriate scaling and item weighting, where applicable.
- Measure is documented to be reliable. The minimal detectable change (MDC) is documented. MDC is the amount of change on a measure required to be confident that true change has occurred that is greater than error.
- Measure is documented to be valid. The minimal clinically important difference (MCID) is documented. MCID is the least amount of change on a scale required to be certain that clinically important change has occurred.
- Measure is documented to be sensitive to valid change. Another term for this is responsiveness.
- Measure is easy to administer with respect to patient and clinician time; also easy to score and record in the medical record.
- Measure is appropriate for wide application to patients in the clinical practice, including patients with different initial functional levels, conditions, diseases, problems and ages.

Step 1: Clinical question

What measures of outcome are appropriate for determining progress and outcome for our patient with chronic mechanical neck pain?

Step 2: The search

By performing a free PubMed search at www.ncbi.nlm.nih.gov/entrez/query.fcgi, we found references on the Patient-Specific Functional Scale (PSFS) (Westaway et al 1998) and Numeric Pain Rating Scale (NPRS) (Stratford & Spadoni 2001). In order to be efficient in further searching for other measures, we then went to two outcome databases available on line. The first is a database sponsored by the Chartered Society of Physiotherapy at www.csp.org.uk/media/publicdomain/omdb; once there, we found the Neck Disability Index (NDI) (Veron & Mior 1991). We then searched a database sponsored by Leeds University at www.leeds.ac.uk/nuffield/infoservices/UKCH/find.html

and found that the SF-36 (McHorney et al 1993, 1994, Ware & Sherbourne 1992) may be applicable to the patient.

Step 3: Do the measures of outcome meet the above criteria?

The Patient-Specific Functional Scale

The Patient-Specific Function Scale (PSFS) was developed by Stratford and colleagues. Its principal goals were to provide a standardized method and measure for eliciting and recording patients' disabilities (Chatman et al 1997, Stratford & Spadoni 2001, Stratford et al 1995). Patients are asked to list up to three important activities they are having difficulty with or are unable to perform. In addition to specifying the activities, patients are asked to rate, on an 11-point scale, the current level of difficulty associated with each activity. Patients are then asked to describe one or two activities with which they are having just a bit of difficulty. The inclusion of these more minor functional limitations allows tracking of any deterioration in the patient's condition. The clinician's role is to read the script (instructions) to the patient and record the activities, corresponding numerical difficulty ratings and the assessment date. At subsequent reassessments, the clinician reads the follow-up script which reminds the patient of the activities she identified previously. Once again, the clinician records the numerical difficulty ratings and the date.

The activities and scores are recorded on the functional goal and outcome worksheet (Fig. 39.2). The scores for the main activities indicated by the patient are averaged together to produce an average score out of 10. The scores for the additional activities with which the patient is having minimal difficulty are also averaged. The functional goal and outcome worksheet was designed to record the PSFS activities and scores, additional functional scale scores, key impairment measures and patient goals at initial assessment and at weekly follow-up.

The reliability, validity and sensitivity to change of the PSFS have been reported for patients with cervical dysfunction (Chatman et al 1997, Stratford & Spadoni 2001, Stratford et al 1995). In these groups, the PSFS was demonstrated to be reliable (test–retest reliability based on average scores and individual activity scores: R = 0.84-0.98). The construct validity of the PSFS was confirmed by comparing patients' PSFS scores with existing measures: the SF-36 in the case of the knee study; the Roland-Morris Back Pain Questionnaire in the case of back pain patients; and the Neck Disability Index in the case of the neck study. Correlation of the PSFS with the relevant comparison scale in each study was adequate to good (r = 0.49–0.83). The sensitivity to valid change of the PSFS was confirmed using a number of different constructs in each of the three studies (Chatman et al 1997, Stratford & Spadoni 2001, Stratford et al 1995). On average, the PSFS took subjects and therapists 4 minutes and 13 seconds (s = 1.9 minutes) to administer (Stratford et al 1995).

With respect to individual patient decision making, the potential error associated with an average score on the PSFS at a given point in time is +/−2 scale points [90% confidence interval (CI)]; the MDC is three scale points (90%CI); and the MCID is three scale points (90%CI) (Chatman et al 1997, Stratford & Spadoni 2001, Stratford et al 1995). This means that at a given point in time, for example initial evaluation, a clinician can be 90% confident that a given PSFS average score out of 10 is within two scale points of the patient's true score. On follow-up, changes in score of at least three scale points can be interpreted with reasonable confidence as true and important patient change.

It appears that the PSFS meets the criteria of established measurement properties and is easy and efficient to administer and incorporate into the clinical record. Our patient's activities and corresponding scores at initial evaluation are found in Figure 39.2. Her average PSFS score is 3/10. These scores can be used to set goals and track progress singly or as an average.

The neck disability index

The Neck Disability Index (NDI) is a condition-specific scale frequently cited in the literature for cervical disorders (Riddle & Stratford 1998, Vernon & Mior 1991). The NDI format was based on the Oswestry scale for patients with low back pain and consists of 10 items, five taken from the original Oswestry. It is a one-page self-administered scale and takes only a few minutes to complete. Scores vary from zero (most desirable state of health) to 50 (least desirable state of health).

The measurement properties of the NDI have been documented in the literature. Test–retest reliability has been reported to be good (r = 0.89) (Riddle & Stratford 1998). In addition, construct validity was found to be acceptable when NDI scores were compared with scores on the McGill Pain Questionnaire scores and on a visual analogue pain scale. Riddle & Stratford (1998) examined the validity and sensitivity to change of the NDI in measuring a variety of cervical conditions. The authors found that the NDI as well as the comparison scale, the physical component score and mental component score of the SF-36, were both adept at measuring change over time in patients with neck conditions.

With respect to individual patient decision making, the potential error associated with a score on the NDI at a given point in time is three scale points (90%CI). The potential error associated with either the MDC or MCID is five scale points (90%CI). This means that at a given point in time, for example initial evaluation, a clinician can be reasonably confident that a given NDI score is within three scale points of the patient's true score. On follow-up, changes in score of +/− 5 scale points or more can be interpreted as true patient change with reasonable confidence.

The NDI meets the criteria for selecting an outcome measure for our patient and, unlike the PSFS, allows comparison between patients or groups of patients on the scale. Our patient has an initial NDI score of 28/50 (see Fig. 39.2).

The SF–36 health status measure

The reliability, validity and sensitivity to change have been well documented for the SF-36 (McHorney et al 1993, 1994, Ware et al 1992). In a comparison of the NDI and SF-36 in patients with cervical spine disorders, substantial overlap on the two measures suggested that use of one of the two measures was appropriate and sufficient (Riddle & Stratford 1998). In light of the time needed to complete the SF-36 and the complexity of scoring, it was decided to administer the NDI rather than the SF-36 in addition to the PSFS to document function.

The numeric pain rating scale

Several measures exist for documenting pain intensity. The NPRS is a simple measure that meets the criteria for selecting an outcome measure. The NPRS is a single-item self-administered measure. Pain is rated on a single 11-point scale from no pain '0' to severe pain '10'. The scale takes only a few seconds to administer and score.

The test–retest reliability has been reported to be in the range of 0.64 to 0.86. In validating the scale in patients with neck dysfunction, the NPRS correlated with the NDI in the range of $r = 0.44$ to $r = 0.52$. With respect to sensitivity to change, NPRS correlates with NDI change ($r = 0.52$).

With respect to individual patient decision making, the potential error associated with a score on the NPRS at a given point in time is two scale points (90%CI). The MDC is three scale points (90%CI) and the MCID is three scale points (90%CI).

Our patient's initial NPRS score is 7/10 (see Fig. 39.2).

Step 4: Application of measures of progress and outcome to patient

Clinicians can use a measure of a patient's initial function, such as that obtained with the NDI, PSFS and NPRS, in order to set functional goals and track the progress of their patients. In order to set short-term and long-term goals based on a functional scale, the clinician must synthesize the clinical history and objective findings of the patient. In addition, the MDC and MDIC of the relevant scale are utilized.

Our patient has an initial NDI score of 28/50, a PSFS score on computer work of 2/10, and a NPRS of 7/10 (see Fig. 39.2). With respect to the NDI, we can be reasonably confident that the true scale score lies between 25 and 31. In setting short-term goals for this patient, we must consider the history and clinical findings as well as the MDC (five scale points) and MCID (five scale points) for the NDI. Since her condition is chronic, and therefore expected to change relatively slowly, we might decide on a 2-week time frame for a change in score of five points. The short-term goal, then, would be to decrease NDI score to less than or

equal to 23/50 in 2 weeks (see Fig. 39.2). On follow-up, for example 1 week later, progress is measured by the amount of change on the scale. In cases where improvement greater than the MDC and MCID occurs, clinicians can be confident that true (MDC) and important (MCID) change has occurred. In cases where there is no change or change is less than the MDC, clinicians can be confident that true change has not occurred. In this case, depending on the clinical picture and the amount of time since the previous assessment, a change in intervention or discharge may be considered.

Figure 39.2 outlines short-term and long-term goals using the NDI, PSFS and NPRS. The functional goal and outcome worksheet provides a section to track impairment measures such as strength and range of motion. In the case of our patient, however, range of motion will be tracked but not utilized as an outcome measure. This is because there are no measures of cervical range of motion that meet the criteria for use as an outcome measure.

In this patient, the long-term goal shows that complete resolution of pain and functional limitation is not expected. Sample week 1 and week 2 scores are shown to illustrate the tracking of progress and goals. Note that at the end of week 2, all short-term goals have been met, the long-term pain goal has been met and range of motion is full. However, the patient continues to have documented functional limitations and further treatment is justified.

The clinical bottom line

There are many benefits to incorporating outcome measurement into practice. The first and most important benefit is enhancement of patient care by focusing on functional goals that are of critical importance to the patient. Patient–clinician communication is improved as patients perceive the physical therapist's interest in their functional limitations. Clinical decision making regarding continuation, change or discontinuation of treatment is improved. Finally, there is clear communication with referral sources and payers regarding patients' functional level and the functional goals and outcomes of physical therapy. Three components affect the successful clinical implementation of a self-report functional measure:

- ease of administration of the questionnaire
- ease of interpretation of the result
- efficient documentation in the medical record.

CONCLUSION

EBP has become an essential critical thinking skill for manual therapists; it is equal to the advanced clinical/manual skill. Persistence and patience are needed when pursuing EBP. Sound clinical judgement and professional experience are essential when integrating evidence based practice into our care processes. So, how did we do in terms of our case

	Initial	Week 1	Week 2	Week 3	Week 4	Week 5	Week 6
Patient Specific Functional Scale (/10)							
1. Using computer	2	4	7				
2. Turning head while driving	4	5	7				
3. Playing flute	3	3	4				
PSFS AVERAGE	3	4	6				
Condition Specific Measure:							
1. NDI (/50)	28	25	19				
Pain Measures:							
1. NPRS (/10)	7	4	2				
Impairment Measures							
1. Right rotation (%)	50	75	Full				
2. Left Rotation (%)	75	75	Full				
Short Term Goals							
Time Frame: 2 weeks							
1. NDI < 23/50			✿✿				
2. PSFS computer > 5/10			✿✿				
3. NPRS < 4/10		✿✿					
Long Term Goals							
Time Frame: 4 weeks							
1. NDI < 5/50							
2. PSFS computer > 8/10							
3. NPRS < 2/10			✿✿				
4. Playing flute > 7/10							

Figure 39.2 Functional goal and outcome worksheet.

scenario? A summary of clinical conclusions and what we will tell the patient follows.

CLINICAL SCENARIO RESOLUTION

Diagnosis Doing pre-manipulative testing of the cervical spine may not increase our ability to find those individuals at risk of serious adverse events following manipulation or mobilization. The current information is based on level IV evidence. We will continue our current practice until stronger evidence becomes available but monitor the literature closely.

Prognosis We cannot offer much specific detail about short-term or long-term outcomes to our patient. The absence of outcome information provides the ideal background for discussions with our patient about our proposed course of treatment, patient goal setting and treatment evaluation with validated outcome measures used in our clinic.

Therapy Mobilizations improve our patient's pain and perceived recovery but may not have functional advantages when compared to GP care. Some advantages exist immediately post-treatment in reducing absenteeism.

Measurement We identified three outcomes that meet criteria for selecting valid outcomes: PSDI, NDI and NRS. We utilized a flow sheet to set goals important to the patient and track change. Using outcomes enhances patient care by focusing on functional goals, clinical decision making and communication of results.

KEYWORDS

mechanical neck disorder	prognosis
dizziness	measurement
diagnosis	clinical judgement
efficacy	

References

Borghouts J A J, Koes B W, Bouter L M 1998 The clinical course and prognostic factors of non-specific neck pain: a systematic review. Pain 77: 1–13

Chatman A B, Hyams S P, Neel J M et al 1997 The Patient Specific Functional Scale: measurement properties in patients with knee dysfunction. Physical Therapy 77: 820–829

Cohen J 1988 Statistical power analysis for the behavioural sciences, 2nd edn. Lawrence Erlbaum, Hillsdale, New Jersey

Côté P, Kreitz B G, Cassidy D, Thiel H 1996 The validity of the extension-rotation as a clinical screening procedure before neck manipulation: a secondary analysis. Journal of Manipulative and Physiological Therapeutics 19(3): 159–164

Feinstein A R 1985 Clinical epidemiology: the architecture of clinical research. W B Saunders, Philadelphia, pp 597–631

Gross A R, Kay T M, Hurley L et al 2001 College of Physiotherapy of Ontario, technical report: clinical practice guidelines on the use of manipulation or mobilization in the treatment of adults with mechanical neck disorders. College of Physiotherapy of Ontario, Toronto available on: http://www.collegept.org; website accessed: Dec 2001

Gross A R, Kay T M, Hurley L et al 2002 Clinical practice guideline on the use of manipulation or mobilization in the treatment of adults with mechanical neck disorders. Manual Therapy 7(4): 193–205

Hoving J L 2001 Thesis. Neck pain in primary care: the effects of commonly applied interventions. Pons and Looijen, Wageningen

Hoving J L, Koes B W, de Vet H C W et al 2002 Manual therapy, physical therapy, or continued care by a general practitioner for patients with neck pain. Annals of Internal Medicine 136(10): 713–759

Hurwitz E L, Aker P D, Adams A H, Meeker W C, Shekelle P G 1996 Manipulation and mobilization of the cervical spine: a systematic review of the literature. Spine 21(15): 1746–1760

McHorney C A, Ware Jr J E, Raczek A E 1993 The MOS 36-item Short-Form Health Survey (SF-36). II: Psychometric and clinical tests of validity in measuring physical and mental health constructs. Medical Care 31: 247–263

McHorney C A, Ware Jr J E, Lu R, Sherbourne C D 1994 The MOS 36-item Short-Form Health Survey (SF-36). III: Tests of data quality, scaling assumptions, and reliability across diverse patient groups. Medical Care 32: 40–66

Riddle D L, Stratford P W 1998 Use of generic versus region-specific functional status measures on patients with cervical spine disorders. Physical Therapy 78: 951–963

Rivett D A, Sharples K J, Milburn P D 1999 Effect of pre-manipulative tests on vertebral artery and internal carotid artery blood flow: a pilot study. Journal of Manipulative and Physiological Therapeutics 22(6): 368–375

Rivett D A, Sharples K J, Milburn P D 2000 Vertebral artery blood flow during pre-manipulative testing of the cervical spine. Abstract 127. In: Singer K P (ed) Program and Abstracts of the Seventh Scientific Conference of the International Federation of Orthopaedic Manipulative Therapists in conjunction with the Eleventh Biennial Conference of the Manipulative Physiotherapists Association of Australia. Centre for Musculoskeletal Studies, University of Western Australia, Perth

Sackett D L, Richardson W S, Rosenberg W, Haynes R B 1997 Evidence-based medicine, how to practice and teach EBM. Churchill Livingstone, New York

Sackett D L, Straus S E, Richardson W S, Rosenberg W, Haynes R B 2000 Evidence-based medicine: how to practice and teach EBM, 2nd edn. Churchill Livingstone, Edinburgh

Stratford P, Spadoni G 2001 The reliability, consistency, and clinical application of a numeric pain rating scale. Physiotherapy Canada 53: 88–91

Stratford P, Gill C, Westaway M, Binkley J 1995 Assessing disability and change on individual patients: a report of a patient specific measure. Physiotherapy Canada 47: 258–262

Stratford P W, Riddle D L, Binkley J M, Spadoni G, Westaway M D, Padfield B 1999 Using the Neck Disability Index to make decisions concerning individual patients. Physiotherapy Canada 51: 107–112

Streiner D L, Norman G R 1995 Health measurement scales: a practical guide to their development and use. Oxford University Press, Oxford

Vernon H, Mior S 1991 The Neck Disability Index: a study of reliability and validity. Journal Manipulation and Physiological Therapy 14: 409–415

Ware Jr J E, Sherbourne C D 1992 The MOS 36-item Short-Form Health Survey (SF-36). I: Conceptual framework and items selection. Medical Care 30: 473–483

Westaway M, Stratford P W, Binkley J 1988 The Patient Specific Functional Scale: validation of its use in persons with neck dysfunction. Journal of Orthopaedic Sports Physical Therapy 27: 331–338

Chapter **40**

Methodological and practical issues in clinical trials on manual therapy

J. L. Hoving, G. A. Jull, B. Koes

INTRODUCTION

In this chapter we discuss some of the specific issues in the field of clinical trials on manual therapy. Examples of practical and methodological issues will be illustrated by two recently completed randomized clinical trials on manual therapy for neck pain (Hoving et al 2002) and cervicogenic headache (Jull et al 2002). The basic design and results of both trials will first be presented in a short introduction. The basic design of a randomized clinical trial in manual therapy can be found elsewhere (Koes & Hoving 1998).

TRIAL ON NECK PAIN

The first randomized clinical trial on manual therapy that we discuss compared the effect of spinal mobilization with two other frequently applied interventions for patients with neck pain in primary care (Hoving et al 2002). A total of 183 patients with non-specific neck pain were randomized into three groups and received 6 weeks of either manual therapy (specific mobilization techniques) once a week, physical therapy (mainly exercise therapy) twice a week, or continued care provided by a general practitioner (analgesics, counselling and education). Figure 40.1 shows the general outline of the randomized clinical trial and the flow of patients through the trial.

The short-term effects were assessed at 3 and 7 weeks, and the long-term effects at 13, 26 and 52 weeks. The primary outcome measures included perceived recovery, physical impairment assessed by a blinded research assistant, pain intensity and disability measured according to the Neck Disability Index (Vernon & Mior 1991). The secondary outcome measures included the severity of the most important functional limitation rated by the patient, cervical range of motion (ROM) and general health status according to the self-rated health index (0–100) of the EuroQol (EuroQol Group 1990).

The success rates, based on perceived recovery after 7 weeks, were 68% for manual therapy, 51% for physical therapy and 36% for continued care, and 72%, 63% and 56%

Figure 40.1 Flow chart describing the progress of patients through the trial. Adapted from Hoving et al 2002.

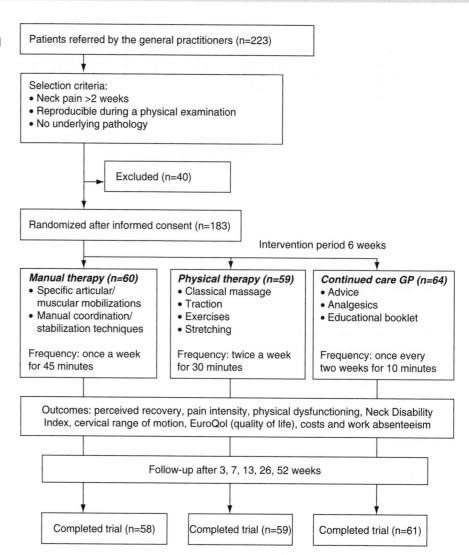

after 52 weeks, respectively. The differences between manual therapy, physical therapy and continued care were substantial just after the intervention period but marginal 1 year after follow-up. Manual therapy scored better than physical therapy and continued care on all primary and secondary outcomes. Physical therapy scored slightly better than continued care by the GP with regard to perceived recovery and severity of impairment, but the differences were, in general, not significant. It was concluded that manual therapy consisting of mainly spinal mobilization was more effective than continued care by a general practitioner and slightly more effective than physiotherapy consisting of exercises.

TRIAL ON CERVICOGENIC HEADACHE

The second randomized clinical trial on manual therapy evaluated the effectiveness of manipulative therapy and a low-load exercise programme for cervicogenic headache when used alone and in combination, as compared with a control group (Jull et al 2002). The headache trial was unique in the sense that it used a 2×2 factorial design. In this study, 200 participants who met the diagnostic criteria for cervicogenic headache were randomized into four groups: manipulative therapy group, exercise therapy group, combined exercise and manipulative therapy group and a control group. Except for simple analgesics or NSAIDs, which were optional in all treatment groups, the control group received no active treatments.

The primary outcome was a change in headache frequency. The other outcomes included changes in headache intensity and duration, the Northwick Park Neck Pain Questionnaire (Leak et al 1994), medication intake and patient satisfaction. Physical outcomes included pain on neck movement, upper cervical joint tenderness, a craniocervical flexion muscle test and a photographic measure of posture. The treatment period was 6 weeks with follow-up assessment after treatment, then at 3, 6, and 12 months.

Both in the short- and long-term follow-up the active treatments (manipulative therapy, exercise therapy and the combined exercise and manipulation therapy) were superior to the control group for the headache frequency and headache intensity (P <0.05 for all). None of the active therapies was superior, but 10% more patients gained greater headache relief with the combination treatment. Effect sizes were at least moderate and clinically relevant. It was concluded that manipulative therapy and exercise can reduce the symptoms of cervicogenic headache, and that these effects are maintained.

Although regarded by many as the gold standard, randomized clinical trials (RCTs) are limited by practical and methodological issues. The interpretation of the design of a randomized clinical trial is not always straightforward. A useful distinction between trial designs is that of explanatory and pragmatic research designs.

DISTINCTION BETWEEN PRAGMATIC AND EXPLANATORY STUDY DESIGNS

Randomized clinical trials in the field of manual therapy are often knowingly, or unknowingly, set up with pragmatic or explanatory study design features. Both study designs have advantages and disadvantages and are relevant for different purposes.

The distinction between these designs explains some of the particular characteristics of manual therapy trials. In reality, many trials have combinations of pragmatic and explanatory designs (see Table 40.1).

Examples of pragmatic and explanatory design features will be discussed throughout this chapter. The two previously discussed manual therapy trials had commonly applied manual therapy treatment options, patient relevant outcome measures and intention-to-treat analysis. These features are usually seen in pragmatic trials. On the other hand, some features were consistent with explanatory

Table 40.1 Characteristics and differences between pragmatic trials and explanatory trials

Pragmatic trial	Explanatory trial
'Effectiveness'	'Efficacy'
Manual therapy in 'usual' daily practice	Manual therapy in 'ideal' situations
Aims to make a decision between treatment alternatives	Aims to test hypothesis aimed at maximizing patient outcomes
Treatment follows general management or guidelines	Treatment follows strict protocol detailing each characteristic
Open selection criteria	Strict selection criteria
Usually patient and therapist not blinded	Blinding of patient and therapist
No placebo	Placebo
All patients, including drop-outs or those not adhering to protocol, are included in 'intention to treat' analyses	Only patients who fully complied with study protocol are included in 'per protocol' analyses

designs, including specific physical selection criteria and physical outcome measures.

Misconceptions arise when pragmatic trials are being judged using criteria which are applicable in explanatory trials or vice versa. Examples of these questions include: 'Why wasn't a placebo group included?'; 'Why were patients with additional complaints included in the trial?'; 'Why was the treatment not standardized in every detail?'; 'Why did the analyses include patients who did not receive the planned treatment or patients who dropped out of the trial?'

Pragmatic trials

The reality in everyday practice is that patients often have additional complaints, do not complete the total number of treatment sessions available to them, receive variations of the same treatment, get other treatment such as massage from a friend, use analgesics, do not perform their home exercises or switch treatment to other (alternative) health care providers for reasons related or unrelated to their current treatment.

In pragmatic trials, one is usually interested in the 'effectiveness' of manual therapy in daily practice and this involves choosing between two or more alternatives available to patients. Pragmatic trials can easily be generalized as situations in this design matched situations encountered in daily practice. However, replication of the exact treatment in this design may prove more difficult due to the more 'open' approach of the pragmatic study. We may find that manual therapy 'works' but we are not exactly sure how and under which optimal conditions.

Because of their applicability in everyday practice, healthcare providers can use evidence from pragmatic trials to make policy decisions (for example, on where patients in primary care should be treated for neck pain). As the design of pragmatic trials aims to inform choices between treatments, its design is well suited to look at the cost-effectiveness (and not cost-*efficacy*) of interventions. Placebos are not generally used in pragmatic trials as they do not usually aim to help clinicians decide between a new treatment and the best current treatment. In a pragmatic approach, the treatment response is the total difference between two treatments, including both treatment and associated placebo effects, as this will best reflect the likely clinical response in practice.

Explanatory trials

In explanatory trials, on the other hand, the focus is on the efficacy of manual therapy under 'ideal' (or laboratory) situations to further scientific knowledge. The treatment protocol usually includes a hypothesis of exactly how the experimental treatment works. In explanatory trials, it is common to have multiple formal hypotheses that are defined in terms of maximizing patient outcomes. As multiple hypotheses can be formulated, many different outcome measures can be used, including pathophysiological outcomes, which have no direct relevance to patients. Often, these are considered as secondary outcomes in pragmatic trials.

Examples of pathophysiological outcomes include measures evaluating cervical joint dysfunction (Jull et al 1997), aerobic capacity (Oldervoll et al 2001), an ability to find the neutral head position (Rogers 1997), fear avoidance beliefs (Linton & Ryberg 2001) and pressure pain thresholds (Vernon et al 1990). Although sometimes used as primary end-point, these outcomes are usually used as intermediate outcomes that help to understand the biological basis of the response to manual therapy.

In both the neck pain and the headache trials it was considered important to assess physical function, which was expected to change in response to the interventions under investigation. In explanatory trials the treatment description involves an exact definition of the treatment parameters and these are to be maintained throughout the trial. In addition, the patients consist of a homogeneous group who, through the hypothesized working mechanism of treatment, could maximally benefit from manual therapy.

Because of their different approaches, generalizations from pragmatic and explanatory trials should be made with caution. Manual therapy may improve segmental mobility and muscle tension but that in itself does not mean the patients feel or function better. In addition, manual therapy tested under ideal conditions may not work in clinical practice or is simply not feasible because of practical limitations.

Conducting a clinical trial has some other specific challenges and issues, specifically related to the field of manual therapy. These will be discussed and the concepts of pragmatic and explanatory designs will be further explored.

ISSUES AROUND THE DEFINITION OF THE MANUAL THERAPY INTERVENTIONS

The body of literature on manual therapy is extensive as is reflected in the impressive number of textbooks and journal articles. However, the literature on manual therapy is highly heterogeneous as there are many different schools of thought. Within these rationales, diagnostic and treatment techniques vary considerably. Whether these philosophical differences have any association with differences in treatment efficacy remains to be seen.

The mechanisms underlying many components of manual therapy rely heavily on theoretical assumption. As described by Gross et al (1996b), mechanisms may include the mechanical alterations of tissue (for example improving mobility in a joint), neurophysiological effects (for example pain modulation) and psychological influences, both through manual contact or 'laying on of hands' and through attention, support and so on. The evidence for these hypotheses is limited and needs to be empirically validated (Farrell & Jensen 1992, Fitzgerald et al 1994).

In general, principles underlying manual therapy are characterized in publications of randomized clinical trials

as 'relieving pain and improving function'. However, it is often not clear what is meant by manual therapy (Hoving et al 2001), what the professional background and experience is of the health professional and whether the manual therapy techniques applied in RCTs are similar to those used in clinical practice.

Studies on implementation and guidelines in the manual therapy literature are scarce. The translation of what works for individual patients into what works for a group of patients suffering from cervical syndromes is difficult. Although it is often possible to describe the combination of treatment components that constitute the treatment strategies, it is much harder to say in which order, intensity, and which specific segmental cervical level was treated because this usually varies per patient and over time.

The number of diagnostic findings that a manual therapist can work from is extensive. To illustrate this, consider the following findings during a physical examination of a specific patient (using segmental motion testing, palpation, inspection, strength testing). 'Manual assessment, including spinal intervertebral motion testing, revealed a localized restriction in joint movement at C2–3 and C3–4, some hypermobility at C4–5 and C6–7, myofascial tightening of the upper back, restricted movement of the upper thoracic vertebrae, forward head posture, tense suboccipital musculature and weak middle and upper trapezius muscles.'

Each of these findings will be addressed in a specific way. Not only will there be different techniques to choose from but the order, intensity, direction, frequency and the decision to change manual therapy techniques over time will also vary between manual therapists. To incorporate all these specific variables into a specific treatment protocol that is applicable in clinical practice is a challenge. A recent survey showed that the top three indications for (a single) cervical spine manipulation were segmental fixation, a stiff but stable joint and internal derangement (indicated by more than 70% of the therapists) (Hurley et al 2002). Unfortunately we do not know how these findings are translated into a treatment plan involving more patients with different clinical presentations.

The reassessment of patients in daily practice and the alteration of treatment techniques according to the patient's response to treatment are essential. However, it has proved difficult to incorporate these into a manual therapy clinical guideline let alone evaluate them in a clinical trial. In addition, the traditional manual therapeutic assessment, for example the assessment of joint play or other manual tests (passive or active), has shown variable intra-rater reproducibility and mostly poor inter-rater reproducibility. Local muscle spasm, the level of patient relaxation or the amount of joint mobility play additional roles which are highly variable. It is easier to establish criteria with more uniformly measurable outcomes such as pain, range of motion, posture or functional activity, but these do not guide the therapist in choosing the correct mobilization or manipulation technique.

Certainly it is possible to set criteria for changing the intensity of treatment by varying the treatment duration or frequency of treatment in broad terms. A few trials, mostly chiropractic (Sloop et al 1982, Vernon et al 1990, Cassidy et al 1992), describe the manipulation technique, but the application of just one manipulation may not be representative of treatment by a manual therapist, but rather more so for chiropractors (Assendelft et al 1992). To overcome detailed rationales and descriptions of a whole range of manual therapy techniques, studies often mention that the manual therapy techniques were provided according to the appropriate textbooks (for example by Maitland, Kaltenborn or Cyriax).

Excellent case studies have been published which include the rationale of the manual therapy procedures and the specific treatment characteristics. Valuable lessons can be learned from these studies. A case study described by Olson & Joder (2001) describes a patient with a common pattern of decreased mobility in the upper and lower cervical and upper thoracic spinal segments and hypermobility of the mid-cervical segments. This case illustrates a treatment approach that combines manual therapy including an array of different techniques on different spinal segments (for example, 'upright C2–3 facet grade IV manipulation'). Manipulation techniques were used to address the limited mobility and low load high repetition exercises were used to treat the (mid-cervical) instability (Olson & Joder 2001). This case study illustrates that many different diagnostic and therapeutic decisions have to be made during the course of treatment, which is typical of manual therapy practice.

There was no common manual therapy guideline for the treatment of non-specific neck pain or cervicogenic headache prior to the commencement of these two clinical trials. Evidence based practice integrates the clinical expertise with the latest evidence. In the absence of clear evidence, clinicians need to gain consensus on the essential elements in the management of cervical syndromes. In clinical practice, reassessment of the patient's condition is normal and helps to alter treatment according to the patient's response to treatment. In the neck pain and the headache trials this was possible. Both trials had a pragmatic approach that allowed the manual therapists to perform their own evaluation and treatment as much as possible. Consequently this was more reflective of manual therapy in usual care. In other words, it is the management protocol (guidelines) that is the subject of the investigation in pragmatic trials, which allows for differences in treatment modes for different patients.

There is an increasing interest in the formulation of clinical guidelines. Even though the evidence base is rather small for most conservative treatments, groups of experts in the field are able to formulate consensus-based guidelines using a systematic process of guideline development. Recently, Scholten-Peeters published clinical guidelines for physiotherapy in the treatment of whiplash-associated disorders in the Netherlands (Scholten-Peeters et al 2002). Additionally, Gross et al (2002b) formulated clinical guidelines for the treatment of neck disorders for the state of Ontario, Canada. However, neither of these guidelines outlines a specific manual therapy protocol.

In the neck pain and the headache trials, there were, a priori, no detailed manual therapy treatment guidelines. However, it was felt that some specific information about the manual therapy treatment needed to be provided. As a result, some of the characteristics were provided after the manual therapy intervention (Jull 2002). This provided some insight into the actual treatments delivered, although due to the limitations described before it was not possible to repeat or describe the exact procedures for a whole group in exact detail.

Manual therapy in the neck pain trial

In the neck pain trial the different treatment variables were recorded in a treatment booklet, for example: the segmental levels being mobilized; whether the technique involved traction, translation, compression or an angular movement; a non-specific or specific (localized) technique; and whether the technique was one-, two- or three-dimensional. In addition, information was recorded regarding the type of (homework) exercises, treatment goals and type of advice. The manual therapy approach was eclectic and incorporated several manual therapy evaluation and treatment techniques. These were described in a handbook (van der El et al 1993) which included the rationale and all specific muscular and articular mobilization techniques.

Mobilization was the main characteristic in the trial and this was defined as 'a form of manual therapy that involves low-velocity passive movements within or at the limit of joint range of motion' (Di Fabio 1999). The active component (involving active participation by the patient) of the treatment consisted of coordination or stabilization techniques. In addition, the manual therapist instructed the patients to perform home exercises.

The patients in the comparison group received a mixture of treatment options frequently applied by physical therapists (Borghouts et al 1999) with an emphasis on exercise therapy, including active exercises and postural exercises, stretching techniques and relaxation exercises. In most treatment sessions some passive form of physical therapy was included, such as massage or manual traction. Of interest is that most manual therapy trials on cervical pain syndromes include multiple treatment elements including exercise, physical agents and education, often referred to as 'multimodal' treatment. This pragmatic approach reflects the current practice of physical therapy.

Manual therapy in the headache trial

The manual therapy treatment in the headache trial was also pragmatic: 'the treating physiotherapists were permitted to select manipulative techniques on the basis of the clinician's clinical reasoning process in physical diagnosis and treatment and in response to the subject's segmental movement dysfunction', according to Maitland et al (2000). Specific techniques consisted of translatory or accessory glides, passive segmental physiological movements (in lateral flexion, rotation, flexion or extension) and combinations of translatory and physiological movements. The manipulative treatment could be augmented with active range of motion exercises and ergonomic advice. Interestingly, in the headache trial the exercise group in combination with manipulative therapy was expected to be the most effective treatment.

Although the specific treatment procedures in the manipulative therapy group were unspecified, the protocol for the exercise group was very detailed. Unlike the manipulative treatment, this protocol described the working mechanism, the type of exercises, the frequencies and the order of each individual treatment component. The detail and the explorative nature of the exercise protocol and the use of intermediate outcomes shows that there was an additional focus on exploring a pathophysiological hypothesis and thus that it had characteristics of an exploratory trial.

ISSUES AROUND IDENTIFYING THE MOST EFFECTIVE TREATMENT COMPONENT

The design of clinical trials is the optimal one to compare the supposed 'specific' treatments effects between groups and keep all other factors comparable. The overall response of a patient treated by a manual therapist may be a combination of components including: the natural course of the disease; the non-specific effects of manual therapy (attention, placebo or so-called 'hands-on' effect); the supposed specific effects of manual therapy techniques (mobilization or manipulation techniques); instruction, advice and counselling by the manual therapist (formal or informal); home exercises; analgesic use (prescription or non-prescription); and other known or unknown contributors.

Interventions in randomized trials should differ sufficiently to show potential differences in the outcomes. Obviously, treatments that are very similar will have less potential to show differences in the clinical outcomes. Control treatments in clinical trials on manual therapy for neck pain consist of other manual therapy techniques (manipulation versus mobilization for example), rest, analgesics, exercise (low or high intensity, using exercise equipment or not, in a supervised group or individual), modalities such as heat or cold, collar, massage and stretching. Other alternatives such as acupuncture have also been used as control treatments (Gross et al 2002a, 2004). Due to the heterogeneity of control treatments, however, it is unclear which combinations of control treatments are effective and which not.

Problems that are faced when setting up a trial are that on the one hand, investigators want to ensure that the treatments under evaluation have a maximal contrast by decreasing treatment overlap, or if this is not possible or desirable, to try to standardize them. On the other hand, the reality in clinical practice is that patients usually receive a combination of manual therapy and other interventions. In most trials there is some trade-off between the desire to optimize contrast and the desire to deliver care that is commonly applied in clinical practice. This is not only because of reasons of contrast; the design of a clinical trial has other restrictions not discussed here. However, treatments in randomized clinical trials are never completely 'pragmatic' (i.e. as in usual clinical practice). This is illustrated in the neck pain and the headache trials.

Treatment components in the headache trial and the neck pain trial

In the literature, none of the single treatment modalities has yet been shown to be superior, and multimodal treatments such as presented in the neck pain and headache trials are more common (Karjalainen et al 2000, Gross et al 2002a, 2004). Due to the pragmatic nature of the neck pain trial, it was difficult to identify the most important contributor to the overall effect for conservative treatments on neck pain, including 'manual therapy'. The advantage of the factorial design in the headache trial was that it allowed an evaluation of the additional value of combining exercises and the manipulation as well as the single use of these modalities.

Although mobilization in the neck pain trial was considered to be dominant in the manual therapy approach, these effects cannot be disentangled from the effects from other treatment components including stabilization exercises, and muscular mobilization techniques, education, advice and home exercises. To ensure a contrast with manual therapy, the physical therapists were not allowed to perform specific mobilization techniques. This hampered, to a certain extent, the pragmatic aspect of this trial because some passive mobilization techniques are used by physical therapists with or without extensive training in manual therapy techniques

ISSUES AROUND THE SELECTION OF THE PATIENT SUITABLE FOR MANUAL THERAPY

Ideally, one wants to select the type of patient that could maximally benefit from manual therapy. Incorporating physical examination procedures into the design of trials on manual therapy can be seen as exploratory. Evidence on which patients are proven to benefit from manual therapy is scarce.

A consensus panel judged cervical mobilization to be appropriate for those patients with neck pain anatomically consistent with a musculotendinous distribution, with no evidence of radiculopathy and no contraindication for manipulation (Coulter et al 1996). Those factors regarded as inappropriate for mobilization (or manipulation) were the presence of substantial trauma, clinical risk factors for neck pain in the absence of radiographs and the presence of disc herniation or spinal canal stenosis. As indicated by the criteria, this still leaves most of the patients with cervical syndromes suitable for cervical mobilization. Moreover, the appropriateness or inappropriateness of manipulation was similar to that of mobilization, though mobilization was rated more favourably.

It is important to perform explorative studies in the absence of evidence of which patient groups benefit from manual therapy. Although this can be done through simple case studies or on a larger scale such as the studies performed by Jull (Jull et al 1988, 1994), this can also be achieved through secondary analyses in randomized clinical trials.

An example of the use of subgroup analyses for generating research hypotheses is provided by the neck pain trial. An interesting finding was that the differences in effect between manual therapy and the other two interventions were significantly more pronounced for patients with severe complaints (more pain and limitation of movement) at baseline. In other words, those patients with a lot of pain and limitation of movement did better with manual therapy than with exercises and counselling. The low severity group showed no distinct differences, although a slight non-significant treatment advantage was observed for exercises by a physical therapist. This can be observed in Figure 40.2.

A new parameter in the neck pain and the headache trials was that these trials checked whether the patients had a mechanical problem in the neck and thus whether these mechanical problems were reproducible during a physical examination. Both trials used a manual therapist to perform a physical examination of the neck to confirm suitability of the patients for the trials, and patients were considered appropriate to receive manual therapy.

The headache trial formulated one of the physical selection criteria as 'symptomatic joint dysfunction in the upper cervical segments (C0–3)'. Thus patients were required to have signs of painful cervical joint dysfunction in at least one of the upper cervical joints detected by manual examination. In previous work, Jull et al (1988) had shown that the examination process was feasible and accurate. This line of work shows that it is possible to explore which type of patient could be suitable for manual therapy.

On a critical note, the practical execution of a trial demands that enough patients are recruited within a certain time frame. Studies, and RCTs in particular, are extremely costly (Koes & Hoving 1998). Most trials in primary care have great difficulty recruiting the desired number of patients. Refining the selection criteria and having very stringent selection criteria may further limit the number of patients actually being recruited. Many trials on manual therapy have small patient samples and lack power to detect a statistically significant treatment effect (Gross et al 2002a, 2004).

In addition, the successful completion of a manual therapy trial starts with the successful recruitment of manual therapists and general practitioners. These factors can easily be overlooked when starting a randomized clinical trial. Every trial should benefit from the experiences of previous trials. Van der Windt et al (2000) summarized the reasons why practitioners may participate in a randomized trial: a relevant research question, knowledge and interest in research methods, minimal time involvement, financial reimbursement, postgraduate training, no burden for the patient, no interference with patient–practitioner relationship, no clear preference for the interventions in the trial, not involved in many other studies (Van der Windt et al 2000). This summary could be used as a checklist for the successful participation of manual therapists and others in future research.

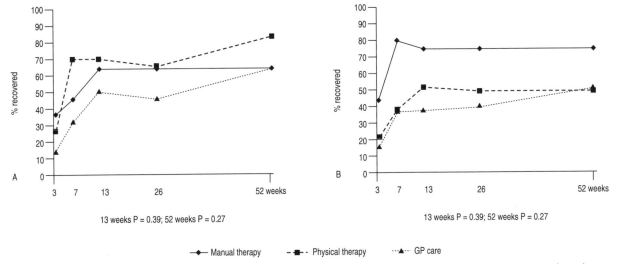

Figure 40.2 A: Perceived recovery 3–52 weeks; subgroup with mild cervical dysfunction. B: Perceived recovery 3–52 weeks, subgroup with severe cervical dysfunction.

To ensure generalizability, pragmatic trials should ideally represent the patients to whom the treatment will be applied. In the neck pain trial, the population was not considered a highly selected patient sample and represents to some extent a general practice population. Similar to a recent Dutch observational study in general practice (Borghouts et al 1999), cervical pain was more frequently found in women, often radiated to the head or radiated below the elbow, and was most prevalent at the age of 45–50 year.

ISSUES AROUND REPORTING ADVERSE EFFECTS

Just as it is important to assess the potential benefits of manual therapy, it is also important to assess potential negative or adverse effects. Manipulation (high velocity thrust techniques) of the cervical spine has been associated with potential severe adverse effects (such as paralysis or death) in a number of case reports in the literature (Assendelft et al 1996). The poor reporting of these incidents and the few studies on this topic make it difficult to assess the available evidence for its validity, importance and relevance to our own patients. It is also unclear whether the side-effect always occurred because of the treatment.

We identified five systematic reviews on manual therapies where the issue of harm was addressed (Vernon 1995, Aker et al 1996, Gross et al 1996b, 2004, Hurwitz et al 1996, Magee et al 2000). Although these review articles addressed complications in general, none reported that manipulation should be discouraged for this reason.

In the neck pain trial, the side-effects reported by patients, including increased pain after treatment, dizziness and headaches, were certainly unpleasant but not severe. These side-effects are well known to physical therapists and manual therapists, especially in patients with cervical syndromes, and are usually transient. Often patients experience these symptoms concurrently with their neck pain. Because these symptoms are frequent it is difficult to assess whether they are a result of the treatment or the disorder. Interestingly, the number of side-effects in the neck pain trial was highest in the manual therapy group, despite the superiority of this treatment.

Likewise in the headache trial, no major adverse events were recorded. The most common side-effect was a temporary aggravation of the headache following treatment. On average 26% of patients reported that treatment aggravated their headache on at least one occasion. Like the neck pain trial, this was marginally higher for the group receiving manual therapy (8.7% of all treatments provoked a post-treatment headache) in comparison to the specific exercise group (5.4%) and the group receiving both manual therapy and exercise (5.2%).

A systematic method for recording adverse reactions is absent in most trials. We found six clinical trials on cervical pain syndromes and manual therapy that reported on adverse events, including more pain, headache, dizziness,

visual disturbances and ear symptoms (Brodin 1984, Cassidy et al 1992, Jensen et al 1995, Bronfort et al 2001; Hoving et al 2001). Although all reported side-effects were relatively benign, thorough examination of all potential side-effects of treatment should be the custom in all randomized trials.

Certainly prevention of serious side-effects must come first and it should be questioned whether any alternative treatments are available with equal benefit. The investigators of the neck pain trial choose to have specific mobilization and not high velocity manipulations in their treatment guidelines. Although the manual therapists performed cervical manipulation routinely, they did not indicate that they believed they would be less successful with their treatment if this possibility were omitted. In contrast, the manual therapists in the headache trial were able to choose to use high velocity manipulations if they considered that this was the preferred technique for their patient, judged on the clinical examination. Nevertheless, this option was not used in 80% of all treatments delivered over the trial period to patients who were assigned to the manual therapy or combined therapies group (Jull 2002). Thus, most commonly, the manual therapists chose to use specific mobilization techniques, but 42% of patients in these groups received a cervical manipulation at some time in the treatment period. This suggests that cervical manipulation was used selectively and relatively conservatively.

The importance of pre-manipulative testing has been stressed in the recent literature (Barker et al 2000, Licht et al 2000) and tests for irritability, stability, vascular and neurological systems have been proposed. Manual therapists have a responsibility to ensure the safe application of manual therapy, especially when performing (rotational) manipulations in the (upper) cervical spine. Both in the neck pain trial and in the headache trial, patients with a perceived risk for manual therapy were excluded and the examination process included a pre-manipulative protocol.

THE COST-EFFECTIVENESS OF MANUAL THERAPY

Virtually no cost-effectiveness studies have been performed in manual therapy trials. There is a clear need to search for the most cost-effective treatment for patient's musculoskeletal disorders and cervical syndromes in particular because of the high costs to society associated with sick leave and disability due to neck complaints.

In the neck pain trial, an economic evaluation was performed to evaluate the cost-effectiveness of manual therapy and the other two treatments (Korthals-de Bos et al 2003). The direct (costs of interventions, additional visits, drugs, professional help) and indirect (work absenteeism) costs were measured by means of cost diaries completed by patients during the intervention period and the 52-week follow-up. The mean total costs in the manual therapy group (447 euros) amounted to approximately one-third of the costs in the physical therapy group (1297 euros) and the continued care group (1379 euros). The differences in total costs between manual therapy and the other two interventions were statistically significant.

Combining the results of the clinical effects with the economical evaluation provides convincing evidence in this study for the benefits of manual therapy in the treatment of patients with cervical pain in primary care. This is an interesting and important finding and could have promise for manual therapy and the use of cost-effectiveness analyses in future trials. The potential cost-effectiveness of manual therapy could change the otherwise mostly inconclusive results reported in previous randomized clinical trials on spinal disorders (Hoving et al 2001, Gross et al 2002a).

BLINDING AND PLACEBO TREATMENTS IN MANUAL THERAPY TRIALS

Cognitions and beliefs can raise expectations about the outcomes in clinical studies which can lead to biased results. 'Blinding' basically means that the treatment allocation is kept hidden and is used to eliminate this bias. Blinding in a randomized clinical trial is theoretically possible at various levels: the patient, the caregiver, the outcome assessor and the person analyzing the data. However, in the case of 'hands-on' therapies such as manual therapy it is difficult, if not impossible, to perform blinding at the level of a patient or therapist. An effective means of blinding the patient, by including a trustworthy placebo therapy, is often not possible in manual therapy trials.

A consequence of a pragmatic study design is that it is impossible to study the effectiveness of any specific effect of the intervention. In the neck pain and the headache trials the observed effects may, to a certain extent, have been the result of the natural course of cervical pain and cervicogenic headache, or they could be attributed to placebo effects of the interventions. The placebo effect is clearly a desirable effect and its use should be maximized. In addition, clinical practice does not normally involve a decision between giving either treatment or a placebo. The aim in clinical practice is to determine which type of treatment should be provided for a patient with neck pain or cervicogenic headache.

CONCLUSION

Until now, there has been no strong evidence to indicate which patients will derive most benefit from manual therapy but it is plausible that manual therapy has different effects on different subsets of patients. An indication for this was seen in the neck pain trial where manual therapy showed a substantially larger treatment effect, especially in patients with more severe neck dysfunction (pain and stiffness). Since manual therapy techniques are specifically (but not exclusively) aimed at restoration of impairments (including improving joint function and pain), this may not be a surprising finding. Preferably, these would be the type of patients to include in a new clinical trial.

It would be useful to develop uniform and internationally accepted classifications, definitions and rationales for the various treatment strategies (components) in the field of manual therapy. It is clear from the reviews on RCTs involving manual therapy that most of the interventions are multimodal and include combinations of several treatment components. Future trials should further investigate which specific treatment components or combinations are the most effective, in which order they are most effective, what the optimal dosage is (number, duration and frequency) and whether multimodal treatments are indeed more effective than single treatment components.

In addition it is important that guidelines are developed in which a set of criteria are developed to guide clinicians in altering their treatment over time. It will be interesting to investigate the effect of a treatment strategy for patients with severe cervical pain involving a clear decision making process (in the form of a decision tree). Current rationales and underlying theories require critical analyses and operationalization.

KEYWORDS	
manual therapy	headache
explanatory design	placebo
pragmatic design	guidelines
methodology	cost-effectiveness
neck pain	adverse effects

References

Aker P D, Gross A R, Goldsmith C H, Peloso P 1996 Conservative management of mechanical neck pain: systematic overview and meta-analysis. British Medical Journal 313: 1291–1296

Assendelft W J J, Koes B W, van der Heijden G J, Bouter L M 1992 The efficacy of chiropractic manipulation for back pain: blinded review of relevant randomized clinical trials. Journal of Manipulative and Physiological Therapeutics 15: 487–494

Assendelft W J, Bouter L M, Knipschild P G 1996 Complications of spinal manipulation: a comprehensive review of the literature. Journal of Family Practice 42: 475–480

Barker S, Kesson M, Ashmore J, Turner G, Conway J, Stevens D 2000 Professional issue: guidance for pre-manipulative testing of the cervical spine. Manual Therapy 5: 37–40

Borghouts A J, Janssen H J, Koes B W, Muris J W M, Metsemakers J F M, Bouter L M 1999 The management of chronic pain in general practice: a retrospective study. Scandinavian Journal of Primary Health Care 17: 215–220

Brodin H 1984 Cervical pain and mobilization. International Journal of Rehabilitation Research 7: 190–191

Bronfort G, Evans R, Nelson B, Aker P D, Goldsmith C H, Vernon H 2001 A randomized clinical trial of exercise and spinal manipulation for patients with chronic neck pain. Spine 26: 788–797

Cassidy J D, Lopes A A, Yong-Hing K 1992 The immediate effect of manipulation versus mobilization on pain and range of motion in the cervical spine: a randomized controlled trial. Journal of Manipulative and Physiological Therapeutics 15: 570–575

Coulter I 1996 Manipulation and mobilization of the cervical spine: the results of a literature survey and consensus panel. Journal of Musculoskeletal Pain 4: 113–123

Di Fabio R P 1999 Manipulation of the cervical spine: risks and benefits. Physical Therapy 79: 50–65

EuroQol Group 1990 EuroQol: a new facility for the measurement of health-related quality of life. Health Policy 16: 199–208

Farrell J P, Jensen G M 1992 Manual therapy: a critical assessment of role in the profession of physical therapy. Physical Therapy 72: 843–852

Fitzgerald G K, McClure P W, Beattie P, Riddle D L 1994 Issues in determining treatment effectiveness of manual therapy. Physical Therapy 74: 227–233

Gross A R, Aker P D, Goldsmith C H, Peloso P 1996a Conservative management of mechanical neck disorders: a systematic overview and meta-analysis. Online Journal of Current Clinical Trials doc no 200–201

Gross A R, Aker P D, Quartly C 1996b Manual therapy in the treatment of neck pain. Rheumatic Disease Clinics of North America 22: 579–598

Gross A, Kay T, Hondras M et al 2002a Manual therapy for mechanical neck disorders: a systematic review. Manual Therapy 7: 131–149

Gross A R, Kay T, Kennedy C et al 2002b Clinical practice guideline (CPG) on the use of manipulation in the treatment of adults with mechanical neck disorders. Technical report of the College of Physiotherapists of Ontario, Toronto, Ontario

Gross A R, Hoving J L, Haines T A et al, 2004 Cervical Overview Group. Manipulation and mobilisation for mechanical neck disorders. Cochrane Library, Issue 1, CD004249

Hoving J L, Gross A R, Gasner D et al 2001 A critical appraisal of review articles on the effectiveness of conservative treatment for neck pain. Spine 26: 196–205

Hoving J L, Koes B W, de Vet H C et al 2002 Manual therapy, physical therapy, or continued care by a general practitioner for patients with neck pain: a randomized, controlled trial. Annals of Internal Medicine 136: 713–722

Hurley L, Yardley K, Gross A R, Hendry L, McLaughlin L 2002 A survey to examine attitudes and patterns of practice of physiotherapists who perform cervical spine manipulation. Manual Therapy 7: 10–18

Hurwitz E L, Aker P D, Adams A H, Meeker W C, Shekelle P G 1996 Manipulation and mobilization of the cervical spine: a systematic review of the literature. Spine 21: 1746–1759

Jensen I, Nygren A, Gamberale F, Goldie I, Westerholm P, Jonsson E 1995 The role of the psychologist in multidisciplinary treatments for chronic neck and shoulder pain: a controlled cost-effectiveness study. Scandinavian Journal of Rehabilitation Medicine 27: 19–26

Jull G 2002 The use of high and low velocity cervical manipulative therapy procedures by Australian manipulative physiotherapists. Australian Journal of Physiotherapy 48: 189–193

Jull G, Bogduk N, Marsland A 1988 The accuracy of manual diagnosis for cervical zygapophysial joint pain syndromes. Medical Journal of Australia 148: 17–20

Jull G, Treleaven J, Versace G 1994 Manual examination: is pain provocation a major cue for spinal dysfunction? Australian Journal of Physiotherapy 40: 159–165

Jull G, Zito G, Trott P, Potter H, Shirley D, Richardson C 1997 Inter-examiner reliability to detect painful upper cervical joint dysfunction. Australian Journal of Physiotherapy 43: 125–129

Jull G, Trott P, Potter H et al 2002 A randomized controlled trial of exercise and manipulative therapy for cervicogenic headache. Spine 17: 1835–1843

Karjalainen K, Malmivaara A, van Tulder M et al 2000 Multidisciplinary biopsychosocial rehabilitation for neck and shoulder pain among working age adults. Cochrane Database Systematic Reviews CD002194

Koes B W, Hoving J L 1998 Masterclass: the value of the randomized clinical trial in the field of physiotherapy. Manual Therapy 3: 179–186

Korthals-de Bos I B, Hoving J L, van Tulder M W et al 2003 Cost effectiveness of physiotherapy, manual therapy, and general practitioner care for neck pain: economic evaluation alongside a randomised controlled trial. British Medical Journal 326: 911

Leak A M, Cooper J, Dyer S, Williams K A, Turner-Stokes L, Frank A O 1994 The Northwick Park Neck Pain Questionnaire, devised to measure neck pain and disability. British Journal of Rheumatology 33: 469–474

Licht P B, Christensen H W, Hoilund-Carlsen P F 2000 Is there a role for premanipulative testing before cervical manipulation? Journal of Manipulative and Physiological Therapeutics 23: 175–179

Linton S J, Ryberg M 2001 A cognitive-behavioral group intervention as prevention for persistent neck and back pain in a non-patient population: a randomized controlled trial. Pain 90: 83–90

Magee D J, Oborn-Barrett E, Turner S, Fenning N 2000 A systematic overview of the effectiveness of physical therapy intervention on soft tissue neck injury following trauma. Physiotherapy Canada 52: 111–130

Maitland G D, Hengeveld E, Banks K, English K 2000 Maitland's Vertebral manipulation. Butterworth, London

Oldervoll L M, Ro M, Zwart J A, Svebak S 2001 Comparison of two physical exercise programs for the early intervention of pain in the neck, shoulders and lower back in female hospital staff. Journal of Rehabilitation Medicine 33: 156–161

Olson K A, Joder D 2001 Diagnosis and treatment of cervical spine clinical instability. Journal of Orthopaedic and Sports Physical Therapy 31: 194–206

Rogers R G 1997 The effects of spinal manipulation on cervical kinesthesia in patients with chronic neck pain: a pilot study. Journal of Manipulative and Physiological Therapeutics 20: 80–85

Scholten-Peeters G, Bekkering G, Verhagen A et al 2002 Clinical practice guideline for the physiotherapy of patients with whiplash-associated disorders. Spine 27: 412–422

Sloop P R, Smith D S, Goldenberg E, Dore C 1982 Manipulation for chronic neck pain: a double-blind controlled study. Spine 7: 532–535

van der El A, Lunacek P B P, Wagemaker A J 1993 Manual therapy: treatment of the spine, 2nd edn. Manuwel, Rotterdam

van der Windt D A, Koes B W, van Aarst M, Heemskerk M A, Bouter L M 2000 Practical aspects of conducting a pragmatic randomised trial in primary care: patient recruitment and outcome assessment. British Journal of General Practice 50: 371–374

Vernon H 1995 Spinal manipulation and headaches: an update. Topics in Clinical Chiropractic 2: 34–47

Vernon H, Mior S 1991 The Neck Disability Index: a study of reliability and validity. Journal of Manipulative and Physiological Therapeutics 14: 409–415

Vernon H T, Aker P, Burns S, Viljakaanen S, Short L 1990 Pressure pain threshold evaluation of the effect of spinal manipulation in the treatment of chronic neck pain: a pilot study. Journal of Manipulative and Physiological Therapeutics 13: 13–16

Chapter 41

Outcomes assessment and measurement in spinal musculoskeletal disorders

R. A. H. M. Swinkels, R. A. B. Oostendorp

INTRODUCTION

In scientific research, instruments have been developed to objectively measure symptoms and signs of various disorders. In the last decade, the use of these instruments, and questionnaires in particular, has been intensively promoted by the authorities in the field of clinimetrics. Names such as 'index', 'scale', 'instrument', 'score' and 'profile' have regularly been applied to the result that emerges from the measurement process. To avoid ambiguity, Feinstein (1987) has suggested 'index' as the preferred term to be used in clinimetrics. Clinimetrics can be described as the domain concerned with indexes, rating scales and other expressions that are used to describe or measure symptoms, physical signs, and other distinctly clinical phenomena (Feinstein 1987). In recent years, the development of clinimetrics has been rapidly progressed with the implementation of evidence based medicine. The main reasons for outcomes management in general are on the one hand to objectify clinical data and on the other to improve quality of care. Outcomes management is a crucial component of improving quality of care without sacrificing cost (Mayer et al 1995). Outcomes management is designed to establish baselines, to document progress (or deterioration), to assist in goal setting and to motivate patients to evaluate the treatment they are receiving (Liebenson & Yeomans 1997). The introduction of evidence based medicine in the last years of the 20th century further stimulated the development and research related to outcome measurement and generated an enormous increase in the number of measurement instruments available. The total number of measurement instruments is now estimated to be between 500 and 600 in the field of musculoskeletal disorders alone. Incorporation of the use of these instruments in clinical settings can seem to take more time than their development. Firstly, the feasibility of the instrument can be an obstacle: required time, costs, availability and problems in interpretation of scores; and secondly, the great number of instruments available can make it difficult to make a good selection. How to sift the wheat from the chaff? For practical purposes, a maximum of 10–15 instruments/questionnaires can be used to describe about 75% of all patients in a regular patient population with musculoskeletal disorders.

The first issue raised is how to choose a clinimetric index. The second concerns the methodological or psychometric properties of the indexes. The European Research Group on Health Outcomes (ERGHO) has published a statement entitled 'Choosing a health outcome measurement instrument' which is applicable to all clinimetrical indexes. In choosing a measurement instrument, the first question to be asked is, 'What is the aim (construct) of the index?' (Chronic) musculoskeletal disorders, and low back pain in particular, clearly are multidimensional problems (Haldorsen et al 1998, Main & Watson 1999). This means that the outcome assessment must also be multidimensional.

The aim of this chapter is to create more clarity in this complex dilemma and to place outcome assessment in a context which is easier to understand. The *International Classification of Functioning, Disability and Health* (ICF) will first be explained in relation to outcome assessment. The relevance of distinguishing several kinds of instruments/ indexes will be explained by discussing the health profile of a patient, based on the ICF. The different kind of instruments will be distinguished. A strategy to choose the optimal index(es) will be presented, followed by a clinical example in the form of a case history.

INTERNATIONAL CLASSIFICATION OF FUNCTIONING, DISABILITY AND HEALTH

A good starting point in dividing domain-specific indexes is the *International Classification of Functioning, Disability and Health* (ICF) (WHO, 2001). The ICF is the result of adaptations of the earlier *International Classification of Impairments, Disabilities and Handicaps* (ICIDH), which was a supplement of the *International Classification of Diseases* (ICD) accepted by the World Health Assembly in 1976 and published by the World Health Organization in 1980 (WHO 1980). The ICF classifies body functions, body structures, activity and participation, environmental factors and personal factors (Fig. 41.1):

1. *Body function* and *body structures* are defined as any loss or abnormality of psychological, physiological or anatomical structure or function. The use of the term 'impairment' does not imply that disease is present or that individuals should be regarded as sick.
2. *Activity* is defined as any restriction or lack (resulting from an impairment) of ability to perform an activity in the manner or within the range considered normal for a human being. The assessment of disability requires judgement of what is normal, which brings together expectations for functioning in physical, psychological and social terms.
3. *Participation* is defined as a disadvantage for a given individual resulting from an impairment or disability

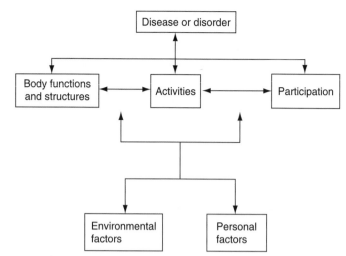

Figure 41.1 Current understanding of interactions and relationships between the dimensions of ICF (WHO 2001).

that limits the fulfilment of a role that is normal for that person, related to age, sex, and social and cultural factors. According to this definition, participation represents the more social consequences which can arise as a result of impairment and disability.

4. *Environmental factors* are organized in six chapters: products and technology; natural environments and man-made changes to environment; support and relationships; attitudes, values and beliefs; services; and systems and policies.
5. *Personal factors* (part of contextual factors) are described as gender, age, other health conditions (co-morbidity), fitness, lifestyle, habits, upbringing, coping styles, social background, education, profession, past and current experience, overall behaviour patterns and character style and individual psychological assets. The environmental factors and personal factors, clustered as external factors, can be positive as well as negative. The external factors can also play a role in the development of disease and act as so-called prognostic factors (Verbruggen & Jette 1994).

The ICF is a good starting point for the first choice of outcome measures and measurement instruments in clinical situations, particularly because diagnostic assessment by physical therapists, other allied healthcare professions and rehabilitation medicine is concerned mainly with functional disorders or consequences that arise as a result of disease (van Triet et al 1990). Furthermore, goals and findings of physical examination and treatment goals are expressed in terms of body functions and structures, activities, participation, and external factors.

HEALTH PROFILE

A very positive contribution of the World Health Organization definition of health is that health is multidimensional. Nowadays the multidimensionality of health is fully accepted and the biopsychosocial model is implemented increasingly, in diagnostics as well as in treatment of patients with musculoskeletal disorders. In the 1990s much research was generated proving that there is a strong relationship between somatic dimensions, psychological dimensions and the social dimension in patients with musculoskeletal disorders. As early as 1989 Loeser had already developed a conceptual model of pain presented in four circles that represent four different dimensions (Fig. 41.2). Tissue damage results in nociception (first circle), leading to pain perception (second circle), which constitutes the somatic dimension. A psychological dimension is reached when pain perception leads to suffering (third circle). Finally a social dimension is added when suffering leads to pain behaviour (fourth circle), preventing the patient from assuming his or her normal social role. In acute or well-managed pain with a normal recovery course, the four circles are of the same size, remain grossly concentric and largely overlap each other. In patients with chronic benign pain these circles are not concentric and there is only a partial overlap, as demonstrated in Figure 41.2.

The consequence of the incorporation of these developments in clinimetrics is that measurable treatment goals cannot be derived from a medical diagnosis but need to be described in terms of a multidimensional health profile of the patient. The implication of this is that either multidimensional indexes are required or more than just one index is needed to gain a complete profile of the patient. When selecting indexes in clinical situations, the health profile should include the following elements:

- complaints and expectations of the patient
- the onset of the current episode
- previous episodes
- course of the current episode, with emphasis on disability and participation level and positive or negative prognostic factors
- impairments
- disabilities
- problems in participation
- external factors

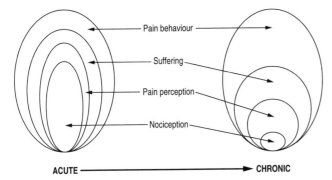

Figure 41.2 The shift from acute to chronic, reflected in the role of nociception, pain perception, suffering and pain behaviour. Adapted from Loeser 1989.

- personal factors
- coping strategy of the patient.

A prognostic health profile characterized by a short duration, low intensity pain with no previous loss of time from work is favourable and has a good prognosis with all chances of an early recovery (Watson et al 1998). McIntosh et al (2000) developed a prognostic model that predicts time receiving workers' compensation benefits in acute low back pain patients. Prognostic factors associated with reduced time of receiving benefits were: intermittent pain, a previous episode of low back pain and values on the Low Back Outcome Score Questionnaire indicating a high level of perceived function. A global prognosis depends on the presence of positive and negative prognostic factors and the possibility of influencing these prognostic factors. Early identification of negative prognostic factors may be important in understanding and possibly preventing chronic low back pain. These factors alter patients' responses to treatment and prognosis.

The factors that influence recovery vary over time. As time passes factors which may not have been important at the onset now have to be considered. Several studies suggest that work and psychosocial factors are stronger predictors of chronicity than any biomedical information (Cats-Baril & Frymoyer 1991, Gatchel et al 1995, Klenerman et al 1995). Neither biomedical factors (such as mobility, strength, the number of previous surgical interventions and medication) nor demographic variables (such as age, sex, marital and employment status) appear to be powerful predictors for return to work (Haldorsen et al 1998). If the patient is not making the expected progress, it is useful to assess the psychosocial prognostic factors. Negative prognostic factors are: beliefs that pain is harmful or potentially severely disabling, distorted ideas about the nature of pain and illness, fear avoidance behaviour, catastrophic thinking, maladaptive coping strategies, reduced activity levels, depressive mood and withdrawal from social interaction (Hasenbring et al 1994, Burton et al 1995, Klenerman et al 1995, Main & Watson 1999, Vlaeyen & Crombez 1999). According to Klenerman et al (1995), fear avoidance predicts 70% of continuing sick-leave after 12 months of treatment. A combination of historic, demographic and fear avoidance factors predicts 85% of return to work. The greater the degree of depressive mood before treatment, the stronger the patient's tendency to avoid social or physical activities (Hasenbring et al 1994). In addition, the greater the patient's tendency to avoid social or physical activities, the higher the probability that the pain will persist. Maladaptive coping strategies such as groaning, rubbing the painful area, grimacing and poor ability to have positive fantasies in coping with pain also increase the risk of chronicity. Burton et al (1995) have shown that inappropriate coping strategies such as catastrophizing are highly predictive of disability and pain. Positive prognostic factors for recovery are young age, male gender and self-efficacy (Beekman et al 1985,

Fredrickson et al 1988, Gatchel et al 1995, Keefe & Kashikar-Zuck 1996). The belief in the patient's own ability to attain a preset goal can improve treatment outcome. Patients with high levels of self-efficacy report an enhanced sense of control over their pain and lower levels of pain and disability.

According to Härkäpää et al (1991), the internal locus of control also affects treatment outcome. Patients who put the responsibility for their health in the therapist's hands or who blame some uncontrollable factor will respond poorly to therapy. Positive as well as negative prognostic factors will influence the patient's recovery rate.

Summarizing, chronic musculoskeletal disorders, and low back pain in particular, clearly are a multidimensional problem (Haldorsen et al 1998, Main & Watson 1999). This also means that outcome assessment must be multidimensional. However, no instruments or questionnaires exist that cover all these aspects. This means that use of questionnaires will always mean a set of questionnaires rather than a single instrument.

TYPES OF INSTRUMENTS

There are an enormous number of measurement instruments available to assess all types of patient variables. To structure this wealth of information it is relevant to divide all instruments on the basis of their properties.

Firstly, there are different kinds of outcome assessment:

1. anthropometric measurement instruments that measure somatic variables by a physical instrument
2. questionnaires to be completed by the patient or the examiner
3. observation lists, to be completed by the examiner.

In relation to musculoskeletal disorders, the great majority are questionnaires, followed by anthropometric instruments. Observation lists are in clinical use, for example for observation of pain behaviour.

Secondly, a distinction is made between generic indexes (measuring general aspects of health or measuring more domains) and non-generic indexes. The latter can be dimension-specific (covering one special dimension of the ICF classification) or disease-specific, intended for a selected group of patients, for example patients with low back pain, rheumatoid arthritis, shoulder problems, cerebrovascular accidents, etc. This distinction recognizes that the central questions to be answered well in advance of selecting a measurement instrument include:

- What is to be measured?
- What information is required from the patient?
- What is the goal of measurement (e.g., diagnostic, discriminative, evaluative)?

It is essential to choose an instrument that serves the desired purpose and that the instrument has the appropriate properties and qualities to fulfil the intended goals. This requires knowledge in the field of clinimetrics in terms of what instruments are available, their intended measure and their qualitative properties.

Searching for the optimal instrument

There are five steps in selecting the appropriate instruments and/or questionnaires.

Step 1. To find the best instruments for a particular clinical situation, the clinician first needs to know exactly what information they need from the patient. What domains need to be measured: body structure and function, activities, problems in participation, environmental factors, personal factors? Depending on the situation, it will often be a combination of several variables.

Step 2. The clinician needs to decide what the aim is in measuring the variable: is it diagnostic or for evaluation of the clinical course? For example, is the information intended to be part of a longitudinal measurement or only for a cross-sectional measurement? This knowledge is relevant to the methodological properties of the instrument, such as responsiveness, sensitivity, specificity, reliability and validity.

Step 3. The clinician needs to consider the methodological quality of the instrument. This requires either knowledge about methodological aspects or the instrument needs to be analysed for methodological quality. Increasing numbers of books are being published which contain data about properties and methodological quality of instruments (Streiner & Norman 1998). An example is the extensive work by Cole et al (1995), describing more than 50 different instruments.

Step 4. The clinician needs to find out how available the desired instruments/questionnaires are. In fact, although some are published commercially and protected by copyright, the great majority of questionnaires are published and freely available in the literature. The main source should be the original questionnaire published by its author(s).

Step 5. The last issue in using questionnaires in clinical settings is the correct interpretation of the results. Sometimes the key to analysis is given (particularly for commercially published questionnaires), but in other cases an extensive literature search is necessary to find out how to analyse the questionnaire. Frequent use of questionnaires generates a lot of data, which makes interpretation more accurate and easier for the clinician.

Figure 41.3 provides an overview of the path for selection of optimal measurement instrument(s), following these five steps.

Properties and methodological quality of instruments

As mentioned in the introduction, one of the challenges for the clinician is to 'sift the wheat from the chaff' in choosing

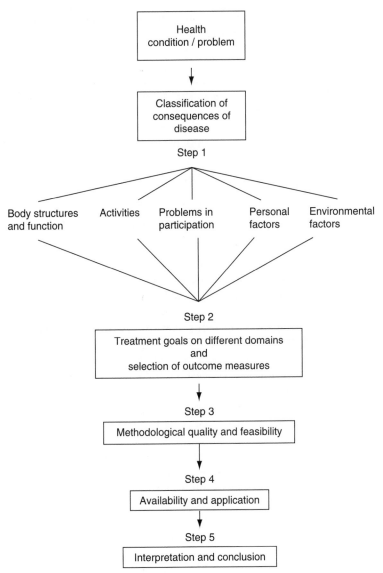

Figure 41.3 Path of selection of optimal indexes.

a measurement instrument. It is essential to examine the methodological quality of the instrument. Aspects of methodological quality are:

1. Standardisation. Is the instrument standardized in order to obtain a reproducible measurement product that can be compared between different patients? Is there an instrument manual available?
2. Reliability. The degree of consistency with which an instrument or rater measures a variable and the degree of reproducibility.
3. Internal consistency or homogeneity, reflecting the extent to which the items of a questionnaire measure the same characteristic. Internal consistency is a form of reliability. A measurement error can be generated when a question is not interpreted in the same way by different patients. To reduce this measurement error, a questionnaire needs to contain an adequate number of questions so that the desired homogeneity is in balance

with an acceptable measurement error. The rule of thumb is that the coefficient of homogeneity should be ≥ 0.80.
4. Validity. Does the instrument measure what it pretends to measure? In establishing validity it is relevant to distinguish criterion validity (validation against a gold standard), concurrent validity (validation by means of simultaneous testing with another and comparable instrument), construct validity (validation against a comparable construct or variable) and face validity (validation against judgement of an authority).
5. Responsiveness or 'sensitivity to change' of an instrument.
6. Sensitivity. A measure of validity of a screening procedure, based on the probability that someone with a disease will test positive.
7. Specificity. A measure of validity of a screening procedure based on the probability that someone who does not have a disease will test negative.

Ideally, all methodological criteria of an index should be established before it is applied in clinical situations or research. However, in reality this may not always be the case. Standardization, good reliability and internal consistency are unconditional and basic requirements for every clinimetrical index. With regard to validity, certain concessions can be accepted depending on the method of validation. A gold standard is not always available, which means that more convergent validation (Convergent validity: an approach in construct validation, assessing the degree to which two different instruments or methods are able to measure the same construct.) or more divergent validation is the relative best that there is. The critical value for accepting or rejecting a validity value is dependent on the method of validation (Is it less or more convergent construct validity? Is it criterion validity? Is it predictive validity? Is it face validity?). Good responsiveness, sensitivity and specificity are not always necessary and are dependent on the user's aim.

Responsiveness is the capacity to detect minimal clinically relevant changes. Obviously this is a particularly relevant characteristic for indexes that are intended to be used for evaluation of clinical health problems. Responsiveness is only relevant in evaluative situations. Sensitivity and specificity are relevant for measurement instruments that are intended to be used for diagnostic purposes.

In judging the properties as well as the methodological quality of an index, a scoring list has been developed (Oostendorp & Elvers 1995) to help make a standardized inventory of these aspects. This list consists of four sections: general description, domain of assessment, methodologic aspects and aspects of use. Methodological aspects can be scored for complete instruments as well as for subscales of questionnaires. Description of the domain of assessment is based on the *International Classification of Impairments, Disabilities and Handicaps* (WHO 1997), a preliminary version of the *International Classification of Functioning, Disability and Health* (ICF). Using this scoring list, it is easy to analyse an article about certain measurement instruments and to detect relevant information about the aim and the quality of that instrument(s) as well as some practical aspects of use. There is a wealth of information available concerning research on properties and qualities of measurement instruments, in particular questionnaires. In order to gain some overview, it may be helpful to reduce research and restrict it primarily to review articles concerning the relevant subject.

APPLICATION OF THE PRINCIPLES OF CLINIMETRICS TO PRACTICE: A PATIENT WITH LOW BACK PAIN

CASE HISTORY

A 30-year-old man with intermittent low back pain since the age of 15 years had a recent relapse of acute low back pain. It started 2 weeks previously when he got out of bed. The previous episode of low back pain was 6 months ago. There is no radiation of pain to his legs. He is limited in activities of daily living and sport (tennis) and on sick leave (blue collar worker in machine factory) for the last 2 weeks. The patient is convinced that continuing work will cause his health to deteriorate and he is worrying about his prognosis. He has not improved and has been referred by his general practitioner for physiotherapy treatment. The physical examination reveals no red flags and it is concluded that the patient has benign a-specific low back pain.

The case can be summarized in terms of the ICF classification and the (prognostic) health profile as follows:

- Body functions and structures: low back pain for 2 weeks, without radiation. No indication of red flags.
- Activities: limited in activities of daily living, sport and work.
- Participation: since this relapse 2 weeks ago he is not participating in sport and he is not working.
- External and personal factors: the patient has some negative cognitions concerning the influence of working and his prognosis.
- Negative prognostic factors:
  - the patient has already had 15 years' intermittent low back pain
  - he has not improved over the last 2 weeks
  - he has not continued working
  - he is worrying about the prognosis
  - there are negative cognitions.

It is assumed that the most important treatment goals for this patient will be pain relief, return to normal activities of daily living and work and prevention of chronicity. That means that the relevant domains for examination and evaluation are impairments in body structures and function (pain), disabilities in daily activities and problems in participation (activities of daily living, sport and work), personal factors (negative cognitions about pain, passive coping strategy). A selection of indexes will be discussed which are based on the flow chart in Figure 41.3). The instruments chosen must be reliable (reproducible results), valid (measure what they intend to measure), and responsive (be able to detect changes over time) to be able to evaluate the effect of treatment. Besides these methodological requirements, feasibility must be acceptable, that is, it should not take too much time to complete a questionnaire, the measurement instrument should not be too expensive and, if it concerns a questionnaire, the questionnaire must be available in the appropriate language. The therapist must be able to interpret the results of the measurement.

For the case history which has been presented the relevant domains to measure are: pain; activities/disabilities; negative prognostic factors; and general perceived health.

Pain

The variable 'pain' can be distinguished as 'sensation of pain' and 'pain behaviour'.

Visual analogue scale (VAS)

The most commonly used measurement instrument for the sensation of pain is the visual analogue scale (VAS). The VAS measures the intensity of pain along a continuous scale. It consists of a straight line, usually 100 mm in length. The ends are defined as 'no pain' and 'the worst pain ever experienced' respectively. The orientation of this line can be either vertical or horizontal. Scoring takes less than 1 minute and training of patient or therapist is not required. Test–retest reliability has been reported with an $r = 0.99$ (P <0.05) (Downie et al 1978, Scott & Huskisson 1979). Concurrent validity based on the correlation between the VAS and the finger dynamometer is $r = 0.87$ (P = 0.001) (Wilkie et al 1990). The finger dynamometer is a device that registers the amount of force exerted that the individual believes is comparable to the pain intensity. A correlation of $r = 0.81$ to 0.87 (P = 0.01–0.001) was found between the VAS and a verbal description scale of pain, (Wilkie et al 1990). Regarding responsiveness of the VAS, it has been found that the VAS is able to detect the 21 levels of just noticeable differences that individuals are able to detect (Carlsson 1983, Langley & Sheppard 1985).

Numeric pain rating scale (NPRS)

The NPRS is a numeric scale to measure the magnitude or intensity of pain. The patient is asked to select a number to represent the intensity of pain at that moment (Cole et al 1995). The scale is 0–10, with 0 being no pain and 10 being the worst pain imaginable. Explanation and administration take less than 5 minutes; training is not required. Test–retest reliability has not been investigated. In relation to concurrent validity, the NPRS and the VAS were found to have a correlation of $r = 0.80$ (P <0.01). The NPRS and the finger dynamometer showed a correlation of 0.47 to 0.68 (P <0.01). Responsiveness of the NPRS has been recently investigated by comparing the changes in the NPRS from baseline to end-point against patients' global impression of change. On average, a reduction of approximately two points or a reduction of approximately 30% in the NPRS represented a clinically important difference (Farrar et al 2001).

McGill pain questionnaire (MPQ)

The McGill Pain Questionnaire (MPQ) is designed to measure the sensory, affective and overall intensity of pain. The MPQ is the most widely used measure of pain in pain research and there has been substantial investigation of its reliability and validity for a number of pain conditions. It is available in many languages (English, Dutch, French, Italian, Norwegian, Spanish). The questionnaire consists of 20 subscales: 10 for sensory-discriminative experience of pain, five subscales for affective modalities of pain and one subscale for cognitive-evaluative aspects of pain. Cumulative calculation results in a pain rating index (PRI). Reliability in terms of correlation between scores before and after treatment were very high (0.80–0.95) (Melzack 1975, Graham et al 1980). The MPQ has been validated, on very different populations, against the VAS for pain with a correlation coefficient varying from $r = 0.45$ to $r = 0.79$ (Mendelson & Selwood 1981, Reading 1982, Walsh & Leber 1983). The MPQ takes 5–10 minutes to complete.

Pain drawing

The pain drawing (Ransford et al 1976) is a screening test thought to determine whether or not further psychological evaluation is required. However, increasing knowledge of the possible presence of abnormal pain processing in the central nervous system in musculoskeletal pain syndromes suggests that caution is required when interpreting pain drawings on a psychological basis alone. For example, Koelbaek-Johansen et al (1999) mapped widespread areas of pain in ipsilateral and contralateral lower limbs following intramuscular saline injection into areas both local (infraspinatus) and remote (tibialis anterior) to the site of pain, which were not evident in asymptomatic subjects. They considered that this widespread pain could be the expression of abnormal pain processing in the central nervous system. The pain drawing assesses the location of the pain and the presence or absence of non-anatomical pain representation and takes about 5 minutes to complete. The scoring systems consists of a five-point Likert scale by rating the drawing on a scale of 1–5 for appropriateness, 1 being completely appropriate and 5 being completely inappropriate (Schwartz & DeGood 1984, Margolis et al 1986).

Reliability of the pain drawing has proven to be good: using the surface area method of scoring, a Pearson product-moment correlation coefficient of $r = 0.85$ was found by Margolis et al (1986). Concurrent validity is explored by comparing the pain drawing to the Minnesota Multiphasic Personality Inventory (MMPI). Overall association of pain drawing and MMPI was found to be 89% (Ransford et al 1976). Responsiveness is not reported (Cole et al 1995).

Activities/disabilities

The questionnaires most used currently for assessment of disabilities in activities of daily living are the Roland-Morris Disability Questionnaire and the Quebec Back Pain Disability Scale (QBPDS).

Roland–Morris disability questionnaire (RDQ)

The RDQ is derived from the Sickness Impact Profile (SIP), a general health questionnaire for several syndromes and patient groups. The RDQ consists of 24 yes/no items from the SIP, adapted specifically for low back pain. There are no specific subscales. Completing this questionnaire takes 5–10 minutes and no specific knowledge or training is required of the examiner. The questionnaire is scored by adding up the number of 'yes' answers, varying from 0 (no disabilities at all) to 24 (severe disabilities). Test–retest reliability for the same day is r = 0.91 and r = 0.83 over a period of 3 weeks. The inter-observer reliability has been demonstrated to be good, with r = 0.92 (Stratford et al 1994). For determination of (construct) validity the RDQ has been correlated with several other indexes and proved to be good (r = 0.80 correlated with the Quebec Back Pain Disability Scale; r = 0.77 correlated with the Nottingham Health Profile, subscale physical mobility; r = 0.64 correlated with VAS pain). Responsiveness is demonstrated by an effect size of 2.02 in the improved group and 0.41 in the not-improved group of patients. The receiver operating characteristic (ROC) or area under curve was 0.93, also demonstrating a very good responsiveness (Beurskens et al 1996).

Quebec back pain disability scale (QBPDS)

The QBPDS is a 20-item questionnaire concerning activities of daily living in relation to low back pain. The items are selected from six relevant sub-domains of functional abilities for patients with low back pain: bed rest, sitting–standing, walking, moving around, bending forward, and lifting heavy objects. The QBPDS is developed in particular for (chronic) low back pain patients. It takes 5–10 minutes to complete the questionnaire and, as with the RDQ, the examiner requires no specific knowledge or training. Scoring (on a Likert scale) is the sum of all items, varying from 0 (no disabilities at all) to 100 (maximally disabled). The internal consistency is good, with Cronbach's alpha varying from 0.95 to 0.96. One week test–retest reliability is r = 0.90 and intra-class correlation coefficient (ICC) = 0.90. Construct validity is calculated at r = 0.80–0.91 when correlated with the Roland Disability Questionnaire (Kopec et al 1995). For responsiveness the correlation with change scores on other questionnaires (longitudinal construct validity) has been calculated: r = 0.60 with the Roland Disability Questionnaire and r = 0.53 with the VAS pain (Schoppink et al 1996).

Negative prognostic factors

These types of factors must be seen in view of threatening development of chronicity.

Acute low back pain screening questionnaire

The Acute Low Back Pain Screening Questionnaire is used to detect psychosocial yellow flags in the acute phase and to identify patients likely to have a poor prognosis. The questionnaire consists of 24 items concerning

psychosocial aspects of persisting low back pain. Five variables are found to be the strongest predictors of sick leave outcome and development of chronicity: fear avoidance work beliefs, perceived improvement, problems with work function, stress and previous sick leave (Linton & Halldén 1998). Completing the questionnaire takes about 5–10 minutes. Ratings are made on a 0–10-scale for each question. The items are weighted differently, and a total score <90 means low risk/expect recovery; 90–105 points means medium risk/pay attention, and a total score >105 means high risk. For validity, an acceptable Pearson product moment on the total score is calculated of 0.83 (range 0.63–0.97). Responsiveness of the Acute Low Back Pain Screening Questionnaire has not as yet been investigated.

Chronic pain grade questionnaire

When there are indications of a more chronic condition of low back pain, the Chronic Pain Grade Questionnaire (CPGQ) can be useful in detecting the chronic stage the patient is in. The CPGQ is a seven-item multidimensional measure of chronic pain severity, initially developed by Von Korff and co-workers (Von Korff et al 1992). The CPGQ is based on measures of pain intensity and pain related disability and is validated on back pain sufferers. The CPGQ includes subscale scores for characteristic pain intensity, disability score and disability points. Scoring results in four hierarchical categories according to pain severity or interference: grade I, low disability – low intensity; grade II, low disability – high intensity; grade III, high disability – moderately limiting; and grade IV, high disability – severely limiting. Reliability has been assessed through internal consistency, with Cronbach's alpha 0.91. Construct validity was assessed by calculating Spearman's correlation coefficients for the CPGQ and the various dimensions of the SF-36. The correlation was highest for pain (r = 0.84) and lowest for mental health (r = 0.38) (Smith et al 1997). Responsiveness was calculated by correlation of changes in chronic pain grade and median SF-36 scores. It has been concluded that changes in chronic pain grades are not merely due to fluctuations but are showing true change over time (Elliot et al 2000).

Tampa scale of kinesiophobia (TSK)

The Tampa Scale of Kinesiophobia was developed by Miller et al (1991) as a measure of fear of movement/reinjury. The questionnaire consists of 17 statements about activities and low back pain and the patient is asked to signal the extent to which they agree with each statement using a four-point Likert scale. The questionnaire takes about 5 minutes to complete. The scores for the items 4, 8,12 and 16 are to be reversed when scoring. Total score varies between 17 and 64. The median score is 37 (37 is normal; >37 is called pathological). There is a moderate internal consistency, with Cronbach's alpha of 0.77 in chronic patients (Vlaeyen et al 1995b) and 0.76 in acute low back pain patients (Swinkels et al 2003). Test–retest reliability reached a Spearman's correlation coefficient of r = 0.76 (Swinkels-Meewisse et al 2003). Construct validity was investigated by calculating Spearman's correlation coefficient between the TSK and the Fear Avoidance Beliefs Questionnaire, resulting in r = 0.53–0.76 (Crombez et al 1999). Validation of the TSK with other psychological instruments resulted in significant correlations (Vlaeyen et al 1995b). In a cross-sectional study of chronic low back pain patients TSK scores were the best predictor of disability (as measured by the Roland-Morris scale) explaining 13% of variance compared to the 4% explained by pain and gender (Vlaeyen et al 1995b).

Pain coping inventory (PCI)

Many questionnaires exist to test the coping strategy of our patient, for example the Coping Strategies Questionnaire (Rosenthiel & Keefe 1983), the VanderBilt Pain Management Inventory (Brown & Nicassio 1987), the Pain Cognition List (Vlaeyen et al 1990) and the Pain Coping Questionnaire (Kleinke 1992). These instruments are tailored to assess coping responses of specific subtypes of chronic pain patients and are characterized by cognitive coping responses. The Pain Coping Inventory (PCI) was developed to assess cognitive as well as behavioural coping strategies across a variety of chronic pain patients (Kraaimaat & Bakker 1994). The PCI is divided into six subscales (pain transformation, distraction, reducing demands, retreating, catastrophizing, resting), which, all together, result in an active coping score or a passive coping score. Completion of the questionnaire takes 10–15 minutes. The internal consistency showed a Cronbach's alpha of 0.62–0.78. Test–retest reliability resulted in Pearson's correlation coefficients of 0.42–0.82 (Kraaimaat et al 1997). Validity of the six PCI scales was assessed by computing Pearson's product moment correlation coefficients between PCI scales and related measures. Seventeen out of 22 predicted relationships were found to be significant (Kraaimaat & Bakker 1994). Responsiveness of the PCI has not been described.

General health

Short form 36 (SF-36)

Many indexes are available to measure general health perception. One of the most intensively investigated and frequently used questionnaires is the SF-36 (Short Form-36). It was designed for medical outcome studies (MOS) and contains eight subscales: physical functioning; role physical; bodily pain; general health; vitality; social functioning; role emotional; mental health. It generates a physical component summary (PCS) and a mental component summary (MCS). Internal consistency was shown to be good (average α = 0.84, varying from 0.66 to 0.93) (Ware et al 1995).

Construct validity of the SF-36 has been tested in many studies and many populations and is, in general, sufficient to good, depending on the method of validation. Responsiveness has also been tested extensively and has been demonstrated to be very acceptable (Wright & Young 1997, Taylor et al 1999). The SF-36 is freely available and can be scored online at www.qmetric.com/forms/permission/ score on-line. The process takes about 5–10 minutes and the result of each subscale in number as well as in histogram related to the reference group is provided.

SELECTION OF INDEXES AND IMPLICATIONS FOR PRACTICE

It must be emphasized that the indexes discussed in this chapter are only a small selection of the enormous number available. However, we have tried to make a selection on the basis of quality and relevance in relation to the case history. In accordance with the five steps described previously, we first analysed the consequences of the low back pain in terms of body functions, activities, participation, personal factors and environmental factors (step 1). In step 2 we set the treatment goals based on different domains. The most relevant treatment goals will be relief of pain, normalizing the level of activities and participation and prevention of chronicity. For the last mentioned goal it is essential to improve the illness insight of this patient.

In step 3 we selected the optimal instruments in relation to these treatment goals, also taking into account the methodological quality and feasibility of the selected instruments. Steps 4 and 5 (availability and interpretation) were more practical and logistical. Based on the analysis of measurement instruments, the visual analogue scale is a very attractive choice to measure and to evaluate pain. It takes little time to complete, is very valid, fits in with the goals, is easy to use and provides a clear interpretation of the results. For the assessment as well as the evaluation of activities related to low back pain, the Roland-Morris Disability Questionnaire and the Quebec Back Pain Disability Scale are both appropriate for the outcome measures desired. There is a slight preference for the RDQ because responsiveness scores are a little bit higher compared to the QBPDS, which is relevant if we also want to evaluate the treatments in relation to the treatment goal.

In relation to the negative prognostic factors in the patient's case history, the most important aspect in view of the treatment goals is the threat of pain becoming chronic. There is no strong indication that the patient is already in the chronic stage, so the Chronic Pain Grade Questionnaire does not seem to be the most relevant index for the moment. Of more prognostic value would be the Acute Low Back Pain Screening Questionnaire, which can be used in this case to obtain an impression of the factors at risk. The Tampa Scale of Kinesiophobia could be a useful addition in relation to the possible negative cognitions.

The VAS and three questionnaires have been used in evaluating the management of this patient. In a clinical situation, the healthcare provider must be careful not to overburden the patient, so the first selection must be well considered. In this case the VAS and the three additional questionnaires provide sufficient material to establish a good treatment plan. Where there is doubt, any other index can be completed at a later stage.

KEYWORDS

Acute Low Back Pain Screening Questionnaire
assessment
Chronic Pain Grade Questionnaire
health profile
ICF
ICIDH
McGill Pain Inventory
measurement
methodological quality
Numeric Rating Scale

outcome assessment
Pain Coping Inventory
pain drawing
Quebec Back Pain Disability Scale
Roland-Morris Disability Questionnaire
SF-36
Tampa Scale of Kinesiophobia
visual analogue scale

References

Beekman C E, Axtell L, Nordland K S, West J Y 1985 Self-concept: an outcome of a program for spinal pain. Pain 22: 59–66

Beurskens A J H M, deVet H C W, Köke A J A 1996 Responsiveness of functional status in low back pain: a comparison of different instruments. Pain 65(1): 71–76

Brown G K, Nicassio P M 1987 Development of a questionnaire for the assessment of active and passive coping strategies in chronic pain patients. Pain 31: 53–64

Burton A K, Tillotson K M, Main C J, Hollis S 1995 Psychosocial predictors of outcome in acute and subacute low back trouble. Spine 20: 722–728

Carlsson A M 1983 Assessment of chronic pain. I: Aspects of the reliability and validity of the visual analogue scale. Pain 16: 87–101

Cats-Baril W L, Frymoyer J W 1991 The economics of spinal disorders. In: Frymoyer J W (ed) The adult spine: principles and practice. Raven Press, New York, pp 85–105

Cole B, Finch E, Gowland C, Mayo N 1995 Physical rehabilitation outcome measures. Williams and Wilkins, Baltimore

Crombez G, Kole-Snijders A M J, Rotteveel A M, Vlaeyen J W S 1999 Pain-related fear is more disabling than pain itself: evidence on the role of pain-related fear in chronic back pain disability. Pain 80: 329–339

Downie W W, Leatham P A, Rhind V M 1978 Studies with pain rating scales. Annals of the Rheumatic Diseases 37: 378–381

Elliot A M, Smith B H, Smith W C, Chambers W A 2000 Changes in chronic pain severity over time: the chronic pain grade as a valid measure. Pain 88(3): 303–308

Farrar J T, Young J P, LaMoreaux L, Werth J L, Poole M 2001 Clinical importance of changes in chronic pain intensity measured on an 11-point numeric pain rating scale. Pain 94: 149–158

Feinstein A R 1987 Clinimetrics. Yale University Press, New Haven

Fredrickson B, Trief P M, Van Beveren P, Yuan H A, Baum G 1988 Rehabilitation of the patient with chronic back pain: a search for outcome predictors. Spine 13: 351–353

Gatchel R J, Polatin P B, Mayer T G 1995 The dominant role of psychosocial risk factors in the development of chronic low back pain disability. Spine 20: 2702–2709

Graham C, Bond S S, Gerkovich M M, Cook M R 1980 Use of the McGill Pain Questionnaire in the assessment of cancer pain: replicability and consistency. Pain 8: 377–387

Haldorsen E M H, Indahl A, Ursin H 1998 Patients with low back pain not returning to work: a 12-month follow-up study. Spine 23: 1202–1207

Härkäpää K, Järvikoski A, Mellin G, Hurri H, Luoma J 1991 Health locus of control beliefs and psychological distress as predictors for treatment outcome in low back pain patients: results of a 3-month follow-up of a controlled intervention study. Pain 46: 35–41

Hasenbring M, Marienfield G, Kuhlendahl D, Soyka D 1994 Risk factors of chronicity in lumbar disc patients. Spine 19: 2759–2765

Keefe F J, Kashikar-Zuck S 1996 Pain in arthritis and musculoskeletal disorders: the role of coping skills training and exercise interventions. Journal of Orthopaedic and Sports Physical Therapy 24: 279–290

Kleinke C L 1992 How chronic pain patients cope with pain: relation to treatment outcome in a multidisciplinary pain clinic. Cognitive Therapy and Research 16: 669–685

Klenerman L, Slade P D, Stanley M et al 1995 The prediction of chronicity in patients with an acute attack of low back pain in general practice setting. Spine 20: 473–477

Koelbaek-Johansen M, Graven-Nielsen T, Schou-Olesen A, Arendt-Nielsen L 1999 Muscular hyperalgesia and referred pain in chronic whiplash syndrome. Pain 83: 229–234

Kopec J, Esdaile J M, Abrahamowicz M et al 1995 The Quebec Back Pain Disability Scale: measurement properties. Spine 20(3): 341–352

Kraaimaat F W, Bakker A H 1994 Pain coping strategies in chronic pain patients: the development of the Pain Coping Inventory (PCI). Third International Congress of Behavioral Medicine, Amsterdam, 6–9 July

Kraaimaat F W, Bakker A H, Evers A W M 1997 Pijncoping-strategieën bij chronische pijnpatiënten: de ontwikkeling van de Pijn-Coping-Inventarisatielijst (PCI). [In Dutch; 'Pain coping strategies in chronic pain patients: the development of the Pain Coping Inventarisation List'] Gedragstherapie 30(3): 185–201

Langley G B, Sheppard H 1985 The visual analogue scale: its use in pain measurement. Rheumatology International 5: 145–148

Liebenson C, Yeomans S 1997 Outcome assessment in musculoskeletal medicine. Manual Therapy 2(2): 67–74

Linton S J, Halldén K 1998 Can we screen for problematic back pain? A screening questionnaire for predicting outcome in acute and subacute back pain. Clinical Journal of Pain 14: 209–215

Loeser J D 1989 Disability, pain and suffering. Clinical Neurosurgery 35: 398–408

McIntosh G, Frank J, Hogg-Johnson S, Bombardier C, Hall H 2000 Prognostic factors for time receiving workers compensation benefits in a cohort of patients with low back pain. Spine 25: 147–157

Main C J, Watson P J 1999 Psychological aspects of pain. Manual Therapy 4: 203–215

Margolis R B, Tait R C, Krause S J 1986 A rating system for use with patient pain drawings. Pain 24: 57–65

Mayer T G, Polatin P, Smith B et al 1995 Contemporary concepts in spine care: spine rehabilitation. Secondary and tertiary nonoperative care. Spine 20: 2060–2066

Melzack R 1975 The McGill Pain Questionnaire: major properties and scoring methods. Pain 1: 277–299

Mendelson G, Selwood T S 1981 Measurement of chronic pain: a correlation study of verbal and nonverbal scales. Journal of Behavioral Assessment 3: 263–269

Miller R P, Kori S H, Todd D D 1991 The Tampa Scale. Unpublished work

Oostendorp R A B, Elvers J W H 1995 Quality scoring list for reading articles. Dutch National Institute for Allied Health Professions, Amersfoort

Ransford A O, Cairns D, Mooney V 1976 The pain drawing as an aid to the psychologic evaluation of patients with low back pain. Spine 1(2): 127–134

Reading A E 1982 A comparison of the McGill Pain Questionnaire in chronic and acute pain. Pain 7: 185–192

Rosenthiel A K, Keefe F J 1983 The use of coping strategies in chronic low back pain patients: relationship to patient characteristics and current adjustment. Pain 17: 33–44

Schoppink L E M, Tulder M W van, Koes B W, Beurskens A J H M, Bie R A de 1996 Reliability and validity of the Dutch adaptation of the Quebec Back Pain Disability Scale. Physical Therapy 76: 268–275

Schwartz D P, DeGood D E 1984 Global appropriateness of pain drawings: blind ratings predict patterns of psychological distress and litigation status. Pain 19: 383–388

Scott J, Huskisson E C 1979 Vertical or horizontal visual analogue scales. Annals of the Rheumatic Diseases 38: 560

Smith B H, Penny K I, Purves A M et al 1997 The Chronic Pain Grade Questionnaire: validation and reliability in postal research. Pain 71(2): 141–147

Stratford P W, Binkley J, Solomon P, Gill C, Finch E 1994 Assessing change over time in patients with low back pain. Physical Therapy 74(6): 528–533

Streiner D L, Norman G R 1998 Health measurement scales: a practical guide to their development and use, 2nd edn., Oxford University Press, Oxford

Swinkels-Meewisse E J, Swinkels R A, Verbeek A L, Vlaeyen J W, Oostendorp R A 2003 Psychometric properties of the Tampa Scale for kinesiophobia and the Fear-avoidance Beliefs Questionnaire in acute low back pain. Manual Therapy 8(1): 29–36

Taylor S J, Taylor A E, Foy M A, Fogg A J 1999 Responsiveness of common outcome measures for patients with low back pain. Spine 24(17): 1805–1812

van Triet E F, Dekker J, Kerssens J J, Curfs E C 1990 Reliability of the assessment of impairments and disabilities in survey research in the field of physical therapy. International Disabilities Studies 12: 61–65

Verbruggen L M, Jette A M 1994 The disablement process. Social Science and Medicine 38: 1–14

Vlaeyen J W S, Crombez G 1999 Fear of movement/(re)injury, avoidance and pain disability in chronic low back pain patients. Manual Therapy 4(4): 187–195

Vlaeyen J W S, Geurts P, Kole-Snijders A M J, Schuerman J A, Groenman N H, Eek H van 1990 What do chronic pain patients think of their pain? Towards a pain cognition questionnaire. British Journal of Clinical Psychology 29: 383–394

Vlaeyen J W S, Kole-Snijders A M J, Boeren R G B, Eek H V 1995a Fear of movement (re)injury in chronic low back pain and its relation to behavioural performance. Pain 62: 363–372

Vlaeyen J W S, Kole-Snijders A M J, Rotteveel A M, Ruesink R, Heuts P H T G 1995b The role of fear of movement/(re)injury in pain disability. Journal of Occupational Rehabilitation 5(4): 235–252

Von Korff M, Ormel J, Keefe F J, Dworkin S F 1992 Grading the severity of chronic pain. Pain 50: 133–149

Walsh T D, Leber B 1983 Measurement of chronic pain: visual analogue scales and McGill Melzack Pain Questionnaire compared. In: Bonica J J et al (eds) Advances in pain research and therapy. Raven Press, New York, vol 5, pp 133–142

Ware J E, Kosinski M, Bayliss M, McHorney C A, Rogers W H, Raczek A 1995 Comparison of methods for the scoring and statistical analysis of SF-36 health profile and summary measures: summary of results from the medical outcome study. Medical Care 33(4): 264–279

Watson P J, Main C J, Waddell G, Gales T F, Purcell-Jones G 1998 Medically certified work loss, recurrence and costs of wage compensation of back pain: a follow-up study of the working population of Jersey. British Journal of Rheumatology 37: 82–86

Wilkie D, Lovejoy N, Dodd M, Tesler M 1990 Cancer pain intensity measurement: concurrent validity of three tools – finger dynameter, pain intensity number scale, visual analogue scale. Hospice Journal 6(1): 1–13

World Health Organization 1980 International classification of impairments, disabilities and handicaps: a manual of classification relating to the consequences of disease. World Health Organization, Geneva

World Health Organization 1997 ICIDH-2 International classification of impairments, activities and participation: a manual of dimensions of disablement and functioning. World Health Organization, Geneva

World Health Organization 2001 International classification of functioning, disabilities and health problems. World Health Organization, Geneva

Wright J G, Young N L 1997 A comparison of different indices of responsiveness. Journal of Clinical Epidemiology 50(3): 239–246

Chapter **42**

Critical appraisal of randomized trials, systematic reviews of randomized trials and clinical practice guidelines

C. G. Maher, R. D. Herbert, A. M. Moseley, C. Sherrington, M. Elkins

INTRODUCTION

Evidence-based practice implies systematic use of best evidence for clinical decision making. The evidence may come in many forms, but the best evidence for making decisions about therapy comes from randomized controlled trials, systematic reviews and evidence-based clinical practice guidelines.

Randomized controlled trials

Randomized controlled trials are experiments on people. In the typical randomized trial, volunteers agree to be randomly allocated to groups receiving one of two conditions. The conditions may be treatment and no treatment, or standard treatment and standard treatment plus a new treatment, or two alternate treatments. The common feature is that the experimental group receives the treatment of interest and the control group does not. At the end of the trial, outcomes of subjects in each group are determined. The difference in outcomes between groups provides an estimate of the size of the treatment effect.

In studies without control groups (such as studies which take measurements before and after treatment on a single group of subjects), a range of factors other than treatment can contribute to the changes observed over the treatment period and these may be mistakenly interpreted as effects of treatment. Factors such as natural recovery, statistical regression (a statistical phenomenon whereby patients selected on the basis of their extremeness become less extreme over time), learning effects and subjects wanting to please the investigator may come together to make treatment appear much more effective than it really is. Controlled studies may be less exposed to these biases. In controlled studies, one group is treated with the experimental treatment and the other is not. Extraneous factors act on both experimental groups so that, in so far as experimental and control groups are comparable, the difference between outcomes of the two groups provides an estimate of the effect of treatment unbiased by factors outside the treatment.

Even controlled studies can be misleading, however, if treatment and control groups are not truly comparable. For example, if subjects in one group have more severe disease or have characteristics that make them more or less responsive to therapies, the comparison between experimental and control groups will reflect these differences as well as the effects of treatment. Thus it is critical to establish comparable groups. Comparability implies that if both groups were to receive the same treatment, or if both received no treatment, both would have the same outcome.

The distinguishing feature of randomized trials is that subjects are randomly allocated to groups. This is important because randomization ensures comparability of groups. In fact, randomization is the only method that can ensure an estimatable level of comparability. Consequently randomized trials are more able than other research designs to differentiate effects of treatment from a range of other extraneous effects. For this reason, randomized trials are generally considered to provide the best method for studying effects of treatment. They should be considered to be the best primary source of information about the effects of manual therapy techniques.

Systematic reviews

Systematic reviews are reviews of the literature conducted in a way that is designed to minimize bias (Petticrew 2001). In the field of health, most systematic reviews assess the effects of health interventions, although a smaller number of systematic reviews assess the accuracy of diagnostic tests (see, for example, Solomon et al 2001) or of prognosis for a particular condition (see, for example, Cote et al 2001). Unlike traditional reviews, systematic reviews explicitly describe the methods used to conduct the review. For example, in systematic reviews there is usually a description of the criteria used to determine which studies will be considered in the review, the search strategy used to locate studies, methods for assessing the quality of the studies and the process used to synthesize the findings of individual studies. Good quality systematic reviews involve comprehensive searches of the literature, and they synthesize the findings of individual studies in a transparent and minimally biased way, so they are often considered the best single source of information of the effects of treatment. They are particularly useful for busy clinicians who may be unable to access all the relevant trials in an area and may otherwise need to rely upon their own incomplete surveys of relevant trials.

Clinical practice guidelines

Clinical practice guidelines are recommendations for management of a particular clinical condition (National Health and Medical Research Council 1999). The production of high-quality evidence-based clinical practice guidelines involves compilation of evidence concerning needs and

expectations of recipients of care, the accuracy of diagnostic tests, effects of therapy and prognosis. Usually this necessitates the conduct of one, or sometimes several, systematic reviews. Recommendations for clinical practice may be presented as clinical decision algorithms. High-quality clinical practice guidelines provide a useful framework upon which clinicians can build clinical practice.

Unfortunately there are not enough randomized trials, systematic reviews and clinical practice guidelines to address all clinical questions. Nor are existing trials, reviews and guidelines of uniformly high quality. The PEDro database (a database of randomized trials and systematic reviews in physiotherapy; available online at: http://www.pedro.fhs.usyd.edu.au lists 1032 trials coded as relevant to the physiotherapy subdiscipline 'musculoskeletal physiotherapy' (search conducted June 2002). Characteristics of these trials, including methodological quality rated on a scale out of 10 (Moseley et al 2002), are given in Figure 42.1. Clearly there are many high-quality trials relevant to musculoskeletal physiotherapy, but there are many more of low quality. Clinicians who are looking for evidence of the effects of manual therapy techniques need to be able to distinguish between high-quality and low-quality trials.

This chapter discusses how clinicians can evaluate and interpret evidence from randomized trials, systematic reviews, and clinical practice guidelines. This process is often referred to as 'critical appraisal'. The methods of critical appraisal described in this chapter are based heavily on the work of the modern pioneers of evidence-based practice (Sackett et al 2000). The process developed and refined by those authors involves asking questions about the presence or absence of key methodological features of individual pieces of evidence. By asking a few relatively simple questions it is often possible to discriminate between high-quality and low-quality evidence.

ASSESSING THE QUALITY OF CLINICAL TRIALS

It may be possible to discriminate between high- and low-quality trials by asking three simple questions:

1. Were subjects randomly allocated to conditions?

Random allocation implies that a non-systematic, unpredictable procedure was used to allocate subjects to conditions. This is best done using a computer-generated list of random numbers, but is sometimes achieved with simple procedures such as coin tossing. Readers of clinical trials can usually ascertain whether random allocation has occurred because, in randomized trials, there is usually reference to random allocation in the title of the paper or in the abstract or the methods section. For example, in the trial of manual therapy for neck pain by Hoving et al (2002) both the title and abstract explicitly describe the study as a ran-

A

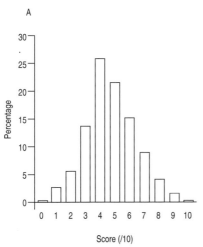

B

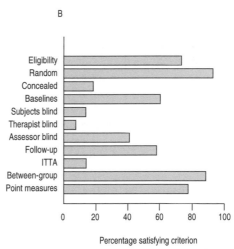

Figure 42.1   Characteristics of all 1032 clinical trials coded as relevant to manual therapy on the PEDro database (11 June 2002). A: Methodological quality scores (/10). B: Percentage of trials satisfying each methodological quality criterion. *Eligibility*, eligibility criteria were specified; *random*, subjects were randomly allocated to groups (or, in a crossover study, subjects were randomly allocated an order in which treatments were received); *concealed*, allocation was concealed; *baselines*, the groups were similar at baseline regarding the most important prognostic indicators; *subjects blind*, there was blinding of all subjects; *therapist blind*, there was blinding of all therapists who administered the therapy; *assessor blind*, there was blinding of all assessors who measured at least one key outcome; *follow-up*, measures of at least one key outcome were obtained from more than 85% of the subjects initially allocated to groups; *ITTA*, all subjects for whom outcome measures were available received the treatment or control condition as allocated or, where this was not the case, data for at least one key outcome was analysed by 'intention to treat'; *between-group*, the results of between-group statistical comparisons are reported for at least one key outcome; *point measures*, the study provides both point measures and measures of variability for at least one key outcome.

domized controlled trial. The title is 'Manual therapy, physical therapy or continued care by a general practitioner for patients with neck pain: a randomized controlled trial' and the abstract reads 'DESIGN: Randomized controlled trial'. Unfortunately, some authors may describe their trial as a randomized trial when a quasi-random process, such as allocation by hospital record number or by alternation, was used. For example, the abstract of the paper by Tuchin & Pollard (1998) states that random allocation was used, but inspection of the methods reveals that subjects were allocated to treatment group according to their employee identification number (a 'quasi-randomized' allocation procedure). Quasi-random allocation may be able to impart the same degree of comparability of groups as random allocation, but it is more easily corrupted (Schulz 1995).

There is evidence that the absence of true randomization is associated with substantial bias (see, for example, Chalmers et al 1983). Consequently, the absence of random allocation should be considered a serious shortcoming. Readers looking for evidence of the effects of manual therapy procedures should be reluctant to base clinical decisions on the findings of non-randomized studies.

Random allocation is not the same as random selection. Random selection refers to the process by which subjects are recruited for the trial, whereas random allocation refers to the process by which subjects are assigned to groups. Selection procedures affect external validity (that is, they determine who the findings can be generalized to) but not the internal validity (whether the effect is due to treatment

or extraneous factors). Random selection is usually impossible and generally is not necessary, whereas random allocation is generally possible and extremely important.

There are several requirements of a good random allocation procedure. Most importantly, allocation should be concealed. Several studies suggest that concealment of allocation is the single most important predictor of bias in randomized clinical trials (Schulz et al 1995, Moher et al 1998). Concealment (not to be confused with blinding) means that the person who is deciding on a patient's eligibility for the trial is not aware, at the time of making that decision, of which group the subject is subsequently to be allocated to. The reason for this is that if the decision to enter or not enter someone into a trial is influenced by the patient's characteristics then there is the possibility of serious bias. In non-concealed studies the person who manages recruitment might consciously or subconsciously choose not to admit to the trial those patients who have a poor prognosis and who would, if admitted to the trial, be subsequently allocated to the control group. In that case the control group would consist of a spectrum of patients with better prognosis than would otherwise be the case and estimates of the effects of therapy (the difference in outcomes of treated and control subjects) would be underestimated. Alternatively, the person managing recruitment might be reluctant to admit those to the trial who have a good prognosis and would be allocated to the control group, as the recruiter might (consciously or subconsciously) prefer that these potential subjects receive the active intervention. This would cause the trial to overestimate the effects of therapy. While concealment of allocation could theoretically produce bias in either direction it has been shown that the overall tendency is to produce bias that tends to inflate estimates of treatment effects (Schulz et al 1995). Randomization is often concealed by keeping each subject's allocation in a sealed envelope that is not opened until the subject is entered into the study (as was done in the trial by Hoving et al 2002), or by keeping the allocation schedule off-site (as was done in the trial by Fritzell et al 2001). This protects the integrity of the allocation process.

Unfortunately, only 18% of the randomized trials of manual therapy indexed on PEDro report concealed allocation (see Fig. 42.1). This low proportion of trials reporting concealed allocation is not a problem unique to manual therapy. We noted a similar problem when we reviewed all trials on PEDro across all subdisciplines of physiotherapy: only 16% of trials reported concealed allocation (Moseley et al 2002). Slightly higher rates of concealment are reported in reviews of medical trials; for example, Schulz et al (1995) noted that 79 of 250 trials they reviewed reported adequate concealment. Fortunately the methodological quality of physiotherapy trials is improving (Moseley et al 2002) and in future more manual therapy trials will report concealment of allocation.

2. Was there blinding of assessors and patients?

It is widely believed that subjects who receive the experimental treatment may experience improved outcomes as a result of knowing that they are getting treated rather than as a direct effect of the treatment itself. Some readers of clinical trials see this as problematic – they would like to know what the effect of treatment is over and above these 'placebo' effects. Other readers are less concerned by placebo effects because they consider that all effects of treatment, placebo and otherwise, are equally worthwhile (Oh 1994).

Some subjects in the experimental group of a clinical trial may report better outcomes than they really experienced because they perceive that this is what is expected from them (Wickstrom & Bendix 2000). In the psychology literature this has come to be known as a 'Hawthorne effect'. The Hawthorne effect is an experimental artifact that is of no clinical utility, so clinical trials are best designed to minimize bias from Hawthorne effects.

In clinical trials it is possible to differentiate the independent effects of treatment from the effects of both placebo and Hawthorne effects by blinding subjects. 'Blinding' (also called 'masking') of subjects implies that subjects cannot discern whether they received the experimental treatment or the control treatment. This is achieved by providing a 'sham' therapy to the control group. The ideal sham therapy is indistinguishable from the experimental therapy but could not have therapeutic effect. An example is provided by McLachlan and colleagues' (1991) randomized trial of

ultrasound. In this trial the sham ultrasound machine was identical to the active unit except the crystal had been removed and replaced with a resistor to produce surface heat only. The machines were simply labelled 'A' and 'B', so subjects were unable to discern if they were being treated with real or sham ultrasound. With this design, placebo and Hawthorne effects can be expected to act equally on experimental and control groups, and the estimate of treatment effect (the difference in outcome of treated and sham-treated subjects) will not be biased by placebo or Hawthorne effects.

In practice it is often not possible to provide a true sham. This is particularly the case for physical therapies such as manipulation and exercise: it is difficult, for example, to provide a convincing sham manipulation. When a sham therapy is not available the best alternative is to provide an intervention that is as similar as possible to the experimental treatment without having any possible therapeutic effect. Examples of control treatments described as sham or placebo in manipulation trials include detuned shortwave diathermy (Glover et al 1974), detuned ultrasound (Pikula 1999) and low force manual contact to mimic an adjustment (Waagen et al 1986) or mobilization (Vicenzino et al 1996). An extreme attempt to blind the patient was reported in Sloop and colleagues' (1982) trial where all patients received an amnesic dose of intravenous diazepam and then either received a cervical manipulation or no treatment. While this approach would certainly blind the patient, the active treatment was probably not a good representation of clinical practice where the therapist typically manipulates a conscious patient and the response of the patient to manual assessment guides the specific manual treatment that is performed. Additionally Sloop and colleagues' method of blinding would be unsuitable for trials where patients are given a course of manual therapy. The more closely the sham therapy resembles the experimental treatment, the better will be the control of placebo and Hawthorne effects. Unfortunately there does not yet seem to be an entirely satisfactory sham manipulation protocol.

It is also desirable that the person who assesses outcomes for each subject is unaware of whether the subject did or did not receive the experimental treatment (Pocock 1983, Schulz et al 1995). When the assessor is blinded, his or her expectations cannot bias measurements of outcomes. For objective measures of outcome, implementation of blinding is usually straightforward: it simply involves getting an independent person to take the measurements. In many trials of manual therapy, outcomes are subjective and must be self-reported. Then blinding assessors requires blinding of patients. Some trials employ blind assessors for some outcome measures (e.g. interpretation of X-rays) and use unblinded assessors for other outcomes (e.g. physical performance or pain).

Trials that do not report double-blinding (i.e. blinding of both subject and assessor) typically report larger treatment effects than those that do (Schulz et al 1995). One interpretation of this finding is that unblinded trials tend to be biased in the direction of reporting exaggerated treatment effects.

3. Was there adequate follow–up?

In most clinical trials of manual therapy techniques, treatment occurs over days, weeks or months, and outcomes may be monitored for up to several years following treatment. Ideally all subjects who enter the trial are subsequently followed up (that is, outcomes are measured in all subjects), but in practice this rarely happens. For all sorts of reasons, subjects are lost to follow-up. This may occur because subjects lose interest in participation in the trial, move house, return to work, become ill, and so on.

When not all subjects are followed up there is a potential for bias. Bias can occur if risk of loss to follow-up is associated with outcome. If subjects with unusually poor outcomes are preferentially lost to follow-up the remaining subjects will have, on average, an unrealistically good outcome. The opposite will occur if subjects with unusually good outcomes are preferentially lost to follow-up. Then any difference in the pattern of drop-outs of treated and control groups will be associated with bias. Unfortunately, as follow-up data are not available for these subjects, it is usually not possible to ascertain if subjects lost to follow-up have atypically good or poor outcomes. Some statistical techniques have been devised to adjust for bias associated with loss to follow-up, but they are not entirely satisfactory (Simes et al 1998). There is always the possibility of significant bias when loss to follow-up is large.

What is a large loss to follow-up, and how much of a loss to follow-up is necessary to significantly bias the findings of a clinical trial? The answers to these questions will vary from trial to trial, but most experts would agree that losses to follow-up of less than 10% are not likely to be associated with serious bias, and losses to follow-up of more than 20% cause potential for serious bias. Perhaps a useful threshold is 15%: as a rule of thumb we might choose to treat the findings of the study with some suspicion if loss to follow-up is more than 15%. Another alternative is to conduct a best case/worst case analysis where subjects lost to follow-up from one group are first presumed to have had a good outcome (e.g. returned to work) and subjects from the other group are presumed to have had a poor outcome. A hypothetical result is then calculated. The process is repeated with the opposite assignments and the results re-calculated. If the results of the study do not materially change under these best and worst case scenarios then the reader can be confident that the loss to follow-up has not introduced a serious bias.

In high-quality trials the loss to follow-up is given explicitly, usually in the first paragraph of the results section. In other studies these data are not given explicitly and the reader may need to calculate loss to follow-up from the number of subjects who entered the trial (that is, the number of subjects randomized to groups) and the number followed up (this number may be found only in results tables in some published papers). In practice, the number of subjects lost to follow-up usually increases with the duration of the follow-up. A trial may have little loss to follow-up in the short-term, but loss to follow-up may increase with time. Such studies may have valid conclusions about the short-term effects of therapy but their conclusions about long-term effects of therapy may be prone to bias.

A related issue concerns how protocol violations are dealt with. In most studies there are some protocol violations. Subjects allocated to receive the experimental treatment may not receive treatment (for example, if the treatment is exercise, subjects may not do their exercises), or subjects in the control group may receive the experimental treatment (for example, subjects in the control group of a study of manipulation may receive manipulation from another therapist). Another common protocol violation occurs when outcome measurements are not taken at the scheduled time, perhaps because the subject missed an appointment or was too ill for the measurements to be taken.

What is the best way to deal with protocol violations? Some experimenters may be inclined not to collect outcome measures from subjects for whom there were protocol violations. The logic is that if the protocol was violated the data may be invalid and should therefore be ignored. Similarly, outcome data might be collected but subsequently discarded. Alternatively, some experimenters may analyse the data according to the treatment actually received (so that data from subjects who did not receive the experimental treatment are analysed as control group data, even though some of these subjects were initially allocated to the treatment group). Neither of these methods is generally recommended because both have the potential to produce serious bias. A better strategy is to collect data from all subjects regardless of whether protocol violations occur, following the protocol as closely as possible, and then analyse the data as if the protocol violations had not occurred. That is, follow-up data are obtained wherever possible and all available data from all subjects for whom data is available are analysed in the groups to which subjects were initially assigned, regardless of protocol violations. This approach, called analysis by intention to treat (ITTA), is generally thought to be the least biased way to deal with protocol violations (Hollis & Campbell 1999).

While it is probably desirable that all studies analyse data by intention to treat, the presence or absence of analysis by intention to treat may not be a particularly useful way to discriminate studies of manual therapy. This is because, as with concealed allocation, relatively few studies of manual therapies explicitly indicate they analysed data by intention to treat. In the 1032 trials we retrieved, only 14% clearly analysed by intention to treat.

In summary, readers of clinical trials should ask three questions to assess validity:

1. Were subjects randomly allocated to conditions?
2. Was there blinding of assessors and patients?
3. Was there adequate follow-up?

The first question might be applied rigorously to filter out evidence. Non-randomized studies of the effects of therapies are exposed to serious bias and probably should not be used for estimating the effects of therapy. The other two questions can probably be applied more judiciously. Studies which do not have blinded patients or assessors may provide useful evidence if the comparison therapy was plausible and the outcomes were measured objectively, and studies with slightly more than 15% drop-outs may be useful if a good case can be made that loss to follow-up was not related to outcome.

Readers wishing to publish a clinical trial should consult the revised CONSORT statement for further details on the reporting of randomized trials (Moher et al 2001).

ASSESSING THE QUALITY OF SYSTEMATIC REVIEWS

Well-designed systematic reviews provide one of the best possible sources of information about the effects of therapy. Fortunately, unlike clinical trials, most systematic reviews are well designed. Systematic reviews performed by the Cochrane Collaboration (www.cochrane.org) are particularly authoritative as these are usually carried out according to strict guidelines.

Readers of systematic reviews can relatively easily detect the few systematic reviews that are of low quality by asking two questions:

1. Was an adequate search strategy described?

One potential source of bias in systematic reviews arises from the search for relevant studies. There is an obvious potential for bias if reviewers review only those studies that they have been involved in, or only those studies whose findings fit with the reviewers' beliefs. A more pernicious problem is publication bias, which arises because studies with the most positive findings are likely to be published in leading journals, and are therefore easily accessed. The result is that an unrepresentatively optimistic subset of trials tends to be reviewed (Stern & Simes 1997). Wherever studies with positive findings are more likely to be reviewed there is the possibility of publication bias.

One way to minimize both these sources of bias is for reviewers to conduct thorough and transparent searches for reports of relevant studies. At the very least, reviewers should search several key databases, using a sensitive search strategy formulated prior to conducting the review. An example of a description of such a search strategy developed by the Cochrane Collaboration Back Review Group is provided by van Tulder and colleagues (1997). A thorough and transparent search strategy will provide

some protection against bias, but probably can not prevent bias altogether.

2. Was the quality of individual trials taken into account when synthesizing the trial findings?

Trials of low quality are potentially biased so they should not be used to draw conclusions about the effects of therapy. Systematic reviews should take trial quality into account when drawing conclusions about the effects of therapy.

Methods for assessing trial quality in systematic reviews are still being developed so it is not yet known how best to assess trial quality or how to incorporate considerations of trial quality into the synthesis of trial findings (Juni et al 1999). Most reviews include only randomized trials. This approach effectively ignores the findings of one particular type of low-quality studies (those that are not randomized). Another potentially complementary approach is to assess the quality of trials using checklists or scales (for reviews of checklists and scales see Moher et al 1995, Verhagen et al 2001) and then consider only those studies which score highly. These approaches appear sensible but have not been empirically validated. In the absence of good information about how trial quality should be assessed and used in systematic reviews, readers should probably be content with any apparently sensible procedure for considering trial quality in systematic reviews.

Readers wishing to publish a systematic review should consult the QUORUM statement for more details on how to report systematic reviews (Moher et al 1999).

INTERPRETING CLINICAL TRIALS AND SYSTEMATIC REVIEWS

Once it is established that a clinical trial or systematic review is of high quality it is necessary to determine what the trial or review means for clinical practice.

It is useful to ask four further questions to assess what randomized trials and systematic reviews mean for clinical practice:

1. Can these findings be used to make inferences about my patients?

Using clinical trials to make inferences about individual patients is potentially problematic because typical subjects in a trial will usually differ in some way from the patients we wish to generalize to. Yet clinical trials and systematic reviews are only useful if they can be used to make inferences about particular patients. Thus the first step in using a clinical trial or review for clinical decision making involves consideration of whether the study's findings can reasonably be applied to a particular patient or group of patients – that is, it is necessary to decide if the patients in the trial were sufficiently like the target patient or patients.

This might require consideration of the method used to select patients, the severity of their presenting problems, co-morbidity rates and other factors that could influence response to treatment. Unfortunately, such considerations can rarely be based on objective evidence about treatment effect modifiers. Instead it is necessary to apply wisdom born of clinical experience.

A degree of caution is required when deciding if the subjects in the trial or review are sufficiently similar to the target patients. The temptation is to dismiss the findings of clinical trials or reviews because of minor differences in the characteristics of patients in the trials or reviews and the target patients. In practice this is probably inadvisable because we can never know with great certainty for whom a treatment will work best. Often the apparent 'subgroups' of responders or non-responders identified in clinical trials are spurious (Yusuf et al 1991). The consequence is that it is hard to know with any certainty what sorts of people are likely to best respond to therapy. Under these circumstances clinicians should be reluctant to dismiss the findings of a clinical trial or review on the basis that the trial population was slightly different to those to whom one wishes to generalize.

We have argued elsewhere (Herbert 2000a) that the best way to apply clinical trials and systematic reviews to individual patients is to take the unbiased global estimates of treatment effects from clinical trials and then to use clinical judgement to adjust these estimates for particular patients.

2.   Was the intervention applied well?

Obviously, clinical trials are most useful when the intervention is applied well. Studies in which the intervention is applied poorly should not be used to make decisions about the effects of the intervention in general. They may, however, provide a useful lower limit to the estimated effect of treatment. It may also be the case that the intervention used in a study was provided in a more intense manner that that able to be offered in the clinical practice of the reader (for example, the therapy administered in a trial may be provided daily over a long time period whereas in practice such intense treatment may not be possible). In this case the reader may need to adjust the effect found in the trial down to predict the average effect on target patients. This, too, requires clinical judgement.

3.   Were the outcomes meaningful?

If a manual therapy is to be useful it must improve quality of life. Consequently it is desirable that all trials of manual therapies measure the effect of the intervention on quality of life.

It is often assumed that changes in measurement of impairment (such as muscle weakness) will automatically translate into changes of quality of life. However, the history of clinical trials says this is not necessarily so. For example, Mannion and colleagues' (2001) trial of exercise for chronic low back pain reported weak relationships between both pain (r^2 = 7%) and disability (r^2 = 25%) and measures of muscle performance at baseline, and no relationship between changes in muscle performance factors and changes in pain or disability. There are other examples where a clinical trial has shown large effects on impairments that have not translated into large effects on quality of life.

When reading clinical trials or systematic reviews ask yourself 'If I was the patient, what would I want out of therapy? Does this trial or review tell me about the things that would matter to me?' If the answer is 'No', the trial or review is probably not likely to assist in clinical decision making.

4.   Was the effect of the intervention big enough to make the intervention worthwhile?

If a treatment is to be useful it must do more good than harm. Potentially, clinical trials and systematic reviews can help us decide if a treatment is useful by helping us assess how much good (and sometimes also how much harm) a treatment can do (Herbert 2000a, 2000b).

Unfortunately, many clinical trials and systematic reviews pay little attention to the size of treatment effects. Instead many are preoccupied with whether the effect of treatment was statistically significant or not. That is unhelpful because the P values used to determine if the effect was statistically significant convey no information about the size of the treatment effect. Sometimes treatment effects are of great clinical significance yet statistically non-significant, and sometimes they are trivial but highly statistically significant. Readers of clinical trials and systematic reviews need to extract clinically useful information about the size of treatment effects, not P values.

Importantly, estimates of the size of treatment effects can only be provided by contrasts between groups. In clinical trials that report mean outcomes for each group, the best estimate of the size of the treatment effect is the difference between group means. This can be illustrated with Faas and colleagues' trial evaluating exercise treatment for acute low back pain (Faas et al 1993). On average, patients receiving exercise entered the trial with a pain rating of 36.1 mm on a 100 mm scale. By the 1-month follow-up, pain had decreased by 19 mm. It may be tempting to view the 50% reduction in pain as evidence of a large benefit of exercise but this would be misleading because the group of patients receiving placebo (minimal dose ultrasound: 5 minutes at 0.1 watts/cm^2) also had a 19 mm reduction in pain. The difference between group means was trivially small. The authors concluded, quite properly, that their data showed exercise is an ineffective treatment for acute low back pain.

The changes that occur within a group over the period of treatment do not provide an estimate of the size of treatment effects because the outcomes of people in that group are determined partly by treatment but also by a range of other factors including natural recovery, statistical regression, placebo effects, Hawthorne effects and so on (Campbell & Stanley 1963, Cook & Campbell 1979). In the trial by Faas and colleagues (1993) these non-treatment factors were responsible for a 50% reduction in pain. (Typically patients interpret pain reductions of this magnitude as 'much improved'; Farrar et al 2001). Thus some treatments may appear spuriously effective if treatment effects are estimated from within-group changes. Unbiased estimates of the size of treatment can only be obtained by contrasting the outcomes of two groups.

The most appropriate descriptor of the contrast between groups, and therefore also of the size of a treatment's effects, will depend on how the outcome is measured. When the outcome is continuous (that is, when the outcome can take on any of many values for a single subject, as it can with visual analogue measures of pain, or measures of disability, or days until return to work) it is appropriate to focus on 'typical' outcomes. Usually typical outcomes are described in terms of the mean (or sometimes median) outcome. The simplest and most useful way of contrasting the mean (or median) outcome of two groups is simply to take the difference between the two groups' means (or medians). Thus, when outcomes are measured on a continuous scale, the best estimate of the size of the treatment effect is usually the difference between group means (or medians).

Other sorts of outcomes cannot take on a range of values – they are events that either happen or do not. These 'dichotomous' variables include outcomes such as recovered/did not recover, recurred/did not recur and returned to work/did not return to work. When outcomes are dichotomous it is not very informative to focus on typical outcomes. Instead we look at the proportion of subjects in whom the event occurs. Conventionally we concentrate on the 'bad' event (the least desirable of the alternative outcomes) and we use the proportion of subjects that experience the bad event as an estimate of the risk of that event. For example, in the trial of specific stabilizing exercise by Hides and colleagues (2001), six of the 20 subjects in the exercise group reported a recurrence of low back pain during the follow-up year compared to 16 out of 19 in the control group. Thus the risk of recurrence was 30% (6/20) in the exercise group and 84% (16/19) in the control group.

As always, the best estimate of the size of the treatment effect is given by contrasting the outcomes of two groups, so when the outcome is measured on a dichotomous scale we need to contrast the risk of that outcome occurring in the two groups. The simplest way to do this is to take the difference in the risk (the 'risk difference' or 'absolute risk reduction'). There are a range of other descriptors that can be used to contrast dichotomous outcomes, such as the number needed to treat, relative risks and odds ratios. These have been described in more detail elsewhere (Herbert 2000b, Sackett et al 2000). In the Hides study (Hides et al 2001) the absolute risk reduction is 84% minus 30%, or 54%. The number needed to treat (in this case the number of subjects needed to be treated with exercise rather than control to prevent one recurrence of low back pain) is calculated by dividing 100 by the absolute risk reduction. Thus the Hides study shows that one recurrence of back pain is prevented for approximately every two subjects treated.

If we are to determine whether benefit outweighs harm, we must also quantify the harm caused by treatment. 'Harm' should be considered in its broadest sense, including the inconvenience, anxiety, discomfort and cost of treatment. The harm of a programme of stabilizing exercise might include the inconvenience associated with attending for several sessions of therapy and performing exercise. In addition, exercise may produce adverse effects in some subjects. How frequent and how serious are these adverse events? Hides et al (2001) did not report any adverse events, but Hoving et al (2002) reported that 11 of 60 patients (18%) in the manual therapy group reported increased neck pain for more than 2 days compared to only 3/64 in the medical care group (5%). Serious adverse responses to manual therapy (such as stroke or death) occur infrequently (Ernst 2002), so it is difficult to obtain accurate estimates of the frequency of such events. Clearly it would be helpful for patient and therapist to be able to accurately estimate the risk of serious adverse events.

Having obtained information about the benefits and harms of therapy, therapists can assist patients to make informed decisions about whether treatment is likely to be worthwhile. If the estimated benefit is perceived to outweigh harm, the therapy is generally indicated. In practice, these sorts of decisions are complex because they are influenced by an individual patient's values and preferences. Some patients consider making several visits to the physiotherapist and following a programme of exercise very inconvenient whereas others enjoy the outing. A very small group may even enjoy doing exercises. Many patients probably do not regard a temporary increase in neck pain as a serious adverse event and many would probably proceed with manual therapy treatment despite some risk of a temporary increase in neck pain. Other patients will be reluctant to submit to treatment if the adverse event could be disabling.

Very often individual clinical trials, particularly small clinical trials with few subjects, provide imprecise estimates of the effects of treatment. It is possible to quantify the precision of the estimate with confidence intervals (see Herbert 2000a and Herbert 2000b for an overview and for details on how to extract confidence intervals about estimates of the size of treatment effects from reports of clinical trials). When this is done it often becomes evident that the estimate is so imprecise that no firm conclusion can be made about whether the treatment produces effects that are big enough to be worthwhile. This is one of the reasons that systematic reviews can be so useful. Sometimes in systematic reviews it is possible to combine the findings of a number of like studies. The pooled estimate can provide a more precise estimate of the size of treatment effects than the estimates provided by the individual studies.

A word of warning is warranted here. There are several ways that the findings of individual clinical trials can be pooled in a systematic review, and some of these ways are quite unsatisfactory. The simplest method, called 'vote-counting', involves tallying up the number of studies with statistically significant findings (see, for example, Brown & Burns 2001). If a majority of studies show statistically significant effects the reviewer concludes that, taken together, the studies provide evidence of an effect of treatment. This is very unsatisfactory, both because it ignores the size of the treatment effect and because it is extremely inefficient (it is likely to conclude that there is no evidence of an effect even when evidence of an effect exists; Hedges & Olkin 1980). Another widely used approach sometimes referred to as 'qualitative synthesis' or 'best evidence synthesis' involves assigning labels to the strength of the evidence (strong evidence, moderate evidence, weak evidence, etc.) on the basis of the number of relevant studies, the quality of the studies and whether or not the individual studies find statistically significant effects (see, for example, van Tulder et al 2000). This approach has the same weaknesses as vote counting and, in addition, suffers from the fact that subtle variations in the definitions of the levels of evidence can profoundly influence how the quality of evidence is classified (Ferreira et al 2002). For these reasons, readers should be reluctant to accept at face value the findings of systematic reviews that synthesize trial findings using vote counting or best evidence synthesis.

The best method for synthesizing findings of like trials in a systematic review is meta-analysis. Meta-analysis involves statistically combining estimates of the size of treatment effects from individual studies to produce a pooled estimate of the size of the treatment effect (Hedges & Olkin 1980, Cooper & Hedges 1994, Egger et al 2001). Often meta-analysis is not possible, either because the individual trials are not sufficiently similar or because the necessary data are not given in the individual trial reports. However, when meta-analysis is possible it provides the best method currently available for obtaining estimates of the size of treatment effects in systematic reviews.

ASSESSING THE QUALITY OF CLINICAL PRACTICE GUIDELINES

Evidence-based clinical practice guidelines are 'systematically developed statements to assist practitioner and patient decisions about appropriate health care for specific clinical circumstances' (Institute of Medicine 1990). Guidelines generally provide a structured summary of all of the options for the management of a particular health problem (e.g. whiplash, urinary incontinence, stroke) along with recommendations for management. They usually consider all diagnosis and treatment options available for the condition and incorporate adverse prognostic indicators (sometimes called 'yellow flags'). Recommendations for management are commonly summarized in a clinical algorithm or pathway.

Ideally, recommendations should be based on high-quality external evidence (i.e. systematic reviews and randomized controlled trials in the case of treatment options). Where there are gaps in the external evidence, recommendations must be based on evidence that is more susceptible to bias (including observational studies and expert consensus). The level of evidence supporting each recommendation should be indicated in the guideline, and could range from very strong (based on a high-quality systematic review of randomized controlled trials showing large treatment effects) to very weak (based on small observational studies with small treatment effects or expert opinion).

Guidelines aim to reduce inappropriate variations in practice, promote the delivery of evidence-based health care and improve health outcomes (Thomas et al 2002). The effects of guideline-directed care have been systematically evaluated in the healthcare system. A Cochrane systematic review has shown that clinical practice guidelines are effective in changing professional practice and improving patient outcomes when used by health professionals allied with medicine (Thomas et al 2002).

As with randomized controlled trials and systematic reviews, guidelines vary in quality and this will influence the validity of the recommendations. Hayward et al (1995) suggest that critical appraisal of guidelines should involve asking the following questions:

1. Are the recommendations valid?

- Were all important options and outcomes clearly specified?
- Was an explicit and sensible process used to identify, select and combine evidence?
- Was an explicit and sensible process used to consider the relative value of different outcomes?
- Is the guideline likely to account for important recent developments?
- Has the guideline been subject to peer review and testing?

2. What are the recommendations?

- Are practical, clinically important recommendations made?
- How strong are the recommendations?
- What is the impact of uncertainty associated with the evidence and values used in the guidelines?

3. Will the recommendations help me in caring for my patients?

- Is the primary objective of the guideline consistent with my objective?
- Are the recommendations applicable to my patients?

The guidelines for the management of whiplash associated disorders (WAD) produced by the Motor Accidents Authority of New South Wales, Australia (Motor Accidents Authority 2001) are used to illustrate the above criteria. This guideline focuses on the early management (first 12 weeks post injury) of WAD grades I, II and III as defined by the Quebec Task Force (Spitzer et al 1995) (i.e. whiplash without vertebral fracture or dislocation).

The WAD guideline considers an important outcome, recovery versus non-recovery. An explicit process was used to identify the external evidence. The recommendations are based on the systematic review of the literature undertaken by the Quebec Task Force in 1993 (Spitzer et al 1995) supplemented by additional searching for evidence published between 1993 and 2000. In terms of values, a multidisciplinary group developed the guidelines but there was limited consumer input and the project was sponsored by the organization responsible for implementing the state's compulsory third party motor vehicle insurance scheme. As indicated above, the guideline could only incorporate developments in the management of WAD up to the year 2000.

The guideline was subject to review by three eminent peer reviewers, but there was limited testing before release.

While the WAD guidelines do make clinically important recommendations, these are framed according to the Quebec Task Force classification of WAD (Spitzer et al 1995) which are yet to be validated. They address management for the first 12 weeks after injury. The level of evidence is provided for each recommendation, but many recommendations are consensus-based rather than evidence-based. An example is the recommendation to use electrotherapies. Interestingly, the Dutch guidelines (Scholten-Peeters et al 2002) used a similar consensus process and did not recommend electrotherapies for acute WAD.

In terms of section three of the critical appraisal process, the primary objective of the WAD guidelines is to change clinical practice. Applicability will be dependent on the health professional using the guideline and the particular patients in question. The guidelines are only relevant to patients who were injured in the preceding 12 weeks. The WAD guidelines appear useful to guide clinical practice but there is sufficient uncertainty to justify formal evaluation of the guidelines.

CONCLUSION

How can clinical trials, systematic reviews and clinical practice guidelines be used in clinical practice? There are many models of clinical practice available to the manual therapist. Our preference is for a revised model of evidence-based practice that has been termed 'research enhanced health care' (Haynes et al 2002). In this model clinical decisions are informed by a consideration of: (i) the research evidence (in this context, trials, reviews and guidelines); (ii) the patient's preferences and actions; and

(iii) the clinical state and circumstances. Importantly the model emphasizes clinical expertise as the means to integrate the first three components in a given clinical situation. An assumption of both the original and revised models of evidence-based practice is that clinical decisions should be made based upon the best evidence. This is a critical issue for the field of manual therapy because the available evidence varies greatly in quality. As a consequence we believe that critical appraisal skills are a prerequisite for contemporary manual therapy practice and should be valued as highly as good practical treatment skills. A summary of the questions to be asked when critically appraising clinical trials, systematic reviews and clinical practice guidelines is given in Box 42.1.

The challenge for manual therapists is to decide what model of practice they will choose to follow. When commenting upon the future for physical therapy, Professor Ruth Grant predicted that 'physical therapy as a profession will prosper in the twenty-first century if physical therapists pay due heed and ensure that their practice integrates the best research evidence with clinical expertise and values' (Grant 2002, p. 420). This advice would seem equally relevant to manual therapy.

Box 42.1 Summary

Questions to ask when assessing the quality of clinical trials
1. Were subjects randomly allocated to conditions?
2. Was there blinding of assessors and patients?
3. Was there adequate follow-up?

Questions to ask when assessing the quality of systematic reviews
1. Was an adequate search strategy described?
2. Was the quality of individual trials taken into account when synthesizing the trial's findings?

Questions to ask when interpreting high quality clinical trials and systematic reviews
1. Can these findings be used to make inferences about my patients?
2. Was the intervention applied well?
3. Were the outcomes meaningful?
4. Was the effect of the intervention big enough to make the intervention worthwhile?

Questions to ask when assessing clinical practice guidelines (Hayward et al 1995)
1. Are the recommendations valid?
2. What are the recommendations?
3. Will the recommendations help me in caring for my patients?

References

Brown G T, Burns S A 2001 The efficacy of neurodevelopmental treatment in paediatrics: a systematic review. British Journal of Occupational Therapy 64: 235–244

Campbell D T, Stanley J C 1963 Experimental and quasi-experimental designs for research. Rand McNally, Chicago, Illinois

Chalmers T, Celano P, Sacks H, Smith H 1983 Bias in treatment assignment in controlled clinical trials. New England Journal of Medicine 309: 1358–1361

Cook T, Campbell D 1979 Quasi-experimentation: design and analysis issues for field settings. Rand McNally, Chicago, Illinois

Cooper H M, Hedges L V (eds) 1994 The handbook of research synthesis. Russell Sage Foundation, New York

Cote P, Cassidy D, Carroll L, Frank J, Bombardier C 2001 A systematic review of the prognosis of acute whiplash and a new conceptual framework to synthesise the literature. Spine 26: E445–E458

Egger M, Davey Smith G, Altman D G (eds) 2001 Systematic reviews in health care: meta-analysis in context. BMJ, London

Ernst E 2002 Manipulation of the cervical spine: a systematic review of case reports of serious adverse events, 1995–2001. Medical Journal of Australia 15: 376–380

Faas A, Chavannes A, van Eijk J, Gubbels J 1993 A randomized, placebo-controlled trial of exercise therapy in patients with acute low back pain. Spine 18: 1388–1395

Farrar J, Young J, LaMoreaux L, Werth J, Poole M 2001 Clinical importance of changes in chronic pain intensity measured on a 11-point numerical pain rating scale. Pain 94: 149–158

Ferreira P, Ferreira M, Maher C, Refshauge K, Herbert R, Latimer J 2002 Effect of applying different 'levels of evidence' on conclusions of Cochrane reviews of interventions for low back pain. Journal of Clinical Epidemiology 55: 1126–1129

Fritzell P, Hägg O, Wessberg P, Nordwall A, Swedish Lumbar Spine Study Group 2001 Volvo Award winner clinical studies. Lumbar fusion versus non-surgical treatment for chronic low back pain: a multicenter randomized controlled trial from the Swedish Lumbar Spine Study Group. Spine 26: 2521–2534

Glover J, Morris J, Khosla T 1974 Back pain: a randomised clinical trial of rotational manipulation of the trunk. British Journal of Industrial Medicine 31: 59–64

Grant R 2002 Reflections on clinical expertise and evidence-based practice. In: Grant R (ed) Physical therapy of the cervical and thoracic spine. Churchill Livingstone, New York, pp 413–421

Haynes R B, Devereaux P J, Guyatt G H 2002 Physicians' and patients' choices in evidence based practice. British Medical Journal 324: 1350

Hayward R S A, Wilson M C, Tunis S R, Bass E B, Guyatt G 1995 Users' guides to the medical literature. VIII: How to use clinical practice guidelines. A. Are the recommendations valid? JAMA 274: 570–574

Hedges L V, Olkin I 1980 Vote-counting methods in research synthesis. Psychological Bulletin 88: 359–369

Herbert R D 2000a How to estimate treatment effects from reports of clinical trials. I: Continuous outcomes. Australian Journal of Physiotherapy 46: 229–235

Herbert R D 2000b How to estimate treatment effects from reports of clinical trials. I: Dichotomous outcomes. Australian Journal of Physiotherapy 46: 309–313

Hides J A, Jull G A, Richardson C A 2001 Long-term effects of specific stabilizing exercises for first-episode low back pain. Spine 26: E243–248

Hollis S, Campbell F 1999 What is meant by intention to treat analysis? Survey of published randomised controlled trials. British Medical Journal 319: 670–674

Hoving J, Koes B, de Vet H et al 2002 Manual therapy, physical therapy or continued care by a general practitioner for patients with neck pain: a randomized controlled trial. Annals of Internal Medicine 136: 713–722

Institute of Medicine 1990 Clinical practice guidelines: directions for a new program. National Academy Press, Washington DC

Juni P, Witschi A, Bloch R, Egger M 1999 The hazards of scoring the quality of clinical trials in meta-analysis. JAMA 282: 1054–1060

McLachlan Z, Milne E, Lumley J, Walker B 1991 Ultrasound treatment for breast engorgement: a randomised double blind trial. Australian Journal of Physiotherapy 37: 23–29

Mannion A, Junge A, Taimela S, Muntener M, Lorenzo K, Dvorak J 2001 Active therapy for chronic low back pain. 3: Factors influencing self-rated disability and its change following therapy. Spine 26: 920–929

Moher D, Jadad A, Nichol G, Penman M, Tugwell P, Walsh S 1995 Assessing the quality of randomized controlled trials: an annotated bibliography of scales and checklists. Controlled Clinical Trials 16: 62–73

Moher D, Pham B, Jones A 1998 Does quality of reports of randomised trials affect estimates of intervention efficacy reported in meta-analyses? Lancet 352: 609–613

Moher D, Cook D, Eastwood S, Olkin I, Rennie D, Stroup D 1999 Improving the quality of reports of meta-analyses of randomised controlled trials: the QUORUM statement. Lancet 354: 1896–1900

Moher D, Schulz K, Altman D 2001 The CONSORT statement: revised recommendations for improving the quality of reports of parallel-group randomised trials. Lancet 357: 1191–1194

Moseley A M, Herbert R D, Sherrington C, Maher C G 2002 Evidence for physiotherapy practice: a survey of the physiotherapy evidence database (PEDro). Australian Journal of Physiotherapy 48: 43–49

Motor Accidents Authority 2001 Guidelines for the management of whiplash-associated disorders. Motor Accidents Authority, Sydney Available online at: http://www.maa.nsw.gov.au

National Health and Medical Research Council 1999 A guide to the development, implementation and evaluation of clinical practice guidelines. National Health and Medical Research Council, Canberra, Australia

Oh V 1994 The placebo effect: can we use it better? British Medical Journal 309: 69–70

Petticrew M 2001 Systematic reviews from astronomy to zoology: myths and misconceptions. British Medical Journal 322: 98–101

Pikula J 1999 The effect of spinal manipulative therapy (SMT) on pain reduction and range of motion in patients with acute unilateral neck pain: a pilot study. Journal of the Canadian Chiropractic Association 43: 111–119

Pocock S 1983 Clinical trials: a practical approach. John Wiley, Chichester

Sackett D L, Straus S E, Richardson W S, Rosenberg W, Haynes R B 2000 Evidence-based medicine: how to practice and teach EBM, 2nd edn. Churchill Livingstone, Edinburgh

Scholten-Peeters G, Bekkering G, Verhagen A et al 2002 Clinical practice guideline for the physiotherapy of patients with whiplash-associated disorders. Spine 27: 412–422

Schulz K F 1995 Subverting randomization in controlled trials. JAMA 274: 1456–1458

Schulz K, Chalmers I, Hayes R, Altman D 1995 Empirical evidence of bias: dimensions of methodological quality associated with estimates of treatment effects in controlled trials. JAMA 273: 408–412

Simes R J, Greatorex V, Gebski V J 1998 Practical approaches to minimize problems with missing quality of life data. Statistics in Medicine 17: 725–737

Sloop P, Smith D, Goldenberg E, Dore C 1982 Manipulation for chronic neck pain a double blind controlled study. Spine 7: 532–535

Solomon D H, Simel D L, Bates D W, Katz J N, Schaffer J L 2001 Does this patient have a torn meniscus or ligament of the knee? Value of the physical examination. JAMA 286: 1610–1620

Spitzer W O, Skovron M L, Salmi L R et al 1995. Scientific monograph of the Quebec Task Force on Whiplash-Associated Disorders: redefining 'whiplash' and its management. Spine 20(Suppl.): 1S–73S

Stern J M, Simes R J 1997 Publication bias: evidence of delayed publication in a cohort study of clinical research projects. British Medical Journal 315: 640–645

Thomas L, Cullum N, McColl E, Rousseau N, Soutter J, Steen N 2002 Guidelines in professions allied to medicine (Cochrane Review). Cochrane Library, issue 2. Update Software, Oxford

Tuchin P, Pollard H 1998 The cost effectiveness of spinal care education as a preventive strategy for spinal injury. Journal of Occupational Health and Safety 14: 43–51

van Tulder M W, Assendelft W J, Koes B W, Bouter L M 1997 Method guidelines for systematic reviews in the Cochrane Collaboration Back Review Group for spinal disorders. Spine 22: 2323–2330

van Tulder M, Malmivaara A, Esmail R, Koes B 2000 Exercise therapy for low back pain: a systematic review within the framework of the Cochrane Collaboration Back Review Group. Spine 25: 2784–2796

Verhagen A, de Vet H, de Bie R, Boers M, van den Brandt P 2001 The art of quality assessment of RCTs included in systematic reviews. Journal of Clinical Epidemiology 54: 651–654

Vicenzino B, Collins D, Wright A 1996 The initial effects of a cervical spine manipulative physiotherapy treatment on the pain and dysfunction of lateral epicondylalgia. Pain 68: 69–74

Waagen G, Hademan S, Cook G, Lopez D, DeBoer K 1986 Short term trial of chiropractic adjustments for the relief of chronic low-back pain. Manual Medicine 2: 63–67

Wickstrom G, Bendix T 2000 The 'Hawthorne effect': what did the original Hawthorne studies actually show? Scandinavian Journal of Work, Environment and Health 26: 363–367

Yusuf S, Wittes J, Probstfield J, Tyroler H A 1991 Analysis and interpretation of treatment effects in subgroups of patients in randomized clinical trials. JAMA 266: 93–98

Chapter 43

Establishing treatment guidelines for manual therapy of spinal syndromes

A. R. Gross, L. Hurley, L. Brosseau, I. D. Graham

INTRODUCTION

Evidence-based clinical practice guidelines (EBCPG) are systematically developed statements about best practice in health care for specific clinical conditions (Woolf 1990, Woolf et al 1999). They can help the clinician and patients to maximize effectiveness and manage costs of care. They should utilize the most current and highest level of evidence-based practice. Potential benefits of their use in clinical practice should outweigh potential harms if guidelines are rigorously developed (Woolf 1990). Typically, EBCPG address a high-cost, high-volume or high-risk area of practice. Treatment of spinal disorders, including manual therapies, meets these criteria. Some evidence suggests there is unexplained variation in clinical practice patterns among physiotherapists practising manual therapy in Ontario (Hurley et al 2002). Manual therapists have concerns that limited resources will reduce the delivery of high-quality care. They also have considerable difficulty in assimilating rapidly evolving scientific evidence into their clinical practice. In fact, some clinicians hesitate to use EBCPG; to some extent these guidelines are perceived to be formulaic and simplistic and to limit autonomy of practice. In spite of these concerns, manual therapists do have interest in EBCPG. This result concurs with another recent survey conducted in Ontario (Brosseau et al 2001). Indeed, over 82% of Ontarian physiotherapists who treat patients with cervical and lumbar syndromes reported having positive or very positive attitudes toward EBCPG. Furthermore, 59.1% of these physiotherapists responded that they use, at least occasionally to almost always, EBCPG in their daily practice. Over 68% of them reported being among the first to adopt innovations in their practice. To become a wise consumer of EBCPG, there are a number of questions a clinician must ask:

1. How are EBCPG developed?
2. How can I identify the best or most valid EBCPG?
3. What should I consider when adopting EBCPG in my practice?

Let us look at a clinical scenario to help work through these questions.

CLINICAL SCENARIO

Your private practice is so busy you can't even think. Four people with spinal disorders (mechanical non-specific neck and low back pain) have entered your clinic for care this morning. You note that you are commonly treating these disorders and believe you provide 'best' practice. But do you? There are a number of EBCPG incorporating manual therapy that you are aware of but have not had a chance to absorb and integrate into your practice environment. What makes them valid and can you use them?

HOW ARE EBCPG DEVELOPED?

There has been much enthusiasm for the establishment of EBCPG to assist in clinical decision making and to improve health outcomes (American Physical Therapy Association 2001, Brosseau & Dubouloz 2001, Helewa & Walker 2000). Evidence suggests that quality of care can be improved through the use of EBCPG (Davis & Taylor-Vaisey 1997, Grimshaw & Russel 1993, Grimshaw et al 1995, Levine et al 1996). Because guidelines are expensive to develop and implement, they should address areas of practice that are high-risk, high-volume or place a heavy burden on the patient and society. The systematic development, implementation, dissemination and evaluation of new EBCPG should be guided by published methods (Cluzeau et al 1999, Graham et al 2001, Philadelphia Panel 2001a, 2001b). The usual steps in guideline development are: forming a development methods group, searching systematically for evidence, grading the evidence, formulating draft EBCPG, forming external multidisciplinary evidence/consensus panels to refine the draft EBCPG, obtaining practitioner feedback and external review, pilot testing the EBCPG, dissemination and implementation of EBCPG and scheduled reviews.

All methods stress the need to develop, implement, disseminate and evaluate the EBCPG. Methods typically use an interdisciplinary, multigroup process. The core steps to

Figure 43.1 The Philadelphia Panel evidence based clinical practice guidelines flow sheet.

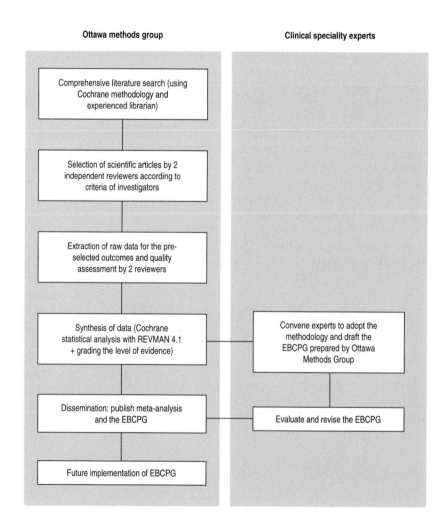

develop a guideline are outlined in Figure 43.1, as illustrated by the Philadelphia Panel (2001a).

Panel development

In preparation for development of the guideline, a guideline coordinating committee should meet to direct the process. This committee could represent the funder, the organization that has identified the need for a guideline, or interested clinicians who are willing to implement the process from start to finish. The coordinating committee chooses a methods group to review the evidence and sets up feedback processes to ensure that clinicians can review and challenge the draft recommendations. Later, an external panel review group will review the quality of the guideline that is developed.

The methods group should include members who are published experts in the evidence of the field (there is no evidence that being published makes a difference, although it is probably preferable), have developed guidelines previously, are experienced in judging levels of evidence, are skilled in using quality review methods for reviewing the evidence and have, or can access, the statistical expertise to extract, pool and analyse the evidence.

The clinician group should be interested in the development of the guideline, participate regularly in the community that will apply the intervention in question and be prepared to challenge the guideline development process to create recommendations that are relevant to front-line practice.

The external panel review group should share expertise similar to that of the methods group, have previous experience in the development of guidelines and include published authors of guidelines, but be independent of the guideline development process and be prepared to independently review the results of the draft guideline development as outlined below.

Selecting and framing the problem

The methods group should convene to refine the question of interest. The question must focus the topic by selecting the patient group, the intervention being studied, the clinically important outcomes and which study designs are of interest. The topic must address a rationale for undertaking the guideline effort. When framing the question, the method group should take into consideration such factors as prevalence of the condition, burden of illness, potential for significant health benefit or risk, relevance to local practice patterns, degree of variation in healthcare practice patterns, likelihood of influencing change in clinical practices, costs and available evidence (Browman et al 1995).

Generating the EBCPG

There are a number of steps in generating EBCPG. The goal is to systematically search for available guidelines and systematic reviews, identify primary studies published subsequent to the last search date, rate the strength of this evidence and generate preliminary recommendations.

Search for existing guidelines

Once the question is refined, the method group does a search for existing guidelines. If they are not current or they do not meet methodological standards, a systematic search for evidence is undertaken.

Gathering and synthesizing the evidence

The search for evidence typically includes meta-analysis, systematic reviews and randomized controlled trials (RCTs) published subsequent to the last search date of the reviews. However, it may additionally include controlled clinical trials, cohort studies and case/control studies, depending on the question. Specific skills and methods are employed when identifying and selecting citations. A research librarian skilled in searching databases and doing systematic reviews should be used. To begin citation identification, the method group first identifies key words and text words related to the population, intervention and study design of interest. The research librarian and investigators design the search strategy for each database. Typical searches include the Cochrane database of systematic reviews, the Campbell collaboration database, MEDLINE, EMBASE, PEDro, CINAHL, Sports Discus, Healthstar, PsychoINFO, Current Contents and the Cochrane Controlled Trials Register. Specific selection criteria are used by two independent raters in two phases. First, citation and abstract postings are screened and key citations are identified. Secondly, full manuscripts of the citations and reviews are retrieved and read. Those meeting the selection criteria are retained for further critique. The methods group then critiques the selected reviews and RCTs, working in pairs for methodological quality using specific rating instruments. Methodological quality rating instruments, such as those described by Jadad et al (1996), assess concealment of random allocation, blinding, and loss to follow-up in RCTs. The rating instruments of Oxman & Guyatt (1991) and van Tulder et al (1997) assess the likelihood of bias in reviews and meta-analyses. Factors such as the comprehensiveness of the search for evidence, the criteria used to decide which studies to include in the meta-analysis, the criteria used to assess the validity of the primary studies and the presentation and analysis of data are critiqued.

Raw data on primary outcomes are extracted by two independent reviewers. Data are analysed using quantitative methods such as meta-analysis and sensitivity analysis or qualitative methods. Primary results are established based on the synthesis of these data and the methodological quality of each trial. The systematic review of the literature is now completed.

Grading the evidence

Levels of evidence apply to individual studies. They are more objective and relate to the study methods. The categorization into levels reflects the susceptibility of the evidence to bias. This may be followed by grading the recommendations. Grades refers to the body of evidence supporting a particular recommendation. Grading is more subjective and decided by the panel. The panel attempts to grade the strength of the evidence supporting a particular recommendation. A number of such classification schemes exist (Browman et al 1995, Canadian Task Force 1986, Cook et al 1992, Guyatt et al 1995, Sackett et al 2000). Examples of the recommended higher levels of evidence based on Cook et al (1992) are:

Level I evidence: *Larger RCTs that are either positive with low risk of false positive conclusions, negative with low risk of false negative conclusions; meta-analyses.*

Level II evidence: *Smaller RCTs that have positive tendencies that are not statistically significant, with high risk of false positive conclusions, or that have no effect with high risk of false negative conclusions.*

Other grading systems used by the Canadian Task Force on the Periodic Health Examination and Shekelle et al (1999) have the ability to grade both the direction of results into smaller subdivisions and the strength of the trial design, as follows:

Levels of Evidence

Level Ia evidence: *A meta-analysis of RCTs.*
Level Ib evidence: *At least one properly done RCT.*
Level IIa evidence: *Well-designed controlled trials without randomization, well-designed cohort or case-control analytic studies, preferably from more than one centre or research group.*
Level IIb evidence: *A quasi-randomized study.*
Level III evidence: *Non-randomized studies.*
Level IV evidence: *Opinions of respected authorities, based on clinical experience; descriptive studies or reports of expert committees.*

Strength of Recommendations

A: *Good evidence to support a recommendation that the intervention be specifically considered.*
B: *Fair evidence to support a recommendation that the intervention be specifically considered.*
C: *Poor evidence regarding inclusion or exclusion of an intervention, but recommendations may be made on other grounds.*
D: *Good evidence that an intervention should not be done.*

Guidelines should use explicit criteria and link these criteria to the recommendations. Lower levels of evidence may be the only evidence available for review, and if this is the case, the guideline is unlikely to meet the criteria for EBCPG development.

Generating and formulating EBCPG

After the large number of initial articles identified has been systematically reviewed and the level of evidence has been established by the methods group, the clinical expert group is convened to interpret the evidence and draft initial recommendations. This group reviews the findings to ensure rigorous methodology, to challenge the findings and to assure relevance to practice. It considers the clinical, public health, policy and payment contexts. The cost-effectiveness of the intervention should also be considered. Feasibility issues such as skill, time, staff and ability of the system to implement the recommendations may also be considered.

Where there is insufficient evidence to answer key questions, the EBCPG panel may proceed to make recommendations based solely on consensus. The process of reaching consensus must be handled objectively and explicitly. This is the area most often challenged by critics of EBCPG. The consensus process must include clinicians as well as methodology experts. The level of evidence in the consensus based recommendations is of a lower level of quality than is found in evidence based recommendations.

Obtaining practitioner feedback and external review

The methods and clinical group is now ready to receive feedback on the initial recommendations. An external methods and clinical expert group should review the process that was used to identify, categorize, and extract the data. The guidelines are pilot tested for readability, feasibility, and ease of implementation.

Using the feedback from this review process, the clinical expert group reconciles and ratifies the evidence based recommendations to produce an EBCPG. Integration of practical and policy issues should also be performed at this stage by the panel. Note that few clinical panels are well positioned to assess policy issues, as the panellists do not have a policy perspective. Implementation is the next step, followed by evaluation to ensure that the guideline will guide and/or change practice. Ideally, the goal should be to achieve the expected health outcome.

Dissemination and implementation of the EBCPG

Guideline attempts have traditionally failed to have an impact on practice because of poor implementation strategies (Basinski 1995, Carter et al 1995, Davis & Taylor-Vaisey 1997, Grimshaw & Russell 1993, Grimshaw et al 1995). The guideline development effort is expensive and time-consuming, and generally absorbs large amounts of goodwill and unpaid time on the part of the methods and feedback groups. However, once these groups have finished their work, the real work on the guideline has just begun.

Most guideline developers disseminate guidelines through journals, association literature, presentations and conferences. While these methods are useful for raising awareness of the guideline, they have not been found to be effective in changing practice (Davis & Taylor-Vaisey 1997, Delitto 1998, Grimshaw & Russell 1993, Grimshaw et al 1995). An implementation strategy is more likely to be effective if it: increases awareness of the guideline; changes attitudes so that the guideline will be accepted; is seen as a means of improving patient care, changes behaviour in clinical practice in accordance with the recommendations of the guideline (Bohannon 1990, 1999, Bohannon & Le Veau 1986, Clemence 1998, Closs & Lewin 1998, Herbert et al 2001); and informs best practice so that quality of care improves (Conroy & Shannon 1995, Lomas 1991).

Any organizational barriers to implementation should be identified. Before implementing an EBCPG, an organization should identify to what degree the EBCPG is different from usual practice, how much the EBCPG challenges established procedures, how much the EBCPG limits practice and whether there is a recommendation to discontinue usual treatment as a result of the evidence.

Effective organizational interventions could include an expanded role for the health professional, financial interventions (for example, professional incentives) and regulatory interventions. Other methods of implementation after dissemination include the use of reminder cards, local champions or organizations to carry the guideline forward, presentations and monitoring and auditing of practice. Strategies are usually multifaceted in nature (Davis & Taylor-Vaisey 1997, Grimshaw et al 1995).

Evaluation

Concurrent with development and implementation, evaluation is necessary to ensure that the EBCPG changes practice. Evaluation is a three-stage process. The first stage, inception evaluation (Basinski 1995), is undertaken when the EBCPG is being developed. It can be a formal or an informal process. It is used to assess the need for an EBCPG and to determine whether the EBCPG actually addresses the stated purpose. This type of evaluation includes assessment of how well clinicians will accept the new EBCPG, how relevant and applicable they will find it to their practice situations, and how clear and practical the new EBCPG appears to them.

The second stage of evaluation occurs once the developed EBCPG has been sent to all stakeholders. Feedback is sought from practitioners on publication, at presentations and conferences, and during informal sharing sessions on the relevance of the EBCPG to practice.

The third stage of the implementation is a scientific evaluation done to assess the effects of the EBCPG on practice and health outcomes. This evaluation looks at areas such as guideline development, format, dissemination and implementation, and provides an evidence basis for further guideline initiatives (Basinski 1995). This third stage evaluation also includes validating the generalizability of the

results and investigating the extent to which changes can be attributed to the guideline.

Updating guidelines

The final step, and part of the accountability process of EBCPG development and implementation, is a commitment by the organization that supported development of the EBCPG to regularly update the evidence.

HOW CAN THE CLINICIAN IDENTIFY THE BEST EBCPG?

Regardless of the strength of the evidence supporting an EBCPG recommendation, it remains the responsibility of the clinician – in this case the manual therapist – to use independent inquiry to interpret the application of an EBCPG (Hurwitz 1999). The clinician exercises customary clinical discretion and judgement, informed by scientific evidence; however, other sources of relevant information and professional experience are required to establish the care needed for an individual patient. Guidelines are a supplement to, not a substitute for, relevant care. The following steps are recognized as fundamental to identifying the best EBCPG in manual therapy: the clinical question should be framed, a search for guidelines should be conducted and the quality as well as their content should be assessed.

Step 1: Framing the clinical question

The clinical scenario presented at the beginning of this chapter will be used to illustrate the process. First, the clinical question is framed. The patient or problem, the intervention of interest and possible comparison interventions and the outcomes of interest are identified. This allows the clinician to identify what kind of evidence to search for.

Step 2: Search for the EBCPG

A search for EBCPG is begun. For this scenario, a brief search is undertaken in Medline and PEDro from December 2001 going back 5 years (this may be sufficient for a busy clinician), and on the Internet for organizational websites using search terms such as publication type: guideline, practice guidelines, and consensus development conference. Note that websites change frequently; new ones are continually being added and old ones disappear. The activity status of the websites should be assessed periodically. Some organizations with useful websites follow (Feder et al 1999, Woolf 1990, and Woolf's detailed article on the British Medical Journal's website <http//:www.bmj.com>):

Europe

- Agence Nationale de l'Accréditation et d'Évaluation en Santé
- Dutch College of General Practitioners
- German Guidelines Clearinghouse

* Royal College of General Practitioners
* Scottish Intercollegiate Guidelines Network
* Swedish Council on Technology Assessment in Health Care

North America
* Agency for Health Care Policy and Research Guidelines
* Alberta Clinical Practice Guidelines
* Canadian Medical Association Infobase: Clinical Practice Guidelines
* College of Physiotherapists of Ontario
* Health Services/Technology Assessment Text
* National Guidelines Clearinghouse
* Philadelphia Panel EBCPGs
* Primary Care Clinical Practice Guidelines
* US EBCPGs Clearinghouse

Australia and New Zealand
* Australian Medical Health and Research Council
* National Health Committee and Accidence Rehabilitation and Compensation Insurance Corporation of New Zealand
* Australian Physiotherapy Association

Feder et al (1999) suggest also using other common bibliographic databases such as CINAHL, Health Star and Embase if a more comprehensive search is desired. Subject headings (MeSh), keywords as well as text words should be used. These include anatomical terms, disorder or syndrome terms, treatment terms and methodological terms. Methodological search terms for Medline should include 'guidelines, consensus development conference' and for CINAHL and EMBASE, terms should include 'practice guidelines' as a publication type or subject heading.

In performing the search, one descriptive study summarizing clinical guidelines for the management of low back pain is found (Koes et al 2001) as well as a number of guidelines. For this exercise, we select and critique three guidelines (Netherlands (Faas et al 1996); Australia (Bogduk 2000); UK (Waddell et al 1999)) which offer differing opinions for low back pain, and two on neck disorders (Australian Physiotherapy Association (APA) and Manipulative Physiotherapy Association of Australia (MPAA) guidelines on pre-manipulative testing of the cervical spine (Magarey et al 2000); the College of Physiotherapy of Ontario (CPO) guidelines on manipulation and mobilization for mechanical neck disorders (Gross et al 2001, 2002)).

Step 3: Assessing the Rigour of EBCPG Development

The clinician has a choice of using a number of criteria checklists or instruments to judge the quality (for example, susceptibility to bias) of the practice guideline (Graham et al 2000). Potential biases of guideline development, the internal and external validity of the resulting recommendations and their feasibility for clinical practice are all impor-

tant issues to assess. The Appraisal of Guidelines for Research and Evaluation (AGREE) Instrument (updated version: 2001; <www.agreecollaboration.org>) provides one framework for judging the quality of EBCPG. Its reliability has been established (Cluzeau et al 1999). The criteria in this tool are based on theoretical assumptions which are consistent with other guides (Hayward et al 1995, Lohr & Field 1992, National Health and Medical Research Council 1999). Its six domains, which include 23 items, cover the following aspects of quality, scope, and purpose in guidelines:

1. scope and purpose (items 1–3)
2. stakeholder involvement (items 4–7)
3. rigour of development (items 8–14)
4. clarity of presentation (items 15–18)
5. applicability (items 19–21)
6. editorial independence (items 22–23).

Each item is rated on a four-point scale where 4 is strongly agree and 1 is strongly disagree. The scale measures the extent to which each item has been fulfilled. A high percentage means most items in that domain have been fulfilled.

As described earlier, classifying the evidence supporting recommendations by levels of evidence is useful. Guidelines derived from level 1a evidence (evidence from meta-analysis of randomized controlled trials) or level 1b evidence (evidence from at least one randomized controlled trial) indicate strong evidence for a particular treatment for a given illness (Shekelle et al 1999).

Table 43.1 depicts the critique of selected guidelines based on the AGREE instrument. To increase the reliability of the appraisal, three authors (LB, AG and IG) critiqued the low back pain and APA and MPAA guidelines on pre-manipulative testing, while two (IG and LB) critiqued the CPO guidelines on mechanical neck disorders; AG abstained due to a conflict of interest. It is noted that typically the scope/purposes and clarity/presentation were well reported for all the EBCPG. However, there was a fair degree of variation between EBCPG in these items: rigour of development, stakeholder involvement and editorial independence. There was consistent lack of information on the applicability of the guidelines; that is, the potential cost implications of applying the recommendations, discussion of organizational barriers to applying the guidelines and key review criteria for monitoring and audit purposes were not noted.

Step 4: Assessing the Reasonableness of the Individual EBCPG

After carefully examining the actual recommendations and the levels of evidence supporting each recommendation, the clinician now exercises customary clinical discretion and judgement, combining the guideline with other sources of relevant information and professional experience to decide on the care needed by an individual patient.

Table 43.1   Critical review of EBCPG based on the AGREE instrument

Author/domain (%)	Scope and purpose	Stakeholder involvement	Rigour of development	Clarity and presentation	Applicability	Editorial independence	Overall assessment
LOW BACK PAIN EBCPG							
Waddell et al 1999	81	88	83	90	25	50	Strongly recommend
Bogduk 1999	69	50	52	79	25	75	Recommend with proviso
Faas et al 1996	53	33	35	60	27	25	Would not recommend
NECK DISORDER EBCPG							
Gross et al 2001	83	50	80	63	33	31	Recommend with proviso
Magarey et al 2000	67	39	36	50	38	25	Recommend with proviso

Key: AGREE Instrument key items organized in six domains with 23 items; the standardized domain score was calculated as follows: (items scores × number of appraisers / total score) × 100 = domain %; a high percentage is better than a low score.

WHAT SHOULD THE CLINICIAN CONSIDER WHEN ADAPTING AN EBCPG INTO THEIR PRACTICE?

Several indicators can influence the actual use of EBCPG in a clinician's daily practice (Logan & Graham 1998):

- the topic of the EBCPG itself and its development process
- the clinician's perceptions and attitudes toward an EBCPG
- the skills needed to apply the EBCPG
- external factors that are generated by the particular clinical environment.

Table 43.2 summarizes potential barriers, implementation strategies, and relevant reminder strategies. Step by step, the clinician can generate relevant clinical questions of interest, systematically search for existing EBCPG and then evaluate them critically with an appraisal instrument in order to provide more effective treatment for the patient. This information can be useful in clinical decision making provided the identified EBCPG have been developed with sufficient methodological rigour and are supported by strong enough evidence to convince the clinician to adopt them.

Once the clinician has decided to adopt specific EBCPG in their practice, their attitude toward these EBCPG can either facilitate or block their intention to use them. The actual use of EBCPG may run counter to their usual practice (for instance, they may require change and thus not be considered advantageous compared to their usual practice), may not be precise, may appear to be complex or difficult to carry out, may not be user-friendly, may be controversial, or may be harder to follow than ones that are compatible with usual practice and not controversial (Grilli & Lomas 1994, Grol et al 1998, Rogers 1995). Reflecting on how you perceive particular EBCPG and the reason for these attitudes may help you identify internal barriers that contribute to your not using the EBCPG (Bohannon 1990, 1999, Bohannon & LeVeau 1986, Clemence 1998, Close &

Lewin 1998, Herbert et al 2001). Other potential barriers to using an EBCPG could relate to the clinician's specific clinical skills or appropriate experience. The EBCPG may not be adopted because of concern that the learning curve may be too steep. A clinician may need to find ways to improve their skills and experience by some means of professional development, such as continuing education, in order to adopt a particular EBCPG (Bohannon 1999, O'Brien 2001, Turner 2001, Turner & Whitfield 1997).

Some of the most difficult barriers to using a EBCPG identified by individual clinicians are the ones created by the practice environment (Bohannon 1999, Clemence 1998, Close & Lewin 1998). A clinician may have limited power to change their practice setting. When adopting an EBCPG, anticipate these external practice setting factors and determine the extent to which you will be able to modify them or find new strategies. Will there be resource issues client issues or organizational issues that could affect your ability to comply with the EBCPG? For example, the use of an EBCPG may be limited because of resources. Does the clinic have the technology required by the EBCPG (e.g. high-tech Cybex exercise equipment for strength training) or will it have to be purchased? Will the recommended procedure be covered by the healthcare system or by the client's insurance? If not, will the client be able to afford to pay for it? Another practice setting issue that might influence the ability to comply with an EBCPG is client preference. How will clients respond to the EBCPG? If the practice is in an organization, does the EBCPG affect other healthcare professionals? How can this effect be limited or managed? Will the clinician need to convince their colleagues of the value of the EBCPG (Logan & Graham 1998)? *The bottom line is that implementing EBCPG takes persistence and patience.*

Evaluation of guideline use can enhance care. The clinician needs to specify the data needed for evaluation prior to implementation of the EBCPG. It should be linked to areas of strong evidence within the guideline. Guidelines can be

Table 43.2 Implementation and evaluation strategies for barriers to professional implementation of EBCPG

Barriers related to	Implementation strategy	Evaluation strategy
THE CPG		
The document is too long and complex	Produce user-friendly algorithm	
THE ADOPTER		
Have not done this before (lack skill or knowledge)	Take course Do workshop Do practicum Observe others doing it	Track the number of patients I use the procedure on Self-assessment against guideline to learn about gaps in performance
My colleagues don't believe it works and they never do it (attitude)	Trial the recommendation and monitor patient progress; this will help you decide if you should retain it in your practice and if you should encourage your colleagues to do the same Local consensus process Educational outreach Bring in opinion leader	Collect information on patient health outcomes
THE PRACTICE SETTING		
Too busy to do it, simply forget to do it, stuck in a routine, culture, or practice pattern	Have reminder system (i.e. prompt sheet/card, cues on chart assessment form, posters in patient treatment rooms) to identify appropriate patients and prompt me to follow recommendation Patient mediated interventions (posters, pamphlets)	Develop tracking system to see if the reminder system is working (i.e. clinical audit group that collects data, does the analysis and feeds back data to the team)
Won't be reimbursed (not insured by payer)	Reminder strategy to prompt query and private pay	
Don't have the necessary equipment	Make budgetary plans Advise patient of circumstance and refer him to an appropriate service/clinic with the equipment	
Patient doesn't want it	Show them evidence to convince them it is beneficial Produce patient pamphlet	Collect information on patient satisfaction to include in pamphlet

used as an instrument for self-assessment or peer review to learn about gaps in your performance. This is especially useful if the guidelines have been turned into specific measurable criteria.

Now, let us use this knowledge and apply it to our case scenario.

Critique of Low Back Pain EBCPG

In terms of low back pain recommendations, it is noted that the UK recommendations scored the highest on the AGREE instrument (see Table 43.1). The other EBCPG did not use a standardized approach to synthesis of the scientific results. This resulted in a lack of clear and precise views of the evidence for intervention efficacy, especially in the face of con-

flicting results on the use of manipulation for acute low back pain found in the guidelines. Some guidelines did not review the raw data of each article using analysis and synthesis set out by the Cochrane Collaboration systematic methodology. In some cases, the scientific results of each study were reviewed separately but no synthesis was carried out. Overall, there were no recent updates; the results of the EBCPG stopped in 1997. However, based on the high validity in the development of the UK EBCPG, if new information does not substantively alter the EBCPG finding on manual therapy and if the patients described as acute and chronic appear similar to their population, the clinician may decide to apply the UK guidelines on a consistent basis in their practice. If so, the clinician will consider manipulative treatment for patients who need additional help with pain relief or who are failing to return to normal activities approximately 2 or 3 weeks post injury. The clinician should judge the application of the guideline on a case-by-case basis, using customary clinical discretion. For example, if the patient prefers not to have manual therapy performed because of associated risks or the patient has other health problems that put him at higher risk of developing side-effects from manual therapy, the clinician may choose not to follow certain aspects of the guideline.

Implementation strategy. The clinician may notice that colleagues in the clinic do not believe that advising activation and monitoring for the need to do manual therapy in the acute phase of LBP works. The clinician may act as a key informant, train other therapists to critique the guidelines and then set up a local consensus process where the therapists critique and debate the guideline findings to heighten their awareness. A group discussion about the impact of these guidelines on current practice is held, an implementation strategy is pre-planned and measurable patient outcomes are identified for tracking. Discussions on clinic barriers, patient barriers and therapist barriers are held, and methods for jogging the therapist's memory are developed. A brief flagging note may be inserted for all acute LBP cases by the intake secretary, using a brief sequence of questions to triage the patients for acute versus chronic LBP. The secretary puts an algorithm into the chart of each patient with acute LBP to cue the therapist. The algorithm should also be readily available in the treatment room for therapist information. Patient information packages and posters could be made available on acute LBP in the waiting room to help influence patient preferences. All therapists should work together to monitor outcomes of pain, function and patient satisfaction, to track the benefit to the patient.

Critique of neck disorder EBCPG

Since the APA EBCPG on pre-manipulative procedures for the cervical spine had low validity as measured by AGREE and was based on level IV diagnostic evidence (Sackett et al 2000), the clinician may consider the recommendations but decide to continue their current practice. They may already work to the minimum standards noted in the guidelines but may not feel that doing detailed testing is worth the time, since the test results do not help either rule in or rule out the signs and symptoms leading to serious consequences. Clearly, this is a personal and difficult decision.

For the CPO guideline on manual therapy for neck disorders, the clinician may accept the EBCPG with provisos. They note that the guideline has appropriate scope, rigour in development, and clarity. However, the provisos are as follows:

- The guidelines were developed for limited clinical practice areas; there was low stakeholder involvement; and the guideline working group was not multidisciplinary.
- There were no measurable criteria noted that could be applied in your clinic.

- The applicability in terms of organizational barriers, costs and key barriers was not discussed.
- Editorial independence was not noted.

The clinician needs to decide if these provisos are influential factors in generalizing the data from the CPO EBCPG to their clinical practice. You are a physiotherapist with advanced manual therapy skills and your typical practice is to use a multimodal management approach. Exercise and manual therapy are key elements in this approach. Other modalities may be used on a case-by-case basis. Typically, it is your goal to achieve a functional change; however, you note that the information from the CPO EBCPG on changing functional outcomes compared to control/comparisons treatments is unclear. You also note that the paucity of information did not allow for treatment differentiation in acute versus chronic mechanical neck disorders, with or without cervicogenic headache. The use of manipulation and mobilization alone seemed less effective than using an exercise and manual therapy based multimodal approach for reducing pain. Because these data can be generalized to your clinical setting, you decide to adopt the guideline but monitor updates closely.

Implementation strategy. Since both guidelines reflect the clinician's current practice, no change in practice pattern is required. The clinician may decide to hold an information session with their colleagues to confirm that their practice is in line with both EBCPG.

RESOLUTION OF CLINICAL SCENARIO

You adopt the UK guideline for acute LBP, thereby limiting the use of manipulation within a needs-based monitoring framework. The CPO guidelines for mechanical neck disorders is adopted with the provisos that you are a manual therapist and your patient population matches the one described in the EBCPG; you note that this guideline does not change your current practice. You reflect on the APA and MPAA guidelines for pre-manipulative testing for the cervical spine. This is a very personal decision as the evidence is not strong (level IV) and the validity of the key diagnostic trials may be flawed. You consider the expert opinion noted in the guideline and decide to continue your current practice pattern since you work to the minimum standards noted in the guideline.

CONCLUSION

EBCPG should be developed using a rigorous scientific process. They require multiple hands and expertise to reach publishable quality. A good place to start developing EBCPG is in high-risk, high-cost or high-volume areas of practice; they should only be developed if a sufficient body of evidence is available. Currently, the methods used to develop EBCPG are much better understood and employed than the methods used to implement EBCPG. Effective implementation strategies are vital to changing practices. Multiple strategies should be used to ensure effective implementation. Three-fold evaluation is necessary: prior to development (a needs analysis), when the EBCPG is first disseminated (relevance to practice), and after the EBCPG has been implemented, to determine if the EBCPG has changed practice.

It is clear that customary clinical discretion and judgement, informed by scientific evidence, must be applied to establish the care needed by an individual patient. Guidelines are a supplement to, and not a substitute for, relevant care.

KEYWORDS

evidence-based clinical practice guidelines
cervical

lumbar
spinal manipulation

Acknowledgement

The authors would like to thank Marla Nayer on behalf of the College of Physiotherapists of Ontario for assistance in manuscript development.

References

American Physical Therapy Association 2001 Guide to physical therapist practice, 2nd edn. Physical Therapy 81: 9–746

Basinski A S H 1995 Evaluation of clinical practice guidelines. Canadian Medical Association Journal 153: 1575–1581

Bogduk N 1999 Draft evidence based clinical guidelines for the management of acute low back pain. National Health and Medical Research Council, Australia. Available online at: http://www.health.gov.au:80/nhmrc/media/2000rel/pain.hlm; website accessed: Oct 2001

Bohannan R W 1990 Information accessing behaviour of physical therapists. Physiotherapy Theory and Practice 6: 215–225

Bohannan R W 1999 Applying research findings to the practice of geriatric rehabilitation. Topics in Geriatric Rehabilitation 14(3): 22–28

Bohannan R W, LeVeau B F 1986 Clinician's use of research findings: a review of literature with implementation for physiotherapists. Physical Therapy 66(1): 45–50

Brosseau L, Dubouloz C J 2001 La pratique fondée sur les faits scientrifiques dans le domains de la réadaptation [Evidence-based practice in rehabilitation]. Les Cahiers Scientifiques de l'ACFAS, no. 98

Brosseau L, Graham I, Longchamps C et al 2001 Determinants of the use of EBCPGs for the treatment of lumbar and cervical pain syndromes among physiotherapists: an Ontario survey. Physiotherapy Foundation of Canada Technical Report

Browman G P, Levine M N, Mahide E A et al 1995 The practice guidelines development cycle: a conceptual tool for practice guidelines development and implementation. Journal of Clinical Oncology 13(2): 502–512

Canadian Task Force on the Periodic Health Examination 1986 The periodic health examination. Canadian Medical Association Journal 134: 172–729. http://wwwctfphcorg/methods.htm; website accessed: Oct 2001

Carter A O, Battista R N, Hodge M J, Lewis S, Haynes R B 1995 Proceedings of the 1994 Canadian clinical practice guidelines network workshop. Canadian Medical Association Journal 153: 1715–1719

Clemence M L 1998 Evidence-based physiotherapy: seeking the unattainable? British Journal of Therapy and Rehabilitation 5(5): 257–260

Closs S J, Lewin B J P 1998 Perceived barriers to research utilization: a survey of four therapists. British Journal of Therapy and Rehabilitation 5(3): 151–154

Cluzeau F, Littlejohns P, Grimshaw J, Feder G, Moran S 1999 Development and application of a generic methodology to assess the quality of clinical guidelines. International Journal for Quality in Health Care 11: 21–28

Conroy M, Shannon W 1995 Clinical Guidelines: Their implementation in General Practice. British Journal of General Practice 45: 371–375

Cook D L, Guyatt G H, Laupacis A, et al 1992 Rules of evidence and clinical recommendations of the use of antithrombotic agents. Chest 102 Suppl:305S-311S

Davis D A, Taylor-Vaisey A 1997 Translating guidelines into practice: a systematic review of theoretical concepts, practical experience and research evidence in the adoption of clinical practice guidelines. Canadian Medical Association Journal 157(4): 408–416

Delitto A 1998 Clinicians and researchers who treat and study patients with low back pain: are you listening? Physical Therapy 78: 705–707

Faas A, Chavannes A W, Koes B W et al 1996 NHG-Standard Lage-Rugpijn. Huisarts Wet 39: 18–31

Feder G, Eccles M, Grol R, Griffiths C, Grimshaw J 1999 Using clinical guidelines. British Medical Journal 318: 728–730

Graham I D, Calder L, Herbert P, Carter A O, Tetroe J M 2000 A comparison of clinical practice guidelines appraisal instruments. International Journal of Technology Assessment in Health Care 16(4): 1024–1038

Grilli R, Lomas J 1994 Evaluating the message: the relationship between compliance rate and the subject of a practice guideline. Medical Care 32(3): 202–213

Grimshaw J M, Russell I T 1993 Effects of clinical guidelines on medical practice: A systematic review of rigorous evaluation. Lancet 342: 1317–1322

Grimshaw J, Freemantel N, Russell I et al 1995 Developing and implementing clinical practice guidelines. Quality in Health Care 4: 55–64

Grol R, Calhuijsen J, Thomas S, in't Veld D, Rutten G, Mokkink H 1998 Attributes of clinical guidelines that influence use of guidelines in general practice: observational study. British Medical Journal 317: 858–861

Gross A R, Kay T M, Hurley L et al 2001 College of Physiotherapy of Ontario, technical report: clinical practice guidelines on the use of manipulation or mobilization in the treatment of adults with mechanical neck disorders. College of Physiotherapy of Ontario, Toronto <http://www.collegept.org>; website accessed: Dec 2001

Gross A R, Kay T M, Hurley L et al 2002 Clinical practice guideline on the use of manipulation or mobilization in the treatment of adults with mechanical neck disorders. Manual Therapy 7(4): 193–205

Guyatt G H, Sackett D L, Sinclair J C et al 1995 User's guides to the medical literature. IX: A method for grading health care recommendations. Journal of the American Medical Association 274(22): 1800–1804

Hayward R S A, Wilson M C, Tunis S R, Bas E B, Guyatt G for the Evidence-Based Medicine Working Group 1995 User's guides to the medical literature. VIII: How to use clinical practice guidelines. A. Are the recommendations valid? Journal of the American Medical Association 274: 570–574

Helewa A, Walker J 2000 Critical evaluation of research in physical rehabilitation. Saunders, Philadelphia

Herbert R D, Sherrington C, Maher C, Moseley A M 2001 Evidence-based practice: imperfect but necessary. Physiotherapy Theory and Practice 17: 201–211

Hurley L, Yardley K, Gross A et al 2002 A survey to examine attitudes and patterns of practice of physiotherapists who perform cervical spine manipulation. Manual Therapy 7(1): 10–18

Hurwitz B 1999 Legal and political considerations of clinical practice guidelines. British Medical Journal 318: 661–664

Jadad A, Moore A, Carrol D et al 1996 Assessing the quality of randomized trials: is blinding necessary? Controlled Clinical Trials 17: 1–12

Koes B W, vanTulder M W, Ostelo R, Burton A K, Waddell G 2001 Clinical guidelines for the management of low back pain in primary care: an international comparison. Spine 26(22): 2504–2514

Levine M N, Browman G, Newman T et al 1996 The Ontario cancer treatment practice guidelines initiative. Oncology 10(Suppl.): 19–22

Logan J, Graham I D 1998 Toward a comprehensive interdisciplinary model of health care research use. Science Communication 20(2): 227–246

Lohr K N, Field M J 1992 A provisional instrument for assessing clinical practice guidelines. In: Riled M J, Lohr K N (eds) Guidelines for clinical practice: from development to use. National Academy Press, Washington DC

Lomas J 1991 Words without action? The production, dissemination and impact of consensus recommendations. Annual Review of Public Health 12: 41–65

Magarey M, Coughlin B, Rebbeck T on behalf of the APA and MPAA. 2000 Australian Physiotherapy Association clinical guidelines for pre-manipulative procedures for the cervical spine. Australian Physiotherapy Association, St Kilda, Victoria

National Health and Medical Research Council 1999 A guide to the development, implementation and evaluation of clinical practice guidelines. Commonwealth of Australia, Canberra

O'Brien M A 2001 Keeping up-to-date: continuing education, practice improvement strategies, and evidence-based physiotherapy practice. Physiotherapy Theory and Practice 17: 187–199

Oxman A D, Guyatt G H 1991 Validation of an index of the quality of review articles. Journal Clinical Epidemiology 44: 1271–1278

Philadelphia Panel (Ottawa Methods Group: Wells G A, Tugwell P, Brosseau L, Robinson V A, Graham I D, Shea B J, McGowan J) 2001a Methodology for the development of the Philadelphia Panel evidence based clinical practice guidelines on selected rehabilitation interventions for musculoskeletal pain. Physical Therapy 81: 1629–1640

Philadelphia Panel (Ottawa Methods Group: Wells G A, Tugwell P, Brosseau L, Robinson V A, Graham I D, Shea B J, McGowan J) 2001b The Philadelphia Panel evidence-based clinical practice guidelines on selected rehabilitation interventions for low back pain. Physical Therapy 81: 1641–1674

Rogers E M 1995 Lessons for guidelines from diffusion of innovations. Joint Commission 21(7): 324–327

Sackett D L, Straus S E, Richardson W S, Rosenberg W, Haynes R B 2000 Evidence-based medicine: how to practice and teach EBM, 2nd edn. Churchill Livingstone, Edinburgh

Shekelle P G, Woolf S H, Eccles M, Grimshaw J 1999 Developing guidelines. British Medical Journal 318: 593–661

Turner P A 2001 Evidence-based practice and physiotherapy in the 1990s. Physiotherapy Theory and Practice 17: 107–121

Turner P A, Whitfield T W A 1997 Physiotherapists' use of evidence-based practice: a cross-national study. Physiotherapy Research International 2(1): 17–29

vanTulder M W, Assendelft W J J, Koes B W, Bouter L M and the editorial board of the Cochrane Collaboration Back Review Group 1997 Method guidelines for systematic reviews in the Cochrane Collaboration Back Review Group for spinal disorders. Spine 22(20): 2323–2330

Waddell G, McIntosh A, Hutchinson A, Feder G, Lewis M 1999 Low back pain evidence review. Royal College of General Practitioners, London. Available online at: http://www.rcgp.org.uk/rcgp/clinspec/guidelines/backpain/index.asp; website accessed: Oct 2001

Woolf S H 1990 Practice guidelines: a new reality in medicine. I: Recent developments. Archives of Internal Medicine 150: 1811–1818

Woolf S H, Grol R, Hutchinson A, Eccles M, Grimshaw J 1999 Potential benefits, limitations and harms of clinical guidelines. British Medical Journal 318: 527–530

Index

W

Y

Z